Principles and Practice
of
Brachytherapy

Edited by

Subir Nag, M.D.

Chief of Brachytherapy
Arthur G. James Cancer Hospital
The Ohio State University
Columbus, Ohio

**Futura Publishing
Company, Inc.**
Armonk, NY

Library of Congress Cataloging-in-Publication Data

Principles and practice of brachytherapy / edited by Subir Nag.
        p.   cm.
    Includes bibliographical references and index.
    ISBN 0-87993-654-1
    1. Radioisotope brachytherapy.   I. Nag, Subir.
    [DNLM: 1. Brachytherapy—methods.   WN 250.5.B7   P957   1997]
RC271.R27P75   1997
616.99'40624—dc21
DNLM/DLC
for Library of Congress   96-46939
                                                                          CIP

Published by
Futura Publishing Company, Inc.
135 Bedford Road
Armonk, New York 10504

LC #: 96-46939
ISBN #: 0-87993-654-1

Dedication

To my parents, Dr. Sunil Nag and Mrs. Bela Nag, who inspired me to start this book, but who passed away before it was completed. This book is dedicated in their memory.

Acknowledgments

I would like to thank the many authors who contributed chapters to this text. No one knows better than they what a daunting task it is to draw together and correlate the contributions of multiple authors. Their hard work and continued cooperation throughout the process of assembling this text are greatly appreciated. I would also like to express my gratitude to Dr. Dimitrios G. Spigos, Chairman of the Department of Radiology, and to Dr. Reinhard A. Gahbauer, Director of the Division of Radiation Oncology, at The Ohio State University Medical Center for their continuing encouragement and support for this project. I am grateful for the encouragement, support, suggestions, and understanding of my colleagues, residents, and staff in the Division of Radiation Oncology at the Arthur James Cancer Hospital and Research Institute. Thanks are also due to Dr. B.C. Goswami, a Visiting Brachytherapy Fellow, for his painstaking proofreading and many helpful comments and to Rita Planitzer for typing many of the manuscripts. This book would not have been completed without the assistance of our technical editor, Mr. David Carpenter, who painstakingly edited the manuscripts, adapting to last minute changes and missed deadlines and working long hours to coordinate the details of publication here at Ohio State. I am indebted to my colleagues in the American Brachytherapy Society for their helpful suggestions in the preparation of this book. Thanks are also due to the staff at Futura Publishing Company, Steven Korn and his associates, whose understanding and patience made timely publication possible. Finally, I want to thank my wife, Sima, and daughters, Sunita and Sumona, for their understanding in the long process of putting this text together and for their unflagging encouragement throughout, despite the many lonely hours that such an endeavor engenders.

Subir Nag, M.D.

Contributors

Andre Abitbol, M.D.
Department of Radiation Oncology
Baptist Hospital of Miami
Miami, Florida, USA

Katherine Albano, M.S.
Medical College of Wisconsin
Department of Radiation Oncology
Milwaukee, Wisconsin, USA

Lowell Anderson, Ph.D.
Department of Medical Physics
Memorial Sloan Kettering Cancer Center
New York, New York, USA

Komanduri Ayyanger, Ph.D.
Radiation Oncology Department
Medical College of Ohio
Toledo, Ohio, USA

J.J. Battermann, M.D., Ph.D.
Department of Radiotherapy
Academic Hospital Utrecht
Utrecht, The Netherlands

Jonathan J. Beitler, M.D., M.B.A.
Department of Radiation Oncology
Montefiore Medical Center
Bronx, New York, USA

John Blasko, M.D.
Department of Therapeutic Radiology
Swedish Hosp./NW Tumor Institute
Seattle, Washington, USA

William R. Bodner, M.D.
New York Medical College
Valhalla, New York, USA

Debra Brown, R.N., B.S.N., O.C.N.
Department of Radiation Oncology
William Beaumont Hospital
Royal Oak, Michigan, USA

Daniel Clarke, M.D.
Northern Virginia Cancer Center
Alexandria, Virginia, USA

Christopher T. Coughlin, M.D., FACP, FACR
Dartmouth Medical School
Lebanon, New Hampshire, USA

Ian Crocker, M.D.
Radiation Oncology
Emory University Hospital
Atlanta, Georgia, USA

Juanita M. Crook, M.D., FRCP(C)
Clinique du Cancer
Hopital General d'Ottawa
Ottawa, Ontario, Canada

David Donath, M.D., FRCP(C)
Department of Radiation Oncology
Centre Hospitalier de l'Université
   de Montréal
Montreal, Quebec, Canada

Kathryn E. Dusenbery, M.D.
Department of Radiation Oncology
University of Minnesota
Minneapolis, Minnesota, USA

Rodney E. Ellis, M.D.
Division of Radiation Oncology
Arthur G. James Cancer Hospital
The Ohio State University
Columbus, Ohio, USA

Beth Erickson, M.D.
Department of Radiation Oncology
Milwaukee County Medical Complex
Milwaukee, Wisconsin, USA

Peter J. Fitzpatrick, M.B., B.S., FRCP(C), FRCR
Radiation Oncology
Cancer Treatment and Research
Halifax, Nova Scotia, Canada

James Fontanesi, M.D.
Gershenson Radiation Oncology Center
Harper Hospital
Detroit, Michigan, USA

Laurie E. Gaspar, M.D.
Gershenson Radiation Oncology Center
Harper Hospital
Detroit, Michigan, USA

Jean-Pierre Gerard, M.D.
Service de Radiotherapie
Centre Hospitalier Lyon-Sud
Lyon, France

Alain Gerbaulet, M.D.
Institute Gustave Roussey
Villejuif Cedex, France

Bruce J. Gerbi, Ph.D.
Department of Radiation Oncology
University of Minnesota
Minneapolis, Minnesota, USA

Michael T. Gillin, Ph.D.
Medical College of Wisconsin
Department of Radiation Oncology
Milwaukee, Wisconsin, USA

Glenn P. Glasgow, Ph.D.
Department of Radiotherapy
Loyola University Medical Center
Maywood, Illinois, USA

Peter D. Grimm, D.O.
Department of Therapeutic Radiology
Swedish Hosp./NW Tumor Institute
Seattle, Washington, USA

William Hanson, Ph.D., FAAPM
M.D. Anderson Hospital
Department of Radiation Physics
Houston, Texas, USA

Louis B. Harrison, M.D.
Department of Radiation Oncology
Memorial Sloan Kettering
New York, New York, USA

Basil S. Hilaris, M.D., FACR
Radiation Medicine
New York Medical College
Our Lady of Mercy Medical Center
Bronx, New York, USA

Nora Janjan, M.D.
Department of Radiotherapy-97
M.D. Anderson Cancer Center
Houston, Texas, USA

Koichi Kaneta, M.D.
Department of Radiation Oncology
Cancer Institute Hospital
Kami-Ikebukuro
Tokyo, Japan

P.C.M. Koper, M.D.
Department of Radiation Oncology
Dr. Daniel Den Hoed Cancer Center
Rotterdam, The Netherlands

Leroy J. Korb, M.D.
West Virginia University Hospitals
Department of Radiology
Medical Center Drive
Morgantown, West Virginia, USA

John P. Lamond, M.D.
Human Oncology
University of Wisconsin Hospitals
Madison, Wisconsin, USA

Eric Lartigau, M.D., Ph.D.
Institute Gustave Roussey
Villejuif Cedex, France

Peter C. Levendag, M.D., Ph.D.
Department of Radiation Oncology
Dr. Daniel Den Hoed Cancer Center
Rotterdam, The Netherlands

Gary Luxton, Ph.D.
Department of Radiation Oncology
USC-Norris Cancer Hosp. & Institute
Los Angeles, California, USA

Alvaro Martinez, M.D., FACR
Department of Radiation Oncology
William Beaumont Hospital
Royal Oak, Michigan, USA

Yosh Maruyama, M.D., FACR (deceased)
Radiation Oncology Department
Harper Hospital
Detroit, Michigan, USA

Dina A. Mastoras
Department of Radiation Medicine
New York Medical College
Valhalla, New York, USA

Minesh P. Mehta, M.D.
Human Oncology
University of Wisconsin Hospitals
Madison, Wisconsin, USA

Ali S. Meigooni, Ph.D.
Chandler Medical Center
Department of Radiation Medicine
University of Kentucky
Lexington, Kentucky, USA

Chitti R. Moorthy, M.D.
Department of Radiation Medicine
New York Medical College
Valhalla, New York, USA

Subir Nag, M.D.
Division of Radiation Oncology
Arthur G. James Cancer Hospital
The Ohio State University
Columbus, Ohio, USA

Ravinder Nath, Ph.D., FACR
Department of Therapeutic Radiology
Yale University School of Medicine
New Haven, Connecticut, USA

Dattatreyudu Nori, M.D.
Radiation Oncology
Booth Memorial Medical Center
Flushing, New York, USA

Colin G. Orton, Ph.D.
Medical Physics
Gershenson Radiation Oncology Center
Harper-Grace Hospitals
Detroit, Michigan, USA

Vladimir Pak, M.D.
Division of Radiation Oncology
Arthur G. James Cancer Hospital
The Ohio State University
Columbus, Ohio, USA

Bhudatt R. Paliwal, Ph.D.
University of Wisconsin CSC
Radiation Therapy
Madison, Wisconsin, USA

Daniel G. Petereit, M.D.
Department of Human Oncology
University of Wisconsin Hospitals
Madison, Wisconsin, USA

Robert Peterson, B.S.
Division of Radiation Oncology
Arthur G. James Cancer Hospital
The Ohio State University
Columbus, Ohio, USA

Lynda Petty, R.N.
Perioperative Education & Training
Arthur G. James Cancer Hospital
The Ohio State University
Columbus, Ohio, USA

Arthur Porter, M.D.
Radiation Oncology Department
Harper Hospital
Detroit, Michigan, USA

Nina Samsami, M.D.
Division of Radiation Oncology
Arthur G. James Cancer Hospital
The Ohio State University
Columbus, Ohio, USA

Cheng B. Saw, Ph.D.
West Virginia University Hospitals
Department of Radiation Oncology
Medical Center Drive
Morgantown, West Virginia, USA

Lynn L. Shih, M.S.
Department of Radiation Medicine
New York Medical College
Valhalla, New York, USA

Penny K. Sneed, M.D.
Department of Radiation Oncology
University of California
San Francisco, California, USA

Burton L. Speiser, M.D.
Department of Radiation Oncology
St. Joseph's Hospital
Phoenix, Arizona, USA

Judith Anne Stitt, M.D.
Department of Human Oncology
University of Wisconsin
Madison, Wisconsin, USA

Patrick S. Swift, M.D.
Department of Radiation Oncology
University of California
San Francisco, California, USA

Bruce R. Thomadsen, Ph.D., FAAPM
Department of Radiation Oncology
University of Wisconsin
Madison, Wisconsin, USA

Cindy Thomason, Ph.D.
Radiation Oncology
Northwestern Memorial Hospital
Chicago, Illinois, USA

Frank A. Vicini, M.D.
Department of Radiation Oncology
William Beaumont Hospital
Royal Oak, Michigan, USA

Bhadrasain Vikram, M.D.
Department of Radiation Oncology
Albert Einstein Medical Center
Bronx, New York, USA

A.G. Visser, Ph.D.
Department of Radiation Oncology
Dr. Daniel Den Hoed Cancer Center
Rotterdam, The Netherlands

Boris M. Vtyurin, M.D., Ph.D.
Department of Brachytherapy
Institute of Medical Radiology
Academy of Medical Sciences of Russia
Obninsk, Kaluga Region, Russia

Ron Waksman, M.D.
Interventional Cardiology
Emory University Hospital
Atlanta, Georgia, USA

Frank M. Waterman, Ph.D.
Department of Radiation Oncology
West Virginia University Hospitals
Morgantown, West Virginia, USA

Jacek G. Wierzbicki, Ph.D.
Radiation Oncology Department
Harper Hospital
Detroit, Michigan, USA

A.J. Wijnmaalen, M.D.
Department of Radiation Oncology
Dr. Daniel Den Hoed Cancer Center
Rotterdam, The Netherlands

J. Frank Wilson, M.D., FACR
Department of Radiation Oncology
Milwaukee County Medical Complex
Milwaukee, Wisconsin, USA

Preface

This text is not intended to be a substitute for performing brachytherapy. It must be stressed that brachytherapy is a procedural speciality; hence no textbook, no matter how well written, can substitute for the experience to be gained in the operating room. Therefore, this book should be used only as a guide to supplement the experience gained during the endless hours in the operating room that practicing the art and science of brachytherapy requires.

The term "brachytherapy," which was coined by Forsell in 1931, refers to a form of radiotherapy that has been used since soon after the discovery of radium by Marie and Pierre Curie in 1898. Its successful application has a number of advantages: 1) brachytherapy provides a high localized radiation dose to a small tumor volume, gives higher local control, and is well tolerated; 2) side effects are minimized; 3) the short duration of brachytherapy treatments prevents proliferation of the tumor tissues and is also more convenient for the patients; 4) continuous radiation by low-dose-rate brachytherapy allows redistribution of the tumor cells within the cell cycle, allowing cells in the less sensitive S-phase to move to more radiosensitive M-phase; 5) with brachytherapy, the nonhomogenous dose distribution in the tumor volume delivers about a 50% higher dose to the center of an implant than to the periphery, thereby preferentially treating the hypoxic central core common to most tumors; 6) continuous low-dose-rate irradiation provides time for re-oxygenation of hypoxic tumor cells during the treatment; 7) brachytherapy is the ultimate form of conformal radiotherapy; and 8) the prescribed dose is usually the minimum dose received within the tumor, with most areas of the tumor receiving a substantially higher dose that increases the effectiveness of the treatment.

Successful application of brachytherapy involves overcoming the disadvantages that have been associated with this mode of treatment. The major disadvantage of brachytherapy in the past, and to a lesser extent today, is the hazard of radiation exposure; however, this hazard has been minimized by the introduction of low energy radionuclides such as iodine-125 and palladium-103 and can be eliminated by the use of remote controlled afterloading techniques. A second disadvantage, brachytherapy often necessitated restriction or hospitalization of the patient, which increased the inconvenience and cost of treatment; this problem has been eliminated by the use of remote controlled high-dose-rate brachytherapy. Third, although brachytherapy has the advantage of giving a localized dose, it does not give a therapeutic dose to the surrounding areas, does not cover a large volume, and, hence, is not suitable for treating larger tumors. Further, the sharp fall-off of the brachytherapy dose makes it less forgiving at the periphery of the treatment volume and can result in underdosing if the implant does not adequately cover the tumor volume. Hence, the astute brachytherapist should be able to integrate external beam irradiation into the treatment program whenever feasible. Fourth, most brachytherapy procedures require a surgical procedure to expose the tumor and hence are associated with surgical trauma. However, newer imaging techniques

xi

(ultrasound, CT scan) can sometimes be used to guide the placement of brachytherapy sources. Fifth, although high doses of low-dose-rate continuous brachytherapy are generally well tolerated, there is a greater risk of late radiation damage if high-dose-rate brachytherapy is improperly used. Hence, it is imperative that the brachytherapist be properly armed with the radiobiological knowledge required for the adequate fractionation needed in high-dose-rate brachytherapy. Finally, acquiring the necessary skill and training for the delivery of brachytherapy has been difficult. Most radiation therapy training programs do not emphasize brachytherapy strongly, few fellowships are available, and most brachytherapy courses are theoretical provide limited practical experience. As a result, lack of expertise in brachytherapy is perhaps the major impediment to the development of brachytherapy at present. We hope that the organization of the text—which begins with basic principles of radiation oncology and brachytherapy, progresses through the various clinical applications of this modality, and concludes with new developments in the field—will make the text readily accessible for users with various purposes and needs.

Principles and Practice of Brachytherapy is intended to serve as a reference text for the radiation oncologists, residents, physicists, dosimetrists, technologists, and other physicians interested in this form of treatment. Our purpose has been to provide a comprehensive overview of the state of the art in brachytherapy that would be accessible to a broad range of clinicians, medical technologists, and researchers. Each chapter has been multi-authored to give a broad view of the approaches to the use of this modality, and each chapter also includes a detailed description of the specific methodology, with the intention of providing the reader step-by-step explanations of the procedures used. The coauthors have both contributed their specific expertise and critically reviewed the entire chapter that includes their contribution. We hope that this approach has produced a comprehensive, detailed, and balanced discussion of the subject.

Background useful in understanding the clinical application of brachytherapy, including brachytherapy principles, basic physics, and radiobiology are described in Part I. Because of their importance in establishing and maintaining a brachytherapy program, treatment planning and radiation safety are discussed in detail. Treatment planning is perhaps the most important component of a successful brachytherapy procedure and includes clinical and physical elements: clinical evaluation; tumor volume determination; target volume determination; treatment volume determination; type of implant; selection of radioisotope; amount of radioactive material; spatial arrangements of the radioactive material in the tumor; and determination of dosimetry. The success of a brachytherapy program depends upon meticulous attention to quality assurance; in fact, quality assurance procedures are even more important for brachytherapy than for external beam radiation therapy (EBRT) since brachytherapy is only occasionally performed at most institutions, and hence the radiation oncology personnel may lack familiarity with those procedures. With afterloading methods, radiation exposure hazards be minimized; however, consistent attention must be paid to radiation protection precautions. This text attempts to provide a description of specific guidelines and procedures to ensure radiation safety in a brachytherapy program.

Brachytherapy can be used either alone or, more commonly, as part of a multi-modality approach with EBRT, surgery, or chemotherapy. This multi-modality approach is emphasized throughout the clinical section of the book, which is divided according to organ site. Common sites implanted by brachytherapy include cervix, endometrium, head and neck, and lung. Brachytherapy is less commonly used in the esophagus, eye, and prostate and is rarely used in biliary sites, the brain, bladder, breast, colorectal, sarcomas, pancreas, and pediatric tumors. This text attempts to provide specific description of each of these various applications.

The final section deals with special topics. The chapter on nursing care discusses the specialized personnel and training necessary for the intensive nursing care requisite to the labor intensive and procedure oriented activities involved in brachytherapy. The chapter on pulsed-dose-rate brachytherapy describes the new technique of pulsing high-dose-rate brachytherapy to simulate low-dose-rate continuous brachytherapy while achieving dose homogeneity throughout an implant volume by dose optimization; clinical results are discussed. A chapter is dedicated to the rationale, methodology, clinical experience, treatment planning, radiobiology, physics, and dosimetry involved in californium-252 brachytherapy, a form of brachytherapy that uses neutrons to treat advanced, bulky, or radioresistant neoplasms. The potential for a synergistic enhancement of treatment efficacy through the application of interstitial thermobrachytherapy makes it an interesting new modality in the field. Intravascular brachytherapy has only recently been proposed as a means of preventing restenosis after coronary angioplasty or stent placement and has produced promising early results in animal studies. If clinical trials prove successful, this modality could become the largest single application of brachytherapy, since 450,000 angioplasties are performed each year in the United States alone.

Perhaps the most persistent and vexing problem facing the brachytherapist today is the lack of standardization and consensus in the field. Regarded by many as more of an art than a science, brachytherapy has evolved from several different schools; therefore, there is wide variation in treatment regimes, techniques, terminology, methodology, dose specification, and dosimetry used. In addition there are few national or international standards or consensus for the practice of brachytherapy. Thus there is an urgent need to develop a common language in the field of brachytherapy so that information and experience can be exchanged. This text is intended to give a specific overview of the state of the art in brachytherapy, both for the practicing clinician and for the resident or therapist for whom learning the application of this treatment modality provides a continuing challenge. We hope that the information provided by this text and the agreements, disagreements, or even controversies that it may engender will contribute to the movement toward a more systematic application of this valuable treatment modality.

With any modern technology, time and use lead to changes and refinements. We expect that the same will be true of brachytherapy; those inevitable changes are certain to necessitate new descriptions of the advances achieved with this modality. Thus, we hope that this book will be only the first of many attempts to provide specific, broad-based understanding of brachytherapy and that this understanding will enable us to treat cancer more effectively. Finally we would be grateful for any comments or criticism the reader might be willing to contribute regarding content, current usefulness, or possible future additions to this text; and with this idea in mind, we have included a questionnaire at the end of the text that can be completed in a few minutes and returned.

Subir Nag, M.D.

Contents

Part I   Basic Principles

Part II Clinical Body Sites

PART I

Basic Principles

Chapter 1

Principles of Brachytherapy

Subir Nag, M.D.

Introduction

The term "brachytherapy" was coined by Forsell in 1931. It is derived from the Greek word *brachio,* meaning short, and refers to "treatment with a radioisotope at a short distance." Other terms, sometimes used interchangeably for the same procedure, are "curietherapy," "endocurietherapy," and "radiation implants." The use of brachytherapy started soon after the discovery of radium by Marie and Pierre Curie in 1898. A detailed discussion of the historical background of brachytherapy is provided in Dr. Basil Hilaris' excellent chapter, "The History of Brachytherapy," in this book.[1]

Principles of Radiation Oncology

An understanding of basic radiation oncology principles is essential to the successful use of brachytherapy as part of a multi-modality approach to the management of the cancer patient. These principles include:

1. The higher the dose delivered to the tumor, the higher the probability of local control of the tumor. Hence, the aim in radiation therapy is to deliver the highest possible dose to the tumor without excessive morbidity to the normal tissues.
2. The lower the radiation dose to the surrounding normal tissue, the lower the associated morbidity. Ideally, one should reduce the dose to the normal tissues while delivering a high dose to the tumor.
3. Larger tumor volumes require higher radiation doses for tumor control. Conversely, small or microscopic tumor volumes require lower doses of radiation for control of the tumor. Therefore, if possible, one should try to irradiate tumors while they are small. Alternatively, rather than uniformly irradiating the entire target area, areas of microscopic tumors could be given modest radiation doses while areas of bulky disease could be boosted to higher doses.
4. Hypoxic tumor cells (usually in the center of a tumor) are radioresistant and require high doses of radiation to achieve cell kill. Surgical removal of hypoxic tumor cells can decrease the dose of radiation required and increase the probability of local tumor control; alternatively, the hypoxic core can be boosted to a higher radiation dose.
5. Potential for morbidity and complications increase if large volumes are irradiated. Conversely, smaller volumes can tolerate higher doses of radiation with less potential morbidity. Hence, the aim is to minimize the volume irra-

From Nag S (ed): *Principles and Practice of Brachytherapy.* © Futura Publishing Co., Inc., Armonk, NY, 1997.

diated while still encompassing the entire tumor volume.

6. Shortening the time interval between radiation treatments reduces the repopulation of tumor cells. Therefore, the aim is to minimize the total duration of treatment.

These basic radiation oncology principles can be used to illustrate the advantages and disadvantages of brachytherapy.

Advantages of Brachytherapy

1. The "introduction of radioactive material into the heart of the tumor" allows for the delivery of a highly localized radiation dose to a small tumor volume. This gives higher local control and is well tolerated.
2. Since the radiation dose attenuates approximately following the inverse square law, there is a sharp fall-off of radiation dose in the surrounding normal tissue. Furthermore, the dose is given at a lower dose rate, and hence the side effects are minimized.
3. The overall duration of brachytherapy is short—generally 2–7 days to deliver 20–70 Gy by removable implant versus 5–7 weeks by external beam radiation therapy (EBRT). This short duration prevents proliferation of the tumor tissues and is also more convenient for the patients. However, permanent implantations deliver the radiation in a few weeks or months, depending upon the half-life of the radionuclide.
4. The continuous radiation by low-dose-rate (LDR) brachytherapy allows redistribution of the tumor cells within the cell cycle, allowing cells in less sensitive S-phase to move to more radiosensitive M-phase, thus providing a radiobiological advantage.
5. With brachytherapy, the dose distribution in the tumor volume is not homogenous. Typically, the center of an implant receives about a 50% higher dose than the periphery. Since the central core of most tumors is hypoxic and, therefore, less radiosensitive, the

higher dose given at the center by brachytherapy is an advantage.

6. Continuous LDR irradiation provides time for reoxygenation of hypoxic tumor cells during the treatment, thus allowing initially radioresistant tumor cells to become more radiosensitive.
7. The dose distribution can be manipulated to match irregular tumor shapes; hence, brachytherapy is the ultimate form of conformal radiotherapy. Furthermore, the chances of geographical miss due to patient movement are reduced, since the radioactive implants are located within the tumor tissues.
8. Since the dose is homogenous in EBRT, the prescribed dose is received throughout the tumor volume. In brachytherapy, the prescribed dose is usually the minimum dose received within the tumor. Most areas of the tumor receive a substantially higher dose than the prescribed dose, hence increasing the effectiveness of brachytherapy compared to EBRT for the same stated dose of brachytherapy.

Disadvantages of Brachytherapy

1. The major disadvantage of brachytherapy in the past and, to a lesser extent, today is the hazard of radiation exposure. The caregivers and family members were fearful of being involved in the care of a radioactive patient and could not spend much time with the patient. However, this hazard has been minimized by the introduction of low energy radionuclides such as iodine-125 and palladium-103 and eliminated by the use of remote controlled afterloading techniques.
2. Another disadvantage associated with the use of brachytherapy is that the patient must be restricted and hospitalized, increasing the inconvenience and cost. This, too, has been eliminated with the use of remote controlled high-dose-rate (HDR) brachytherapy.
3. While brachytherapy has the advantage of giving a localized dose, it does

not give a therapeutic dose to the surrounding areas or adjacent lymph draining areas, which may have microscopic or gross disease. Furthermore, it does not cover a large volume and, hence, is not suitable for treating larger tumors.

4. The delivery of brachytherapy requires special skill and training. While most radiation oncologists have expertise in delivering EBRT, the training in brachytherapy (other than intracavitary gynecological applications) is rather limited at most centers. This has hampered the growth of the specialty of brachytherapy. There are few fellowships available. Most brachytherapy courses are theoretical and provide limited practical experience. Initiatives taken by the American Brachytherapy Society on providing brachytherapy workshops are a good start. However, the lack of expertise in brachytherapy is perhaps the major impediment to the development of brachytherapy at present.

5. While brachytherapy is effective if it encompasses the entire tumor volume, its sharp fall-off makes it less forgiving at the periphery and will result in underdosing of the tumor if the implant does not adequately cover the tumor volume.

6. Most of the brachytherapy procedures require a surgical procedure for exposure of the tumor, and hence is associated with its resultant surgical trauma. However, new techniques using fluoroscopic, ultrasound, or CT scan guidance, minimize these traumas.

7. While high doses of LDR continuous brachytherapy are generally well tolerated (due to the reasons stated above), there is a greater risk of late radiation damage if HDR brachytherapy is given with inadequate fractionation.

Types of Brachytherapy

There are various ways to categorize brachytherapy. It may be categorized by the location of the implant, the type of loading, the dose rate, the duration treatment, or type of emission.

Categorization by the Location of the Radioactive Material in Relation to the Tumor

Intracavitary Techniques

Intracavitary techniques involve placing radioactive material into body cavities. This is especially useful in gynecological tumors where the radioactive material is placed in the uterine cavity and vagina. This is the most common form of implant done. It is performed in 71% of all centers in the United States.[2] A subcategory of the intracavitary technique is the intraluminal technique whereby the radioactive material is inserted in the lumen of the bronchus, esophagus, or bile duct, and is performed in 29% of centers[2] in the United States.

Interstitial Brachytherapy

Interstitial brachytherapy involves placing the radioactive material within tissues. Thus, most nongynecological implants are performed using interstitial techniques. This is the most common form of nongynecological brachytherapy procedure, performed in 51% of all radiation oncology centers.[2]

Surface Applications (Molds or Plaques)

In this technique, the radioactive material in the form of molds or plaques is placed on the surface of the tumor rather than being placed inside the tumor. This technique is not very commonly used (used in only 14% of the centers).[2]

A summary of these techniques and the equipment related to their use is given in Table 1.

Categorization by Type of Loading

Manual "Hot" Loading

When brachytherapy was first introduced, the radiotherapy material was directly introduced into the tumor, hence subjecting the operator to the adverse effects of radiation.

Table 1.
Brachytherapy Instruments and Techniques

Interstitial Brachytherapy		
Permanent	Removable	
1. Single seed applicator 2. Mick applicator 3. Scott applicator 4. Absorbable sutures 5. Gelfoam/surgical	1. "Standard" plastic tube technique: a. Steel needles (#14 and #17 gauze) b. Catheters (blind-ended, single- ended, double-ended, buttoned) c. Buttons (plastic, metal, domed) 3. Hair-pin/guide gutter	2. Templates: a. Syed Neblett Gyn b. MUPIT c. Porter d. Prostate, rectal e. Custom made 4. Swage on

Intracavitary Brachytherapy		
Preloaded Gyn	Afterloaded Gyn	Intraluminal
1. Stockholm 2. Paris 3. Manchester 4. Fletcher 5. Ernest	1. Fletcher (and modifications) 2. Henschke 3. Kumar Cervical 4. Botstein Zacharopoulous 5. Simon-Heyman capsules 6. Hilaris Endometrial Applicator 7. Delcos vaginal cylinders	1. Esophageal 2. Endobronchial 3. Biliary

Plaques and Molds	Remote Brachytherapy
1. Eye plaques (Cobalt, Ruthenium, I-125) 2. Strontium eye applicator 3. Custom made	1. Brachytron (LDR Co-60) 2. Cathetron (LDR Co-60) 3. Selectron (LDR Cs-137) 4. Microselectron (HDR Ir-192) 5. Gamma-Med (HDR Ir-192)

LDR = low-dose-rate; HDR = high-dose-rate.

Direct "hot" loading is almost never used now because of its radiation hazards.

Manual Afterloading

Since the middle of this century, most brachytherapy procedures have been performed using afterloading techniques whereby hollow needles, catheters, or applicators are first inserted into the tumor area. Once the position of the carrier is confirmed, the radioactive material is introduced manually into the catheter or applicator, usually in the patient's room. This procedure improves accuracy while reducing the radiation exposure to the medical caregivers.

Remote Afterloading

Although the manual afterloading technique mentioned above reduces radiation exposure for the staff, some associated radiation exposure to caregivers and visitors remains. This exposure can be virtually eliminated by the use of remote controlled afterloading, in which the radioactive material is loaded into the applicator by remote control while the caregivers are in an adjacent room. The various advantages of remote afterloading, especially remote HDR brachytherapy, have made this technique very popular. Our recently published textbook provides further details.[3]

Categorization by Dose Rate

Brachytherapy can be delivered at different dose rates. These have been arbitrarily divided into low-, medium-, and high-dose-rates. The International Commission for Radiation Units (ICRU), Report No. 38 defines dose rates as follows:

1. *Low-Dose-Rate (LDR)—0.4 to 2.0 Gy per hour:* Brachytherapy was tradi-

tionally performed using LDR techniques. These are generally manually loaded, although LDR remote afterloaders are also available in a few centers.

2. *Medium-Dose-Rate (MDR)—2 to 12 Gy per hour:* This is also called "intermediate-dose-rate." This dose rate is rarely used since it gives excessive exposure if manually loaded and does not have the advantages of outpatient brachytherapy afforded by the HDR technique when loaded by remote control.

3. *High-Dose-Rate (HDR)—more than 12 Gy per hour:* Since HDR brachytherapy is associated with high radiation exposure, it is only used by remote control techniques rather than being manually loaded. The usual dose rate used in current HDR brachytherapy units is about 100–300 Gy per hour, allowing the treatments to be given in only a few minutes on an outpatient basis. The use of HDR remote brachytherapy has provided new impetus to brachytherapy, and hence we have devoted a separate book to HDR brachytherapy.[3]

Categorization by Duration of Brachytherapy

Permanent Implants

In a permanent implant, the radioactive sources are permanently implanted into the tumor and allowed to decay. Hence, neither the dose nor the dose distribution can be changed after the initial insertion. It is, however, a simple procedure, and some of them can be done on an out-patient basis. Other advantages of the permanent implant are that, in deep-seated tumors, it is safer because of the lower risk of infection and that a second operation for its removal is not required. Permanent implantations are performed with relatively short half-life radioisotopes like iodine-125, palladium-103, or gold-198.

Removable (Temporary) Implants

In a removable implant, the radioactive material is temporarily implanted into or close to the tumor and is removed once the desired radiation dose has been delivered. Therefore, there is better control of the total dose and the dose distribution. Removable implants are more time consuming. Their principal indication is in the treatment of accessible tumors where the aim is cure, or at least long-term palliation.

The decision to use either temporary and permanent implantation depends upon the judgment of the practitioner. With skill and experience, a brachytherapist can use either modality at different locations.

Categorization by Type of Emission

Gamma Emitters

Most brachytherapy uses radioisotopes (such as radium, cobalt, cesium, gold, iridium, etc.) with high energy gamma emissions that penetrate deeply and also require radiation protection for the safety of the caregivers and the patient's family. Brachytherapy with low energy gamma emitters, like I-125 and Pd-103, require less radiation protection.

Beta Emitters

These are commonly used as unsealed sources for systemic brachytherapy. Beta emissions are absorbed within a few millimeters in tissues. Hence, they require minimal radiation precautions unless there is spillage. These sources include phosphorous-32, ruthenium-106, and strontium-89 and yttrium-90.

Neutron Emitters

The only neutron emitter of practical importance is californium-252. The advantage of neutron emitters is that they are more effective against hypoxic tumors because they have a higher linear energy transfer than gamma emitters. They are, however, associated with far greater radiation hazards and therefore are not commonly used. Further details are given on californium-252 neutron brachytherapy in Chapter 35 by Dr. Yosh Maruyama.

Indications for Brachytherapy

Brachytherapy can be used to advantage in most areas of the body if a radiation therapist is interested, innovative, and skillful. It can be used either alone or, more commonly, as part of a multi-modality approach with EBRT, surgery, or chemotherapy. The following are general guidelines for use of brachytherapy:

1. In small, localized tumors (e.g., prostate carcinoma), brachytherapy can be used alone.
2. In more bulky tumors, EBRT is used to treat the lymphatics and to shrink the tumor, and brachytherapy is used to boost the area of gross tumor.
3. In tumors recurrent after EBRT, where other alternatives do not exist, brachytherapy can be given alone or combined with chemotherapy, surgery, or hyperthermia.
4. In palliative cases, brachytherapy can be used to reduce the overall treatment time of 4–5 weeks associated with EBRT.

Common sites implanted by brachytherapy include the cervix (67%), endometrium (54%), head and neck (34%), and lung (33%). Brachytherapy is less commonly used in the esophagus (22%), eye (20%), and prostate (20%).[2] Rare sites for implants include biliary, brain, bladder, breast, colorectal, sarcomas, pancreas, and pediatric tumors. Details of its use in different organs are in separate chapters in *Section II: Clinical Sites* in this book.

Brachytherapy Treatment Planning

Treatment planning is perhaps the most important component of a successful brachytherapy procedure and includes clinical and physical elements. The physical elements are detailed in Chapter 8 of this book.[4]

1. Clinical Evaluation: One has to determine whether the tumor is suitable for brachytherapy as per the indications given above, and if so, whether we need to combine it with any other modality.
2. Tumor Volume Determination: This can be done clinically or, more commonly, with the aid of radiographic (plain x-rays, CT scan, MRI, ultrasound) and other studies. Tumor volume determination is dealt with in detail in Chapter 9.[5]
3. Target Volume Determination: This is the region to which we plan to deliver the radiation dose and includes the tumor and some margin (usually about 1 cm) but should avoid any major radiosensitive structures.
4. Treatment Volume Determination: This is the region into which the radioactive materials are placed to deliver the desired dose to the target volume. Ideally, the treatment volume should be equal to the target volume; but, in practice, this equivalence is rarely achieved.
5. Type of Implant: Namely, permanent or removable, and whether planar (single or double) or a volume implant.
6. Selection of Radioisotope: The selection of radioisotope will depend upon whether it is to be used for permanent or removable implants. The characteristics of radionuclides commonly used in brachytherapy are given in Table 2. Radionuclides used for permanent implants generally have a lower energy emission and short half-life. In general, radionuclides used for removable brachytherapy have an intermediate or long half-life and can have either high energy emissions (requiring greater radiation protection) or a low energy (to minimize radiation exposure). Beta emitters are generally used when limited penetration is required.
7. Amount of Radioactive Material: A nomogram can be used to estimate the amount of radioactive material required for permanent implantation or for removable implants. Alternatively, a computerized preplan can be performed. The necessary amounts of radioactive material must be ordered in advance if they are not already in stock.
8. Spatial Arrangements of the Radioactive Material in the Tumor: This is the actual implantation procedure. The radioactive materials are usually placed parallel to each other if possi-

Table 2.
Radionuclides Commonly Used for Brachytherapy

Nuclide (symbol)	Half-Life	Therapeutic Emission	Energy (keV)	Half Value Layer
Californium-252 (^{252}Cf)	2.65 years	neutron	2350	5 cm of water
Cesium-137 (^{137}Cs)	30 years	gamma	662	6 mm of lead
Cobalt-60 (^{60}Co)	5 years	gamma	1173–1332	12 mm of lead
Gold-198 (^{198}Au)	2.7 days	gamma	412	3 mm of lead
Iodine-125 (^{125}I)	60 days	x-ray	27–32	0.02 mm of lead
Iridium-192 (^{192}Ir)	74 days	gamma	340	3 mm of lead
Palladium-103 (^{103}Pd)	17 days	x-ray	20–23	0.01 mm of lead
Phosphorus-32 (^{32}P)	14 days	beta	1710	minimal
Ruthenium-106 (^{106}Ru)	367 days	beta	2390–3550	minimal
Strontium-90 (^{90}Sr)	28.1 years	beta	2280 max	minimal

ble, and equally spaced (Quimby system) or follow the recommendation of the Patterson-Parker system, which results in a more uniform dose distribution. The radioactive materials are inserted using needles, catheters, or specialized applicators as detailed in the chapter entitled, *Instrumentation and Equipment*.[6] Care must be taken to adequately implant the target volume.

9. Determination of Dosimetry: This can be done by the Patterson-Parker system, the Quimby system, or the Paris system. Most modern centers however, use a computerized dosimetry to determine isodoses at multiple transverse planes and from there, determine the minimum and maximum dose rates to the tumor, the dose at the sensitive tissues, and the dose distribution. From these, the duration and total dose of the implant are established.

Quality Assurance

A brachytherapy program will only be successful if meticulous attention is paid to quality assurance, both to ensure the best possible outcome in tumor control (which is of course of primary importance to the patient and the practitioner) and to prevent loss of radioactive material (which could result in undesirable consequences for all involved, including the institution itself). Attention to quality assur-

ance procedures is even more important for brachytherapy than for EBRT since brachytherapy is only occasionally performed at most institutions, and hence the radiation oncology personnel may lack familiarity with those procedures. Adherence to quality management procedures is also essential to meet with federal and institutional guidelines. Details of quality assurance and quality management programs are given in Chapter 7.[7] It is mandatory for anyone performing brachytherapy procedures to have a quality assurance and quality management program in place before they start their procedures. Licensing requirements must be met. There should be adequate physics support to maintain quality assurance as well as to perform dosimetry. All treatments should be adequately documented and a flow chart maintained. Examples of checklists and forms to help in quality assurance are also given in Chapter 7.[7]

Radiation Safety

With afterloading methods, the radiation exposure hazards are minimized. Several precautions are listed here and detailed in Chapter 10.[8] These are to be kept in mind by anyone handling radioactive isotopes.

1. Distance: The longer the distance from the source, the lower the exposure; therefore, close contact should take place only when absolutely necessary. Radioactive material should al-

ways be handled using long-handled instruments.

2. Shielding: Whenever possible, caregivers should stay behind the lead shields while handling the radioactive sources or patients.

3. Time: The shorter the time spent near the radioactive patient, the lower the radiation exposure. However, we encourage frequent short visits to the patient to counteract the development of sensory deprivation syndromes that ultimately lead to more complications and, as a result, greater radiation exposure to the caregivers in the long run, since they must spend more time in close proximity to the patient dealing with these complications. These precautions are mainly required for the removable implants. The permanent iodine-125 and palladium-103 implants usually do not pose any major radiation hazards. With the proper precautions, the radiation exposure is minimal, well within the recommended limits of 5 rems/year for occupationally exposed personnel.

Standardization and Consensus in Brachytherapy

Brachytherapy is regarded by many more as an art than a science. Brachytherapy has evolved from several different schools and hence there is wide variation in treatment regimes, techniques, terminology, methodology, dose specification, and dosimetry used among different brachytherapists. There is controversy about the radionuclide and techniques, as well as dosing, dose rate, and fractionation of brachytherapy to be used. The methodologies for dosimetry and prescription point also vary among different users. This idiosyncratic approach to the application of brachytherapy hinders discussion of technique and results, and limits communication between investigators. There is paucity of national or international standards or consensus.

Stating that "a tumor received 50 Gy radiation by brachytherapy" is meaningless because such a statement can be interpreted in a number of ways:

1. It could refer to the minimum dose at the periphery of the tumor;
2. It could be the average dose delivered to the tumor;
3. It could be a dose at a certain distance, e.g., 0.5 cm, or 1 cm from the source;
4. It could be given to the surface of the tissue;
5. It could be the dose given at a depth of 0.5 cm within the tissue;
6. It could be given at any of the above points at an LDR over a few days;
7. It could be given as a permanent implant over a few months; or
8. It could be given as HDR brachytherapy in a few minutes.

The biological effects of this same dose (50 Gy) will vary by a factor of several hundred percent, depending on the interpretation taken. Hence, major errors in therapy can occur depending on how it is interpreted. There is an urgent need to develop a common language in the field of brachytherapy and to come to some preliminary consensus. There have been some attempts at developing some consensus opinion in brachytherapy by the High Dose Rate Working Group (HIBWOG), the American Brachytherapy Society, and the ICRU. Although the initial steps have been taken, there is an urgent need for more consensus and standardization in brachytherapy for the specialty of brachytherapy to prosper. It is highly recommended that these guidelines be followed whenever they are available.

Another factor hindering the training has been the lack of a comprehensive textbook in brachytherapy. Several articles or monographs on brachytherapy are available,[9–17] as are a number of abstracts and presentations in proceedings of meetings. This book attempts to provide comprehensive coverage in all aspects of brachytherapy.

References

1. Hilaris B, Mastoras DA, Shih LL, et al. History of brachytherapy: The years after the discovery of radium and radioactivity. In: Nag S (ed). Principles and Practice of Brachytherapy. Futura Publishing Co., Armonk, NY, 1996.
2. Nag S, Owen JB, Farnan N, et al. Survey of brachytherapy practice in the United States: A

report of the clinical research committee of The American Endocurietherapy Society. Int J Radiat Oncol Biol Phys 1995;31:103–107.

3. Nag S. High Dose Rate Brachytherapy: A Textbook. Futura Publishing Co., Armonk, NY, 1994.

4. Thomadsen BR, Ayyangar K, Anderson L, et al. Brachytherapy treatment planning. In: Nag S (ed). Principles and Practice of Brachytherapy. Futura Publishing Co., Armonk, NY, 1996.

5. Paliwal BR, Thomadsen BR, Petereit DG. Imaging applications in brachytherapy. In: Nag S (ed). Principles and Practice of Brachytherapy. Futura Publishing Co., Armonk, NY, 1996.

6. Saw CB, Waterman FM, Meigooni A, et al. Instrumentation and equipment. In: Nag S (ed). Principles and Practice of Brachytherapy. Futura Publishing Co., Armonk, NY, 1996.

7. Gillin MT, Albano K. Quality assurance in brachytherapy. In: Nag S (ed). Principles and Practice of Brachytherapy. Futura Publishing Co., Armonk, NY, 1996.

8. Samsami N, Peterson R, Nag S. Radiation protection. In: Nag S (ed). Principles and Practice of Brachytherapy. Futura Publishing Co., Armonk, NY, 1996.

9. George EW. Modern Interstitial and Intracavitary Radiation Management. Masson Publishing, New York, 1981.

10. Goffinet DR, Cox RS, et al. Brachytherapy. Am J Clin Oncol (CCT)1988;11(3):342–354.

11. Hilaris BS. Handbook of Interstitial Brachytherapy. Memorial Sloan Kettering Cancer Center, Publishing Sciences Group, Acton, MA, 1975.

12. Hilaris BS, Nori D, Anderson LL. An Atlas of Brachytherapy. Macmillan Publishing Co., New York, 1988.

13. Hilaris BS, Nori D, Anderson LL. New approaches to brachytherapy. In: DeVita VT, Hellman S, Rosenberg SA (eds). Important Advances in Oncology. J.B. Lippincott, Philadelphia, PA, 1987.

14. Phillips TL, et al. Brachytherapy. Cancer Treatment Symposium 1984;1:119–126.

15. Pierquin B, Wilson JF, Chassagne D. Modern Brachytherapy. Masson Publishing, New York, 1987.

16. Interstital Colaborative Working Group (eds). Interstitial Brachytherapy: Physical, Biological, and Clinical Consideratons. Raven Press, New York, 1990.

17. Sauer R (ed). Interventional Radiation Therapy Techniques—Brachytherapy. Springer-Verlag, Berlin, 1991.

Chapter 2

History of Brachytherapy:
The Years After the Discovery of Radium and Radioactivity

Basil S. Hilaris, M.D., FACR, Dina A. Mastoras,
Lynn L. Shih, M.S., William R. Bodner, M.D.

Introduction

Brachytherapy, the treatment of cancer by radioactive elements placed at a short distance from a tumor, was born shortly after Henri Becquerel's discovery of radioactivity in Paris (1896) and Marie Curie's extraction of a tiny amount of radium from tons of pitchblende ore at her laboratory in the outskirts of Paris (1898). Marie and her husband Pierre Curie (Figure 1), soon afterwards had loaned a small radium tube to Danlos at St. Louis Hospital in Paris, who treated a patient with lupus. In 1903, Becquerel and the Curies were jointly awarded the Nobel Prize in Physics for the discovery of radioactivity.

In 1903, H. Strebel instituted an interstitial afterloading radium technique following an unsuccessful attempt to treat a patient with lupus using a radium surface applicator in Munich.[1] Just about the same time, Goldberg and London successfully treated two patients with basal carcinoma of the face in St. Petersburg.[2] In 1905, Robert Abbe, chief surgeon at St. Luke's Hospital, New York (Figure 2) obtained two tubes containing radium from the Curies in Paris and used it as an adjuvant to surgery. After resection of a tumor, he positioned tubes into the tumor bed and later inserted radium sources, thus pioneering the afterloading technique of radium therapy in the United States.[3]

In 1906, Wickham and Degrais, two Parisian physicians, established the Biological Laboratory of Paris (Radium Institute of Paris) (Figure 3), a center for radium therapy with Dominici as clinical director. After the tragic, accidental death of Pierre Curie in 1906, Marie Curie pursued her research of radium, determining its atomic weight in 1907, and subsequently succeeding in isolating it in a pure state. In 1911, as a consequence of this later work, she received a second Nobel Prize in Chemistry.

Early Attempts of Radium Therapy and the Development of Radon Sources in the United States

William Duane, a former associate of Mme Curie, had perfected a radium emanation (radon) extraction and purification plant in use in his laboratory at Harvard University.

From Nag S (ed): *Principles and Practice of Brachytherapy.* © Futura Publishing Co., Inc., Armonk, NY, 1997.

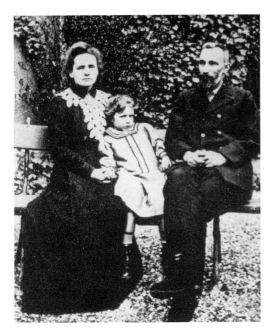

Figure 1. Pierre and Marie Curie and daughter Irene (1901).

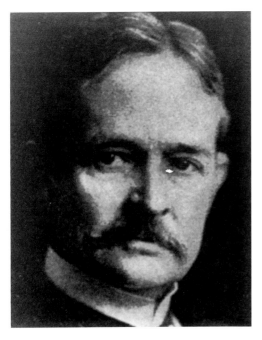

Figure 2. Robert Abbe (1905) (courtesy of Juan del Regato).

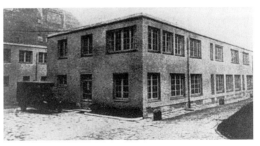

Figure 3. Radium Institute of Paris (1910) (courtesy of Juan del Regato).

Duane agreed to install a model of his plant at Memorial Hospital in New York (Figure 4).

A Radium Department was established at Memorial Hospital in 1915 with Henry H. Janeway, a surgeon, as its director (Figure 5). The first staff of this Radium Department included J.S. Sheerer, professor of Physics at Cornell, as a consulting physicist; H.C. Bailey, a gynecologist, B.S. Barringer, a urologist, S. Brown, an assistant physician, and R.S. Bosworth, a full time physicist.[4] In 1915, Gioacchino Failla joined as an assistant physicist to take care of the radon plant and study methods of improving radon applications in cancer treatment (Figure 6). Failla[5] learned to operate the plant, but he also learned everything

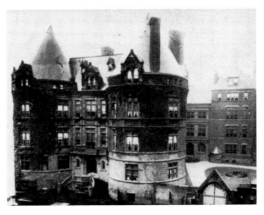

Figure 4. Old Memorial Hospital located at 100th Street and Central Park West in New York. Known as the "Bastille" due to its architecture, or the "Radium Hospital" because of the extensive use of radium (1930s).

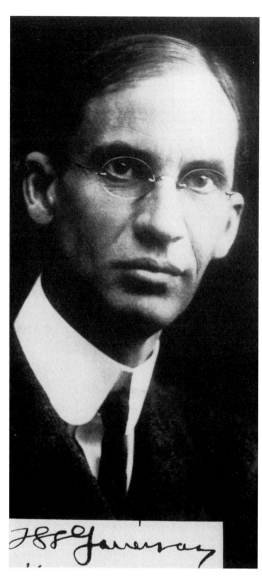

Figure 5. Henry H. Janeway (1915).

known about radioactivity and its medical uses. It became possible to compress radon into capillary glass tubes. At first, the glass containers of radon were placed in contact with accessible tumors in the same manner as surface applications of radium.[5] Janeway provided surgeons with the radon sources for the treatment of malignant tumors of various parts of the body (Figure 7).

Just about the same time, John Joly and Walter C. Stevenson[6] of Dublin were success-ful in placing capillary containers into the lumen of ordinary steel serum needles. This not only provided desirable filtration but, in addition, permitted the interstitial implanta-tion of the radioactive sources into the tu-mors. Barringer adopted this innovation in order to implant radon into carcinomas of the prostate with local anesthesia through the perineum. In 1917, Janeway, Barringer, and Failla[7] coauthored a book, *Radium Therapy in Cancer*, a report of the early efforts at the Memorial Hospital (Figure 8). The first 50 pages of this book were devoted to a didactic discussion of the physics of radioactivity by Failla; Janeway gave details of his experience with cancer of the skin and oral cavity; and Barringer gave the results of the irradiation of 25 patients with cancer of the bladder and 30 patients with cancer of the prostate. In the process, Barringer also contributed the tech-nique of the valuable procedure of perineal needle biopsy of the prostate. In 1918, small capillary glass tubes containing radium ema-nation were introduced for the first time into the tissues through fine trocar needles and left in place permanently thus adopting the prin-ciple of permanent interstitial radiation.[7]

In 1919, at the insistence of Janeway, Me-morial Hospital created a department of phys-ics of which Failla was appointed as director. In the same year, Edith H. Quimby (1891–1982) joined as an assistant to Failla. She would write later, "I was fortunate enough to apply and be accepted for the posi-tion, and thus started an association which was terminated only when we both reached retirement age in 1961. A few really extensive studies on dose distribution had been carried out, notably that by Kroenig and Friedrich, in Germany, with the first water phantom and horn ionization chamber. Regaud, in France, had called attention to the need of differen-tiating between radiation emitted from a source and that received by cells exposed to this beam, but had done nothing about it. Russ, in England, and Ghilarducci, in Italy, were making advances into the field that later developed into radiation biophysics, but there was very little work relating directly to medical radiological problems."[8]

In the 1920s, Stenstrom at the New York State Institute for the Study of Malignant Dis-ease at Buffalo (later, Roswell Park Memorial

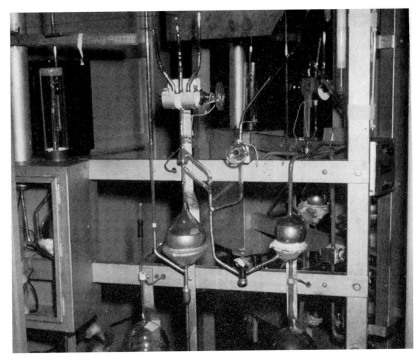

Figure 6. Radon plant pump at Memorial Hospital installed by Failla (1915).

Institute), Weatherwax at the Philadelphia General Hospital, and Glasser and Fricke at the Cleveland Clinic, began the development of radiation physics departments that steadily contributed to the science of radiology. During the same period, Sievert in Sweden, Mayneord in England, and Dessauer in Germany organized their laboratories. The former two having since dominated the field. Henry H. Janeway's experience with the interstitial use of radon seeds was published in the American Journal of Roentgenology in 1920.[9] Janeway recommended the use of radon in combination with external irradiation in lip and intraoral tumors, in rectal lesions, in cancer of the cervix, prostate, bladder, breast "when it is desired to avoid surgical removal," primary and metastatic tumors involving lymph nodes, and finally in sarcomas of the extremities.

During this period, radium had been used clinically in the form of tubes for surface or intravaginal and uterine applications; and needles for interstitial implantation. The alternative to keeping radium stock was to use radon seeds. The use of radon seeds ("la methode americaine," according to Regaud) became very popular in the United States as they were available commercially to physicians.[10]

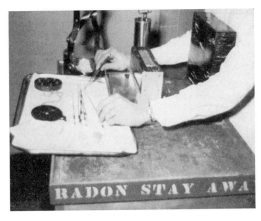

Figure 7. Manual loading in the operating room of radon "gold seeds" into needles for permanent implantation (1959).

RADIUM THERAPY IN CANCER

AT THE MEMORIAL HOSPITAL NEW YORK

(FIRST REPORT: 1915 - 1916)

BY

HENRY H. JANEWAY, M.D.

WITH THE DISCUSSION OF TREATMENT OF CANCER OF THE
BLADDER AND PROSTATE

BY BENJAMIN S. BARRINGER, M.D.

AND AN INTRODUCTION UPON THE PHYSICS OF RADIUM

BY GIOACCHINO FAILLA, E.E., A.M.

NEW YORK
PAUL B. HOEBER
1917

Figure 8. Cover of book entitled, "Radium Therapy in Cancer" by Janeway, et al. (1917).

Radium Treatment of Uterine Cancer

Wickham can be properly referred to as the father of the radium treatment of uterine cancer. He began his work in 1906 and published the results of the treatment of a thousand cancer cases in 1910 and 1913.[11]

In France

In 1907, Dominici demonstrated the different biological effects of the various qualities of rays emanated by radium salt and found that the superficial burn caused by a radioactive substance was due to beta and soft alpha rays. In 1909, Dominici reported that in 25% of his inoperable cases of uterine carcinoma he had obtained such local improvement of the tumor and infection, that these inoperable cases were regarded as operable after the treatment. Wickham and Degrais took up the problem of filtration and introduced tubes with a small thickness of 2 and 3 mm of lead. They were also the first to introduce systematic cross-fire radiation. By 1913, Cheron and Rubens-Duval had treated a large number of patients with cervical carcinoma using larger doses of radium than before, and demonstrated the necessity of a stronger filtration when the radium content of the applicators was increased. Among 50 inoperable cases, they obtained clinical cure of the growth affecting the cervix in 18 cases. The subsequent years brought further reports mainly from Regaud and Lacassagne, who painstakingly perfected techniques and dosimetry for intracavitary applications of radium for cancer of the cervix (Figure 9).

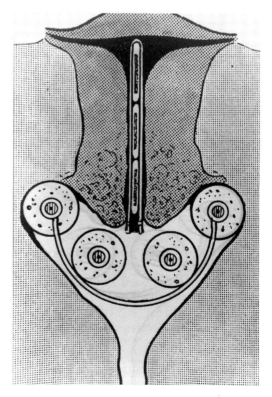

Figure 9. The Paris System (originally developed by Regaud) of intracavitary irradiation for carcinoma of the cervix (courtesy of Juan del Regato).

In Germany

The main pioneers of gynecological radiation therapy were: Doderlein, the director of the Gynecology Clinic in Tubingen and later in Munich; Kroenig, the director of Gynecology in Freiburg; Bumm, the director in Berlin; Gauss, the director in Wurburg; Menge, the director in Heidelberg; and Seitz, the director of Gynecology in Erlangen. In 1912, Kroenig presented several cases of breast and cervical carcinoma at the International Gynecologic Congress in Berlin and demonstrated the histologic eradication of these tumors with radiotherapy. This presentation stimulated the German Society of Obstetrics and Gynecology to choose as its main theme at its Congress in Halle in 1913, "the Radiotherapy of Uterine Cancer." This meeting became the milestone in the move to radiation therapy in carcinoma of the cervix following the reports of Doederlein, Kroenig, Gauss, and Bumm. They caused enormous interest not only among physicians, but also among lay people and were published throughout the world. Professor Veit closed the Congress with the cautious words, "Today we are unable to judge finally the impact of this new method, but let us continue the work for two years and then meet again." The impression that the Congress made was, however, best characterized by Janeway who wrote in 1919, that "while it is just to give to Kroenig the credit of the introduction of the use of radium in gynecology, it was Doederlein's and Bumm's reports before the German Society in Halle, in May 1913, and the papers by Cheron and Rubens-Duval, Schauta, Schindler, Scherer and Keley, Latzko and Schueller, all in 1913, that furnished the great impetus to treat cancer of the uterus by radium."[11,12] The outstanding physics department in Germany at this time was in the gynecology clinic in Freiburg, for which Kroenig secured the services of Walter Friedrich, a pupil of Roentgen, whose work with Lane and Knipping on the "nature of the x-rays" had been awarded the Nobel prize in 1911. Another famous physics department of this period was that of the gynecology clinic in Munich, under Doderlein, which was staffed in succession by Voltz, Neef, and Henschke.

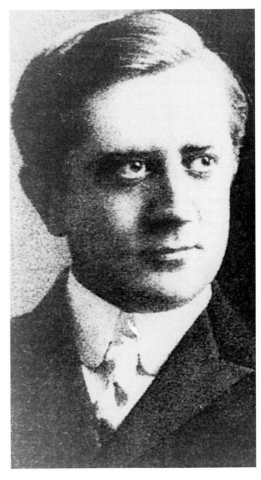

Figure 10. Gosta Fossell (1910) (courtesy of Juan del Regato).

In Sweden

Radium treatment of carcinoma of the cervix was started by Gosta Forssell[13] (Figure 10) in 1910, when a separate radiotherapy department, Radiumhemmet (the Radium House) was established (Figure 11). According to Heyman, the first years were devoted to experiments (Figure 12). The institution consisted of Forssell and one nurse with only 16 beds and 120 mg of radium in their possession. Forssell began treating inoperable patients only. When the technique of treatment had been firmly established and favorable experience gained, he also adopted treatment of borderline cases. Operable cases were not submitted to radium therapy until it had been

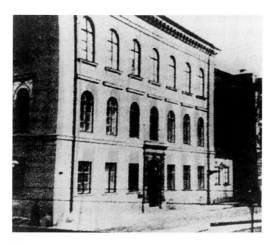

Figure 11. The Radiumhemmet (1916) (courtesy of Juan del Regato).

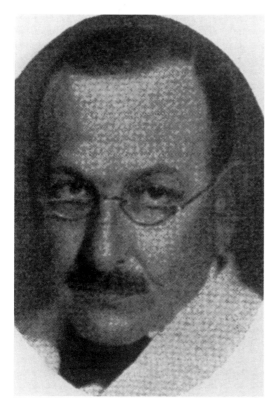

Figure 12. James E. Heyman (1930) (courtesy of Juan del Regato).

demonstrated that radium therapy in borderline cases gave equally favorable results as surgical methods. He published the first results of the primary treatment of carcinoma of the female genitalia by radium, in 1912.[13] In 1914, the Radiotherapy Department was divided into a gynecology section under James Heyman and a general section under Elis Berven. At this time, Forssell had realized the importance of keeping in contact with treated patients in order that experience gained by repeated follow-up examinations might contribute to progress. In 1917, the government began to cover the travel expenses of all cancer patients, thus making it possible to systematically study the late as well as the early reactions of irradiation. Since 1917, gynecological radiotherapy in Sweden has been considered a specialty in its own right, requiring competence in both gynecology and radiotherapy. The practice and development in this field following these developments centralized to three and later to seven clinics in Sweden. The brachytherapy methods for treatment of carcinoma of the cervix are usually referred to as "the Stockholm technique" and the method for the treatment of carcinoma of the uterus as the "Heyman packing technique." The amount of radium applied in Stockholm was two to three times higher than in Paris and its modification in Manchester, but the total number of milligram-hours of radium was very similar. The dose rate was, therefore, higher in Stockholm than in Paris and Manchester during the two or three fractions of protracted irradiation which normally were given.[14]

In England

Neville S. Finzi[15] was one of the outstanding pioneers (Figure 13). In 1913, he wrote Radium Therapy, summarizing his 4-year experience using radium. Up to that time, radiotherapy was used only in inoperable patients and with very poor results.[15] Mills at the Cancer Hospital in London was unable to report any cures following radium therapy until 1921, and Rowntree's experience was likewise not encouraging in spite of the comparatively large amounts of radium used. Whitehouse, in reporting the results of treatment of patients treated at six clinics in Eng-

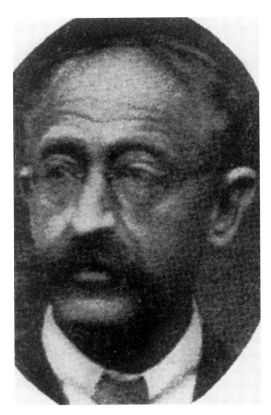

Figure 13. Neville S. Finzi (1940) (courtesy of Juan del Regato).

lation of two million in northwest England, and was treating over 2000 patients with cancer each year. Paterson held to the view that radiotherapy should be left to radiotherapists. Gradually his view prevailed.[16]

In the United States

The oldest claim to the use of radium in cervical cancer is that of Margaret A. Cleaves,[17] a New York gynecologist, who used a combination of x-rays and radium. During the first decade of this century in the United States, radium had to compete with another newly advanced method of treatment, Percy's thermotherapy. Percy's method was based on laboratory experiments that showed that cancer cells could not be successfully transplanted after exposure to 45°C

land during the period 1921–1926, counted only 507 patients, of whom 56 had no recurrence at 5 years. During this period, the Holt Radium Institute was established in Manchester and in 1931 Ralston Paterson was appointed its director (Figure 14). Paterson brought the Holt Radium Institute to the forefront of therapeutic radiology attracting students from around the world. Treatments were standardized for the same type of tumor. Paterson, Tod, and Meredith introduced changes in the classic concepts of irradiation of cancer of the cervix. Regaud's cylindrical colpostat radium containers were replaced by ovoids with the shape of the isodose curve of the radium rays. They introduced two arbitrary points, A and B, to integrate x-ray doses given from outside with gamma doses administered internally. Paterson pioneered the randomization of cases for scientific comparison by clinical trials. The Institute served a popu-

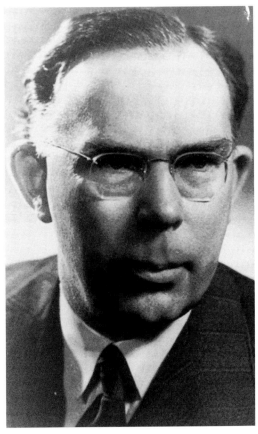

Figure 14. Ralston Paterson (1950) (courtesy of Juan del Regato).

for 10 minutes, while normal tissue cells could stand a temperature from 55°-60°C without being devitalized. In the case of cervical carcinoma, he applied an electrically heated iron to the cancerous field, introducing it through a specially devised water cooled vaginal speculum. Through a laparotomy, an assistant grasped the uterus and tumor and judged when the heating was sufficient. By this procedure, large tumors were removed at one sitting, but at times, several operations were required. This method, however, was quickly abandoned because of the frequent later hemorrhages and fistulae and because of the simultaneous progress in radium techniques. Kelly began radium therapy at Johns Hopkins, in Baltimore, in 1908. At the beginning, he only treated inoperable cases and recurrences after surgery, but as early as 1913 he extended the treatment to operable cases, giving prophylactic treatment before hysterectomy. In 1908, he reported a case, still surviving, who had an inoperable carcinoma in 1906. In 1915, Bailey and Healy began systematic radiotherapy of carcinoma of the cervix at Memorial Hospital in New York. These reports stimulated wide use of radiation therapy in cancer of the cervix. During the same period, Janeway's work at Memorial Hospital with radium in uterine cancer was most notable. He was the first man in this country to advocate radium as the agent of choice in cervical carcinoma. The technique of burying radium emanation in the cervix was developed by him and, in fact, all his work with radium emanation needles was primarily original. His work on conservative surgery plus radium was recognized early and his paper on the treatment of uterine carcinoma became a classic work.[11]

The Development of Radium Therapy Dosimetry: The Quimby and Manchester Dosage Systems

To quote Quimby, "It was understood almost from the beginning that any biological change brought about by radiation must result from a transfer of energy to the affected cells. It was also recognized that any definite number of milligrams of radium always emits the same amount of energy per hour. Thus, the number of milligrams employed and duration of treatment could lead to a dosage specification in terms of milligram hours. This formula was used for some time." In the 1920s, Quimby, at Memorial Hospital in New York, calculated the exposure in terms of milligramhours, which would produce a faint erythema with any of the applicators in use at Memorial Hospital.[18] In the 1930s, several dosage systems were developed, notably those of Quimby in New York and Paterson and Parker in Manchester.[19,20] The latter gave the doses in terms of roentgens. The roentgen as an ionization unit for x-rays had been found satisfactory, and it was natural to express radium doses in terms of the same unit. Accordingly, by means of a correction factor, the Memorial Hospital tables were transcribed into roentgens. Soon after the development of the external applicators dose tables, dose tables for interstitial therapy were also developed. They allowed the determination of the amount of radium required to give 1000 roentgens. A plan of the distribution of radium in the treated area or throughout the treated volume was obtained by the use of distribution rules. Radium techniques were devised to ensure the precise implementation of the so-called Quimby or Paterson and Parker dosage systems, and to make the most efficient use of radium.

Decline of Brachytherapy and the Introduction of Afterloading

In the 1940s, all was not easy for radiotherapy in general and brachytherapy in particular. Juan del Regato (Figure 15), one of the pioneers of radiotherapy gives the following account of that era in the United States: "the Memorial Hospital surgeons who had pioneered the use of radium remained the acknowledged arbiters of what was right or wrong in the treatment of cancer. Moreover, general radiologists were unable to accept the notion of anyone practicing radiotherapy exclusively: they feared dismembering the specialty of radiology."

In the 1950s, professional concern regarding the harmful effects of radiation caused a serious decline in the field of brachytherapy.

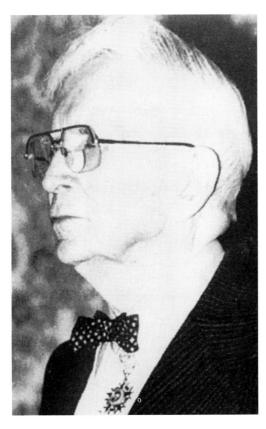

Figure 15. Juan del Regato.

developed further by Ulrich K. Henschke (Figure 16), initially, at Ohio State University (Figure 17) and beginning in 1955 at Memorial Sloan-Kettering Cancer Center (MSKCC) in New York City. The principle of afterloading consists of two steps: the insertion of unloaded tubes or applicators; and the afterloading with radioactive sources.[21]

One of us recalls the bewilderment of the participants of the 10th International Congress of Radiology in the summer of 1962 in Montreal when, following Henschke's presentation on the principle and applications of afterloading, a young woman in the front row suddenly stood up and started singing, "Afterloading hits the spot, saves your skin from getting hot, keeps your friends and fingers too, afterloading is the thing for you." The startled audience paused for a few seconds and then exploded into loud applause over this planted maneuver.

On another occasion, one late evening in 1962, we had just finished inserting afterloading plastic tubes in the operating room, tired and skeptical that we would be able to complete the hand dose calculations on time, prior to the insertion of the radioactive sources. Then we heard Henschke asking one of our physicists, Bill Siler, to try to use the

Radium, hermetically sealed in tubes, needles, or capsules, allowed the development of well established techniques that produced satisfactory clinical results. However, since the radium salt was in the form of fine powder, rupture of the sealed container resulted in the dispersal of the active material, with disastrous results owing to the long half-life of radium and its high radiotoxicity. The gamma rays emitted by radium sources were of sufficiently high energy to present serious problems in personnel exposure. During the same period, spectacular technical developments in external beam therapy and improvements in surgical techniques contributed to further declines in brachytherapy.

It has already been mentioned that afterloading of radioactive sources was used in 1903 by Strebel in Munich and soon afterwards by Abbe in New York. The principle was reintroduced and the method refined and

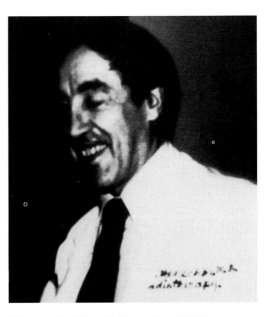

Figure 16. Ulrich K. Henschke (1970).

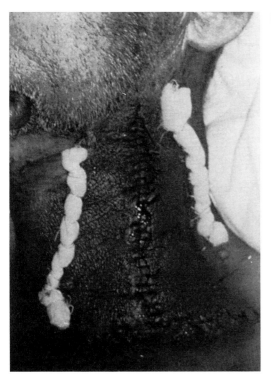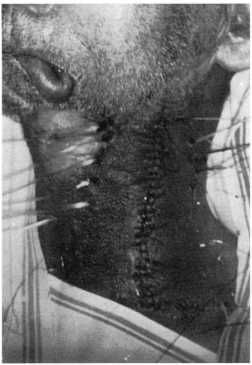

Figure 17. The first patient treated with postoperative afterloading by U.K. Henschke.

Bendix computer in the basement of the hospital to do the calculations. The next morning, at the usual 8 o'clock meeting, he triumphantly showed us the planes of the computed calculations, which Siler had obtained while working through the night. The first application of computer dosimetry in conjunction with afterloading had taken place.

Atomic Era and the Development of Substitute Sources for Radium and Radon

Despite good clinical results, professional concern regarding the harmful effects of radium exposure, technical difficulties related to source construction and availability, and laborious dose calculations limited the use of brachytherapy to major centers. Many radiation workers felt that the disadvantages of radium warranted the investigation of other radionuclides for clinical use, which had become possible with the development of nuclear reactors. Increased production of artificial radionuclides resulted in a variety of commercially available sources for brachytherapy, each with certain advantages and disadvantages.

Gold-198 was introduced in 1947, followed by Cobalt-60 in 1948, Iridium-192 in 1954, Yttrium-90 in 1956, and Cesium-137 in 1957, which in the 1960s and 1970s became the radionuclide of choice in intracavitary therapy, replacing Radium-226.

Iridium-192, in the form of wires and/or seeds, was introduced in 1955 by Henschke as a substitute for radium needles and/or radon seeds.[22] In the mid-1960s, however, the US Atomic Energy Commission imposed several restrictions, and, as a result, its use for permanent implantation was abandoned. Iridium-192 seeds for temporary implantation became commercially available in nylon ribbons and completely replaced radium needles. Because of concern over possible radioactive contamination, the use of Iridium-

192 wires was also restricted in the United States, while it became standard practice in Europe.

Introduction of Low Energy Radionuclides for Interstitial Brachytherapy

The use of low energy radionuclides for interstitial brachytherapy was investigated by our group at Memorial Hospital in New York in the early 1960s. Three such isotopes with their main lines around 30 kV, were investigated: Xenon-133 (in cooperation with Leonard Packer), Cesium-131, and Iodine-125, the last two in cooperation with Donald Lawrence.[23,24]

Low energy Iodine-125 sources were commercially produced and introduced at Memorial Hospital in 1965 as a substitute for Gold-198 and Radon-222 sources for permanent implantation. Their soft radiation had the advantage of being well localized and not exposing distant portions of the bone marrow. Localization and dosimetry procedures were developed specifically for these sources and contributed to their wide use for cancer therapy. The first clinical study was carried out at Memorial Hospital from 1966 through 1967 by Hilaris and Holt. A more detailed study by Hilaris, Holt, and St. Germain followed in the years 1968–1971.[25] Grants from the National Center for Radiological Health of the PHS supported both studies. In 1972, Anderson replaced Holt and became instrumental in developing the dosimetry for Iodine-125. The Atomic Energy Committee removed the Iodine-125 seeds from the investigational procedure list in June 1975. In November 1975, excerpts from the final report of the study, *Cancer Therapy by Interstitial and Intracavitary Radiation*, conducted at Memorial Hospital from 1968–1971 was published by the US Department of Health, Education and Welfare, Food and Drug Administration, "to encourage medical facilities to participate in the evaluation of a potentially safer and more effective therapeutic agent (Iodine 125)".

Remote Afterloading: The Turning Point in Brachytherapy

Conventional radium applications were complicated and time consuming. They involved radiation hazard to hospital personnel and, for the patient, necessitated general anesthesia during the insertion of the applicator, followed by a day or two in an isolation room. Remote afterloading with small cobalt sources of high activity moving back and forth to simulate sources of different longer active lengths was proposed by our group as an alternative technique. "Moving source remote afterloaders can be useful with all gamma emitting radioisotopes, but Cesium 137 appears most suitable except in the case of short treatment times, for which Cobalt 60 and Iridium 192 are preferable because of their higher specific activity, which in turn permits smaller sources and applicators."[26]

Our first model at MSKCC in New York was commercially marketed by the Atomic Energy of Canada Limited under the name Brachytron, and was installed in several medical centers such as the University of California in San Diego, the University of Southern California in Los Angeles, and the Cancer Institute of Beijing. This remote afterloader remained in use at MSKCC from 1964 until 1979 when it was replaced by a commercial unit (Gamma Med II). The early results were reported by us in 1974.[27]

In England, the TEM Company produced the Cathetron, and in Japan, the Ralston was produced commercially.[28,29] In Germany, the Buchler Company produced a remote afterloader, which used a high activity oscillating Iridium-192 source. Clinical experience with this machine was presented by Rotte.[30]

Low activity remote afterloaders were initially favored in Sweden, France, and Switzerland. The pioneer work of Walstam in this field resulted in two commercially produced machines, the Cervitron and the Curietron.[31] With these machines, the usual treatment times of 7 days were used (Paris technique). The sources were retracted before anyone entered the patient's room. Clinical experience with the Curietron was reported by Chassagne, Delouche, Rocoplan, Pierquin, and Gest.[32]

Galloping Towards the 21st Century: Computer Technology and High-Dose-Rate Brachytherapy Units

The role of brachytherapy in the last few years is dramatically changing, driven by extensive technological developments, including the introduction of computer produced dose distributions and three-dimensional planning, commercially produced high-dose-rate units, and finally CT and ultrasound-based, real time planning. New radionuclides are being investigated or have already become available as alternatives to existing radionuclides.

The rationale for the use of brachytherapy with conservative surgery is based on the premise of organ preservation. Current goals include refinements of technique and identification of patients to be benefitted according to stage and histologic type. The realization of these goals will enable a broader use of brachytherapy both as a primary treatment and in combination with other cancer treatment modalities.

References

1. Strebel H. Vorschlaege zur radiumtherapie. Deutsche Medizinal Zeitung 1903;24:11–45.
2. Goldberg SW, London FS. Zur Frage der Beziehungen zwischen Becquerelstrahlen und Hautaffectionen. Dermatologische Zeitschrift 1903; 10:457.
3. Abbe R. Radium in surgery. J Am Med Assoc 1906;47:183.
4. Archives of Memorial Hospital, Radium Department. Memorial Hospital, New York, 1917.
5. Failla G. Design of a well protected radium "pack." Am J Roentgenol 1928;20:128–141.
6. Stevenson WC. Preliminary clinical report on a new and economical method of radium therapy by means of emanation needles. Br Med J 1914;2:9–10.
7. Janeway HH, Barringer BS, Failla G. Radiation therapy in cancer at the Memorial Hospital, New York. Paul B. Hoeber, Division of Medical Books, Harper & Brothers, New York, 1917.
8. Quimby EH. Medical radiation physics in the United States. Radiology 1962;78:518–522.
9. Janeway HH. The use of buried emanation in the treatment of malignant tumors. Am J Roentgenol 1920;7:325–327.
10. del Regato JA. Claudius Regaud. In: Radiological Oncologists: The Unfolding of a Medical Specialty. Radiology Centennial, Inc, Reston, VA, 1993, pp. 53–63.
11. Janeway HH. The treatment of uterine cancer by radium. Surg Gynecol Obstet 1919;29: 242–265.
12. Baier K, Sauer O, Rotte K. From radium to remote afterloading: German gynecological

13. Forssell G. Radium behandling av maligna tumorer i kvinnliga genitalia. Hygiea 1912;74: 445–450.
14. del Regato JA, Gosta Forssell. In: Radiological oncologists: The Unfolding of a Medical Specialty. Radiology Centennial, Inc, Reston, VA, 1993, pp. 37–44.
15. Finzi NS. The early days of radiology. Clin Radiol 1961;12:143–146.
16. del Regato JA. Ralston Paterson. Int J Radiat Oncol Biol Phys 1987;13:1081–1091.
17. Cleaves M. Radium—with a preliminary note on radium rays in the treatment of cancer. Med Rec 1903;64:601–606.
18. Quimby EH. The development of dosimetry in radium therapy. In: Hilaris BS (ed). Afterloading: 20 Years of Experience, 1955–1975. Proceedings of the 2nd International Symposium on Radiation Therapy. Memorial Sloan-Kettering Cancer Center, New York, 1975, pp. 1–6.
19. Quimby EH. The grouping of radium tubes in packs and plaques to produce the desired distribution of radiation. Am J Roentgenol 1932; 27:18.
20. Paterson R, Parker HM. Dosage system for gamma-ray therapy. Br J Radiol 1934;7: 592–632.
21. Henschke UK, Hilaris BS, Mahan GD. Afterloading in interstitial and intracavitary radiation therapy. Am J Roent Radium Ther Nucl Med 1963;90:386–395.
22. Henschke UK. The treatment of cancer with small sources of radioactive iridium. In: Pack GT, Ariel IM (eds). Treatment of Cancer and Allied Diseases. Second Edition. Paul B Hoeber, Inc, Division of Harper Books, New York, 1958, Vol 1, pp. 431–434.
23. Henschke UK, Hilaris BS. Afterloading for interstitial gamma-ray implantation. In: Fletcher GH (ed). Textbook of Radiotherapy. Lea & Febiger, Philadelphia, PA, 1966, pp. 39–44.
24. Henschke UK, Lawrence DC. Cesium 131 seeds for permanent implants. Radiobiology 1965;6:1117–1119.
25. Hilaris BS, Henschke UK, Holt GH. Clinical experience with long half-life and low-energy encapsulated radioactive sources in cancer radiation therapy. Radiology 1968;91: 1163–1167.
26. Henschke UK, Hilaris BS, Mahan G. Remote afterloading for intracavitary radiation therapy. In: Ariel IM (ed). Progress in Clinical Cancer. Grune & Stratton, Inc, New York, 1966, pp. 127–136.
27. Hilaris BS, Ju H, Lewis JL, et al. Normal and

neoplastic tissue effects of high intensity intracavitary irradiation: Cancer of the corpus uteri.
Radiology 1974;110:459–462.

28. O'Connel D, Joslin CAF, Howard N, et al. The
treatment of uterine carcinoma using the Cathetron: Part I: Technique. Br J Radiol 1967;40:
882–887.

29. Wakabayashi M. High dose intracavitary radiotherapy using the Ralston. I: Treatment of carcinoma of the uterine cervix. Nippon Acta Radiol 1971;31:340–378.

30. Rotte K. The intracavitary radiation of cervical
cancer using an afterloading device with an
iridium 192 pinpoint source. Meeting Proceedings. Cancer of the Uterus in Developing
Areas. Rio de Janeiro, 1973, pp. 274–282.

31. Walstam R. Remotely controlled afterloading
apparatus. Acta Radiol (Ther) 1965;(Suppl 23):
84.

32. Chassagne D, Delouche G, Rocoplan JA, et al.
Description et premiers essais du Curietron. J
Radiol Electrol 1969;50:910–913.

Radiobiology

Colin G. Orton, Ph.D.

Introduction

There is really no difference in principle between teletherapy and brachytherapy in the way radiation kills cells, damages normal tissues, and destroys tumors. The basic radiobiology is the same. What is different is the physics, specifically spatial and temporal distributions of dose. This chapter presents an overview of the radiobiological principles of radiotherapy, with special emphasis on the aspects of radiobiology associated with the unique spatial and temporal attributes of brachytherapy.

The central issues that control the effectiveness of brachytherapy treatments are the dose-rate effect at low-dose-rate (LDR) and the fractionation effect at high-dose-rate (HDR).

The Dose-Rate Effect and Fractionation

With LDR brachytherapy there is ample clinical evidence to demonstrate that, for a given dose, an increase in dose rate leads to an increase in biological effect. Hence higher dose rates are an advantage for tumor control but a disadvantage with regard to risk of complications. For example, it has been shown that, for interstitial breast implants, local control is improved as dose rate is increased (Figure 1).[1] Similar dose-rate effects have been observed for the induction of complications

in normal tissues. Of special interest as far as complications are concerned are the results of a randomized clinical trial in which two low dose rates (0.38 and 0.73 Gy/hr) were compared for the intracavitary treatment of cervical carcinoma.[2] As shown in Figure 2, the cumulative incidence of complications after 6 months was higher at 0.73 Gy/hr. So also were serious injuries, although for these the difference was not statistically significant. Similar effects of *fractionation* on complication rates observed with HDR treatments for cervical carcinoma are illustrated in Figure 3.[3]

The basic radiobiological reasons for these dose-rate and fractionation effects are best illustrated in terms of the 4Rs of radiotherapy: Repair; Repopulation; Reassortment; and Reoxygenation.[4,5]

The 4Rs of Radiotherapy

Repair

Repair relates to the ability of a cell to recover from damage to its vital genetic structure before further damage renders recovery impossible. This is illustrated in Figure 4 by the curvature of the low linear energy transfer (LET) cell-survival curve, which would be a straight line if there were no repair possible, such as with high LET radiation (α particles, heavy ions, slow electrons). With high LET radiations, the density of ionization within an individual target molecule in the cells is high

From Nag S (ed): *Principles and Practice of Brachytherapy.* © Futura Publishing Co., Inc., Armonk, NY, 1997.

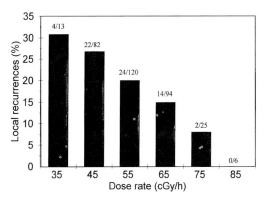

Figure 1. Influence of dose rate on local control of breast cancers treated with an Ir-192 boost dose of 37 Gy. Different dose rates were used primarily because of different source strengths available at the time of each implantation.[1]

enough to make the resulting damage so devastating that repair cannot be accomplished. On the other hand, with low LET the damage is more subtle, such as scission of a single strand of the DNA molecule (or single arm of a chromosome). Then repair can be achieved by a series of enzymatic processes by which the damaged part of the DNA molecule is excised and replaced by an identical genetic se-

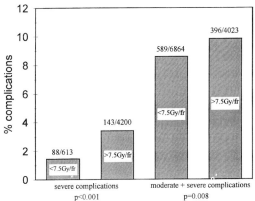

Figure 3. The effect of dose/fraction to Point A on complication rates observed in a nonrandomized, retrospective analysis of HDR intracavitary brachytherapy for the treatment of cervical carcinoma. Had this been a randomized clinical trial the effect of dose/fraction would have been highly statistically significant for both severe and moderate plus severe complications.[3]

quence obtained by synthesis of a copy of the information from the opposite, undamaged, strand. This process takes time, usually of the order of many minutes up to several hours. It is also a function of dose rate, since the higher the dose rate the more likely it is that the second strand of the DNA molecule will be damaged before the repair of the first strand has been initiated. This is the major cause of the

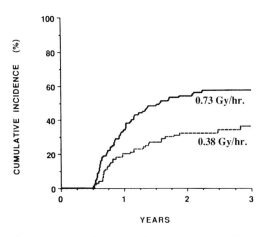

Figure 2. Cumulative incidence of late complications observed in a randomized clinical trial comparing two dose rates, 0.38 Gy h⁻¹ (lower curve) and 0.73 Gy h⁻¹ (upper curve) for the treatment of cervical carcinoma. The difference was highly significant (P<0.001). (Reproduced with permission[2]).

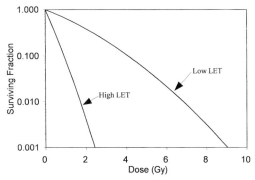

Figure 4. Typical log cell surviving fraction curves for high LET (α particles, heavy ions, slow electrons) and low LET (x-rays, γ rays, fast electrons) radiations for short irradiation times, i.e., acute exposures (or HDR).

dose-rate effect: the lower the dose rate, the more likely it is that repair will occur, and hence the cell-survival curve will become shallower. This is shown in Figure 5. In the limit when the dose rate is low enough for all repairable lesions to be repaired during the irradiation, the survival curve approaches a straight line. Note that this is not a horizontal straight line, even though complete repair has been accomplished. This is because some of the damage even for low LET radiation such as x or γ rays, is irreparable. The reason for this is that some ionizing particles traversing the DNA molecule will damage both arms simultaneously. This is especially likely if the particles are relatively slow electrons (delta rays), which always make up a small fraction of the electrons present when x or γ rays interact with biological tissue.

Repair takes place with both tumor and normal tissue cells but there is a difference that is vitally important in radiotherapy. Specifically, late-reacting normal tissue cells tend to be more capable of repair than the cells of tumors and early-responding normal tissues. This is illustrated in Figure 6, which shows that cell-survival curves for late reacting normal tissues tend to be "curvier" than those for tumor cells, and to have shallower initial slopes.[5] This means that at low doses (before the crossover point in Figure 6) more tumor cells will be killed than late reacting normal tissue cells. This is why conventional radio-

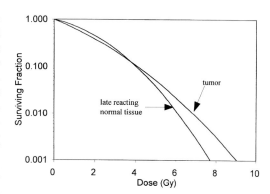

Figure 6. Log cell surviving fraction curves for late-reacting normal tissue cells tend to be "curvier" and have a shallower initial slope at low doses than those of tumor cells.[5] This difference is vitally important in radiotherapy and is the major reason for the need to fractionate with HDR treatments, or to use low dose rate for LDR.

therapy is fractionated, keeping each fraction at a dose below this crossover point. Similarly, low dose rates, which maximize repair, will benefit normal tissue more than tumors, and this is the major rationale for LDR brachytherapy.

Repopulation

Whereas "repair" represents intracellular recovery from radiation damage, "repopulation" represents extracellular recovery. Specifically, cells that have escaped damage, divide and replace "killed" cells. This can either occur at the normal rate of cell division in a dividing population of cells, whereby it is referred to as *repopulation* (or regeneration) or, if in response to damage caused by irradiation the undamaged cells cycle faster than normal, then *accelerated repopulation* occurs.[5] In either case this phenomenon takes a great deal of time to be accomplished, usually many days up to weeks, or even months.

A good example of how this effects the results of radiotherapy is illustrated in Figure 7, which shows that tumor control achieved by a course of intracavitary brachytherapy plus teletherapy for the treatment of cervix cancer is significantly reduced as overall time is increased.[6] Apparently, as treatment time is increased, tumor cells are able to repopulate

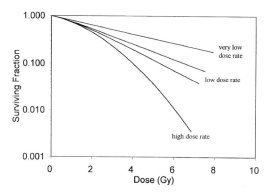

Figure 5. Typical log cell surviving fraction curves for low LET radiation as a function of dose rate. As the dose rate is reduced, cells become more resistant to irradiation and the surviving fraction curve becomes more linear.

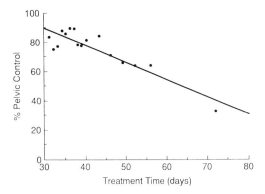

Figure 7. The effect of overall time on local control for the combined intracavitary brachytherapy/teletherapy treatment of cervical carcinoma. All 621 patients in this single institution nonrandomized, retrospective study received 45 Gy in 20 fractions by external beam plus 40 Gy to Point A via intracavitary LDR brachytherapy. The reasons for the wide variations in overall treatment times were primarily individual physician preferences, changes in treatment policies, or untoward breaks in treatment caused by machine breakdowns, holidays, travel problems, intercurrent disease, or acute toxicity. (Reproduced with permission[6]).

faster than the radiation is able to destroy them. This is especially important when the potential doubling time of the viable cancer cells (T_{pot}) is short, since the cells of late-responding normal tissues repopulate very slowly, if at all, and therefore benefit little from repopulation. The cells of acutely responding normal tissues do repopulate rapidly, however, so increasing the length of a course of radiotherapy reduces acute reactions and decreases local control, but has little effect on late reactions. As far as brachytherapy is concerned, repopulation should only be of significance for long treatments such as permanent implants of long-lived radionuclides, or courses of combined teletherapy/brachytherapy.

Reassortment

Reassortment (or redistribution) relates to the cell-cycle effect of radiation, whereby cells vary in sensitivity depending upon where they are in the cell cycle at the time of irradiation. Specifically, cells in the late G_2- and M-phases of the cell cycle tend to be most sensitive, and cells in late S-/early G_2-phases are most resistant. Hence, immediately following irradiation there will be a bolus of surviving cells in the resistant phase of the cell cycle, and these will tend to produce a partial synchrony in the dividing cell population, i.e., the cells are "redistributed" in the cell cycle.

Whereas repair and repopulation have demonstrable significance in radiotherapy, the importance of redistribution is equivocal. There has been no clinical demonstration that redistribution influences the effect of either LDR or HDR brachytherapy (or teletherapy), although an apparent "inverse dose-rate effect" observed in a few in vitro experiments, where increase in dose rate caused a decrease in cell survival over a limited dose-rate range,[7] has been explained as being due to reassortment. However, since such cell-survival effects have only been observed rarely in vitro, and never in vivo, and since no clinical effects have been demonstrated, redistribution will not be discussed further in this chapter.

Reoxygenation

Reoxygenation relates to the oxygen effect, whereby cells deprived of oxygen are more radioresistant than well oxygenated cells, and there is ample evidence to demonstrate that a significant proportion of human tumors contain regions of hypoxia. However, it is known that at least some of these hypoxic regions "open-up" during a course of radiotherapy, thus enabling previously hypoxic cells to "reoxygenate." It might be argued that hypoxic cells are unimportant in radiotherapy because of this phenomenon of reoxygenation, although there is much clinical data to refute this, at least for some cancers. Of special interest here is the data from the Princess Margaret Hospital, Toronto, on the effect of blood transfusions on anemic cervix cancer patients treated with intracavitary brachytherapy and teletherapy. This was a randomized prospective study, and they found that blood transfusions significantly improved local control of the tumor and they interpreted this as the failure of hypoxic cells to spontaneously reoxygenate in anemic patients.[8] However, in a nonrandomized study at the Institute Gustave-Roussy, blood transfusions during therapy were found *not* to improve local control, so the effect of reoxygenation remains somewhat equivocal.[9]

Another aspect of reoxygenation is the effect of time. Reoxygenation is a time-consuming process, so the longer the course of radiotherapy, the greater the opportunity for hypoxic regions of the tumor to reoxygenate. Another time-dependent factor relates to the oxygen effect itself. Specifically, the oxygen enhancement ratio (OER) (ratio of doses under hypoxic and well oxygenated conditions to produce the same biological effect) is thought to be lower at lower dose rates than at higher dose rates. This might be due to reoxygenation, but could also be related to the cell-cycle effect. Cells in the most sensitive phases of the cell cycle are known to have fairly straight cell-survival curves and hence exhibit little repair.[10] These cells would therefore be little affected by the absence of oxygen, because one of the mechanisms by which oxygen sensitizes cells is prevention of repair (O_2 "fixes" single-strand breaks in the DNA molecule, which otherwise might be repaired). Hence, the most sensitive cells will have a low OER, and these are the cells that will be most affected by irradiation at low doses and low dose rates. Probably the only time that this might significantly influence the effectiveness of brachytherapy is at very low dose rates, such as with permanent I-125 implants. For any other application of brachytherapy the effect of dose rate on OER is probably negligible.

Overall Effect

The overall effect of the 4Rs on the effectiveness of a course of brachytherapy can be summarized as follows. *Repair* is the major reason for the dose-rate effect, and at low doses and dose rates it favors late-responding normal tissues relative to tumors and thus provides the rationale for fractionation and LDR brachytherapy. *Repopulation*, on the other hand, benefits tumors more than late-reacting normal tissues, especially tumors with short potential doubling times. It is especially important when overall treatment time is long. The effect of *reassortment* is not so obvious and is probably of little consequence in radiotherapy and, even if it were, it would be very

difficult to utilize to advantage. Finally, *reoxygenation* is probably important for many tumors. However, experiments to demonstrate reoxygenation have shown that it varies tremendously from one type of tumor to the next and is, therefore, highly unpredictable.[11] To quantitate the effect of reoxygenation on a course of brachytherapy is not possible at this time, so it will be ignored in the following discussion of radiobiological models.

Biological Models of Radiation Effect

Biological modeling of the effects of radiation is important in order to define, in mathematical terms, the shapes of cell-survival curves, and to quantify the effectiveness of a course of radiotherapy.

Shape of the Cell-Survival Curve

With low LET radiations such as x and γ rays, cell-survival curves for short "acute" exposures tend to have a characteristic shape that has two distinct components (Figure 8). At low doses, the log cell-survival curve is linear with a negative slope but, as dose increases, it becomes progressively curvier. At

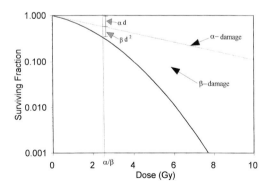

Figure 8. Typical log cell surviving fraction curve for late-responding normal tissue cells. The upper (dashed) line represents irreparable, (or α-type) damage, and between this line and the overall survival curve is a region of repairable (or β-type) damage. The dose at which α-damage equals β-damage (i.e., $\alpha d = \beta d^2$) is α/β which, in this example of a late-responding normal tissue, is about 2.5 Gy.

least, this is the shape according to the linear-quadratic (L-Q) model of cell-survival,[12–14] which has become popular because, unlike its major competitor, the "target theory," it can be readily explained in terms of the physical interactions of radiation on cells. Specifically, the L-Q model is based on the premise that double-strand breaks in DNA molecules are the lesions mainly responsible for cell lethality. The linear (low dose) part of the cell-survival curve is explained as being due to interactions where double-strand breaks in DNA molecules (or two arm breaks in chromosomes) are caused by the passage of single ionizing particles. The probability of such an interaction will be a linear function of dose, since only one ionizing particle is involved. Then the mean number of such events in each cell of a population of cells irradiated to a dose d can be represented by the expression (αd), where α is the average probability per unit dose that such an event will occur. Then, according to Poisson statistics, the probability of cells escaping any such α-type lethal events, i.e., the cell-surviving fraction, S_α, is given by[15]:

$$S_\alpha = e^{-\alpha d}$$

By similar argument, the mean number of double-strand breaks caused by the independent interactions of two separate ionizing particles is (βd^2), where β is the average probability per unit (dose)^2 that such interactions will occur. In this case the probability is a function of (dose)^2 because it is the product of the probabilities that each separate event occurs, each of which is proportional to dose. Then the fraction of cells surviving such β-type lethal events is given by:

$$S_\beta = e^{-\beta d^2}$$

Combining these expressions, the overall probability of survival, S, is given by:

$$S = S_\alpha \, S_\beta = e^{-(\alpha d + \beta d^2)}$$

Then, taking natural logs of both sides of this equation, gives:

$$-\ln S = \alpha d + \beta d^2 \qquad (1)$$

This is the relationship that gives the cell-survival curve its characteristic shape shown in Figure 8, which illustrates how two components of cell killing, α-damage and β-damage, combine to form the resultant cell-survival curve. Of special interest is the dose at which α-damage equals β-damage, i.e., $\alpha d = \beta d^2$ or d = α/β. This parameter α/β thus represents the curviness of the cell-survival curve: the straighter the cell-survival curve the higher the α/β value. Then tumor cells will tend to have a higher α/β ratio than cells from late-reacting normal tissues. For example, typical values of α/β for tumor and late-responding normal tissue cells are 10 Gy and 2.5 Gy, respectively, and these were the values used to plot the cell-survival curves in Figures 6 and 8.

So far, only repair has been considered in the development of the L-Q formula (Equation 1) but, at least as far as tumor and early responding tissue cells are concerned, repopulation is also important. Since repopulation is a function of time, this means that a time-dependent parameter needs to be introduced. This should be a function of both the irradiation time, T, and the potential doubling time, T_{pot}, and the most accepted form of this repopulation parameter is $0.693\,T/T_{pot}$. This will *decrease* the effectiveness of a course of therapy, so the L-Q equation becomes[16]:

$$-\ln S = \alpha d + \beta d^2 - \frac{0.693\,T}{T_{pot}} \qquad (2)$$

Note that T is the overall time for the course of therapy, not just the time of a brachytherapy treatment. Both T an T_{pot} are normally expressed in days. In the derivation of Equation 2 it has been assumed that repopulation continues at a constant rate throughout the course of treatment, otherwise the equation becomes more complicated. For example, if accelerated repopulation is assumed to start at a "kick-in" time T_k after the initiation of a course of treatment, then T needs to be replaced by (T-T_k) for T>T_k in Equation 2, with no (or reduced) repopulation assumed for T≤T_k.

Equation 1 represents shape of the cell-survival curve at HDR when no repair of potential β-type damage is possible during the short exposure time. However, as the dose rate is reduced, repair begins to occur *during* the irradiation and the fraction, G, of the β-type damage that is expressed begins to decrease, where G is a function of the irradiation time and the rate of sublethal damage repair.[14] The shape of the cell-survival curve is thus represented by the expression:

$$-\ln S = \alpha d + G\beta d^2 - \frac{0.693T}{T_{pot}} \quad (3)$$

Note that the two extreme values of G are G = 1 (all β-damage expressed) for irradiation times $t\mapsto0$, and G = 0 (all β-damage repaired) for $t\mapsto\infty$. For intermediate irradiation times, the equation for G is[13,14]:

$$G = \frac{2}{\mu t}\left[1 - \frac{1 - e^{-\mu t}}{\mu t}\right]$$

where t is the irradiation time for each exposure (LDR or HDR). It is represented here as a lower case t to distinguish it from the upper case T used in Equation 3, which is the overall time for the course of therapy. The t in the above equation is usually expressed in hours, and μ, the repair rate constant for the tissue cells, is in units of h^{-1}. The reciprocal of μ is the mean time for repair, and $0.693/\mu$ is thus the repair half-time. Experiments to determine such repair half-times have demonstrated wide variations between cell types[17] so, for demonstration purposes it has become common practice to use "generic" values for specific tissues. For example, it is most frequently assumed that a good representative value for the half-time for repair of late-responding normal tissue cells is 1.5 hours, or a μ value of 0.46 h^{-1}. For tumor cells, preferred half-times range from 0.5–1.5 hours, which correspond to μ values of 1.4–0.46 h^{-1}.

Following are some examples of the use of the L-Q model to demonstrate some important radiobiological principles of brachytherapy.

Applications of the Linear-Quadratic Model

Comparison of Low-Dose-Rate and High-Dose-Rate

Figure 6 illustrated the important differences in shapes of the survival curves for

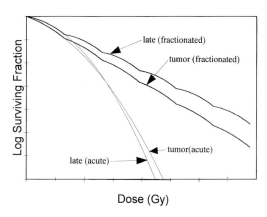

Figure 9. Illustration of how fractionation, with dose/fraction below the crossover point of the late-responding normal tissue and tumor cell-survival curves for short (acute) exposures, results in higher cell survival for the late-responding normal cells.

tumor and late-responding normal tissue cells. It was explained that fractionation at doses/fraction below the crossover point made it possible to destroy more tumor cells than those of normal tissues. This is demonstrated in Figure 9. Each fraction is assumed to reduce the log cell-survival in equal increments, so the L-Q equation for fractionated radiotherapy becomes:

$$-\ln S = N(\alpha d + G\beta d^2) - \frac{0.693T}{T_{pot}} \quad (4)$$

when N = number of fractions each of dose d (= Rt). It is similarly possible to take advantage of the different shapes of the cell-survival curves by the use of low dose rate. Comparable LDR cell-survival curves are illustrated in Figure 10. The separation between the tumor and normal-tissue curves in Figures 9 and 10 increases with decrease in dose/fraction or dose rate, respectively. Indeed, if a dose/fraction beyond the crossover point of the acute irradiation curves is used, the fractionated curves are reversed in position, and cell damage becomes greater for the normal tissues compared to tumor, as shown in Figure 11. The same effect occurs with increase in dose rate and the tumor and normal tissue curves can actually crossover (Figure 12), much like the acute exposure curves. However, whether

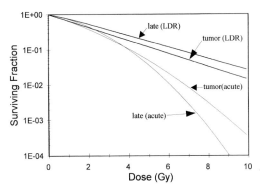

Figure 10. Illustration of how low dose rates can be utilized to take advantage of the favorable higher cell survival for late-responding normal cells at low doses (before the crossover point of the acute exposure curves). L-Q model parameters used for these curves are: $\alpha_t = 0.4$ Gy^{-1}, $(\alpha/\beta)_t = 10$ Gy, $\mu_t = 1.4$h^{-1}, $\alpha_\ell = 0.22$ Gy^{-1}, $(\alpha/\beta)_\ell = 2.5$ Gy, $\mu_\ell = 0.46$h^{-1}. The LDR dose rate was 0.4 Gy h^{-1}.

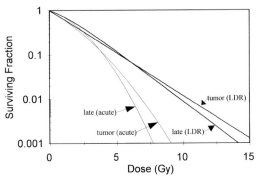

Figure 12. Demonstration of how the LDR tumor/late reacting normal tissue cell-survival curves can cross over if the dose rate is too high. The same L-Q parameters as in Figure 10 have been used but with the dose rate increased to 0.8 Gy h^{-1}.

they ever cross or, if they do, the crossover dose, is highly dependent upon the L-Q model parameters assumed. Figures 9–12 demonstrate the important radiobiological principal that the best advantage of repair is achieved by the use of low dose/fraction with HDR, or low dose rate with LDR.

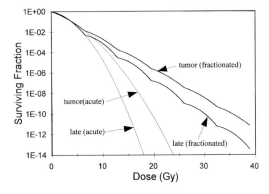

Figure 11. Demonstration of how the use of too high a dose/fraction for fractionated HDR treatments, above the crossover point of the acute irradiation curves, leads to higher survival of tumor compared to late-reacting normal tissue cells. For this example, the HDR dose/fraction was 6.5 Gy and the L-Q parameters used were the same as for Figure 10.

There have been many studies published using the L-Q model to determine the HDR equivalent of an LDR regime. As was the case with Figures 9–12, the result is highly dependent upon the L-Q model parameters assumed. For example, if the same repair rates are assumed for normal tissue and tumor cells, and the same dose is delivered to both, it has been shown that to replace a 60-Gy, 72-hour LDR application would require as many as 15–20 HDR fractions.[14,18–21] This reduces to only about seven fractions if it is assumed that tumor cells repair faster than normal tissue cells. Furthermore, even fewer fractions are needed if it is assumed that there is some "geometrical sparing" of normal tissues with brachytherapy, which is not an unreasonable assumption, since one of the major advantages of brachytherapy is that the radiation is put in or around the tumor.[14,18–21] This geometrical sparing has a very significant effect on the crossover point of normal tissue and tumor cell-survival curves, as illustrated in Figure 13. This considerably increases the dose/fraction of HDR that can be used to mimic a course of LDR therapy. This is illustrated in Figure 14, which shows that six HDR fractions of 6.5 Gy can be used to replace a 72-hour LDR application at 0.8 Gy/hr if only a modest 20% geometrical sparing is assumed, where the geometrical sparing is represented by the parameter f defined as:

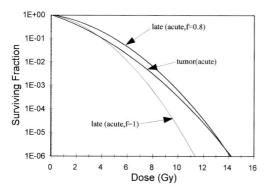

Figure 13. Illustration of how the crossover point for acute irradiations moves to considerably higher tumor doses if there is some "geometrical sparing" of the normal tissues. In this example, even with a modest 20% sparing of normal tissues (geometrical sparing factor f = 0.8), the crossover point moves from about 4 Gy out to 14 Gy. The L-Q parameters assumed are the same as for Figure 10.

geometrical sparing factor, f

$$= \frac{\text{effective normal tissue dose}}{\text{effective tumor dose}}$$

However, it must be realized that this number of HDR fractions is highly dependent upon the geometrical sparing and the L-Q model parameters assumed, especially the repair rate constant, μ. It also depends on whether or not some extra geometrical sparing can be realized when converting from LDR to HDR, such as by better retraction/packing as with cervix Ca intracavitary brachytherapy, or improved dose distributions obtainable with optimization of dwell times achievable with an HDR remote afterloader. Figure 15 illustrates how these three parameters, f, μ, and f' (the extra geometrical sparing factor HDR vs LDR) can combine to make a five fraction HDR course equivalent to a 72-hour, 60-Gy LDR schedule. The top line shows the combinations of f and f' needed to make these HDR and LDR regimes equivalent (breakeven) when the repair rate constant for tumor, μ_t, is 1.4h^{-1}. Any combination of f and f' below this line makes HDR better than LDR, and for anything above the line, LDR is better. Note that if HDR offers no additional geometrical

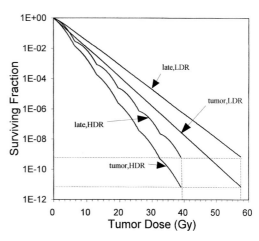

Figure 14. Demonstration of how six HDR fractions of 6.5 Gy/fraction can be equivalent, both for late reacting normal tissue and tumor cells, to a 72-hour LDR regime at 0.8 Gy h^{-1}. The L-Q model parameters used for this example are the same as were used in Figure 10, and a geometrical sparing factor of 0.8 has been assumed.

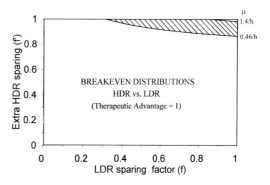

Figure 15. Combinations of geometrical sparing factor, *f*, and extra HDR sparing factor, *f'*, which make it possible to replace a 60 Gy, 72-hour LDR regime by a course of five HDR fractions. For "breakeven," the effects on both late-responding normal tissues and tumor are identical, HDR versus LDR. If μ_t = 0.46 h^{-1}, for all combinations of *f* and *f'* below the shaded region, HDR will be better than LDR. If μ_t = 1.4 h^{-1}, for all combinations *above* the shaded area, LDR will be better. These conclusions are highly dependent upon the L-Q parameters assumed, which are the same as for Figure 10.

sparing ($f=1$), HDR becomes equal to or better than LDR only when f is less than about 0.8. If $\mu=0.46$ h^{-1} the situation is not as favorable for HDR, as illustrated by the lower line in Figure 15, which shows that if $f=1$, then f needs to be below about 0.3 before HDR becomes better than LDR. However, even a modest extra geometrical sparing factor of 0.85 causes HDR to be always better than LDR. This is probably the main reason for the lower complication rates reported with HDR for cervix cancer brachytherapy without reduction in local control.[3,22,23]

All of the above calculations and graphs have been generated using the L-Q model without the repopulation factor 0.693T/T$_{pot}$ in Equation 4. This is reasonable for comparison of HDR and LDR regimes because it is relatively easy to keep the overall treatment time fairly constant, especially when each is combined with a course of teletherapy. The situation with permanent implants is, however, quite different, and repopulation plays an important role in the determination of outcome.

Permanent Implants

The two most commonly used sources for permanent implants today are I-125 and Pd-103. Others have been used in the past, Rn-222 and Au-198 being the best examples, and others are being considered for the future, such as Yb-169 (see Chapter 4). The major reason for changing from Rn-222 and Au-198 has been radiation safety, since all the newer sources emit radiations of considerably lower energy, so shielding is simpler and in some cases even unnecessary. However, due to their different half-lives, they are quite different radiobiologically when used as permanent implants. Ling[24] has used the L-Q model, modified to account for decreasing dose rate with time, to demonstrate these radiobiological differences and some of his results are shown in Figure 16. His analysis shows that for rapidly proliferating tumors (short T$_{pot}$), Pd-103 implants are more effective than I-125 (Figure 16A), but the reverse is true for slowly growing tumors (Figure 16B). This demonstrates mathematically what would be expected intuitively from the different half-lives of I-125 and Pd-103 of 60 days and 17 days,

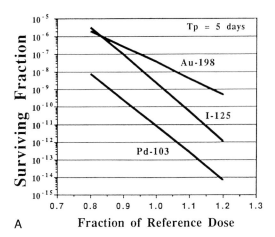

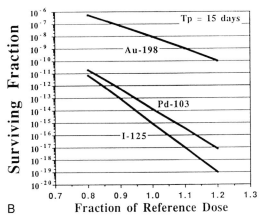

Figure 16. Tumor cell surviving fraction curves for permanent implants of Au-198, Pd-103, and I-125. A reference dose of 1.0 indicates the typical total doses to complete decay used in clinical practice of 60 Gy, 120 Gy, and 160 Gy, respectively.[24] L-Q model parameters used were: $\alpha = 0.3$ Gy^{-1}; $\alpha/\beta = 10$ Gy; and $\mu = 0.693$ h^{-1}. (A) Potential doubling time T$_{pot}$ = 5 days; (B) T$_{pot}$ = 15 days. (Reproduced with permission[24]).

respectively, since I-125 will take better advantage of the differences in repair capacities of normal tissues and tumors, whereas Pd-103 will minimize the effect of tumor cell repopulation. The L-Q model does a good job illustrating how these radiobiological principles might influence the relative effectiveness of these permanent implants. However, this is a good example of why the L-Q model needs to be used with caution, because quite different conclusions could result if different parameters had been used in the equations. For example, Ling showed that, for permanent prostate implants, Au-198 should produce more late complications than I-125, for the same tumor effect, whereas Dale[25] drew exactly the opposite conclusion, because he used different L-Q model parameters. Hence, results obtained using the L-Q model, and any other mathematical model that attempts to represent the highly complex events that occur in irradiated tissues in a "simple" equation, have to be treated with a certain degree of skepticism. Such models are useful for the qualitative description of radiobiological principles, but they will never replace good hard clinical data. In the absence of such data, however, they provide a means to delve into the un-

known. A good example of such an application is pulsed brachytherapy (PB).

Pulsed Brachytherapy

A major advantage of HDR is the ability to create an almost infinite array of dose distributions, especially with the most common single source remote afterloading systems. Indeed, the extra geometrical sparing of normal tissues that can be achieved by the optimization of such dose distributions could well be the major reason why HDR brachytherapy for cervix cancer seems to exhibit a therapeutic advantage over LDR. The objective of PB is to provide a similar advantage to LDR treatments (see Chapter 33).

In the absence of clinical, or even animal,

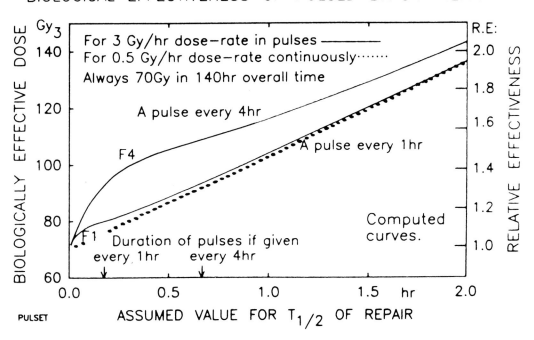

Figure 17. Variation of Biologically Effective Dose (BED) or Relative Effectiveness (RE) with the assumed half-time for repair for continuous LDR therapy (140 h at 0.5 Gy h^{-1}) shown by the dotted line, and for two pulsed brachytherapy (PB) schedules (one pulse every hour or every 4 hours), where BED = (-ln S)/α and RE = BED/(total dose).[26] The curves are for late-responding normal tissues (α/β = 3 Gy). At a repetition frequency of 1 pulse/hour, PB and LDR are essentially equivalent, whereas at 1 pulse every 4 hours, PB is more damaging than LDR. However, it is also more damaging to tumor cells and Fowler has demonstrated that the effect this has on the therapeutic ratio depends on the μ-values assumed. (Reproduced with permission[27]).

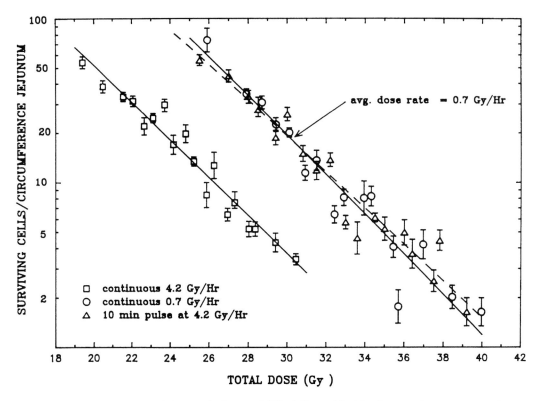

Figure 18. Demonstration of the equivalence of PB, delivered in 10-minute pulses, once-per-hour, and LDR at the same average dose rate of 0.7 Gy h[-1]. Shown are the surviving stem cells/circumference of mouse jejunum for overall exposure times of 30–60 h. (Reproduced with permission[28]).

data to demonstrate the effectiveness of PB, several studies using the L-Q model to predict biological effects of PB have been undertaken.[17,26,27] For example, Fowler and Mount[26] predicted that with pulses delivered every hour, the biological effectiveness of PB should not be significantly different from conventional brachytherapy regardless of the half-time for repair (Figure 17). However, with pulses given every 4 hours, PB becomes significantly more biologically damaging. Interestingly, the equivalence of PB and conventional LDR has since been demonstrated for once-per-hour pulses by in vivo experiments using crypt-cell survival in the mouse jejunum as the biological end-point (Figure 18).[28]

Fowler has taken his L-Q model calculations one step further by suggesting that there might even be a potential therapeutic advantage of PB if tumor cells repair sublethal dam-age faster than the cells of late-responding normal tissues.[27] Specifically, he has shown that if the half-times for repair of tumor and late reacting normal tissue cells are 0.5h and 1.5h, respectively, then the ratio of the biological effect on tumor to that on normal tissues should be slightly higher for PB than for continuous LDR. However, this is highly conjectural since it is not possible to count on such favorable repair half-times. The differences are also "slight," so it is unlikely that they will be exploitable.

Modification of Clinical Regimes

The L-Q model is widely used for the determination of iso-biologically effective treatment schedules when conventional regimes are modified, either in routine clinical practice or for the design of new protocols.[12–14] For this purpose it is convenient to rearrange the cell-survival L-Q equation (Equation 4), by dividing both sides by α to form the expression for the so-called Biologically Effective Dose (BED)[16]:

$$(-\ln S)/\alpha = NRt\left(1 + G\frac{Rt}{\alpha/\beta}\right) - kT \quad (5)$$

where $0.693/(\alpha T_{pot})$ has been replaced by k because, in retrospective analyses of clinical data, it is easier to determine the single repopulation parameter k than the two separate parameters, α and T_{pot}. Here k is the extra BED per day necessary to combat repopulation.

In order to expedite calculation of BEDs, a set of tables for LDR at different dose rates and overall times has been generated for various combinations of μ and α/β (Tables 1–3). These should be sufficient for the solution of most problems, provided the user is willing to accept generic μ and α/β values. For HDR just one table of BEDs/fraction for various α/β values should suffice (Table 4). To use these tables, simply read off the BED for a particular dose rate and time (or for a specific BED/fraction for HDR and multiply by the number of fractions), using the α/β and μ values appropriate for the tissue in question: for late-responding normal tissues use $\alpha/\beta = 2.5$ Gy and $\mu = 0.46$ h^{-1}; for early-responding tissues or tumors use $\alpha/\beta = 10$ Gy and μ either 0.46 h^{-1} or 1.4 h^{-1} and, if necessary, subtract the repopulation correction kT.

The following examples illustrate use of these Tables.

Modification of LDR Dose Rate

A radiation oncologist considers the standard regime for a particular Ir-192 temporary interstitial implant to be 48 hours at 0.8 Gy h^{-1}. The Ir-192 sources are of lower activity than usual, such that the dose rate is only 0.4 Gy h^{-1}. What is the implant time needed in order for the effect on the tumor to be unchanged?

Assume $\mu = 1.4$ h^{-1} so, using Table 1 and interpolating between 40 and 50 hours, the planned BED = 42.7. Then looking down the 0.4 Gy h^{-1} column to find a BED of 42.7 shows that between 100 (42.3) and 110 (46.5) hours are required. Interpolation yields 101

hours. Note that, because the correction for repopulation is likely to be small, especially if this is just a boost dose for a course of teletherapy, it has been ignored in this calculation.

Modification of HDR Fractionation

What HDR dose/fraction in four fractions is equivalent to six fractions of 5 Gy/fraction as far as late-reacting normal tissues are concerned?

Assume that the α/β for late-reacting normal tissue cells is 2.5 Gy. Then, from Table 4, the BED/fraction for $\alpha/\beta = 2.5$ Gy and 5 Gy/fraction is 15.00, so the total BED is 6x15.00 = 90. Then in four fractions, the required BED/fraction is 90/4 = 22.5. Looking down the $\alpha/\beta = 2.5$ Gy column it is observed that the required dose/fraction lies between 6 (20.40) and 6.5 (23.40) Gy. Interpolation yields 6.35 Gy/fraction. Again, repopulation correction has been ignored for simplicity.

Conversion of LDR to HDR for Cervix Cancer Brachytherapy

It is required to convert an intracavitary regimen of 70 hours at 0.8 Gy h^{-1} (Point A) to a five fraction HDR regimen. Ignoring repopulation corrections, what dose/fraction is necessary in order to maintain the same tumoricidal effect, and how will this effect risk of complications assuming a geometrical sparing factor of 0.8 and no extra HDR sparing?

Assume $\mu_t = 1.4$ h^{-1} and that Point A represents tumor. Then Table 1 yields a tumor BED for 70 hours at 0.8 Gy h^{-1} of 62.3. For a five fraction HDR regime, the BED/fraction is therefore 12.46. Looking down the $\alpha/\beta = 10$ Gy column of Table 4 shows that the dose/fraction lies between 7 (11.90) and 7.5 (13.13) Gy, and interpolation gives 7.23 Gy/fraction.

For the late-responding normal tissues, $f = 0.8$, so the LDR dose rate is 0.8x0.8 = 0.64 Gyh^{-1}, and the HDR dose/fraction is 7.23x0.8 = 5.78 Gy. From Table 3, the BED for 70 hours at 0.64 Gy h^{-1} is, by interpolation between 0.6 (84.5) and 0.7 (106.8) Gy h^{-1}, equal to 93.4. From Table 4, looking down the $\alpha/\beta = 2.5$ Gy column, the BED/fraction lies between 17.60 (5.5 Gy/fraction) and 20.40 (6 Gy/fraction). Interpolation to 5.78 Gy/frac-

Table 1.
Biologically Effective Doses

Time (hours)	Dose Rate (Gy/hour)																			
	0.1	0.2	0.3	0.4	0.5	0.6	0.7	0.8	0.9	1.0	1.1	1.2	1.3	1.4	1.5	1.6	1.7	1.8	1.9	2.0
10	1.0	2.1	3.1	4.2	5.3	6.5	7.7	8.8	10.1	11.3	12.6	13.9	15.2	16.6	18.0	19.4	20.8	22.3	23.8	25.3
20	2.0	4.1	6.2	8.4	10.7	13.0	15.4	17.8	20.2	22.8	25.3	28.0	30.7	33.4	36.2	39.1	42.0	44.9	48.0	51.0
30	3.0	6.2	9.4	12.7	16.0	19.5	23.1	26.7	30.4	34.2	38.1	42.0	46.1	50.2	54.4	58.7	63.1	67.6	72.1	76.8
40	4.1	8.2	12.5	16.9	21.4	26.0	30.8	35.6	40.6	45.6	50.8	56.1	61.5	67.0	72.6	78.4	84.2	90.2	96.3	102.5
50	5.1	10.3	15.6	21.1	26.8	32.5	38.5	44.5	50.7	57.0	63.5	70.1	76.9	83.8	90.9	98.0	105.4	112.8	120.4	128.2
60	6.1	12.3	18.8	25.4	32.1	39.1	46.2	53.4	60.9	68.5	76.3	84.2	92.3	100.6	109.1	117.7	126.5	135.5	144.6	153.9
70	7.1	14.4	21.9	29.6	37.5	45.6	53.9	62.3	71.0	79.9	89.0	98.3	107.7	117.4	127.3	137.4	147.6	158.1	168.8	179.6
80	8.1	16.5	25.0	33.8	42.8	52.1	61.6	71.3	81.2	91.3	101.7	112.3	123.2	134.2	145.5	157.0	168.8	180.7	192.9	205.4
90	9.1	18.5	28.1	38.0	48.2	58.6	69.3	80.2	91.3	102.8	114.4	126.4	138.6	151.0	163.7	176.7	189.9	203.4	217.1	231.1
100	10.1	20.6	31.3	42.3	53.5	65.1	77.0	89.1	101.5	114.2	127.2	140.4	154.0	167.8	181.9	196.3	211.0	226.0	241.3	256.8
110	11.2	22.6	34.4	46.5	58.9	71.6	84.7	98.0	111.7	125.6	139.9	154.5	169.4	184.6	200.2	216.0	232.2	248.6	265.4	282.5
120	12.2	24.7	37.5	50.7	64.3	78.1	92.4	106.9	121.8	137.1	152.6	168.6	184.8	201.4	218.4	235.7	253.3	271.3	289.6	308.2
130	13.2	26.7	40.7	55.0	69.6	84.7	100.1	115.8	132.0	148.5	165.4	182.6	200.2	218.2	236.6	255.3	274.4	293.9	313.7	334.0
140	14.2	28.8	43.8	59.2	75.0	91.2	107.8	124.7	142.1	159.9	178.1	196.7	215.7	235.0	254.8	275.0	295.6	316.5	337.9	359.7
150	15.2	30.9	46.9	63.4	80.3	97.7	115.5	133.7	152.3	171.3	190.8	210.7	231.1	251.8	273.0	294.7	316.7	339.2	362.1	385.4
160	16.2	32.9	50.1	67.6	85.7	104.2	123.2	142.6	162.5	182.8	203.6	224.8	246.5	268.6	291.3	314.3	337.8	361.8	386.2	411.1
170	17.2	35.0	53.2	71.9	91.1	110.7	130.9	151.5	172.6	194.2	216.3	238.9	261.9	285.4	309.5	334.0	359.0	384.4	410.4	436.8
180	18.3	37.0	56.3	76.1	96.4	117.2	138.6	160.4	182.8	205.6	229.0	252.9	277.3	302.3	327.7	353.6	380.1	407.1	434.6	462.6
190	19.3	39.1	59.4	80.3	101.8	123.7	146.3	169.3	192.9	217.1	241.8	267.0	292.7	319.1	345.9	373.3	401.2	429.7	458.7	488.3
200	20.3	41.1	62.6	84.6	107.1	130.3	154.0	178.2	203.1	228.5	254.5	281.0	308.2	335.9	364.1	393.0	422.4	452.3	482.9	514.0

Table of biologically effective doses (BEDs) for low-dose-rate brachytherapy. This table is for tumors and uses $\alpha/\beta = 10$ Gy and repair-rate constant $\mu = 1.4$ h^{-1}, i.e., half-time for repair of 0.5 hours.

Table 2.
Biologically Effective Doses

Time (hours)	Dose Rate (Gy/hour)																			
	0.1	0.2	0.3	0.4	0.5	0.6	0.7	0.8	0.9	1	1.1	1.2	1.3	1.4	1.5	1.6	1.7	1.8	1.9	2
10	1.0	2.1	3.3	4.5	5.9	7.2	8.7	10.2	11.8	13.4	15.1	16.9	18.8	20.7	22.7	24.7	26.9	29.1	31.3	33.6
20	2.1	4.3	6.7	9.2	11.9	14.8	17.8	21.0	24.3	27.8	31.4	35.2	39.1	43.2	47.4	51.8	56.4	61.1	66.0	71.0
30	3.1	6.5	10.1	13.9	18.0	22.4	26.9	31.7	36.8	42.1	47.6	53.4	59.4	65.7	72.2	79.0	86.0	93.2	100.7	108.4
40	4.2	8.7	13.5	18.6	24.1	29.9	36.1	42.5	49.3	56.4	63.9	71.7	79.8	88.2	97.0	106.1	115.5	125.3	135.4	145.8
50	5.2	10.8	16.9	23.3	30.2	37.5	45.2	53.3	61.8	70.8	80.2	89.9	100.1	110.8	121.8	133.2	145.1	157.4	170.1	183.2
60	6.3	13.0	20.3	28.0	36.3	45.1	54.3	64.1	74.4	85.1	96.4	108.2	120.5	133.3	146.6	160.4	174.7	189.5	204.8	220.6
70	7.3	15.2	23.7	32.7	42.4	52.6	63.5	74.9	86.9	99.5	112.7	126.5	140.8	155.8	171.4	187.5	204.2	221.6	239.5	258.0
80	8.3	17.4	27.0	37.4	48.5	60.2	72.6	85.7	99.4	113.8	128.9	144.7	161.2	178.3	196.1	214.6	233.8	253.6	274.2	295.4
90	9.4	19.5	30.4	42.1	54.5	67.7	81.7	96.4	111.9	128.2	145.2	163.0	181.5	200.8	220.9	241.8	263.4	285.7	308.9	332.7
100	10.4	21.7	33.8	46.8	60.6	75.3	90.8	107.2	124.5	142.5	161.5	181.3	201.9	223.4	245.7	268.9	292.9	317.8	343.6	370.1
110	11.5	23.9	37.2	51.5	66.7	82.9	100.0	118.0	137.0	156.9	177.7	199.5	222.2	245.9	270.5	296.0	322.5	349.9	378.2	407.5
120	12.5	26.0	40.6	56.2	72.8	90.4	109.1	128.8	149.5	171.2	194.0	217.8	242.6	268.4	295.3	323.2	352.1	382.0	412.9	444.9
130	13.6	28.2	44.0	60.9	78.9	98.0	118.2	139.6	162.0	185.6	210.3	236.0	262.9	290.9	320.1	350.3	381.6	414.1	447.6	482.3
140	14.6	30.4	47.4	65.6	85.0	105.6	127.4	150.4	174.5	199.9	226.5	254.3	283.3	313.5	344.8	377.4	411.2	446.2	482.3	519.7
150	15.6	32.6	50.8	70.3	91.1	113.1	136.5	161.1	187.1	214.3	242.8	272.6	303.6	336.0	369.6	404.5	440.8	478.3	517.0	557.1
160	16.7	34.7	54.2	75.0	97.2	120.7	145.6	171.9	199.6	228.6	259.0	290.8	324.0	358.5	394.4	431.7	470.3	510.3	551.7	594.5
170	17.7	36.9	57.6	79.7	103.2	128.3	154.8	182.7	212.1	243.0	275.3	309.1	344.3	381.0	419.2	458.8	499.9	542.4	586.4	631.9
180	18.8	39.1	61.0	84.4	109.3	135.8	163.9	193.5	224.6	257.3	291.6	327.3	364.7	403.5	444.0	485.8	529.5	574.5	621.1	669.3
190	19.8	41.3	64.4	89.1	115.4	143.4	173.0	204.3	237.2	271.7	307.8	345.6	385.0	426.1	468.8	513.1	559.0	606.6	655.8	706.7
200	20.9	43.4	67.7	93.8	121.5	151.0	182.1	215.0	249.7	286.0	324.1	363.9	405.4	448.6	493.5	540.2	588.6	638.7	690.5	744.1

Table of tumor biologically effective doses (BEDs) for low-dose-rate brachytherapy with $\alpha/\beta = 10$ Gy and $\mu = 0.46$ h^{-1}, i.e. half-time for repair of 1.5 hours.

Table 3.
Biologically Effective Doses

Time (hours)	Dose Rate (Gy/hour)																			
	0.1	0.2	0.3	0.4	0.5	0.6	0.7	0.8	0.9	1	1.1	1.2	1.3	1.4	1.5	1.6	1.7	1.8	1.9	2
10	1.1	2.5	4.2	6.2	8.4	10.9	13.7	16.7	20.1	23.6	27.5	31.7	36.1	40.8	45.7	50.9	56.4	62.2	68.3	74.6
20	2.3	5.2	8.8	13.0	17.8	23.2	29.2	35.8	43.1	51.0	59.5	68.6	78.4	88.8	99.8	111.4	123.6	136.4	149.9	164.0
30	3.5	7.9	13.4	19.7	27.1	35.4	44.7	55.0	66.2	78.4	91.6	105.7	120.8	136.8	153.9	171.9	190.9	210.8	231.7	253.6
40	4.7	10.6	17.9	26.5	36.4	47.7	60.2	74.1	89.3	105.8	123.6	142.7	163.2	184.9	208.0	232.4	258.1	285.1	313.5	343.1
50	5.8	13.3	22.5	33.3	45.8	59.9	75.8	93.2	112.4	133.2	155.6	179.8	205.6	233.0	262.1	292.9	325.4	359.5	395.3	432.7
60	7.0	16.0	27.1	40.1	55.1	72.2	91.3	112.4	135.5	160.6	187.7	216.8	248.0	281.1	316.3	353.4	392.6	433.8	477.0	522.3
70	8.2	18.7	31.6	46.9	64.5	84.5	106.8	131.5	158.5	188.0	219.7	253.9	290.3	329.2	370.4	414.0	459.9	508.2	558.8	611.8
80	9.4	21.4	36.2	53.7	73.8	96.7	122.3	150.6	181.6	215.3	251.8	290.9	332.7	377.3	424.5	474.5	527.2	582.5	640.6	701.4
90	10.5	24.1	40.7	60.4	83.2	109.0	137.8	169.8	204.7	242.7	283.8	327.5	375.1	425.4	478.7	535.0	594.4	656.9	722.4	791.0
100	11.7	26.8	45.3	67.2	92.5	121.2	153.4	188.9	227.8	270.1	315.9	365.0	417.5	473.5	532.8	595.5	661.7	731.2	804.2	880.5
110	12.9	29.5	49.9	74.0	101.9	133.5	168.9	208.0	250.9	297.5	347.9	402.0	459.9	521.5	586.9	656.1	728.9	805.6	885.9	970.1
120	14.0	32.2	54.4	80.8	111.2	145.8	184.4	227.1	274.0	324.9	379.9	439.1	502.3	569.6	641.1	716.6	796.2	879.9	967.7	1059.6
130	15.2	34.9	59.0	87.6	120.6	158.0	199.9	246.3	297.1	352.3	412.0	476.1	544.7	617.7	695.2	777.1	863.5	954.3	1049.5	1149.2
140	16.4	37.6	63.6	94.4	129.9	170.3	215.4	265.4	320.2	379.7	444.0	513.2	587.1	665.8	749.3	837.6	930.7	1028.6	1131.3	1238.8
150	17.6	40.3	68.1	101.1	139.3	182.6	231.0	284.5	343.2	407.1	476.1	550.2	629.5	713.9	803.4	898.1	998.0	1103.0	1213.1	1328.3
160	18.7	43.0	72.7	107.9	148.6	194.8	246.5	303.7	366.3	434.5	508.1	587.2	671.9	762.0	857.6	958.7	1065.2	1177.3	1294.9	1417.9
170	19.9	45.7	77.3	114.7	158.0	207.1	262.0	322.8	389.4	461.9	540.2	624.3	714.3	810.1	911.7	1019.2	1132.5	1251.6	1376.6	1507.5
180	21.1	48.4	81.8	121.5	167.3	219.3	277.5	341.9	412.5	489.3	572.2	661.3	756.6	858.1	965.8	1079.7	1198.8	1326.0	1458.4	1597.0
190	22.3	51.1	86.4	128.3	176.7	231.6	293.1	361.1	435.6	516.6	604.2	698.4	799.0	906.2	1020.0	1140.2	1267.0	1400.3	1540.2	1686.6
200	23.4	53.8	91.0	135.0	186.0	243.9	308.6	380.2	458.7	544.0	636.3	735.4	841.4	954.3	1074.1	1200.7	1334.3	1474.7	1622.0	1776.2

Table of biologically effective doses for late-responding normal tissues, with $\alpha/\beta = 2.5$ Gy and $\mu = 0.46$ h^{-1}.

Table 4.
BED per Fraction

Dose/fr (Gy)	α/β													
	1	1.5	2	2.5	3	4	6	8	10	12	14	16	18	20
0.5	0.75	0.67	0.63	0.60	0.58	0.56	0.54	0.53	0.53	0.52	0.52	0.52	0.51	0.51
1	2.00	1.67	1.50	1.40	1.33	1.25	1.17	1.13	1.10	1.08	1.07	1.06	1.06	1.05
1.5	3.75	3.00	2.63	2.40	2.25	2.06	1.88	1.78	1.73	1.69	1.66	1.64	1.63	1.61
2	6.00	4.67	4.00	3.60	3.33	3.00	2.67	2.50	2.40	2.33	2.29	2.25	2.22	2.20
2.5	8.75	6.67	5.63	5.00	4.58	4.06	3.54	3.28	3.13	3.02	2.95	2.89	2.85	2.81
3	12.00	9.00	7.50	6.60	6.00	5.25	4.50	4.13	3.90	3.75	3.64	3.56	3.50	3.45
3.5	15.75	11.67	9.63	8.40	7.58	6.56	5.54	5.03	4.73	4.52	4.38	4.27	4.18	4.11
4	20.00	14.67	12.00	10.40	9.33	8.00	6.67	6.00	5.60	5.33	5.14	5.00	4.89	4.80
4.5	24.75	18.00	14.63	12.60	11.25	9.56	7.88	7.03	6.53	6.19	5.95	5.77	5.63	5.51
5	30.00	21.67	17.50	15.00	13.33	11.25	9.17	8.13	7.50	7.08	6.79	6.56	6.39	6.25
5.5	35.75	25.67	20.63	17.60	15.58	13.06	10.54	9.28	8.53	8.02	7.66	7.39	7.18	7.01
6	42.00	30.00	24.00	20.40	18.00	15.00	12.00	10.50	9.60	9.00	8.57	8.25	8.00	7.80
6.5	48.75	34.67	27.63	23.40	20.58	17.06	13.54	11.78	10.73	10.02	9.52	9.14	8.85	8.61
7	56.00	39.67	31.50	26.60	23.33	19.25	15.17	13.13	11.90	11.08	10.50	10.06	9.72	9.45
7.5	63.75	45.00	35.63	30.00	26.25	21.56	16.88	14.53	13.13	12.19	11.52	11.02	10.63	10.31
8	72.00	50.67	40.00	33.60	29.33	24.00	18.67	16.00	14.40	13.33	12.57	12.00	11.56	11.20
8.5	80.75	56.67	44.63	37.40	32.58	26.56	20.54	17.53	15.73	14.52	13.66	13.02	12.51	12.11
9	90.00	63.00	49.50	41.40	36.00	29.25	22.50	19.13	17.10	15.75	14.79	14.06	13.50	13.05
9.5	99.75	69.67	54.63	45.60	39.58	32.06	24.54	20.78	18.53	17.02	15.95	15.14	14.51	14.01
10	110.00	76.67	60.00	50.00	43.33	35.00	26.67	22.50	20.00	18.33	17.14	16.25	15.56	15.00
10.5	120.75	84.00	65.63	54.60	47.25	38.06	28.88	24.28	21.53	19.69	18.38	17.39	16.63	16.01
11	132.00	91.67	71.50	59.40	51.33	41.25	31.17	26.13	23.10	21.08	19.64	18.56	17.72	17.05
11.5	143.75	99.67	77.63	64.40	55.58	44.56	33.54	28.03	24.73	22.52	20.95	19.77	18.85	18.11
12	156.00	108.00	84.00	69.60	60.00	48.00	36.00	30.00	26.40	24.00	22.29	21.00	20.00	19.20
12.5	168.75	116.67	90.63	75.00	64.58	51.56	38.54	32.03	28.13	25.52	23.66	22.27	21.18	20.31
13	182.00	125.67	97.50	80.60	69.33	55.25	41.17	34.13	29.90	27.08	25.07	23.56	22.39	21.45
13.5	195.75	135.00	104.63	86.40	74.25	59.06	43.88	36.28	31.73	28.69	26.52	24.89	23.63	22.61
14	210.00	144.67	112.00	92.40	79.33	63.00	46.67	38.50	33.60	30.33	28.00	26.25	24.89	23.80
14.5	224.75	154.67	119.63	98.60	84.58	67.06	49.54	40.78	35.53	32.02	29.52	27.64	26.18	25.01
15	240.00	165.00	127.50	105.00	90.00	71.25	52.50	43.13	37.50	33.75	31.07	29.06	27.50	26.25

Table of biologically effective doses (BEDs) per fraction (fr) for different values of α/β and dose/fraction for acute irradiations, i.e., high-dose-rate brachytherapy or fractioned teletherapy. To determine a BED, simply multiply the value in this table (for the desired α/β) by the number of fractions.

tion yields 19.17 BED/fraction. Then in five fractions, the total BED is 95.8. This, compared with the LDR BED of 93.4, shows that the HDR regime should be slightly more toxic.

Hence, in order not to increase toxicity, six fractions of HDR should be used (repeating the above calculations shows that six fractions should lead to a slight reduction in toxicity, HDR vs LDR) or, alternatively efforts should be made to gain some extrageometrical sparing with the HDR regimen. Repetition of the above calculations for a five fraction HDR regime with only a 2% extrageometrical sparing ($f = 0.98$) shows that this is sufficient to equalize the complication risks, HDR versus LDR.

Conclusions

Radiobiological effects induced by both teletherapy and brachytherapy irradiations are both governed by the 4Rs of radiotherapy: repair; repopulation; reassortment; and re-

oxygenation. However, because of the unique spatial and temporal distributions of dose inherent with brachytherapy, the way in which the 4Rs influence outcome can be different.

Because of the different repair capacities of tumor and late-reacting normal tissue cells, dose rate (with LDR) and fractionation (with HDR) play a vital role in brachytherapy. If either the dose rate or the dose fraction is too high, cell kill in normal tissues can exceed that in tumors, thus making it impossible to gain local control without exceeding tolerance. Fortunately, "geometrical sparing" of normal tissues is often possible with brachytherapy and this significantly increases the dose rate and dose/fraction limits below which uncomplicated control is achievable.

The effect of repopulation in brachytherapy is little different from that in teletherapy, especially since brachytherapy is frequently an adjunct to a course of teletherapy and, most often, the length of the brachytherapy component is relatively short. Hence, the effect of repopulation is essentially driven by the length of the course of teletherapy. The exception will be when brachytherapy is the primary radiotherapy treatment, especially permanent implants where it is probably better to tailor the half-life of the radionuclide used to the proliferation rate of the tumor cells. This can be demonstrated using the L-Q model, although detailed information on exactly which isotope to use when, is equivocal due to lack of knowledge of the proper L-Q parameters to use.

The roles of reassortment (cell-cycle effect) and reoxygenation (oxygen effect) in influencing the outcome of a course of brachytherapy are more ill-defined. There is some clinical indication that oxygenation of tumors can modify local control in brachytherapy, and some radiobiological evidence that the oxygen enhancement ratio might be reduced at the very low dose rates inherent with permanent implants, but both these concepts need further investigation. Reassortment, on the other hand, has not yet been demonstrated to be of much concern in clinical brachytherapy.

The L-Q model is useful for the study of several interesting brachytherapy problems, especially the comparison of HDR and LDR, and pulsed brachytherapy. The model demonstrates that HDR can be equivalent to LDR, provided enough fractions are delivered, but the appropriate number of fractions is highly dependent upon the parameters assumed, especially the repair rate constant for tumor cells, and the geometrical sparing factor for normal tissues. Clinical evidence indicates that equivalence to LDR is achievable with a reasonable number of HDR fractions for the intracavitary treatment of carcinoma of the cervix, but information for other sites is not yet available for analysis. With pulsed brachytherapy, the L-Q model indicates that equivalence to continuous LDR should be achievable with pulses once every hour, and this has been confirmed in a few radiobiological experiments.

References

1. Mazeron JJ, Simon JM, Crook J, et al. Influence of dose rate on local control of breast carcinoma treated by external beam irradiation plus iridium 192 implant. Int J Radiat Oncol Biol Phys 1991;21:1173–1177.
2. Lambin P, Gerbaulet A, Kramar A, et al. Phase III trial comparing two low dose rates in brachytherapy of cervix carcinoma: Report at two years. Int J Radiat Oncol Biol Phys 1993;25:405–412.
3. Orton CG, Seyedsadr M, Somnay A. Comparison of high and low dose rate remote afterloading for cervix cancer and the importance of fractionation. Int J Radiat Oncol Biol Phys 1991;21:1425–1434.
4. Withers HR. The four R's of radiotherapy. Adv Radiat Biol 1975;5:241–247.
5. Hall EJ. Radiobiology for the Radiologist. Fourth Edition. Lippincott, Philadelphia, PA, 1994, pp. 212–229.
6. Keane TJ, Fyles A, O'Sullivan B, et al. The effect of treatment duration on local control of squamous carcinoma of the tonsil and carcinoma of the cervix. Semin Radiat Oncol 1992;2:26–28.
7. Mitchell JB, Bedford JS, Bailey SM. Dose-rate effects on the cell cycle and survival of S3 HeLa and V79 cells. Rad Res 1979;79:520–536.
8. Bush R. The significance of anemia in clinical radiation therapy. Int J Radiat Oncol Biol Phys 1986;12:2047–2050.
9. Girinski T, Pejovic-Lenfant MH, Bourhis J, et al. Prognostic value of hemoglobin concentrations and blood transfusions in advanced carcinoma of the cervix treated by radiation therapy: Results of a retrospective study of 386 patients. Int J Radiat Oncol Biol Phys 1989;16:37–42.
10. Sinclair WK, Morton RA. X-ray and ultraviolet sensitivity of synchronized Chinese hamster cells at various stages of the cell cycle. Biophys J 1965;5:1–25.
11. Rockwell RS, Moulder JE. Biological factors of importance in split-course radiotherapy. In: Paliwal BR, Herbert DE, Orton CG (eds). Optimization of Cancer Radiotherapy. Am Inst Phys, New York, 1985, pp. 171–182.
12. Barendsen GW. Dose fractionation, dose rate and isoeffect relationships for normal tissue responses. Int J Radiat Oncol Biol Phys 1982;8:1981–1997.
13. Dale RG. The application of the linear-quadratic dose-effect equation to fractionated and protracted radiotherapy. Br J Radiol 1985;58:515–528.
14. Orton CG, Brenner DJ, Dale RG, et al. Radiobiology. In: Nag S (ed). High Dose Rate Brachytherapy: A Textbook. Futura Publishing Company, Inc., Armonk, NY, 1994, pp. 11–25.
15. Casarett AP. Radiation Biology. Prentice-Hall, Englewood Cliffs, NJ, 1968, pp. 136–144.

16. Fowler JF. The linear-quadratic formula and progress in fractionated radiotherapy. Int J Radiat Oncol Biol Phys 1992;62:457–467.

17. Brenner DJ, Hall EJ. Conditions for the equivalence of continuous to pulsed low dose rate brachytherapy. Int J Radiat Oncol Biol Phys 1991;20:181–190.

18. Dale RG. The use of small fraction numbers in high dose-rate gynecological afterloading: Some radiobiological considerations. Br J Radiol 1990;63:290–294.

19. Brenner DJ, Hall EJ. Fractionated high dose rate versus low dose rate regimens for intracavitary brachytherapy of the cervix I: General considerations based on radiobiology. Br J Radiol 1991;64:133–141.

20. Stitt JA, Fowler JF, Thomadsen BR, et al. High dose rate intracavitary brachytherapy for carcinoma of the cervix: The Madison System: I. Clinical and radiobiological considerations. Int J Radiat Oncol Biol Phys 1992;24:335–348.

21. Scalliet P, Gerbaulet A, Dubray B. HDR versus LDR gynecological brachytherapy revisited. Radioth and Oncol 1993;28:118–126.

22. Orton CG. High dose rate versus low dose rate brachytherapy for gynecological cancer. Semin Radiat Oncol 1993;3:232–239.

23. Patel FD, Sharma SC, Negi PS, et al. Low dose rate vs high dose rate brachytherapy in the treatment of carcinoma of the uterine cervix: A clinical trial. Int J Radiat Oncol Biol Phys 1994;28:335–341.

24. Ling CC. Permanent implants using Au-198, Pd-103 and I-125: Radiobiological considerations based on the linear quadratic model. Int J Radiat Oncol Biol Phys 1992;23:81–87.

25. Dale RG. Radiobiological assessment of permanent implants using tumour repopulation factors in the linear-quadratic model. Br J Radiol 1989;62:241–244.

26. Fowler JF, Mount M. Pulsed brachytherapy: The conditions for no significant loss of therapeutic ratio compared with traditional low dose rate brachytherapy. Int J Radiat Oncol Biol Phys 1992;23:661–669.

27. Fowler JF. Why shorter half-times of repair lead to greater damage in pulsed brachytherapy. Int J Radiat Oncol Biol Phys 1993;26:353–356.

28. Mason KA, Thames HD, Ochran TG, et al. Comparison of continuous and pulsed low dose rate brachytherapy: Biological equivalence in vivo. Int J Radiat Oncol Biol Phys 1994;28:667–671.

—— Chapter 4 ——————————————————————

Basic Physics of Brachytherapy

Ali S. Meigooni, Ph.D., Ravinder Nath, Ph.D.,
Cheng B. Saw, Ph.D.

Introduction

Brachytherapy refers to the treatment of cancer by inserting sealed radioactive sources into the patient's natural body cavity (intracavitary) or into the tumor (interstitial). This radiation treatment modality has been used since the discovery of radium by Marie Curie in 1898. In early days, selections of treatment time and source strengths were based on clinical observations of changes in irradiated tissues. However, in the 1930s this technique was revised, a change attributed in part to the introduction of the radiation unit, the Roentgen, and to the formulation of the Manchester system by Paterson and Parker.[1A] Since then, many man-made radionuclides, such as Cs-137, Ir-192, and I-125, have been introduced for brachytherapy treatments to optimize the absorbed dose to the target region and to minimize the radiation dose to surrounding tissues. Brachytherapy treatments are categorized as low-dose-rate (LDR) for dose rates <100 cGy per hour or high-dose-rate (HDR) for dose rates >600 cGy per hour or 10 cGy per minute. This chapter deals with the basic physics of LDR brachytherapy and includes discussion of the physical characteristics of brachytherapy sources, the specification of source strength, the absorption and scattering of the radiation through the matter in the brachytherapy energy range, and traditional and current dose calculation formalisms for brachytherapy treatment.

Physical Characteristics of Brachytherapy Sources

Though radium and radon have been used extensively in the past, they are virtually unused today, primarily because of the hazards of chemical and radioactive toxicity of radium and its by-products and because of the high energy of photons emitted by these sources. The high energy of the photons makes it difficult to shield health professionals and the others from radiation exposure. For these reasons, several lower energy photon emitters have been introduced. Table 1 shows the physical characteristics of brachytherapy sources that are available for brachytherapy implants. These radioisotopes are encapsulated in sealed, nontoxic capsules made of titanium or stainless steel (Figure 1). The physical characteristics of some of the commonly used brachytherapy are described below.

Radium-226

Radium-226 (Ra-226) is the sixth member of the uranium series that starts with U-238 and ends with stable Pb-206. Radium decays into radon, with a half-life of about 1622 years; radon is a heavy inert gas that in turn

From Nag S (ed): *Principles and Practice of Brachytherapy.* © Futura Publishing Co., Inc., Armonk, NY, 1997.

Table 1.
Physical Characteristics of Radionuclides Used in Brachytherapy Sources

Isotope	Exposure Rate Constant (Γ_δ)$_x$ (R cm^2 mCi^{-1} hr^{-1})	Mean Photon Energy (MeV)	Half-Life	HVL* (mm of Pb)	Permanent (P)/ Temporary (T) Implants	f$_{muscle}$** (cGy/R)
^{60}Co	13.07	1.25	5.26 years	10.2	T	0.962
^{226}Ra	8.26‡	1.03	1622 years	14.0	T	0.962
^{137}Cs	3.28	0.662	30.0 years	5.57	T	0.962
^{192}Ir	4.69	0.380	73.83 days	2.5	T	0.962
^{198}Au	2.35	0.412	2.70 days	2.68	P	0.962
^{169}Yb	1.58	0.093	32 days	0.48	T	0.960
^{241}Am	0.12	0.0595	432.2 years	0.126	T	0.937
^{145}Sm	0.78	0.043	340 days	0.060	T	0.922
^{125}I	1.45	0.028	59.6 days	0.025	P and T	0.920
^{103}Pd	1.48	0.021	17 days	0.004	P	0.920

‡ The exposure rate constant for all the radionuclides except radium-226 is for a bare point source with no filtration. For radium, this value is for a source with 0.5 mm platinum filtration and it is expressed in units of (R cm^2 mg^{-1} hr^{-1}).

* Half value layer thickness.

** Exposure in air to dose in muscle conversion factor.

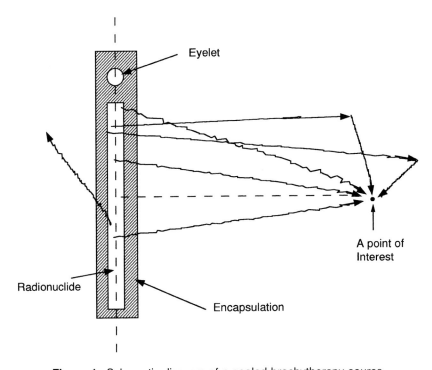

Figure 1. Schematic diagram of a sealed brachytherapy source.

disintegrates into its daughter products. As a result of the decaying processes from Ra-226 to Pb-206, at least 49 photons are emitted, with energies ranging from 0.184–2.45 MeV. The average energy of the γ-rays from radium in equilibrium with its daughter products and filtered by 0.5 mm of platinum is 0.83 MeV. There are also some high energy β-particles and α-particles emitted by this isotope that are absorbed by the encapsulation material. The half-value-layer (HVL) of this radioisotope is about 14 mm of lead.

The radioactive material was supplied mostly in the clinical form of radium sulfate or radium chloride mixed with inert filler and loaded into cells about 1 cm long and 1 mm in diameter. A radium source might contain 1–3 cells depending on the source length. Radium sources were manufactured as needles or tubes in a variety of lengths and activities. As mentioned earlier, radium sources are no longer used in clinical practice.

Cesium-137

Cesium-137 (Cs-137) is a by-product of fission in nuclear reactors. It has a half-life of about 30 years and decays through β-emission (93.5%) to the metastable state of Ba-137 (half-life 2.5 minutes) and then through γ-ray emissions to its ground state. The γ-rays emitted have a photon energy of 662 keV. The HVL for this radioisotope is about 5.5 mm of lead.

The radioactive material is supplied in the form of insoluble powders or ceramic microspheres labeled with cesium and doubly encapsulated in stainless steel for both needles and tubes. The β-particles and low energy characteristic x-rays are totally absorbed by the stainless steel encapsulation, making the clinical source a pure γ-emitter. The active length of the tube sources manufactured by Amersham International (Amersham, England) is normally 13.5–14.0 mm (external size = 20 mm long and 2.65–3.05 mm in diameter). For the needles, the active length ranges from 15–54 mm and the external length from 24.5–55 mm. The needles are available from Amersham in two diameters, 1.65 mm and 1.85 mm.

Cs-137 sources are less hazardous and require less shielding compared to that required for Ra-226 sources. Although the half life of Cs-137 is much less than that of Ra-226, the cesium sources can be used clinically for about 7 years without replacement. In clinical use, the activity of the sources must be adjusted for the decay of Cs-137 over time. Cs-137 sources have been used in both interstitial and intracavitary brachytherapy.

Iridium-192

Iridium-192 (Ir-192) is a reactor-produced radioisotope via neutron capture by stable Ir-191. Ir-192 has a half-life of 73.83 days and decays primarily by β-emission and electron capture to excited states of Pt-192 and Os-192. Subsequently, the daughters decay to the ground states by γ-ray emission. Ir-192 has a very complicated γ-ray spectrum. The average energy of γ-ray spectrum is about 0.38 MeV. Because of the lower γ-ray energy than radium or cesium, Ir-192 sources require less shielding. The HVL thickness for this radionuclide is about 2.5 mm.

In the United States, Ir-192 sources are available in the form of small sources placed in nylon ribbons for safety purposes. Two different source designs are commercially available in the United States. The sources offered by Best Medical International (Springfield, VA, USA) have an inner core alloy composed of 30% iridium and 70% platinum, encapsulated in stainless steel (Figure 2, left). However, the sources offered by Alpha Omega Services Inc. (Bellflower, CA, USA), have an inner core alloy composed of 10% iridium and 90% platinum surrounded by a 0.1-mm thick cladding of platinum (Figure 2, right). Both source types are 3 mm long and 0.55 mm in diameter; they are press-fitted, normally at 1-cm intervals, into nylon ribbons with an outer diameter of about 0.8 mm.

In Europe, Ir-192 sources are commonly available as wires composed of an alloy of 25% iridium and 75% platinum enveloped in pure platinum. The wires are available in two sizes with outer diameters of 0.3 mm and 0.5 mm.

Ir-192 wires and sources in ribbons are particularly suitable for afterloading technique. These sources are used for temporary brachytherapy implants only, because their high average photon energy has the potential to pro-

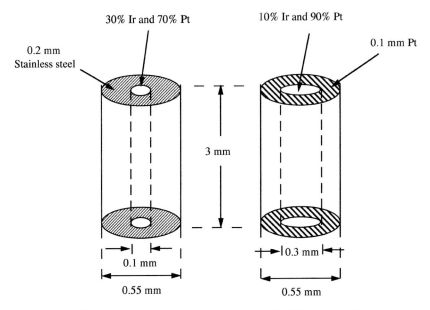

Figure 2. Schematic diagrams of a platinum-encapsulated Ir-192 source (right) and a stainless-steel-encapsulated Ir-192 source (left).

duce radiation protection problems if used in permanent implants. High intensity Ir-192 sources are also available for the HDR remote afterloader units. The high intensity sources are described in Chapter 5.

Gold-198

Gold-198 (Au-198) is produced in a reactor by bombarding a gold target with neutrons. Au-198 has a half-life of 2.7 days and emits a monoenergetic γ-ray with an energy of 0.412 MeV and β-rays with a maximum energy of 0.96 MeV. A typical gold seed, also known as a gold "grain," is encapsulated in 0.1 mm of platinum, which is sufficient to absorb the β-rays emitted by Au-198. The outside dimensions of a Au-198 source are 2.5 mm long and 0.8 mm in diameter. Because of their short half-life, Au-198 seeds are used in permanent implants only. Although commonly used in Canada, the Au-198 sources have been used only sparsely in the United States.

Iodine-125

Iodine-125 (I-125) has a half-life of 59.6 days decaying exclusively by electron capture

process to an excited state of Te-125 followed by spontaneous decay to the ground state with the emission of 35.5 keV γ-rays. Characteristic x-rays in the range of 27–35 keV are also emitted as a consequence of the electron capture and internal conversion processes. One of the advantages of this radioisotope over radon and gold is the lower energy of the photons that it emits, which makes reducing radiation exposures around the patient much easier. The HVL thickness for this radionuclide is about 0.025 mm of lead.

Two models of the I-125 seeds are provided by Amersham (Figure 3). In model 6711, the I-125 is adsorbed on a 3-mm long silver rod that is the central core of the source. The rod is encapsulated in 0.5 mm of titanium; the resultant seed is 4.5-mm long and 0.8 mm in

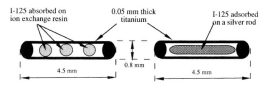

Figure 3. Schematic diagrams of Model 6702 (left) and Model 6711 (right) I-125 seeds.

diameter. In model 6702, the seed consists of a titanium tube containing 2–4 ion exchange resin spheres I-125. Titanium encapsulation serves to absorb low energy electrons and x-rays. The ion exchange resin beads are impregnated with I-125 in the form of iodide ion. This technique offers an efficient absorption of I-125, which allows fabrication of higher activity sources than is possible with model 6711. The titanium tube is welded at both ends to form a cylindrical 4.5 mm × 0.8 mm capsule. Except for their use in I-125 eye plaques, Model 6711 I-125 seeds are used principally for permanent implants, because the activity is insufficient for use in temporary implants. Model 6702 can be used for both permanent or temporary implants.

Californium-252

Californium-252 (Cf-252) has a half-life of 2.65 years decaying via nuclear fission. It emits neutrons with a spectrum of neutron energies similar to that of a fission reactor and with an average energy of 2.15 MeV. A significant number of γ-rays with an average energy of 0.7–0.9 MeV are also emitted from the fission events and from the decay of fission products.

The Cf-252 source, developed at the University of Kentucky, has a central core consisting of a ceramic metal mixture of Cf-252 oxide and palladium. This core is encapsulated with platinum (10% Ir) to limit the combined γ-ray and β-ray dose to one third the effective neutron dose. The seed is about 6 mm long and 0.8 mm in diameter. Cf-252 sources are intended for use as temporary implants.

Palladium-103

Palladium-103 (Pd-103) is produced in a nuclear reactor when stable Pd-102 captures a thermal neutron. With a half-life of 17 days, it decays via electron capture process with the emission of characteristics x-rays in the energy range of 20–23 keV and Auger electrons. The HVL photons emitted from Pd-103 are 0.004 mm of lead.

The Pd-103 sources manufactured by Theragenics Corporation (Atlanta, GA, USA) consist of a cylindrical titanium tube sealed at both ends with laser welded titanium end cups (Figure 4). Enclosed in the tube are two Pd-103 graphite cylinders and a lead rod x-ray marker for radiographic identification. The cylindrical tube is about 4.5 mm long and 0.81 mm in diameter. The Pd-103 seeds are presently used for permanent implants.

Strontium-90

Strontium-90 (Sr-90) decays with a half-life of 28.9 years to Yttrium-90 and yields β-rays

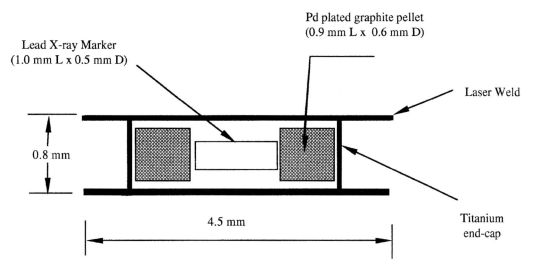

Figure 4. Schematic diagram of a Pd-103 source.

with a maximum energy of 0.5 MeV. It is a pure β-ray emitter suitable for treatment of superficial lesions. The Sr-90 ophthalmic applicators are described in the instrumentation and equipment chapter in this text.

Other Radioisotopes

Other radioisotopes that have been used in brachytherapy include Cobalt-60 (Co-60), Tantalum-182, Ruthenium-106, Rhodium-106, Americium-241, Samarium-145, and Ytterbium-169.[1B]

The long half-life of Am-241 and the intermediate photon energy of about 60 keV indicate that this radionuclide may be well suited for intracavitary use in which custom designed shielding may be required.[2] The Sm-145 has a half-life of 340 days and photon energies in the range of 38–45 keV. With its low energy and relatively long half-life, Sm-145 is being considered as a substitute isotope for removable interstitial implant.[3]

Source Strength Specification

At present, there are four measures for specifying the source strength: 1) activity of a radionuclide; 2) exposure rate at a reference point in space; 3) equivalent mass of radium; and 4) air-kerma rate at a reference point in free space. These specifications have been addressed in American Association of Physicists in Medicine (AAPM) report No: 21[4] and are briefly reviewed here.

Activity of a Radionuclide

The rate of disintegration of a radioactive material is known as "activity." This quantity, A, is proportional to the number of the radionuclide atoms, N, present in a sample as:

$$A = dN/dt = -\lambda N \qquad (1)$$

where λ is the decay constant expressed in s^{-1}. Equation 1, can be rewritten as:

$$dN/N = \lambda \, dt \qquad (2)$$

Solving this differential equation leads to:

$$N = N_o \, e^{-\lambda t} \qquad (3)$$

where N_o and N are the initial and decayed number of radionuclide, respectively, in the source. In one half-life, $T_{1/2}$, of the source, the number of radionuclide decays into half of its initial value. Substituting these parameters in Equation 3, leads to the relation between the decay constant, λ, and half-life as:

$$\frac{1}{2} N_o = N_o e^{-\lambda T_{1/2}} \qquad (4)$$

Dividing both sides of this equation by N_o and applying the natural logarithmic will lead to:

$$\ln \left(\frac{1}{2} \right) = -\lambda \, T_{1/2} - 0.693 = -\lambda \, T_{1/2} \lambda$$
$$= \frac{0.693}{T_{1/2}} \qquad (5)$$

Comparison of Equations 1 and 3 shows that the source activity also decays exponentially with time as:

$$A = A_o e^{-\lambda t} \qquad (6)$$

where A_o and A are the initial and decayed activity, respectively, of the source.

Two commonly used units of activity are the *Curie* (Ci) and the *Becquerel* (Bq). The reference for the older of the two units, the Curie, is the decay rate of 1 g of Ra-226, which at the time this unit was adopted had been determined to be 3.7×10^{10} dps (disintegration per second). With modern instruments, it has been determined that the decay rate of 1 g of Ra-226 is 3.61×10^{10} dps; therefore, 1 Ci has been redefined to be equal to 3.7×10^{10} dps. This definition is applicable for all of the radionuclides. The commonly used submultiples of Curie, mCi and μCi, are equal to 3.7×10^7 dps and 3.7×10^4 dps, respectively. The modern unit of activity is the Becquerel, which is defined to be 1 dps. Therefore, one millicurie is equal to 3.7×10^7 Bq or 37.0 Mbq.

The radiation emitted by a radioactive source can be absorbed or attenuated by the enclosing materials. Since this absorbed radiation does not reach the tumor, it should not be considered in radiation therapy. Therefore, to account for this effect, vendors have used "content activity" and "apparent activity" to describe the activity of sources.

Content Activity

Content activity is the activity of the actual radionuclide within a brachytherapy source, as opposed to apparent activity, which is described in the following section. Direct measurement of the content activity is a difficult procedure. National standards for the radioactivity measurements of many radionuclides are not available. Moreover, exposure rate constants must be determined in order to perform brachytherapy dosimetry based on activity. The content activity of a source does not take into account the distribution of the radioactivity within the source and the source geometry. The exposure rate of an encapsulated linear source is normally less than the expected value from a bare point source. To account for the variation of the source geometry and also attenuations of the photons by the source structure, an effective source activity or apparent activity has been defined.

Apparent Activity

The apparent activity of a real source is equivalent to the activity of a bare point source that produces the same exposure rate at a reference point. For example, if exposure rate at 1 cm from an I-125 source is 145 R/hr, the apparent activity is equivalent to 100 mCi of the bare point source. In order to produce the resulting exposure rate, the activity inside the source encapsulation must be about 70% more, because the content activity is attenuated by this amount by the encapsulation and by self-absorption. The manufacturers of the brachytherapy sources usually provide both content and apparent activity of the sources. For high energy photon emitters, the difference between the content and apparent activity is small (<2%). However, for low energy photon emitters such as I-125 and Pd-103, the differences are large and depend on the type and thickness of the encapsulation material.

Exposure Rate at a Reference Point in Free Space

Strength of a brachytherapy source can be expressed in terms of the exposure rate at a specified distance (usually 1 m) along the perpendicular bisector of the source. This specification is a measured quantity that can be directly traceable to the national standard. Dose rate in tissue is more closely related to the knowledge of exposure rate than to the activity in an encapsulated source.

Equivalent Mass of Radium

The source strength can also be expressed in terms of equivalent mass of radium. This is particularly useful in the case of Cs-137 used in intracavitary application. The equivalent mass of radium is defined as the mass of radium encapsulated in 0.5-mm Pt that produces the same exposure rate at a reference distance as the source to be specified. The relationship between the equivalent mass of radium and the source activity is:

$$\text{mgRaeq} = \frac{A_{app}\Gamma}{\Gamma_{Ra}} \quad (7)$$

where A_{app} is the source activity, Γ is the exposure rate constant for the radionuclide, and Γ_{Ra} is the exposure rate constant for radium encapsulated with 0.5-mm Pt (Table 1). In addition to intracavitary application, this expression for source strength also facilitates the use of radium dosage tables that had been well established and widely used. As the philosophy on the planning of brachytherapy evolves with the routine use of computers, the use of these tables may be declining. As such, the usage of this source strength unit may decline as well.

Air-Kerma Rate at a Reference Point in Free Space

The source strength can also be expressed in terms of air-kerma rate at a specified distance (usually taken as 1 m) along the perpendicular bisector of a line source. The air-kerma strength is defined as the product of the air-kerma rate in free space and the square of the distance of the calibration point from the source center along the perpendicular bisector. Unit of the air-kerma strength is μGy-m^2 h^{-1}, which is numerically equivalent to cGy-cm^2 h^{-1}. This unit has been defined by the symbol U. Thus $1U = 1\ \mu$Gy-m^2 h$^{-1} = 1$

cGy-cm^2 h^{-1}. The air-kerma strength is related to the exposure rate of the source at a reference point in free space as:

$$S_k = K \cdot d^2 \qquad (8)$$

where:

$$K = X (W/e) \qquad (9)$$

where X is the exposure rate and (W/e) is the average energy required to produce an ion pair in dry air, which is 0.876 cGy/R.

The air-kerma based quantities have been recently advocated by the scientific committees like AAPM,[5] British Committee on Radiation Units and Measurements,[6] and French Committee on Radioisotopes.[7A] This usage also appears in the International Commission on Radiological Units and Measurements in its report[7B] for intracavitary therapy. Manufacturers have also initiated the use of air-kerma strength or reference air-kerma rate for specifying the source strength instead of apparent activity or equivalent mass of radium.

During this transitional period, it is convenient to use the conversion factors for selective radionuclides set forth by the AAPM task group 32,[5] such as I-125 (1.270 U mCi^{-1}), Ir-192 (7.227 U mg Ra Eq^{-1}), and Pd-103 (1.293 U mCi^{-1}).

Basic Dose Calculation Techniques

Dose distribution around a brachytherapy source is a complex function of the source geometry, emitted radiation, and surrounding media. In general, dose calculations for an implant are performed assuming a homogenous water equivalent medium, using either point source approximations (seeds) or linear source approximation. The following sections present a brief review of traditional and current dose calculation techniques.

Conventional Formalism

Point Source Approximation

Dose at distances larger than twice the active length of the source can be estimated using point source approximation. Under this approximation, the dose rate at a distance r from the source center in water medium is given by:

$$\dot{D}(r) = A_{app} \cdot (\Gamma_\delta)_x \cdot f_{med} \cdot \frac{T(r)}{r^2} \, \bar{\phi}_{an}$$

$$(10)$$

where A_{app} is apparent activity in mCi, $(\Gamma_\delta)_x$ is exposure rate constant in R $\cdot$ cm^2 $\cdot$ h^{-1} $\cdot$ mCi^{-1}, f_{med} is exposure-to-dose conversion factor in cGy $\cdot$ R$_{-1}$, T(r) is the tissue attenuation factor, and ϕ_{an} is the anisotropy factor. Apparent activity has been explained above. Other parameters are discussed below.

Inverse Square Law. The inverse square law refers to the change of the dose rate inversely proportional to the change of the distance between the source of radiation and point of interest. Therefore, dose rates are reduced to one quarter and one ninth if the distances are increased to double or three times, respectively. The impact of inverse square law is more critical in brachytherapy than teletherapy. For example, a 1 cm increase in distance in teletherapy may reduce the dose rate by about 2%. However, in brachytherapy, dose rate from a single source reduces by about 75%, by increasing the distance from 1 cm to 2 cm. This phenomenon implies that the dose gradient is steeper in brachytherapy than teletherapy.

Exposure Rate Constant, $(\Gamma_\delta)_x$. Exposure rate constant, $(\Gamma_\delta)_x$ of a brachytherapy source is defined as the exposure rate at a reference point (1 m) along the transverse axis of a unit apparent activity source. Exposure rate constant is one of the physical characteristics of the radionuclide. It is independent of the source design or encapsulation. The tabulated exposure rate constants (Table 1) are expressed in R cm^2 mCi^{-1} h^{-1}, which refers to apparent activity (except for Ra-226, which is in R cm^2 mg^{-1} h^{-1}, which refers to content activity in milligram of radium).

Tissue Attenuation Factors, T(r). In addition to the inverse square law, dose rates from a brachytherapy source in a medium depend upon the effects of absorption and scattering

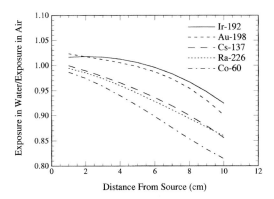

Figure 5. Ratios of exposure in water to exposure in air (selected data from reference 13 with permission) for several brachytherapy sources.

of photons in tissue. Normally, for energies above 100 keV, the scattered photons in tissue compensate for the absorption of photons in tissue. However, absorption of lower energy photons by the photoelectric process outweighs the contribution of the scattered dose. Meisberger et al.[2] have measured the effective attenuation of gamma rays emitted by several brachytherapy sources in water. They compared the measured ratios of exposure rates at distances ranging from 1–10 cm in water to the calculated values. The average values between the measured and calculated data (Figure 5) were selected for clinical applications. A third order polynomial fit to these ratios were obtained as:

$$T(r) = \frac{\dot{X}(water)}{\dot{X}(air)} = A + Br + Cr^2 + Dr^3$$

(11)

The coefficients of this polynomial are known as Meisberger's coefficients. Some of the treatment planning systems require Meisberger's coefficients as input data.

Exposure-to-Dose Conversion Factor, f_{med}. Dose distribution around a brachytherapy source can be calculated from the exposure rates using the exposure-to-dose or roentgen-to-rad conversion factor, f_{med}. This conversion factor is an energy dependent parameter and is defined as:

$$f_{med} = 0.873 \left(\frac{\bar{\mu}_{en}}{\rho}\right)_{air}^{med}$$

(12)

Table 1 shows the f_{muscle} for the commonly available brachytherapy sources.

Anisotropy Factor. Exposure distribution around a brachytherapy source is not isotropic due to the attenuation of photons by the encapsulation of the source and also distribution of radioactivity within the source. The nonuniformity of exposure distribution around a brachytherapy source is expressed using the anisotropy function. This function is defined as the ratio of exposure rate at any point in the space relative to the exposure rate at the same distance from the source center, along the transverse axis of the source. Some computer-assisted brachytherapy treatment planning systems model the exposure distribution around the interstitial sources as a one-dimensional isotropic distribution. For an implant with a large number of randomly oriented seeds, dose distribution is obtained by summing the dose contributions from each seed and can be accurately obtained with the isotropic point source approximation technique. In this technique, exposure rate at any distance is approximated by the 4π averaged exposure rates as:

$$\dot{X}(r) = \frac{1}{4\pi}\int_{4\pi} \dot{X}(r,\theta) \cdot d\Omega$$

(13)

In clinical dosimetry, this is achieved by applying the anisotropy factor, ϕ_{an}, to the measured exposure rate constant. This anisotropy factor is obtained by averaging exposure rate, at each fixed distance, with respect to solid angle and normalized to the transverse-axis exposure rate.

$$\phi_{an} = \frac{\int \dot{X}(r,\theta)d\Omega}{4\pi \, \dot{X}(r,\pi2)}$$

(14)

The anisotropy factor is generally assumed to be independent of distance from the source center.

Linear Source Approximation

For dose calculations using extended sources (for example linear sources) distribution of radioactivity within the source should be considered. The conventional formalism for calculation of dose rates at a distance of r from a linear source center in water is given by the Sievert Integral.

Sievert Integral. Exposure rate distribution around a linear brachytherapy source can be calculated using an integral, introduced by Rolf Sievert[8] in 1921. In this method a linear source with an active length of L is divided into several segments (Figure 6) with the active length of dx such that they can be considered as a point source in calculating the exposure rate at a point $P(x_o, y_o)$. The photons emitted by these source segments are filtered by the materials in the encapsulation before

they reach the point of interest. Note that this method does not incorporate the attenuation of the photons by self-absorption in the radionuclide itself. Exposure rate from the source segments are calculated as:

$$d\,\dot{X}(x_o, y_o) = \frac{A\,\Gamma\,dx}{L\,r_o^2}\,e^{-\mu t\,\sec\theta} \quad (15)$$

where t is the thickness of the filtration, dx is the active length of the source segments, r_o is distance between the source center and point $P(x_o, y_o)$, θ is the angle between the source axis and the line connecting the point $P(x_o, y_o)$ to the source segments, A is the source strength, and μ is the effective attenuation coefficient of the filtration material. Total ex-

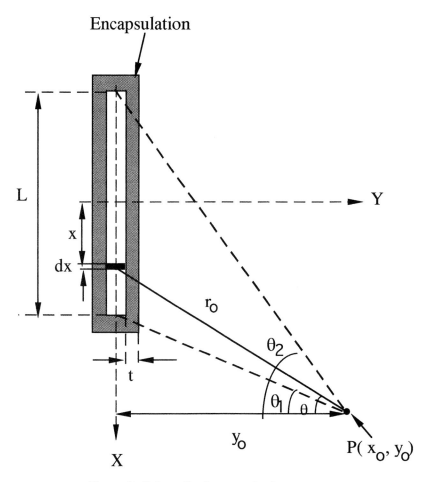

Figure 6. Schematic diagram of a linear source.

posure rate, $X(x_o,y_o)$, at point $P(x_o,y_o)$ is then calculated by integrating contributions from each source segment, as:

$$\dot{X}(x_o,y_o) = \frac{A\Gamma}{L} \int \frac{1}{r_o^2} e^{-\mu t \sec\theta} dx \quad (16)$$

This equation can be simplified by knowing that:

$$r_o = y_o \sec\theta$$
$$x_o - x = y_o \tan\theta \quad (17)$$
$$dx = -y_o \sec^2\theta\, d\theta$$

Therefore:

$$\dot{X}(x_o, y_o) = \frac{A\Gamma}{Ly_o} \int_{\theta_1}^{\theta_2} e^{-\mu t \sec\theta} d\theta \quad (18)$$

Solving this equation using numerical analysis is a trivial task for modern computers.

Calculations of dose-rate distributions around a linear source using the exposure rate obtained by the Sievert integral method consists of several assumptions. For example, this method does not incorporate the attenuation of radiation by the encapsulation material. Also, most of the treatment planning systems normally apply a single tissue attenuation correction for the given distance between the source-center and point of interest, independent to the active length of the source. This assumption introduces an error for long source such as Ir-192 wires.

AAPM Formalism

Recently a new formalism was introduced by the Interstitial Collaborative Working Group[9,10] and endorsed by the AAPM Task Group 43[11] for all interstitial brachytherapy sources. This formalism is applicable for calculation of two-dimensional dose distribution around any cylindrically symmetric source. Dose rate at any point in or around the source is calculated as:

$$\dot{D}(r,\theta) = S_K \cdot \Lambda \cdot \frac{G(r,\theta)}{G(r_o,\theta_o)} \cdot F(r,\theta) \cdot g(r)$$
$$(19)$$

where S_K = source strength in terms of air-kerma strength in units of U where $1U = 1$ $\mu Gy\ m^2\ h^{-1} = 1\ cGy\ cm^2\ h^{-1}$. $G(r,\theta)$ = geometry function in units of cm^{-2}. $G(r,\theta)$ describes the dose fall-off about an extended source solely due to the effects of inverse square law at $P(r,\theta)$. It depends on the spatial distribution of radioactivity within the source but ignores the effects of absorption and scattering in the source and the surrounding medium. In the general three-dimensional case:

$$G(\vec{r}) = \frac{\int \frac{\rho(\vec{r}')}{|\vec{r}' - \vec{r}|^2} \cdot dV'}{\int \rho(\vec{r}') \cdot dV'} \quad (20)$$

where $\rho(\vec{r})$ represents the density of radioactivity at the point $\vec{r} = (x, y, z)$ within the source in units of Bq/cm^3. The geometry factor is used to suppress variation in anisotropy profiles and transverse axis dose distributions due to inverse square law variations with respect to distance and angle. Especially near the source, this greatly improves the accuracy of two-dimensional interpolation and permits use of sparse data matrices. When the distribution of radioactivity can be approximated by a cylindrically symmetric line source or a point source $G(r,\theta)$ reduces to:

$$G(r,\theta) = \begin{cases} r^{-2} & \text{Point Source} \\ \dfrac{\beta}{L \cdot r \cdot \sin\theta} & \text{Line Source of active} \\ & \text{length L} \end{cases} \quad (21)$$

where β is the angle subtended by the active source with respect to the point $p(r,\theta)$ shown in Figure 7.

$P(r_0,\theta_0)$ = the reference point near the source where the dose distribution is normalized to unity. $P(r_0,\theta_0)$ is assumed to lie on the transverse bisector of the source at a distance of 1 cm from its center, i.e., $r_0 = 1$ cm and $\theta_0 = \pi/2$. Λ = the dose-rate constant for the source and surrounding medium and has units of $cGy\ h^{-1}\ U^{-1}$:

$$\Lambda = \frac{\dot{D}(r_o,q_o)}{S_k} \quad (22)$$

This constant depends on the medium sur-

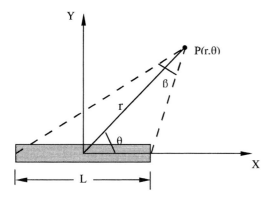

Figure 7. Geometry of linear source with an active length of L, subtended by an angle β from a calculation point, $P(r,\theta)$.

rounding the source and includes the effects of source geometry, spatial distribution of radioactivity, encapsulation, self-filtration in the source, and absorption and scattering of photons in the surrounding medium. It also depends on the standardization measurements to which the air-kerma strength calibration of the source is traceable. Table 3 shows the dose-rate constant for the most common brachytherapy source.[16-19]

g(r) = Radial dose function of the brachytherapy sources, which are defined as:

$$g(r) = \frac{\dot{D}(r,\theta) \times G(r_o,\theta_o)}{\dot{D}(r_o,\theta_o) \times G(r,\theta)} \quad (23)$$

where the point $p(r_0,\theta_0)$ is defined as a reference point on the transverse axis of the source (normally $p(r_0 = 1\,cm, \theta_0 = \pi/2)$). By definition radial dose function is unity at the reference point. This parameter represents the dose fall-off along the transverse axis of the source due to the absorption and scattering of photons in the medium. The Monte Carlo calculated radial dose function[12] of monoenergetic photons in the energy range of 30–1000 keV is shown in Figure 8. These data indicate a large dose fall-off for 30 keV, where the photoelectric absorption is the dominant photon interaction with tissue. However, at higher energies, dose fall-off converts to dose build-up with a maximum build-up at about 80 keV. This effect reverses again at higher energies and it is about unity for 1000 keV photons. The variation of radial dose function as a function of photon energy is experimentally verified for several brachytherapy sources (Figure 9), which indicates an excellent agreement with the Monte Carlo Calculated data.[12] Also, the variation of radial-

Table 2.
Dose-Rate Constants of Several Brachytherapy Sources

Source	Λ (cGy h^{-1} U^{-1})	Active Length Assumed for G(r,θ)
^{192}Ir* (Fe Clad)	1.12	3 mm
^{125}I (Model 6702)*	0.93	3 mm
^{125}I (Model 6711)*	0.88	3 mm
^{125}I (Model 6712)†	0.79	3 mm
^{125}I (Model 2300)‡	0.86	point source
^{103}Pd**	0.74	point source

* Data from reference 15.
† Data from reference 16.
‡ Data from reference 14.
** Data from references 17 and 18.

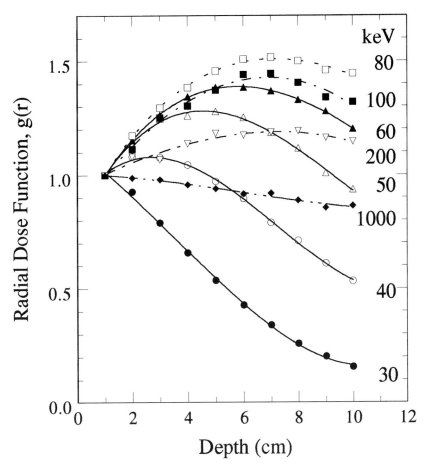

Figure 8. Monte Carlo Calculated radial dose function for monoenergetic photons in the energy range of 30–1000 keV.

dose function with photon energy at distances of 2, 5, and 10 cm from the source center are shown in Figure 10. Note that this variation is more pronounced at depths of 5 and 10 cm. Radial dose function is similar to a normalized transverse axis tissue attenuation factor or absorbed dose-to-kerma in free space ratio. Table 3 shows the radial dose function for the most commonly used brachytherapy sources.[16–19]

F(r,θ) = This two-dimensional function gives the angular variation of dose about the source at each distance from the source center as:

$$F(r,\theta) = \frac{\dot{D}(r,\theta) \times G(r_o,\theta_o)}{\dot{D}(r,\theta_o) \times G(r,\theta)} \quad (24)$$

where $\theta_0 = \pi/2$, are the polar coordinates of the reference point. This nonuniformity of dose distribution is due to self-filtration, oblique filtration of primary photons through the encapsulating material, and photon attenuation and scattering in the surrounding medium. The role of the geometry distribution in Equation 24 is to suppress the influence of inverse square law on the angular dose distribution arising from the spatial distribution of radioactivity within the source. Anisotropy function is a dimensionless quantity that takes a value of unity at $\theta = \pi/2$. Figure 11 shows the anisotropy function for I-125, Models 6711 and 6702,[13] and I-125, Model 2300,[14] and also for Pd-103[13] and Ir-192[13] sources. These data indicate a much larger nonuniformity of dose distributions for Pd-103, I-125, (mean energies of

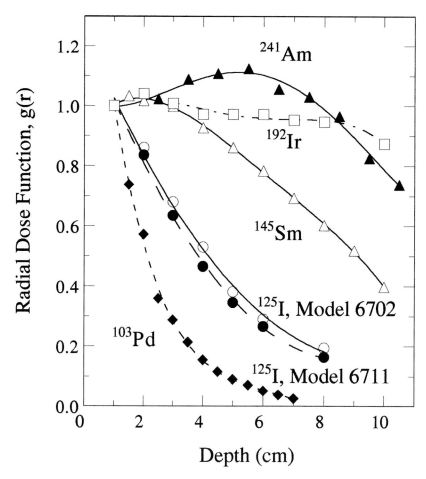

Figure 9. Measured radial dose function for several brachytherapy sources. (Reprinted with permission[12]).

about 20 keV and 30 keV, respectively) relative to Ir-192 (mean energy of about 370 keV). Table 4 shows the anisotropy factor for the most commonly used brachytherapy sources.[13]

Anisotropy Factor, $\phi_{an}(r)$ and Anisotropy Constant, $\dot\phi_{an}$

Most computer-assisted brachytherapy treatment planning systems model the dose distribution about interstitial sources as a one-dimensional isotropic distribution. In this approximation, dose depends only on the distance from the source center. If the number of sources is large and their axes are randomly oriented, the dose contribution from each

source can be accurately approximated by the average radial dose estimated as follows:

$$\dot D(r) = \frac{1}{4\pi} \int_{4\pi} \dot D(r,\theta) \cdot d\Omega \qquad (25)$$

In clinical dosimetry, this is achieved by applying the anisotropy factor, $\phi_{an}(r)$, to the isotropic point source model. This factor is obtained by averaging the dose, at each fixed distance, with respect to the solid angle and normalized to the transverse axis dose rate.

$$\phi_{an}(r) = \frac{\int_0^\pi \dot D(r,\theta) \cdot \sin\theta \cdot d\theta}{2 \cdot \dot D(1,\pi/2)} \qquad (26)$$

Combining Equations 19 and 26 leads to:

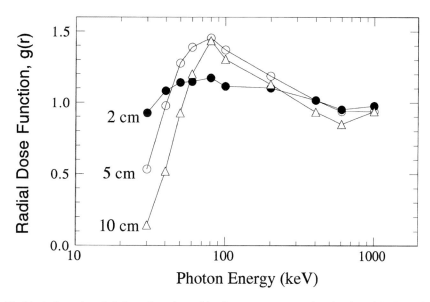

Figure 10. Variation of radial dose function with photon energy at the depths of 2, 5, and 10 cm in water. (Reprinted with permission[12]).

Table 3.
Radial Dose Function, g(r), of ^{192}Ir, ^{125}I (Models 6702, 6711, and 2300), and ^{103}Pd Brachytherapy Sources

Distance, r (cm)	Radial Dose Function, g(r)				
	^{103}Pd* Model 200	^{125}I† Model 6711	^{125}I† Model 6702	^{125}I‡ Model 2300	^{192}Ir†
0.5	1.29	1.04	1.04	1.06	0.994
1.0	1.00	1.00	1.00	1.00	1.00
1.5	0.765	0.926	0.934	0.92	1.01
2.0	0.576	0.832	0.851	0.84	1.01
2.5	0.425	0.731	0.760	0.76	1.01
3.0	0.310	0.632	0.670	0.68	1.02
3.5	0.224	0.541	0.586	0.60	1.01
4.0	0.165	0.463	0.511	0.52	1.01
4.5	0.123	0.397	0.445	0.46	1.00
5.0	0.0893	0.344	0.389	0.40	0.996
5.5		0.300	0.341	0.34	0.985
6.0		0.264	0.301	0.29	0.972
6.5		0.233	0.266	0.25	0.957
7.0		0.204	0.235	0.21	0.942
7.5					0.927
8.0					0.913
8.5					0.900
9.0					0.891

* Data from references 17 and 18.
† Data from reference 19.
‡ Data from reference 14.

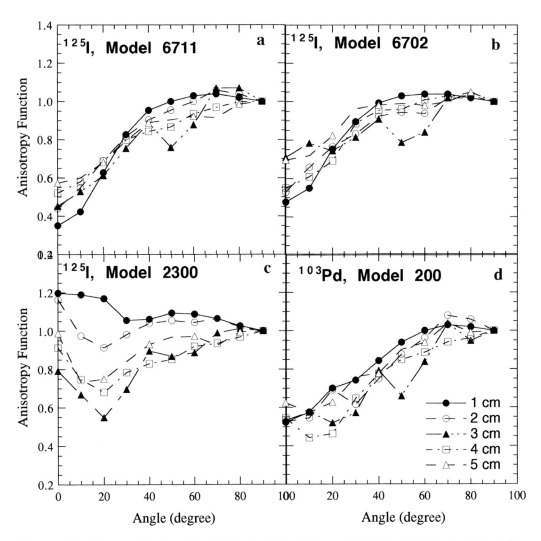

Figure 11A. Anisotropy function of I-125, Model 6711, 6702, and I-125, Model 2300, Pd-102 brachytherapy sources.

$$\dot{D}(r) = S_k \cdot \Lambda \cdot \frac{G(r,\theta)}{G(1,\pi/2)} \cdot g(r) \cdot \phi_{an}(r)$$

$$(27)$$

At distances larger than two active lengths of the source, the dose computational model is further simplified:

$$\dot{D}(r) = \frac{S_k \cdot \Lambda}{r^2} \cdot g(r) \cdot \phi_{an}(r) \qquad (28)$$

For an isotropic point source, $\phi_{an}(r)$ is unity at all distances. However, for a real brachytherapy source, $\phi_{an}(r)$ is less than unity and varies slightly with distance,[13] as shown in Table 4. Since $\phi_{an}(r)$ varies only slightly with radial distance, the anisotropy function may be approximated by a distance-independent constant, called the anisotropy constant and represented by the symbol ϕ_{an}. For I-125, note that the recommended anisotropy factor differs significantly from the conventional values of 0.86 and 0.87 for the Models 6702 and 6711 sources, respectively. These older values are based upon the polar angular dependence

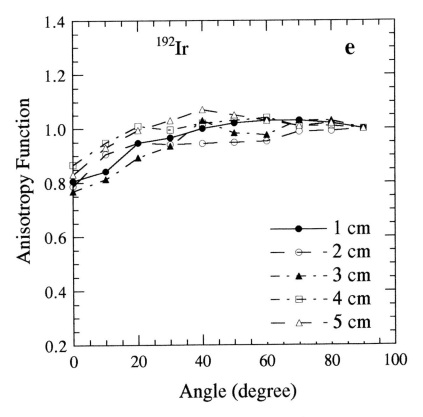

Figure 11B. Anisotropy function of Ir-192 brachytherapy sources.

Table 4.
Anisotropy Factors, $\phi_{an}(r)$, and Anisotropy Constants, Φ_{an}, for Interstitial Sources

| Distance, r (cm) | Anisotropy Factors, $\phi_{an}(r)$ | | | |
	^{103}Pd Model 200	^{125}I Model 6711	^{125}I Model 6702	^{192}Ir
1	0.921	0.944	0.968	0.991
2	0.889	0.936	0.928	0.947
3	0.820	0.893	0.897	0.970
4	0.834	0.887	0.942	0.989
5	0.888	0.884	0.959	0.998
6		0.880	0.891	0.949
7		0.901	0.907	0.965
8				0.955
9				0.974
Anisotropy constant Φ_{an}	0.90	0.93	0.95	0.98

Reprinted with permission.[11]

of energy fluence in air.[15] These estimates exaggerate anisotropy effects by as much as 10% because they ignore the smoothing effect of photon scattering in the medium, which is much more isotropically distributed than the primary dose component.

References

1A. Merridith WJ (ed). Radium Dosage, The Manchester System, Livingstone, Ltd., Edinburgh, 1967.

1B. Nath R, Gray L. Dosimetric studies on prototype ^{241}Am sources for brachytherapy. Int J Radiat Oncol Biol Phys 1987;13:897–905.

2. Meisberger LL, Keller RJ, Shalek RJ. The effective attenuation in water of gamma rays of gold 198, iridium 192, cesium 137, radium 226, and cobalt 60. Radiology 1968;90:953.

3. Fairchild RG, Kalef-Ezra J, Packer S. Samarium-145: A new brachytherapy source. Phys Med Biol 1987;32:847–858.

4. AAPM Report No: 21 Sepcification of brachytherapy strength. American Iistitute of Physics, New York, 1987.

5. Williamson JF, Nath R. Clinical implementation of AAPM Task Group 32 recommendations on brachytherapy source strength specifications. Med Phys 1991;18:439–448.

6. British Committee on Radiation Units and Measurements. Specification of brachytherapy sources. Br J Radiol 1984;57:941.

7A. Comite Francais Measure des Rayonnements Ionisants. Recommendations Pour la Determination Des Doses Absorbee En Curietherapie. CFMRI Report No: 1, 1983.

7B. ICRU Report 38. Dose and volume specification for reporting intracavitary therapy in gynecology.

8. Sievert RM. Die Intensitätsverteilung der primären, γ-Struhlung in der Nähe medizinischer Radiumpräparate. Acta Radiol 1921;1–89.

9. ICWG: Interstitial Collaborative Working Group (ICWG). In: Anderson LL, Nath R, Weaver KA, et al. (eds). Interstitial Brachytherapy: Physical, Biological, and Clinical Considerations. Raven Press, New York, 1990.

10. Weaver KA, Anderson LL, Meli JA. Source Characteristics. In: Anderson LL, Nath R, Weaver KA, et al. (eds). Interstitial Brachytherapy: Physical, Biological, and Clinical Considerations. Raven Press, New York, 1990, pp. 3–13.

11. AAPM Task Group 43: (1995) Dosimetry of interstitial brachytherapy sources: Recommendations of AAPM Radiation Therapy Task Group No 43. Med Phys 1995;22:209–234.

12. Meigooni AS, Nath R. A comparison of radial dose function for ^{103}Pd, ^{125}I, ^{145}Sm, ^{241}Am, ^{169}Yb, ^{192}Ir, and ^{137}Cs brachytherapy sources. Int J Radiat Oncol Biol Phys 1992;22:1125–1130.

13. Nath R, Meigooni AS, Muench P, et al. Anisotropy function for ^{103}Pd, ^{125}I, and ^{192}Ir interstitial brachytherapy sources. Med Phys 1993b:1465.

14. Nath R, Melillo A. Dosimetric characteristics of a double wall ^{125}I source for interstitial brachytherapy. Med Phys 1993a:1475–1483.

15. Williamson JF. Comparison of measured and calculated dose rates in water near ^{125}I and ^{192}Ir seeds. Med Phys 1991a:776–786.

16. Ahmad M, Fontaenla DP, Chiu-Tsao ST, et al. Diode dosimetry of models 6711 and 6712 ^{125}I seeds in water phantom. Med Phys 1992;19:391–399.

17. Meigooni AS, Sabnis S, Nath R. Dosimetry of Pd brachytherapy sources for permanent implants. Endocurither Hypertherm Oncol 1990;6:107–117.

18. Chiu-Tsao ST, Anderson L. Thermoluminecent dosimetry for ^{103}Pd seeds (model 200) in solid water. Med Phys 1991;18:449–452.

19. Meli JA, Anderson LL, Weaver KA. Dose distributions. In: Anderson LL, Nath R, Weaver KA, et al. (eds). Interstitial Brachytherapy: Physical, Biological, and Clinical Considerations. Raven Press, New York, 1990, pp. 21–32.

Instrumentation and Equipment

Cheng B. Saw, Ph.D., Frank M. Waterman, Ph.D., Ali Meigooni, Ph.D., Leroy J. Korb, M.D.

Introduction

This chapter describes the various instruments and applicators that are commonly used for implanting radioactive sources into or in the immediate vicinity of tumors. The instruments and applicators serve to create pathways for the insertion of radioactive sources into the tumor and/or to retain the sources in fixed geometry for the course of the radiation treatment. Internally, applicators are fabricated to maintain the geometric position of radioactive sources relative to each other and externally to conform to the anatomical structures of the human body. Instrumentation used for inventory and transport of radiation sources will be discussed in the radiation safety chapter. Instrumentation used for the calibration of radioactive sources will be discussed in the source calibration section.

Associated with the brachytherapy procedure is the concern for the safe handling of radioactive sources. Major advancements in brachytherapy radiation safety occurred with the introduction of afterloading devices and more recently remote afterloading units. The remote afterloading unit is a computerized system that automatically loads radioactive sources into the appropriate locations in specialized applicators for the appropriate times per treatment prescription. The design and

function of the remote afterloading units will also be described.

Interstitial Brachytherapy

Interstitial brachytherapy implants are performed by directly placing sealed radioactive sources into tumors instead of through natural body openings or cavities (see intracavitary brachytherapy and intraluminal brachytherapy sections). These implants may be either permanent or temporary. In a permanent implant, radioactive sources are either sutured or injected into the tumor where they remain for the full decay of their radioactivity. On the other hand, in a temporary implant, radioactive sources are loaded into applicators and/or specialized catheters that are embedded within the tumor, and are removed after delivering the prescribed dose. The instrumentation used for the implantation is briefly reviewed in the following sections.

Permanent Implants

Single-Seed Needle

Loose radioactive sources such as I-125, Au-198, and Pd-103 seeds can be implanted into tumors using 10- to 20-cm long 14- to 17-gauge stainless steel needles. Each needle is

From Nag S (ed): *Principles and Practice of Brachytherapy.* © Futura Publishing Co., Inc., Armonk, NY, 1997.

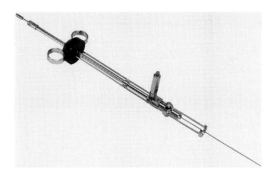

Figure 1. The Mick applicator, Model 200 with attached magazine and stylet in place. (Courtesy of Mick Radio-Nuclear Instruments, Inc.)

for different tumor sites, such as 20-cm needles for perineal implants, 15-cm needles for prostate implants, and 9-cm needles for superficial implants. Different types of Mick applicators as depicted in Figure 3 are commercially available (Mick Radio-Nuclear Instruments, Inc., Bronx, NY, USA). The applicator shown on the right of Figure 3 is a Mick 200, which is a more recent version specifically designed for transperineal prostate implants. The Mick applicator is fixed to the end of one of the implanted needles, and I-125 seeds are deposited, one at a time at specified intervals along the needle track as the needle is withdrawn by the applicator. An advantage of this applicator is that the needle is with-

loaded with a seed in the operating room for implantation. To prevent the seed from falling out, the tip is sealed with sterile bone wax prior to loading. An obturator is inserted into the needle to inject the seed into the tumor. After inserting the needle, the proximal end of the obturator is held fixed in space while the needle is withdrawn over it to ensure the seed remains inside the tumor. In selective cases, curved needles may be used to better access some tumors.

Mick Applicator

For many years interstitial implants were performed using a loose single-seed needle guided technique. To increase the efficiency and accuracy in implanting multiple seeds, modern applicators such as the Mick applicator or Mick "Gun" are used (Figure 1). In using this device, either I-125 or Pd-103 seeds are preloaded into spring-loaded cartridges or magazines (Figure 2). After the loading, the cartridge is attached to the applicator for implantation. Various needle lengths are used

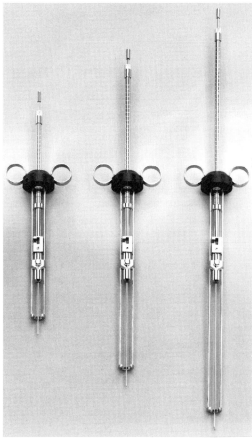

Figure 3. Various sizes of Mick applicators: mini-Mick (left); regular Mick applicator (center); and Mick 200 (right). (Courtesy of Mick Radio-Nuclear Instruments, Inc.)

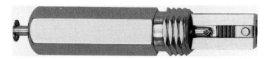

Figure 2. A magazine loaded with seeds for all types of Mick applicators. (Courtesy of Mick Radio-Nuclear Instruments, Inc.)

drawn between the implantation of each seed in precisely controlled distances that should, in principle, produce a track of uniformly spaced seeds. Depth of the implanted seeds is determined using a grid handle attached to the needle.

Scott Applicator

A column of prearranged radioactive sources and spacers can be implanted using the Scott Applicator (Lawrence Soft-Ray Corp., San Jose, CA, USA [Note: the Scott Applicator is no longer in production).[1] The Scott applicator depicted in Figure 4 has a needle holder (collar) that glides along a 0.4-cm square rail that is about 17 cm long. At one end, the rail is bent perpendicular with a hole to allow an obturator to pass through. At the other end, a flat V-shaped metallic piece (foot) is attached to the rail for placing onto the tissue surface. The collar has a pressure depressor to either grip or allow the needle to pass through a hole. During implantation, the needle is preloaded and inserted into the tumor. To load the needle, the tip is first occluded with a small amount of sterile bone wax. The seeds are then loaded with a spacer between each seed to maintain a distance of 1 cm between the centers of the seeds. Absorbable surgical suture materials are commercially available for this spacer purpose. After completing the loading of sources, the end of the needle is capped with bone wax again. The Scott applicator is then set in a fashion that the needle is gripped by the collar and within the V-shaped metallic piece. The obturator is inserted into the empty end of the implanted needle and locked to the applicator. To implant the seeds, the collar is slid along the rail away from the patient resulting in the retraction of the needle. During retraction, the obturator prevents the seeds and spacers from moving with the needle. The applicator should be held rigidly during implantation otherwise the track length can be either foreshortened or elongated.

An updated version of implanting a column of prearranged sources and spacers is the Quick Seeder System offered by Mick Radio-Nuclear Instruments, Inc. In this system, empty 18-gauge needles are inserted into the target. The seeds and spacers are preloaded into a cartridge constructed of a stainless steel housing with a polysulfone core. To transfer the preloaded sources and spacers, the cartridge is attached to the coupler on one end and the other end to the needle. The column of sources and spacers are pushed into the needle via a stylet. With the stylet locked in place, the sheath or needle is retracted leaving behind the column of seeds and spacers.

Gold-Grain Gun

The Manchester gold-grain gun device was developed at Royal Marsden Hospital for injecting activated gold grains into tumors.[2] The

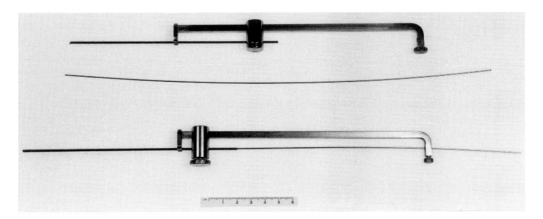

Figure 4. The assembly of Scott applicators. The obturator is placed outside the assembly in top applicator. The needles are locked to the collar.

gold grains can be purchased in a cartridge of 14 seeds and loaded into the gun for use. Needles with various curvatures can be attached to the gun to gain access to the tumor. After placing the needle tip at the precise location, the gun trigger is pulled causing a single gold grain to be ejected into the tumor. This process is repeated until the implantation is complete.

Absorbable Sutures

I-125 seeds in absorbable sutures are used for implanting shallow depth tumors or deeper tumor beds during surgery.[3] These seeds held to Vicryl (polyglactin) absorbable sutures are available from Medi-Physics, Inc. (Arlington Heights, IL, USA). A half-circle taper point needle is attached to one end of the suture. The distal end containing the sources is housed within a stainless steel ring. The Model 6720, I-125 seeds in a carrier, consists of ten I-125 seeds spaced 1 cm center-to-center in the suture. The usual activity for the ten seeds ranges from 0.40–0.42 mCi. Other seed activity in the range of 0.2–1.0 mCi may be available from the vendor. In addition, other configurations up to 20 seeds or spacing between 0.5–1.5 cm center-to-center can be made available at special request. The stainless steel ring, which provides radiation shielding, is sealed in a moisture resistant foil bag that is enclosed in a Steri-Lok gas sterilization bag. As described, the Model 6720, I-125 seeds in a carrier, is sterile when shipped.

Gelfoam

Technical difficulties are involved with the placement of brachytherapy seeds into tumors adjacent to critical structures such as blood vessels, vertebral column, or brain and also into resected tumor beds with limited normal tissues for seed anchoring. These implants can be performed by placing the seeds into a layer of absorbable Gelfoam about 7 mm thick with dimensions covering the target area, which is then either sewn or draped in place.

Temporary Implants

Standard Plastic-Tube Techniques

There are currently available four different types of nylon catheters for temporary inter-stitial implants (Figures 5 and 6), as described below.

Single Leader Catheters. This single leader or blind-end catheter is normally placed in the tumor bed during surgery and may be fixed in place using loosely tied sutures.[4] The closed end of the catheter remains within the patient's body, in or near the tumor. The thinner portion of the catheter or "leader" is passed through the skin using a straight or a curved stainless steel needle of 17–18 gauge. These catheters are then anchored to the patient's skin using either metallic or plastic buttons. These buttons are normally sutured to the patient's skin after closing the wound. The leaders (about 20 cm long) are used to thread the buttons and should not be cut until the button is in place. Typically the length of the single leader catheter is about 30 cm long.

Double Leader Catheters. Double leader or double-ended catheters are normally used for implanting unresected tumor sites in the breast, head, and neck, or tumors that need to be loaded from two ends such as in the base of the tongue. The double leader catheter is identical to the single leader catheter except the leaders are at both ends. The leader passes through the skin using a straight or a curved stainless steel needle of 17–18 gauge. These catheters are also anchored to the patient's skin using either metallic or plastic buttons.

Buttoned Catheters. These catheters are similar to the blind-end catheters except for the buttons that are fixed to the closed-end for anchoring the catheter to the patient's skin. This technique requires two skin punctures for each catheter. These catheters are anchored to the patient's skin using either metallic or plastic buttons as above.

Flexible Guides. The flexi-needles or catheters that are more rigid than nylon catheters are used in any application that requires stainless steel needle guides (Figure 6A). Although the flexi-needles are typically 20 cm long, custom length can be made available upon request from Best Medical International (Springfield, VA, USA). Depending on the application, the flexi-needles with a pointed or

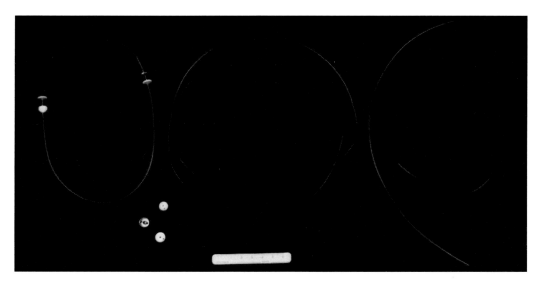

Figure 5. Three different types of nylon tubes or catheters used in temporary implants. From left to right are the buttoned catheter, double leader catheter, and single leader catheter. A metal button and radio-opaque buttons are shown on the left.

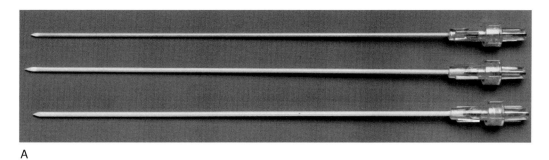

A

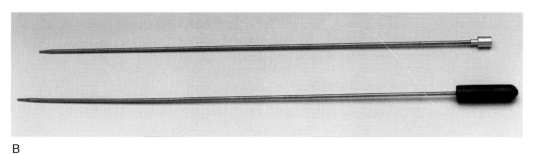

B

Figure 6. (A) Flexiguide needles with two different types of stylets for 14- and 17-gauge needles. (B) Two different types of stylets used with the flexiguides. (Courtesy of Best Medical International).

blunt closed end may be used. A metallic stylet (Figure 6B) placed inside the catheter helps to keep the catheter rigid during insertion. These catheters are secured to the patient's skin using plastic buttons. A small amount of surgical glue will hold the catheter and button together. Also, the flexi-guide catheters are often used with templates as discussed below. Caps are available to slip over the loaded flexi-needle to hold the sources in place during irradiation.

Templates

A large variety of templates have been fabricated to facilitate the implantation of radioactive sources with the intent of obtaining a homogeneous dose distribution in interstitial brachytherapy. The commonly used templates and their characteristics are described below.

Syed-Neblett Template. This template consists of two plastic plates joined by six screws that tighten to fix in place as many as 38 afterloading, stainless steel needles. It is primarily used for gynecological and perineal implantation. Six additional needles can be fitted into the grooves made around the 2-cm diameter plastic vaginal cylinder. These needles can be arranged in concentric circles or arcs with a minimum spacing of 1 cm between adjacent needles. Commonly, 20 cm long 17-gauge needles are used for these implants.

Several different modified Syed-Neblett templates for gynecological, rectal, prostate, and urethral implants are commercially available from Best Medical International. These templates hold the needles tightly in place without using any buttons. A sample of this template is depicted in Figure 7A. Figure 7B shows two different types of plastic vaginal cylinders for the Syed-Neblett applicator.

MUPIT Template. The Martinez Universal Perineal Interstitial Template (MUPIT) was designed as a generalized template for interstitial-intracavitary applications.[5] This template has been used in the treatment of cervix, vagina, female urethra, perineum, prostate, and anorectal region. The MUPIT consists of two sets of acrylic cylinders, a flat acrylic tem-

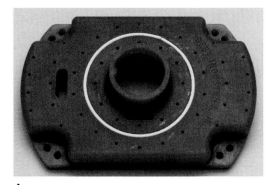

A

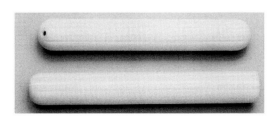

B

Figure 7. (A) A modified Syed-Neblett template. (B) Two different vaginal cylinders to be used with Syed-Neblett template. (Courtesy of Best Medical International).

plate with a predrilled array of holes, a flat acrylic cover plate, obturators, screws, and sets of stainless needles of various lengths. Along the centerline of the template are three large holes to allow the passage of a Foley catheter and accommodate either a vaginal cylinder or a rectal cylinder or both as needed. An array of symmetric predrilled holes about the centerline on the template serves as a guide for needle placements. Some of the predrilled holes are angled outward for parametrial or pararectal irradiation as well as to prevent the needles from striking the ischium. The cylinders have an axial hole large enough to accommodate the central tandem or allow the drainage of secretions. In addition to the central hole, each cylinder has a flange that carries an array of eight holes for needle placements. The holes are drilled in a circle slightly smaller than the diameter of the cylinder and continue as grooves along the length of the cylinder. This design facilitates the irradiation of the vaginal or rectal wall. As designed, the MUPIT allows for both intracavi-

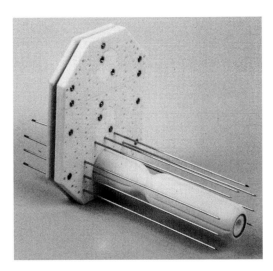

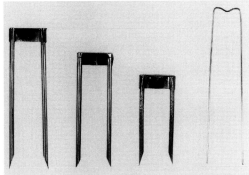

Figure 9. Different size twin gutter guides for Ir-192 hairpin implants. An Ir-192 hairpin is shown on the right.

Figure 8. MUPIT template adapted for use with remote afterloading unit. (Courtesy of Nucletron Corporation, Columbia, MD, USA).

tary placement of Cs-137 tubes as well as interstitial placement of Ir-192 ribbon sources. When in use, the cylinder inserted into the vagina and/or rectum is fastened to the template. This rigid geometry preserves the relationship of the target volume and normal structures to the source placements. The resulting dose distribution remains constant throughout the course of treatment. The MUPIT has been adapted for use with Nucletron remote afterloading units (Figure 8).

Breast Template. In addition to the gynecological and rectal-perineal implants, templates have also been used for breast implantation. The breast template consists of two plastic plates held together like a clamp. During implantation, the breast is pressed together by the two plates. Needles are inserted into predrilled holes on one plate, through the breast and into the other plate.

Hairpin Gutter Guides

Interstitial implants using Ir-192 wires in smaller tumors located in the oral cavity or anal region can be performed using the hair-

pin gutter guide.[6] Figure 9 shows three different length twin gutter guides and an Ir-192 hairpin. The gutter guide consists of two parallel tubes having an external diameter of 1.8 mm with internal diameter of 1.4 mm. The two parallel tubes that are separated by 12 mm are joined at the superior end by a metallic plate 5 mm tall with a small lip on its external side providing a surface that can be firmly gripped by the instruments used during implantation. In addition to the twin gutter guides, single gutter guides are also available. The single gutter guide is essentially a single tube, either straight or curved with an attached metallic plaque 10 mm in diameter at the superior end to permit a firm grip. During implantation, Ir-192 hairpin ends are inserted along the gutters that are held in place with a fine-tip clamp. After the insertion, the gutter guide is removed. The gutters provide the rigidity needed for uniform and predictable insertion of Ir-192 wires for the delivery of a more homogeneous dose distribution across the tumor.

Intracavitary Brachytherapy Applicators

Uterine Cervix

At least four commercially available low-dose-rate (LDR) applicators are currently being used to irradiate cancers of the uterine cervix. These include: 1) the rectangular handle Fletcher-Suit afterloading applicator; 2) the round handle Fletcher-Suit-Delclos (FSD) afterloading applicator; 3) the Delclos mini-ovoid afterloading applicator; and 4) the Henschke afterloading applicator. The first three of these applicators evolved from the preloaded ovoid and tandem applicators that were developed by Gilbert H. Fletcher and his collaborators in the late 1940s and early 1950s.[7] The basic design of the original applicator has been retained so that present day applicators produce essentially the same radiation dose distribution. Because this design has been so successful, it is fitting to begin by reviewing the characteristics of the original applicator.

Early systems for treatment of uterine cervix cancer were developed in Stockholm, Paris, and Manchester. Examples of these early radium systems are shown in Figure 10. Each system used a T-shaped arrangement of radium sources, although there was considerable variation in the source strengths and treatment times used. The Manchester system was also different in that it used large diameter (2.0, 2.5, or 3.0 cm) rubber ovoids capable of accommodating a single radium source to increase the radium to mucous membrane distance.

The development of the Fletcher applicator was strongly influenced by the Manchester technique, which used a rubber uterine tandem and rubber ovoids separated by a rubber spacer. The original Fletcher applicator[7,8] consisted of two 2-cm diameter by 3-cm high cylindrical ovoids (colpostats) fastened to separate handles, which were locked together at a scissor joint. The cylindrical shape was an intentional departure from the oval shape of the Manchester ovoids, which were designed to have the shape of an isodose surface. Each ovoid was preloaded with a single radium source and then held in position with its axis in an anterior-posterior direction, or approximately perpendicular to the tandem. Tungsten buttons were inserted in each end of the ovoid to shield the anterior rectal wall and trigone of the bladder, without decreasing the radiation in the direction of the cervix, uterosacral ligaments, and broad ligaments. Plastic jackets were added to the ovoids whenever feasible to increase their diameter to 2.5 or 3.0 cm, thereby reducing the radiation dose to the mucous membrane. The uterine tandem was a separate tubular device, supplied in lengths to hold one, two, or three radium sources.

A problem with the original applicator, as well as with all the applicators of the era, was that the ovoids and tandem had to be preloaded with radium sources before inserting

EARLY RADIUM SYSTEMS FOR CERVIX CANCER

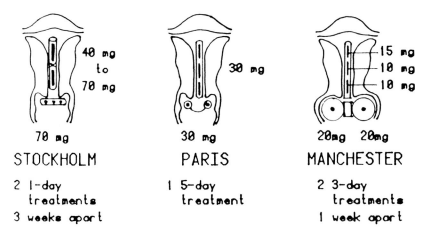

Figure 10. Uterine cervix systems from Stockholm, Paris, and Manchester. (Courtesy of Hilaris, et al.[14])

into the patient in the operating room. As a result, the physicians and other operating room personnel received significant radiation exposure during the insertion and packing of the tandem and ovoids. Hence, the development of an applicator that could be afterloaded was a major improvement. The first afterloading cervix applicator was introduced by Henschke in 1960.[9] This was soon followed by an afterloading version of the original Fletcher applicator introduced by Suit et al. in 1962.[10]

Rectangular Handle Fletcher-Suit Applicator

The rectangular handle Fletcher-Suit applicator[11] was the first afterloading applicator of the Fletcher-type. Afterloading of the ovoids was achieved by inserting the sources through the handle. This seemingly simple solution is complicated by the fact that the axis of an ovoid is nearly perpendicular to the handle, with the consequence that the source must undergo a sharp bend upon entering the ovoid. Entry into the ovoid was achieved by designing a source carrier with a double hinged "bucket" that allowed the bucket with the source to undergo the sharp bend. The tandem was simply extended in length so that the source could be afterloaded with a Teflon tube containing the radium. Tandems with different curvatures are available to adapt to the curvature of the cervix. A flange, adjustable along the length of the tandem, is set flush against the cervical os.

The outer dimensions of the ovoids are identical to the original Fletcher ovoids except they are 1 mm longer. However, it was necessary to rotate the shielding at the ends of the ovoids medially, as shown in Figure 11 in order to accommodate the afterloading feature. Except for the changes caused by the rotation of the shielding, this applicator produced essentially the same dose distribution as the original applicator; however, it was heavier and bulkier.[11] This applicator is no longer commercially available.

Round Handle Fletcher-Suit-Delclos Applicator

A round handle afterloading version of the original Fletcher applicator was developed by

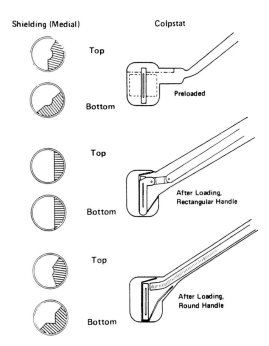

Figure 11. Fletcher ovoids. (Courtesy of Delclos, et al.[15])

Green et al.[12] around 1964. It differed from the Fletcher-Suit applicator in three significant aspects: 1) the handles of the colpostat were fabricated from thin tubing, which reduced the bulkiness and weight of the applicator; 2) the shields in the ovoids were reoriented to their positions in the original Fletcher applicator; and 3) the sources were afterloaded into the ovoids via a rubber plunger and retrieved via a suture attached to the source. This applicator does not appear to have gained widespread use and is not commercially available.

The FSD applicator, shown in Figure 12, is a commonly used round handle afterloading version of the original Fletcher applicator.[10] Introduced in 1968, it is very similar to the rectangular handle Fletcher-Suit applicator, except that the colpostat handles are round, making it less bulky, lighter, and simpler to load. Also, the shields in the ovoids were returned to their configuration in the original Fletcher design. The FSD applicator also retained the "bucket" type of source carriers for afterloading the ovoids. This applicator is commercially available.

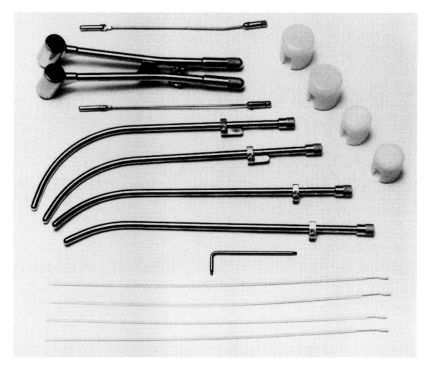

Figure 12. Fletcher-Suit-Delclos applicator. (Courtesy of Best Medical International).

Delclos Mini-Ovoid Applicator

The Delclos mini-ovoid applicator, shown in Figure 13, was designed for the patient with a narrow or distorted vagina that will not accomodate the standard FSD colpostat.[13] The mini-ovoids have a radius of 0.8 cm and have a flat inner surface. In the original design, the mini-ovoids did not have shielding because of the lack of space. Shielding is now available in some mini-ovoids constructed for smaller cesium sources.

The specifications of two commercially available Delclos mini-ovoid applicators differ somewhat from the original design. The ovoids of an applicator available from Best Medical International have a diameter of 1.2 cm, and contain no shielding. However, shielding is included in plastic caps that can be added to the ovoids to increase their diameter to 2.0, 2.5, or 3.0 cm. The ovoids of a similar applicator available from Medi-Physics, Inc. have a diameter of 1.6 cm and contain shielding. This applicator also comes with plastic caps that can be used to increase the

diameter of the ovoids to 2.0, 2.5, and 3.0 cm. An advantage of the mini-ovoid applicator is its adaptability to a wide range of clinical situations. It can be used with the mini-ovoids or configured to simulate the FSD applicator.

Henschke Cervix Applicator

The Henschke applicator,[9] introduced in 1960, was the first afterloading cervix applicator. The ovoids consisted of nylon balls with attached afterloading tubes that extended through the vagina to the outside. These tubes and the central tandem passed through holes in an alignment plate located immediately behind the ovoids, which maintained the positions of the ovoids relative to the tandem. The afterloading tubes did not change direction upon entering the ovoids. Hence, the source axis was approximately parallel to the tandem. Whereas in Fletcher-type applicators, the source axis is approximately perpendicular to the tandem. Because of the difference in the shape to the ovoids and the source orientation, the dose distribution obtained with

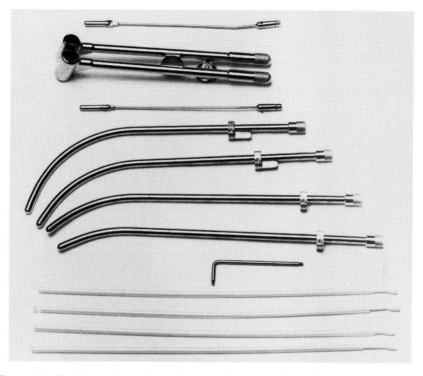

Figure 13. Delclos mini-ovoids applicator. (Courtesy of Best Medical International).

the Henschke and Fletcher-type applicators is somewhat different. Comparison of the dose distributions of these two types of applicators have been published.[14,15]

Figure 14 shows a commercially available Henschke applicator. Although this applica- tor maintains most of the basic features of the original Henschke applicator, some differ- ences do exist. Most notably, the ovoids are hemispheres instead of spheres and the align- ment plate has been replaced by a metal yoke. The nylon ovoids are 2.0 cm in diameter, but

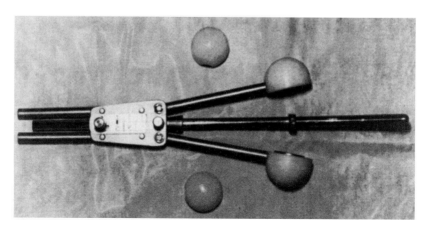

Figure 14. Henshke applicator. (Courtesy of Hilaris, et al.[14])

can be increased to 2.5 or 3.0 cm by adding hemispherical nylon caps. Removable tungsten inserts can be used to shield the bladder and rectum if needed.

High-Dose-Rate Cervix Applicators

Many different cervix applicators are available for high-dose-rate (HDR) brachytherapy, some of which are based on the design of the Fletcher-Suit applicator, while the others are of European origin. A physical difference between these HDR applicators and the LDR versions is the significantly smaller (3.2 mm) diameter of the tandem. Ovoid caps made of plastic with different diameters are available, as well as tandems of different curvatures. Shielding material for the HDR applicator is stainless steel instead of tungsten. With this material, the dose to the bladder and rectum

may be higher compared to LDR applications. However, tailoring of dwell times with dose constraints may minimize the dose difference. Like LDR, the HDR applicators also have the added safety feature of noninterchangeability of the transfer tubes for FSD applications.

Vaginal Cylinders

Vaginal cylinders used to irradiate the vaginal cuff or the whole vagina are simple in design compared to afterloading cervix applicators. Consequently, they are often fabricated in-house at institutions having a machine shop. A variety of commercially produced vaginal cylinders are also available, some of which offer considerable flexibility.

In its simplest form, a vaginal cylinder consists of a plastic cylinder into which cesium, radium, or iridium sources can be inserted

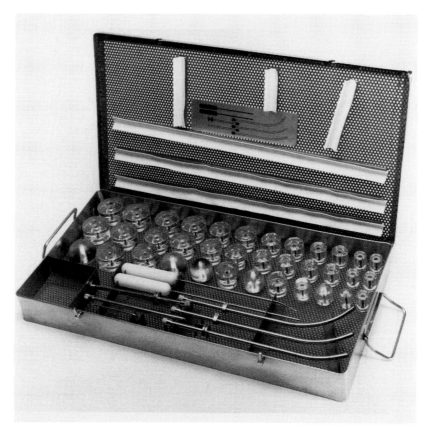

Figure 15. Uterine vaginal afterloading applicator. (Courtesy of Best Medical International).

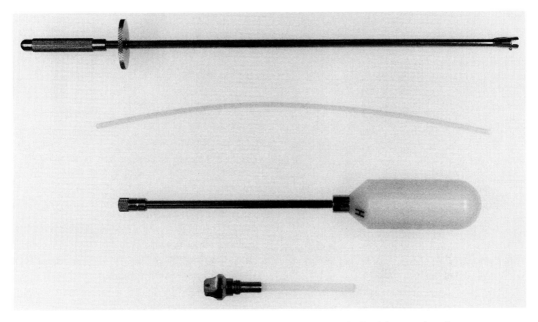

Figure 16. Burnett applicator. (Courtesy of Best Medical International).

along its axis. The distal end of the cylinder is usually rounded or dome shaped for ease of insertion and to better fit the vagina. The radioactive sources are generally held in a metal tube that extends outside the body so that the cylinder can be afterloaded. In some vaginal cylinders, the metal tube extends beyond the tip of the cylinder so that the uterine cavity can be treated as well.

Figure 15 shows a commercially available uterine vaginal afterloading applicator and dome assembly developed by Delclos et al.[10] In this applicator, the vaginal cylinder is segmented to permit adjustment of the length and diameter of the cylinder. Each segment is 2.5 cm long and has steel pins for identification on film. Six sets of cylinders with incremental diameters from 2.0–4.5 cm in steps of 0.5 cm are included along with three uterine tandems and one vaginal tandem. The first cylinder mounted on the tandem is dome shaped.

Figure 16 shows a commercially available uterine vaginal afterloading applicator of a somewhat different type developed by Burnett in 1957.[16] The Burnett applicator consists of a set of eight cylinders with fixed length and diameter, in contrast to the segmented cylinder of the Delclos type. The appropriate cylinder without a tandem is first inserted into the patient. The tandem, loaded with a linear array of sources and spacers, is afterloaded into the cylinder. The Burnett applicator was originally used with radium sources, but is now more commonly used with Cs-137 or Ir-192 sources.

Vaginal cylinders of the Delclos and Burnett type are also commercially available for use with Ir-192 HDR units. Shielding is available with an applicator of the Burnett type for vaginal (or rectal) treatments when partial shielding is required. Longitudinal shielding of 90°, 180°, or 270° can be achieved using either tungsten alloy or stainless steel shields.

Simon-Heyman Capsules

Packing of the uterus with capsules of radium was originally described by Heyman et al.[17] in 1934 for the treatment of the cancer of the endometrium. The capsules inserted through the cervix were typically 0.4–1.0 cm in diameter. These capsules were preloaded with radium prior to insertion. They were removed by means of a wire cable attached to each capsule.

Afterloading was made possible later through the introduction of the Simon afterloading Heyman applicators. This applicator consisted of a hollow plastic tube (0.2-cm outer diameter) with a bulbous end. The bulbous end, designed to simulate a Heyman capsule, was produced in various lengths and diameters. A wire obturator inserted into the applicator provides the rigidity necessary for insertion into the uterus. This system allows the radiation oncologist to pack the uterus with the applicators in the operating room, take radiographs with dummy sources, and make any positioning adjustments. Miniaturized Cs-137 sources attached to thin steel rods are commonly used with Heyman applicators, but they are no longer commerically available. Instead of Cs-137 sources, Ir-192 sources are now available for use with Heyman applicators (Best Medical International). Figure 17 shows a Heyman applicator that is used for LDR Ir-192 brachytherapy and a dummy source. The dummy and actual source consist of three seeds placed end-to-end encapsulated in a nylon tube along a wire cable leader. It should be mentioned that the arrangement of dummy and actual sources can be customized. A similar applicator, referred to as a Norman Simon applicator, is available for HDR application.

Ophthalmic Applicators and Eye Plaques

Strontium-90 Applicators

Ophthalmic applicators with Sr-90 radioactive sources have been used to irradiate postresection pterygium and other benign diseases of the surface of the eyes. As depicted in Figures 18 and 19, the applicator consists of either a flat or concave distributed source of strontium-90 in equilibrium with yttrium-90 bonded in silver foil attached to a metallic cylindrical rod. The source is covered with a 0.05-mm thick polythene plastic and sealed by a double hermetic seal. Low energy beta rays are absorbed by the foil and plastic. The metallic rod serves as a means of holding the radioactive source while the lucite disk on the shaft of the rod serves to shield the hand from the beta-rays. The maximum energy of the emitted electrons is 2.27 MeV and the half-value thickness in tissue is about 1 mm. The active area of the source in a commercially available applicator is typically circular with diameter in the range of 5–9 mm and an overall diameter of about 12–13 mm.[18,19]

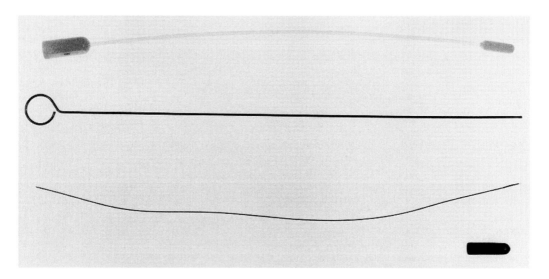

Figure 17. Heyman applicator. (Courtesy of Best Medical International).

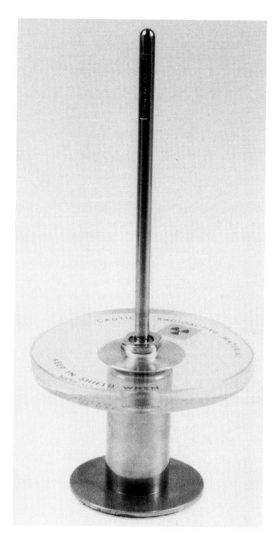

the Collaborative Ocular Melanoma Study (COMS) for this form of therapy are depicted in Figure 20. This COMS eye plaque consists of an outer gold plaque and a flexible inner plastic insert also called plaque or carrier engraved with slots to accommodate the I-125 seeds as shown in Figure 21. After the seeds have been inserted into the groove, they are glued to the outer plaque using surgical glue. As such, the seeds are sandwiched between the outer plaque and the insert to minimize dislodgment as well as defining the distance to the sclera. In some institutions, the seeds are directly fixed to the inner surface of the gold plaque. The eyelets on the outer gold plaque allow for suturing to the eyeball. Since the geometrical seed positions are defined for each plaque, the dose distributions are the same for the patients using the same size plaque with the same number of sources. Saw et al.[26] have constructed simple tables for different seed activity delivering a defined dose to the tumor for a treatment time period of 4 and 5 days.

COMS also recommends the use of a dummy plaque. This plaque is identical to the actual except that it is made of a silver outer rim with eyelets and central portion of lucite.

Figure 18. Sr-90 ophthalmic applicator placed on a shield before being used for treatment.

Eye Plaques

Localized intraocular malignancies like retinoblastoma and choroidal melanoma have been treated using eye plaque therapy. This technique involves the fabrication of a small curved plaque that conforms to the shape of the globe of the eye as well as the tumor. Radioactive eye plaques with either Rn-222, Co-60, Ir-192, I-125, or Ru-106/Rh-106 have been used.[20–26]

Though different types of plaques exist, standardized size plaques recommended by

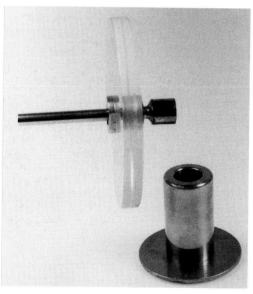

Figure 19. This view shows the size of the Sr-90 ophthalmic applicator. The plastic plate provides radiation shielding to the hand.

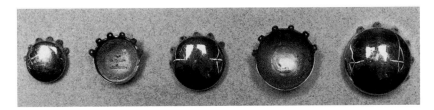

Figure 20. Standardized COMS eye plaques whose sizes are 12, 14, 16, 18, and 20 mm in diameter.

The transparent window allows for visual inspection of the location of the plaque and suturing area on the eyeball with respect to the tumor.

Molds

Molds are usually custom made and hence are unique to each treatment. As such, a mold is an elegant type of applicator that can be shaped to snugly fit almost any anatomical structure. Molds can be easily manipulated to hold afterloading catheters and/or radioactive sources in a fixed geometry. The fabrication of a mold typically requires the skill and time of local personnel.

Before a mold can be fabricated, a detailed impression of the surface cavity must be made. This impression of a body cavity may be difficult to obtain. Therefore, fabricating intracavitary molds is tedious and time consuming compared to surface molds. The impression is usually made with the dental impression alginate. The alginate consists of a powder which, when mixed with water, produces a creamy mixture that sets in a few minutes to form an elastic rubbery compound. A positive impression is obtained by

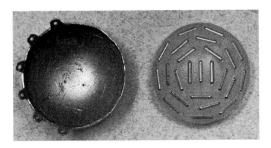

Figure 21. Each eye plaque consists of an outer gold plaque and a flexible inner plastic mold engraved with slots to accommodate I-125 seeds.

filling the alginate with plaster or dental stone to form a replica. Like the alginate, the dental stone is a powder that when mixed with water forms a creamy mixture that sets and hardens in about 2–3 hours. A negative impression of the replica is then made using transparent acrylic to form the mold. Afterloading catheters are embedded within the mold to create pathways for the insertion of radioactive sources. These catheters are often designed to be at predetermined distances from the target area and each other to deliver a uniform distribution of dose. Shielding material can be included to reduce radiation exposure to the patient and/or personnel. Surface molds are generally fabricated to lie over the surface of the tumor and adjacent region while intracavitary molds fit snugly into the cavity. For intracavitary molds, afterloading catheters are longer and externally accessible for radioactive source loading. Various straps, hooks, and string tying techniques are used to anchor the mold to the patient.

Intraluminal Brachytherapy Applicators

Intraluminal brachytherapy involves the placement of radioactive sources into natural anatomical structures that are tubular in shape. This type of brachytherapy is commonly used in tumors of the lung/bronchus, esophagus, nasopharynx, biliary tree, and occasionally ureters.

The bronchial tube is typically used for LDR intraluminal irradiation. This tube is a closed ended afterloading nylon tube with a cable guide wire and marker, as shown in Figure 22. The guide wire enables the tube to bend without kinking as the tube is being pushed through anatomical curvatures. The marker serves to show the position of the tube with

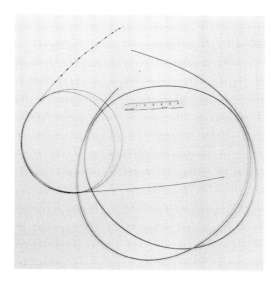

Figure 22. A bronchial tube with cable and a dummy seeds cable for seed verification.

respect to the tumor and/or anatomical structures in a radiograph. Depending on the clinical needs, the bronchial tube can be purchased commercially in lengths of 120, 150, 180, and 240 cm.

In addition to its usage in endobronchial treatments, the bronchial tube can be utilized as an afterloading catheter for bile duct treatment. The catheter is usually introduced into the bile duct postoperatively via an external biliary drain in the abdominal wall or naso-oral cavity during fiberoptic scoping of the bile duct.

A simple esophageal applicator can be fabricated by creating a hole 60 cm from the bottom of the nasogastric (NG) tube to accept the bronchial tube.[27] The bronchial tube is usually inserted to the bottom of the NG tube. The NG tube is inserted into the patient's esophagus. This type of applicator is also commercially available (Best Medical International). Another type of esophageal applicator consists of a flexible tube with six afterloading catheters or channels circumferentially placed 3 mm from the central axis of the applicator to accommodate Ir-192 sources.[28,29] This applicator is about 60 cm long with an outer diameter of 1.0 cm (Figure 23).

Specialized nasopharyngeal applicators are also commercially available. These include integral immobilization devices for fixation in the nasal/pharynx cavities. Many users prefer to use a Foley urinary catheter for afterloading nasopharynx treatment. The Foley balloon is inflated for immobilization.

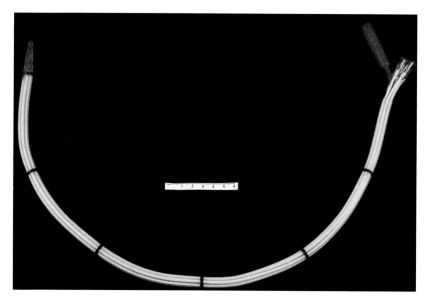

Figure 23. An esophageal applicator with six lumens. (Courtesy of Alpha-Omega Services, Inc., Bellflower, CA, USA).

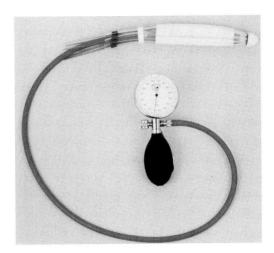

Figure 24. HDR intraluminal applicator with adjustable and immobilization capabilities. Courtesy of Nucletron Corp.

Intraluminal applicators used in conjunction with remote afterloading units have essentially the same basic structure, i.e., the long tubular form. However, the length and size of the afterloading catheters may be different depending on the type of afterloading device used. Also coupling devices are used to ensure the proper transfer of the source from the HDR unit to the treatment catheters. Some HDR intraluminal applicators have also been designed to be adjustable and have immobilization capabilities (Figure 24).

Remote Afterloading Brachytherapy Equipment

The manufacturers of remote afterloading brachytherapy equipment have developed several different, but equally eloquent, solutions to a basic problem, i.e., how to remotely introduce a radioisotope into precise position within the patient's body, keep it in place for a predetermined length of time, and finally remove the source to a safe location when the radiation treatment is completed. The goals of this type of treatment are to maximize tumor doses while minimizing personnel exposure to radiation. Additionally, because some remote afterloading machines use a high activity radioisotope and hence are HDR, the treatment times are dramatically shortened over conventional LDR brachytherapy. It should be

mentioned that the significantly different biological effects of HDR treatments in both tumors and normal tissue require dose and fractionation schemes different from those used in LDR treatments.

In general, all remote afterloading units share several common features[30] (Figure 25). These include:

1. Small radioactive sources of either Ir-192, Cs-137, or Co-60.
2. An integral shielded safe made of either lead, tungsten, or depleted uranium to house the sources when not in use. This results in a small and insignificant amount of radiation exposure to personnel in the treatment room.
3. A driving mechanism to transport the source from the safe to the tumor through source-guide tubes via a steel cable or pneumatic techniques.
4. An indexer to allow the same sources be directed into different guide tubes or channels as the clinical need requires.
5. Specially designed applicators for almost any conceivable body site requiring treatment. These applicators are typically smaller than conventional brachytherapy catheters and hence are more comfortable and better tolerated by the patient.
6. A microprocessor to monitor and control the source travel between the safe and the dwell positions, as well as treatment times. This unit also prints a summary of the treatment delivered.
7. A separate treatment planning computer system to optimize treatment doses and volumes. Most systems run on either an IBM/DOS/Windows or UNIX platform.
8. Emergency back up systems for source retraction in the event of a power failure, as well as door interlocks and emergency stop buttons.
9. Dummy sources or pellets that travel to the applicator prior to the actual treatment to verify the integrity of the treatment path.

Different units are available to provide either LDR brachytherapy in the range of

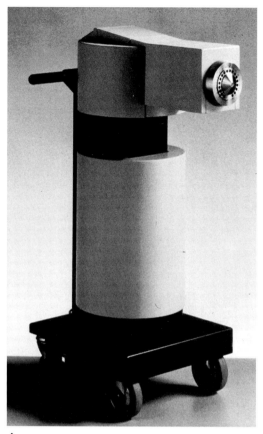

A

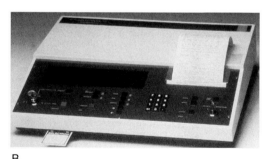

B

Figure 25. (A) External view of a MicroSelectron HDR unit. B) MicroSelectron HDR treatment console. Courtesy of Nucletron Corp.

40–200 cGy per hour or medium dose rate or HDR brachytherapy at dose rates >200 cGy per minute.[31] Additionally, a microSelectron pulse-dose-rate (PDR) remote afterloading device is commercially available that has the

similar features of the microSelectron HDR unit except for the source strength. The PDR has a maximum source strength of 1 Curie of Ir-192. This unit has been configured to simulate LDR brachytherapy by programming the source to dwell in the treatment area for a short period every hour and then be retracted. The treatment and retraction processes referred to as pulsing are repeated throughout the treatment time to deliver an equivalent dose effect similar to LDR brachytherapy.

Small pellets of radioactive sources with an active diameter under 1 mm and length <5 mm are used in the HDR unit. This small source, which carries a high radioactive strength of about 10 Ci of Ir-192, is securely attached to the end of a flexible thin steel cable. The attachment can be part of or welded to the cable. Before any radiation treatment is performed, a dummy source is used to check the channels and pathways for any obstruction. During treatment, the source is either pushed out of or pulled into the safe using the cable depending on the type of HDR unit. The dwell positions and dwell times based on treatment planning data are dictated by a stepping motor under the microprocessor control. Since the HDR treatment modality is a computerized unit, it maintains an internal clock that permits automatic decay correction of the source strength; therefore, the planned treatment times often may be different from the actual treatment times as printed out by the HDR treatment unit. The indexer sets the proper channel permitting the source to enter into the appropriate part of the applicator through the proper guide tube. Such is the case when multiple guide tubes are used; for example, in endobronchial treatment using two catheters, the source is withdrawn after treating the first catheter and then sent into the next treatment tube and catheter by automatic movement of the indexer. The source transfer tubes that connect the remote afterloader to the applicators are available in different lengths and are equipped with quick release couplings to simplify hook-up. Since the HDR source and drive cable are so thin, the applicators can be made small, thereby minimizing patient discomfort and further allowing the source to navigate relatively sharp bends in the treatment applicators and catheters. The latter feature leads to the fabrication

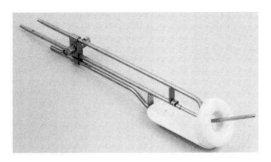

Figure 26. An HDR ring applicator. Courtesy of Nucletron Corp.

of unique applicators, which is not possible with conventional LDR brachytherapy. As an example, the ring and tandem cervical applicator set replaces the ovoids with a continuous movement of the source through a circular applicator as shown in Figure 26.

In contrast, the LDR remote afterloaders use either a fixed chain of either Ir-192 or Cs-137 sources (microSelectron LDR) or multiple pellets of active and dummy Cs-137 sources (Selectron). In the microSelectron LDR unit, up to a maximum of 48 sources can be stored in the main safe. However, up to 15 sources can be moved through 15 channels to the intermediate safe and thereafter to the treatment area. The intermediate safe serves as temporary storage and hence allows the withdrawal of the sources as required to eliminate exposure to the staff or public visiting the patient. These sources are essentially manipulated via cables attached to them. This afterloader can be used with Ir-192 for interstitial or Cs-137 for gynecological applications. The Selectron LDR unit has either three channels or six channels for the treatment of two patients in adjoining rooms. The sources in this unit are driven via pneumatic pressure. This unit is used mainly for gynecological or esophageal applications. In this unit, the intermediate safe serves as the location where the actual and dummy sources are sequenced for a proper predetermined configuration of dose distribution. Grisby et al.[32] have reported combinations of these pellets that simulate Cs-137 tube sources.

HDR and PDR treatment units allow tailoring of the dose distribution. In the HDR unit, this is accomplished by varying the dwell time and the distance between dwell positions.

The minimum increment between dwell positions is 1 mm for the GammaMed 12i and 2.5 mm for the Nucletron microSelectron units. In the microSelectron unit, the maximum number of dwell positions is 48 per channel, which may limit the treatment length. Through manipulation of dwell times and positions, dose distributions can be made to conform to many different and complex tumor volumes or may be configured to produce essentially the same dose distribution as a LDR applicator loaded with cesium, or modified, if necessary, to improve the dose distribution. When multiple channels are used, the dose homogeneity can be optimized even when channels touch or are in close proximity.

The heart of any HDR remote afterloading unit is its computerized treatment planning system. From the input data, the planning system provides data (dwell position, dwell times, number of channels) for entry into the HDR treatment unit. The treatment planning softwares are vendor specific and are user friendly with graphical interfaces, three-dimensional treatment planning, and other enhancements. The data for each treatment are drawn from a variety of sources, including digitization of films with applicators loaded with dummy sources, dose constraint points (minimum and maximum doses), prescription points, and step spacing, as well as the source activity at the time of treatment. The data entry is typically by keyboard and/or film digitizer. With the availability of sophisticated software, different film techniques, such as variable angle films aided by a localization box, can be used to reconstruct the dwell positions. The program will attempt to optimize the dose constraints primarily by varying the dwell times. Output of the dose distributions can be viewed in many formats, at points, in planes, and, in some cases, with three-dimensional enhancement. Additional data such as dose volume histograms and radiobiological models for PDR to emulate the conventional LDR brachytherapy are available in some software modules. After planning, treatment data are transferred to the treatment machine either by floppy disk, EPROM card, or hard wired network where they are verified prior to the actual treatment.

Acknowledgments: Even though it has already been mentioned above, we would like to acknowledge the vendors' contributions to this chapter. Below are the addresses of the vendors should there be an interest in the appropriate products by the readers.

Best Medical
  International
7643 Fullerton Road
Springfield, VA 22153

Alpha-Omega
  Services, Inc.
PO Box 789
Bellflower, CA 90706

Medi-Physics, Inc.
3350 N. Ridge Avenue
Arlington Heights, IL
  60004

Nucletron Corporation
7080 Columbia
  Gateway Drive
Columbia, MD 21046

Mick Radio-Nuclear
  Instruments, Inc.
PO Box 99
1470 Outlook Avenue
Bronx, NY 10645

References

1. Scott WP. Rapid injector for permanent radioactive implantation. Radiology 1972;105:454–455.
2. Jones CH, Taylor KW, Stedeford JBH. Modifications to the Royal Marsden Hospital gold grain implantation gun. Br J Radiol 1965;38:672.
3. Scott WP. Surgical radiation therapy with vicryl ^{125}I absorbable sutures. Surg Gynecol Obstet 1976;142:667–670.
4. Cano E, Janecka I, Saw CB, et al. Surgical resection followed by brachytherapy for malignancies involving the base of the skull. Skull Base Surg 1993;3:141–145.
5. Martinez A, Cox RS, Edmundson GK. A multiple-site perineal applicator (MUPIT) for treatment of prostatic, anorectal, and gynecologic malignancies. Int J Radiat Oncol Biol Phys 1984;10:297–305.
6. Pierquin B, Wilson JF, Chassange D (eds). Modern Brachytherapy. Masson Publishing, New York, 1987.
7. Fletcher GH, Shalek RJ, Wall JA, et al. A physical approach to the design of applicators in radium therapy of cancer of the cervix uteri. Am J Roentgenol 1952;68:935–947.
8. Fletcher GH. Cervical radium applicators with screening in the direction of bladder and rectum. Radiology 1953;60:77–84.
9. Henschke UK. "Afterloading" applicator for radiation therapy of carcinoma of the uterus. Radiology 1960;74:834.
10. Suit HD, Moore EB, Fletcher GH, et al. Modification of Fletcher ovoid system for afterloading using standard sized radium tubes (milligram and microgram). Radiology 1963;81:126–131.
11. Haas JS, Dean RD, Mansfield CM. Dosimetric comparison of Fletcher family of gynecologic colpostats 1950–1980. Int J Radiat Oncol Biol Phys 1985;11:1317–1321.
12. Green A, Broadwater J, Hancock J. Afterloading vaginal ovoids. Am J Roentgenol 1969;105:609–613.
13. Delclos L, Fletcher GH, Moore EB, et al. Minicolpostats, dome cylinders, other additions and improvements of the Fletcher-Suit afterloadable system: Indications and limitation of their use. Int J Radiat Oncol Biol Phys 1980;6:1195–1206.
14. Hilaris BS, Nori D, Anderson LL. Intercavitary brachytherapy planning and evaluation. In: Atlas of Brachytherapy. Macmillan Publishing Co., New York, 1988, pp. 96–110.
15. Delclos L, Fletcher GH, Sampiere VA, et al. Can the Fletcher gamma ray colpostat be extrapolated to systems? Cancer 1978;41:970–979.
16. Burnett HW. A vaginal radium applicator. Radiology 1965;84:859–860.
17. Heyman J, Reuterwall O, Benner S. The radiumhemmet experience with radiotherapy in cancer of the corpus of the uterus. Acta Radiol 1941;22:14.
18. Ali MM, Khan FM. Determination of surface dose from a ^{90}Sr ophthalmic applicator. Med Phys 1990;17:416–421.
19. Johns HE, Cunningham JR. The Physics of Radiology. Charles C Thomas Publishing, Springfield, IL, 1983, pp. 493–494.
20. Moore RF. Choroidal sarcoma treated by the intraocular insertion of radon seeds. Br J Ophthalmol 1930;14:145–152.
21. Stallard HB. Radiotherapy for malignant melanoma of the choriod. Br J Ophthalmol 1966;50:147–155.
22. Packer S, Rotman M. Radiotherapy of choroidal melanoma with iodine-125. Ophthalmology 1980;87:582–590.
23. Lommatzsch PK. β-irradiation of choroidal melanoma with ^{106}Ru/^{106}Rh applicators: 16 years experience. Arch Ophthalmol 1983;101:713–717.
24. Luxton G, Astrahan MA, Liggett PE, et al. Dosimetric calculations and measurements of gold plaque ophthalmic irradiators using Iridium-192 and Iodine-125 seeds. Int J Radiat Oncol Biol Phys 1988;15:167–176.
25. Lederman M. Radiotherapy in the treatment of orbital tumors. Br J Ophthalmol 1956;40:592–610.
26. Saw CB, Seidel M, Pawlicki T, et al. Seed strength determination for eye plaque therapy. Med Dosm 1993;18:33–37.
27. Moorthy CR, Nibhanupudy JR, Ashayeri E, et

al. Intraluminal radiation for esophageal cancer: A Howard University technique. J Nat Med Assoc 1982;74:261–266.

28. Saw CB, Korb LJ, Cano ER, et al. Dosimetric considerations of commercially fabricated esophageal applicators. Radiother Oncol 1994; 31:184–186.

29. Saw CB, Pawlicki T, Wu A, et al. Dose volume analysis of commercially fabricated nasopharyngeal applicators. Endocuriether Hypertherm Oncol 1994;10:35–41.

30. AAPM Report No: 41: Remote afterloading technology. American Institute of Physics, New York, 1993.

31. ICRU Report No: 38: Dose volume specification for reporting intracavitary therapy in gynecology. International Commission on Radiation Units and Measurements, Bethesda, MD, 1985.

32. Grigsby PW, Williamson JF, Perez CA. Source configuration and dose rates for the selectron afterloading equipment for gynecologic applicators. Int J Radiat Oncol Biol Phys 1992;24: 321–327.

Chapter 6

Calibration of Brachytherapy Sources

Cindy Thomason, Ph.D., Glenn P. Glasgow, Ph.D.

Introduction

Uniformity of absorbed dose calculation is essential for any meaningful assessment of clinical results. Integral with this goal is consistency in brachytherapy source specification and calibration. Particularly essential is traceability of source calibration to a national standard. The strength (defined later) of a brachytherapy source should be known with an accuracy better than ± 5% prior to its medical use.[1-4] It is, therefore, important that the user be able to determine source strength within this accuracy, since reliance on manufacturer's calibration is not advised.[4]

While these objectives are analogous to those already realized in external photon beam therapy, a number of problems exist that are either unique to or more extreme for measurement of output (defined later) from a brachytherapy source. These problems include:

1. The low energy of photons emitted by brachytherapy sources. Energies are typically lower than those encountered in external beam therapy. Ionization chambers may not have calibrations from a standards laboratory at appropriate energies and uncertainty may exist concerning required chamber wall thickness. Sources with extremely low energies, such as I-125, may require a different ionization chamber than is used for external beam therapy.

2. The low-dose-rate of most sources. It is often not possible to use a small volume stem type ionization chamber such as used for external beam calibrations because ionization current will be very low with respect to leakage and background. A large volume stem type ionization chamber may be needed. However, a large volume stem type ionization chamber will have poor spatial resolution and suffer the effects of photon fluence gradient as discussed below. A reentrant (well) type ionization chamber suffers from other geometrical effects.

3. The steep photon fluence gradient surrounding brachytherapy sources, especially at distances close to the source. Due to inverse square law fall-off, positioning of both the source and ionization chamber requires fractional millimeter precision. While measurements made at distances far from the source would minimize the problem, they may be precluded by low signal intensity. In addition, a fluence gradient correction must be made due to

From Nag S (ed): *Principles and Practice of Brachytherapy.* © Futura Publishing Co., Inc., Armonk, NY, 1997.

the variation in photon fluence across the ionization chamber.[5] This correction is often difficult to determine and is approximate. Use of a small volume chamber would minimize this correction but may not provide sufficient signal intensity.

4. Detector energy dependence. The photon spectrum from an encapsulated source typically is not well known. Small changes in encapsulation may make significant changes in attenuation and scatter. Measurement configuration may also have an effect on the spectrum. Spectrum changes in phantom may be particularly severe.

5. Increased difficulty in establishing traceability to a standards laboratory. The short half-life of some sources as well as to the large number of sources that may be used precludes establishing direct traceability.

Choice of detector type and size as well as measurement configuration for source calibration represents a trade-off between such effects. While much progress has been made in establishing traceability to standards laboratories in the last 10 years, continued efforts are needed by standards laboratories and source manufacturers.

Source Specification

"Strength" is used as a general term that applies to any quantity that describes either the amount of radioactivity contained in a source or the amount of radiation it emits, often referred to by another general term, output. The strength of a brachytherapy source may be specified in several ways using a variety of units. Activity and mass of radium, described below, are two measures of the amount of radioactivity contained within the source. These quantities are typically obtained by a direct measure of radioactivity within the source without consideration of self-absorption or filtration by source encapsulation. Other quantities, equivalent mass of radium, apparent activity, and reference exposure rate, described below, are source output quantities, the values of which are typically obtained by measurement of source output in air or in phantom.

There has been much discussion in the literature as to the optimum method of source strength specification.[6–11] The most recent recommendations are those presented by the American Association of Physicists in Medicine (AAPM).[12] However, compliance with this recommendation has been slow, and there are still numerous quantities for source specification in use.

Equivalent Mass of Radium

The first standardized brachytherapy source strength occurred in 1911 when Madame Curie prepared a radium standard that consisted of 21.99 mg of radium chloride in a glass tube.[13] Source specification in terms of milligrams of radium together with thickness of wall filtration (mm of Pt) has a strong historical basis and, although not recommended, is still in use. Mass of radium was a convenient quantity for specification when only radium sources were used in brachytherapy. When the radium substitutes Cs-137 and Co-60 were introduced in the 1960s, the concept of equivalent mass of radium was introduced. This source specification allows dose tables and systems of calculation developed for radium to be used for radium substitutes as well as aiding in application of medical experience gained with radium, which was typically in terms of mg hr. (Mg hr is the product of the total milligrams of all sources in an implant and treatment time in hours.)

The equivalent mass of radium, in units of either mg or mg Ra eq, is defined as that mass of Ra-226 encapsulated by some filtration of platinum (Pt), typically 0.5 mm, that gives the same output as the source of interest at the same distance along their perpendicular bisector. The mg Ra eq, M_{eq}, of a radioactive source is given by:

$$M_{eq} = \frac{(\dot{X}_S)M_{Ra}}{(\dot{X}_{Ra})}$$

where $\dot{X}_S$ is the exposure rate from the source of interest and $\dot{X}_{Ra}$ is the exposure rate from a mass M_{Ra} of radium measured under the same geometric conditions. Traditionally, output was exposure rate; however, airkerma rate may just as easily be used. Of course, this relationship holds only if the instrument reading is independent of or corrected for source energy dependence.

For dosimetry purposes, the general quantity of interest is source output. The exposure rate from a source may be calculated from the mass of radium or the equivalent mass of radium as follows:

$$\dot{X}_S = \frac{(\varGamma_\delta)_{Ra}(M_{Ra})}{r^2}$$

$$= \frac{(\varGamma_\delta)_{Ra}(M_{eq})_S}{r^2}$$

where r is the distance between the source and point of interest.

Equivalent mass of radium may be calculated from source activity, A_S, by the following relationship:

$$A_S \varGamma_\delta)_S = M_{eq})_S \; \varGamma_\delta)_{Ra}$$

where $\varGamma_\delta)_S$ and $\varGamma_\delta)_{Ra}$ are the exposure rate constants of the source of interest and radium, respectively. (Historically, the specific gamma rate constant expresses the exposure rate ($R \; h^{-1}$) per unit activity (mCi) at a specified distance (1 cm) for a source of specific wall encapsulation and the exposure rate constant express the same concept for an unencapsulated point source. More recently, the term exposure rate constant has been used rather than the more correct specific gamma ray constant.) Typically $\varGamma_\delta)_{Ra}$ is for a radium needle source filtered by 0.5 mm Pt and has a historical value of 8.25 R cm²/h mg.[14]

There are a number of reasons why this method of source specification is no longer satisfactory:

1. The concept of equivalent mass of radium does not consider any of the physical characteristics of the radium substitute such as energy or source configuration. Many of the presently used sources are very different from radium source in size, design, and encapsulation. Identical exposure rate at a point in air along the perpendicular bisector of the radium and substitute source does not ensure similar dose distributions in air or in tissue. Differences in energies cause different dose distributions. Even Cs-137 needles or tubes, the substitute closest in energy to radium, exhibit dose distributions near the ends of the sources quite different than a radium source. These differences may or may not be within acceptable limits for medical purposes.

2. Errors may be introduced in measurement of exposure or air-kerma rate from a radium substitute relative to that measured from a radium standard. If the energies and, less importantly, encapsulation of the two sources are not the same, the ionization chamber used for these measurements can exhibit a different response for each for which corrections must be made.

3. As discussed above, equivalent mass of radium of the substitute can be determined from its activity by application of the ratio of exposure rate constants of the substitute to that of radium. Conversely, activity of the substitute source may be determined from its equivalent mass of radium using the inverse of that ratio. However, there is still uncertainty in the values of the exposure rate constants. Jayaraman and Lanzl[8] point out that exposure rate constants recommended by various authors over a 20-year period have varied by 5% for Cs-137 and 20% for Ir-192 even though the value for commonly used Ir-192 seeds is now known.[15–17] In addition, the value of equivalent mass or activity is supplied by a vendor and may have been determined using a different exposure rate constant than is subsequently applied by the user, leading to errors.

4. Finally, because radium is no longer widely used in North America, specification in terms of its equivalent mass is no longer convenient or necessary. There is now a broad medical experience of treatment with radium substitutes so application of clinical experience in terms of mg hrs is no longer necessary. With the advent of source specific computerized brachytherapy

isodose computations, radium dosage tables and calculation systems are no longer widely used except for pre-planning.

Activity

Source strength can be specified in terms of activity, A, which is the rate at which spontaneous nuclear transitions occur within a source in disintegrations per second (dps). The International System of Units (SI) unit of activity is the becquerel (Bq), which is one disintegration per second (1 Ci = 3.7×10^{10} dps = 3.7×10^{10} Bq).

Activity contained within a source has little practical value for several reasons. Source output, not activity, is the quantity of interest for dosimetry. Unfortunately, to determine output from contained activity, corrections for self-absorption and filtration that are not straightforward must be applied. Contained activity itself is difficult to determine accurately as the source is encapsulated. Contained activity has no direct role in dosimetry and is useful only for radiation safety purposes such as source inventory.

To remedy this situation, the quantity apparent activity, A_{app} was introduced to describe relative output of a source, somewhat analogous to equivalent mass of radium. Apparent activity of an encapsulated source is the activity of an unfiltered point source of the same radionuclide that produces the same exposure or air-kerma rate as the encapsulated source. It typically is determined from an exposure rate or air-kerma rate measurement by dividing by the exposure rate or air-kerma rate constant, respectively, for a source of defined encapsulation.

$$A_{app} = \frac{\dot{X}_S r^2}{(\Gamma_\delta)_S}$$
$$= \frac{\dot{K}_S r^2}{(\Gamma_K)_S}$$

where $\dot{X}_S$ is the exposure rate from the source of interest, $(\Gamma_\delta)_S$ is the exposure rate constant, $\dot{K}_S$ is the air-kerma rate, $(\Gamma_K)_S$ is the air-kerma rate constant (both for a source of defined encapsulation), and r is distance between the center of the source and point of measure-

ment. Apparent activity often is called compensated activity or equivalent activity and has the same units as contained activity. Because of self-absorption and filtration, apparent activity is always less than contained activity.

The most significant problem involved with specification of source strength in terms of apparent activity involves its determination from a measurement of exposure or air-kerma rate for a source of defined encapsulation and subsequent application of an exposure rate or air-kerma rate constant for that same source. Application of these constants is needed conversely for determination of exposure from a given activity. The comments made above regarding uncertainty in the exposure rate constant for a source of defined encapsulation apply equally here.

Another problem arises if apparent activity is determined by a comparison of ionization produced by a given source to that produced by a standard source of the same radionuclide. To make a valid comparison, the two sources must be similar in encapsulation and design; otherwise, corrections must be made.

Reference Exposure Rate

To avoid these problems in source specification, in 1974 the National Council on Radiation Protection and Measurement (NCRP)[9] recommended use of exposure rate at one meter from and perpendicular to the long axis of a source at its center for source specification. This quantity is known as reference exposure rate, R_x and has units of R m^2 h^{-1}. Specification of brachytherapy sources in terms of reference exposure rate has a number of advantages:

1. As stated above, the user is ultimately interested in exposure rate from the source, not its activity or its equivalent mass of radium. Source specification in terms of reference exposure rate gives the desired quantity directly, eliminating the previous steps with their uncertainties and potential errors. Exposure rate at any distance from the source can easily be calculated from reference exposure rate.

2. Reference exposure rate is more directly related to absorbed dose rate in

tissue than either activity or equivalent mass of radium.

3. Self-absorption and effects of source encapsulation are included in the directly measured quantity and need not be estimated by approximate methods. Therefore, precise knowledge of the photon spectrum of the source is not needed when strength is specified in terms of reference exposure rate.

4. Specification in terms of exposure is consistent with external beam therapy. In 1964, the ICRU[18] recommended that high activity gamma ray sources, such as used in external beam therapy, be specified in terms of exposure rate at a reference point one meter from the front surface of the source capsule.

5. If apparent activity is needed for radiation protection purposes or by regulatory agencies, it may still be determined from reference exposure rate in the manner described above. Equivalent mass of radium also may be determined.

6. Reference exposure rate is a measured quantity that may be directly traceable to a National Institute of Standards and Technology (NIST) (formerly NBS) exposure standard.

Certain conditions must be met for measurement of reference exposure rate. Again, the measurement must be made at sufficient distance along the perpendicular bisector of the source to minimize effect of any anisotropy along the long axis of the source. The measurement distance need not be the same as the reference distance but it must be large with respect to the dimensions of both the source and detector so they both may be considered points. Effect of oblique transmission of photons through the source encapsulation also is minimized at this distance. NCRP[9] also specifies that the measurement be made with an ionization chamber that has a calibration in the appropriate energy range traceable to NIST exposure standards. In addition, this ion chamber should have an air equivalent response and walls of proper thickness to establish electronic equilibrium. Corrections must

be made for air attenuation and radiation scattered from the surroundings.

The reference exposure rate is given by:

$$R_x = \dot{X}_0 r_0^2$$

where $\dot{X}_0$ is exposure rate in free space (i.e., corrected for air attenuation and scattering) on the perpendicular bisector of the source at the reference distance, r_0 from its center. Again, the reference distance is one meter.

Reference Air-Kerma Rate

Following the adoption of SI units, the recommended quantity for source specification became the reference air-kerma rate, R_K,[10,11,19] in units of μGy m^2 h^{-1}. It is analogous to reference exposure rate and carries with it the same advantages; however exposure rate is replaced by air-kerma rate. The reference air-kerma rate can be defined as the product of air-kerma rate $\dot{K}_0$ in free space (i.e., corrected for air attenuation and scattering) along the perpendicular bisector of the source and the reference distance r_0, usually one meter, as follows:

$$R_K = \dot{K}_0 r_0^2$$
$$= \dot{X}_0 (W/e) r_0^2$$

where W/e is the mean energy expended per unit charge created in dry air (33.97 J C^{-1} or 86.7 Gy/R[20]). As with reference exposure rate, corrections must be included for air attenuation and radiation scattered from the surroundings. The measurement distance need not be the same as the reference distance but it must be sufficiently large that both the source and detector may be treated as points.

Air-Kerma Strength

More recently, the AAPM[12] has recommended the special term air-kerma strength, S_K, for specification of brachytherapy source strength. Air-kerma strength is numerically equal to the reference air-kerma rate:

$$S_K = R_K = \dot{K}_0 r_0^2$$

All of the caveats listed above for reference air-kerma rate apply equally to air-kerma strength. Again, the recommended reference distance for air-kerma strength is one meter. The recommended units of air-kerma strength are μGy m^2 h^{-1}, which are often denoted by the symbol U[21]:

$$1\ U = 1\ \text{Unit of air kerma strength}$$
$$= 1\ \mu\text{Gy m}^2\text{h}^{-1}$$
$$= 1\ \text{cGy cm}^2\text{h}^{-1}$$
$$= 1\ \text{rad cm}^2\text{h}^{-1}$$

Relationship Between Quantities

Air-kerma strength may become the predominant method of source specification in the United States in the future. However, there has been a reluctance in brachytherapy to change long established methodology and even to adopt SI units. Since the AAPM has adopted a term at variance with the SI term, it is important to understand the relationship between the different quantities used.

Air-kerma strength for a source of specific encapsulation may be related to mass of radium and equivalent mass of radium source of specific encapsulation.

$$S_K = M_{Ra}\Gamma_\delta)_{Ra}(W/e)$$
$$S_K = M_{eq}\Gamma_\delta)_{Ra}(W/e)$$

Air-kerma strength for a source of specific encapsulation also can be related to activity and apparent activity.

$$S_K = A\Gamma_\delta)_S(W/e)E(d)$$
$$S_K = A_{app}\Gamma_\delta)_S(W/e)$$

E(d) is a factor that accounts for the effects of attenuation and scattering of radiation in the source core and encapsulation. E(d) is very dependent on source geometry and construction and no simple method exists, applicable to all types of sources, for its evaluation. Uncertainties arise in approximate methods of its evaluation.

Reference exposure rate is related to air-kerma strength by the following:

$$S_K = R_x(W/e) = X_0 r_0^2(W/e)$$

In all cases, these relationships assume that the correction for radiative loss due to electrons released by photons is negligible, which is valid in the energy ranges commonly used in brachytherapy.

Discussion

Adoption of a single quantity of source strength specification, air-kerma strength, which is applicable to all photon emitting sources, should simplify brachytherapy dosimetry as well as improve accuracy. Further details regarding the implementation of the AAPM recommendations[12] have been discussed in the literature.[21]

Most commercially available computerized treatment planning systems still require source specification in terms of apparent activity or equivalent mass of radium. Users may derive either value from air-kerma strength by application of an air-kerma or even exposure rate constant for sources of specific encapsulation. As long as the same value is used in the treatment planning system as is used as a constant in dose calculations, the rate constant for source of specific encapsulation acts as a dummy variable and is canceled out. However, the brachytherapy community should exert pressure on manufacturers of treatment planning systems to make the revisions necessary for consistency with current recommendations for source specification.

Measurement of Source Strength at a National Standards Laboratory

The International Measurement System (IMS) is a system of primary measurement standards located at the large national standard laboratories throughout the world and at the International Bureau of Weights and Measures (Bureau International des Poid et Mesures, BIPM) located in Paris.[22] It is through this system that a user of brachytherapy sources can ensure traceability to standards for radiation dosimetry. In the United States, NIST provides this traceability, which is important to ensure the highest quality of medical treatment. Due to the range of half-lives as well as the large number of sources often used, establishing traceability to NIST standards is not as simple as it is for external beam therapy. AAPM Report 21[12] has defined two levels of traceability.

Establishment of the first level, *direct traceability*, occurs when a brachytherapy source is calibrated at NIST. Establishment of *secondary traceability* occurs when a source is calibrated by comparison with a source of the same type that has been calibrated by NIST. It is recommended that for long half-life sources this comparison be done using either a stem or a well type ionization chamber. For short half-life sources, NIST recommends a well type ionization chamber that has been calibrated using a directly traceable source. A long half-life source should then be used to assure constancy of the well chamber.

For situations where large numbers of sources are used, *secondary traceability by statistical inference* has been recognized. This is established for a group of sources when a random sample of that group has been calibrated by comparison with a directly traceable source. Comparison of the random sample should be performed similarly as for secondary traceability. *Remote traceability* occurs if the calibration provided by the manufacturer is used as the only standard.[4] This calibration may or may not be traceable to a national standard and may be used for newer radionuclides for which no national standard exists.

NIST presently offers calibration of Co-60, and Cs-137 brachytherapy sources similar in construction to the NIST standards and of Ir-192 and I-125 brachytherapy sources of the same type as NIST standards.[23] The range of acceptable air-kerma strengths sources is given in Table 1. NIST does not offer calibration for brachytherapy sources of Pd-103, Au-198, or Am-241 and no longer offers calibration for Ra-226 sources. Calibration services also are offered by the AAPM Accredited Dosimetry Calibration Laboratories (ADCLs), which are discussed below.

Prior to Oct 1, 1987, NIST provided calibrations in terms of exposure rate at one meter perpendicular to the long axis of the source corrected for air attenuation, build-up, and room scatter. Since that time, calibrations have been provided in terms of air-kerma strength, S_K in units of μGy m^2/h following the recommendation of the AAPM.[12]

In general, brachytherapy source calibra-

Table 1.
Range of Exposure Rates and Air Kerma Strengths of Brachytherapy Sources Acceptable for Calibration for the National Institute of Standards and Technology[24]

Radionuclide	Range of Acceptable Exposure Rates (μR m^2/s)	Range of Acceptable Air-Kerma Strengths (μGy m^2/h)
^{60}Co	0.3 to 50	10 to 1500
^{137}Cs	0.3 to 50	10 to 1500
^{192}Ir	0.004 to 1	0.1 to 30
^{125}I	0.004 to 1	0.1 to 30

tion is accomplished by comparison of the user's source with a NIST source that has in turn been compared with an exposure standard.[24] For sources with a long half-life, calibration is by direct comparison with the NIST working standard source while for sources with a short half-life, calibration is indirect using a reentrant ionization chamber that itself was calibrated against a NIST working standard source.

Long Half-Life Sources: Cs-137 and Co-60

Working standards of Cs-137 and Co-60 sources are calibrated using a series of spherical graphite cavity ionization chambers.[25,26] Calibrations are performed in air at distances of one meter or less and corrected to one meter. Measurements are also corrected for air attenuation, build-up, and room scatter. Six spherical chambers with volumes from 1–50 cm^3 are used and the NIST air-kerma standard is based on the mean response of all.[24]

The source to be calibrated is then compared to the working standard. The radiation detector used for this comparison for both Co-60 and Cs-137 is a 2.8 L spherical aluminum ionization chamber.[24] Calibration is carried out in a concrete calibration range at distances between 0.5 and 1 m, depending on source strength. With this setup a significant amount of scattered radiation reaches the detector and is assumed to be the same for measurement of both the unknown source and working standard source. Since calibration of the working standard is corrected for room scatter using the replacement method described below, calibration of the unknown source is relative to scatter-free conditions. However, the assumption of equal scatter for measurement of the unknown and standard is only valid if the sources are of the same radionuclide and similar in configuration. Variations in size, shape, and encapsulation give rise to differences in the amount and distribution of radiation scattered from the concrete calibration range. NIST can provide information on the specific types of Cs-137 and Co-60 sources that can be calibrated. To avoid uncertainty due to potential nonuniformity of the unknown source, it is rotated 90° between measurements so that the final value represents the mean of four orientations.

Long half-life sources sent to NIST are calibrated by the replacement method that consists of measurement of air-kerma rate from a standard source, S, replacement of the standard source with an unknown source, U, of the same radionuclide, followed by measurement of air-kerma rate from the unknown. Measurement of air-kerma rate of the standard and the unknown source must be done under the same conditions, that is, using the same source holder and source to detector distance (SDD). Air-kerma rate or strength from the unknown source, $\dot{K}_U$, is related to that from the standard source, $\dot{K}_S$, by the following:

$$\dot{K}_U = \frac{273.15 + T_U}{273.15 + T_S} \frac{P_S}{P_U} \frac{I_U - b}{I_S - b} \dot{K}_S$$

where I_U is the mean signal for the unknown source and I_S is the mean signal for the standard source, both of which are corrected for background, b, temperature, T, and pressure, P.

NIST follows the recommendation of the Comitê International des Poids et Mesures in assessment of uncertainty in brachytherapy source calibration.[24] There are two kinds of uncertainty estimates that make up overall uncertainty. "Type A" consists of statistical estimates of random uncertainties (i.e., standard deviations of the mean) while "Type B" consist of subjective estimates based on experience of the calibration staff. The estimates of

each type are combined to give an overall uncertainty that is considered to have the approximate significance of a 95% confidence limit. More specific details can be found in reference 24. The uncertainty estimate for long half-life sources is made up of two components: 1) uncertainties involved in determination of the air-kerma rate of a NIST working standard source; and 2) uncertainties involved in determination of the air-kerma rate of the unknown source by the replacement method. The overall uncertainty quoted by NIST in calibration of both Cs-137 and Co-60 brachytherapy sources is 2%.

Short Half-Life Sources: Ir-192 and I-125

As these sources exhibit lower air-kerma rate and shorter half-lives, calibration is indirect, using a reentrant ionization chamber that itself is calibrated against an NIST working standard source.

Standardization of Ir-192 was carried out using the same spherical graphite cavity ionization chambers used for standardization of Cs-137 and Co-60. Because current per unit volume of air produced by a single source of Ir-192 of the activity (56 MBq) used by NIST is significantly less than leakage current for a good electrometer, an array of approximately 50 sources was used[27] for each of two types of Ir-192 sources. Reference air-kerma rate in free air (i.e., corrected for room scatter and air attenuation) was determined for each array. Each seed in the array was then measured individually in the reentrant ionization chamber described below and the sum of the individual ionization currents combined with air-kerma rate from the composite array to establish the calibration of this chamber.

The procedure for standardization of I-125 is primarily the same as that used for Ir-192. However, since photon energies of I-125 are too low for the use of the spherical graphite cavity chambers, a free-air chamber (FAC) was used instead.[28] The FAC used was designed by Ritz[29] and is the standard chamber used for all NIST instrument calibrations in the 20- to 100-kV x-ray range. To achieve a reasonable signal-to-noise (SNR) ratio for the activity of seeds used by NIST, air-kerma rate was determined for an array of four to six seeds of each of the three types of I-125 seeds. Measurements were corrected for air attenuation and room scatter to obtain reference air-kerma rate in free space. As with Ir-192, each seed was then measured individually in the reentrant ionization chamber and the sum of individual ionization currents combined with air-kerma rate from the composite array to establish calibration of this chamber. Due the anisotropy of the I-125 seeds, it is important, both at this step and when calibrating an unknown source, to remove and replace a seed a number of times in order to randomize its orientation.

Kubo[30] and Williamson[31] both have reported that the contribution to measured air-kerma rate from the low energy (4.5 kev) titanium (Ti) characteristic x-rays generated in the encapsulation of I-125 seeds can be significant and that the NIST standard of air-kerma strength may be in error by as much as 10% due to error in estimation of air attenuation. These x-rays contribute to air-kerma rate measured using the FAC but would be absorbed near the surface of the seed when implanted in tissue and thus have negligible effect on the dose distribution. NIST is aware of this potential source of error and is reviewing this standard to determine whether a change is necessary in the calibration factor of the reentrant chamber.

The radiation detector used for the calibration of both Ir-192 and I-125 seed sources is a spherical aluminum reentrant (well) type ionization chamber[24] illustrated in Figure 1. It has an internal volume of 3.44 L and is vented to the atmosphere. To ensure the constancy of the chamber over time, it is tested with a Ra-226 working standard source before each use. The reentrant tube used for Ir-192 source calibration is made of brass. Because of attenuation of low energy photons, the brass reentrant tube could not be used for I-125 sources. Instead, a tube fabricated of aluminum is used. For both Ir-192 and I-125, air-kerma strength is determined from repeated placements of the seed in the tube to be representative of random source orientation.

Reentrant chamber calibration factors have been determined for two types of Ir-192[27]:

1. Ir-192 seed with a 0.3-mm diameter core of 90% Pt/10% Ir and 0.1-mm thick Pt encapsulation;

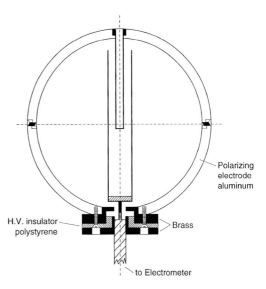

Figure 1. Spherical aluminum reentrant ionization chamber used by NIST for the calibration of ^{192}Ir and ^{125}I seeds. (Courtesy of the National Institute of Standards and Technology).

2. Ir-192 seed with a 0.1-mm diameter core of 70% Pt/30% Ir and 0.2-mm thick stainless steel encapsulation.

Both sources have an outside diameter of 0.5 mm and a length of 3 mm. Type of encapsulation must be specified when a user submits an Ir-192 source since calibration factors for the reentrant chamber differ by approximately 3% for the two types of seeds. Calibration factors also have been determined for three types of I-125 seeds:[28]

1. Model 6701, gold marker with I-125 adsorbed on two resin balls;
2. Model 6702, no marker with I-125 adsorbed on three resin balls;
3. Model 6711, silver wire with I-125 adsorbed on silver wire.

All three sources have an 0.8-mm outside diameter and are 4.5 mm long and are encapsulated by Ti. Again, the source model must be specified since the reentrant chamber calibration factors differ for each of the three models with a spread of approximately 20%.

The uncertainty estimate for the short half-life sources is made up of three components: 1) uncertainties involved in determination of air-kerma rate of the array of sources; 2) uncertainties involved in the use of the array of sources to standardize the reentrant chamber; and 3) the uncertainty in measurement of the unknown source in the reentrant chamber. The I-125 seeds are not as reproducible and each type exhibits different uncertainties. The overall uncertainty estimate quoted by NIST is 7% for Model 6701, 5% for Model 6702, and 6% for Model 6711.

Au-198

While NIST does not offer calibration for brachytherapy sources of Au-198, it does offer calibration of Au-198 in solution in terms of activity in Bq. A sample of Au-198 dissolved in aqua regia and in the chemical form of $KAu(CN)_4$ contained in a special glass ampoule provided by NIST may be submitted for calibration in a $4\pi\ \gamma$ ionization chamber.

Regional Calibration Laboratories

The AAPM Accredited Dosimetry Calibration Laboratories (ADCLs) offer brachytherapy source calibration following the guidelines of the AAPM Regional Calibration Laboratories Accreditation Subcommittee. In general, their procedures are similar to NIST and involve comparison of the user's source with a NIST source. Again, comparison is direct for sources with a long half-life and indirect for sources with a short half-life. Not all ADCLs offer all source calibrations. Some ADCLs also offer calibration of well type chambers for brachytherapy sources. The individual ADCL should be contacted for a listing of services provided.

Measurement of Source Strength by the Manufacturers

For many years, manufacturers of brachytherapy sources specified their strength in either apparent activity or equivalent mass of radium even though the original calibration was in exposure rate. As discussed above, conversion by the user of either quantity to exposure rate had the potential for error by application of a different exposure rate constant for sources of specific encapsulation

than was originally used by the manufacturer. Fortunately, the present situation is much improved. Source specification in terms of air-kerma strength or air-kerma rate at one meter is common. Those manufacturers who continue to quote source strength in terms of apparent activity or equivalent mass of radium at least provide exposure rate constants for sources of specific encapsulation used in the conversion so the user may apply the same values. Still other manufacturers provide both air-kerma strength and apparent activity or equivalent mass of radium.

In general, all manufacturers calibrate sources following methods typically done in the field that provide traceability to national standards as discussed below. Calibration techniques used by some of the brachytherapy source manufacturers are discussed below. This discussion is not meant to be complete but simply to provide a representative sampling of techniques.

Best Industries, Inc. (Springfield, VA, USA) individually calibrates a random selection of 5–10 Ir-192 seeds from a large batch of seeds after their irradiation.[32] This is done in a well chamber (Capintec Isotope Calibrator Model CRC-5R), which has itself been calibrated against a NIST calibrated Ir-192 seed. The batch seed sources are then loaded in ribbons, each ribbon is calibrated individually. Only those ribbons whose total activity agrees within ±5% of the average activity are sent. A calibration certificate gives mean activity of the random selection of individually calibrated seeds in terms of mg Ra eq as well as maximum and minimum activities all of which have a quoted accuracy of better than ±5%.[33] While sources are not specified in terms of air-kerma strength, values of the specific gamma ray constants of Ir-192 and Ra-226 that were used to determine mg Ra eq are given.

Each Ir-192 seed sold by Radiation Safety & Nuclear Products, Inc. (RSNP) (Salt Lake City, UT, USA) is individually assayed in one of two ways.[34] One method uses a reentrant ionization chamber while the other uses a pressurized stem type ionization chamber that is used in a fixed geometry. The latter method is used routinely since it is quicker than using the well ionization chamber. A NIST calibrated Ir-192 source was originally used to obtain calibrations for both chambers while a Ra-226 source is currently used as a constancy standard.

All Cs-137 sources sold by Medi-Physics, Inc. (Arlington Heights, IL, USA) are calibrated against a NIST/ADCL calibrated source of Cs-137 to an accuracy of $\pm 5\%$ and are provided with a certificate of measurement that documents traceability to national standards.[35] Sources are specified in terms of air-kerma strength, i.e., air-kerma rate at one meter (μGy/hr at 1 m).

Each production seed of I-125 sold by Medi-Physics, Inc. is measured by comparison in a reentrant chamber in a fixed geometry with an I-125 seed of the same model that has been NIST calibrated.[35] The NIST source is also sent to an ADCL as a second check. Production sources are provided with a certificate that specifies the source in terms of air-kerma strength in μGy m^2/h and quotes overall uncertainty in calibration to be $\pm 4\%$. Apparent activity of the source is also provided as well as the exposure rate constant that was used for its determination.

The high-dose-rate Ir-192 sources used in remote afterloaders manufactured by Nucletron Corporation (Columbia, MD, USA) are made in Germany and are measured in a well chamber that has a calibration traceable to German standards as well as to the University of Wisconsin ADCL.[36] Specification is provided to the user in terms of apparent activity in Bq and Ci; however, the factor used for conversion from air-kerma strength is given.

RTS Technology (North Andover, MA, USA) who manufacturers high-dose-rate Ir-192 for the Gammamed remote afterloader have a thimble chamber mounted inside of the hot cell where sources are made.[37] The chamber is located inside a lead shield so that it is looking at a small collimated beam from each source in a fixed geometry. These values are compared with those obtained placing a previously calibrated source with the same fixed geometry in the cell. Their standard source was measured using the same thimble chamber in air at a distance of approximately 20 cm. They specifically recommend against use of their value for medical treatment and claim that it is only measure of activity for safety purposes.

The calibration of Au-198 sources sold by RSNP is based upon a source that was originally measured by them and was then sent to NIST.[34] NIST dissolved the source and provided a value of contained activity. Since NIST maintains no standards for Au-198 in the form used for brachytherapy sources, this is the closest possible means to provide traceability.

NIST maintains no standard for calibration of Pd-103 sources. To provide an indirect means of traceability, Theragenics Corporation (Atlanta, GA, USA) calibrates their Pd-103 sources by reference to a source of Cd-109 whose calibration is directly traceable to NIST.[38] This is done using the replacement method and a thin NaI crystal. Since the average energy of Cd-109 (approximately 23 keV) is similar to that of Pd-103 (approximately 21 keV), detector efficiency calculated for Cd-109 may be applied to determination of source strength of Pd-103. More specifically, the photon spectrum emitted in air at large distance along perpendicular bisector of the Pd-103 source axis is measured using the NaI detector that has been calibrated using the Cd-109 source.[39] The spectrum is integrated to obtain total number of photons in the energy range of 20–23 keV and corrected for detector efficiency. The number of disintegrations per second can then be calculated knowing the number of photons produced per disintegration (0.74), yielding apparent activity.

While traceability to national standard typically now is established by the manufacturer, it is not recommended that the user rely on this value.[2,40]

Measurement of Source Strength in the Field

It has been recommended[12] that brachytherapy sources have calibrations that establish either direct or secondary traceability to NIST or an ADCL. It is also recommended that source users have the ability to independently verify the source strength provided by the manufacturer.[4] Long half-life sources should be calibrated by the user while traceability by statistical inference may be used for short half-life sources, depending upon the number of seeds or ribbons under consideration. For only a few seeds or ribbons, it is recommended that all be calibrated. For a large number of seeds, a random sample of at least

10% should be calibrated. For a large number of ribbons, a minimum of 10% or two ribbons, whichever is larger, should be calibrated.

It is, therefore, essential that each user have the capability to measure brachytherapy source strength. The recommended device for accurate calibration is a reentrant type ionization chamber; however, a stem type ionization chamber also may be used. Reentrant chambers tend to be simplest to use and need fewer corrections. Either type ionization chamber can be used for high activity sources in remote afterloaders. While a reentrant chamber is preferable for calibration of low-dose-rate sources, stem type ionization chambers also have been used successfully.[41–45] If appropriate dosimetric corrections are made, either type of chamber should give equivalent results.[46] In general, any chamber may be used as long as it has a stable response and a SNR sufficiently large for the source of interest. The methods detailed below are applicable to the calibration of either high-dose-rate or low-dose-rate brachytherapy sources. (For a discussion of calibration applicable only to high-dose-rate sources, see references 46 and 47.)

Whichever type of chamber is used, its calibration should be traceable to NIST or an ADCL. For a reentrant chamber, this is most commonly done by use of one or more NIST or ADCL calibrated sources. For stem type chambers, calibrated sources can be used; however, it may be possible to obtain a chamber calibration factor directly from NIST or an ADCL for the radionuclide of interest. The most obvious way to obtain a calibrated source is to send the source of interest to NIST or to an ADCL for calibration.[43] This may take several months for NIST but typically may be completed within a month from an ADCL. Alternatively, an individual calibrated source may be ordered directly from the manufacturer who will provide a calibration traceable to NIST. This is not generally recommended. If a user has access to a chamber with factors directly traceable to NIST, it may be used to obtain a calibrated source, however, no more than one transfer of calibrations factors should be made. It may also be possible to borrow a NIST calibrated source from another user.

Reentrant (Well) Type Ionization Chambers

A reentrant or well type ionization chamber offers a convenient method of source calibration for either high- or low-dose-rate brachytherapy sources. These chambers, an example of which is shown in Figure 2, have a source well that is surrounded by a spherical or cylindrical gas filled ion collection volume, approximating 4π measurement geometry. The gas may be air or pressurized argon. Commercially available well ionization chambers may be either a nuclear medicine dose calibrator or a chamber designed specifically for brachytherapy. Nuclear medicine dose calibrators are traditionally used for assay of liquid radiopharmaceuticals. Calibration factors obtained using nuclear medicine standards, which are in the form of a liquid contained within a glass vial or syringe, cannot be used for brachytherapy sources as will be discussed below. These calibrators typically are filled with argon gas under high pressure and can be used for low-dose-rate sources with activities ≤ 37 GBq (1 Ci). More recently, well chambers that are specific for brachytherapy use have been developed or adapted from nuclear medicine dose calibrators. Some of the brachytherapy well chambers have the

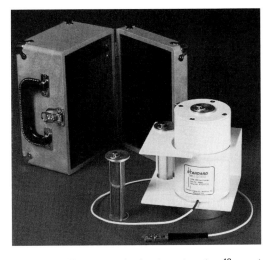

Figure 2. Reentrant ionization chamber[48] used for calibration both low- and high-dose-rate sources in the field. (Courtesy of Standard Imaging, Middleton, WI, USA).

capability to measure only low-dose-rate sources, while others[48] can measure both low- and high-dose-rate sources. They are typically open to the atmosphere necessitating air density corrections. Properties of any reentrant chamber must be thoroughly investigated prior to its use for source calibration. Factors that must be taken into account will be discussed below.

Precision/Response Stability: It has been recommended that the reproducibility of the reentrant chamber should be better than 2%.[4] Since response of these chambers is dependent on source orientation and position in the well,[40] a source holder that will keep the source in a reproducible, vertical position must be devised. Long-term stability can be determined by measuring a long half-life source such as Cs-137 or Ra-226 prior to each use. This measurement has the added benefit of acting as a quality assurance check of the entire system.

Scale Factors/Linearity: The reentrant chamber should respond linearly over the desired measurement range of each scale. It is recommended that a single scale or radionuclide setting be used for all types of radionuclides calibrated.[2] If the scale linearity cannot be determined independently, a short half-life source may be measured as it decays.[40]

Ion Collection Efficiency: Collection efficiency should, in general, be better than 99% for commercial well chambers and conventional brachytherapy sources.[4] This can be verified by making measurements at different polarizing voltages[49] using a source of the highest intensity expected to be calibrated. Due to the large volume of these chambers, a correction for ion recombination losses may be necessary, particularly for high-dose-rate sources.

Some of the commercially available reentrant chambers, typically nuclear medicine dose calibrators, do not allow a change in polarizing voltage for measurement of collection efficiency. However, most do provide the range of source strengths that can be measured. However, any differences in collection efficiency for different strength sources should be seen when doing the above test of linearity. While it may not be possible to separate linearity from collection efficiency, a

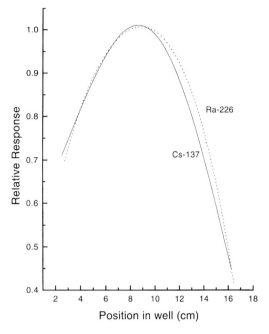

Figure 3. Relative response versus position within the well of a reentrant ionization chamber.

combined correction factor may be determined.

Geometry and Length Dependence: As mentioned above, a reproducible source holder must be used since chamber response is dependent on source orientation due to source anisotropy. Source response also varies with position within the well and with source length. The magnitude of this variation may be determined in two ways.[50] One method involves moving a short source through the active volume of the chamber and integrating sensitivity over the measurement regions. The other method involves making measurements as a long source (wire or seed assembly) is physically shortened. Geometry dependence may be a function of radionuclide so the variation should be determined for each type of source to be calibrated. Figure 3 shows a graph of relative response as a function of position within the chamber well determined for the reentrant chamber discussed in reference 50.

Energy Dependence: Prior to use for source calibration, energy dependence of a reentrant chamber must be investigated. In general, re-

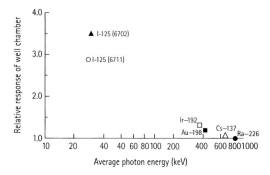

Figure 4. Energy dependence of a reentrant ionization chamber, RADCAL Corporation, Model 4050. (Courtesy of Raven Press, Ltd.).[40]

sponse/unit air-kerma rate of all reentrant type chambers will vary with photon energy due to absorption and scatter of photons and secondary electrons both in the chamber walls and gas volume.[40–42,51] Figure 4 shows the energy dependence of an Ar filled well chamber (RADCAL Corporation, model 4050 [Monrovia, CA, USA]).[40] As can be seen, chamber response varies by a factor of approximately 3.5 over the energy range of commonly used sources.

In addition, changes in energy spectrum due to filtration and absorption by source encapsulation have been shown to affect chamber response.[41,51] Williamson et al.[51] found the effects of source construction to range from 2%–10%. Figure 4 shows a difference of approximately 20% in chamber response between two different model I-125 seeds.

Chamber Calibration Factors: Because of energy and encapsulation dependence of reentrant ionization chambers discussed above, calibration factors must be determined for each radionuclide and type of source encapsulation. This means that a calibrated standard source is required for each. In addition, calibration factors obtained for a dose calibrator using nuclear medicine standards cannot be used for brachytherapy sources due to differences in construction mentioned previously.

Calibration Procedure: The following procedure should be followed when using a reentrant ionization chamber for brachytherapy source calibration.[2,50] The reentrant chamber should be identified and its electrical

and radiological characteristics investigated. These characteristics include: precision and response stability; scale factor and linearity; ion collection efficiency; geometry and length dependence; and energy dependence. Correction factors should be determined if necessary.

For long half-life sources: One source of each radionuclide and encapsulation should be identified as a standard. Sources should be marked so that they may be identified at a later date. These sources should be sent to NIST or an ADCL for calibration. They may then be used to calibrate similar sources using the replacement method described above.

For short half-life sources: One source of each radionuclide and encapsulation should be identified as a reference source. Again, sources should be marked so that they may be identified at a later date. These sources should be sent to NIST or an ADCL for calibration. They may then be used determine a calibration factor for that source type for the reentrant chamber. Since the reference source has a short life time, a long half-life standard source should be identified and used as a constancy check for the chamber prior to each use. Alternatively, a ratio of chamber response of the reference source to the standard source may be determined experimentally.

Stem Type Ionization Chambers

In theory, stem type ionization chambers may be used for source calibration. However, in practice, such measurements are difficult and time consuming and require close attention to detail. At the present time, stem type ionization chambers are more commonly used for calibration of high activity sources.[52–54] Measurements with a stem ionization chamber may be made either in-air or in-phantom. Measurements made in-air have the advantage of a larger signal for low energy sources since there is no phantom attenuation. Therefore, for low energy sources, measurements may be made at larger SDDs and/or using a smaller volume chamber than in-phantom, both of which minimize the gradient correction factor that need be applied. In addition, small errors in measured SDD have less of an effect when this distance is large. There is little difference between signal intensity measured in-air and in-phantom for sources of higher energy. Measurements made in-air have the disadvantage of poor mechanical stability necessitating use of some type of a calibration jig. Measurements in a phantom have the advantage that no correction for room scatter or for air attenuation and multiple scatter need be applied. In addition, positional reproducibility of a solid phantom is better than an in-air calibration jig. However, due to phantom attenuation, it may be necessary to use shorter SDDs and larger chamber volumes, both of which increase the magnitude of the gradient correction that must be applied. The decision as to whether to perform calibrations in-air or in-phantom is purely a matter of choice. Again, if appropriate dosimetric corrections are made, both techniques should give equivalent results.[53] Techniques for both types of calibrations follow.

In-Air Calibration

In spite of low signal from low strength sources, a stem type ionization chamber can be used for calibration of low-dose-rate sources as well as for high-dose-rate sources. Williamson et al.[41] used a 30-cm³ chamber that was itself calibrated by comparison with a Farmer type chamber in-air. Values determined for Ra-226, Cs-137, and Ir-192 sources agreed with NIST values to within ± 1.7%. Boyer et al.[42] used a 630-cm³ tissue equivalent ionization chamber for the measurement of Ir-192. Ling et al.[45] reported the use of a modified low energy ionization chamber made for radiation protection measurements used in a fixed geometry for calibration of I-125 seeds. Kubo[44] reported on the use of large volume mammography chamber that had calibration traceable to a standard air ionization chamber for measurement of I-125 seeds and found agreement with NIST to within 5%. Meertens[55] used a 0.6-cm³ Farmer type chamber for calibration of Cs-137 sources.

Based on considerations discussed below, a geometrical configuration for source calibration should be decided upon and investigated thoroughly. After determination of the various correction factors, the configuration and its position within a particular room should be kept constant for all subsequent measurements.

Precision: Precision, or response stability, of a stem type ionization chamber and its associated electrometer must be investigated prior to its use for calibration of brachytherapy sources. Measurements made in-air are less stable than those made in a phantom, necessitating fabrication and use of some sort of a calibration jig to guarantee reproducible measurements. A device that will hold both the chamber and source in a fixed orientation and at a fixed distance from each other should be made using the least possible amount of low density plastic to minimize scatter.[46]

One of the most important considerations in the use of stem type ionization chambers for source calibration is SNR and is the reason why these chambers are most commonly used for measurement of high activity sources. Ezzell[53] has reported a current of approximately 5 pA at 20 cm and 20 pA at 10 cm from a 300 GBq (8.1 Ci) source of Ir-192 using a Farmer type chamber with leakage current of ≤0.01 pA. This gives SNRs of approximately 500 and 200 at distances of 10 and 20 cm, respectively, which are adequate. From these values, the SNR of a 0.5 MBq (1.5 mCi) source of Ir-192 at 10 cm from the same chamber can be estimated as approximately 4:1. It is obvious that a larger volume chamber should be used. Leakage becomes particularly important with the long integration times that are typically used. It has been recommended[4,56] that SNR be at least 100:1. Leakage should be integrated over the same duration as the measurement and, even with a high SNR system, subtracted from the integrated current from the source. Techniques to minimize leakage include use of low noise cables and allowance of long electrometer warm-up times.[46] It should be possible to obtain both short-term and long-term precision to be better than 2%.[56]

Ion Collection Efficiency: Ion collection efficiency should be determined from measurements made at different polarizing voltages[49] using a source of the highest intensity that is expected to be calibrated. A correction should be applied if necessary.

Air Attenuation and Multiple Scatter: NIST calibrations are in terms of air-kerma strength in free air, i.e., corrected for air attenuation and multiple scattering of photons. Read et al.[57] have reported a figure of 0.2% per meter correction for air attenuation and multiple scatter for Ra-226, Co-60, and Cs-137, justifying the neglect of this correction for these radionuclides at distances used for source calibration (5–100 cm). An estimate of this correction factor based on mass energy absorption coefficient, μ_{en},[58] and a fluence weighted average energy of 347 keV for Ir-192 is approximately 0.3% per meter, again justifying its neglect. (While there are many low energy lines in the spectrum of Ir-192, which would be subject to greater attenuation, they represent a small fraction of the total.) A similar estimate for I-125 gives a correction of approximately 2.5% per meter. Since measurements for such low energy sources are often made at short SDDs, the correction may be negligible but must be evaluated for the specific geometry used.

Fluence Gradient Corrections: The photon fluence gradient across the finite volume of an ionization chamber due predominately to inverse square law fall-off, necessitates a correction to a point detector. This correction is largest when using a large volume chamber close to a source and decreases with both chamber size and increasing SDD. The correction for spherical chambers is smaller than that for cylindrical chambers, which should always be used with their longest dimension parallel to the long axis of the source to minimize this effect. Both Dove[59] and Kondo and Randolph[60] have developed methods for calculating a multiplicative correction factor.

Dove[59] assumes a cylindrical chamber with a cavity of radius a and length 2h located at a distance X from the source and the geometry shown in Figure 5. The measured air-kerma rate, $\dot{K}(X,a,2h)$, is related to the air-kerma rate, $\dot{K}$, by:

$$\frac{\dot{K}(X,a,2h)}{\dot{K}(X)} =$$
$$\left[\begin{array}{l} 1 - 1/X^2(h^2/3 - a^2/2) \\ + 1/X^4(h^4/5 - 2h^2a^2/3 + a^4/3) \\ - 1/X^6(h^6/7 - 7h^4a^2/20 + h^2a^4/9 - a^6/4) \end{array}\right]$$

under the condition that:

$$h^2 < X\,[(2X^2 + 4a^2) - (X^2 + a^2)]^{-1/2}$$

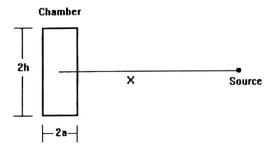

Figure 5. Configuration of source and detector used by Dove[59] for estimation of fluence gradient correction factors.

Correction factors due to Kondo and Randolph[60] are similar to those of Dove[59] except for short SDDs where both are most uncertain. SDDs this short should not be used. In addition, both provide corrections for additional geometries. Gradient correction factors for a 0.6-cm³ Farmer type chamber and source in the geometry shown in Figure 5 are given in Table 2. AAPM Report 41[46] provides a table of factors applicable to other cylindrical chambers. Recent Monte Carlo calculations and experimental results of Bielajew[61] are in agreement with these factors.

While the correction discussed above[59–61] assumes a point source, Boyer[5] has presented an analytical expression that takes source geometry into account. More recently, Tolli and Johansson[62] have presented an experimental methodology that is valid both in-air and in-

Table 2.
Gradient Correction Factors for a Farmer-Type Chamber with its Longest Dimension Aligned Along the Long Axis of a Brachytherapy Source

Source to Chamber Distance (cm)	Gradient Correction Factor	
	Dove[59]	Kondo and Randolph[60]
1.0	1.338	1.93
2.0	1.107	1.107
5.0	1.019	1.017
7.5	1.013	1.011
10.0	1.006	1.005
15.0	1.003	1.002
20.0	1.001	1.001

phantom and that takes into effect source geometry and source energy dependence. Their method, however, is time consuming and requires very precise knowledge of SDDs. The complexity and approximations involved in determination of gradient correction factor encourages use of a reentrant type chamber for source calibrations.

Room Scatter: The contribution to measured air-kerma strength from scatter from all surfaces, including chamber holder, must be evaluated. To minimize this effect, the source and chamber should be kept approximately two meters from all surfaces, including the floor, at which point room scatter can be assumed to be independent of SDD.[46] With this "good geometry," room scatter is typically <0.5% of the total measured charge necessitating careful measurement for its determination.

Ezzell[63] detailed one method of measuring room scatter. By assuming that room scatter is independent of SDD and contributes a constant value at all distances:

$$K = K_0(d_0/d)^2 + K_{RS}$$

where

d = distance from the source to point of measurement

d_0 = distance from the source to a reference point

K = total air-kerma (primary plus room scatter) at d

K_0 = primary air-kerma at d_0

K_{RS} = room scatter air-kerma (assumed to be constant for all d)

K_0 and K_{RS} may be determined by making measurements of equal duration at a number of distances and applying regression analysis to K versus $(d_0/d)^2$. Before analysis, measurements must be corrected for all distance dependent factors such as gradient effects. Corrections for timer error may be avoided by using a separate timer.

Goetsch et al.[64] modified this technique to include a correction for effective distance between source and detector centers. If the measured distance, d, is in error by a constant amount:

$$d' = d + c$$

where

d' = effective source to detector distance
d = true source to detector distance
c = error in distance.

Again, it is assumed that room scatter is independent of SDD and contributes a constant value at all distances, M_s such that:

$$M_d = M'_d + M_s$$

where M_d is the integrated charge reading at d and M'_d is the integrated charge reading due only to primary radiation. A constant may be defined at each distance:

$$f = M'_d \cdot d'^2 = (M_s - M_2)(d + c)^2$$

If measurements are made at least at three distances, the above equation may be used to solve for the three unknowns, f, c, and M_s.

Timer Error: Corrections for timer error need only be made when calibrating sources in a remote afterloader and then only if the remote afterloader timer is used, a practice which is not recommended. Methods standard for external beam therapy may be used without modification. However, with a remote afterloader, timer error is a function of SDD and must be determined at each point of measurement. Its effect is minimized with long integration times and short SDDs where total signal is large.

Timer error, which is defined as the difference between real exposure time, $(t + \epsilon)$ and set exposure time, t, may be determined experimentally from the integrated chamber response for two different timer settings. True response rate for different settings is equivalent, therefore:

$$\epsilon = \frac{M_1 t_2 - M_2 t_1}{M_2 - M_1}$$

Timer error also may be obtained by linear regression analysis of integrated chamber response collected for a number of different timer settings. The slope of the resulting line is ϵ.

With both methods, timer error is determined from a series of measurements at a constant distance. Therefore, correction factors for gradient effect or room scatter need not be applied. It is preferable to use a separate timer in connection with the electrometer. This avoids the need for timer error corrections by allowing multiple measurements to be made while the source is in a fixed position.

Calibration Factors: Calibration factors for an ionization chamber with appropriate build-up cap may be obtained directly from NIST or an ADCL for Co-60 or Cs-137. NIST offers a large number of beam qualities in the diagnostic energy range. For lower energy sources such as I-125, it should be possible to obtain N_x at beam qualities closely bracketing the energy of the desired radionuclide to at least determine an indirect calibration factor for the desired radionuclide. Chamber wall plus cap must be sufficiently thick to ensure electronic equilibrium for the radionuclide being measured. This can be determined by slowing increasing the total thickness until no further increase in signal is produced.

The AAPM has recently approved the use of an interpolative technique for determination of a chamber calibration factor for Ir-192.[64] At the present time, at least two ADCLs (UW ADCL and K&S Associates, Inc. [Nashville, TN, USA]) can provide N_x for Ir-192. To determine the factor, the chamber, which must have a build-up cap of at least 0.3 g/cm^2, is calibrated for Cs-137 and 250 kVp. N_x is determined by interpolating between these two values as follows:

$$(N_x)_{Ir} = (1 + x)[(N_x)_{250\,kVp} + (N_x)_{Cs}]/2$$

where

$$x = 0.0037\,(t/9.3 \times 10^{22})$$
and

$(N_x)_{Ir,\,250\,kVp,Cs}$

= chamber calibration factors (R/C) for ^{192}Ir, 250 kVp x-rays and ^{137}Cs, respectively.

t = wall plus cap thickness (electron/cm^3)

9.3×10^{22} = the number of electrons/cm^3 in 0.31 g/cm^2 of graphite.

0.0037 = correction for attenuation by a wall plus cap thickness of 0.31 g/cm^2.

Perhaps the simplest way to assign a chamber calibration factor for a particular radionuclide is to measure a NIST calibrated source. Calibration factors may be transferred to the ionization chamber as described above.

Air-kerma rate in free air, $\dot{K}(r)$, at a distance, r, from a source calibrated in-air using a stem type ionization chamber is given by:

$$\dot{K}(r) = \dot{M}(r) \cdot C_{TP} \cdot A_{ion} \cdot P_{ion} \cdot C(r)_{grad}$$
$$\cdot C_{RS} \cdot C_{att} \cdot W/e$$

where

$$\dot{M}(r) = \frac{M(r)}{(t + \epsilon(r))}$$

and

$\dot{M}(r)$ = accumulated charge (coulombs) corrected only for leakage

t = duration of charge collection (seconds).

$\epsilon(r)$ = timer error (seconds) for remote afterloading systems. If a separate timer is used or for conventional sources, this error is taken as zero.

C_{TP} = correction for temperature and pressure.

A_{ion} = correction for collection efficiency of chamber/electrometer at time of their calibration.

P_{ion} = correction for collection efficiency of chamber/electrometer at time of measurement

$C(r)_{grad}$ = correction factor for fluence gradient

C_{RS} = correction for room scatter.

C_{att} = correction for air attenuation and multiple scattering, typically taken as unity.

W/e = mean energy expended per unit charge created in dry air (33.97 J C^{-1} or 86.7 Gy/R^{20}).

Air-kerma strength, S_K, may then be determined by correcting measured air-kerma rate to a distance of one meter by application of inverse square law.

In-Phantom Measurements

In-phantom calibrations using a stem type ionization chamber, in general, are not recommended except for high activity sources. However, in-phantom calibrations with stem type ionization chambers have been successfully performed.[43,55,66,67] Because of attenuation by the phantom for low energy sources, signal strength may be significantly less for calibrations done in a phantom than in air.

Again, a geometrical configuration for source calibration in phantom should be decided upon after consideration of concerns addressed below. Corrections should be determined and the geometrical configuration kept constant for subsequent measurements. The discussions above concerning precision, ion collection efficiency, chamber calibration, and timer error may be directly applied to measurements made in-phantom. Corrections for air attenuation and multiple scattering as well as for room scatter, are not necessary. The fluence gradient correction factor also may be directly applied. However, expressions determined by both Dove[59] and Kondo and Randolph[60] consider only primary radiation and, therefore, are more approximate when applied to measurements made in-phantom. If possible, measurements should be made at source to chamber distances of at least 5 cm to minimize this correction.

Water Equivalence of Solid Phantom Materials: It may be more convenient, as well as more accurate with respect to reproducible positioning, to perform source calibrations in a solid phantom rather than a water phantom. However, all phantom materials may not be water equivalent for the radionuclide of interest. Water equivalence of solid phantom materials used with Cs-137 and Co-60 sources may be determined following current external beam therapy protocols.[65] For these radionuclides, a scaling factor, which is a ratio of mean linear attenuation coefficient of water to that of the solid phantom material, is applied to the physical source to chamber distance to obtain water equivalent depth. For example, this factor is 0.99 for polystyrene

and 0.88 for polymethylmethacrylate (PMMA) for Co-60. Meli et al.[68] showed that polystyrene, PMMA, and solid water all may be used for calibration of Ir-192 sources under conditions of full scatter. However, only polystyrene and solid water may be used for conditions with partial scatter. Both experimental and Monte Carlo calculations of Meigooni et al.[69] showed that polystyrene and PMMA are not suitable phantom materials for use with I-125, while solid water may be used. However, data of Williamson[70] does not support the water equivalence of solid water for I-125. In this case, measurements are best done in water using only small amounts of a solid material, preferably solid water, for immobilizing source and detector.

Conditions of Full Scatter: In order to apply corrections for phantom attenuation and scatter that are discussed below, conditions of full scatter must be approximated. It has been shown that dose at any point in a phantom is practically independent of boundary effects provided the boundary of that phantom is at least one photon mean free pathlength from the point of interest.[71] Conservatively, a phantom of 30x30x30 cm³ should be used since the mean free pathlength is approximately 9 cm for Ir-192 and 12 cm for Cs-137. Smaller phantoms may be used for lower energy radionuclides such as I-125, however, their dimensions must be determined based on mean free pathlength for that radionuclide.

Phantom Attenuation and Scatter: Corrections for phantom attenuation and scatter take the form of a tissue-air-ratio. The values of Meisberger et al.[72] are typically used, however radial dose factors of others[73–75] may also be used.

Displacement Effect: The displacement effect occurs when a part of a solid phantom is replaced by the low density cavity of an ionization chamber causing less photon attenuation than in the original volume. Therefore, the average electron fluence is higher in the air cavity. One may apply a correction to dose determined at the center of the cavity or by determining dose at an effective point of measurement. Tolli and Johansson[76] have shown that the displacement effect exists close to Co-60 and Ir-192 sources for cylindrical chambers but, due to steep dose-rate gradients, it is much smaller than for external photon beams.

They found that the shift in effective point of measurement is only a few percent of the internal radius of cylindrical chambers and that it is dependent on the source to chamber distance. The shift is typically only a fraction of a millimeter for chambers studied and will have minimal effect of calibration for SDDs commonly used.

Air-kerma rate in free air, $\dot{K}(r)$, at a distance r from a source calibrated in-phantom is given by:

$$\dot{K}(r) = \dot{M}(r) \cdot C_{TP} \cdot A_{ion} \cdot P_{ion}$$
$$\cdot C(r)_{grad} \cdot (C_{AS})^{-1} \cdot (f_{med})^{-1} \cdot W/e$$

$$\dot{M}(r) = \frac{M(r)}{(t + \epsilon(r))}$$

and

where

$M(r) =$ accumulated charge (coulombs) corrected only for leakage.

$t =$ duration of charge collection (seconds).

$\epsilon(r) =$ timer error (seconds) for remote afterloading systems. If a separate timer is used or for conventional sources, this error is taken as zero.

$C_{TP} =$ correction for temperature and pressure.

$A_{ion} =$ correction for collection efficiency of chamber/electrometer at time of their calibration.

$P_{ion} =$ correction for collection efficiency of chamber/electrometer at time of measurement

$C(r)_{grad} =$ correction factor for fluence gradient

$C_{AS} =$ correction for attenuation and scatter in the phantom.

$f_{med} =$ (0.00876 Gy/R) $(\mu_{en}/\rho)_{med}/(\mu_{en}/\rho)_{air}$.

$W/e =$ mean energy expended per unit charge created in dry air (33.97 J C^{-1} or 86.7 Gy/R[20]).

Air-kerma strength, S_K, may then be determined by correcting measured air-kerma rate to a distance of one meter by application of the inverse square law.

Other Detectors

There are many other types of dosimeters that can be used for measurement of brachytherapy source strength. They exhibit varying degrees of accuracy and precision and, in general, are not recommended for routine calibration of sources. Some of the techniques involved are complex and time consuming and traceability to a national standard is not possible in most cases. The techniques briefly mentioned below are more applicable to measurement of relative dose distribution surrounding a source than its calibration.

Photographic Film: Much of the early dosimetry for brachytherapy sources was performed using photographic film.[77,78] Film is easy to work with and has excellent spatial resolution. However, film also has an energy-dependent response and may be nonlinear. While a calibration curve for the film must be produced, it is not possible to achieve any type of traceability to NIST. Variation from batch to batch of film must be accounted for and, depending on the type of film used, reciprocity failure may be a problem at the low-dose-rates sometimes encountered with brachytherapy sources. Film dosimetry is still used in certain circumstances[79,80] but its use should not be attempted for source calibration.

Thermoluminescent Dosimeters (TLDs): TLDs also have been in use for many years for brachytherapy dosimetry.[81,82] While they are more commonly used for determination of relative dose distributions,[17,73,83–85] they more recently have been used for absolute dose measurement.[86,87] While TLDs offer excellent spatial resolution due to their small size, they exhibit energy dependence[88,89] and are time consuming to use. To achieve accuracy comparable to that quoted in the literature, 3%–6%,[86,89] careful attention to detail is needed. Again, traceability of calibration to a national standard is a problem.

Solid State Detectors: Diode detectors are attractive because of their small size and high signal, and again, have been used by many authors for relative dose measurement.[79,90,91] However, they exhibit an angular dose response as well as energy dependence. Traceability of calibration to NIST cannot clearly be established.

Scintillation Detectors: Scintillation detectors have been used extensively,[80,92,93] particularly in early years,[78,94] for dosimetry of brachytherapy sources. Again, since traceability of calibration to NIST cannot clearly be established, it is recommended to limit their use to relative measurements.

Spectral Detectors: This method of source calibration was briefly discussed above as the way activity of Pd-103 seeds are assessed by the manufacturer. It is particularly useful for sources that are not calibrated by a national standards laboratory and has been used extensively in the past for I-125 and Ir-192 prior to the establishment of NIST standards for those radionuclides.[42,95–99] Measurements may be done with NaI, Si(Li), and high purity germanium detectors, among others, and a multichannel analyzer to determine energy spectrum for the radionuclide in question. Total number of photons from each energy level must be corrected for intrinsic efficiency of the detector, which is dependent on energy. Activity, A, in Bq, can then be determined from the gamma ray spectrum using the following equation for each energy peak.[97]

$$A = \frac{C}{t \cdot \epsilon \cdot f \cdot G \cdot \exp(-\mu x)}$$

where

  C = net counts for a particular energy peak
  t = counting time in seconds
  ϵ = intrinsic efficiency of detector
  f = number of unconverted photons emitted per disintegration
  G = geometry factor
    = $\dfrac{S}{4\pi r^2}$
  S = area of detector face
  $\exp(-\mu x)$ = attenuation for air and detector window.

The activity obtained by this method is apparent activity. Again, source calibration as per this method is not traceable to NIST. The technique, which is complex, should be reserved for special circumstances.

Calibration of Sr-90 Ophthalmic Applicators

In comparison to calibration of photon emitting sources, calibration of sources emitting beta particles, namely Sr-90 ophthalmic applicators, is not as well established. While these applicators are in fairly widespread use, many are quite old and have not been recalibrated since being manufactured. Initial calibrations were often in terms of quantities with questionable validity—reps per second, beta roentgens, exposure rate—and only more recently in terms of Gy/s. Originally distributed by a number of manufacturers, there is now only one commercial vendor, Amersham International (Amersham, England).

Measurement of surface dose from a beta source is more difficult than measurement of photon emitting sources due to the higher probability for interaction in the media between source and detector and resulting change in beta particle spectrum with measurement configuration and, therefore, in detector response.[100] Because of these difficulties, it is not common for calibration to be done by the user. While NIST only performs a small number (5–8) of these calibrations per year,[101] a difference of approximately 35% in dose-rate calibration between Amersham International and NIST was recently noted, which has lead to revision of the NIST calibration procedure.[102]

NIST has offered calibration of Sr-90 planar ophthalmic applicators since 1977.[103,104] These sources are calibrated in terms of surface absorbed dose rate to water averaged over the active area of the source in Gy/s. Applicators calibrated typically range from 370 MBq (10 mCi) to 7.4 GBq (200 mCi) with corresponding approximate average surface absorbed dose rates from 0.1–2 Gy/s.

The NIST calibration procedure uses an extrapolation chamber[105] to measure ionization current per unit mass of air. Measurements are made with the applicator at several distances from the center of the chamber air gap and extrapolated to zero distance to obtain a value at the surface of the applicator.[103,104] First, a small area collecting electrode with a small fixed air gap is used to look at variations in dose rate across the surface and to measure the active area of the applicator. The active area, A, is taken to be the full width at half maximum current points of the profile obtained by scanning across the applicator face. Next, the collecting electrode is replaced with one that is at least two beta particle ranges larger than the active area of the source. The total current per unit air gap at the source surface, $(I/d)_0$, is measured by the method described above. The average surface absorbed dose rate, $\dot{D}_{water}$, is directly proportional to the ratio of $(I/d)_0/(\rho A)$ where ρ is the density of air at reference temperature and pressure.

Finally, Bragg-Gray cavity theory is used to convert this ratio into absorbed dose rate.

$$\dot{D}_{water} = \frac{(I/d)_0}{\rho A}\,(W/e)\,\frac{(\bar{S}/\rho)^{water}}{(\bar{S}/\rho)^{air}}\,k_{back}\,k_{foil}$$

where $(\bar{S}/\rho)$ is average collision mass stopping power of water and air, k_{back} corrects for a difference in backscatter between the collecting electrode and water, and k_{foil} corrects for attenuation or build-up in the high voltage electrode.

Uncertainties in absorbed dose include instrumental (0.3%), average energy per ion pair (0.4%), stopping power ratio (3%), rate of change of current (3%), backscatter correction (1%), attenuation correction (<0.1%), source surface area (6%), which combine in quadrature to give 7%.[103,104] Doubling this value and rounding off gives an overall uncertainty ±15%, which can be interpreted as having the approximate significance of a 95% confidence limit.

In 1988, the ADCL at the University of Wisconsin (UW) was asked by the Amersham Corporation to calibrate one of their Sr-90 ophthalmic applicators.[102] This applicator had previously been calibrated both by the manufacturer and by NIST. The UW ADCL measured a dose rate that was 48% higher than that measured by the manufacturer while the NIST value was 57% higher. To try to resolve these differences, NIST held a nationwide workshop on calibration of Sr-90 applicators in March of 1989 and in June of the same year it suspended source calibrations until this issue had been thoroughly explored and a consistent method of calibration established. The procedure used by Amersham International for calibration of their internal standards uses an extrapolation chamber and

is, in principle, similar to that used by NIST.[101] The fundamental difference between the two methods appears to be that in contrast to the NIST extrapolation chamber, the collecting electrode of the Amersham chamber is much smaller than the active area of most applicators. It is, therefore, not surprising that discrepancies existed since Goetsch and Sunderland[101] have shown that measured dose rate is itself a function of construction of the extrapolation chamber and, in particular, of diameter of the collecting electrode. Other differences include effective depth of measurement and range of air gap widths over which the limiting ionization current versus air gap slope was measured.[106]

After much review, as well as blind intercomparisons between NIST, Amersham International and other laboratories, and measurements made using other detectors such as radiochromic dye films and TLD, NIST has published a revised approach to their calibration procedure for ophthalmic applicators.[107] Revision of the procedure has brought their measured dose rates down from between 5%–15%; however, the Amersham method still gives a calibration approximately 21% lower than that of NIST. This discrepancy is reduced to approximately 10% by using NIST constants and applying a 7% correction to the Amersham calibration for transmission factor between the surface and quoted depth of measurement. With the NIST overall uncertainty now quoted as ±12%, this agreement is felt to be satisfactory.

The discovery of the discrepancy between NIST and Amersham has had a very positive effect of standardization of calibration for Sr-90 applicators. In addition to procedural review by NIST, other laboratories have published results of measurements with extrapolation chambers,[101] radiochromic dye films,[108] and TLD,[109] which have appeared to agree with NIST. While these reports lend weight to the NIST procedure, the extrapolation chamber is still the only detector used that does not require calibration with other radiation sources. In addition, a calibration facility for Sr-90 ophthalmic applicators has been established at the UW ADCL. Their procedure is similar to that followed by NIST with some modifications.[101] Instead of ionization current measurements, an autoradiograph is used to determine the active area of the applicator. Also, three different commercially available chambers are used instead of the custom made extrapolation chamber used at NIST.

At the present time, NIST provides no calibration service for concave Sr-90 applicators. Unfortunately, many Sr-90 applicators in clinical use are concave. Recently, several groups have presented techniques for determination of surface absorbed dose. Reft et al.[109] have used TLDs to measure surface dose for both concave and planar applicators. Their value for the planar applicator was consistent with NIST and they conclude that TLDs provide an accurate method of measuring output from Sr-90 applicators. Soares[110] used radiochromic foils to determine the average absorbed surface dose rate for concave applicators and compared his results with values determined by Amersham International using a calibrated scintillator probe. Values determined using the radiochromic foils, which had an uncertainty of ± 15%, were approximately 10% higher than those determined by Amersham International and, therefore, consistent with NIST.

Conclusion

Consistent brachytherapy source specification and calibration is essential for high quality patient treatment. While for many years the issue of source specification was controversial, it is now clear that air-kerma rate or air-kerma strength are the recommended methods and all brachytherapy source users and manufacturers should strive to comply with these recommendations.

No longer can the user rely on brachytherapy source calibrations provided by the manufacturer. The user himself must be able to measure source strength with an accuracy better than ± 5%. In addition, the user must be able to ensure traceability to a national standards laboratory. This should be achievable using techniques detailed in this chapter.

References

1. International Commission on Radiation Protection (ICRP). Protection of the patient in radiation therapy: ICRP Publication 44. Pergamon Press, Oxford, 1985.

2. American Association of Physicist in Medicine (AAPM). Physical aspects of quality assurance in radiation therapy: AAPM Report No. 13. American Institute of Physics, New York, 1984.

3. World Health Organization (WHO). Quality Assurance in Radiotherapy. WHO, Geneva, 1984.

4. Kutcher GJ, Coia L, Gillin M, et al. Comprehensive QA for radiation oncology: Report of AAPM Radiation Therapy committee Task Group 40. Med Phys 1994;21:581–618.

5. Boyer AL. A fundamental accuracy limitation on measurements of brachytherapy sources. Med Phys 1979;6:454–456.

6. Dutreix A. Un nouvell methode de specification des sources radioactive en curietherapie. J Radiol d'electrologie et de Medicine Nucleaire 1974;55:781–784.

7. Dutreix A, Wambersie A. Specification of gamma-ray brachytherapy sources. Br J Radiol 1975;75:1034–1035.

8. Jayaraman S, Lanzl LH. An overview of errors in line source dosimetry for gamma-ray brachytherapy. Med Phys 1983;10:871–875.

9. National Council on Radiation Protection and Measurement (NCRP). Report No. 41: Specification of gamma-ray brachytherapy sources. NCRP Publications, Washington, D.C., 1974.

10. British Committee on Radiation Units and Measurements. Specification of brachytherapy sources. Br J Radiol 1981;57:941–942.

11. Comite Francois pour la mesure des rayonnements ionisants. Rapport CFMRI no. 1: Recommandations pour la determination des doses absorbees en curietherapie. Bureau National de Meterologie, Paris, 1983.

12. AAPM Task Group 32. AAPM Report No. 21: Specification of brachytherapy source strength. American Institute of Physics, New York, 1987.

13. Bjarngard BE. Early brachytherapy dosimetry. In: Shearer DR (ed). Recent Advances in Brachytherapy Physics. American Institute of Physics, New York, 1981, pp. 1–5.

14. Payne WH, Waggener RG. A theoretical calculation of the exposure rate constant for radium-226. Med Phys 1974;1:210–214.

15. Glasgow GP, Dillman LT. Specific γ-ray constant and exposure rate constant of ^{192}Ir. Med Phys 1979;6:49–52.

16. Glasgow GP. Exposure rate constants for filtered ^{192}Ir sources. Med Phys 1981;8:502–503.

17. Weaver KA, Smith V, Huang D, et al. Dose parameters of ^{125}I and ^{192}Ir seed sources. Med Phys 1989;16:636–643.

18. International Commission on Radiation Units and Measurements. ICRU Report 18: Specifi-

cation of high activity gamma-ray sources. International Commission on Radiation Units and Measurements, Washington, DC, 1970.

19. International Commission on Radiation Units and Measurements. ICRU Report No. 38: Dose and Volume Specification for Reporting Intracavitary Therapy in Gynecology. International Commission on Radiation Units and Measurements, Washington, DC, 1985.

20. Boutillon M, Perroche-Rous AM. Re-evaluation of the W value for electrons in dry air. Phys Med Biol 1987;32:213–219.

21. Williamson JF, Nath R. Clinical implementation of AAPM Task Group 32 recommendations on brachytherapy source strength specification. Med Phys 1991;18:439–448.

22. Loevinger R. The role of the standards laboratory in brachytherapy. In: Shearer DR (ed). Recent Advances in Brachytherapy Physics. American Institute of Physics, New York, 1981, pp. 22–31.

23. Simmons JD (ed). NIST calibration services user guide 1991: NIST special publication 250. US Government Printing Office, Washington, DC, 1991.

24. Weaver JT, Loftus TP, Loevinger R. Calibration of gamma-ray-emitting brachytherapy sources: NBS Special Publication 250–19. US Government Printing Office, Washington, DC, 1988.

25. Loftus TP, Weaver JT. Standardization of ^{60}Co and ^{137}Cs gamma-ray beams in terms of exposure. J Res NBS 1974;78A:465–476.

26. Loftus TP. Standardization of cesium-137 gamma-ray sources in terms of exposure units (roentgens). J Res Natl Bur Stands 1970; 74A:1–6.

27. Loftus TP. Standardization of iridium-192 gamma-ray sources in terms of exposure. J Res Natl Bur Stands 1980;85:19–25.

28. Loftus TP. Exposure standardization of iodine-125 seeds used for brachytherapy. J Res Natl Bur Stands 1980;89:295–303.

29. Ritz VH. Standard free-air chamber for the measurement of low energy x rays (20 to 100 kilovolts-constant-potential). J Res Natl Bur Stands 1960;64C:49–53.

30. Kubo H. Exposure contribution from Ti K x rays produced in the titanium capsule of the clinical I-125 seed. Med Phys 1985;12: 215–220.

31. Williamson JF. Monte Carlo evaluation of specific dose constants in water for ^{125}I seeds. Med Phys 1988;15:686–694.

32. Yalamanchili R. Private communication. Springfield, VA: Best Industries, Inc., 1994.

33. Yalamanchili R. Source Calibration Certificate. Springfield, VA: Best Industries, Inc., 1994.

34. Johnson E. Private communication. Salt Lake City: Radiation Safety & Nuclear Products, Inc, 1994.

35. Langton MA. Private communication. Arlington Heights, IL: Medi-Physics, Inc., 1994.

36. Speck T. Private communication. Columbia, MD: Nucletron Corporation, 1994.

37. Monroe J. Private communication. North Andover, MA: RTS Technology, 1994.

38. Renton D. Private communication. Atlanta: Theragenics Corporation, 1994.

39. Meigooni AS, Sabnis S, Nath R. Dosimetry of palladium-103 brachytherapy sources for permanent implants. Endocuriether/Hyperther Oncol 1990;6:107–117.

40. Weaver KA, Anderson LL, Meli JA. Source calibration. In: Interstitial Collaborative Working Group. Interstitial Brachytherapy. Raven Press, New York, 1990.

41. Williamson JF, Khan FM, Sharma SC, et al. Methods for routine calibration of brachytherapy sources. Radiology 1982;142:511–516.

42. Boyer AL, Cobb PD, Kase KR, et al. ^{192}Ir hospital calibration procedures. In: Shearer DR (ed). Recent Advances in Brachytherapy Physics. American Institute of Physics, New York, 1981, pp. 82–103.

43. Diffey BL, Klevenhagen SC. An experimental and calculated dose distribution in water around CDC K-type caesium-137 sources. Phys Med Biol 1975;20:446–454.

44. Kubo H. Comparison of two independent exposure measurement techniques for clinical I-125 seeds. Med Phys 1985;12:221–224.

45. Ling CC, Anderson LL, Biggs PJ, et al. Activity assay of ^{125}I implant seeds. In: Shearer DR (ed). Recent Advances in Brachytherapy Physics. American Institute of Physics, New York, 1981, pp. 115–125.

46. AAPM Task Group 41. Remote afterloading technology. American Institute of Physics, New York, 1993.

47. DeWerd LA, Ezzell GA, Williamson JF. Calibration priciples and techniques. In: Nag S (ed). High Dose Rate Brachytherapy: A Textbook. Futura Publishing Company, Inc., Armonk, NY, 1994, pp. 63–80.

48. Goetsch SJ, Attix FH, DeWerd LA, et al. A new re-entrant ionization chamber for the calibration of iridium-192 high dose rate sources. Int J Radiat Oncol Biol Phys 1992;24:167–170.

49. Holt JG, Stanton RE, Sell RE. Ionization collection efficiency of some ionization chambers in pulsed and continuous radiation beams. Med Phys 1978;5:107–110.

50. Berkley LW, Hanson WF, Shalek RJ. Discus-

sion of the characteristics and results of measurements with a portable well ionization chamber for calibration of brachytherapy sources. In: Shearer DR (ed). Recent Advances in Brachytherapy Physics. American Institute of Physics, New York, 1981, pp. 38–48.

51. Williamson JF, Morin RL, Khan FM. Dose calibrator response to brachytherapy sources: A Monte Carlo and analytic evaluation. Med Phys 1983;10:135–140.

52. Flynn A, Workman G. Calibration of a Microselectron HDR iridium 192 source. Br J Radiol 1991;64:734–739.

53. Ezzell GA. Evaluation of calibration techniques for the microSelectron-HDR. Activity 1989;1:10–14.

54. Park HC, Almond PR. Evaluation of the buildup effect of an ^{192}Ir high dose-rate brachytherapy source. Med Phys 1991;19:1293–1297.

55. Meertens H. In-phantom calibration of Selectron-LDR sources. Radiother Oncol 1990;17:369–378.

56. Khan FM. The Physics of Radiation Therapy. Williams and Wilkins, Baltimore, 1994.

57. Read LR, Burns RA, Liquorish AC. Exposure rate calibration of small radioactive sources of ^{60}Co, ^{226}Ra and ^{137}Cs. Int J Appl Radiat Isot 1978;29:21–27.

58. Hubbell JH. Photon mass attenuation and energy-absorption coefficients from 1 keV to 20 MeV. Int J Appl Radiat Isot 1982;33:1269–1290.

59. Dove DB. Effect of dosimeter size on measurements close to a radioactive source. Br J Radiol 1959;62:202–204.

60. Kondo VS, Randolph ML. Effect of finite size of ionization chambers on measurements of small photon sources. Rad Res 1960;13:37–60.

61. Bielajew AF. An analytic theory of the point-source non-uniformity correction factor for thick-walled ionization chambers in photon beams. Phys Med Biol 1990;35:517–538.

62. Tolli H, Johansson KA. Quality assurance in brachytherapy: Principles for ionization chamber measurement of absorbed dose close to brachytherapy sources. Phys Med Biol 1993;38:1475–1483.

63. Ezzell GA. Evaluation of calibration techniques for a high dose rate remote afterloading Iridium-192 source. Endocuriether/Hyperther Oncol 1990;6:101–106.

64. Goetsch SJ, Attix FH, Pearson DW, et al. Calibration of ^{192}Ir high-dose-rate afterloading systems. Med Phys 1991;18:462–467.

65. AAPM Task Group 21. A protocol for the determination of absorbed dose from high-energy photon and electron beams. Med Phys 1983;10:741–771.

66. Serago CF, Houdek PV, Pisciotta C, et al. Scattering effects on the dosimetry of iridium-192. Med Phys 1991;18:1266–1270.

67. Meredith WJ, Greene D, Kawashima K. The attenuation and scattering in a phantom of gamma rays from some radionuclides used in mould and interstitial gamma-ray therapy. Br J Radiol 1966;39:280–286.

68. Meli JA, Meigooni AS, Nath R. On the choice of phantom material for the dosimetry of ^{192}Ir sources. Int J Radiat Oncol Biol Phys 1988;14:587–594.

69. Meigooni AS, Meli JA, Nath R. A comparison of solid phantoms with water for dosimetry of ^{125}I brachytherapy sources. Med Phys 1988;15:695–701.

70. Williamson JF. Comparison of measured and calculated dose rates in water near I-125 and Ir-192 seeds. Med Phys 1991;18:776–786.

71. Ellett WH. Specific absorbed fractions for photon point sources within a scattering medium. Phys Med Biol 1969;14:615–626.

72. Meisberger L, Keller R, Shalek R. The effective attenuation in water of the gamma rays of gold 198, iridium 192, cesium 137, radium 226 and cobalt 60. Radiology 1968;90:953–957.

73. Thomason C, Mackie TR, Lindstom MJ, et al. The dose distribution surrounding ^{192}Ir and ^{137}Cs seed sources. Phys Med Biol 1991;36:475–493.

74. Dale RG. A Monte Carlo derivation of parameters for use in the tissue dosimetry of medium and low energy nuclides. Br J Radiol 1982;55:748–757.

75. Meli JA, Anderson LL, Weaver KA. Dose distribution. In: Interstitial Collaborative Working Group. Interstitial Brachytherapy. Raven Press, New York, 1990, pp. 21–32.

76. Tolli H, Johansson KA. Quality assurance in brachytherapy: The displacement effect in the vicinity of ^{60}Co and ^{192}Ir brachytherapy sources. Phys Med Biol 1993;38:1485–1492.

77. Tochilin E. A photographic method for measuring the distribution of dosage from radium needles and plaques. Am J Roentgenol Radium Therapy Nucl Med 1964;73:265–274.

78. Horsler AFC, Jones JC, Stacey AJ. Caesium 137 sources for use in intracavitary and interstitial radiotherapy. Br J Radiol 1964;37:385–390.

79. Metcalfe PE. Experimental verification of cesium brachytherapy line source emission using a semiconductor detector. Med Phys 1988;15:702–706.

80. Nath R, Gray L. Dosimetry studies on proto-

type [241]Am sources for brachytherapy. Int J Radiat Oncol Biol Phys 1987;13:897–905.

81. Grotenhuis IM, Martin TJ, Hilger MS, et al. Experimental comparison of radium, cesium-137 and cobalt-60 tissue doses. Am J Roentgenol Rad Therapy Nucl Med 1964;86: 145–146.

82. Punnunni Kartha KI, Kenney GN, Cameron JR. An experimental determination of the absorption and buildup factor in water for radium, cobalt 60, and cesium 137 gamma rays. Am J Roentgenol Rad Therapy Nucl Med 1966;96:66–69.

83. Chiu-Tsao S-T, Anderson LL. Thermoluminescent dosimetry for [103]Pd seeds (model 200) in solid water phantom. Med Phys 1991;18: 449–452.

84. Thomason C, Higgins P. Radial dose distribution of ^{192}Ir and ^{137}Cs seed sources. Med Phys 1989;254–257.

85. Gillin MT, Lopez RW, Grimm DF, et al. Comparison of measured and calculated dose distributions around an iridium-192 wire. Med Phys 1988;15:915–918.

86. Hartmann GH, Schlegel W, Scharfenberg H. The three-dimensional dose distribution of ^{125}I seeds in tissue. Phys Med Biol 1983;28: 693–699.

87. Nath R, Meigooni AS, Meli JA. Dosimetry on transverse axes of ^{125}I and ^{192}Ir interstitial brachytherapy sources. Med Phys 1990;17: 1032–1040.

88. Meigooni AS, Meli JA, Nath R. Influence of the variation of energy spectra with depth in the dosimetry of ^{192}Ir using LiF TLD. Phys Med Biol 1988;33:1159–1170.

89. Weaver KA. Response of LiF powder to ^{125}I photons. Med Phys 1984;11:850–854.

90. Schell MC, Ling CC, Gromadzki ZC, et al. Dose distributions of model 6702 I-125 seeds in water. Int J Radiat Oncol Biol Phys 1987; 13:795–799.

91. Scarbrough EC, Sanborn GE, Anderson JA, et al. Dose distribution around a 3.0-mm type 6702 I-125 seed. Med Phys 1990;17:460–463.

92. Schulz RJ, Chandra P, Nath R. Determination of the exposure rate constant for ^{125}I using a scintillation detector. Med Phys 1980;7: 355–361.

93. McCullough KP. A scintillation detector for the calibration of individual seeds within an Ir-192 ribbon. Int J Radiat Oncol Biol Phys 1992;24(Suppl 1):288.

94. Ter-Pogossian M, Ittner WB, Samira MA. Comparison of air and tissue doses for radium gamma rays. Nucleonics 1952;10:50–52.

95. Ling CC, Gromadzki ZC, Rustgi SN, et al. Directional dependence of radiation fluence from ^{192}Ir and [198]Au. Radiology 1983;146: 791–792.

96. Hashemi AM, Mills MD, Hogstrom KR, et al. The exposure rate constant for a silver wire ^{125}I seed. Med Phys 1988;15:228–234.

97. Cobb PD, Chen TS, Kase KR. Calibration of brachytherapy iridium-192 sources. Int J Radiat Oncol Biol Phys 1981;7:259–262.

98. Ling CC, Yorke ED, Spiro IJ, et al. Physical dosimetry of ^{125}I seeds of a new design for interstitial implant. Int J Radiation Oncol Biol Phys 1983;9:1747–1752.

99. Ling CC, Anderson LL, Shipley WU. Dose inhomogeneity in interstitial implants using ^{125}I seeds. Int J Radiat Oncol Biol Phys 1979;5: 419–425.

100. Pruitt JS, Soares CG, Ehrlich M. Calibration of beta-particle radiation instrumentation and sources: NBS special publication 250–21. US Government Printing Office, Washington, DC, 1988.

101. Goetsch SJ, Sunderland KS. Surface dose rate calibration of Sr-90 plane ophthalmic applicators. Med Phys 1991;18:161–166.

102. Goetsch SJ. Calibration of Sr-90 ophthalmic applicators. Int J Radiat Oncol Biol Phys 1989; 16:1653.

103. Pruitt JS. Calibration of beta particle emitting opthalmic applicators: NBS Special Publication 250–9. US Government Printing Office, Washington, DC, 1987.

104. Pruitt JS. Calibration of beta-particle opthalmic applicators at the National Bureau of Standards. J Res Natl Bur Stands 1986;91: 165–170.

105. Loevinger R, Trott NG. Design and operation of an extrapolation chamber with removable electrodes. Int J Appl Rad Isotopes 1966;17: 103–111.

106. Deasy JO, Soares CG. Extrapolation chamber measurements of [90]Sr + [90]Y beta-particle ophthalmic applicator dose rates. Med Phys 1994;2:91–99.

107. Soares CG. Calibration of ophthalmic applicators at NIST: A revised approach. Med Phys 1991;18:787–793.

108. Sayag JA, Gregory RC. A new method for characterizing beta ray ophthalmic applicator sources. Med Phys 1991;18:453–461.

109. Reft CS, Kuchnir FT, Rosenberg I, et al. Dosimetry of Sr-90 ophthalmic applicators. Med Phys 1990;17:641–646.

110. Soares CG. A method for the calibration of concave [90]Sr + [90]Y ophthalmic applicators. Phys Med Biol 1992;37:1005–1007.

Chapter 7

Quality Assurance in Brachytherapy

Michael T. Gillin, Ph.D., Katherine Albano, M.S.

Introduction

The International Standards Organization has developed basic definitions relating to quality assurance. The Report of the American Association of Physicists in Medicine (AAPM) Radiation Therapy Committee Task Group 40, Comprehensive QA for Radiation Oncology, adapted these definitions to radiation oncology.[1] Quality is defined as the totality of features and characteristics of a radiation therapy process that bear on its ability to satisfy stated or implied needs of the patient. Quality assurance is defined as all those planned or systematic actions necessary to provide adequate confidence that a product or service will satisfy given requirements for quality. Quality control is defined as the operational techniques and activities used to fulfill requirements of quality.[2]

Quality assurance is an essential part of brachytherapy, both in order to provide appropriate brachytherapy services that satisfy the needs of the patient and to comply with federal and/or state regulations which, at least in theory, protect the patient and the general public. At most institutions brachytherapy procedures are performed far less frequently than external beam procedures and thus quality assurance and quality control are even more important. Scientific and professional

organizations have published specific recommendations on brachytherapy quality assurance and quality control. AAPM Report No. 13, Physical Aspects of Quality Assurance in Radiation Therapy, devotes an entire chapter to brachytherapy that contains explicit recommendations for calibration of brachytherapy sources.[3] The Report of AAPM Task Group 40, which is entitled Comprehensive Quality Assurance for Radiation Oncology, is an update to Report No. 13 and has a section entitled Brachytherapy. This section has major subdivisions on sealed sources, treatment planning and dosimetry, and remote afterloading. The American College of Radiology (ACR) has published a document entitled "Physical Aspects of Quality Assurance" that addresses brachytherapy and unsealed source therapy procedures.[4] As part of their series of published standards, the ACR is working on a separate standard for brachytherapy. The development of high-dose-rate (HDR) devices with their inherent complexity has reenforced the need for good brachytherapy quality assurance procedures. The recommendations of these scientific and professional organizations supplement the requirements imposed upon institutions providing brachytherapy services, namely licensees, by the U.S. Nuclear Regulatory Commission (USNRC [NRC]) through their

From Nag S (ed): *Principles and Practice of Brachytherapy.* © Futura Publishing Co., Inc., Armonk, NY, 1997.

published regulations, Title 10, Chapter 1, Code of Federal Regulations, Part 35, Medical Use of Byproduct Material, and through specific conditions imposed on individual licenses or the individual agreement of states through their regulations.[5]

Regulatory Quality Assurance Requirements

The Atomic Energy Act of 1954, and its amendments, provides the legal authority of the USNRC to issue licenses for use in medical therapy. As a consequence there are many regulations concerning brachytherapy. The NRC defines an authorized user as a physician, dentist, or podiatrist who is identified as an authorized user on a Commission or Agreement State license that authorizes the medical use of by-product material.[6] The radiation oncology brachytherapist as an authorized user has special obligations and responsibilities that are detailed in the federal regulations. In addition, these regulations form the basis of a brachytherapy quality assurance program. There may be some slight differences between the federal regulations and those of the individual agreement states. However, the basic requirements are essentially the same.

Quality Management Programs

In the early 1990s, the NRC expanded its regulations when it published and implemented its rules on Quality Management Programs (QMP). The stated purpose of the QMP is "to provide high confidence that . . . radiation from byproduct material will be administered as directed by an authorized user physician."[5] This sounds remarkably like the purpose of a quality assurance program. The QMP regulations defined a "written directive" as an order in writing for a specific patient, dated and signed by an authorized user prior to the administration of therapy, which must contain specifically defined details. For low-dose-rate (LDR) brachytherapy, the written directive is two-fold and must contain, prior to the loading of the sources, the radioisotope and the source strength and total number of sources and, prior to the completion of the procedure, the treatment site, the isotope,

total source strength, and time of implant or equivalently the total dose. For HDR, the written directive, which again is an order in writing for a specific patient, must state the treatment site, the isotope, and the total dose.[7] A footnote to Paragraph 35.32 addresses medical emergencies and states that an oral directive is acceptable in such an event to be followed within 24 hours by a written directive.[7]

The QMP has five objectives:

1. Preparation of a written directive before administration;
2. Identification of the patient, by more than one method, as the individual named in the written directive before each administration;
3. Accordance of the final plans of treatment and related calculations with the written directive;
4. Accordance of each administration with the written directive;
5. Identification and evaluation of any unintended deviation from the written directive and implementation of appropriate action.[7]

Thus, the written directive is a prescription written by the radiation oncologist to provide guidance to the supporting staff. The written directive should represent a summary of the brachytherapy procedure in that it contains the basic set of information that describes the brachytherapy application, namely, the treatment site, the isotope, the number and activity of sources, the implant pattern, and the dose to be delivered to one point or the total time of the implant. The written directive is a document that can be reviewed at a later date and compared against the plan of treatment as stated in the patient's chart. In fact, such a review is required at least annually by the NRC.[7] The Regulatory Guide 8.33 (Task DG-8001), QMP describes a method to determine the number of patient cases to be reviewed.[8] This method is based upon statistical acceptance sampling principles. For all but the largest practices, an annual review of all brachytherapy cases would not require much time. This review must compare the written directive to the actual procedure performed, as documented in the patient's chart. It is our experience that this review has not revealed any problems at our institution. This is not surprising given the close cooperation between oncologists and support staff. It is helpful to prepare separate written directive forms for each major type of implant, e.g., interstitial head and neck, perineal templates, HDR tandem and ovoids, eye plaques, etc. These forms are tailored to the unique requirements of that implant and can serve as useful tools in communication between the radiation oncologist and the physics/planning staff and in documenting specific details of the treatment. Figure 1 contains two examples of written directive forms, one used for an HDR procedure and the other used for an LDR procedure. The written directives can be an important component of any brachytherapy quality assurance program if designed pragmatically.

The Regulatory Guide 8.33 (Task DG-8001), QMP contains extensive requirements/recommendations of a quality assurance nature to implement the QMP.[8] The QMP is a 'performance based program' and thus the methods of developing and maintaining a QMP are left to the individual institution. The recommendations contained in this guide are offered by the NRC as suggestions and individual licensees are free to propose alternative approaches. It should be noted that most of the recommendations in this guide have not been developed by the NRC but represent a summary of recommendations found in the literature.

The QMP requires acceptance testing before the clinical use of each treatment planning or dose calculating computer program for both HDR and LDR programs. Such acceptance testing should be based upon the institution's specific needs and applications.[9] This requirement has been a long-standing recommendation and is good practice.[10]

In addition, the QMP requires that each individual plan be checked before the delivery of treatment for HDR or before the total prescribed brachytherapy dose has been administered for LDR.[11] In fact, for HDR such a requirement is now found in many licenses. There are separate recommendations for manual and computer generated dose distributions, which are essentially the same for HDR and LDR.[11] This regulatory guide recommends that manual dose calculations be checked for arithmetic errors, that appropriate data has been used in the dose calcula-

tions, and that the calculations are consistent with the written directive. It also recommends that computer generated dose distributions be checked by either examining the output to verify that correct data for the patient, based upon the written directive, was used or by performing a manual calculation to a single point and comparing the computer and manual results.[11]

There are now several years of experience with the QMP. The initial review by the NRC of each licensee's QMP has been completed. NRC inspectors are reviewing compliance with the QMP in great detail. As part of the inspection process, the charts on selected brachytherapy patients are being reviewed. The apparent net effect of the QMP has been to emphasize quality assurance in brachytherapy.

Quality Assurance Requirements of Part 35

In addition to the QMP requirements, Part 35 of Title 10 of the Code of Federal Regulations, Medical Use of Byproduct Material, contains sections on General Administrative and Technical Requirements as well as a section entitled Subpart G, Sources for Brachytherapy. There are many required quality assurance and control measures in this section. In this current version of Part 35, HDR remote afterloading devices are not mentioned.

The most well publicized elements in Part 35 are the regulations requiring the user to either document or report quality assurance failures as part of the NRCs misadministration rules. In 1991, the NRC modified its definition of misadministration and introduced a new category, the recordable event.[5] In brachytherapy, a recordable event occurs when radiation is administered without a written directive or when the calculated administered dose differs by >10% from the prescribed dose. A misadministration occurs when the radiation is administered to the wrong patient or with the wrong isotope or wrong treatment site, or with a sealed source that is leaking, or when one or more sealed sources are not removed upon completion of a temporary implant, or when the calculated administered dose differs from the prescribed dose by >20%. The 1991 modifications did not change

Low Dose Rate Written Directive For Tandem and Ovoids Using Cs-137 Sources

Patient: Date:

Staff: Resident:

Site: Cervix or Endometrium
Active Length Tandem
Ovoid Diameter

Drawing:

Initial Plan

Dose Prescription Points: Pt. A   cGy/h

                                   Ovoid Surface   cGy/h

                                   Other _____

Projected Total Time: hours

Modifications During Treatment: YES   No

Actual Total Time: hours

Staff   Date

_____ , M.D.   _____

If plan has changed, a written order describing the change must be made.

Figure 1A. Example of a low-dose-rate written directive.

**High Dose Rate Written Directive For Vaginal Cylinders For
Ir-192 Source**

Patient   Date:

Staff: Resident:

Site:

Applicator Diameter: Active Length

Initial Plan
Number of fractions: Dose per fraction:

Dose Prescription Points: Surface of Applicator including apex

                           Other _____

Actual Treatments

	Changes		Staff
Date			
First Fraction:	No	Yes _____ , MD	_____
Second Fraction:	No	Yes _____ , MD	_____
Third Fraction:	No	Yes _____ , MD	_____
Fourth Fraction:	No	Yes _____ , MD	_____
Fifth Fraction:	No	Yes _____ , MD	_____
Sixth Fraction:	No	Yes _____ , MD	_____

If plan has changed, a written order describing the change must be
made.

Figure 1B. Example of a high-dose-rate written directive.

the requirements for reporting misadministration to the NRC, the referring physician, and possibly even the patient.[12] There are also requirements for the documentation of recordable events.[12]

Paragraph 35.400 lists the NRC approved uses for various sources. Co-60 and Cs-137 are approved in the form of needles and applicator cells for topical, interstitial, and intracavitary treatment of cancer. Ir-192 seeds encased in nylon ribbon, Pd-103, I-125, and Au-198 seeds are approved for interstitial treatment of cancer.[13] Thus to use Ir-192 for intraluminal or intracavitary cases or to use I-125 in eye plaques, it is advisable to amend your license to explicitly permit these applications. Source manufacturers have applied for the specific uses for their sources, which are defined in paragraph 35.400. It is the position of the NRC that other uses, such as the intraluminal use of an Ir-192 ribbon, may not be safe as it has not been reviewed by the NRC.

The NRC requires strict accounting in the form of a paper trail for all sources used for an implant. The goal is to be able to determine the location of all brachytherapy sources all of the time. Thus for a specific implant a record must be made that includes the patient's name and room number, the number and activity of the sources removed from storage together with the time and date they were removed, the number and activity of sources remaining in storage, and the initials of the individual who removed the sources from storage. Immediately after implanting the sources in a patient, a survey must be performed of the patient and the area to confirm that no sources have been misplaced. Immediately after removing the last source from the patient at the end of the implant, the patient must be surveyed with a radiation detection survey instrument to confirm that all sources have been removed. (It is difficult to believe that patients have been discharged with brachytherapy sources still in them. However, patients have been discharged while still containing both HDR and LDR sources.) Upon returning the sources to storage, a record must be made of the patient's name and room number, number and activity of the sources returned, the time and date that the sources were returned, the number and activity of sources in storage after the sources were returned, and the initials of the individual who returned the sources.[14] As noted above, the net result is a paper trail of all the brachytherapy sources at all times.

The NRC requires a list of the names of all the individuals who are permitted to handle brachytherapy sources.[14] It does not specify any requirements for these individuals, however. The NRC has training and experience requirements for authorized users of brachytherapy sources.[15] These requirements are either board certification by appropriate boards or 200 hours of classroom and laboratory training plus 500 hours of supervised work experience under the supervision of an authorized user. The NRC does not have any requirements for a brachytherapy physicist, even for HDR. (They do have requirements for a teletherapy physicist, however.[16]) Appropriate training and experience of brachytherapy support staff remains an ongoing quality issue.

The NRC has regulations relative to radiation safety instruction for all personnel caring for the brachytherapy patient.[17] These instructions must include the size and appearance of the brachytherapy sources, safe handling and shielding instructions in the case of a dislodged source, procedures for patient and visitor control, and a procedure to notify the radiation safety officer if the patient dies or has a medical emergency. The NRC also has regulations relative to appropriate posting of the patient's room, the measurements of radiation levels in contiguous restricted and unrestricted areas, and visitation by family members.[18] For a permanent implant, the NRC requires that the patient be provided "with radiation safety guidance that will help to keep radiation dose to household members and the public as low as reasonably achievable before releasing the patient."[18] Again, these regulations represent an attempt to ensure that the entire procedure satisfies all of the needs of the patient, the family, and the support staff.

For brachytherapy purposes, the NRC requires two different portable radiation survey instruments. One is a detection survey instrument capable of detecting dose rates within a range of 0.1–100 millirem per hour. This would typically be a G-M type instrument whose purpose is to identify the presence of small radiation fields. The other is a measurement survey instrument capable of measuring dose rates from 1.0–1000 millirem per hour.[19] An ionization type meter is what is intended and is useful in quantifying the radiation fields around an HDR unit. The NRC has regulations relative to the calibration and operational checks of such survey instruments.[20]

The NRC has specific requirements for the possession of brachytherapy sources, even if these sources are not used.[21] These requirements include leak testing at intervals not to exceed 6 months, quarterly physical inventory of all sources in its possession, and quarterly measurement of the ambient dose rates in all areas where such sources are stored. The inventory records must contain the model number of each source, the serial number, the identity of source radionuclide and its nominal activity, the location of each source, and the signature of the radiation safety officer. This requirement applies to Cs-137 sources. Most sources with short half-lives are either returned to the manufacturer or placed in permanent storage before the inventory or leak test requirements can be applied.

In summary, the federally mandated QMPs are quality assurance plans designed to eliminate errors resulting from sloppy procedures in brachytherapy, while the requirements contained in Part 35 are detailed quality control procedures. Any error is generally interpreted by the regulators to mean that an institution did not follow their written procedures and thus makes the institution liable to be publicly criticized or fined or both. The NRC has a record of misadministrations that have been reported over the last 15 years. The most famous misadministration involves the discharge of a patient who contained a HDR Ir-192 source. Clearly there are quality assurance failures in some brachytherapy procedures. The QMP can be helpful in developing and maintaining quality assurance and quality control.

Nonregulatory Recommendations

The federal regulations form the basis of a necessary but not sufficient quality assurance program in brachytherapy. Quality assurance in brachytherapy is discussed in detail in several recent references, such as the report of AAPM TG 40, Comprehensive QA for Radiation Oncology, and in *Modern Clinical Brachytherapy Physics*, the 1994 AAPM summer school.[22,23] The report of TG 40 is quite detailed and discusses both LDR and HDR. The brachytherapy portion of this report has major subsections on sealed sources, treatment planning and dosimetry, remote afterloading units, and safety. It recommends frequencies and tolerances of specific quality assurance tests for brachytherapy sources, Table IX, for brachytherapy source calibrators, Table X, and for brachytherapy applicators, Table XI.[24–26] It also has recommendations for procedure specific brachytherapy parameter verification, Table XII.[27] This report notes that an uncertainty of ± 15% in the delivery of the prescribed dose for intracavitary and plaque therapy is a realistic goal, while there are even larger uncertainties for multiplane interstitial implants.[27]

Some quality assurance recommendations of the report from TG 40 and other such documents are worth highlighting. These topics include source calibration and calibrators, patient dose calculations, treatment preparation and delivery, documentation of treatment, and HDR remote afterloading devices.

Source Calibration

It is the responsibility of each institution providing brachytherapy services to ensure that the activity of each brachytherapy source used for a patient is correct so that the prescribed dose can be delivered. There are many units in which source activity can be expressed including milligram radium equivalents, curies, and air-kerma in air. Different treatment planning computer systems have different requirements to describe source activity. There is ample opportunity for confusion. All dose calculation schemes rely on some statement of source activity. License conditions require the calibration of HDR sources. While there is currently no federally mandated requirement to calibrate LDR brachytherapy sources, there are numerous recommendations that each institution providing brachytherapy services "have the ability to independently verify the source strength provided by the manufacturer."[28] A comprehensive approach to source calibration was presented in AAPM Report 13.[29] The Report of the Interstitial Collaborative Working Group, *Interstitial Brachytherapy*, has a chapter on source calibration and recommends in its chapter on quality assurance that the activity of all high activity sources be checked and that for large, LDR implants a "minimum of 10% of the batch, or 10 seeds, whichever is larger, should be measured."[30] The Report of AAPM Task Group 40 contains explicit recommendations on source calibration and brachytherapy source calibrators.[31] For a modest amount of money, it is possible to develop a brachytherapy calibration system that establishes direct traceability of source calibrations for most sources used in brachytherapy to either the NIST or an AAPM accredited dosimetry calibration laboratory. There are several well established approaches to calibrate HDR sources, including a dedicated reentrant ion chamber or appropriately calibrated thimble chambers.[32,33]

Quality Assurance of Calculational Approaches

There are many methods for calculating the dose rate for a specific implant, such as look up tables, unfiltered line source calculations, and Sievert integrals. Every approach depends upon an accurate knowledge of the source location and activity. Most calculational approaches depend upon characteristics of the individual sources, such as encapsulation material or source construction. Every method used should be thoroughly evaluated for accuracy. AAPM Report No. 13 contains the following recommendation: "In implementing new or unfamiliar computer programs for brachytherapy dose calculations, it is advisable: (1) to compare results for an idealized (e.g. single source) configuration with the results of hand calculations, and (2) to compare results for one or more typical clinical applications with those obtained using an established computing system, perhaps at another institution."[10]

Basic parameters for source descriptions and dose-rate tables can be found in *Interstitial Brachytherapy* or in Chapter 12 of *Principles and Practice of Radiation Oncology*.[34,35] In addition to the calculation algorithm, tests

should be made of the data input system, e.g., is the software correctly demagnifying the films; and the data output system, e.g., is the computer and output device accurately placing the dose calculational points. It should be remembered that the NRC QMP mandates such tests. HDR planning systems impose new requirements over the older calculational systems. Each new software version should be treated independently of previous versions and rigorously reviewed and tested prior to its first clinical use. Van Dyk et al.[36] have recently published a comprehensive article on the quality assurance of treatment planning computers. They suggest a 5% criteria of acceptability for single point and single line source dose calculations between 0.5 and 5.0 cm away from the source. (For the line sources, the points of calculation that meet this criteria should be normal to the central 80% of the active length of the source.)

Detailed dosimetric information on Ir-192, I-125, and Pd-103 has recently been published by AAPM Task Group 43 in a report entitled "Dosimetry of Interstitial Brachytherapy Sources."[37] This comprehensive report recommends the same dose calculational formalism as the Interstitial Collaborative Working Group. It contains recommendations for various dosimetry parameters including anisotropic factors. Table XIII of this report presents the average dose rate times distance squared for distances ranging from 0.5–9.0 cm, assuming a point source approximation, for Pd-103, I-125 both models 6711 and 6702, and Ir-192.[38] This table should be used as a reference to compare against the results of the treatment planning computer. This report states that "the overall uncertainty in determination of dose rate at a point around a source using the recommended protocol is estimated to be about 10%."[39]

A thorough independent review for each implant including the dose calculation to at least one critical point should be an established practice and has been recommended.[40] The critical point should be a point of dose specification or a point that if it were underdosed or overdosed may result in complications to the patient. Independent checks should start with the written directive and the implant films. The implant films should display not only the applicator and dummy sources in the patient but also the location of specific points of dose calculation, such as the rectum and bladder. The independent check should also include a review of the statement of the activity of the sources from the vendor, the institution's measured activity, and the activity input into the planning system. The independent check can use simplified calculational approaches, such as along and away tables or the unfiltered line source calculation. It has been our experience that errors most likely occur in the input parameters to the calculation. Therefore, the distances of points of interest should be checked on the film and compared to the distances shown on the treatment plan. A 15% agreement between the independent check calculation and the initial calculation has been recommended as the appropriate level for agreement.[27]

The Special Case of I-125 Calculations

Williamson[23] has recently summarized the data for I-125 interstitial dosimetry and reports that conventional dose calculations for I-125 seeds overestimate the absorbed dose rates in water by 13%–20%. He states that approximately one third of this discrepancy is due to contaminant x-rays in the I-125 NIST air-kerma strength standard, while the rest may be due to differences in seed construction and encapsulation between the various model I-125 seeds. In any event, it is reasonable to anticipate that there will be major changes in basic dosimetric data pertaining to I-125 calculations over the next 5 years with subsequent recommendations to update institutions' calculational approaches. Great care will be required in the physical and clinical implementation of these changes.

Quality Assurance in the Delivery of Brachytherapy Treatments

The preparation for and the delivery of the brachytherapy treatment should have a high degree of quality control, i.e., the operational techniques and activities for treatment preparation and delivery should provide for monitoring of the process and eliminating causes of errors in order to achieve an effective result. Communication between the radiation oncologist and the support staff is crucial. The written directive should help in basic communication of the details for the application to be performed. It is possible to change the written directive both before and during the implant, which could reflect a continuing reevaluation of the clinical situation. The NRC QMP explicitly requires a policy "for all workers to seek guidance if they do not understand how to carry out the written directive."[41]

Preplanning complicated implants helps the oncologist refine his/her questions and concerns. A brief meeting between the radiation oncologist and the support staff can review the clinical problem, different approaches to the clinical problem, the equipment needed for each approach, and the desired dose distribution and dose rates. Such a meeting will help ensure that appropriate equipment has been sterilized and brought to the operating room. Preplanning for the unusual case will help the planners to determine appropriate source activities to obtain the desired dose rate. (In fact, a preplanned dose distribution, perhaps as part of a library of dose distributions, can serve as another independent check of the final dosimetry.) Preplanning will also help the radiation oncologist decide the level of support required by a particular implant. The report of Task Group 40 recommends that "physics representatives should be in the operating room during custom-planned interstitial procedures and/or challenging dosimetric problems."[42]

In many institutions, it is the physicist who will provide the technical continuity for the entire implant. For even a simple brachytherapy treatment, the options available to the radiation oncologist are quite numerous. For a more complicated treatment, the options can be truly staggering. Thus, there needs to be close cooperation between those individuals providing support and the oncologist. The NRC QMP requires "a procedure to have the authorized user or a qualified person under the supervision of an authorized user, verify that the radioisotope, the number of sources, source strengths, and, if possible, loading sequence of the sources to be used are in agreement with the written directive and the plan of treatment before implanting the radioactive sealed sources."[43]

Documentation of Treatment

Documentation of brachytherapy procedures serves as an important element in ensuring quality. A detailed report of the brachytherapy application has been recommended by the ICRU for intracavitary procedures and will soon be recommended by the ICRU for interstitial procedures.[44,45] The recommended documentation includes a description of the sources, a description of the technique and source pattern used, the total time of dose delivery, the total air-kerma, a description of the dose that includes the prescribed dose, the dose at the periphery of the target volume, a central dose, and regions of high or low dose, isodose distributions, and other dose summary information. The NRC refers to a treatment plan and requires that the patient's chart contain documentation that indicates that the written directive and the treatment plan are consistent with what was delivered to the patient. There is an advantage to having separate reports written by the physicist dealing with source calibration, dose calculations, and analysis of the dose distributions.[46] The technical details, such as the planning software and the calculational approach used, can be reviewed by the radiation oncologist.

Quality Assurance of Remote Afterloading Units

AAPM Report No. 41, *Remote Afterloading Technology*, contains a section on quality assurance that provides some general recommendations for remote afterloading units.[47] Quality assurance for LDR afterloading units has been recently presented by Slessinger.[48] Table 3 of his work presents recommendations for daily, quarterly, and annual quality control activities for these units. Quality assurance for HDR brachytherapy has been addressed by multiple authors.[49,50] The recent textbook, *High Dose Rate Brachytherapy*, contains a chapter on quality assurance.[51] This work summarizes the experience at three different institutions, each of which have substantial HDR experience. Major sections include Safety of the Patient and the Public, Positional Accuracy, Temporal Accuracy, Dose Delivery Accuracy, and Periodic Quality Assurance. Tables are presented that discuss daily, monthly, quarterly, and annual quality assurance, as well as quality assurance for the planning system. This chapter is very comprehensive and represents an excellent reference for both experienced and new HDR users. Quality assurance for pulsed-dose-rate systems has recently been addressed by Williamson.[52]

The unique quality assurance and quality control challenges associated with HDR procedures should be emphasized. Typically, an HDR procedure utilizes special applicators, its own treatment planning system that calculates dose based upon specific source locations, time, and optimization approach, a microprocessor-based control console that requires input from the planning system, and a remote treatment delivery unit with a short lived isotope. The entire procedure, namely applicator insertion, treatment planning and review, and treatment delivery is to be performed in <4 hours. The potential for errors caused by working with complicated equipment under such time constraints is high. All quality assurance and review activities must be completed prior to the initiation of treatment as the treatment times are very short. AAPM Report No. 41 addresses this situation in the following paragraph:

"Preparation and use of well-planned pretreatment forms and check lists for each anatomic site commonly used is recommended. A generic checklist could include, but would not be limited to, the following items: Have the pretreatment functional QA tests been done? Is the prescription (written directive) completed and signed? Has the prepared treatment plan (prescription, target volume specification, dose, dose rates, number of sources, their spatial positions, etc.) been independently reviewed, e.g., will the planned use of the device yield the desired dose and dose distribution? Have the treatment parameters keyed by the operator into the microprocessor controlling the unit been reviewed by a second individual? Are all pre-treatment forms completed and signed prior to treatment? Do pre-treatment autoradiographs, if any, confirm the proposed treatment is correctly entered into the console?"[47]

Each institution must develop their own approach to delivering HDR treatments. Given

Table 1.
High-Dose-Rate Final Check List

Before the treatment is initiated, the following conditions will be verified by the physicist delivering the treatment:

1. QA tests have been performed and are satisfactory.
2. The patient has been identified in redundant fashion.
3. The Written Directive has been signed for this treatment or fraction.
4. The source transfer tube length has been established.
5. A treatment plan has been prepared and independently reviewed

   or

   Source decay from an earlier treatment has been calculated and compared to increase in treatment time between the earlier and current fraction.
6. The treatment parameters, as printed by the control console, including the number of catheters, the dwell positions, and each dwell time, have been compared with the treatment plan and the written directive.
7. The authorized user and other required personnel are present.
8. The connection of each catheter to the applicator has been reviewed.

pear in the form of individual NRC releases or summarized in special publications, e.g., isoTopics.[53] Many of these events involve either LDR and HDR brachytherapy procedures. Such publicity is both educational and inspirational. It emphasizes the detailed nature of brachytherapy procedures and the consequences of failing to attend to each detail. Communication and training are emphasized as important areas if misadministrations are to be avoided. Federal regulations are essentially demanding zero defect brachytherapy procedures. If institutions decide to offer brachytherapy procedures to their patients, then it is in their best interest to ensure that there are adequately trained staff and appropriate equipment to support this decision. The brachytherapist, together with the physicist, treatment planners, and nursing staff, should analyze and prepare for each different type of brachytherapy procedure. Part of this analysis and preparation should involve quality assurance and quality control. Federal regulations are not making clinical judgments relative to brachytherapy patients, but they are defining standards of practice for all of us involved in delivering these services.

our modest workload of 3–5 treatments per week, we have decided that treatments will be planned and delivered by physicists who have been given complete responsibility for all technical aspects of the treatment. Treatments will not be delivered until the physicist delivering the treatment is satisfied with all the technical aspects of the treatment. Our pretreatment check list is presented in Table 1.

Together the radiation oncologists and the physicists have developed a site specific in-house planning guide so that all HDR patients are being planned in a similar fashion with a consistent definition of dose specification points. This planning guide is included in a GYN Handbook for Residents used at our institution. This handbook serves multiple purposes, including being a repository of specific details relating to brachytherapy.

Within the last several years, the NRC has begun to publicize the abnormal occurrences that have been reported to it. These may ap-

References

1. Kutcher GJ, et al. Comprehensive QA for radiation oncology: Report of AAPM Radiation Therapy Committee Task Group 40. Med Phys 1994;21:581–618.
2. Kutcher GJ, et al. Comprehensive QA for radiation oncology: Report of AAPM Radiation Therapy Committee Task Group 40. Med Phys 1994;21:614–615.
3. Svensson GK, et al. Physical Aspects of Quality Assurance in Radiation Therapy, AAPM Report No. 13. American Institute of Physics, New York, 1984.
4. United States Nuclear Regulatory Commission, Rules and Regulations, Title 10, Chapter 1, Code of Federal Regulations—Energy, Part 35.
5. United States Nuclear Regulatory Commission, Rules and Regulations, Title 10, Chapter 1, Code of Federal Regulations—Energy, para 35.2.
6. Federal Register, Vol 56, No 143, Thursday July 25, 1991, para 35.32(a).
7. United States Nuclear Regulatory Commission, Rules and Regulations, Title 10, Chapter 1, Code of Federal Regulations—Energy, Part 35, para 35.32.

8. U.S. Nuclear Regulatory Commission Regulatory Guide 8.33 (task DG-8001), Quality Management Program, 1991.

9. U.S. Nuclear Regulatory Commission Regulatory Guide 8.33 (task DG-8001), Quality Management Program, 1991, para 3.19 and 3.2.13.

10. Svensson GK et al. Physical Aspects of Quality Assurance in Radiation Therapy, AAPM Report No. 13. American Institute of Physics, New York, 1984, p. 45.

11. U.S. Nuclear Regulatory Commission Regulatory Guide 8.33 (task DG-8001), Quality Management Program, 1991, para 3.1.6 and 3.2.10.

12. United States Nuclear Regulatory Commission, Rules and Regulations, Title 10, Chapter 1, Code of Federal Regulations—Energy, para 35.33.

13. United States Nuclear Regulatory Commission, Rules and Regulations, Title 10, Chapter 1, Code of Federal Regulations—Energy, para 35.400.

14. United States Nuclear Regulatory Commission, Rules and Regulations, Title 10, Chapter 1, Code of Federal Regulations—Energy, para 35.406.

15. United States Nuclear Regulatory Commission, Rules and Regulations, Title 10, Chapter 1, Code of Federal Regulations—Energy, para 35.940.

16. United States Nuclear Regulatory Commission, Rules and Regulations, Title 10, Chapter 1, Code of Federal Regulations—Energy, para 35.961.

17. United States Nuclear Regulatory Commission, Rules and Regulations, Title 10, Chapter 1, Code of Federal Regulations—Energy, para 35.410.

18. United States Nuclear Regulatory Commission, Rules and Regulations, Title 10, Chapter 1, Code of Federal Regulations—Energy, para 35.415.

19. United States Nuclear Regulatory Commission, Rules and Regulations, Title 10, Chapter 1, Code of Federal Regulations—Energy, para 35.420.

20. United States Nuclear Regulatory Commission, Rules and Regulations, Title 10, Chapter 1, Code of Federal Regulations—Energy, para 35.51.

21. United States Nuclear Regulatory Commission, Rules and Regulations, Title 10, Chapter 1, Code of Federal Regulations—Energy, para 35.59.

22. Kutcher GJ, et al. Comprehensive QA for radiation oncology: Report of AAPM Radiation Therapy Committee Task Group 40. Med Phys 1994;21:599–607.

23. Williamson JF, et al. Modern Clinical Brachytherapy Physics, 1994 AAPM Summer School, American Institute of Physics, New York, 1994.

24. Kutcher GJ, et al. Comprehensive QA for radiation oncology: Report of AAPM Radiation Therapy Committee Task Group 40. Med Phys 1994;21:601.

25. Kutcher GJ, et al. Comprehensive QA for radiation oncology: Report of AAPM Radiation Therapy Committee Task Group 40. Med Phys 1994;21:602.

26. Kutcher GJ, et al. Comprehensive QA for radiation oncology: Report of AAPM Radiation Therapy Committee Task Group 40. Med Phys 1994;21:603.

27. Kutcher GJ, et al. Comprehensive QA for radiation oncology: Report of AAPM Radiation Therapy Committee Task Group 40. Med Phys 1994;21:605.

28. Kutcher GJ, et al. Comprehensive QA for radiation oncology: Report of AAPM Radiation Therapy Committee Task Group 40. Med Phys 1994;21:599.

29. Kutcher GJ, et al. Comprehensive QA for radiation oncology: Report of AAPM Radiation Therapy Committee Task Group 40. Med Phys 1994;21:600.

30. Interstitial Collaborative Working Group. Interstitial Brachytherapy Physical, Biological, and Clinical Considerations. Raven Press, New York, 1990, p. 297.

31. Kutcher GJ, et al. Comprehensive QA for radiation oncology: Report of AAPM Radiation Therapy Committee Task Group 40. Med Phys 1994;21:600–603.

32. Goetsch SJ, et al. Calibration of high-dose-rate afterloading systems. Med Phys 1991;18:462–467.

33. Ezzell GA. Evaluation of Calibration Techniques for the MicroSelectron HDR. Brachytherapy 2: Proceedings of the 5th International Selectron User's Meeting. Leersum: Nucletron, 1989, pp. 61–69.

34. Interstitial Collaborative Working Group. Interstitial Brachytherapy Physical, Biological, and Clinical Considerations. Raven Press, New York, 1990, pp. 3–31.

35. Perez CA, Brady LW. Principles and Practice of Radiation Oncology. Second Edition. Lippincott, Philadelphia, PA, pp. 265–299.

36. Van Dyk J, et al. Commissioning and quality assurance of treatment planning computers. Int J Radiat Oncol Biol Phys 1993;26:261–273.

37. Nath R, et al. Dosimetry on interstitial brachytherapy sources: Recommendations of the AAPM Radiation Therapy Committee Task Group No. 43. Med Phys 1995;22:209–234.

38. Nath R, et al. Dosimetry on interstitial brachytherapy sources: Recommendations of the

AAPM Radiation Therapy Committee Task Group No. 43. Med Phys 1995;22:218.

39. Nath R, et al. Dosimetry on interstitial brachytherapy sources: Recommendations of the AAPM Radiation Therapy Committee Task Group No. 43. Med Phys 1995;22:219.

40. Svensson GK, et al. Physical Aspects of Quality Assurance in Radiation Therapy, AAPM Report No. 13. American Institute of Physics, New York, 1984, p. 33.

41. U.S. Nuclear Regulatory Commission Regulatory Guide 8.33 (task DG-8001), Quality Management Program, 1991, para 3.2.4.

42. Kutcher GJ, et al. Comprehensive QA for radiation oncology: Report of AAPM Radiation Therapy Committee Task Group 40. Med Phys 1994;21:605–606.

43. U.S. Nuclear Regulatory Commission Regulatory Guide 8.33 (task DG-8001), Quality Management Program, 1991, para 3.2.5.

44. International Commission on Radiation Units and Measurements. Dose and Volume Specification for Reporting Intracavitary Therapy in Gynecology, Report No. 38. Washington DC: ICRU, 1985.

45. Hanson WF. ICRU recommendations on dose specification in brachytherapy. In: Modern Clinical Brachytherapy Physics, 1994 AAPM Summer School. American Institute of Physics, New York, 1994.

46. Gillin MT, et al. Practical considerations for interstitial brachytherapy. In: Advances in Radiation Oncology Physics Dosimetry, Treatment Planning, and Brachytherapy, Medical Physics Monograph No. 19. American Institute of Physics, New York, 1992, pp. 703–727.

47. Glasgow, et al. Remote Afterloading Technology, A Report of AAPM Task Group No. 41. American Institute of Physics, New York, 1993, pp. 61–62.

48. Slessinger ED. Clinical implementation of low dose rate remote afterloading brachytherapy. In: Modern Clinical Brachytherapy Physics, 1994 AAPM Summer School. American Institute of Physics, New York, 1994.

49. Baltas D. Quality assurance in HDR brachytherapy. In: International Brachytherapy. Veenendaal: Nucletron, 1992, pp. 240–247.

50. Jones CH. Quality Assurance in Brachytherapy Using the Selectron LDR/MDR and MicroSelectron-HDR. Selectron Brachytherapy J 1990;4: 48–52.

51. Williamson JF, et al. Quality assurance for high dose rate brachytherapy. In: Nag S (ed). High Dose Rate Brachytherapy: A Textbook. Futura Publishing Company, Armonk, NY, 1994.

52. Williamson JF. Clinical physics of pulsed dose rate (PDR) remotely afterloaded brachytherapy. In: Modern Clinical Brachytherapy Physics, 1994 AAPM Summer School. American Institute of Physics, New York, 1994.

53. IsoTopics, NUS, Aikeen, South Carolina.

Chapter 8

Brachytherapy Treatment Planning

Bruce Thomadsen, Ph.D., FAAPM,
Komanduri Ayyangar, Ph.D., Lowell Anderson, Ph.D.,
Gary Luxton, Ph.D., William Hanson, Ph.D., FAAPM,
J. Frank Wilson, M.D., FACR

Introduction

Brachytherapy treatment planning consists of many individual steps that lead to and past the physical application of the radionuclides to the patient. The grouping of the steps, and even the steps themselves, may differ for individual patients or for a given individual's practice. However, contents of the steps as outlined below fit into all brachytherapy cases. This discussion addresses the steps in a common chronological order.

Modality

The first decision involves selection of the modality best suited to the clinical circumstances of the patient. Usually, the oncologist chooses between high-dose-rate (HDR), temporary low-dose-rate (LDR), or permanent applications. Advantages of HDR brachytherapy over LDR include the following:

1. Easier and more precise optimization of the dose distribution to the needs of the individual patient, including reduction of dose to critical organs;

2. More precise delivery of the planned dose, through immobilization;
3. The ability to move some normal tissue structures away from the source to reduce their doses during treatment;
4. Treatment on an out-patient basis;
5. Elimination of radiation exposure to personnel;
6. The ability to treat patients with intercurrent medical conditions that prohibit prolonged hospitalization or bedrest for the duration of an LDR treatment.

Unfortunately, HDR brachytherapy carries with it the following disadvantages:

1. Increased normal tissue effect compared with tumor effect (i.e., decreased therapeutic ratio) for a given dose.
2. Increased probability of executing an error before detection.
3. Increased time and personnel requirements.

Some of the factors involved in deciding between HDR or LDR applications include:

From Nag S (ed): *Principles and Practice of Brachytherapy.* © Futura Publishing Co., Inc., Armonk, NY, 1997.

1. History of previous irradiation: If the normal tissues previously received doses approaching tolerance, LDR brachytherapy may provide some tissue sparing.
2. Need for precision delivery of the dose: A sensitive structure lying near a target may be spared from radiation exposure because of the precision delivery and dose tailoring capabilities of HDR brachytherapy.
3. A patient's need for frequent attention: If the patient's medical condition requires intensive nursing, HDR treatments eliminate the problem of limiting the time nurses may spend caring for the patient.
4. Cost of in-patient care: In the context of rising costs of in-patient care, HDR *may* provide a less expensive alternative. However, due to the cost of the equipment and the increased number of personnel required for the procedure, the price advantage does not always hold.

The different biological effectiveness of HDR brachytherapy for tumor and for normal tissue makes using the advantages of the modality particularly important, for example, adding distance between the source and the rectum by keeping a speculum in the vagina during gynecological applications. The differences in biological effectiveness also imply that simply duplicating with HDR brachytherapy those patient dose distributions used with LDR treatments gives different relative biological effectiveness distributions. For example, LDR treatments with a tandem and ovoid delivering 145% of the Point A dose to the vaginal surfaces biologically equates to HDR treatments of 3.7 Gy per fraction to Point A with 140% of the point A dose to the vaginal mucosa. Were 9.0 Gy fractions to Point A used, this same relative biological effective dose to the vaginal surface would be 135%. Practitioners initiating an HDR program may want to consult *High Dose Rate Brachytherapy: A Textbook*[1] for more detailed discussions on the modifications of LDR practices required with the change in modalities.

Choosing LDR brachytherapy requires another decision: to implant sources permanently or temporarily. Permanent implants use either radioactive materials with short half-lives, so that the patient requires only a brief radiation isolation, or materials with low penetration (beta emitters or low energy photons) so that no isolation is required. Since no in-dwelling applicators are used and only the small sources (often called seeds) remain in the patient, permanent implants usually prove more comfortable for the patient and entail less risk of infection than most temporary implants. Through careful selection of the particular radionuclide used, the treatment duration can be matched to the biological characteristics of the tumor cells (delivering the dose over about a year for I-125, about 3 months for Pd-103, or about 2 weeks for Au-198). On the other hand, permanently implanted sources tend to migrate (sometimes even being lost if implanted near conduits such as the urethra or bowel); and, even if the sources are well anchored in tissue, the relative geometry changes with tumor regression or normal tissue atrophy. Because of the short duration of the treatment using Au-198 seeds, the dose is not affected; however, such changes add uncertainty to the dose calculations for the long-lived radioisotopes such as I-125. Migration becomes a major source of concern with implants in locations such as muscles (e.g., the tongue), where there is sustained contraction and relaxation.

In temporary implants, needles and templates hold the sources in their intended positions for the duration of treatment, thereby offering better precision and control of the dose to the target. Even though the patient remains in isolation during the course of therapy, the applicators used in temporary implants hold the seeds in place and reduce the probability of losing sources. LDR remote afterloaders eliminate radiation exposure to personnel, and LDR implants deliver the dose to the target at a controlled, uniform (or nearly uniform) rate that can be chosen to correspond to the considerable reported experience that exists with this modality.

Source Material

The choice of modality often dictates the source material. However, although different materials may fit the major criteria for a given implant, each may provide a different characteristic to the dose distribution. For example, I-125, Pd-103, or Au-198 may be used for permanent implants; however, because of their lower energies, the I-125 or Pd-103 would deliver a more restricted dose distribution than that seen with Au-198. In addition, the time course of the therapy would be very different in all three cases. Likewise, in temporary implants, using Ir-192 results in a different dose distribution than that seen with I-125. The biology of the tumor is also an important variable in the isotope selection. All of these variables must be considered in this basic step in treatment planning.

Coverage

The physician must determine the extent of the tumor. The tools for this determination include careful physical examination with or without special procedures such as endoscopy, x-ray, CT-scan, MRI, ultrasound (US), endoscopy or, less frequently, more conventional radiographic modalities such as mammography, arteriography, or simple radiographs. Often, imaging fails to completely delimit the true extent of the tumor. For example, bronchoscopy aids in positioning an endobronchial catheter and identifies the proximal end of the tumor, but usually provides no information on the distal end or the diameter of the target. If no other study demonstrates the complete extent of the tumor, the physician must use "clinical judgment." From the limits of the tumor, the physician determines the target volume, i.e., the volume to be raised to the prescribed treatment dose. Conventional terminology includes the following formal definitions:[2]

Tumor Volume: the volume containing known, clinically evident tumor.
Target Volume: the volume intended to receive the prescribed dose, that includes the tumor volume and any margin around the tumor volume that might harbor tumor cells.
Treatment Volume: the volume raised to at least the treatment dose.
Reference Volume: the volume enclosed by a specified, reference isodose surface (not necessarily the treatment isodose surface), used mostly for comparison between patients or facilities.
Irradiated Volume: the volume raised to a dose considered significant compared to tissue tolerance.

Ideally, the treatment volume conforms to the target volume. In brachytherapy, anatomical limitations often prevent this. For example, restricting the dose to the anterior rectal wall or the urethra around a prostate implant may result in the treatment volume not covering the prostate (i.e., the target volume) completely. In many instances, the treatment volume must be adjusted to encompass nonevident disease, and the target volume may also include some margin for uncertainty in the application technique.

The International Commission on Radiological Units and Measurements (ICRU) has provided the following stratification of the progression from tumor volume to target volume:[3]

Gross Tumor Volume (GTV): The volume containing known, clinically evident tumor, comparable with the conventional tumor volume.
Clinical Tumor Volume (CTV): The volume of gross disease plus a margin to include likely sites of occult cells.
Planning Tumor Volume (PTV): The CTV plus a margin to account for uncertainties in the delivery of the treatment, which serves as the conventional target volume.

While in some cases, this decision on the target volume awaits examination of the patient under anesthesia at the time of an implant, it must precede (with some exceptions) the placement of the applicators. Before placement of the applicator, the physician further translates from the target volume to the volume included in the distribution of the radioactive material, called the implanted volume. Protocols help limit the range of possible arrangements of radioactive material. Protocols with some specific characteristics form a *system*. Characteristics of a system include:

1. *A Goal*. The goal usually involves the dose distribution. For example, as its goal, the Manchester system for inter-

stitial implants strives to deliver a uniform dose to the treatment volume.[4] Some systems leave the goal implicit and the result of the application of the system.

2. *A Type of Applicator and Sources.* For a given system the relevant applicator may be explicit, such as the latex tandem and hard rubber ovoids used with the original Manchester system for gynecological brachytherapy,[5] or obvious as with the radium needles for their interstitial system. The use of a system with an applicator other than that for which it was designed may yield unexpected and undesirable results.

3. *Application Rules.* The rules describe the use of the applicator. Some systems, such as the Paris system,[6] have very detailed rules, while others (e.g., the Quimby system)[7] summarize the rules in a few sentences.

4. *Prescription Definitions.* Any application gives rise to a complex dose distribution including multiple dose levels within the implanted volume, large dose gradients, and low doses distant to the sources. Describing the dose distribution in detail usually requires considerable data or multiple graphics. When combined with the distribution rules, defining particular points of interest or dose relationships allows a shorthand way to refer to the amount of radiation delivered to the patient. Examples include the Manchester Point A for gynecological insertions and the Paris system's reference dose (both discussed below).

5. *Doses for Given Conditions (optional).* Some systems, such as the Manchester system for gynecological insertions, specify dose as part of the protocol description. Most of the interstitial systems make no assumption about the types of cases implanted, and, thus, offer no guidance for the dose to be prescribed. An interstitial system may, however, specify a range of dose rates that will result from following the system's rules.

While some of the systems originated before computers made dosimetry calculations commonplace, their rules still prove useful during the planning phases. In any event, dosemetric calculations should be based upon the source pattern actually achieved, rather than a conceptual ideal if serious treatment complications are to be avoided.

Having determined the target volume, the physician must decide on the placement of the sources for LDR brachytherapy or the source track for a stepping source, remote afterloader used with middle-dose-rate (MDR), HDR, or pulsed-dose-rate (PDR) brachytherapy. A system usually specifies the positioning of the sources with respect to the edge of the target volume and throughout the interior. The main decision involves placing the sources at the edge of the target volume or slightly inside of the volume. Placing the sources at the edge of the volume *can* give a more uniform dose to the target than placing the sources within the volume, but at the expense of a larger dose outside of the target. Placing the sources appropriately within the volume allows the beginning of the rapidly decreasing dose region (the equivalent of the field penumbra in external beam) to begin at the interface between the target and normal tissue.

Each of the systems has its advantages for given situations. However, doses as specified in one system can mean a very different amount of radiation delivered to the patient as compared to the same dose stated for a different system. *Within a department, switching between systems should be avoided for a given type of patient.*

For discussion purposes, a brief description of several systems is presented below, with the caution that the reader should consult the original sources, or better, study under a practitioner of one of the systems, before attempting to use the system in practice. Of necessity, the presentations here only abstract the systems; many important details and recent modifications remain unstated.

Systems for Interstitial Implants

The Manchester System

Paterson and Parker presented the first rationalized system for brachytherapy, the Manchester System, for interstitial brachytherapy in 1934. This system is still used today and has influenced all subsequent systems. Its goal is to deliver a "uniform" dose to the implanted volume (which defines the target volume in this system). "Uniformity" in this case means the prescribed dose ± 10%, not counting corners, where the dose may fall below the criterion. To achieve this goal, the framers developed rules for the distribution of the radioactive material. The rules fall into two categories: those for planar implants and those for volume implants (basically cylinders, spheres, and cubes). They also address more exotic applications, such as rings for penis treatments, but these will not be presented in this short summary.

Planar Applications

The rules for any planar application derive from those for a surface application. Surface applicators allow essentially complete access for the distribution of the radioactive material in any way in order to achieve the uniform dose. A surface applicator consists of tissue-equivalent material, called a mold, placed on the patient's skin or mucosal surface, with the radioactive material arranged on the opposite side of the mold. Figure 1 shows two possible molds for use with a certain patient's lesion.

The dose rate that a mold delivers depends on the distance from the radioactive sources and the area covered by those sources. Originally the conversion from mg to dose rate used graphs; but a table, such as Table 1, replaced the graphs in a 1967 summary exposition of the system.[8] The values in the table, here called $R_A(A,h)$, give the number of mg hr of radium required to deliver 1000 R to a point in the middle of the area A, and at a distance h. The reader will notice immediately that the table explicitly applies to radium filtered with 0.5-mm Pt and that it expresses the "doses" in "R," for roentgen. Both of these points will be discussed below. The dose rate at distance h follows:

$$\dot{D}(h) = S/R_A(A, h). \quad (1)$$

where S equals the source strength in mg of radium.

Looking at Figure 1, the dose at the bottom of the lesion compared to the dose at the skin, the fractional depth dose (FDD), is given by:

$$FDD = \frac{\dot{D}(h_d)}{\dot{D}(h_s)} = \frac{R_A(A, h_s)}{R_A(A, h_d)}. \quad (2)$$

For the example in Figure 1, for a 36-cm² area distribution of radium and 0.5 cm between the skin and the deepest extent of the lesion, the FDD for the 0.5-cm thick mold equals 0.63, while that for the 3.0-cm mold equals 0.83, illustrating the general rule that the FDD increases with the thickness of the mold. Thus, the first decision following the determination of the area of the lesion concerns the thickness of the mold, and the depth of the deep edge of the target; and the sensitivity of any underlying structures must be taken into account. In this case, the "uniformity" of the goal refers not to the dose throughout the entire volume, but rather to the uniformity of the dose *in the plane at distance h*. As seen from the FDD values in the above example, the dose *will* vary by more than ± 10% from the skin to some locations at the depth.

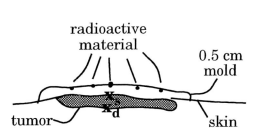
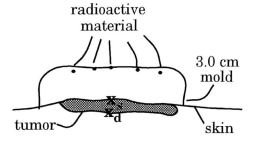

Figure 1. Two possible surface molds for treatment of a skin lesion.

Table 1.
Milligram-Hours per 1000 R for Different Areas and Various Treating Distances

Filtration = 0.5 mm Platinum

Area ↓	Treating Distance in cm									
	0.5	1.0	1.5	2.0	2.5	3.0	3.5	4.0	4.5	5.0
Sq. cm.										
0	30	119	268	476	744	1071	1458	1904	2412	2976
1	68	171								
2	97	213	375	598	865	1197	1595	2043	2545	3117
3	120	247								
4	141	278	462	698	970	1305	1713	2168	2665	3243
5	161	306								
6	177	333	536	782	1066	1405	1822	2286	2778	3360
7	192	359								
8	206	384	599	855	1155	1500	1924	2395	2883	3472
9	221	408								
10	235	433	655	923	1235	1590	2020	2500	2987	3580
11	248	456								
12	261	480	710	990	1312	1673	2112	2603	3087	3682
13	274	502								
14	288	524	764	1053	1386	1753	2200	2698	3185	3785
15	302	546								
16	315	566	814	1113	1460	1830	2283	2790	3280	3883
17	328	585								
18	342	605	863	1170	1525	1905	2363	2879	3370	3985
19	355	623								
20	368	641	910	1225	1588	1979	2445	2965	3461	4080
22	393	674	960	1280	1650	2049	2522	3047	3550	4174
24	417	707	1008	1335	1712	2117	2598	3126	3639	4267
26	442	737	1056	1388	1768	2188	2670	3200	3724	4356
28	466	767	1100	1438	1826	2254	2742	3275	3804	4446
30	490	795	1142	1487	1880	2320	2817	3348	3883	4534
32	513	823	1185	1537	1936	2380	2888	3420	3966	4620
34	537	854	1226	1587	1992	2442	2956	3490	4047	4700
36	558	879	1268	1638	2048	2502	3022	3559	4125	4783
38	581	909	1308	1685	2100	2562	3088	3627	4198	4863
40	603	934	1346	1732	2152	2620	3150	3695	4273	4942
42	624	962	1384	1780	2203	2677	3215	3762	4348	5020
44	644	990	1420	1825	2255	2733	3275	3826	4423	5096
46	665	1015	1457	1870	2305	2788	3335	3890	4494	5174
48	685	1043	1490	1915	2354	2843	3395	3954	4565	5250
50	705	1072	1522	1958	2402	2897	3455	4018	4633	5327
52	725	1098	1554	2004	2450	2950	3513	4080	4702	5400
54	744	1125	1588	2047	2500	3003	3569	4142	4768	5475
56	762	1152	1618	2092	2548	3055	3625	4205	4835	5548
58	781	1177	1650	2137	2597	3106	3678	4267	4903	5620
60	800	1206	1682	2180	2646	3160	3735	4328	4970	5690
62	818	1230	1712	2222	2692	3212	3790	4389	5037	5760
64	837	1260	1740	2262	2736	3262	3845	4447	5105	5830
66	855	1285	1769	2302	2782	3310	3900	4505	5171	5900
68	873	1313	1798	2342	2828	3360	3950	4562	5232	5967
70	890	1340	1827	2380	2875	3410	4001	4618	5294	6033
72	908	1367	1857	2420	2922	3460	4053	4675	5355	6098
74	927	1394	1887	2455	2968	3510	4105	4733	5417	6162
76	945	1421	1915	2490	3013	3560	4158	4791	5480	6225
78	963	1446	1941	2527	3058	3608	4210	4846	5542	6288
80	981	1473	1966	2562	3103	3657	4260	4900	5600	6350
84	1016	1524	2020	2630	3192	3755	4360	5014	5720	6473
88	1052	1572	2075	2698	3282	3849	4462	5126	5838	6598
92	1087	1620	2130	2765	3371	3943	4560	5235	5954	6720
96	1122	1668	2186	2828	3459	4033	4657	5340	6068	6842
100	1155	1716	2238	2890	3545	4120	4750	5445	6180	6956

Larger Areas
Treating Distance in cm

Area ↓	0.5	1.0	1.5	2.0
Sq. cm.				
120	1307	1960	2510	3180
140	1463	2194	2788	3470
160	1608	2412	3055	3736
180	1746	2617	3312	4010
200	1880	2820	3560	4288
220	2008	3008	3805	4554
240	2132	3200	4045	4824
260	2256	3383	4288	5095
280	2372	3560	4530	5360
300	2495	3747	4760	5630
320	2622	3924	4984	5892
340	2737	4105	5200	6145
360	2853	4280	5427	6388
380	2968	4455	5630	6623
400	3080	4620	5840	6864

Some Filtration Correctors

Filter Used	Correction to Radium Used
0.3 mm. Pt	+4%
0.6 mm. Pt	−2%
0.7 mm. Pt	−4%
0.8 mm. Pt	−6%
1.0 mm. Pt	−10%
1.5 mm. Pt	−20%

Two Plane Separation Factors

Separation	Factor
1.5 cm.	1.25
2.0 cm.	1.4
3.0 cm.	1.5

As an example, assume as a target a surgical scar in a 10 MV external photon beam treatment field delivering 60 Gy to the peak depth of 2.5 cm. The tissues 1 cm deep received a dose of at least 54 Gy from the external treatments; but, because the facility did not use bolus, the scar received only 30 Gy superficially and 45 Gy at a depth of 0.5 cm. Using the 0.5-cm thick mold and the FDD calculated above, the scar at the skin surface could be given an additional 24 Gy to bring it to 90% of the target dose of 60 Gy, with the dose to the deep portion of the scar of 15 Gy from the surface application, also for a total of 60 Gy. The surface application delivers 44% of the surface dose to the point 1 cm deep, or 10.5 Gy, for a combined total at that point of 64.5 Gy.

After establishing the thickness of the mold, the strength of the radium is determined using Equation 1 and Table 1. The original tables require some corrections, as discussed by Shalek and Stovall[9]:

1. *Correction for* Γ: At the time of calculation, the accepted value for the Γ for radium was 8.4 R cm^2/mg hr. It now seems that 8.25 R cm^2/mg hr better approximates the value. Multiplying the table entries by 1.018 corrects for this change.

2. *Conversion to dose*: The tables use exposure in "R" to express the quantity of radiation given to the patient. Currently, dose in Gy serves that function. Inclusion of the f-factor to muscle tissue of

$$f = 0.00961 \text{ Gy/R} \qquad (3)$$

converts to the current, customary units and corresponds to multiplying the table's entries by 104. This operation results in extremely large numbers in the table because the entries would then be the mg hr to deliver *1000 Gy*. To obtain more fathomable entries, multiplying by 0.104 produces values of mg hr to deliver 1 Gy, which not only yields more normal looking numbers, but eliminates having to carry factors of 1000 for R

"doses" or 10 when the tables are expressed as mg hr/10 Gy.

3. *Correction for oblique filtration*: The manner of the original calculations neglected the effect of some of the rays traveling obliquely through the walls of the radium needles. Mitchell[10] estimates this effect would require a 2%–4% increase in the values of R$_A$ listed in the table, depending on the geometry, with the largest correction applying to the shorter distances and the larger areas.

4. *Correction for tissue attenuation and scatter*: Paterson and Parker calculated the table values for sources in air, assuming that an increase in dose due to scatter cancels the decrease due to attenuation. The correction for the effect of tissue on the radiation amounts to increasing the table values by about 1%/cm.

Shalek notes that the last two corrections work in opposite directions and that, for distances of 3 cm or less, a constant correction factor works well. His table for various distances from typical size areas (adjusted for changes in the values accepted for the f-factor since its publication) is reproduced with permission as Table 2. As a further correction, as the ratio of the longest dimension to the shortest dimension increases, the radiation from the more distant regions of the mold contributes less to the dose in the middle, and an elongation correction must be included if the ratio of these dimensions differs significantly from unity. For the example case, the strength of radium including corrections for a

Table 2.
Corrections for the Manchester System's Planar Implant Table (Based on Shalek, Stovall, and Sampiere[12])

Distance (cm)	"1000 R" in the Tables Equals (Gy)
0.5–2.5	9.03
3.0	8.94
3.5	8.84
4.0	8.74
4.5	8.64
5.0	8.54

Table 3.
Surface Applicator Distribution Rules

Circles with a diameter of D, percent of the radium placed in compartment

Compartment	D/h				
	<3	3–6	6	7.5	10
Outer circle (diameter D)	100	95	80	75	70
Inner circle (diameter D/2)	0	0	17	22	27
Center	0	5	3	3	3

    Rectangles with a smaller side, width, of w and a linear radium density (amount of radium/
      perimeter) around the outside of ρ_p.
1. The spacing between lines in the w direction shall not exceed 2h.
2. If lines need to be added to keep the separation < 2h, the linear radium density
    of the added,
      inside lines, ρ_i, shall be:
  a. $\rho_i = 1/2\ \rho_p$ for one added line.
  b. $\rho_i = 2/3\ \rho_p$ for more than one added line.

typical LDR application using 0.6 Gy/hr to the skin becomes:

$$S = \dot{D} \cdot R_A \qquad (4)$$

$$= (0.6\,\text{Gy/hr})(558\,\text{mg}\cdot\text{hr}/1000\,\text{R}) \qquad (4a)$$

$$(1R/0.00903\text{Gy}) \qquad (4b)$$

$$= 37.1\,\text{mg}$$

The distribution of the radium on the mold follows specific rules. To achieve uniformity, some of the radium goes on the periphery of the treatment shape, and some may fill in the area in the interior, depending on the ratio of the shortest side to the treatment distance, referred to as h. Table 3 gives the rules.

Figure 2 shows a top view of the example mold. In this example, the mold requires four interior lines, each with 2/3 the linear radium density of the periphery lines. The distribution then comes from solving:

$$(\text{Periphery} \times \rho_p)$$
$$+\ (\text{No. interior lines} \times \text{length/line} \times \rho_i)$$
$$= \text{Strength} \qquad (5)$$

$$\text{or}$$

$$(24\ \text{cm} \times \rho_p)$$
$$+\ (4\ \text{lines} \times 7\ \text{cm/line} \times 2/3\ \rho_p)$$
$$= 37.1\ \text{mg.} \qquad (5a)$$

From this,

$$\rho_p = 0.87\ \text{mg/cm and } 2/3$$
$$\rho_p = 0.58\ \text{mg/cm.} \qquad (5b)$$

The challenge comes in obtaining the distribution using standard radium needles that came as "full strength," with 0.66 mg/cm, and "half strength," with 0.33 mg/cm, and with active lengths of 1.5, 3.0, and 4.5 cm (called short, medium, and long, respectively). To achieve this loading, the needles could be distributed as shown in Figure 3.

With this arrangement, the periphery carries 21.8 mg, with a linear radium density of 0.91 mg/cm (4.3% too high), and the interior needles carry 15.84 mg, with a linear radium density of 0.57 mg/cm (2.5% too low). The actual dose rate for this mold becomes $\dot{D} = (21.8 + 15.84)$ mg/(61.79 mg hr/Gy) $= 0.609$ Gy/hr.

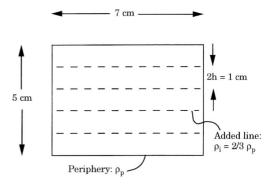

Figure 2. A view looking down onto the top of the example mold showing the arrangement of the lines for the loading of the radioactive materials.

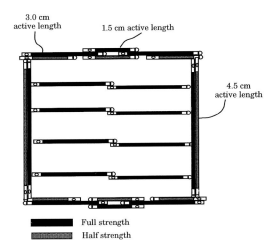

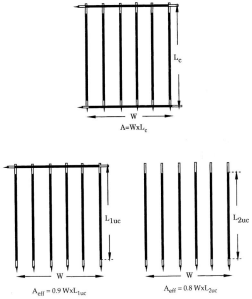

Figure 3. A top view of the example mold showing the distribution of the radioactive material.

Figure 4. The different possibilities for crossing the ends of a needle plane.

Planar Implants

The Manchester system considers planar implants as limited versions of planar molds. These implants are limited primarily by their inability to accommodate the required linear radium density. In the example mold considered above, several of the lines depended on tandem needle placement, one after the other in line. Needles in implants cannot be sunk deeply, each on top of its predecessor. Thus, the distribution may be less than ideal. The rules become simpler according to Table 4.

Because many implants run from the skin surface deep into the patient, the periphery must often be left incomplete; frequently, the needle plane covers only three sides of a rectangle, the deep side remaining incomplete (uncrossed in Manchester terms). Figure 4 shows the three possible situations for a plane. Without the crossing needle on one

end, the treatment area at depth retracts from where the crossing needle would have been to the distal active end. Even at that, the treatment area between the needles withdraws farther into the volume. Thus, when finding the R_A, the reference area becomes

$$A_{ref} = 0.9 \ b \ c \qquad (6a)$$

Because neither end is crossed (a rare situation with radium needles, but common with iridium), the loss in area occurs on both ends, and

$$A_{ref} = 0.8 \ b \ d \qquad (6b)$$

In practice, the target determines the treatment depth or length. If either end remains uncrossed, the active length or depth of insertion must compensate. In general, to cover the target with a plane with one uncrossed end, the depth of insertion to the active end, c, becomes

$$c = target \ depth/0.9. \qquad (6c)$$

Quimby and Castro[11] suggest that the im-

Table 4.
Distribution Rules for Planar Implants

Area of plane (cm²)	Fraction of the radium	
	On Periphery	Over the Interior
>25	2/3	1/3
25–100	1/2	1/2
>100	1/3	2/3

planted length from the skin to the active end extend as

$$c = \text{target depth}/0.8 \qquad (6d)$$

to assure coverage of the target between the needles at the depth. The area used to find R_A would still follow from $A_{eff} = 0.9$ c b.

The Manchester system always considers the treatment distance for a single plane to be 0.5 cm. Treating farther than that requires an excessively high dose in the implant plane. According to the distribution rules for a mold, the needle separation should be 2h or 1 cm between needles for h = 0.5 cm. Because they are included in the system as a special case of planar molds, implants use the same table of R_A values.

For lesions between 0.5 and 2.5 cm thick in their smallest dimension, the system uses a two plane implant, but provides an important caveat. The dose with two planes *still refers to a distance 0.5 cm from one plane, in the direction of the other plane, not at midplane.* For separations >1.5 cm between planes, the dose on the midplane falls below the 10% criterion. Table 5 gives some sense of how doses at midplane compare with the stated doses. As seen in the table, the deficit decreases with increased planar area. Thus, a two plane implant with a separation of 2 cm may adequately treat an implant with an area of 35 cm², but not one with 20 cm² (the latter would benefit from a three plane implant). For no

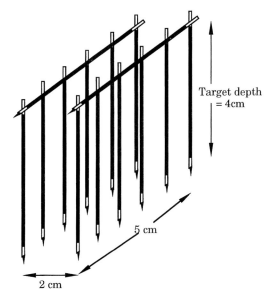

Figure 5. Two plane implant with target dimensions of 5 cm long, 4 cm deep, and 2 cm thick.

area does the midplane dose fall within 10% of the nominal dose for planes with separations of 2.5 cm².

The dose rate for a given amount of radium divided evenly between two identical planes separated by 1 cm equals that for a single plane, since both cases use the same distance between the plane of calculation and the source plane. But as the separation between the two planes increases and the calculation plane remains 0.5 cm from one of the implant planes, the distance from the opposite implant plane and the calculation plane increases. Thus, the dose rate to the calculational plane decreases with separation. The system compensates for this decrease in dose rate by using separation factors (S.F.) to increase the R_A. These factors can be found appended to Table 1.

For example, consider an implant as shown in Figure 5. The implant brackets the target volume, that is 5 cm long, 4 cm deep, and 2 cm thick. The deep end lying in the patient precludes that crossing, but a needle running just subcutaneously crosses the superficial end. To compensate for the loss in treatment depth, the distal active end must fall between 4.44 cm (i.e., 4 cm/0.9) and 5 cm (i.e., 4 cm/

Table 5.
Midplane Dose for a Two-Plane Manchester Implant Compared to the Nominal Dose

Area (cm²)	Midplane Dose as Percent of Nominal Dose	
	Separation of Planes	
	2.0 cm	2.5 cm
10	− 20.1	− 31.1
16	− 19.7	− 28.8
24	− 16.6	− 25.9
36	− 11.8	− 22.5
50	− 10.1	− 20.1
− 64	− 10.3	− 18.5
80	− 11.1	− 17.5
100	− 11.2	− 16.5

0.8) from the surface. The 4.5-cm active length needles serve adequately as the "vertical" sources. Either a single 4.5-cm needle or a combination of a 2-cm and a 3-cm needle in tandem may serve for crossing the top. That decision awaits the distribution calculation. The amount of radium on each plane comes from the follwing equation:

$$S = \dot{D} \cdot {}_{eff} R_A(A_{eff}, h = 0.5 \text{ cm})$$
$$\cdot \text{ S.F.}/2 \text{ planes.} \qquad (7)$$

The effective area remains the same as the target area since

$$A_{eff} = 0.9 \ A_{implant} = 0.9 \ (A_{target}/0.9)$$
$$= 20 \text{ cm}^2. \qquad (8a)$$

If we use a typical dose rate of 0.55 Gy/hr, the strength becomes

$$S = (0.55 \text{ Gy/hr})$$
$$\times [(368 \text{ mg hr}/1000r) \ (1r/0.00903 \text{ Gy})]$$
$$\times (1.4)/2 \text{ planes} = 15.7 \text{ mg/plane.} \qquad (8b)$$

From the distribution rules, two thirds of the radium, or 10.5 mg, belongs on the periphery, with the remaining one third or 5.2 mg, in the interior. The periphery consists of three sides. Using 4.5-cm active length, full strength needles (2.97 mg each) gives 8.91 mg. The four vertical, interior needles would carry 5.94 mg if half strength. In this case, the total would equal 14.85 mg, or 95% of what the plan called for, with 60% (instead of 67%) on the periphery and 40% (instead of 33%) in the interior. This example would have worked out better if the bottom end could have been crossed, but in real life, such a crossing is often not possible. Although interstitial implants limit the possibilities for "creative" distributions more than surface applicators do, in a case like this one, the vertical, peripheral needle position could use parallel full strength and half strength needles. This side-by-side arrangement would give 11.88 mg on the periphery (33%), keeping 5.94 mg in the interior (67%), for a total of 17.82 mg. With this loading, the proportions on the periphery and the interior work out exactly, but the total

becomes 13.5% too high, giving a dose rate of 0.62 Gy/hr. The two dose rates would probably give equivalent results, thus giving preference to the second distribution.

Volume Implants

For lesions larger than accommodated by a two plane implant, the Manchester system suggests the use of volume implants. Their volume implants come in several subclasses, the most common being multiple plane implants.

Multiple Plane Implants. Multiple plane implants follow the same rules as two plane implants, except that instead of dividing the radium equally between the two planes (or directly in proportion to their areas), the weighting of the radium in each outside plane to that on each inside plane follows a ratio of 3:2. One centimeter should separate each plane.

Cylindrical Implants. Cylindrical implants consist of four sections: needles parallel to the altitude around the outside of the cylinder, called the belt; interior needles parallel to the altitude with half the diameter of the belt, called the core; and a plane of needles perpendicular to the belt capping off each end of the cylinder, called the ends.

Table 6 gives the rules for distribution for a cylindrical implant. The "Parts" refers to the fraction of the radium carried in the section. For example, assume a cylindrical, perineal volume 4 cm in diameter and 4 cm long implanted with needles running mostly along the body axis, then the superficial end of the

Table 6.
Distribution Rules for Cylindrical Implants

Section	Minimum, Number of Needles	Parts
Belt	8	4
Core	4	2
End	as needed	1 each (crossed at active end) 2 each (crossed at physical end)

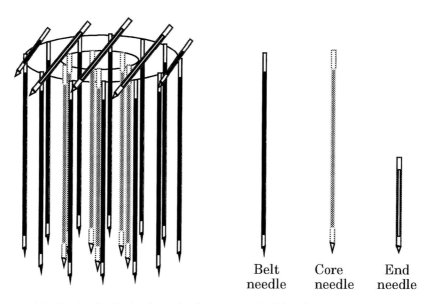

Figure 6. An idealized cylindrical volume implant as per the Manchester system.

cylinder can be crossed, but not the deep end. As with the planar implants, such an uncrossed end results in the loss of treatment length compared to that achieved with a crossing end, the only difference being the use of a 0.925 multiplier times the length for each uncrossed end instead of 0.9 as is used in planar implants. In the example, the circumference of the belt, 4 cm $\times \pi = 12.6$ cm, could accommodate 12 needles with about 1 cm between. The core could carry six needles. Covering the ends takes a bit more consideration. Figure 6 shows the implant. The crossing needles should match the circular projection of the cylinder. In this case, for the outer crossing needles, two short needles (active length of 1.5 cm) just inside the edge of the cylinder provide more than adequate coverage. The next crossing needles falls 1 cm inside the edge, where the chord length equals about 3.5 cm. The medium needles (active length of 3.0 cm) leave a little space at their ends uncovered, but the Manchester system allows "corners" to run a little cold; and the next size up, the long needles with an active length of 4.5 cm, certainly would extend too far beyond the edge of the cylinder. The middle crossing needle covers the full diameter, requiring a long needle. Al-

though not as common as the short, medium, and long needles, medium-short and medium-long needles, with active lengths of 2.0 and 4.0 cm, respectively, often prove useful, as they would in this example.

The needles used in the core and the belt must not only cover the treatment length, but also must make up for the absence of the bottom crossing needle. From the skin to the deep active end, c must satisfy

$$c = \frac{\text{treatment length}}{0.925}$$

$$= \frac{4 \text{ cm}}{0.925} = 4.3 \text{ cm}. \qquad (9)$$

This depth requires the long needles; however, with their active length 4.3 cm deep, the superficial active end as well as the inactive end sticks out of the skin. A small plastic sheet with holes drilled for each needle position (a crude form of a template) could provide protection for the ends and hold the needles at their proper depth. Particular attention must be paid to the dose to the skin in such situations, to avoid skin necrosis. Another option would be to extend the needles farther, so that the suture hole lines up with the skin. In this case, the depth, c, would equal the 4.5

cm active length plus about 3 mm of inactive end, giving a treatment depth of 0.925x4.8 cm = 4.4 cm. Depending on underlying structures, the additional 4 mm probably would make no clinical difference; and, based on Quimby's suggestion, it would help to move the deep end of the implant into the more uniform region. Again, this is a situation where medium-long needles would provide just the right tool. This example also demonstrates some of the restrictions of brachytherapy practice using radium or cesium needles.

The dose calculations follow the same model as the planar implants. The Manchester R_V values come from an equation:

$$R_V = 34.1V^{2/3}e^{0.07(E-1)}, \qquad (10)$$

where V = the volume of the implant, and
 E = the longest principal axis/shortest principal axis.

Again, these values require correction for the same four reasons as did the R_A table. From the equation, for an effective volume of $(2 \text{ cm})^2 \pi$ 0.925x4.8 cm = 55.8 cm^3, the $R_V = 505$ mg hr/9.03 Gy = 55.9 mg hr/Gy. A dose rate of 0.55 Gy/hr requires 30.76 mg of radium. The first step in calculating the distribution of the radium entails summation of the "parts" used. The belt gets four parts, the core two parts; and, because the crossing takes place at the active ends in line with the skin, the end gets one part. Thus, the implant divides the total amount of radium into seven parts, with each part equal to 30.76 mg/7 parts = 4.39 mg/part. Portioning the radium by parts gives: Belt 17.57 mg; Core 8.79 mg; and End 4.39 mg. The lower activity needles, half strength, at 0.33 mg/cm, carry 1.49 mg each on the belt, for a total of 17.82 mg. The six needles in the core carry 8.91 mg. The half strength needles on the end supply 4.46 mg. This combination carries 31.19 mg and delivers a dose rate of 31.19 mg/(55.9 mg hr/Gy) = 0.56 Gy/hr, just slightly above the desired dose rate.

Using afterloading Ir-192 seeds in this example, with a seed separation of 0.5 cm separation center-to-center, each needle would

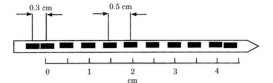

Figure 7. The distribution of Ir-192 seeds in a needle for the cylindrical implant example.

carry a configuration as shown in Figure 7. The first and last seed in each needle is added to those that form the belt or core, and they abut the next seed. These end seeds form the "ends" of the cylinders. Since the cylinder has two ends now, the total radium equivalent divides into eight parts. Not counting the first and the last seeds in the belt needles (we will come back to the end seeds), each of the equally spaced seeds could contain the equivalent of (30.76 mg x 4 parts/8 parts)/(12 needles x 9 seeds/needle) = 0.142 mg Ra eq. Because the core contains half the activity in half the number of needles, the same strength seeds serve there also. Since each end contains 3.845 mg Ra eq spread over 18 seeds (one for each needle), the end seed activity equals 0.214 mg Ra eq. Because the end seeds act as crossing planes, the active length need not increase beyond the 4 cm of the target.

Spherical Implants. The most common application for spherical implants is for permanent seed placements. The division of the radioactive material follows: Shell (the outer surface): 6 parts; and Core: 2 parts. The material in the core should be distributed as uniformly as possible; and, for both divisions, the separation between seeds should be between 1 and 1.5 cm.

Consider the example of a 3 cm x 3 cm x 3.5 cm organ implanted with Au-198 seeds as a 20 Gy boost after external beam therapy. Originally, the Manchester system treated radon seeds the same as radium sources and gold seeds as radon seeds except for correction for the specific exposure rate constant and half-life. Shalek, Stovall, and Sampiere[12] found that seeds give a slightly different R_V up to about 100 cm^3. Table 7 gives their suggested values. For our example, the approximately 16.5 cm^3 volume gives $R_V = 276.8$ mg hr/9.03 Gy = 30.65 mg hr/Gy.

Table 7.
Volume Implants of Radioactive Seeds

Volume in Cubic Centimeters	*mg hr/1,000 r
1	80.9
2	102
3	118
4	132
5	142
10	209
15	263
20	309
25	344
30	379
40	442
50	502
60	560
70	616
80	670
90	723
100	772

Above 100 cm³, Paterson and Parker volume tables are valid for seed volumes implanted on a 1 cm cubic lattice.

* Calculated for radon with a filtration of 0.5 mm Pt; corrections should be made for particular types of seeds.

The procedure for the seed implants follows the steps below:

1. Solve the problem as if using radium. The 20 Gy boost requires

$$N_{Ra} = 20 \text{ Gy} \times 30.65 \text{ mg hr/Gy}$$

$$= 613 \text{ mg hr} \quad (11a)$$

2. Convert the required number of disintegrations of radium into number of disintegrations of gold:

$$N_{Au} = N_{Ra} \left(\frac{\Gamma_{Ra}}{\Gamma_{Au}} \right)$$

$$= 613 \text{ mg hr}$$

$$\times [(8.25 \text{ R cm}^2/\text{mg hr})$$

$$/(2.32 \text{ R cm}^2/\text{mCi hr})]$$

$$= 2180 \text{ mCi hr.} \quad (11b)$$

3. Find the initial activity to implant to provide the required number of disin-

tegrations. Assume that each radioactive nucleus implanted eventually disintegrates. In that case,

$$A_{Au} = \lambda N_{Au} \quad (11c)$$

$$= \frac{0.693}{T_{1/2}} N_{Au}. \quad (11d)$$

In this case,

$$A_{Au} = 0.693 \times 2180 \text{ mCihr}$$

$$/(2.7 \text{ d} \times 24 \text{ hr/d})$$

$$= 23.3 \text{ mCi.} \quad (11e)$$

The harder part of the problem involves the seed placement. The peripheral seeds forming the shell should fall about 1 cm from each other.

Figure 8 shows the implant schematically. The shell can start with a seed in the tip of the long axis. A distance of about 1 cm along the surface from the first seed forms a circle. This circle holds five seeds spaced at 1 centimeter intervals. One centimeter further along the surface forms a circle holding eight seeds at 1 centimeter intervals. The actual positioning of the circles makes the implant symmetrical from tip to end. This placement results in the use of 28 seeds in the shell. The activity for each seed becomes

$$A_{Au}/\text{seed}$$

$$= (23.3 \text{ mCi}/28 \text{ seeds})$$

$$\cdot (6 \text{ parts on shell}/8 \text{ parts on shell})$$

$$= 0.62 \text{ mCi/seed} \quad (11f)$$

Spreading the remaining activity over the interior becomes more arbitrary. Usually, the implant uses same strength seeds for the interior and the shell to prevent mistaken applications. With this policy, the interior gets

No. of seeds

$$= (23 \text{ mCi}/0.62 \text{ mCi per seed})$$

$$\cdot (2 \text{ parts in core}/8 \text{ parts total})$$

$$= 9 \text{ to } 10 \text{ seeds} \quad (11g)$$

The "X" marks in Figure 8 indicate some possible locations for the core seeds as seen on the end view. Although, for simplification,

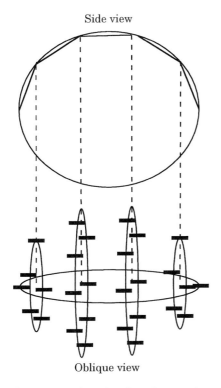

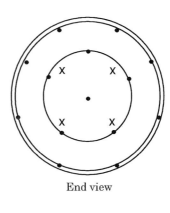

Figure 8. The distribution of radioactive seed type sources in the example ellipsoidal implant using the Manchester system.

they are not shown on the oblique view, the two sets of the square pattern would each fall just toward the ends of the larger shell seed planes, with one additional core seed in the very center of the ellipsoid, as seen in the end view.

One practical problem with this implant, or most Manchester spherical implants, involves the number of needle tracks required. This case uses 18 tracks for the 37 seeds, all falling in a 3 cm diameter. The delivery of the seeds becomes intense and difficult.

The initial dose rate for this implant can be found as

$$\dot{D}_0 = 0.693D/T_{1/2}. \tag{12}$$

$$= 0.693 \times 20 \text{ Gy}/$$

$$(2.7 \text{ d} \times 24 \text{ hr/d}) \tag{12a}$$

$$= 0.21 \text{ Gy/hr}. \tag{12b}$$

The dose rate, of course, decreases from the time of implantation. The LDR corresponding to low total doses may limit the usefulness of such implants for boosts based on biological response models.

The Quimby System

Originating just after the development of the Manchester system, the Quimby system addressed a desire for a system that differed from the Manchester system in three ways:

1. *Loading*: The Quimby system used uniform distribution of the radioactive material, rather than following complex distribution rules.
2. *Source strength*: The Quimby system allowed for the use of the higher strength radium needles commonly in use in the United States at the time (typically with a linear radium density of 1.0 mg/cm compared with those used with the Manchester system that

had a denisty of 0.66 and 0.33 mg/cm).

3. *Dose distribution*: The uniform loading results in an inhomogenous dose distribution, delivering a higher dose in the center of an implant than to the periphery.

Quimby did not depreciate uniform dose throughout a target, but observed that achieving the uniform dose often became impractical and that, for some tumors, an increased dose in the center may be beneficial (due to their hypoxic, radioresistant core).

While the Manchester system attempted to keep a consistent method of dose specification for all implants (i.e., dose specified 10% above the minimum dose either in the volume or on a plane of interest), the form of dose specification in the Quimby system depends on the type of application.

Planar Implants and Molds

For planar applications, the Quimby system defines the dose in the *center* of the parallel plane at the treatment distance. For the uniform loading of the implant source plane, the specified dose corresponds to the *maximum* dose on the plane of interest. Unlike the Manchester system, but as with the Johns variation of that system, for a two planar implant, the Quimby system would most likely state the dose on the midplane rather than a plane 0.5 cm from a source plane, although it is not clear that the planar implant tables were ever actually intended for use with two plane implants. The method of calculation follows the same pattern in both systems, multiplying R_A factors times a dose rate to find the quantity of radium for the application. Using the original Quimby table requires corrections, as did the Manchester table, for changes in the specific

Table 8.
R_A Table for Planar Applications for the Quimby System Values of mgRaeq/Gy

Distance (cm)	Circular Applicators (Diameter in cm)					
	1	2	3	4	5	6
0.5	4.68	7.98	10.97	18.10	23.42	35.13
1.0	14.55	18.83	23.54	32.10	39.59	48.47
1.5	30.43	34.84	43.01	51.18	60.43	73.22
2.0	53.59	58.56	65.59	75.63	85.90	99.19
1.5	79.03	85.48	93.00	102.7	124.2	136.0
3.0	118.9	125.5	133.1	144.0	156.0	170.8

Distance (cm)	Square Applicators (Diameter in cm)					
	1	2	3	4	5	6
0.5	4.90	8.52	12.24	20.97	26.61	37.26
1.0	15.09	20.11	25.46	34.99	43.33	54.67
1.5	31.72	37.09	44.62	54.94	64.51	79.03
2.0	54.02	61.59	69.69	80.71	92.38	108.0
1.5	78.49	85.48	96.23	108.6	122.6	147.3
3.0	118.9	125.5	138.6	151.7	165.8	182.2

Distance (cm)	Rectangular Applicators (Diameter in cm)					
	1×1.5	2×3	3×4	4×6	6×9	8×12
0.5	5.4294	10.965	15.224	30.554	60.682	101.7
1.0	15.834	22.896	29.315	45.577	77.674	118.8
1.5	32.041	39.782	50.104	67.092	101.61	145.7
2.0	54.673	63.749	77.255	94.002	133.98	180.4
1.5	77.521	90.316	106.44	122.57	163.43	215.0
3.0	121.11	129.84	145.66	165.84	210.58	272.8

Derived from Quimby's Table 13-3 in reference 9, multiplied by 0.1059, and then increased by 1%/cm distance.

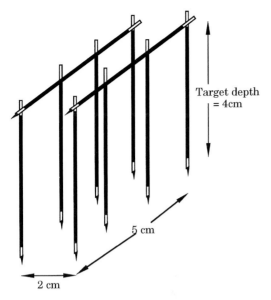

Target depth = 4cm

5 cm

2 cm

Figure 9. The example two plane implant approached through the Quimby system.

exposure rate constant, conversion from exposure (R) to dose (Gy), and tissue attenuation and scatter; because of the difference in the methods used to calculate the tables, the Quimby tables include the effect of oblique filtration. Table 8 gives the R_A values for use with the Quimby system, including the three corrections. The reductions in the effective length (because ends of planes cannot be crossed) follow those for the Manchester system. The Quimby system allows more leeway in the spacing of the needles, permitting 1–2 cm between needles.

Consider the two plane implant worked as an example for the Manchester system. Two centimeters separated the two 4 cm x 5 cm planes; and, to make up for the uncrossed bottom end of the planes, the 4 cm length was extended to 4.5 cm. In this case, the 0.55 Gy/hr target dose rate falls halfway between the two planes, so h = 1 cm. Interpolating between the square 4x4 cm^2 and 4x6 cm^2 values for R_A gives 40.3 mg hr/Gy. The ideal quantity of radium becomes 40.3 mg hr/Gy x 0.55 Gy/hr = 22.14 mg, or 11.07 mg/plane. Figure 9 shows the implant, each plane with four parallel 4.5-cm needles (separated by 1.7 cm) and one 4.5-cm needle as a crosser. Ideally, each of the five needles contains the same amount

of radium; therefore, each of the five needles would contain 2.21 mg (11.07 mg/5 needles = 2.21 mg/needle). This corresponds to a linear radium density of 0.49 mg/cm, approximately the 0.5 mg/cm used in the early, American half strength needles. In the 1953 article, Quimby states that many departments in the United States had only the 1.0 mg/cm needles that, in this example, would deliver the dose at approximately 1.12 Gy/hr, significantly faster than the usual British dose rate. Biologically, the difference required modification of the total dose. As with examples above, the current use of iridium sources, other custom supplied isotopes, or HDR units eliminate the restrictions imposed by the old style radium source inventory.

Volume Implants

While the Quimby system specified the dose for a planar implant as the *maximum* on the plane of interest, for volume implants the stated dose corresponds to the *minimum* dose in the implanted volume, usually found on the periphery between the sources. As Quimby points out and as was seen in the cylindrical implant example above, the Manchester rule requiring eight needles in the belt and four in the core causes problems with small implants, and the uniform distribution becomes more practical. For larger volumes, the two systems use very similar distributions. However, even though the distributions match, the total amount of radiation the patient receives differs markedly because the dose specification differs. Again, consider the examples given above.

Cylindrical Implants. The example cylinder had a diameter of 4 cm and used needles with the active end 4.8 cm below the skin, with the deep end uncrossed. For the Quimby implant, from Table 9, the 55.8 cm^3 effective volume gives $R_V = 78$ mg hr/Gy, for a quantity of radium of $S = R_V \dot{D} = 42.9$ mg. Using a larger separation between the crossing needles, four medium needles cover the end. "Uniform distribution" becomes difficult to define for the cylindrical volume, but the basic belt and core concept works well. Using about 1.5 cm separation between needles in the belt results in eight needles, and four needles in the core

Table 9.
Rv Table for Planar Applications for the
Quimby System Values of mgRaeq/Gy

Volume (cc)	Rv	Diameter of a Sphere (cm)	Rv
5	21.4	1.0	4.45
10	34.3	1.5	11.39
15	41.8	2.0	20.97
20	47.2	2.5	33.37
30	58.1	3.0	47.51
40	66.8	3.5	59.12
60	81.0	4.0	73.09
80	94.1	4.5	87.59
100	108	5.0	104.6
125	122	6.0	147.3
150	136	7.0	200.2
175	151		
200	164		
250	184		
300	197		

Derived from Quimby's Table 13-3 in reference 9, multiplied by 0.1059, and then increased by 1%/cm of average distance to the center of the volume.

would fill approximately the volume, as shown in Figure 10. The total length for this implant equals 66 cm, and the ideal linear radium density becomes 42.9 mg/66 cm = 0.65 mg/cm, or almost exactly that of the (not early American) standard full strength needle. If full strength needles were used, the dose rate would become 0.56 Gy/hr.

When performing the implant using iridium seeds, double loading the ends simulates crossing (as with the Manchester implant), so the length need not be extended. The distribution of seeds along the needle then looks identical to Figure 7, containing 11 seeds. The activity of each seed equals 42.9 mg/132 seeds = 0.33 mg/seed.

Spherical Implant. Looking at the spherical, permanent gold seed implant considered previously, the distribution with the Quimby system could look like that shown in Figure 11. This distribution uses only 12 needle tracks, compared with the 18 of the Manchester, simplifying the delivery. The seeds fall between

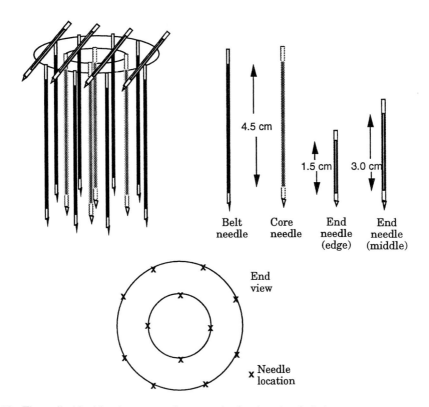

Figure 10. The cylindrical implant example as worked using the Quimby system.

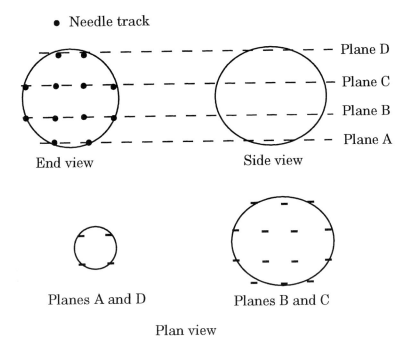

• Needle track

End view   Side view

Plane D
Plane C
Plane B
Plane A

Planes A and D   Planes B and C

Plan view

Figure 11. The example ellipsoidal implant using the Quimby system.

1 and 1.2 cm from the next nearest seed. The distance could have been stretched to 1.5 cm, reducing the number of needle tracks to 7, but markedly diminishing the uniformity and coverage. Sticking with the 12 needle track implant, the application uses 36 seeds. From Table 9, the R_V comes from the value approximating a sphere for the average diameter of 3.17 cm, giving 44.8 mg hr/Gy. Following the same procedures as before, the 20 Gy dose uses

$$\text{Act/seed} = \frac{0.693}{T_{1/2}} \frac{\Gamma_{Ra}}{\Gamma_{Au}} \frac{DR_V}{\text{No. of seeds}} \quad (13)$$

$$= 34 \text{ mCi/36 seeds} \quad (13a)$$

$$= 0.947 \text{ mCi per seed.} \quad (13b)$$

Memorial Systems

Systems developed at Memorial Hospital in New York have addressed mainly interstitial implants. The first of these, based on computer calculations by Laughlin et al.,[13] applied to rectangular matrices of equal activity seeds. Dose was calculated in planes 1 cm apart that

were 0.5 cm from source planes within the implant and that extended to 5 cm beyond the implant. The system defined the terms:

Reference Maximum Dose: the highest dose found in the implanted volume,
Minimum Peripheral Dose: the lowest dose found in peripheral seed planes (along lines of intersection with perpendicular dose planes),
Centerline: a line passing through the reference maximum dose point (at the center of the matrix or 0.5 cm from the center) and parallel to a side of the matrix,
Centerline Peripheral Dose: the dose found at the intersection of the centerline and the periphery of the matrix.

From their calculations, the authors derived tables, similar to the Manchester tables, of mg · hr for 1000 rad for planar implants with the dose specified on a plane 0.5 cm from the implant plane (Table 10) and for volume implants (Table 11). The calculations explicitly include tissue attenuation and scatter for radon seeds; but, through conversion using the ratio of exposure rate constants, the tables could be applied with little error to planning implants of standard Ir-192 ribbons or Au-198 seeds. Figure 12 shows that, as "shells" of seeds are added, at 1 mg · hr/seed, the reference maximum dose increases linearly (for volume implants) with the cube root of the number of seeds. This relationship prevails because the number of seeds in each shell is roughly proportional to the square of the distance from the center and therefore is balanced by inverse square law reduction of the dose, making the plot essentially one of "number of shells" versus "distance from center," the distance being proportional to the cube root of the number of seeds. The plot for planar implants would have been linear had the data been plotted versus the square root of the number of seeds.

A system to facilitate planning for tumor bed implants of Ir-192 seeds in ribbons was

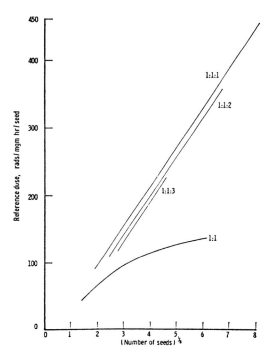

Figure 12. "Reference dose" as a function of the cube root of the number of seeds in a rectangular array. The straight lines correspond to three-dimensional arrays with the specified ratios of the number of seeds on a side; the curved line corresponds to a planar array. (From Laughlin JS, Siler WM, Holondy EI, Ritter FW. A dose description system for interstitial radiation therapy. Am J Roentgenol Radium Ther 1963;89:470–490 with mission.)

Table 10.
Plane Implants Milligram-Hours to Deliver 1,000 RADS at Designated Point

Area (cm^2)	(1) Minimum Peripheral Dose Point	(2) Reference Maximum Dose Point	Ratio (1)/(2)
1	95	84	1.13
2	116	94	1.23
3	138	107	1.29
4	165	124	1.333
5	189	138	1.367
6	211	152	1.39
7	236	166	1.42
8	256	178	1.44
9	280	193	1.45
10	300	204	1.47
12	342	228	1.50
14	380	250	1.52
16	419	272	1.54
18	454	291	1.56
20	488	311	1.57
25	570	354	1.61
30	650	399	1.63
35	734	442	1.66
40	812	485	1.675
45	892	528	1.69
50	973	569	1.71

Dose points are defined in a plane 0.5 cm from plane of implant. The sources are assumed uniform in strength and located on a 1 cm grid.

developed subsequently in the form of a nomograph.[14] Given the active length, width, and seed strength of a planar implant, the user of the nomograph (Figure 13) could quickly find the number (and hence the spacing) of catheters required to achieve a dose rate of 10 Gy/day at a peripheral reference point. Within a treatment plane 0.5 cm from the source plane, this reference point was located 1.5 seed spacing units (i.e., 1.5 cm for standard Ir-192 ribbons) inward from the end source of a ribbon and 0.5 intercatheter spaces inward from the edge ribbon. Relative to the Manchester system planar implant table, the total source strength required to produce a given dose rate at the nomograph reference point was 96% for an area of 10 cm^2, 114% for 100 cm^2, and 133% for 400 cm^2, not a

Table 11.
Volume Implants Milligram-Hours to Deliver 1,000 RADS at Designated Point

Volume (cm³)	(1) Minimum Peripheral Dose Point	(2) Center Line Peripheral Dose Point	(3) Reference Maximum Dose Point	Ratio (1)/(3)	Ratio (2)/(3)
1	95	95	84	1.13	1.13
5	184	165	145	1.27	1.14
10	254	214	185	1.37	1.155
15	322	263	225	1.43	1.165
20	378	301	255	1.48	1.18
25	433	339	285	1.52	1.19
30	472	366	305	1.55	1.20
40	560	424	350	1.60	1.21
50	640	478	390	1.64	1.225
60	719	544	430	1.67	1.235
80	865	625	500	1.73	1.25
100	1,000	715	565	1.77	1.265
120	1,130	800	625	1.81	1.28
140	1,240	875	680	1.83	1.285
160	1,365	952	735	1.86	1.295
180	1,475	1,020	785	1.88	1.30
200	1,575	1,090	830	1.90	1.31
250	1,840	1,250	945	1.95	1.32
300	2,080	1,400	1,050	1.98	1.335
350	2,310	1,550	1,155	2.00	1.34
400	2,540	1,690	1,255	2.20	1.35

The sources are assumed uniform in strength and located on a 1 cm grid.

surprising comparison in view of the uniform ribbon spacing required by the nomograph system. Although, by permitting decay compensation for an in-house stock of Ir-192, this nomograph served a worthwhile purpose initially, it has fallen into disuse because of the current overnight availability of Ir-192 seeds at nearly any specified strength.

Using the nomograph for the planar mold example worked previously for the Manchester system—drawing a line from the 7 cm length through the 5 cm width to the tie line provides a pivot. From this pivot point, a line to the Number of Ribbons scale value of 6 (the same number of lines as the Manchester system used) passes approximately through 0.53 mg Ra eq. This nomograph gives configurations to produce 10 Gy/day = 0.417 Gy/hr. To obtain 0.6 Gy/hr requires seed strengths of (0.6/0.417)x0.53 mg Ra eq = 0.76 mg Ra eq. Since each line carries eight seeds, the six lines contain a total of 0.76 mg Ra eq/seedx8 seeds/linex6 lines = 36.5 mg Ra eq (vs 37.1 mg Ra eq for the Manchester system).

For permanent volume implants of I-125 seeds, Henschke and Cevc[15] applied the system of *dimension averaging* in which the total seed strength to be implanted is taken to be proportional to the average, d_a, of three mutually perpendicular target dimensions measured at the time of surgery. This system had initially been applied to Rn-222, for which the activity to implant was taken to be

$$A(mCi) = 10d_a. \qquad (14)$$

The total dose in gray for the permanent implant is calculated from the relationship approximated by Quimby volume implant data,[7]

$$D = \frac{1.44AT_{1/2}C}{\sqrt{V}}, \qquad (15)$$

with the activity in mCi, time in hours, and the volume in cm³, and where the constant C = 0.1 for Rn-222. Determination of the volume uses either

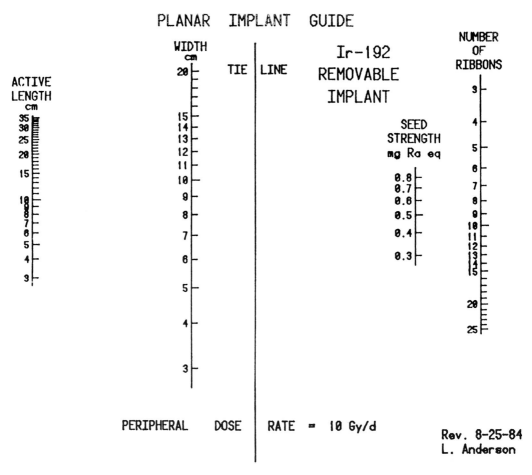

Figure 13. A nomograph from planning an Ir-192 interstitial planar implant, used particularly for intraoperative application given the available sources with a specific strength.

$V = abc$ for rectangular implants (16a)

or

$V = \left(\dfrac{\pi}{6}\right) f_e^3 d_a^3$ for ellipsoidal implants, (16b)

where $f_e = a/c$. For the example ellipsoidal implant using radon seeds, the activity from Equation 14 becomes $A = 10$ mCi/cm×3.17 cm = 31.7 mCi, giving a dose of

$D = 1.44 \times 31.7$ mCi $\times 93.3$ hr

$\times 0.1/(16.5 \text{ cm}^3)^{0.5} = 104.8$ Gy (17a)

The activity to deliver 20 Gy would just be in proportion to the doses,

$A = (20 \text{ Gy}/104.8 \text{ Gy})$

$\times 31.7$ mCi = 6.05 mCi (17b)

Finally, to convert this to the activity of gold seeds requires the ratios of the exposure rate constants and the half-lives, as

$A_{Au} = \left(\dfrac{8.25 \text{R·cm}^2/(\text{mCi·hr})}{2.32 \text{R·cm}^2/((\text{mCi·hr})}\right)\left(\dfrac{91.9\text{hr}}{64.8\text{hr}}\right)$

$\times 6.05$ mCi$_{Rn}$ = 30.5 mCi (17c)

For I-125, the constant of proportionality was determined empirically to be 5 mCi per cm. A nomograph developed by Anderson[16] incorporated the arithmetic to determine the number of seeds (of a given strength) to be used and offered limited guidance on spacing (assumed to be uniform in all directions).

A consequence of the unmodified average dimension method was that the dose decreased as the treatment volume increased. At Memorial, dose evaluation for I-125 volume implants of individual seeds involves determining the *matched peripheral dose* (MPD), i.e., the dose for which the isodose contour occupies the same volume as the target volume (which usually is approximated as the volume of an ellipsoid having the same orthogonal dimensions). It was evident from actual patient data that MPDs not only decreased with implant volume, but that they

decreased more rapidly for I-125 than for Rn-222, because of the lower photon energies of I-125. In a subsequent version of the nomograph, the total strength was made proportional to power functions of the average dimension, with the power increasing from 1.0 for $d_a < 2.4$ cm, to 1.29 for 2.4 cm $< d_a < 3.2$ cm, and to 1.58 for $d_a > 3.2$ cm.[15,17] The 1.29 power was derived, by fitting patient MPD data, as that required to restore the dose fall-off with volume to that which had been obtained with Rn-222 seeds. For $d_a < 2.4$ cm, the original rule was left in place to take advantage of the higher radiation tolerance of smaller volumes and permit higher doses to more curable le-

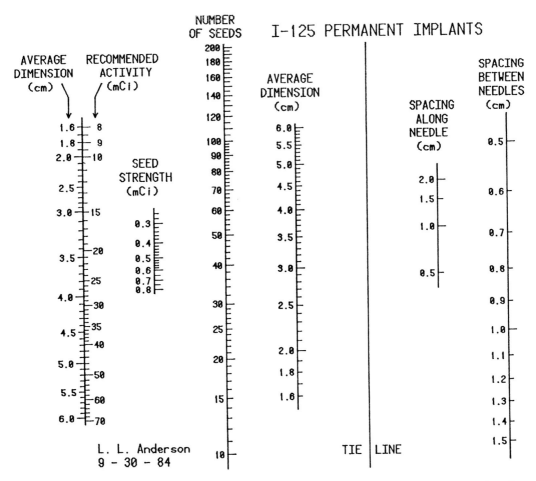

Figure 14. A nomograph for planning an I-125 volume implant. The nomograph was designed to give a matched peripheral dose of 160 Gy based on conventional dosimetry calculations. New data and the new dosimetry protocol would change the dose to approximately 140 Gy.

sions. For $d_a > 3.2$ cm, another 0.29 was added to the power in order to try to improve tumor control rates for larger volumes relative to the Rn-222 experience. This nomograph also provided more realistic spacing guidance, taking into account the fact that commonly used applicators afford spacing options (along the needle track) in 0.5-cm increments.

The current version of the Memorial I-125 nomograph (Figure 14) is still based on the average dimension, but now reflects total seed strength proportionality to the 2.2 power of average dimension, the fitted power value required for the MPD to be constant (at 160 Gy using the conventional dosimetry data and protocol; at approximately 140 Gy using the new radial dose function and anisotropy function and the new dosimetry protocol) as a function of implant volume.[17] Interestingly, the Manchester relationship between dose and volume corresponds to a 2.0 power of average dimension, so the extra 0.2 may be attributed to the photon energy difference between radium and I-125. In a nomograph developed in the same manner for Pd-103 seed implants, the power is 2.56, reflecting an even lower photon energy (Figure 15).[18] In both the I-125 and the Pd-103 nomographs, the original direct proportionality rule is retained for $d_a < 3.0$. The clinical decision to make the dose constant with volume was based on the failure to observe unacceptable complications over many years of experience with the preceding dose prescription formulas.

Considering the example seed implant worked for the Manchester and Quimby sys-

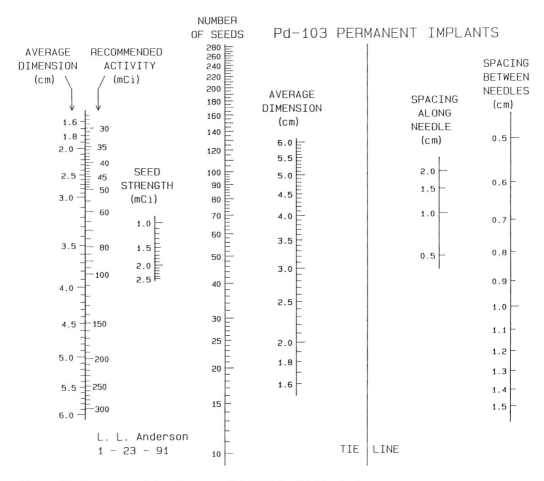

Figure 15. A nomograph for planning a Pd-103 interstitial implant.

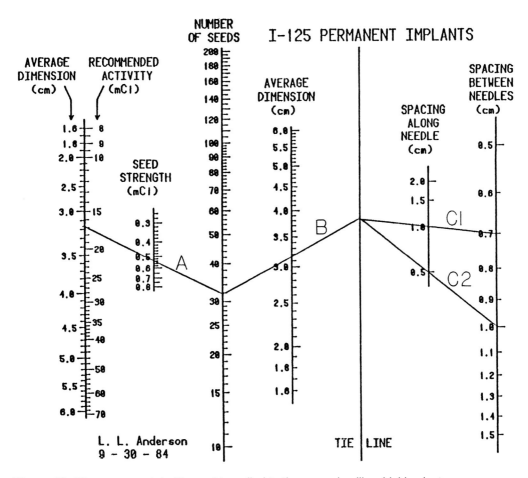

Figure 16. The nomograph in Figure 14 applied to the example ellipsoidal implant.

tems, with the Memorial system using I-125 seeds, the implant's average dimension is (3.5 cm + 3.0 cm + 3.0 cm)/3 = 3.17 cm. From the nomograph, an activity of 16.9 mCi is required to deliver 160 Gy. If we assume that the seeds available have an activity of 0.54 mCi each, the number of seeds required is 32 (line A in Figure 16). Spacing options are given by drawing line B through the same average dimension to a point on the tie line (which represents an intermediate result in the calculation) and drawing lines C1 and C2, to find that one may either place the seeds on 0.5 cm centers along the needle track and the needles 1 cm apart, or place the seeds on 1.0 cm centers and the needles 0.7 cm apart. Figure 17 shows one possible configuration of such an implant.

The Paris System

Pierquin's description of the basic Paris system[19–21] rules and application physics spans 34 pages in one of his texts[22]; thus, any synopsis here necessarily abbreviates the subject tremendously. The design of the system assumes the use of solid Ir-192 wire, although the authors accept uniformly loaded seeds in ribbons. The wires should be arranged in uniformly spaced, straight or curved lines.

As with any system, the rules depend on the specification of "dose." Figure 18 shows some sample source arrangements. For each arrangement, the minimum dose in the midtransverse plane between a set of neighboring needle tracks defines a quantity called basal dose. For the entire arrangement, the average

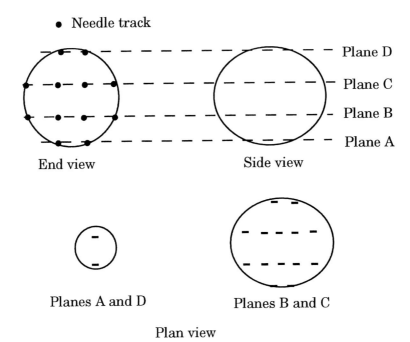

Figure 17. Source configuration for the example ellipsoidal implant using the Memorial system.

of all of the basal doses forms *the* basal dose. The prescribed dose corresponds to a quantity called the reference dose, defined as

$$RD = 0.85 \, BD. \qquad (18)$$

Notice in Figure 19 that the reference dose extends *outside* the boundary limited by the implant needles. The Paris system also considers the volume raised to a "high dose" defined as twice the reference dose.

Due to the uniform activity along each line and the absence of crossing needles, the source material must extend *beyond* the target volume to provide adequate doses at the margin. The active length follows the general rule:

$$\text{Active length} = 1.43 \, \text{Target length}, \qquad (19)$$

although the actual factor varies from 1.54 for 1 cm lengths to 1.33 for 10 cm lengths. The definition of the treatment length has changed through the years from the minimum of the lengths to the average (Figure 19). The configuration for the needles in an implant depends on the number of planes.

Single Plane Implant for Thicknesses of <1.2 cm

The spacing between the lines for a single plane follows from the relationship between the treatment thickness and the interneedle spacing:

$$\text{Thickness} = 0.5 \, \text{Spacing for two}$$
$$\text{needle tracks}, \qquad (20a)$$
$$= 0.6 \, \text{Spacing for more than}$$
$$\text{two needle tracks}. \qquad (20b)$$

As with the treatment length, the definition of the treatment thickness has changed from the minimum of the thicknesses to their average (Figure 19).
Solving for the spacing gives:

$$\text{Spacing} = 2 \times \text{target thickness for}$$
$$\text{two needle tracks}, \qquad (21a)$$
$$= 1.67 \times \text{target thickness}$$
$$\text{for more than two}$$
$$\text{needle tracks}. \qquad (21b)$$

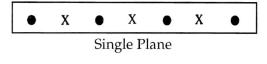

Single Plane

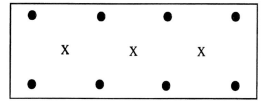

Two Planes - square configuration

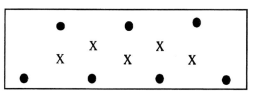

Two Planes - triangular configuration

● Catheter tracks
(into the page)

X Basal Dose Points

Figure 18. Some needle track arrangements and the associated basal dose points as per the Paris system.

Given a spacing, the treatment width becomes:

Treatment width = 1.75 Spacing for two

lines in a plane,   (22a)

= (N − 0.32)

Spacing for more

than two lines,   (22b)

where N = the number of needle tracks. Performing these calculations and solving for the number of needles gives

$$N = \frac{0.6 \cdot \text{(target width)}}{\text{thickness}} + 0.32. \quad (23)$$

Just as with the Manchester system, where the 1 cm spacing between needles yields only integer treatment widths, the treatment width in the Paris system usually exceeds the target width.

Following this spacing rule gives a lateral margin (the distance between the lateral most needle track and the lateral most extent of the treatment dose, as shown in Figure 19) of:

Lateral margin = 0.37 Spacing for two

needle tracks,   (24a)

and

= 0.34 Spacing for

more than

two needle tracks,   (24b)

In no case should the spacing between lines exceed 2.2 cm, limiting the high-dose volume to 1 cm diameter around a 10-cm long line. Although the system suggests a minimum separation of 1.2 cm, based on anatomical limitations and "what actually happens during the implant," needles may lie as close as 0.5 cm apart.

Two Plane Implants: For Thicknesses >1.2 cm

Two plane implants may either form patterns of squares or equilateral triangles. Again, the first step determines the spacing of the needle tracks based on the target thickness from the relationships:

Spacing ≅ 0.64 · (target thickness)

for square patterns   (25a)

≅ 0.77 · (target thickness)

for triangular patterns.   (25b)

With two plane implants, the relationships depend on whether the needle tracks form squares or triangles. The concept of *safety margin*, the average of the minimal distances between the needle boundary and the reference isodose line, replaces lateral margin, as illustrated in Figure 19, and varies with needle spacing as

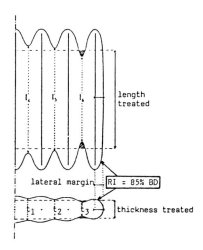

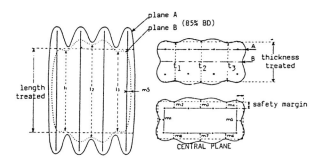

Figure 19. An illustration showing the relation between the reference dose to the implant geometry. (Reprinted with permission from Modern Brachytherapy by B. Pierquin, J.F. Wilson, D. Chassagne. Masson Publishing USA, Inc.)

Safety margin = 0.27 Spacing for square

patterns   (26a)

= 0.20 Spacing for triangular

patterns   (26b)

The authors of the system note that the margin on the lateral aspects of the implant usually are smaller than those on the other sides, and suggest that the implanted width should actually cover the target width.

Volume Implants

For cylinders, the Paris system recommends using not more than five needle tracks to form the peripheral surface of the cylinder (the belt in Manchester parlance) with no needle tracks in the interior. With a 2.1-cm spacing limitation, the maximum possible treatment diameter becomes 4 cm.

Examples

Turning again to the two plane implant example given above, the planes would probably take on a different appearance in the Paris system. For the 5-cm long, 4-cm deep, 2-cm thick target volume implanted in a square pattern, the spacing between needle tracks equals the separation between planes, and comes from Equation 25a. In this case, the spacing = 0.64x2 cm = 1.28 cm≈1.3 cm. With the safety margin of 0.27 cm around the implant, five needles would only cover

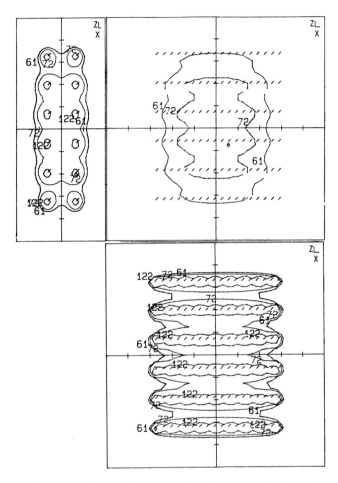

Figure 20. The two plane example considered previously, now worked as a Paris system implant: a) perpendicular to the planes through the middle of the implant; b) parallel to the planes midway between the planes; and c) parallel to the planes through a needle plane. The lines shown represent the basal dose, the reference dose, and the high-dose region.

$$(N - 1) \cdot 1.3 \text{ cm} + 2(0.27 \text{ cm}) = 4.74 \text{ cm} \tag{27a}$$

which fails to treat all of the target width. Thus, each plane requires six needle tracks, treating a width of approximately 6 cm. The length is 5.7 cm (4 cm/0.7), with the active ends extending 0.9 cm beyond the target volume.

Figure 20 shows the configuration. This implant has five basal dose points, each in the midplane centered between the squares formed by adjacent needle pairs, with doses as follow:

Point	Dose (Gy/hr)/(mCi/cm)
A	0.67
B	0.75
C	0.76
D	0.75
E	0.67
Average	0.72

While these values came from a computerized planning system, older Paris system references include figures (escargot curves) to assist in this calculation. Figure 20 displays the isodose curves in the central, transverse

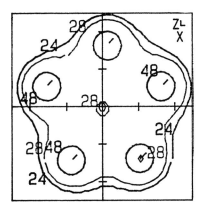

Figure 21. The isodose distribution in the mid-transverse cut for the example cylindrical volume implant as a Paris system implant.

plane, the midplane, and one of the implant planes, showing the basal isodose, reference isodose, and high-dose isodose lines. The reference isodose line corresponds to

$$0.85 \times 0.72 \ (Gy/hr)/(mCi/cm)$$
$$= 0.61 \ (Gy/hr)/(mCi/cm) \quad (27b)$$

To obtain a reference dose rate of 0.55 Gy/hr, the iridium wire's linear activity should be

$$(0.55 \ Gy/hr)/[0.61 \ (Gy/hr)/(mCi/cm)]$$
$$= 0.90 \ mCi/cm \quad (27c)$$

The total lengths of the 12 needles equals 68.4 cm. Thus, the total activity becomes 61.6 mCi.

For the example cylindrical implant used above (4 cm diameter, 4 cm long), the Paris system would use five needles only, in the configuration the Manchester system called the belt. Using the center of the implant as the basal dose point and experimentally placing the needle tracks at radii of 1.7 cm gave a reference isodose curve with minimum radii of 2 cm, thus covering the target volume in the central plane, as shown in Figure 21. The basal dose with this configuration equals 0.28 (Gy/hr)/(mCi/cm) and the reference dose 0.24 (Gy/hr)/(mCi/cm). The one basal dose point falls in the center of the implant and coincides with the minimum in the central transverse plane. In the longitudinal direction, the center forms the maximum with the

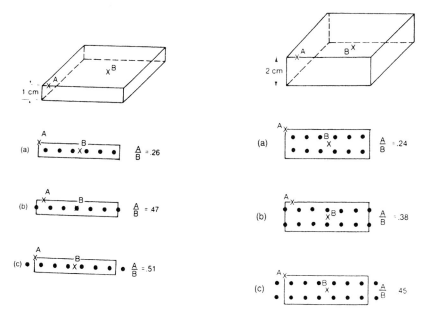

Figure 22. Illustration of the definition of the minimum (A) and maximum (B) target doses for a Kwan system implant: right. single plane; left. two plane. (Reprinted with permission from Kwan et al.)

dose falling toward the ends. A dose rate of 0.55 Gy/hr comes from a source strength of

$$\rho = (0.55 \text{ Gy/hr})/[0.24 \text{ (Gy/hr)}/(\text{mCi/cm})]$$
$$= 2.29 \text{ mCi/cm} \quad (27\text{d})$$

Kwan System

Noting that the Quimby system fails to address the minimum dose for planar implants, Kwan et al.[23] suggested a modification for use also with uniformly loaded planes. Kwan et al. particularly investigated Ir-192 seed implants, and defined two points of interest (Figure 22): A, the point of minimum dose in the target volume; and B, the point of maximum dose. Computer simulations established that the "uniformity," as measured by the ratio of A to B, improves when the outer most radioactive sources fall at the periphery of the target volume (configuration "b" in Figure 23)

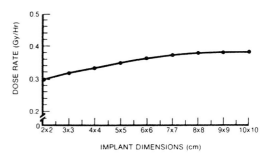

Figure 24. A graph giving the dose rate for a Kwan system, single plane implant as a function of planar area. (Reprinted with permission from Kwan et al.)

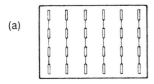

(a)

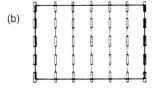

(b)

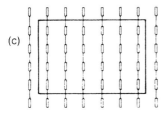

(c)

Figure 23. Three usual relationships between seed placement and target volumes for planar implants. (Reprinted with permission from Kwan et al.)

or beyond (configuration "c"); but because configuration c increases the doses outside of the target, the system uses configuration b. Based on the uniformity derived from the simulations, the system specifies the geometry for the seed placement as described in Table 12.

Figures 24 and 25 give the dose rate to the point of minimum dose in terms of (Gy/hr) for a 0.5-mg Ra eq seed strength, through a target thickness of 2 cm. For thicknesses of 2.5 cm, the dose rates for 2 cm thickness are multiplied by 0.87. For rectangular implants, the equivalent square formula from external beam therapy applies, where

$$\text{Equivalent square} = \frac{2 \cdot (\text{length} \times \text{width})}{(\text{length} + \text{width})}. \quad (28)$$

Applying this system to our two plane example (a target volume of 4 cm deep, 5 cm wide, and 2 cm thick) immediately forces a decision either to follow the separation guidance for needle tracks and implant a 4.5 cm width (configuration "a" in Figure 23) or 6 cm (configuration "c"), or follow the geometric guidance and use a needle track separation of 1 cm (configuration "b"). Following the separation guidance, the decision to implant 4.5 or 6 cm depends on the surrounding structures and the need to extend the treatment dose fully to the corner. Picking an implant width of 4.5 cm, each plane contains four needle tracks of five seeds each (which doesn't exactly follow configuration "a"),

Table 12.
Kwan System Seed Placement Geometry

Implant	Needle Track Separation (cm)	Source Separation (cm)	Plane Separation (cm)
Single plane (target thickness = 1 cm)	1	1	—
Two Plane (target thickness = 2–2.5 cm)	1.5	1	1.5

making no adjustment for the lack of crossing ends. From Figure 25, a square equivalent 4.4 cm field with 1.5 cm separation between needle tracks and 0.5 mg Ra eq seeds yields a minimum dose rate of 0.35 Gy/hr. To achieve a dose rate of 0.55 Gy/hr requires a seed strength of 0.786 mg Ra eq, for a total strength of 31.44 mg Ra eq.

Following configuration "b" uses six needle tracks per plane, with five seeds per track, for a total of 60 seeds. Again from Figure 25, the same equivalent square gives a minimum dose rate of 0.455 Gy/hr for 0.5-mg Ra eq seeds. To obtain the 0.55 Gy/hr dose rate takes 0.60-mg Ra eq seeds, for a total strength of 36.26-mg Ra eq.

Zwicker System

Similarly to the Kwan system, the Zwicker et al.[24] system addresses uniformly loaded, Ir-192 seed, planar implants. While the reference isodose surface in the Kwan system covers all of the rectangular, implanted volume, that dose surface also extends well beyond the target width in the middle of the implant. Since most tumors are roundish, Zwicker notes, extending the dose into the corners serves no therapeutic purpose. This system defines the reference isodose surface as shown in Figure 26. In Figures 26a and 26b, the reference isodose surface in the midplane coincides with the edge of the implanted volume in the middle of each edge. This system uses a 1 cm separation between needle tracks and also between seeds along a needle track for all implants in order to reduce the high-dose volume as compared to larger separations.

Two Plane Implants

The separation between planes depends on the area of the implanted planes, as given in Table 13. For rectangular implants, the equivalent square formula of Equation 28 gives the side of the square for the table, but

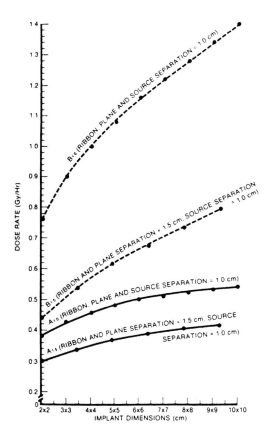

Figure 25. A graph giving the dose rate for a Kwan system, two plane implant as a function of planar area. (Reprinted with permission from Kwan et al.)

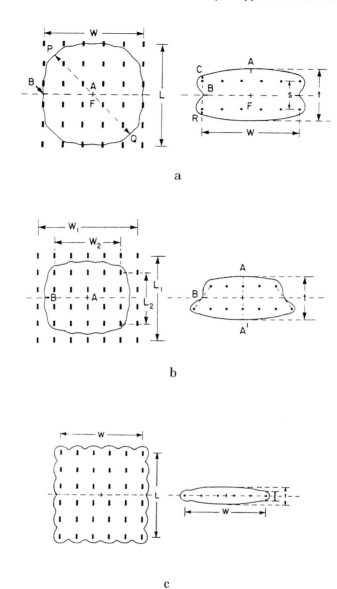

a

b

c

Figure 26. Dose specification points in the Zwicker system, for: a) two plane, square grid implant; b) two plane, triangular grid implant; and c) single plane implant. (Reprinted with permission from Zwicker et al.)

the separation between the planes should be reduced by 1 mm. The 1 mm reduction in the separation of the planes also applies for any implant where the two source planes have different dimensions (as in Figure 26b), in which case the equivalent square formula uses the average of the two lengths and the average of the two widths. Table 13 also gives the reference dose rate corresponding to a seed strength of 1 mCi. The example two plane implant studied previously (again, a target volume 4 cm deep, 5 cm wide, and 2 cm thick) with the Zwicker system, each of the source planes contain six needle tracks and each track carries five seeds. The table gives the separation for the 4.4-cm equivalent

Table 13.
Dose Rates (Ḋ) and Plane Separations (s) for Various Treatment-Volume Thickness (t) and Implant Areas (A), from Ir-192, Two-Plane Implants

t(cm)	2.0		2.5		3.0		3.5	
A (cm)	s	D	s	D	s	D	s	D
3 × 3	1.2	61	1.5	53	1.8	46	2.1	40
4 × 4	1.2	69	1.5	60	1.7	53	2.0	47
5 × 5	1.1	79	1.4	69	1.7	61	1.9	55
6 × 6	1.1	84	1.3	75	1.6	67	1.9	60
7 × 7	1.0	92	1.3	81	1.5	73	1.8	66
8 × 8	1.0	96	1.2	87	1.5	78	1.7	71
9 × 9	0.9	103	1.2	91	1.4	83	1.7	75
10 × 10	0.9	107	1.1	97	1.4	87	1.6	80

Double-plane implant, seed activity = 1.0 mCi.

Note 1: For rectangular implants, use equivalent square field size from formula:

$$\text{Eq. Sq.} = \frac{2 \cdot L \cdot W}{L + W}.$$

Note 2: For planes of different size, take average of linear dimensions (L and W) and use these in equivalent square formula.

Note 3: For either rectangular implants or planes of different size, reduce interplanar spacing by one millimeter.
A = implant dimensions (length L × width W); t = thickness of treatment volume; s = spacing between planes (cm); D = reference dose rate (cGy/hr) for seed activities of 1.0 mCi. Ribbon spacing = 1.0 cm, seed spacing = 1.0 cm.

square of 1.15 cm through interpolation. Because of the rectangular shape of the implant, as opposed to a square shape, the actual planar separation becomes 1.05 cm, which could be rounded to 1 cm. For this geometry, the tabulated dose rate equals 73 cGy/hr per mCi. The desired target dose rate of 0.55 Gy/hr requires

$$\text{Activity} = \frac{0.55 \text{ Gy/hr}}{0.73 \text{ Gy/hr}} \cdot \frac{1 \text{ mCi}}{\text{seed}}, \quad (29a)$$

$$= 0.75 \text{ mCi/seed}, \quad (29b)$$

$$= 0.42 \text{ mg Ra eq./seed}. \quad (29c)$$

The 60 seeds contain a total of 25.2-mg Ra eq.

Single Plane Implants

Since the system fixes the needle track separation at 1 cm for a given implanted area, changing only the source strength changes the distance the treatment length falls from the implant plane. Because of the uniform loading, the reference isodose surface bulges in the middle and narrows toward the edge. This is not necessarily bad; tumors may also follow this pattern. Table 14 gives the reference dose rate per mCi seed activity and the thickness of the treated volume at the edge of the implant as a function of the implant area and the target thickness.

With the Zwicker system, the example problem worked above could have been treated using a single plane. In this case, the seed strength becomes

$$\text{Strength} = \frac{0.55 \text{ Gy/hr}}{0.32 \text{ Gy/hr}} \quad (30)$$

$$\cdot \frac{1 \text{ mCi}}{\text{seed}} \cdot \frac{1 \text{ mg Ra eq.}}{1.79 \text{ mCi}}$$

$$= 0.96 \text{ mg Ra eq/seed}, \quad (30a)$$

for a total strength for all 30 seeds of 28.8-mg Ra eq. Table 14 also indicates that the implant provides a 1.4 thickness at the lateral edge.

Comparison of Systems

Because the different systems refer to doses at different locations and under different con-

Table 14.

Dose Rates ($\dot{D}$) and Lateral-Edge Thicknesses (z) for Various Treatment-Volume Thickness (t) and Implant Areas (A), from Ir-192, Single-Plane Implants

t(cm)	1.0		1.5		2.0		2.5	
A (cm)	$\dot{D}$	z	$\dot{D}$	z	$\dot{D}$	z	$\dot{D}$	z
3 × 3	41	0.8	32	1.1	26	1.6	21	2.0
4 × 4	46	0.7	37	1.1	30	1.5	25	1.9
5 × 5	52	0.6	43	1.0	35	1.3	30	1.7
6 × 6	55	0.5	46	0.9	39	1.2	33	1.6
7 × 7	60	0.5	50	0.8	43	1.1	37	1.5
8 × 8	63	0.4	53	0.8	46	1.1	40	1.4
9 × 9	66	0.3	56	0.7	49	1.0	43	1.3
10 × 10	—	—	59	0.7	51	1.0	45	1.3

Single-plane implant, seed activity = 1.0 mCi.

Note: For rectangular implants, use equivalent square field size from formula:

$$\text{Eq. Sq.} = \frac{2LW}{L + W}.$$

A = implant dimensions (length L × width W); t = treatment volume thickness at center (cm); z = treatment volume thickness at lateral edge; $\dot{D}$ = reference dose rate (cGy/hr) for seed activities of 1.0 mCi. Ribbon spacing = 1.0 cm, seed spacing = 1.0 cm.

ditions, comparing them is difficult at best and misleading at worst. Quimby[11] compared the Manchester and Quimby system for the total (mg · hr)/1000 R required for a specified dose for volume implants and found the ratio varied from a factor of 2 for small volumes to 1.31 for 150 cm[3]. Shalek, Stovall, and Sampiere[12] compared both systems to calculations they performed for regular lattices of seed sources, and found that their R_V values fell between those of the Manchester and Quimby systems for small implants, but followed closely the Manchester tables for larger volumes. Laughlin et al.[13] also compared several sets of tables, producing Figure 27. In these comparisons, the authors assumed that the configuration for all systems differed negligibly. Gillin et al.[25] compared the Manchester and Paris systems for the same target volumes, using implants appropriate for each system, and found that for the same activity on two planes, the nominal dose rate for the Manchester implant matched the basal dose rate for the Paris system. Such a match indicates that for the same *reference* dose, the Paris system would use more radioactive material by about 15%.

Comparison of implants performed using the different systems cannot consider only the activity used in each case, but must also consider the distribution of the dose. In the example considered by Gillin et al.,[25] both the dose through the volumes and the volumes treated by the two systems differed markedly. Still, it proves interesting to look at the total activity suggested by each system. Table 15 lists the total source activity from the examples included in the discussion of each system above.

A Final Word on Systems

With the exception of the Manchester system, each of the systems considered above specifically applies to uniformly loaded implants. This reflects the reality of the practice at the time of the system's creation. With LDR Ir-192 seeds, and particularly with HDR remote afterloaders, variation of the integrated source strength with position in the implant to produce a uniform dose distribution has become commonplace. The Paris system lends itself to modification for use with an optimized application. van der Laarse[26] describes such a modification called the Stepping Source Dosimetry System, where instead of just defining the doses in the central trans-

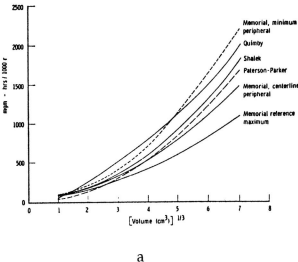

a

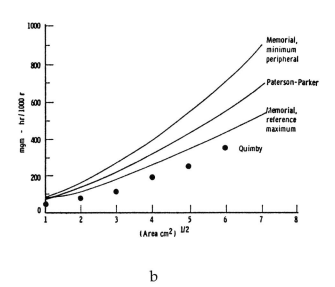

b

Figure 27. Comparisons of the mg·hr/1000 "r" specified by some interstitial implant systems for: a) volume implants (particularly using "seed" type sources); and b) planar implants. (Reprinted with permission from Laughlin et al.)

versal plane, basal dose points fill the treated volume. With optimization, the sources no longer must extend beyond the target volume. Other systems, such as the Quimby system, serve little purpose and offer no guidance for optimized treatments. The concepts of these systems are useful as a means of highlighting the practitioner's requirements and as a basis for discussion and comparison. The foregoing are systems for interstitial implants only. There are many systems for intracavitary insertions as well, particularly for the treatment of cervical cancer. Later chapters on the treatment sites will consider these.

Table 15.
Source Strengths for the Systems Considered for the Example Cases

System	Source Strength for the Example		
	Two-plane Implant (mg Ra eq./0.55 Gy/hour)	Cylindrical Implant	Permanent Ellipsoid (mCi ^{198}Au)
Manchester	31.4	30.76	23.3
Quimby	22.4	42.9	34.0
Memorial			30.5
Paris	34.4	36.5	
Kwan	36.3 (31.4)		
Zwicker	25.2		

Dose Specification and Prescription

Dose specification for brachytherapy is far from standardized. The above discussion of the various dosimetry systems lists various studies that found different systems to yield different numerical results. In a study of clinical practice in the United States, Olch et al.[27] report differences in dose prescription (specification) that differs by as much as a factor of 3 for treatment of the same clinical target. It appears important that some efforts be made to standardize the specification and reporting of dose in brachytherapy.

The American Endocurietherapy Society (now the American Brachytherapy Society) published a standard in 1991.[28] The ICRU has recently completed a report on "Dose and Volume Specification for Reporting Interstital Therapy," due to be published soon. The philosophy of the ICRU report can be summarized in the following statements:

1. Clinicians should *not* change their present implant practices; however, they should adopt the ICRU notations and report implant doses and volumes following the ICRU recommendations.
2. More than one dose value is necessary to adequately describe the dose distribution from an implant.
3. Not all clinics have the same degree of calculation sophistication, so a hierarchy of parameters to report are specified in the ICRU report.
4. In brachytherapy the dose distribution includes steep dose gradients, particularly near each source. However, there are regions within the target volume where the dose distribution approximates a plateau.
5. To provide the minimum dose distribution information, isodose distributions should be presented in at least one plane, the plane through approximately the center of the implant perpendicular to the main direction of the sources. This plane is referred to as the central plane.
6. To properly compare implants from different institutions using different "systems," dose should be specified and reported in a systematic manner.
7. A region of plateau dose (low-dose gradient) is a place where the dose can be calculated reproducibly and compared easily by different facilities.

Four dose related terms are described in the protocol: peripheral dose, mean central dose, high-dose regions, and low-dose regions. Two dose homogeneity indices are also described.

Peripheral Dose is the minimum dose at the periphery of the clinical target volume and should be the minimum dose decided upon by the clinician as adequate to treat the target. This dose is similar to the typical "prescribed dose" used by many American clinicians.

A Low-Dose Region is a region within the clinical target volume where the dose is <90% of the peripheral dose. The maximum dimensions of this volume are reported. This obviously relates to an underdosed volume of the target and so should correlate with treatment failure.

A High-Dose Region should correlate with complications. The high-dose region is defined as the volume encompassed by the isodose line equal to 150% of the mean central dose. The maximum dimensions of this volume in all planes calculated should be reported.

The Mean Central Dose is defined as the arithmetic mean of the local minimum doses between all adjacent sources in the implant. This concept approximates the basal dose in the Paris system.

It is intuitively obvious that the dose halfway between two equal strength brachytherapy sources is the dose minimum. Likewise as seen in Figure 28, for three equal strength

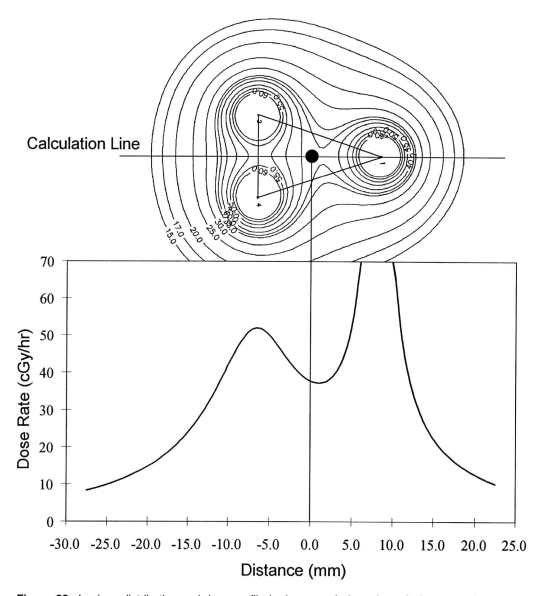

Figure 28. Isodose distribution and dose profile in the central place through three equal strength, 5 cm long Ir-192 sources. The region of low-dose gradient between the three sources is obvious from the isodose distribution and shown quantitatively in the dose profile.

sources forming a triangle, the dose minimum passes through the geometric center of the triangle (the intersection of the perpendicular bisectors of the sides of the triangle). In practice, to account for unequal weighting of sources or the presence of other sources in the implant, the mean central dose is determined by the arithmetic mean of the dose halfway between adjacent source lines in the implant, considering the dose contribution from all sources. For multiple plane implants, the mean central dose is the arithmetic mean of the local minimum doses between each set of three adjacent source lines within the implant. Three practical methods are described for determining the mean central dose. These include:

1. Identification of local minimum doses. For implants with nearly parallel lines in the central plane, identify all triangles formed by the source lines, choosing as many acute triangles as possible. The mean of the doses at the centroids of such triangles is the mean central dose.

2. Evaluation of dose profiles. Calculate dose profiles along one or more lines expected to pass as close as possible to expected dose minimum. Obtain the dose minima by inspection and form the mean of the local minimum doses. This may be the preferred method for permanent seed implants.

3. Inspection of dose distribution. An isodose distribution is plotted in 5%–10% (relative dose) increments in the central plane. The local minimum dose between adjacent sources can be

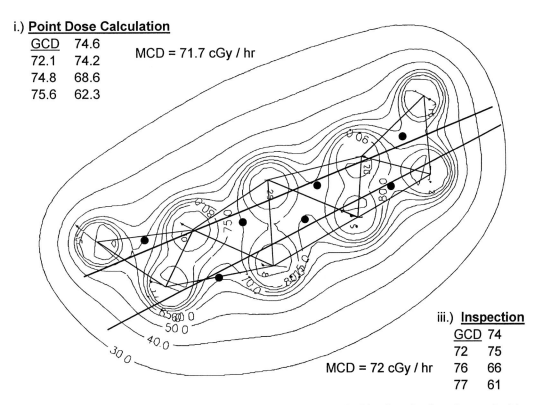

i.) Point Dose Calculation

GCD	74.6
72.1	74.2
74.8	68.6
75.6	62.3

MCD = 71.7 cGy / hr

MCD = 72 cGy / hr

iii.) Inspection

GCD	74
72	75
76	66
77	61

Figure 29. Isodose distribution in the central plane of a typical double plane implant (breast, in this case). The choice of triangles formed by the source lines is shown. The large dots represent the geometric centers of the triangles where the local minimum doses are determined. The two dose calculation lines shown are adequate to pass near all of the geometric centers. The local dose minima and mean values obtained are shown for methods i. and iii.).

observed by inspection and the mean formed.

An example of a two plane breast implant is shown in Figures 29 and 30. All three methods of estimating the mean central dose are included. All three methods achieve the same value within 5%.

Two dose homogeneity parameters are also proposed by the ICRU: The *spread* in the individual local minimum doses (expressed as a percent of the mean central dose) and the ratio of the peripheral dose to the mean central dose. The first gives a measure of nonuniformity within the implant and may be a measure of how well the implant was accomplished. The second is related to proper spacing of the source lines relative to the peripheral "reach" of the implant.

The ICRU report cautions that each of the dose definitions has been used in some form, but the combination has not been extensively clinically tested. Therefore, clinicians are encouraged not to change their methods of prescribing dose but rather to perform the dose calculations specified by the ICRU in addition to present methods. These reported values would provide a uniform dose specification system for interstitial implants.

Dosimetry I: Calculation Algorithm

Basic Algorithms

Dose rate to a point in tissue from a number of discrete radioactive seeds can be expressed as the sum of the dose rates to that point from each of the individual seeds. This assumes that the interseed effect of one source absorbing and scattering radiations from another may be neglected. Dose-rate computation is based on tables of dose-rate distribution for standard strength brachytherapy sources, and the calculation is reduced to providing seed strengths and standard dose-rate tables to a computer program. For each calculation point, a computer program sums the contribution to the dose rate from each source.

Traditionally, a one-dimensional approximation for relative dose rate has been used for seed sources. In this approximation, the dose rate per unit seed strength depends only on the distance to the center of the seed. For

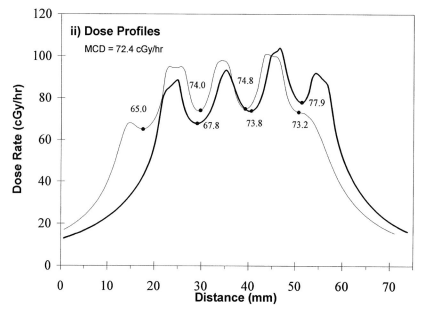

Figure 30. Dose profile along the two calculation lines in the central plane through the implant in Figure 29. The local dose minima taken from the curves are listed.

gynecological intracavitary applications, however, extended linear sources, typically 0.5- to 3-cm active length encapsulated tubes or needles of Ra-226 or Cs-137, have been used. Clinical dose-rate calculations for these sources are generally based on the use of tables of two-dimensional relative dose-rate distributions for each source.

Conventional Point Source Model

The traditional point source approximation for the dose rate at a distance r from a brachytherapy source is given by[29]

$$\dot{D}(r) = A_{app} \cdot \Gamma \cdot f_{med} \cdot (1/r^2) \cdot T(r) \cdot \phi_{an} \tag{31}$$

where
A_{app} is the apparent activity of the source (mCi),
Γ is the specific gamma ray constant for the radioactive species contained in the source, $(R\ cm^2\ mCi^{-1}\ h^{-1})$,
$T(r)$ is the tissue scatter attenuation factor, defined by the ratio

$$\frac{\text{exposure in tissue}}{\text{exposure in air}} = \frac{\text{dose rate in tissue}}{\text{dose rate in free space}} \tag{32}$$

at distance r from the point source, along the transverse axis of the seed,
f_{med} is the tissue-kerma to exposure ratio,

$$0.876 \frac{(\mu_{en}/\rho)_{med}}{(\mu_{en}/\rho)_{air}} \text{ cGy/R} \tag{33}$$

where $(\mu_{en}/\rho)_{med}$ is the mass energy absorption coefficient for the tissue medium. The number 0.876 is equal to the air-kerma in cGy per roentgen exposure.
ϕ_{an} is the anisotropy constant, defined as the dose rate at some reference distance averaged over all directions, divided by the dose rate at the same distance along the transverse axis of the seed. The reference distance is generally taken to be 1 cm.

If the seed were truly a point source, then ϕ_{an} would be identically equal to 1 by definition, and no reference to direction relative to the seed would be required in the definition of $T(r)$. We see that the conventional point source methodology does partially account for anisotropy through the use of an average correction factor to determine the effective source strength. In this conventional approach, if $\phi_{an}<1$ the actual dose rate along the transverse direction from a seed is larger than the nominal dose rate given by Equation 31.

The most commonly used data for the scatter attenuation factor of seeds of Au-198, Ir-192, Cs-137, Ra-226, and Co-60 for the point source model are those for water given by Meisberger et al.[30] in 1968. Meisberger et al.[30] expressed $T(r)$ as a third order polynomial of the distance. Some more recent data calculated by Monte Carlo methods are available, including data for different media.[31–33]

A problem that has been noted with the traditional point source model expressed by Equation 31 is that the dose rate is expressed in terms of the quantities A_{app}, Γ, and f_{med}, all of which refer to an idealized source rather than to an actual seed design. Thus, actual source geometry, encapsulation, and calibration methodology are not taken into account by the traditional formalism. Furthermore, according to the recommendations of American Association of Physicists in Medicine (AAPM) Report 21, source strength calibrations should be specified in terms of the air-kerma rate rather than in terms of activity.[34]

Another problem with the traditional point source model is the markedly anisotropic distribution of the radiations from some low energy radiation seed sources, even small radionuclide seeds, such as those of model 6702 and model 6711 I-125 seed designs. These anisotropies can be significant, particularly in specialized treatment planning applications such as ophthalmic plaque dosimetry.[35] To take these asymmetries into account, the traditional spherically symmetric point source model for seeds (Equation 31) must be replaced by a two-dimensional model. Since seeds are manufactured with an axis of symmetry, a two-dimensional model is sufficient.

Conventional Line Source Models

The dose rate $\dot{D}(x,y)$ from a cylindrically symmetric brachytherapy source at distance x in the direction along the symmetry axis of the source, and distance y in the direction perpendicular to the axis is given by

$$\dot{D}(x,y) = A_{app} \cdot R(x,y) \qquad (34)$$

where A_{app} has the same meaning as in Equation 31, and $R(x,y)$ is the dose rate at point (x,y) from a source of unit activity. The relative dose distribution, $R(x,y)/R(x_o,y_o)$ for some reference point (x_o,y_o) is frequently modeled as the distribution from a filtered line source, specifically as the integral of the attenuated primary fluence over the length of the source. The primary fluence from a differential line segment is proportional to its activity multiplied by the attenuation factor multiplied by $1/r^2$. For each photon energy in the energy spectrum of the source, the integral of this quantity for direct attenuation along a slant path along the line of sight through an effective encapsulation thickness gives rise to a Sievert integral. The attenuation factor in this case is $\exp(-\mu t/\cos\theta)$, where μ is the linear attenuation coefficient, t is the effective wall thickness, and θ is the angle between the line of sight direction and the direction of the transverse to the seed axis. Since not all interactions in the wall result in the complete absorption of the energy of the photon, it has been conventional to use μ_{en}, the linear energy absorption coefficient, instead of μ, the linear attenuation coefficient.[36] Tables of Sievert integrals over different ranges of the angle θ for various values of the attenuation parameter μt are given by Shalek and Stovall.[36] A computer program can readily be devised to use these tables of the Sievert integral for a particular tube or needle design to calculate the two-dimensional function $R(x,y)$ in Equation 34.

A more sophisticated model for $R(x,y)$ could be devised by introducing the previously discussed point source scatter attenuation factor, $T(r)$ of Equation 31, as a factor under the integral sign. The resulting expression would not be a Sievert integral, but individual seed designs could readily be calculated numerically by computer.

The data for $R(x,y)$ can in principle, be measured, although practical difficulties make it difficult to achieve measurements within a few millimeters of the source. A Monte Carlo model calculation does not have this limitation. The Monte Carlo is needed to take into account the multiple secondary electrons and photons produced in the medium by the primary radiations of the physical source. Williamson[37] has tabulated Monte Carlo calculated values for $R(x,y)$ for several designs of Cs-137 sources.

AAPM TG-43 Recommended Dose Computation Model

There is a need to standardize available dosimetry information about brachytherapy sources, particularly for use in computer dose-rate calculations. Partly in response to the perception of this need, a formalism has emerged that takes into account the detailed measured and calculated properties of standard brachytherapy seeds. The new formalism is a convenient method for including the effect of nonisotropic radiations of the radioactive seeds used for brachytherapy.

Following the recommendations of AAPM Report 21, the formalism refers to source strength only in terms of air-kerma rate, which is directly measurable.[34] Absolute dose rate in tissue is obtained from source strength by reference to a dose-rate constant λ. The quantity λ, which is different for different media, represents the dose rate to a tissue like medium at a standard distance ($r_o = 1$ cm) from a standard practical source of known strength. λ is measurable in principle.

The new formalism is expressed in Equation 35 below. The two-dimensional dose rate is broken down into the product of several quantities. One quantity, $G(r,\theta)$, called the geometry factor, is a function representing the behavior of an idealized geometric source. This factor describes the approximate effect of the inverse square behavior for the contributions to dose rate from the individual volume elements in the source. The geometry factor neglects photon absorption and scatter both in the source and in the medium. For a point source, this is $1/r^2$. For a line source of length L, the geometry factor turns out to be $\beta/(Lr\sin\theta)$, where b is the angle subtended by the active source with respect to the point (r,θ) (Figure 31).

The utility of extracting the geometry factor is that the remaining factors more closely represent any special character of the particular seed design. The neglect of scatter and absorption in the idealized geometric source is for the purpose of simplicity. The residual

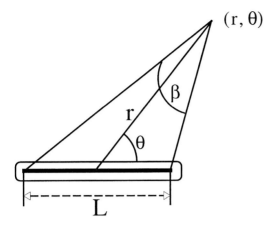

(r, θ)

Figure 31. Graphical representation of the coordinate system showing (r, θ), the point for which the dose rate is calculated. The distance from the calculation point to the center of the line source of active length L, is shown as r.; β is the angle subtended at point (r, θ) by the line source. The geometry factor for a line source is $\beta/(Lr \sin\theta)$. The geometry factor is $1/r^2$ for a point source.

two-dimensional dose distribution is described by the product of the radial dose function g(r), and an anisotropy function, $F(r, \theta)$. The dose rate at the point (r, θ) is given by[29]:

$$\dot{D}(r, \theta) = S_k \cdot \Lambda \cdot \frac{G(r, \theta)}{G(r_0, \theta_0)} \cdot g(r) \cdot F(r, \theta)$$

(35)

where S_K is air-kerma strength of the source in $U(cGy\ cm^2\ h^{-1})$, Λ is the dose-rate constant for the source in tissue medium in $(cGy\ h^{-1}\ U^{-1})$, $G(r, \theta)$ is a purely geometrical factor that describes the dependence of the dose rate on the distribution of radioactive material, ignoring scatter and attenuation. This quantity is defined as the volume averaged distribution of radioactive material, weighted by the inverse square factor. G has the dimensions of $1/(distance)^2$. $g(r)$ is the radial dose function (dimensionless) normalized so that $g(r_0) = 1$, where r_0 is a standard reference distance, universally taken to be 1 cm. $F(r, \theta)$ is a dimensionless anisotropy function, that describes the angular dependence of the dose rate, with the geometry factor $G(r, \theta)$ extracted, normalized so that $F(r, \theta_0) = 1$.

The dimensionless radial dose function g(r)

represents the dependence on distance for $\theta = \pi/2$, after the geometry factor has been extracted. This factor is determined by the photon energy spectrum of the source and the material of the medium. This can be calculated for all sources and media by Monte Carlo methods. This function corresponds to T(r), the Meisberger polynomial, in the traditional dose calculation formalism.

The anisotropy function, $F(r, \theta)$, is a dimensionless function of the angle variable, θ, the angle between the seed axis and the line joining the center of the seed with the calculation point (r, θ) (Figure 31). $F(r, \theta)$ is normalized so that $F(r, \theta_0) = 1$. By convention and by symmetry for a cylindrical source, this direction is taken to be transverse to the seed axis of symmetry, i.e., $\theta_0 = \pi/2$.

The isotropic point source approximation has wide practical utility, and the point source model may be adequate for many, or even most clinical dose calculations. The two-dimensional model contains this as a special case, viz., $G(r, \theta) = 1/r^2$, $F(r, \theta) = 1$.

A spherically symmetric approximation that nevertheless allows for an averaged anisotropy that can depend on r may be written as[29]

$$\dot{D}(r, \theta) = S_k \cdot \Lambda \cdot r^{-2} \cdot g(r) \cdot \phi_{an}(r) \quad (36)$$

where $\phi_{an}(r)$ is the anisotropy factor averaged over all solid angles

$$\phi_{an}(r) = \frac{\int \dot{D}(r, \theta) \sin\theta\ d\theta}{2\dot{D}(r, \theta_0)} \quad (37)$$

where the integration is over the range 0 to π.

Tables of the anisotropy function $F(r, \theta)$, the radial dose function g(r), and the anisotropy factor $\phi_{an}(r)$, for Ir-192, I-125 (models 6702 and 6711), and Pd-103 are given in reference 29 for Solid Water as a medium, taken from measurements reported by Nath et al.[38] Monte Carlo calculated radial dose functions g(r) for liquid water are given by Williamson for Ir-192 and I-125, and by Luxton for I-125 and Pd-103.[31,33]

Tissue Effects and Inhomogeneities

The dose rate in tissue differs from the idealized formula of Equation 34 in several ways: 1) tissue is not an infinite medium and the dose rate may be decreased from that due to the relative lack of full scatter; 2) different tissues are characterized by different dose-rate constants and different radial dose functions g(r), particularly for low energy isotopes such as I-125 and Pd-103; and 3) tissues are not homogeneous. These issues are generally not addressed at present in routine clinical treatment planning calculations.

Localized shielding may be introduced to provide differential radioprotection near the target volume, such as in the relatively standard use of ovoid shields in gynecological brachytherapy to provide some sparing of the rectum and bladder. Measurement of the dosimetric effects of these shields have been reported by Mohan et al.[39] Prasad, Bassano, and Kubsad[40] have measured the effect of 2-cm thick slabs of different materials on the dose rate at a distance of 5 cm from a Cs-137 source. Meigooni and Nath[41] have developed measurement data and a model for the effect of uniform cylindrically symmetric inhomogeneities. Williamson et al.[42,43] have proposed an analogue to the scatter summation algorithm familiar from external beam dose calculations as an approach to a general methodology for dealing with localized inhomogeneities. These efforts to deal with the general problem of tissue heterogeneities may lead to algorithms that will enable brachytherapy dose calculations of the future to routinely include the effects of shielding and inhomogeneities, thereby making possible more quantitatively informed evaluation of clinical treatment plans.

Dose and Treatment Duration

After the dose rate from a source configuration is established, the problem usually becomes determining the treatment duration. Generally, the following equation relates the dose and the dose rate:

$$D = \int_{t=0}^{t} \dot{D} \cdot dt \qquad (38)$$

where $t = 0$ represents the time when the source or sources first come into position (usually source insertion for LDR brachytherapy). The general solution for this expression,

assuming only exponential decay of the source activity as a cause of change in the dose rate becomes

$$D = \frac{\dot{D}_0}{\lambda} (1 - e^{\lambda t}) \qquad (39)$$

where $\dot{D}_o$ = the initial dose rate (the dose rate at time $t = 0$), and

$$\lambda = \frac{0.693}{T_{1/2}} \qquad (40)$$

and $T_{1/2}$ signifies the half-life of the isotope used. Equation 39 applies directly when using Ir-192 over durations of longer than about 5 days, after which the dose rate has decreased by approximately 5% from the initial dose rate. The delivery of most brachytherapy takes place over durations that simplify Equation 39:

1. Durations that are very short with respect to the isotopic half-life. Treatments using Cs-137 over a period of a week, or HDR treatments using Ir-192 lasting a few minutes fall into this category. In this case, the $1 - e^{\lambda t}$ factor becomes, to the first order, λt, and the equation for the dose

$$D = \dot{D}_0 t \qquad (41)$$

2. Permanently implanted sources. Permanently implanted sources assume delivery of the dose through the decay of all of the radioactive nuclei implanted, i.e., as the treatment time becomes very much longer than the half-life of the isotope. In this case, the exponential term goes to zero, and Equation 39 becomes

$$D = \frac{\dot{D}_0}{\lambda} . \qquad (42)$$

HDR units warrant special consideration. While the movement of LDR sources into position usually takes <0.1% of the treatment duration, the 4–8 seconds required for an HDR source to come to the dwell positions may equal several percent of the total dwell time. The dose delivered during this transit depends strongly on the geometry of the applications and the distance from the applicator to the point of interest. Houdek et al.[44] and Bastin et al.[45] assessed the dose under several situations. For the most part, the transit dose becomes significant only for implants with large numbers of catheters, such as a template, and then mostly for low target doses. It is harder to generalize about the doses delivered by the source moving between dwell positions because different units treat this time differently; and, if the dwell positions remain relatively close, the dose during the movement closely resembles the planned dose and the time often becomes incorporated into the dwell time of the position to which the source moves.

Dosimetry II: Three-Dimensional Planning

Benefit of Three Dimensions over Two Dimensions

The potential benefit of three-dimensional planning is that of more accurate and obvious characterization of the dose distribution with respect to the target volume and normal tissues at risk than with two-dimensional planning. This improved characterization may result not only in better tumor control but also a lower probability of complications. The documentation and further analysis of a patient data base using volumetric three-dimensional dose analysis should result in better protocols for effective therapy and a better understanding of dose related responses.

Implementation of Three-Dimensional Treatment Planning

Some noteworthy articles on the implementation of three-dimensional treatment planning include: Warszawski et al.[46] describing a technique to combine two-dimensional film and three-dimensional CT for HDR and external beam; McShan et al.[47] describing an integrated brachytherapy three-dimensional treatment planning system; and Ayyangar et al.[48] describing a comprehensive planning system for external beam and three-dimensional brachytherapy. The application of three-dimensional techniques for brachytherapy involves three-dimensional: 1) displays; 2) coregistration; 3) optimization; and 4) special calculation/analysis methods as described below.

Three-Dimensional Displays

One of the major advantages of three-dimensional planning systems over two-dimensional systems is the ability to visualize the relative orientations of the radioactive sources, applicators, target and critical structures, and isodose surfaces in three dimensions, and to manipulate the objects on the computer terminal for viewing from any direction. This requires highly interactive computer hardware and software with special graphics capabilities.

Hardware Requirements. In addition to a fast CPU (Central Processing Unit), large memory, and adequate disk space, three-dimensional display requires special graphics hardware, a graphics board, and a color monitor that can display each pixel (picture element) in color (typically 1280x1024 graphics resolution). In true color mode, this means 24 bit planes arranged as 8 bits per color for the three primary colors, i.e., red, green, and blue, which when mixed can give 16.7 million color combinations. Display of pixels is not adequate by itself; the hardware must be able to quickly calculate the pixel values of a scene and send that information to the display board as three-dimensional vectors (lines) and polygons. In radiation therapy and other scientific visualization, one can measure the graphics performance by how fast one can render, rotate, and manipulate the objects in three dimensions that involves thousands of pixels per second.

Software Methods. To use the special graphics hardware for radiation therapy, one needs to adapt the data into a displayable format. In one method, target contours are drawn on transverse images on the computer screen or digitized from films and other relevant structures (outer contour or skin), arranged according to the z-values (defined in the superior to inferior direction of patient) and connected by tiling or triangulation.[48]

The x, y, and z coordinates of all contour points and the tiling scheme are stored as a file on disk, called the geometry file. The graphics programs written for visualization display the geometry files and render the triangles in color, giving them a three-dimensional appearance. The programs manipulate the data using a mouse or a knob-box along with several other geometry files. Thus, moving the mouse or rotating a knob translates or rotates the object in real time on the screen.

Three-Dimensional Coregistration

The tumor outlines are not always fully differentiated in any particular imaging modality; therefore, information from different sources has to be combined for accurate description. Coregistration allows the combining of the results of different imaging modalities. Typically, target and critical structures from MRI can be transferred to a CT image set that has the skin and other structures digitized. Coregistration is usually accurate enough if the relative positions of all structures involved in both the sets overlie. Coregistration works well in the head (a relatively rigid frame). However, the spatial distortion from MRI can introduce error. Coregistration in the abdomen requires more care and always involves some error due to movement of the soft tissue.

It is not entirely necessary to have the digital images from all modalities in the computer. For example, it is possible to digitize contours outlined on film and then to coregister with other data. Coregistration between two image sets of data from different modalities can be performed: 1) in visual graphics; or 2) by computation and minimization of the differences between a set of variables that define the agreement of the two sets. In the visual graphics technique[48] the two object sets represented by two geometry sets are matched by translating and rotating one object with respect to the other. The transformation coordinates are obtained, and a new object is created using the translation and rotation parameters. The computational method minimizes the mean distance between the two sets.[49] In addition to the translation and rotation, one needs to correct for distortion.

Three-Dimensional Plan Optimization

Extensive literature exists for optimization in three dimensions and this is addressed elsewhere in the chapter. Annweiler et al.[50] and Niemierko et al.[51] address optimization methods specifically for three-dimensional brachytherapy treatment planning. Three-dimensional plan optimization provides important information before the patient undergoes irradiation. For example, for a brain implant, a preplan is usually needed to order the radioactive material, catheters, and other apparatus. This order is based upon available diagnostic information. Preplan information can also be obtained using nomograms; however, the approach and the number of catheters that can be physically placed sometimes require a preplan. On the day of the implant, another plan with optimization is needed either before or after the catheters are placed. A post-implant dose calculation is needed for dose-rate prescription and analysis. Typical methodology used for brain implants is described by Ayyangar et al.[52]

Special Calculation/Analysis Methods

Three-dimensional dose calculations can be performed for a set of two-dimensional matrices or a single three-dimensional matrix. The dose thus calculated is used to display isodose surfaces or calculate dose volume histograms (DVH). In some instances, calculations are performed in three dimensions for plan optimization. Also, it is possible to take all the dose volume information and analyze it with a radiobiological model, as demonstrated by Ling et al.[53] A scatter subtraction model for heterogeneity correction of brachytherapy has been developed by Williamson et al.[54] One method (used by Ayyangar) to calculate DVH using multiple two-dimensional sections follows:

1. Choose a dose matrix size to enclose the structure (target or any structure) in all planes and calculate the dose throughout the matrix. To save computational time, dose can be calculated in a relatively larger grid interval, typically a 2–5 mm increment in brachytherapy.
2. Select a dose matrix for any or each

plane of calculation and the corresponding structure contour. Interpolate the dose matrix to a matrix with a 1-mm interval.

3. Check every point in the interpolated dose matrix to see if the structure encloses the point. If the point is within the contour, increment the corresponding DVH dose bin by 1 count. The LDR DVH dose bin size is typically 1 cGy/hr, and the dose search is conducted from 1–200 cGy/hr.
4. Repeat the steps 2 and 3 for all planes.
5. Normalize the dose bins by the total number of points in the entire structure to represent 100% volume. The dose bins can be integrated to generate integral DVH. An advantage of this method is that it is not sensitive to the slice-to-slice distance, as long as the distance remains uniform throughout the structure.

The smaller the number of points in the contours and the smaller the number of planes in which the contours are drawn, the faster the DVH calculation. Typically, the calculation of DVH for a brain target drawn in ten slices takes <1 minute with the current hardware (ARDENT1500) at the institution of one of the authors (Medical College of Ohio, Toledo).

Examples

The following clinical examples illustrate the importance of three dimensions in brachytherapy.

Brain Implant with I-125

Brain implants commonly use temporary placement of HDR I-125 seeds, although some other isotopes (Pd-103, Ir-192) also find use. Three-dimensional planning of brain

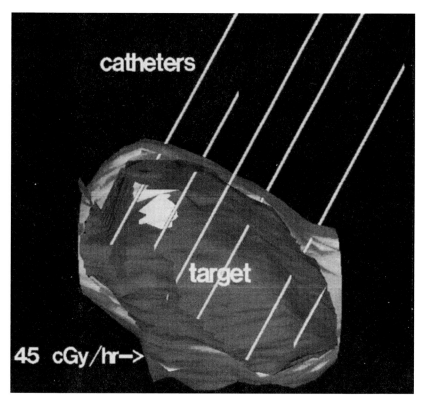

Figure 32. A three-dimensional representation of brain implant showing target, catheters, and a 45 cGy/hr dose surface. Notice that the dose coverage to posterior region is tight.

implants requires specialized computer software (Ayyangar et al.,[52] Ten Haken et al.[55]). Brachytherapy optimization differs from external beam therapy optimization and is somewhat more complex due to each source of radiation having a location dictated by three position parameters, viz. x, y, and z, as well as a source intensity. In addition, one needs to optimize on the number of catheters used and the needle direction. Few studies have been done on optimization of brain implants (see Bauer-Kirpes et al.[56] for an example). Planning and optimizing remains difficult and developmental.[57]

Figure 32 shows a brain implant case. The target volume is derived from CT scans. The figure shows the catheters, target volume, and the 45 cGy/hr isodose rate surface in three dimensions. It can be seen that the coverage of this isodose rate surface around the target nearly conforms to the shape of the target volume. Although better coverage is obtained with a lower isodose rate surface that covers the posterior part of the target volume, this isodose rate surface was selected by the physician to avoid hot spots in the target volume. An interactive program displays the information in real time. It should be noted that some institutions use a very small number of higher activity seeds (as high as 40 mCi) and hence

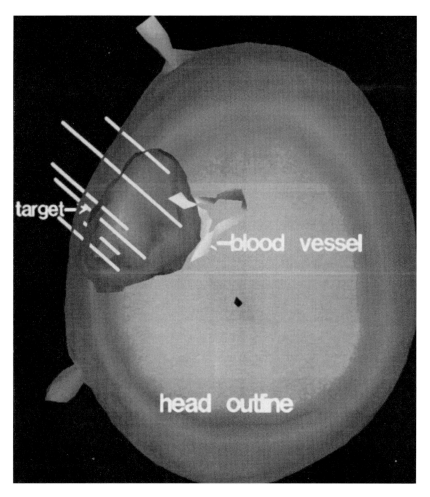

Figure 33. A typical brain implant demonstrating the ability to place catheters optimally in target while avoiding critical structures.

treat to a combination of nearly spherical volumes. The example shown, however, is an example of conformal brachytherapy, somewhat similar to multi-isocentric radiosurgery.

One of the advantages of three-dimensional planning over two-dimensional is that the coverage of a given isodose rate surface can be assessed quickly and a prescription dose rate selected. Another advantage is that critical structures can be outlined and avoided. Figure 33 shows a blood vessel that has been outlined. The placement of catheters is designed to avoid hitting the blood vessel while planning the radiation to conform to the target volume.

Floor of the Mouth Implant

Parsai et al.[58] give an example of a recurrent cancer in the gingiva treated using a specially fabricated dental acrylic appliance. In this example, a replica of the floor of the mouth, gums, and teeth was constructed using a hydrocolloidal impression material. To localize the surface and periphery of the tumor, four metal wires 0.5 cm long were embedded in the fabricated appliance. The appliance was molded to hold Ir-192 wires in near-contact with the target surface and to allow afterloading. A specially designed lead shield was embedded onto the dorsal surface of the appliance to reduce dose to the tongue and maxillary structures of the mouth. CT scans and simulation films were obtained to digitize the location of all structures and catheters. Three-dimensional treatment planning was used to generate isodose distributions and to allow preplanning. The dose calculation algorithm was modified to account for the attenuation of the lead shield. For each point of calculation, the path length of the radiation emanating from each seed is followed; if the ray intercepts the lead shield, the calculation includes the attenuation factor based on that path length through the shield. This calculation ignores scatter changes, but developing algorithms could include this component of the dose. This method of calculation produces an accurate and effective means to display the dose delivered to the target volume as well as to partially shielded critical normal structures as shown in Figure 34.

In contrast, two-dimensional methods allow one to calculate dose to some specific points. In this example the attenuating effect of the irregular lead could be approximated only by visually determining if the ray to the point of calculation is intercepted by the lead shield.

Ir-192 Implantation for Head and Neck

Hayes et al.[59] reported using CT and three-dimensional planning for Ir-192 for head and neck implants. They described a technique of using simulation film derived source positions and isodose distributions superimposed on CT images. Figure 35 shows the orthogonal images for a treatment of a recurrent squamous cell carcinoma of the neck from the Medical College of Ohio. The dosimetric reconstruction of the implant was obtained using orthogonal films. Subsequently, the patient underwent CT examination. The 6 cm x 4 cm x 3 cm implant was afterloaded using 12 Ir-192 ribbons of 1.0 mCi/cm linear activity. The catheter locations on CT images were digitized on all contiguous slices using special software that joins each end of the catheter segment to the corresponding segment on the adjoining CT slice. Since it is necessary to account for the catheter sections that were not loaded, the film derived sources were coregistered with the catheter segments from CT. Thus, the radioactive segments were identified on CT slices, and the dose was calculated in three dimensions. Figure 36 shows a CT image with isodose rates displayed. Figure 37 shows a three-dimensional representation of the implant with the 50 cGy/hr dose-rate surface, the radioactive source segments, and the outer surface of patient's neck. The three-dimensional distribution allows better visualization of the dose to the critical structures and facilitates dose summation with external beams.

Breast Implant Using Ir-192 Ribbons

Some institutions routinely use Ir-192 breast implants with catheters placed at the time of lumpectomy. Mansfield et al.[60] reported on the advantages and clinical results of this modality compared to electron boost. Lee et al.[61] presented an example of three-dimensional reconstruction using CT. Figure

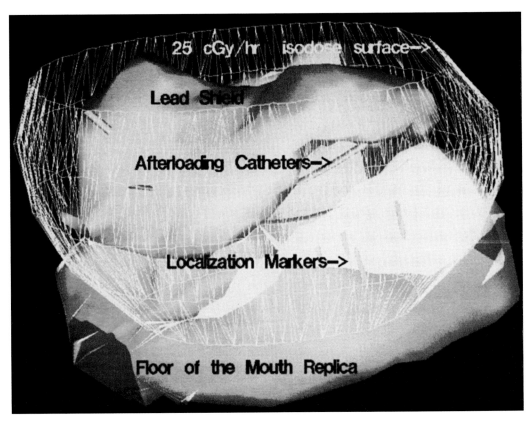

Figure 34. A three-dimensional reconstruction of Ir-192 implant for the treatment of alveolar ridge of the mandible.

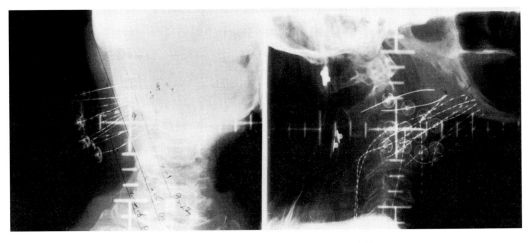

Figure 35. A head and neck implant reconstructed from orthogonal films.

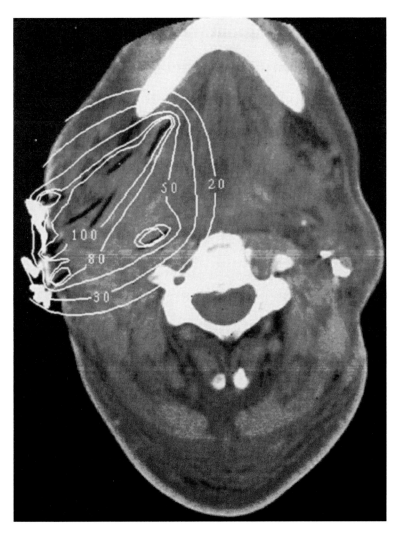

Figure 36. A CT scan of the head and neck implant in Figure 35. The numbers reflect dose rate in cGy/hr.

38 shows such a reconstruction with Ir-192 dosimetry using CT information. The physician has drawn a target volume based on the breast tissue around the lumpectomy site. The figure also shows the location of the lung. The breast implant contains two planes, with six catheters in the anterior plane and seven catheters in the lower plane. The figure shows the prescription isodose rate lines of 36 cGy/hr and 18 cGy/hr, demonstrating rapid dose fall-off. The advantage of three dimensions in this case is the ability to calculate dose volume histograms for the target and the lung.

Treatment of Prostate Using Ultrasound Guided I-125 Implantation

Avizonis et al.[62] described a three-dimensional application of an Au-198 implant for prostate cancer. Niroomand-Rad and Thomadsen[63] described a three-dimensional reconstruction technique for seed implants. Ayyangar et al. described a method that combines CT images with radiographic localization of seeds in an ultrasound guided permanent prostate implant.[57] This technique provides accurate seed location and dose dis-

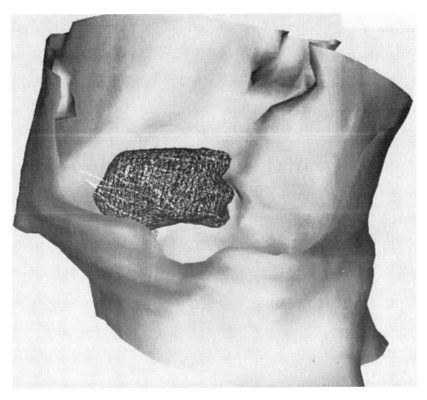

Figure 37. A three-dimensional representation of 50 cGy/hr isodose rate surface for the head and neck implant in Figure 35. The radioactive wire segments and the outer surface of the neck can also be seen.

tribution data in relation to the three-dimensional localization of target volume and critical organs at risk, viz., the bladder and rectum. The accurate determination of radioactive seed locations in permanent implants from CT images is limited by the pixel size and the slice thickness. The image of a single seed may appear in more than one consecutive CT image. Ayyangar described a method of removing this artifact using a tolerance diameter around a seed center determined in the previous CT slice. To further improve the accuracy of defining the seed positions and orientations, the reconstructed seed coordinates derived from the three-film technique were transformed into CT coordinates for dose distribution computations. Ayyangar recommended that the three-film method be used in conjunction with CT to improve the accuracy of seed localization and thereby improve accuracy of dose volume histograms of critical structures.

Figure 39 shows a three-dimensional representation of prostate, bladder, rectum, and a 80 Gy dose surface reconstructed from the seed positions derived using the three-film technique.

Cs-137 in Gynecological Applicators

Figure 40 shows a three-dimensional reconstruction of a dose-rate surface for a Fletcher-Suit-Delclos applicator. The data have been generated using conventional AP and lateral films where the points were marked on both films. The application of three dimensions in this case allows not only for dose evaluation for brachytherapy, but also for combination with external beam treatment planning. However, in some instances, the points chosen on two-dimensional films may not represent the maximum dose to critical structures, as demonstrated by Schoeppel et al.,[64] who compared dose to

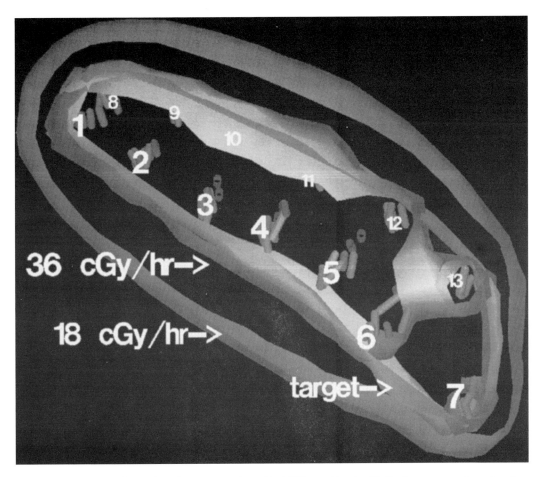

Figure 38. A three-dimensional reconstruction of Ir-192 breast implant in the transverse view showing seven ribbons in the lower plane and six ribbons in the upper plane.

critical structures using CT and traditional film techniques and three-dimensional calculations and analysis, using a Fletcher-Suit applicator specially designed for CT and three-dimensional planning.[65] Figure 41 shows a sagittal reconstruction of such an application using CT data. The value of CT in this example is clearly demonstrated in that using the traditional orthogonal film method could underestimate the dose maxima for rectum and especially for the bladder since the Foley balloon need not be at the closest point with respect to the high-dose region. The use of CT and three-dimensional reconstruction allows one to achieve accurate assessment of doses to the critical structures.

Gynecological Treatment Using a Syed-Neblett Template

Some gynecological treatments use a Syed-Neblett applicator, varying the source intensity and configuration to achieve the desired dose distribution. The applicator allows the simultaneous use of a conventional tandem and sources. A clinical example of three-dimensional reconstruction of sources and the 60 cGy/hr isodose rate surface is shown in Figure 42. As with the breast example, combining this information with CT data would allow the use of three-dimensional capabilities to calculate dose volume histograms and assess dose to critical structures.

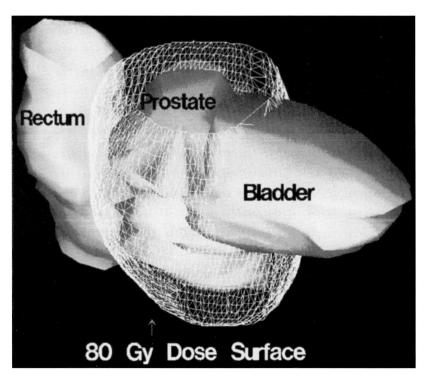

Figure 39. A three-dimensional reconstruction of a prostate implanted with permanent I-125 seeds.

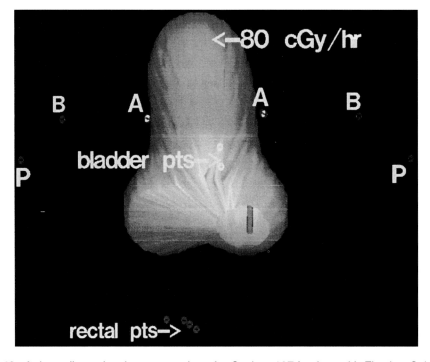

Figure 40. A three-dimensional reconstruction of a Cesium-137 implant with Fletcher-Suit-Delclos applicator.

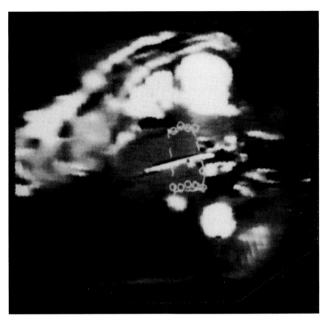

Figure 41. Sagittal reconstructed CT images with the cervix outlined. The borders of the cervix can often be better visualized with this view. (Reprinted from Schoeppel SL, et al. Three-dimensional treatment planning of intracavitary gynecologic implants: Analysis of ten cases and implications for dose specification. Int J Radiat Onc Biol Phys 1994;28:277–283 with kind permission from Elsevier Science Ltd., United Kingdom.)

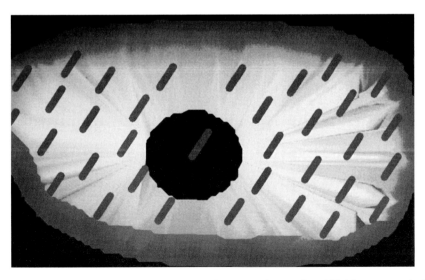

Figure 42. A three-dimensional reconstruction of sources from a Syed-Neblett gynecological template. Also shown is the 60 cGy/hr isodose rate surface.

Dosimetry III: Optimization

The process of weighting the strength of individual sources, dwell times, or source positions in order to produce a desired dose distribution defines "optimization." The decision of whether to optimize the dose distribution interrelates with the decisions on source position (as discussed under "Coverage") and dose specification and prescription. None of these parameters can be decided without consideration of the others. Operating under a system determines whether to apply optimization.

At the beginning of treatment planning one must decide whether to attempt to cover the treatment volume with a uniform dose or to allow (or aim for) a higher dose in the center of the volume. Using a system usually determines this issue. The definition of "uniform dose" remains open for discussion. Some systems provide definitions, while others leave the term vague. Even the most uniform dose distributions have extremely high doses near the sources. For the most part, these small regions of high dose have no clinical significance, as long as they remain small and isolated. The section on "Evaluation" discusses the issue of uniformity.

A decision to deliver a nonuniform dose usually accompanies a concomitant decision to use a uniform distribution of the radioactive material through the target volume. The latter decision precludes delivery of a uniform dose; however, the Paris system, which uses uniform loading, contains rules for source spacing designed to mitigate the volume raised to high doses.

Delivery of a uniform dose to the target volume requires differential distribution of the radioactive material throughout the volume. Establishing the relative spatial or temporal distribution of the source material is the process of optimization. Optimization strategies fall into four general categories:

1) *Optimization based on rules:* The Manchester system of interstitial implants forms a simple optimized system based on rules, without the need for computer-based calculations. The rules in this approach are generalizations derived from calculations of dose for various situations. When applied to situations similar to those that formed the basis for the calculations, the rules yield very good results. As the clinical implant deviates from the geometry of the idealized model, so does the dose uniformity. This approach works well with highly symmetric implants, but fares more poorly as the implant conforms to the shape of odd tumor volumes. In general, the dose uniformity resulting from application of the Manchester rules ($\pm 10\%$ within the implanted volume, not counting corners) falls short of that achievable using computer-based algorithms—although for some regular, symmetric volumes (mostly cylindrical) the uniformity surpassed the system's goal.

2) *Optimization based on geometry:* Geometric optimization[66] assumes that the sources or dwell positions follow the target. The approach further assumes that a given source contributes strongly to the target near the source, but little individually to the target in the vicinity of other sources. From these assumptions, the optimization procedure starts by calculating the contribution to the dose at the position of a source from all sources *except* the source occupying that position. The weight (or relative strength) of that source becomes the inverse of the calculated dose contribution from all other sources.

The assumption that distant sources contribute little to the dose at the position occupied by a given source begins to fail for other nearby sources that begin to dominate the weighting function. The calculation of the dose from all other sources often excludes the contribution from adjacent sources in the same needle track or catheter, or sources in neighboring tracks within some specified distance from the source being optimized. A criterion often used eliminates from consideration those sources in the same catheter closer than the next closest other catheter. While avoiding the problem of domination by nearby sources, ignoring these contributions compromises the accuracy of the process. Edmunson[67] suggests separating the sources along a catheter by the same distance that separates catheters, physically matching the calculational procedures. The cost of this maneuver is an increase in the local dose near the sources.

Geometric optimization separates into two subsets based on the goal of the treatment: *Volume optimization* where the uniform dose distribution fills the volume between all catheters. This option excludes the contribution from all of the sources in the same catheter when calculating the weight for a source; and *Distance optimization* where the uniform dose distribution follows the path of the catheter at a fixed distance or radius. This option includes the contribution from all of the sources in the same catheter (except those closer than the closest other catheter or other exclusion criteria) when calculating the weight for a source. Including these sources tends to produce isodose surfaces that follow the catheters.

3) *Optimization based on specified dose points*: With dose-point optimization, the operator designates specific points that should receive specified doses. The calculational algorithm then attempts to vary the source strengths to satisfy the desired dose conditions. In the most basic form,[68,69] the specified doses and the source strengths establish a set of simultaneous equations of the form

$$D_i = C_{ij}S_j \qquad (43)$$

where D_i = the dose specified to point i, S_j = the strength of source at position j, and C_{ij} = the factors that give the dose contribution at i due to the source at j, with the sum over all sources. The source strength at each source position forms a variable (unknown), and each dose specification point yields an equation. The dose specification points also go by the term optimization points.

Figure 43 shows a simple example of a vaginal cylinder treatment prescribed to give a uniform dose along its surface. In this situation, the number of specified doses equals the

number of source positions. Thus, the set of equations characterized by Equation 43 contains the same number of variables and equations, and the source strengths have single, exact values. Equal numbers of sources and dose points form a *determined* system.

In more complex cases, there may be more optimization points than source positions, resulting in an *overdetermined* system (more equations than variables). In this situation, the source strengths can be varied to minimize the square of the differences between the desired and calculated doses at the optimization points.

At the other extreme, a case may have more source positions than optimization points (more variables than equations), resulting in an *underdetermined* system. In this situation, the source strengths have no well defined values. Minimizing the differences between adjacent source strengths proves to be a useful additional constraint, providing an additional equation of the form

$$X = (S_j - S_{j+1})^2. \qquad (44)$$

The additional constraint of minimizing Equation 44 also proves useful in the determined system (and sometimes the overdetermined system) to prevent the generation of negative strengths from the calculation, a condition that often falls out of the arithmetic but corresponds to an impossible physical situation. An additional condition for underdetermined systems selects solutions that minimize the total radiation to the patient.

The results of the optimization procedure depend critically on the selection of the optimization points. Using too few points or the concentrating of points in certain locations while leaving other parts of the target unspecified easily leads to inappropriate dose distributions. The dose distributions may satisfy the specifications established for the optimization points, but leave portions of the target without dose specification points untreated. Similarly, placement of points at a position of an expected large dose gradient can produce unexpected and inappropriate results from the optimization routine.

Large numbers of optimization points or source positions, or both, increase the time required to run the program solving the equa-

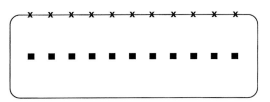

x Optimization points
■ Source position

Figure 43. A vaginal cylinder treatment prescribed to give a uniform dose along its surface at the indicated dose points.

tions. Curve-fit approximations cut the calculational time greatly without significantly compromising the accuracy of the final dose distribution, particularly in cases with a large number of source positions. Several other mathematical approaches have been described in the literature.[70-74]

4) *Optimization based on trial and adjustment:* Without a computer algorithm available for optimization, a practitioner desiring a uniform dose distribution throughout a target volume must resort to *optimization based on trial and adjustment.* Optimization based on rules provides a starting condition in many cases, but may not provide adequate uniformity, particularly for irregularly shaped volumes.

Optimization calculations compute relative dose distributions and require only spatial dose information. After the shape of the dose distribution is established, the entire distribution must be raised or lowered to give the correct absolute dose or dose rate to a specified point, or the average at a number of specified points. This process requires some evaluation of the dose distribution.

Dosimetry IV/Dose Specification II: Evaluation of the Planned Dose Distribution

Interstitial Implants

The planning process may have produced multiple plans for a given application. Choosing between optimized and nonoptimized plans may be as simple as deciding to use a uniform dose distribution or one with high-dose regions in the center. Sometimes the decision entails choosing between several plans optimized using different methods, or with different features. In addition, after selecting a plan, the physician still must select an isodose level for the prescription. Neither the selection of a plan nor the prescription isodose are unambiguous, which accounts for the various techniques developed to aid in this decision-making procedure.

Systems

Following a system may relieve the user from much of the task of evaluating a treatment plan. For example, under the Manchester system the only evaluation required for an implant entails seeing that the needles follow the intended paths and, if they do not, recalculating the treatment duration for the actual implanted volume. The same holds true for a Manchester gynecological insertion. This, of course, fulfills the intent of the system: to allow high quality brachytherapy in facilities lacking in high power physics support. The M.D. Anderson system of brachytherapy for uterine cervix also requires no evaluation of the resultant dose distribution, only the application.[75] Both of these systems prescribe the loadings for use in any given case on the premise that following the rules yields the expected results.

The Paris system gives rules to follow like the Manchester system, but requires dose calculations after the execution of the implant to assess the basal dose. Although this system defines the dose with a rule (the prescribed dose, called the reference isodose, $RI = 0.85$ basal dose), it includes a definition for the high-dose volume as that volume enclosed by the isodose surface equal to 1.7 basal dose, but gives no guidance regarding acceptable values for the high-dose volume.

Isodose Surface I

The conventional approach to evaluating a treatment plan involves visual inspection of the isodose surfaces. With this approach, the radiation oncologist judges which isodose level covers the target and whether the dose inside the implanted volume (and to neighboring structures) remains within tolerances. Normalizing isodose surfaces differently often displays the information in different perspectives. For example, normalizing the prescription isodose surface to 100% highlights the relative doses and simplifies assessment of the high-dose regions. Alternatively, expressing the isodose levels in terms of total dose for the application may accentuate volumes where the doses exceed tolerance. A dose-rate presentation tends to be the most common for LDR and shows at a glance where the dose rates may slip out of the normal range (approximately 0.2–1.2 Gy/hr) and biological models should be invoked. This discussion of inspection of isodose surfaces will continue after considering other modalities used for evaluation of brachytherapy applications.

Volume-Dose Histograms

Several very different presentations of very different information fall under the category of VDH, which is itself divided into two basic subdivisions: integrated and differential volumes.

Integrated VDHs come in two types: absolute and relative. Figure 44 shows an absolute, integral VDH for a 6 cm diameter, 10 cm long cylindrical interstitial implant. The graph displays dose delivered on the abscissa and the volume receiving *at least* that dose on the ordinate. As expected, the curve shows large volumes receiving low doses and small volumes (eventually just surrounding the needles) enclosing high doses. The "absolute" nature of the histogram merely reflects that the graph displays all of the volume in-

cluded within an isodose surface without respect to any specified targets or structures. In using such histograms to judge the "quality" of an implant, the features to observe (moving from the right to the left) include:

1. That the long, high-dose tail runs close to the axis. This tail corresponds to the high-dose regions within the treatment volume. Large volumes taken to doses significantly above the treatment dose can cause complications. A "good" implant keeps these high-dose volumes small.
2. A rise from the high-dose tail to a target volume plateau leading to the reference dose. For the target volume to receive a near-homogeneous dose without excessive high-dose volumes requires a rapid rise.
3. A low sloping, low-dose shoulder. These doses correspond to the doses

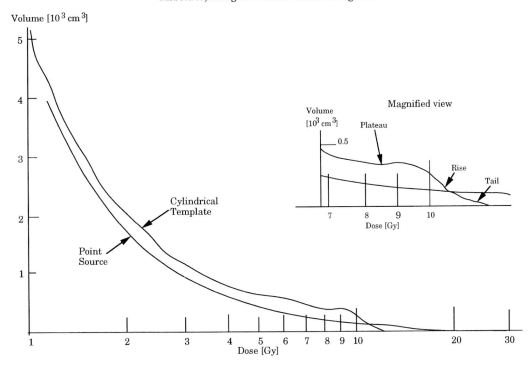

Figure 44. An absolute, integral VDH: for a 6 cm diameter, 10 cm long cylindrical interstitial implant compared with a point source of the same activity. The insert shows a magnified view of the curves near the reference dose end with the features indicated.

outside the target volume. Ideally, the implant should minimize the doses to the surrounding tissues.

The rise in volume included in the high-dose region to the target reference dose (feature 2) and the flattened shoulder of the low-dose volumes (feature 3) indicate the concentrating of the dose in a volume. These differ from the constant upward sweep (from right to left) characteristic of a single point source at the center of the treatment volume, which corresponds to the worst source distribution for the treatment.

Figure 45 shows a relative, integrated VDH. While the absolute integrated VDH presented information on the implant in the patient as a whole, a relative integrated VDH's display deals with specific sites. The abscissa again marks dose, but the ordinate records the percentage of the structure that receives at least the indicated dose. The histogram in Figure 45 comes from a CT-based, custom designed, temporary prostate implant using Ir-192. For the target structure, the curve should follow the 100% (or 1.00) level (top of the graph) from the low doses on the left through the target dose, indicating that all of the target receives at least the target dose. Beginning at the target dose the curve should fall. For an implant designed to deliver a uniform dose throughout the target volume, the curve falls rapidly since no large volumes should receive doses much higher than the target dose. For uniformly loaded implants such as those that sometimes are used for permanent prostate implants, the curve falls more slowly, indicating that much of the target receives relatively high doses. Figure 46 shows the relative integrated VDH for the permanent prostate implant from Figure 39. As with the absolute integrated VDH, the high-dose tails show the high-dose volumes concentrated around the sources. Where the curve begins to fall with respect to the target dose depends on the method used to specify the dose. If the target dose means the minimum dose to the target, then the curve should still be at 1.00 at that dose. However, if the dose is specified as a matched peripheral dose, or as in the Manchester system as 10% greater than the minimum (peripheral) dose in the implanted volume, then the curve begins to decrease at doses lower than the target dose.

Figures 45 and 46 also show curves for the rectum. Just as for the target, the histogram displays the fraction of the organ receiving a given dose. A simpler criterion applies for evaluating the curves for nontarget structures than for the target: the curve should show minimal doses to all of the structure. Unfortu-

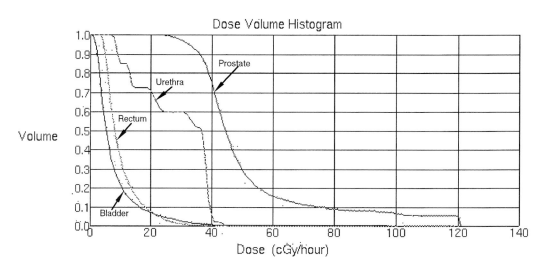

Figure 45. A relative, integral VDH for a customized, temporary prostate template treatment. The curves show the volumes taken at least to the specified dose for the target (the prostate), the urethra, the rectum, and the bladder.

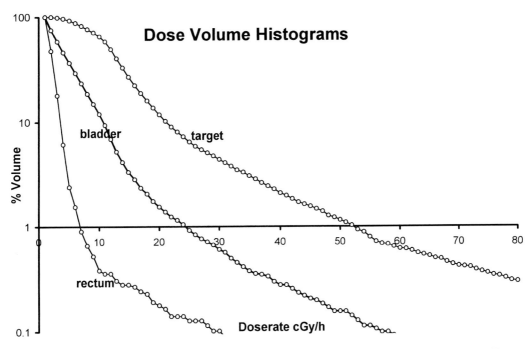

Figure 46. A relative dose volume histogram for the permanent prostate implant shown in Figure 39 with the curves for the target (the prostate), bladder, and rectum.

nately, in many treatments, normal structures fall too close to the target to be avoided entirely, as in this example. The histogram can give an idea of how much of the organ may be at risk for complications. In general, relative histograms, such as the one shown, give fractions of a structure (as contoured) raised to at least the dose on the abscissa. Although the whole bladder may have been outlined on the entire CT study, contours for the rectum stop shortly beyond the CT cuts showing the prostate. Thus, the histogram only includes part of the organ at most. Controversy still surrounds the issue of how to define the important variable relating exposed volume to the probability of complication for the rectum or bowel. Most likely, the absolute volume irradiated (rather than the fractional volume) and the general pattern of the irradiation dictate the biological effect. To reflect such a relationship would require a hybrid VDH describing the absolute volume as a function of dose for the given, contoured organ.

The most elementary differential VDHs display something akin to the volume taken to

a specific dose, rather than to all doses above a given dose, as does the integral VDH. The abscissa gives dose ranges, and the ordinate gives the volume included in that range. If the histogram is refined by letting the dose bins become infinitesimal, the ordinate becomes the change in volume for a change in dose, dV/dD. Figure 47 shows such a histogram for the example cylindrical implant. Compared with the integrated VDH, the differential VDH shows the concentration of the dose in the implanted volume more prominently. Figure 47 shows an "absolute" VDH since no reference is made to a target volume. Differential VDHs also come in "relative" versions with respect to a specified volume, as shown in Figure 48, that refers to the intracavitary insertion displayed in Figure 40. At present, relative differential VDHs find little application. The *relative* differential VDH displays much of the information relevant to the treatment plan, i.e., what doses actually fall in the target (or other) volumes.

Differential VDHs often illustrate differences between competing treatment plans

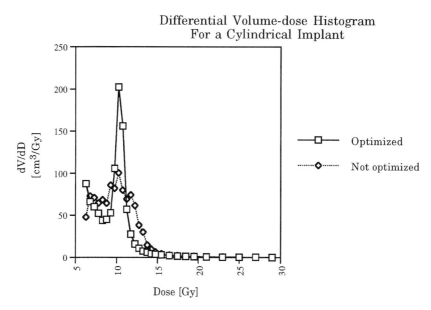

Figure 47. A differential VDH for the cylindrical implant considered in Figure 44 for optimized and nonoptimized distributions.

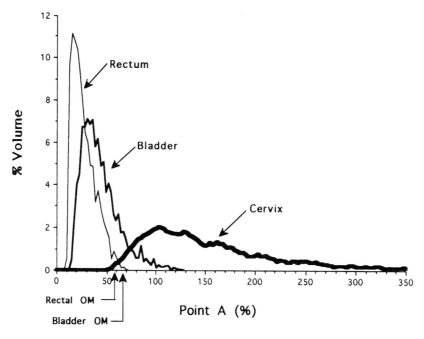

Figure 48. A relative, differential dose volume histogram of cervix, bladder, and rectum. The dose is normalized as a percentage of Point A. The dose maxima derived using orthogonal films are marked OM on the x-axis. (Reprinted from Schoeppel SL, et al. Three-dimensional treatment planning of intracavitary gynecologic implants: Analysis of ten cases and implications for dose specification. Int J Radiat Oncol Biol Phys 1994;28:277–283 with kind permission from Elsevier Science Ltd., United Kingdom.)

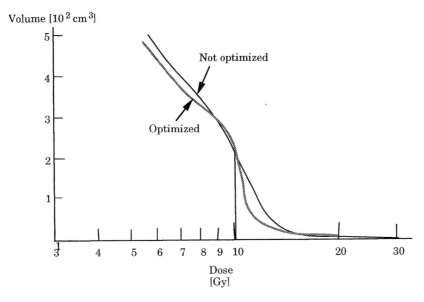

Figure 49. An absolute, integral VDH for the cylindrical implant considered in Figure 44 for the optimized and nonoptimized distributions.

better than integral VDHs. Figure 49 plots the integral VDH for the same implant as Figure 47. The differential VDH shown in Figure 47 shows much more clearly the bunching of the volume elements around the treatment doses for the optimized plan. Both the differential and the integral show the decrease in the volume taken to high doses with the optimized plan.

Geometry (basically the inverse square law) dominates most brachytherapy applications. The inverse square law gives the VDH the characteristic general shape of decreasing volumes with increasing doses. This sloping underlying baseline tends to obscure the significance of small superimposed peaks. Anderson[76] proposed a new form for such histograms, called the "natural" VDH, that removes the effect of the inverse square law. For details on the derivation, the reader should consult Anderson or Thomadsen et al.[77] Briefly, a point source yields a dose distribution for which dV varies with $D^{-3/2}$. Plotting the histogram as $dV/d(D^{-3/2})$ yields a horizontal line for a point source and also for the unconcentrated portion of dose from any implant. With

such an approach, bunching of the dose at a relatively constant value over an extended volume stands out as a marked peak rising over a flat baseline. Figure 50 displays the natural VDH for the example cylindrical implant.

Differential VDHs often make use of specially defined points along the curve. Some commonly used terms include:

Low Dose: The dose midway between the dose corresponding to a peak and that of the "limit value" on the low-dose side. The "limit value" means the dose where the peak falls back into the point-dose-like background. On a normal differential VDH the limit value may be difficult to establish accurately due to the slope of the background and the peak. Use of the natural VDH simplifies finding the limit value because the background forms a horizontal line.

High Dose: The dose midway between the dose corresponding to a peak and that of the "limit value" on the high-dose side.

Target Dose: The dose prescribed for the implant.

The VDH provides much information on an implant, both in general (the absolute) and

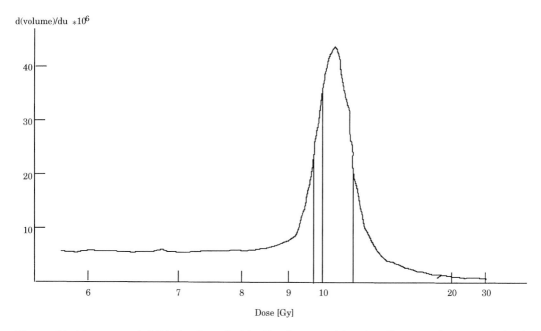

Figure 50. The "natural" VDH for the cylindrical implant considered in Figure 44 for the optimized dose distribution.

with respect to the target (the relative). However, distilling the importance or meaning of the information remains difficult. That a histogram has a pronounced peak fails to delineate where along the curve the "ideal" reference dose falls. The selection depends in part on the clinical objectives. Several quantitative measures assist in assessing of the "quality" of an implant or in deciding between optional treatment plans. Saw and Suntharalingam[78] give a good review and example of some of these quantities. Some of these quantities include:

High-Dose Volume: The volume raised to a dose significantly higher than the target dose. The Paris system defines the high-dose volume as containing doses exceeding the target dose by a factor of 2. Saw and Suntharalingam suggest a factor of 1.5. Zwicker and Schmidt-Ullrich[79] makes the factor a variable, p, used during optimization.

Uniformity Index: A measure of the uniformity of the dose delivered over the treated volume, defined as

$$UI = \frac{V(TD - HD)}{TD^{-3/2} - HD^{-3/2}} 2 \frac{V(TD)}{TD^{-3/2}} . \quad (45)$$

The uniformity index indicates a relative quantity, depending on the target dose selected, although not relating to any preselected target volume. This index also can be applied using high dose defined as the high-dose volume (i.e., the dose above an arbitrary factor times target dose) rather than as the volume defined in the differential VDH. With the high-dose volume definition, Zwicker points out that uniformity index depends not only on the target dose picked, but also on the value, p, used to define the high-dose volume.

Quality Index: A measure of the concentration of dose in the implant, defined as

$$QI = \frac{V(TD - HD)}{LD^{-3/2} - HD^{-3/2}} \bigg| \frac{V(LD)}{LD^{-3/2}} . \quad (46)$$

The quality index forms an absolute quantity, being independent of the target dose selected, but depending only on the geometry of the implant.

Volume Gradient Ratio: A measure of how the implant dose distribution differs from that of a point source. For the assessment a volume encloses the implant with a specified margin (usually 1 cm) and the highest dose on the surface of the box is found. The algorithm then matches this maximum dose to that for a point source in the center of the confined volume and plots the differential histograms for each source configuration. Between any two dose levels, D_1 and D_2, the *volume ratio, VR(D_1-D_2)*, equals the area under the plot for the implant (i.e., the volume enclosed) between the two dose levels divided by the area under the plot for the point source between the same limits. The volume gradient ratio then is defined as

$$VGR = \frac{VR(D_{95} - D_{105})}{\sqrt{VR(D_{85} - D_{95}) \times VR(D_{105} - D_{115})}}. \tag{47}$$

The volume gradient ratio gives the ratio of the volume raised to the target-dose range (target dose ±5%) to the geometric mean of the volumes taken to 10 percentage points less and 10 percentage points greater than the target dose. Larger values of this ratio indicate a greater concentration of the dose in the treatment volume; however, it makes no comparison with the target volume.

Coverage Index: A measure of the fraction of the target volume receiving a dose equal to or greater than the target dose. The coverage index corresponds to the value on the relative integrated VDH for the target dose (see Figure 45).

Dose Nonuniformity Ratio: The ratio of the high-dose volume to that taken to at least the target dose.

External Volume Index (EI): A measure of radiation to normal tissue. The external volume index equals the volume of nontarget tissue receiving doses equal to or greater than the target dose, as a fraction of the target volume.

Relative Dose Homogeneity Index (HI): A measure of the uniformity of the dose through the target volume. The homogeneity index equals the fraction of the target volume receiving a dose between the target dose and the high-dose level.

These quantities sort into categories as shown in Table 16. All of the differential quantities are also absolute, although the integral quantities are relative. Both quadrants contain a mixture of quantities that depend on the target dose or independent of the target dose. The table illustrates why analysis of an application needs to consider many of these quantities and why no single index summarizes all aspects.

None of these quantities tells the whole story for a given implant. A mixture of absolute and relative quantities can help in evaluating an implant and selecting the target dose. Most of the published work on the use of these indices concerns selecting a dose or dose-rate isodose surface to use for the prescription. Saw and Suntharalingam illustrate the use in a graph such as that in Figure 51. This figure shows the listed quantities for a 8 cm x 8 cm x 1.5 cm two plane implant, with

Table 16.
Indices and Quantities

	Absolute		Relative	
	Independent of TD	Dependent on TD	Independent of TD	Dependent on TD
Differential	LD HD QI	HDV UI VGR		
Integral			Volume of organ	CI DNR EI HI

TD = target dose; LD = low dose; HD = high dose; QI = quality index; HDV = high-dose volume; UI = uniformity index; VGR = volume gradient ratio; CI = coverage index; DNR = dose nonuniformity ratio; EI = external volume index; HI = homogeneity index.

COMPARISON OF QUANTITIES

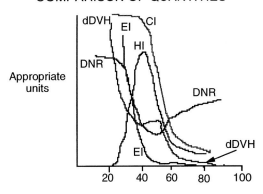

Figure 51. A comparison of various indices for a specific implant as a function of the dose rate (isodose line) selected for the prescribed dose. (Adapted from Saw and Suntharalingam.[80])

a source spacing of 1.5 cm. Inspecting the figure shows that a dose rate of 40 cGy/hr maximizes the relative dose homogeneity index, while 45 cGy/hr minimizes the dose nonuniformity ratio. Any dose rate above 35 cGy/hr sacrifices coverage of the target volume (reduces the coverage index from 100%), but the external volume index continues to decrease significantly with selected dose rate through about 48 or 50 cGy/hr. In this case, the ideal dose rates for the various criteria range across a ±17% span to either side of the median dose (42.5 cGy/hr), and any selection entails some serious compromises. The example illustrates why no single index or quantity perfectly characterizes an implant: evaluation requires consideration of many different aspects, not all of which optimize for the same conditions. Any or all of the quantities provide useful information, but final decisions require consideration of the large overview of the implant.

Isodose Surfaces II

After considering the various graphical and numerical tools available for evaluation of the dose distribution from a treatment plan, visual inspection of the isodose distribution again becomes an essential activity. Some tools exist to assist in evaluation of isodose surfaces also. The first consideration is coverage. What the coverage index evaluates numerically, isodose surfaces address pictorially. The isodose

plot for an implant with a CI of 1.00 would also show complete coverage. However, in some cases, complete coverage may be impossible or undesirable when the total effects are considered. Take for example a transperineal prostate and seminal vesicle implant. The target may be the organs and some margin, but constraints due to dose limiting structures and the inverse square law may prohibit complete coverage. In particular, the treatment may require holding the dose to the urethra in the center of the target to some tolerance value. Such a limitation would affect the dose to the surrounding prostate. A numerical index tells only that some of the target remains at doses below the target dose while the isodose surface plots show where this deficiency occurs.

Two complementary tools assess the uniformity of the doses in the isodose distribution. The *maximum significant dose* refers to the highest level isodose surface that encompasses more than one needle track. Conceptually, the dose around each needle track becomes astronomical, but the body seems to tolerate these local near-singularities. The maximum significant dose provides a convenient criterion indicating when small, high-dose volumes become "significant" and likely to produce biological consequences. For an implant taken to normal tissue tolerance, the maximum significant dose corresponds to the tolerance dose. The experience at the University of Wisconsin-Madison indicates that the maximum significant dose should not exceed 110% of the reference dose for such tolerance implants.

Neblett et al.[80] developed a technique for assessing the uniformity in the interior of an implant by contiguous volume analysis. With this technique the system calculates the dose distribution over a three-dimensional grid of voxels and then calculates contiguous volumes for the various isodose levels. The criterion specifies that contiguous voxels for a given isodose level share a common side and contain a dose at least equal to the specified isodose level. The surface/volume ratio for the largest contiguous volume for a given isodose level and its associated surface area is compared with the ratio for a cube with the same volume as an indication of how compact the volume is. Plotting the isodose level as a function of the maximum contiguous volume for that level, Neblett suggests that the more horizontal the resulting curve is the more homogeneous (better) the implant. A related quantity, the *maximum contiguous dose* specifies the highest isodose level not to break into separate distributions around needle tracks or groups of needle tracks. The maximum contiguous dose can prove particularly useful during planning prior to an implant when choosing needle placement. For fixed source strengths, spreading the needle tracks tends to decrease the maximum contiguous dose, while at the same time increasing the high-dose volume. The maximum contiguous dose becomes very sensitive to the position of peripheral needle tracks. Potentially, for planar implants or for customized irregular implants, placing peripheral needle tracks with the same separation as that between interior tracks often produces low doses in their neighborhoods; this characteristic is exhibited as isodose levels that surround all other needle tracks as a whole, but form separate surfaces around the outside needles. Moving the peripheral needles slightly inwards leads to the isodose surfaces coalescing and to an increase in the maximum contiguous dose.

Intracavitary

Visual inspection of isodose plots remains the primary method of evaluating dose distributions for intracavitary insertions. Techniques involving measuring uniformity or concentration of dose fail because intracavitary applications almost always place the source material at some distance from the target, or at least from the distal most point of the target, and accept the large gradient in dose thoughout the treatment volume. With such a configuration, the VDH looks much like those for a single line source: essentially featureless. Judging if the application satisfies the treatment intentions requires a clear prescription of the dose distribution desired and actual isodose distributions in all relevant planes or three dimensions.

For example, consider a treatment for an inoperable stage II cancer of the endometrium. A conventional approach uses a Heyman packing of the corpus possibly with a tandem in the cervical canal and ovoids in the vaginal fornices. The prescription may call for an application of 7000 mg Ra eq hr in two fractions. Older, stainless steel Heyman cap-

sules usually prevented localization films from showing the source locations and therefore prohibited meaningful dosimetry. Although newer, afterloading capsules allow accurate source localization and dose calculation, the treatment never makes use of the information. Evaluation simply becomes checking the films to see if the applicators appear to be in the correct position. Variations in source geometry produce differences in the dose to various parts of the organ and to the superior bowel, rectum, and bladder. These variations in dose may be responsible for some complications and treatment failures. However, without clear cut specifications of dose limits for the target or normal structures, no evaluation can determine whether a particular application satisfies the treatment criteria or not. A lack of dose criteria becomes a larger problem when changing a treatment pattern, such as converting from manual afterloading to remote afterloading or, to an even greater degree, going to a HDR regimen. Even the conversion from radium-loaded, steel capsules to cesium-loaded plastic applicators should include consideration of the dose distribution differences between the two systems and specification of doses to the target and organs.

As discussed earlier, optimization provides for a more uniform dose through the target volume with less exposure to normal tissue *outside* the target volume, but not without a price. Weighting of the ends of needle tracks within the target volume shortens the active length. Around the ends, the doses near the needle tracks become larger than those for uniformly loaded needles. Thus, although less normal tissue receives significant radiation doses, the total volume taken to high doses (usually defined as 1.5 or 2.0 times the target dose) increases. "Optimization" produces a uniform dose only at specific points or under specific conditions. Outside those conditions, the dose distribution may be less uniform. For example, consider the intraluminal application in Figure 52. The left-hand side shows the dose from a uniform weighting along the catheter, while the right-hand side indicates the dose for optimized weightings. Both deliver the same dose over the target length at the target distance. The uniformly loaded catheter needs to extend well beyond the target end-points to avoid underdosing the ends. The source for the optimized cathe-

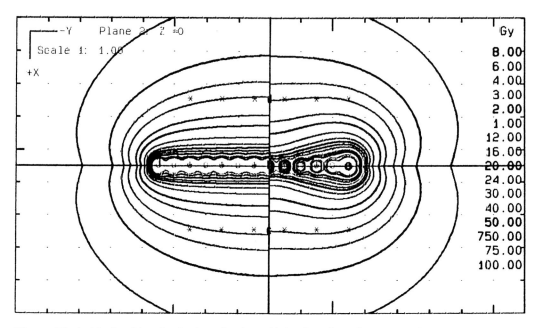

Figure 52. In idealized intraluminal application with isodose lines from an optimized (left half) and uniform (right half) loading patterns.

ter stops within the target volume. Figure 53 shows the integrated VDH for the applications.

Localization and Reconstruction

Correct delivery of the dose to the targets requires accurate localization (imaging) and reconstruction (rendering to spatial coordinates) of the source material and patient anatomy (for some rigid applications, source and/or anatomical information may be obtainable by direct measurement), and some form of immobilization to ensure that the relative positions used during dose calculations remain constant during treatment. Although each of the processes has its own considerations, each depends on the other two. Chapter 9 on Imaging Systems discusses the requirements and equipment available for localization in detail and should be read in conjunction with this chapter.

Execution of the Planned Treatment

The accurate execution of a planned treatment depends on the proper placement of the sources and their immobilization in the patient.

Proper Placement of the Sources

Proper placement of the sources depends on the situation. At one extreme fall tumors that can be assessed in their entirety only under general anesthesia. In such cases, the oncologist or surgeon goes into the operating room with only a general conception of the implant layout, and "proper placement" becomes trying to place the needles or catheters in a good, evenly spaced geometry. In such cases, the planning comes after the fact.

For many interstitial implants, the target volume is well known from physical examination, CT studies, or other localization techniques. In such cases, the success of the implants depends on duplicating the geometry used during the generation of the plan. Templates provide a tremendous aid in correct placement. For treatment of deep seated lesions, single plate templates serve to position the needle entry points, guide the needle direction, and hold the needles in place. To satisfy these requirements, the templates must be thick enough to guide the needle in the

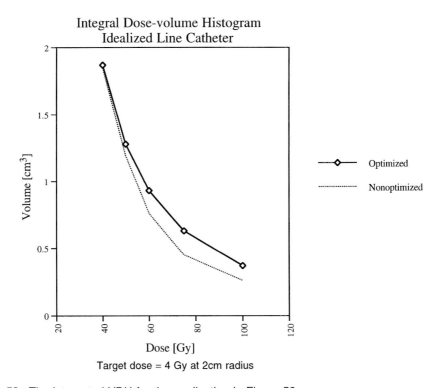

Figure 53. The integrated VDH for the application in Figure 52.

desired direction during insertion. Generally, this guidance requires template thicknesses greater than one centimeter. Most templates use one of two methods to stabilize the needles during the treatment: 1) using set screws to lock each needle in place; or 2) using a material around the needles that grabs and holds them under certain conditions. The latter method is more common and particularly useful for templates with large numbers of needles. In one form, such a template consists of two plates that sandwich a rubbery material through which the needles pass. After completion of the implantation, the two sides of the template are pressed together (often by screws connecting the two template

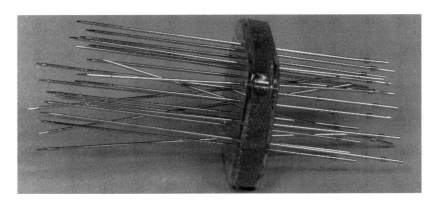

Figure 54. A custom designed template for a prostate patient based on CT treatment planning.

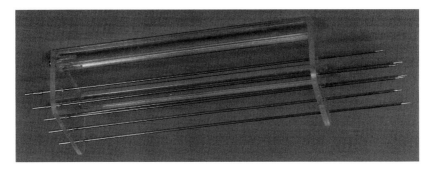

Figure 55. A set of template sheets used for a breast implant.

sheets), compressing the intervening material, which in turn tightly grabs the needles and prevents them from slipping. The rubbery material may be o-rings around each needle or a single slab of Superflab™ (Soule Protection Perfection, Tampa, FL, USA) covering the whole template. For pelvic applications, several commercial templates exist.[81,82] For prostate implantation, bones often obscure parts of the target when it is approached straight from the perineal surface requiring that some needles approach from different angles. Some commercial prostate templates contain swiveling ball-in-socket joints that allow needles to angle behind bones or bowel. Custom cut templates may have angled holes for this purpose. Figure 54 shows a template custom designed for a prostate patient based on CT treatment planning.

If implant catheters enter and exit the patient, such as with most breast and head and neck cases, thinner templates situated on the entrance and exit surfaces hold the needles or catheters in place better than a single, thick template on one end. For breast implants, two plastic sheets often stand as parallel planes held in place by bracing struts, as shown in Figure 55. With LDR implants, the needles can be crimped on the outside surface of the template sheets for stabilization. In HDR cases, the distal ends may be crimped, but the proximal ends require a clear opening for the source passage. A floor of mouth implant may use a custom molded template fabricated from clear dental impression material used for athletic mouth guards.

Proper execution in intracavitary insertions usually has less to do with duplication of a previously generated plan than with simply placing the applicator in the proper anatomical location, with the various parts of the applicator correctly oriented and located with respect to each other. With gynecological applications using a tandem and ovoids, the tandem should bisect the ovoids as seen in the AP and lateral images (fluoroscopic or radiographic); and the top of the tandem should not curve to either side (an indication of a rotation of the tandem). The ovoids should touch the tandem on their medial side, and the whole system should rest about midway between the bladder and the rectum. A significant spread of the ovoids from the tandem indicates a need for a larger size cap. Depending on the system being used, the tandem should abut the fundus or extend a specified distance above the cervical os depending on the depth sounded. Fixed geometry applicators, with the tandem and colpostat(s) yoked, simplify execution to the extent that applicator orientation remains correct with respect to itself (although possibly not adapting to the patient's anatomy as well). In all cases, the main problems involve correctly describing the insertion with the reconstruction and immobilizing the applicator with respect to the patient during the period between localization imaging and completion of the treatment.

References

1. Nag S (ed). High Dose Rate Brachytherapy: A Textbook. Futura Publishing Company, Inc., Armonk, NY, 1994.
2. International Commission on Radiation Units and Measures (ICRU) Report 38: Dose and vol-

ume specification for reporting intracavitary therapy in gynecology. ICRU, Bethesda, 1985.

3. International Commission on Radiation Units and Measurements (ICRU). ICRU Report No. 50, Prescribing, recording, and reporting photon beam therapy. ICRU, Washington, DC, 1993.

4. Paterson R, Parker H. A dosage system for gamma-ray therapy. Br J Radiol 1934;7: 592–632.

5. Tod M, Meredith W. A dosage system for use in the treatment of cancer of the uterine cervix. Br J Radiol 1938;11:809–824.

6. Pierquin B, Chassagne DJ, Chahbazian CM, et al. Brachytherapy. Warran H. Green, Inc., St. Louis, MO, 1978.

7. Quimby EH. Dosage calculations with radioactive materials. In: Glasser O, Quimby EH, Taylor LS, et al. (eds). Physical Foundations of Radiology. Third Edition. Hoeber Medical Division, Harper & Row, New York, 1963, pp. 336–381.

8. Meredith WJ (ed). Radium Dosage: The Manchester System. E and S Livingstone, LTD., Edinburgh, 1967.

9. Shalk RJ, Stovall M. Brachytherapy dosimetry. In: Kase KR, Bjarngard BE, Attix FH (eds). The Dosimetry of Ionizing Radiation. Volume III. Academic Press, Inc., San Diego, 1990, pp. 259–321.

10. Mitchell RG. Effect of oblique filtration in radium dosimetry. Br J Radiol 1956;29:631.

11. Quimby EH, Castro V. The calculation of dosage in interstitial radium therapy. Am J Roentgenol 1953;70:739–743.

12. Shalek RJ, Stovall MA, Sampiere VA. The radiation distributions and dose specification in volume implants of radioactive seeds. Am J Roentgenol Radium Therapy Nucl Med 1957;77: 863–868.

13. Laughlin JS, Siler WM, Holodny EI, et al. A dose description system for interstitial radiation therapy. Am J Roentgenol Radium Ther 1963; 89:470–490.

14. Anderson LL, Hilaris BS, Wagner LK. A nomograph for planar implant planning. Endocuriether/Hypertherm Oncol 1985;1:9–15.

15. Henschke UK, Cevc P. Dimension averaging a simple method for dosimetry of interstitial implants. Rad Biol Ther 1968;9:287–298.

16. Anderson LL. Spacing nomograph for interstitial implants of I-125 seeds. Med Phys 1976;3: 48–51.

17. Anderson LL, Nath R, Weaver KA, et al. Interstitial Brachytherapy: Physical, Biological and Clinical Considerations. Raven Press, New York, 1990.

18. Anderson LL, Moni JV, Harrison LB. A nomo-

graph for permanent implants of Pd-103 seeds. Int J Radiat Oncol Biol Phys 1993;27:129–136.

19. Dutreix A, Marinello G, Wambersie A. Dosimetrie en Curietherapie. Masson, Paris, 1982.

20. Perquin B, Wilson JF, Chassagne DJ. Modern Brachytherapy. Masson Publishing, Inc., New York, 1987.

21. Perquin B, Dutreix A, Paine CH, et al. The Paris System in interstitial radiation therapy. Acta Radiol Oncol 1978;17:33–48.

22. Perquin B, Chassagne DJ, Chahbazian CM, et al. Brachytherapy. Warren H. Green, Inc., St. Louis, MO, 1978.

23. Kwan DK, Kagan AR, Olch AJ, et al. Single- and double-plane iridium-192 interstitial implants: Implantation guidelines and dosimetry. Med Phys 1983;10:456–461.

24. Zwicker RD, Schmidt-Ullrich R, Schiller B. Planning of Ir-192 seed implants for boost irradiation to the breast. Int J Radiat Oncol Biol Phys 1985;11:2163–2170.

25. Gillin MT, Kline RW, Wilson JF, et al. Single and double plane implants: A comparison of the Manchester system with the Paris system. Int J Radiat Oncol Biol Phys 1984;10:921–925.

26. van der Laarse R. In: Thomadsen BR, Houdek PV, van der Laarse R, et al. Treatment planning and optimization. In: Nag S (ed). High Dose Rate Brachytherapy: A Textbook. Futura Publishing Co., Inc., Armonk, NY, 1994, pp. 85–91.

27. Olch AJ, Kagan AR, Wollin M, et al. Multi-institutional survey of techniques in volume iridium implants. Endocuriether/Hypertherm Oncol 1986;2:193–197.

28. American Endocurietherapy Society (Anderson L, Nath R, Olch A, et al. Authors). American Endocurietherapy Society recommendations for dose specification in brachytherapy. Endocuriether/Hypertherm Oncol 1991;7:1–12.

29. American Association of Physicists in Medicine, Task Group No. 43: Nath R, Anderson LL, Luxton G, et al. Dosimetry of interstitial brachytherapy sources: Recommendations of the AAPM Radiation Therapy Task Group No. 43. Med Phys 1995;22:209–234.

30. Meisberger LL, Keller R, Shalek RJ. The effective attenuation in water of the gamma rays of AU-198, Ir-192, Cs-137, Ra-226, and Co-60. Radiology 1968;90:953–957.

31. Williamson JF. Comparison of measured and calculated dose rates in water near I-125 and Ir-192 seeds. Med Phys 1991;18:776–786.

32. Williamson JF. Monte Carlo and analytic calculation of absorbed dose near Cs-137 intracavitary sources. Int J Radiat Oncol Biol Phys 1988; 15:227–237.

33. Luxton G. Comparison of radiation dosimetry in water and in solid phantom materials for I-

125 and Pd-103 brachytherapy sources: EGS4 Monte Carlo study. Med Phys 1994;21: 631–641.

34. American Association of Physicists in Medicine, Report No. 21. Specification of brachytherapy source strength. American Institute of Physics, New York, 1987.

35. Astrahan MA, Luxton G, Jozsef G, et al. Optimization of I-125 ophthalmic plaque therapy. Med Phys 1990;17:1053–1057.

36. Shalek RJ, Stovall M. Dosimetry in implant therapy. In: Attix FH, Roesch WC, Tochilin E (eds). Radiation Dosimetry. Second Edition. Academic Press, New York, 1969, pp. 743–807.

37. Williamson J. Monte Carlo and analytic calculation of absorbed dose near Cs-137 intracavitary sources. Int J Radiat Oncol Biol Phys 1988;15: 227–237.

38. Nath R, Meigooni AS, Meunch P, et al. Anisotopy functions for Pd-103, I-125, and Ir-192 interstitial brachytherapy sources. Med Phsy 1993;20:1465–1473.

39. Mohan R, Ding IY, Martel MK, et al. Measurements of radiation dose distributions for shielded cervical applicators. Int J Radiat Oncol Biol Phys 1985;11:861–868.

40. Prasad SC, Bassano DA, Kubsad SS. Buildup factors and dose around a Cs-137 source in the presence of imhomogeneities. Med Phys 1983; 10:705–708.

41. Meigooni AS, Nath R. Tissue inhomogeneity correction for brachytherapy sources in a heterogeneous phantom with cylindrical symmetry. Med Phys 1992;19:401–408.

42. Williamson JF, Li Z, Wong JW. One-dimensional scatter-subtraction method for brachytherapy dose calculation near bounded heterogeneities. Med Phys 1993;20:233–244.

43. Williamson JF, Perera H, Li Z, et al. Comparison of calculated and measured heterogeneity correction factors for I-125, Cs-137, and Ir-192 brachytherapy sources near localized heterogeneities. Med Phys 1993;20:209–222.

44. Houdek PV, Schwade JG, Wu X, et al. Dose determination in high dose-rate brachytherapy. Int J Radiat Oncol Biol Phys 1992;24: 795–801.

45. Bastin K, Podgorsak M, Thomadsen B. The transit dose component of high dose rate brachytherapy: Direct measurements and clinical implications. Int J Radiat Oncol Biol Phys 1993;26:695–702.

46. Warszawski N, Bleher M, Bratengeier K, et al. The use of isodose curves on radiographs and on CT scans in interstitial brachytherapy. Clin Oncol 1992;4:228–231.

47. McShan DL, Ten Haken RK, Frass BA. 3-D treatment planning: IV integrated brachytherapy planning. In: Bruinvas IAD, et al. (eds). Use of Computers in Radiation Therapy, Proceedings of the Ninth International Conference on Computers in Radiotherapy, Scheveningen, The Netherlands June 1987. Elsevier Science Pub, New York, 1987, pp. 249–252.

48. Ayyanger K, Yeung D, Suntharalingam N, et al. Three-dimensional radiation treatment planning system based on stardent supergraphic workstation. Proc. of 10th Intl. Conf. on Computers in Radiation Therapy, Lucknow, India, Nov. 11–14, 1990. Medical Physics Bulletin, Special Issue, 16, 1991, pp. 36–43.

49. Chen GT, Pelizzari CA, Levin DN. Image correlation in oncology. In: DeVita VT, Hellman S, Rosenberg SA (eds). Important Advances in Oncology. J.B. Lippincott Company, Philadelphia, 1990, pp. 131–141.

50. Annweiler H, Albrecht G, Tabor P, et al. Three dimensional optimization of the dose distribution of interstitial and intracavitary afterloading methods. Strahlentherapia Und Oncologie 1988;82:78–82.

51. Niemierko A, Urie M, Goitein M. Optimization of 3D radiation therapy with both physical and biological end points and constraints. Int J Radiat Oncol Biol Phys 1992;23:99–108.

52. Ayyangar K, Saw CB, Tupchong L, et al. Planning system for stereotactic brain implants. Endocuriether/Hypertherm Oncol 1990;6: 245–250.

53. Ling CC, Roy J, Sahoo N, et al. Quantifying the effect of dose inhomogeneity in brachytherapy: Application to permanent prostatic implant with 125I seeds. Int J Radiat Oncol Biol Phys 1994;28:971–978.

54. Williamson JF, Li Z, Wong JW. One-dimensional scatter-subtraction method for brachytherapy dose calculation near bounded heterogeneities. Med Phys 1993;20:233–244.

55. Ten Haken RK, Diaz RF, McShan DL, et al. From manual to 3-D computerized treatment planning for 125-I stereotactic brain implants. Int J Radiat Oncol Bio Phys 1988;15:467–480.

56. Bauer-Kirpes B, Sturm V, Schlegel W, et al. Computerized optimization of 125-I implants in brain tumors. Int J Radiat Oncol Biol Phys 1988;14:1013–1023.

57. Ayyangar K, Gupta S, Dobelbower RR, et al. Radioactive seed localizations from computed tomography imaging technique. J Med Phys 1994;19:121–126.

58. Parai E, Ayyanger K, Bowman D, et al. 3-D reconstruction of Ir-192 implant dosimetry for irradiating gingival carcinoma on the mandibular alveolar ridge. Oral Surg Oral Med Oral Pathlo Oral Radiol Endod 1995;79:787–792.

59. Hayes JK, Moeller JN, Leavitt DD et al. Com-

puted tomography treatment planning in Ir-192 brachytherapy in the head and neck. Int J Radiat Oncol Biol Phys 1992;22:181–189.

60. Mansfield CM, Krishnan L, Komarnicky L, et al. A review of the role of radiation therapy in the treatment of patients with breast cancer. Semin Oncol 1991;18:525–535.

61. Lee KR, Dwyer SJ, Mansfield CM. Radiation therapy treatment planning. In: Mansfield C (ed). Therapeutic Radiology. Elsevier, Amsterdam, 1989, pp. 95–126.

62. Avizonis VN, Hussey DN, Anderson KM, et al. Three-dimensional viewing of and dosimetic calculations in Au-198 implants of the prostate. Radiology 1992;184:275–279.

63. Niroomand-Rad A, Thomadsen BR. Evaluation of the reconstruction of seed positions from stereo and orthogonal radiographs for routine radiotherapy planning. Radiat Med—Med Imag Radiat Oncol 1990;8:145–151.

64. Schoeppel SL, LaVigne ML, Martel MK, et al. Three-dimensional treatment planning on intracavitary gynecologic implants: Analysis of ten cases and implications for dose specification. Int J Radiat Oncol Biol Phys 1994;28:277–283.

65. Schoeppel SL, Frass BA, Hopkins MP, et al. A CT-compatible version of the Fletcher system intracavitary applicator: Clinical applicaton and 3-dimensional treatment planning. Int J Radiat Oncol Biol Phys 1989;17:1103–1109.

66. Edmundson GK. Geometry based optimization for stepping source implants. Activity—The Setectron user's newsletter 1991;5:22.

67. Edmundson GK. Geometric optimization: An American view. In: Mould RF (ed). International Brachytherapy. Nucletron International BV, Veenendaal, The Netherlands, 1992, p. 256.

68. van der Laarse R. Optimization of high dose rate brachytherapy. Activity—The Selectron user's newleter 1989;2:14–15.

69. van der Laarse R, Edmundson GK, Luthmann RW, et al. Optimization of HDR brachytherapy dose distributions. Activity—The Selectron user's newsletter 1991;5:94–101.

70. Sloboda RS. Optimization of brachytherapy dose distributions by simulated annealing. Med Phys 1992;19:955–964.

71. Sloboda RS, Pearcey RG, Gillan SJ. Optimized low dose rate pellet configuration for intravaginal brachytherapy. Int J Radiat Oncol Biol Phys 1993;26:499–511.

72. Holms TW. A model for the physical optimization for external beam radiotherapy. Thesis: University of Wisconsin.

73. Luenberger DG. Linear and Nonlinear Prograuming. Second Edition. Addison and Wesley, Reading, MA, 1989, Chapter 9.

74. Holms TW, Mackie TR. A comparison of three inverse treatment planning algorithms. Phys Med Biol 1994;39:91–106.

75. Fletcher GH, Hamberger AD. Female pelvis (treatment technique according to size of the cervical lesion and extension). In: Fletcher GH (ed). Textbook of Radiotherapy. Third Edition. Lea and Febiger, Philadelphia, 1980, pp. 732–772.

76. Anderson LL. A "natural" volume-dose histogram for brachytherapy. Med Phys 1986;13:899–903.

77. Thomadsen BR, Houdek PV, van der Laarse R, et al. Treatment planning and optimization. In: Nag S (ed). High Dose Rate Brachytherapy: A Textbook. Futura Publishing Co., Inc., Armonk, NY, 1994, pp. 79–145.

78. Saw CB, Suntharalingam N. Quantitative assessment of interstitial implants. Int J Radiat Oncol Biol Phys 1991;20:135–139.

79. Zwicker RD, Schmidt-Ullrich R. Dose uniformity in a planar interstitial implant system. Int J Radiat Oncol Biol Phys 1995;31:149–155.

80. Neblett D, Syed AMN, Puthawala AA, et al. An interstitial implant technique evaluated by contiguous volume analysis. Endocurietherapy/Hyperthem Oncol 1985;1:213–221.

81. Fleming P, Syed AMN, Neblett D, et al. Description of an afterloading Ir-192 interstitial-intracavitary technique in the treatment of carcinoma of the vagina. Obstet Gynecol 1980;55:525–530.

82. Martinez A, Cox RS, Edmundson GK. A multiple-site perineal applicator (MUPIT) for treatment of prostatic anorectal and gynecological malignancies. Int J Radiat Oncol Biol Phys 1985;1:25–34.

Chapter 9

Imaging Applications in Brachytherapy

Bhudatt R. Paliwal, Ph.D.,
Bruce R. Thomadsen, Ph.D.,
Daniel G. Petereit, M.D.

Introduction

The ability to deliver curative doses to the tumor while sparing normal tissues due to the rapid dose fall-off is the major advantage of brachytherapy. The availability of small sealed sources of variable strength permits the spatial control of radioactivity distribution, and thus, the dose distribution. This, however, can only be as good as our ability to localize all radioactive sources in the body and their spatial relationship with respect to each other, the target volume and all other anatomical landmarks, as well as the surrounding normal structures pertinent to the treatment setup. Some examples of the relative effect of spatial uncertainty on the calculated dose is shown in Table 1. Very often these objectives present a serious challenge to the variety of imaging tools commonly required. Presence of metallic sources or applicators produce artifacts in a CT image or prohibit the use of MRI whereas in the diagnostic radiographic and fluoroscopic procedures, small seeds often are shadowed by the high density bony structures. In this review of the imaging applications in brachytherapy, an attempt is made to address some of these issues.

Imaging

Interstitial and intracavitary brachytherapy, whether using high-dose-rate (HDR) or low-dose-rate (LDR), have unique characteristics with respect to localization, immobilization, and applicators used. However, in either system, localization proceeds through standard phases, although in particular cases (or practices), steps may coalesce.

Preplanning Imaging

This first phase identifies the target volume and possible approaches for the procedure. On one extreme falls the stereotactic procedures where localization utilizes a rigid frame coupled to a CT or MRI unit and a computer suggests the approach (needle tracks). An example of such an application of preplanning imaging in prostate implant is shown in Figures 1, 2, and 3. A volume rendered display of skeletal anatomy and the needle tracks in and around the prostate, created from CT images, is shown in Figure 1. Figure 2 shows software generated locations of the needle tracks for a prostate template. Figure 3 shows corresponding digitally reconstructed lateral and AP views as well as the preplanned radia-

Table 1.
Percent Error Due to Source Position

To a Point at a Distance (mm) of	Percent Change in Dose from a Point Source for an Error in Distance (mm) of		
	1	2	5
10	21	44	225
15	14	28	78
20	10	21	56
30	7	14	36

tion dose distributions for a preselected loading. Gynecological implants are often the other extreme where standard applications and doses are delivered without individual preplanning. Separation of preplanning imaging from the procedure in space and time compromises the value of the information gained. Thus, the imaging should precede the planning and execution by as little time as compatible with the planning and include any possible immobilization to keep the patient in the same orientation between the two.

Procedural Imaging

Imaging during the procedure assists in executing the planned application. For most brachytherapy, fluoroscopy serves for live-

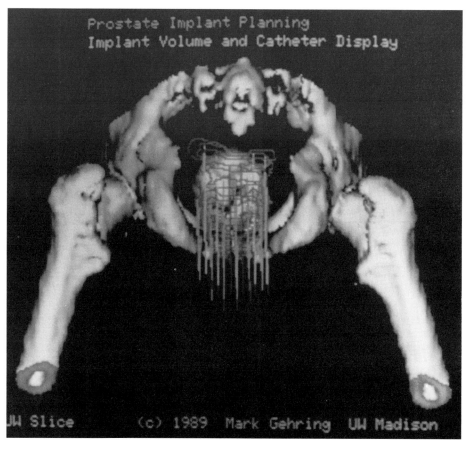

Figure 1. A volume rendered display of skeletal anatomy and the needle tracks in and around the prostate—created from CT images.

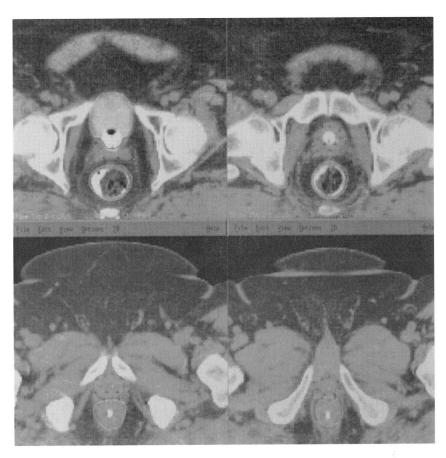

Figure 2. Software generated locations of the needle tracks for a prostate template.

time evaluation of the application geometry. For example, fluoroscopy in the procedure room for a gynecological insertion permits adjustment of the applicators to obtain symmetry of the tandem with respect to ovoids or changes in the packing to displace the bladder or rectum without waiting for films and making changes. With some procedures such as ultrasound-guided prostate implants, the implantation takes place interactively with the procedural imaging. Examples of ultrasound-guided localization of the bladder, uterus, and the Foley catheter as well as the tandem are shown in Figures 4 and 5. In recent years, several publications[1–3] have documented the contribution of ultrasonic imaging in gynecological brachytherapy. It is a valuable aid in the accurate determination of the thickness of the uterine wall in uterine cancer and it also

provides immediate feedback on misplacement of the applicators or inadvertent uterine perforation.

Postprocedural or Localization Imaging

The last phase of imaging serves to identify/verify source positions and anatomy for dosimetry after completion of the source/applicator placement procedure. Most temporary implants use afterloading dummy sources to identify source positions, whereas in permanent implants, the sources themselves are imaged to perform this function. An example of a typical gynecological application imaging a tandem with cylinders is shown in Figures 6, 7, and 8. Figure 6 shows a photograph of an applicator assembly made with 4-cm diameter cylinder segment and a

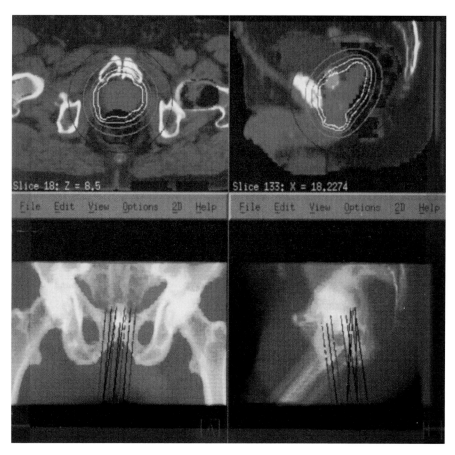

Figure 3. Digitally reconstructed lateral and AP views as well as the preplanned radiation dose distributions for a preselected loading in needle tracks shown in Figure 2.

stainless steel tandem. The stainless steel disks between each cylinder segment and the sets of size indicating markers in each cylinder segment is imaged to accurately determine the vaginal applicator dimensions and geometry from the radiographs shown in Figures 7 and 8. In some situations, for example a template using stainless steel needles for the loading of ribbons, radiographic or CT imaging may be performed. For CT imaging, it is desirable to have nonmetallic needles to avoid artifacts. Figure 9 shows such a CT verification image of needles implanted transrectally in the prostate with minimal artifact.

While many applications follow the above described order of imaging, some notable exceptions deserve comment: 1) Permanent implants with long-lived radionuclides, such as I-125, may change with time. The operative procedure may cause edema and long-term radiation fibrosis may cause shrinkage. To more accurately represent the dose, localization films may be delayed for a specific duration. This delay usually makes no impact on the patient management since neither the position of the sources nor the duration of the implant can be changed very easily, if at all. As the geometry of the implant varies due to radiation changes in the tissue, seed migration, or loss, follow-up imaging and dosimetry adjust the calculated dose to more accurately assess the actual dose delivered; 2) Large volume, template-guided implants can suffer a significant number of needles deviating from the intended location and trajectory without markedly changing the dose distribution. As a

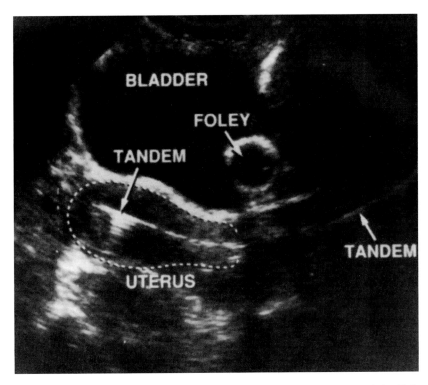

Figure 4. A lateral of ultrasound-guided localization of the bladder, uterus, and the Foley catheter as well as the tandem.

result, the postprocedure imaging simply may verify the execution of the planned implant with no revision of the dosimetry. Actual identification of dummy locations for dosimetry in implants with a large number of needles poses a challenge under the best of situations; 3) Very well controlled situations, such as surface molds, may require no imaging other than photography for documentation.

Source Localization Techniques

The form of imaging for each of the above discussed steps depends on the intention and the system used. Preplanning images increasingly tend to be CT or MRI. Many "homegrown" computer planning systems now allow for implant planning based on such images, but such capability in commercial systems still remains a rarity. Postimplant analysis of an implant when using the Manchester system requires only assessment of areas or volumes, probably derived from orthogonal films. The use of a computer for dose calculation often imposes the form of imaging and may demand strict conformity to a protocol. By far, the most common forms of localization remains plane film radiographs from more than one vantage, localizing structures by triangulation.

General Technical Considerations

First, the radiographic film imaging system needs to clearly display dummy seeds, which indicate the locations of possible dwell positions. Consider the common situation of gynecological, radiographic imaging. In anterior or anterior oblique projections the seeds often fall either behind a Foley balloon containing contrast medium, or above the bowel, likewise containing contrast, or between both opaque structures. Dilution of the contrast medium reduces the impact of the contrast in the anatomy: in the Foley 5–7 cc of Hypaque™ (Nycomed, Inc., New York, NY,

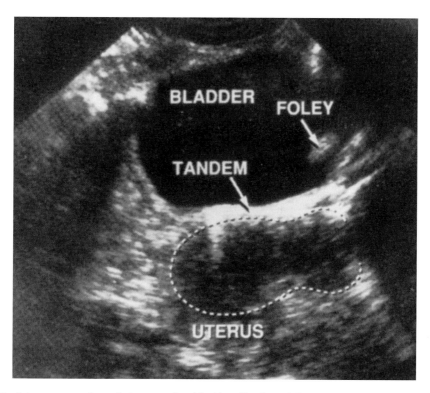

Figure 5. A transverse view of ultrasound-guided localization of the bladder, uterus, and the Foley catheter as well as the tandem.

USA) iodine and in the rectum approximately 50 cc of 20% Polarbar™ (E.2. EM, Inc., Westbury, NY, USA) barium sulfate suspension in water suffices. The contrast in the Foley bulb could be diluted further if imaging becomes impossible. An anterior film requires a high kVp to penetrate the patient and provide adequate contrast. On a lateral film, the dummy seeds seldom coincide with any of the contrast filled structures, but often fall between the femoral heads or other pelvic bones. While the bones do increase the radiographic density, the major problem is patient thickness. Pelvic thicknesses of 45–50 cm commonly fill the space between the source and the receptor. Since obesity is a risk factor in the development of uterine cancer, imaging the applicators in these patients is often problematic. These large pelvic girths strain the x-ray tube to penetrate and generate large quantities of scatter that cloud the film's image. Careful collimation helps prevent some scatter production, but for facilities that calculate the doses to lymph nodes using the lymphatic-trapezoid method, extensive collimation excludes imaging necessary to utilize these nodal points.[4,5] Highly effective grids markedly improve the image contrast, but increase the skin dose to the patient.

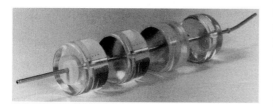

Figure 6. A photograph of an applicator assembly made with a 4-cm diameter cylinder segment and a stainless steel tandem. The cylinders are sandwiched with thin stainless steel disks to determine the cylinder size and its location in the radiographs shown in Figures 7 and 8.

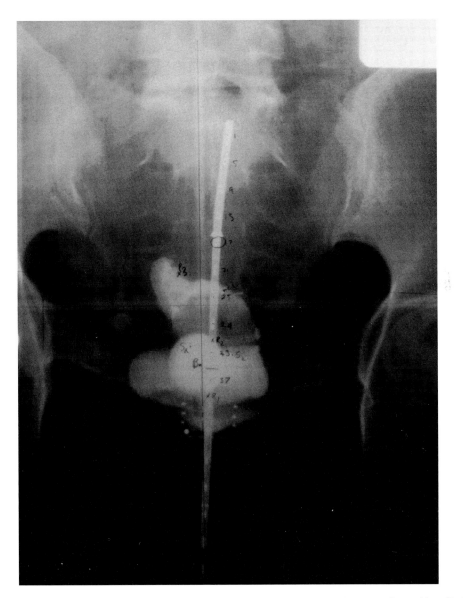

Figure 7. An AP radiograph of a typical gynecological application imaging a tandem with cylinders. The set of three dots indicates the size (3 cm) of the cylinders used.

Some of the specialized methods of localization and related mathematical equations are discussed below.

Orthogonal Films Technique

In this method, orthogonal radiographs are taken at right angles with the central axes of the x-ray beams meeting approximately in the middle of the implant. Typically, AP and lateral films taken isocentrically (Figures 7 and 8, respectively) create the needed geometry shown in Figure 10. Given the geometry in Figure 10, the equations for the x, y, and z coordinates follow from demagnification of the coordinates on the radiographs, x' and z' on the AP, and y' and z'' on the lateral, as:

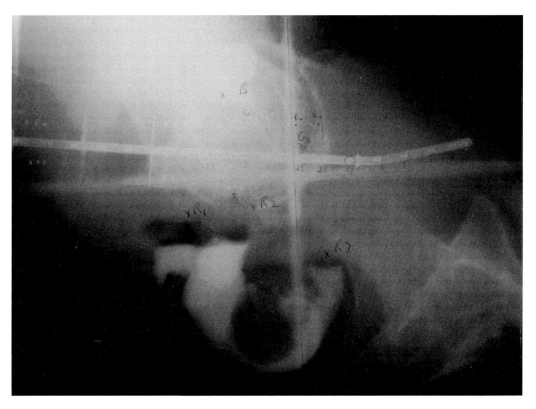

Figure 8. A lateral radiograph of a typical gynecological application imaging a tandem with cylinders. The set of three dots indicates the size (3 cm) of the cylinders used.

$$x = x' \frac{FAD_{ap} - y}{FFD_{ap}} \quad (1a)$$

$$y = y' \frac{FAD_{lat} - x}{FFD_{lat}} \quad (1b)$$

$$z = z' \frac{FAD_{ap} - y}{FFD_{ap}} \quad (1c)$$

Solving for the unknown true coordinates in terms of the known film coordinates and the beam distances gives:

$$x = \frac{x' \left(\frac{FAD_{ap}}{FFD_{ap}}\right) - \frac{x'y'}{FFD_{ap}} \left(\frac{FAD_{lat}}{FFD_{lat}}\right)}{1 - \frac{x'y'}{FFD_{ap} \cdot FFD_{lat}}} \quad (2a)$$

$$y = \frac{y' \left(\frac{FAD_{lat}}{FFD_{lat}}\right) - \frac{x'y'}{FFD_{lat}} \left(\frac{FAD_{ap}}{FFD_{ap}}\right)}{1 - \frac{x'y'}{FFD_{ap} \cdot FFD_{lat}}} \quad (2b)$$

$$z = \frac{z'}{FFD_{ap}}$$

$$\left[FAD_{ap} - \frac{y' \left(\frac{FAD_{lat}}{FFD_{lat}}\right) - \frac{x'y'}{FFD_{lat}} \left(\frac{FAD_{ap}}{FFD_{ap}}\right)}{1 - \frac{x'y'}{FFD_{ap} \cdot FFD_{lat}}} \right]. \quad (2c)$$

Solving first for x, then for y, and then for z allows use of the equations for y and z given first. Measurement of the focal axis distance (FAD) for a beam may prove difficult, in which case the distance can be derived from a magnification ring placed on the patient's skin at the entry point for the other film in the set. For the given film the relation is

$$\frac{FAD}{FFD} = \frac{\text{true ring diameter}}{\text{maximum image diameter}}. \quad (3)$$

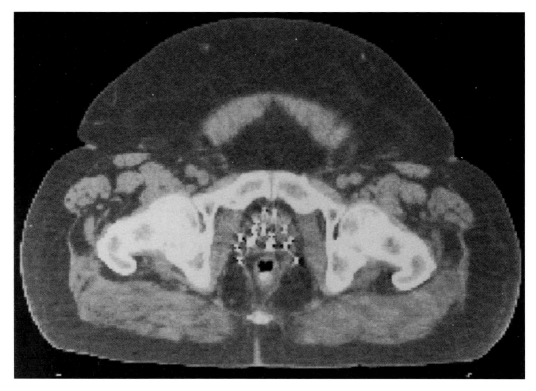

Figure 9. CT image of needles implanted transrectally in the prostate with minimal artifact.

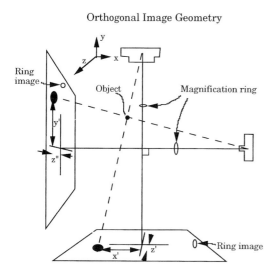

Orthogonal Image Geometry

Figure 10. The geometry of radiographs used for source localization in the orthogonal technique.

The orthogonal film technique assumes that the beam axes fall orthogonal to each other, that each film lies normal to its respective beam, and the focal film/focal axis distances are highly precise. As the setup deviates from orthogonality or measurement of the distances becomes uncertain, the accuracy of the final calculation becomes compromised.

Stereo-Shift Technique

The stereo-shift technique is less demanding on the x-ray equipment than the orthogonal film technique. First, the technique requires only anterior films so the generators need to provide less power to penetrate the patient. Second, the movement between films, being linear only, requires precise movement in fewer directions on the part of the tube support system. In fact, using the single film/double exposure technique insists only that the support of the tube housing remain stable between exposures. A two film

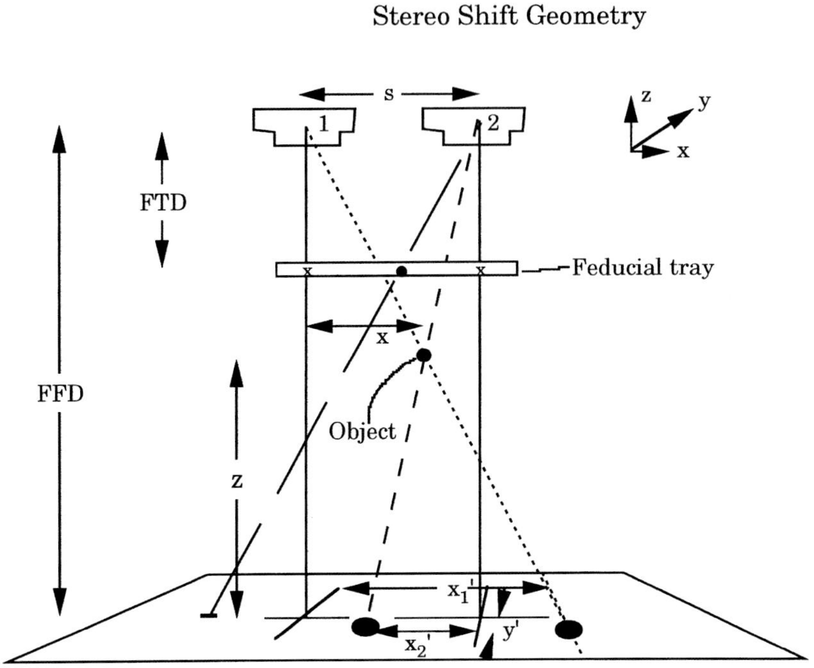

Stereo Shift Geometry

Figure 11. The geometry of radiographs used for source localization in the stereo-shift technique.

technique additionally requires a means of registering the images. A feducial plate over the patient with marks for the centers of each exposure can provide such information and, if placed at a fixed distance, can also yield the other required information, the focal film distance (FFD).

The stereo-shift method of source localization requires two radiographs of the same view, but the x-ray tube is shifted about 20 cm between the two exposures. This configuration is shown in Figure 11.

Given the geometry in Figure 11, the expressions for the coordinates become:

$$x = x_1' \left(\frac{s}{i + s} \right) \qquad (4a)$$

$$y = y_1' \left(\frac{s}{i + s} \right) \qquad (4b)$$

$$z = \frac{i \cdot FFD}{i + s} \qquad (4c)$$

where i indicates the shift in the image in the x direction, and

$$i = x_1' - (x_2' + s) \qquad (5)$$

The uncertainty in reconstructing the stereo-shift technique depends on the image separation and size of the shift. Using a large shift (usually interpreted as 25 cm or greater) and a short FFD (about 80 cm) gives good accuracy. Shortening the FFD too much can begin to compromise the z-axis reconstruction. Several articles address the accuracy and the requirements for accurate reconstruction when using stereo-shift techniques.[6–9]

Knowing the distance from the source to the feducial tray to within a small uncertainty by construction, the magnification of the mark in the center of the tray, M_m in Figure 11, yields the FFD through Equation 6:

$$FFD = M_m FTD \qquad (6)$$

Semiorthogonal Technique

Depending on the construction of the equipment, this technique has two major subcategories. One of these geometries is shown in Figure 12.

$$\text{FFD} = \frac{c_L c_S s}{c(c_L - c_S)}, \qquad (7)$$

where c_L = the size of the larger image of the crosshairs on the film; c_S = the size of the smaller image of the crosshairs on the film; and c = the actual size of the crosshairs in the feducial box. The distance from the nearest crosshairs to the film, d, is given by:

$$\delta = \text{FFD}\left(1 - \frac{c}{c_S}\right). \qquad (8)$$

Looking at the semilateral projection, the temporary coordinate system has the origin at the center of the larger crosshair, with the y' direction along the veritcal arm of the crosshair and the z'' direction along the horizontal arm. The quantity Dy' defines the y' component of the distance between the centers of the crosshair images. From these measured and derived variables, the true coordinates of the x-ray focal spot become:

$$x_2 = \text{FFD}_2 - \delta_2 - s_2, \qquad (9a)$$

$$y_2 = \frac{\Delta y'[\text{FFD}_2 - (\delta_2 + s_2)](\text{FFD}_2 - \delta_2)}{(\delta_2 + s_2)[(\text{FFD}_2 - \delta_2)(1 - \delta_2) + s\delta_2]}, \qquad (9b)$$

$$z_2 = \frac{\Delta z''[\text{FFD}_2 - (\delta_2 + s_2)](\text{FFD}_2 - \delta_2)}{(\delta_2 + s_2)[(\text{FFD}_2 - \delta_2)(1 - \delta_2) + s\delta_2]}. \qquad (9c)$$

Similarly, using the complimentary definition for the semianteroposterior image, the coordinates for the semivertical focal spot become:

$$x_1 = \frac{\Delta x'[\text{FFD}_1 - (\delta_1 + s_1)](\text{FFD}_1 - \delta_1)}{(\delta_1 + s_1)[(\text{FFD}_1 - \delta_1)(1 - \delta_1) + s\delta_1]}, \qquad (10a)$$

$$y_1 = \text{FFD}_1 - \delta_1 - s_1, \qquad (10b)$$

$$z_1 = \frac{\Delta z'[\text{FFD}_1 - (\delta_1 + s_1)](\text{FFD}_1 - \delta_1)}{(\delta_1 + s_1)[(\text{FFD}_1 - \delta_1)(1 - \delta_1) + s\delta_1]}, \qquad (10c)$$

Knowing the coordinates of the focal spots, the coordinates of the object can be found by writing the equations of the lines connecting each focal spot with its respective image of the object and solving for the intersection. For the semilateral, the projection of the line through the object in the x,y plane follows:

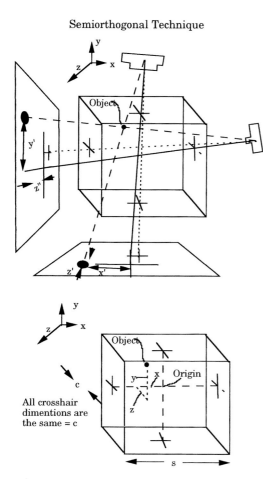

Semiorthogonal Technique

All crosshair dimentions are the same = c

Figure 12. The geometry of radiographs used for source localization in the semiorthogonal technique.

In this manifestation of the technique, the films lie parallel to the sides of the feducial box holding the crosshairs. The first step in the reconstruction finds the position of the x-ray tubes' focal spots in space based on the center of the box as the origin of the coordinate system. Since no a priori relationship exists between the x-ray units and the coordinate system (that is, after all one of the draws of the technique, one can just point and shoot without care), reconstruction requires a "temporary" coordinate system based on the larger projection of a crosshair on each film. For either projection, the FFD comes from the equation:

$$\text{slope}_2 = m_2 \tag{11a}$$

$$= \frac{\Delta y' - y' + y_2 \left(1 + \dfrac{\delta_2}{\text{FFD}_2 - \delta_2}\right)}{\text{FFD}_2},$$

and

$$\text{intercept}_2 = b_2 \tag{11b}$$

$$= y' + \text{slope}_2 \cdot \left(\frac{s_2}{2} + \delta_2\right),$$

and for the semivertical:

$$\text{slope}_1 = m_1 \tag{11c}$$

$$= \frac{\text{FFD}_1}{\Delta x' - x' - x_1 \left(1 - \dfrac{\delta_1}{\text{FFD}_1 - \delta_1}\right)},$$

and

$$\text{intercept}_1 = b_1 = \text{slope}_1$$

$$\cdot \left(\Delta x' - x' - \frac{\delta_1 x_1}{\text{FFD}_1 - \delta_1}\right) - \left(\frac{s_1}{2} + \delta_1\right). \tag{11d}$$

Once these values have been calculated, the equation for the intersection of the two lines becomes:

$$x = \frac{b_2 - b_1}{m_1 - m_2}, \tag{12a}$$

$$y = \frac{m_1 b_2 - m_2 b_1}{m_1 - m_2}, \tag{12b}$$

$$z = \left[\frac{z' + \Delta z' + \left(\dfrac{\delta_1}{\text{FFD}_1 + \delta_1}\right) z_1}{\text{FFD}_1}\right.$$

$$\left. \times \left(\text{FFD}_1 - \delta_1 - \frac{s}{2} - y\right)\right] - z_1. \tag{12c}$$

Dosimetric Quantities

Applying the equations above to a linear source determines the coordinates of the tip (x_t, y_t, z_t) and the end (x_e, y_e, z_e) of the source.

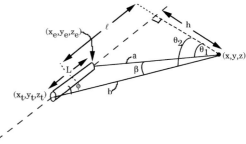

Figure 13. The geometry of a linear source used for dosimetry calculations.

Calculation of the dose to a point (x,y,z) often requires some of the following parameters, as shown in Figure 13.

The length of lines a and b can be expressed as:

$$a = \sqrt{(x - x_e)^2 + (y - y_e)^2 + (z - z_e)^2}, \tag{13a}$$

and

$$b = \sqrt{(x - x_t)^2 + (y - y_t)^2 + (z - z_t)^2}, \tag{13b}$$

From the law of cosines,

$$\cos \phi = \frac{-a^2 + b^2 + L^2}{2bL}. \tag{14}$$

But, from the definition of cosine,

$$\cos \phi = \frac{L/2 + \ell}{b}. \tag{15}$$

Thus,

$$\frac{L/2 + \ell}{b} = \frac{-a^2 + b^2 + L^2}{2bL}, \tag{16}$$

so that

$$\ell = \frac{b^2 - a^2}{2L}. \tag{17}$$

From

$$h^2 = b^2 - (L/2 + \ell)^2, \tag{18}$$

substituting for ℓ gives

$$h = \sqrt{b^2 - \left(\frac{L^2 - a^2 + b^2}{2L}\right)^2}. \quad (19)$$

From the definition of tangent,

$$\theta_1 = \tan^{-1}\left(\frac{\ell - L/2}{h}\right), \quad (20a)$$

and

$$\theta_2 = \tan^{-1}\left(\frac{\ell + L/2}{h}\right). \quad (20b)$$

Thus,

$$\beta = \theta_2 - \theta_1 \quad (21)$$

or

$$\beta = \tan^{-1}\left(\frac{\ell + L/2}{h}\right) - \tan^{-1}\left(\frac{\ell - L/2}{h}\right). \quad (22)$$

Automated Reconstructions[10–13]

Conceptually, computer programs could correlate a seed's image on two images. The usual process involves sorting seed images by their axial coordinate and matching as many seeds as possible with identical and unique values. A third image at an intermediate position between the two main images often serves to provide an additional perspective to sort among seeds with the same axial coordinate. These routines often work well for small implants, but fail with large implants where the number of seeds with coincident axial coordinates becomes large (about 100 seeds).[14]

Immobilization and Imaging

The accuracy of the dosimetry based on the imaging discussed above assumes that the radioactive material remains flexed with respect to the patient between all steps and throughout the course of treatment. Many implants immobilize themselves. For example, large volume template implants move very little and, as mentioned above, small changes in the positions of some needles make little difference in the doses delivered. Planar implants using plastic catheters pose more of a problem. The positions of seeds in a catheter in a breast implant move relative to the patient and also with respect to the other catheters as the patient moves. For this reason, many practitioners use metal needles held in place by rigid plastic templates for such applications.

While interstitial cases often tend to self-immobilize, nothing inherently holds intracavitary applications in place. In LDR treatment for cervical cancer, tandem and ovoids are held in place with vaginal gauze packing. King et al.[15] reported on a comparison of localization images taken at the end of therapy to those used for dosimetry. Movements up to a few centimeters were documented at the end of treatment. Such shifts invalidate the otherwise high accuracy of the dosimetric calculations and may account for unexpected complications as the applicator moves toward a sensitive structure or even treatment failure due to geographic miss. HDR gynecological applicators are locked into table brackets that fix in place during planning and treatment. The fixation assures a high correlation between the calculated and delivered dose. Thomadsen et al.[16] reported an average movement of 2.6 mm between dosimetry films and posttreatment films. Movement of the patient between imaging and treatment even on immobilization board compromises this precision. Intraluminal applications lend themselves less well to immobilization. The usual assumption with LDR treatments for endobronchial or endoesophageal insertions is that the treatment catheter follows a narrow tube, so once fixed at the insertion point (usually a naris), the position along the tube remains constant. For many patients this assumption appears to hold, yet for some, there seems to be movement. This becomes most noticeable for patients localized recumbent, but treated sitting upright (Personal communication, B.R. Thomadson). This movement is even more pronounced when the catheter is in place for a number of days. In addition, for endobronchial applications, deep, heavy coughs can dislodge a catheter not inserted deeply into the bronchial tree. Undetected, such a major movement can result in the mistreatment of incorrect locations or even the wrong bronchus. One HDR unit manufacturer

(Varisource by Varian Associates, Palo Alto, CA, USA) developed a releasable hooking mechanism for the tip of an intraluminal catheter to anchor the distal end.

Equipment Considerations

Imaging equipment often limits the ability to visualize necessary information.

1. Using a portable unit brought into the room used for the insertion: Portable x-ray units seldom have the power to penetrate adequately on the lateral projection. In addition, they suffer from geometric instability problems further discussed below.
2. Moving the patient to the radiotherapy simulator: Simulators provide some of the most powerful radiographic imaging systems, but their use involves moving the patient, a practice to be avoided, again as discussed below.
3. Using overhead or C-arm x-ray tubes: Most diagnostic type overhead tube systems fall in-between the portables and simulators in power, probably being just adequate for the lateral imaging. As with the portable units, most diagnostic sets are not made for highly precise and accurate setting of angles and distances.

Geometrical Considerations

Accurate assessment of the dose to the normal structures depends critically on accurate reconstruction through imaging. For the reconstruction to render the coordinates of the sources and anatomical structures correctly, the criteria for the type of localization used must be met. For example, when using orthogonal films, the axes must be very close to truly orthogonal, both axes must be completely contained in a single plane (i.e., the central rays must fall in a given transverse cut), and the films must be perpendicular to their central rays. Also for each film, the FFD and the FAD (the distance from the focus to the intersection of the two axes) must be known to a high degree of accuracy. Each film needs to show the crosshairs indicating the central ray. Failure of any of these criteria

markedly decreases the accuracy of the dose calculation, which could lead to inappropriate doses and therefore compromise treatment results. Adams[17] presents an excellent discussion of localization accuracy and its dependence on proper input. For a portable x-ray unit, the distances often are difficult to know accurately, particularly the FAD. Often, a ring of a known diameter placed on the entrance location for one of the laterals provides the magnification at the isocenter on the opposite film in the set, usually in the AP set and vise versa. This requires including at least one of the skin surfaces on each set of films, thereby generating more scatter in the larger volume and decreasing film visibility. In addition, moving the unit between the two images makes it difficult to keep the axes intersecting. During the time it takes for this movement, the patient also may move, again reducing reconstruction accuracy. This also holds true for most overhead and column mounted x-ray units. C-arm units that rotate between a lateral and posterior axis frequently have trouble holding steady as film cassettes are inserted and removed. This is due to the large lever-arm torque at the cassette holder. In addition, the mounting on most C-arm units restricts their movements to only a posterior and a lateral for orthogonal views.

A Practical Approach

At the University of Wisconsin, a ceiling mounted C-arm was bolted in the lateral projection and a surplus overhead tube and housing was attached at the apex of the "C." This forms an orthogonal pair of x-ray beams that can be lowered over the patient. Figure 14 shows the arrangement. In this configuration, the orthogonal set no longer requires moving the patient between films and thus reduces the time for imaging and possible uncertainties. The particular arrangement uses a single generator to power both tubes, allowing only for sequential rather than true simultaneous exposures. However, tests with film in both receptors during either exposure indicate that the patient generates too much scatter to the orthogonal film to permit simultaneous exposures. Unlike scatter generated grossly along the beam direction that a grid attenuates,

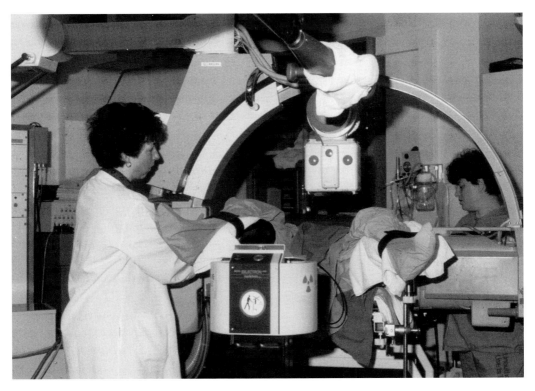

Figure 14. A ceiling mounted C-arm with two orthogonal x-ray tubes and fluoro system.

much of the scatter from the orthogonal beam falls into the grid's acceptance angle.

An added advantage of the C-arm system is that it allows for fluoroscopy. Such live-time imaging shows the physician if changes in the applicator placement should precede filming. When the applicator needs adjustment, the changes can be monitored and corrected the first time. Considering the time involved with taking and processing the films, prefilming fluoroscopy often considerably reduces the time the patient spends on the table.

Clinical Applications

The use of CT and MRI is limited in gynecological brachytherapy since most applicators are not compatible with either imaging modality. As previously discussed, a rigid immobilization system is utilized in HDR brachytherapy at the University of Wisconsin. This facilitates the accurate delivery of a single, large radiation fraction. Moving the patient between the brachytherapy suite and a CT or

MRI scanner would most likely result in applicator movement that would preclude accurate dose delivery. In addition, tandem and ovoids can be accurately placed clinically since the tumor is usually visualized and palpated. CT or MRI may have a role in interstitial brachytherapy where the entire tumor extent may not be clinically determined. Also, these imaging modalities may be helpful after the needles have been inserted to verify that the tumor has been implanted and that normal tissue structures are out of the implant volume.

Ultrasound is very helpful in HDR gynecological brachytherapy. For patients with either surgically or medically inoperable uterine cancer, the exact uterine length is pivotal for curative therapy. We treat a number of patients with medically inoperable uterine cancer due to morbid obesity. The average weight exceeds 300 lbs with an occasional patient over 400 lbs. In these patients, the fundal height cannot be determined clinically. We routinely obtain a pelvic ultrasound, either before the insertion or at the first insertion, to determine the uterine length. The ultrasound in Figure 4 indicates the tandem tip needs to be advanced another 1–2 cm. While it is not critical that the tandem be at the very top of the uterus for patients with cervical cancer, it is essential for patients with uterine cancer since a geographic miss may result.

Ultrasound is also very helpful to rule out a perforation in patients with bulky cervical cancer and in patients with uterine cancer that grossly invades the cervix. McGinn et al.[3] reported the use of ultrasound in our initial 51 HDR patients at the University of Wisconsin. Ultrasound was used in 3% (7/237) of the insertions. Figure 5 demonstrates a uterine perforation in a patient with a necrotic cervical cancer. Figure 4 is the same patient after the tandem has been readjusted and placed in the uterine cavity. The decision to obtain an ultrasound is a clinical one. If there is a concern that the lower uterine segment or fundus has been perforated an ultrasound is obtained. The typical scenario is a patient with a necrotic cervical cancer in which the endocervical canal is not easily cannulated and many false passages are created. Also, the HDR tandem is 3.2 mm in diameter as opposed to the LDR tandem, which is 6.4 mm. This means the chance of perforating a cervix replaced with tumor and being outside of the uterine cavity is potentially greater with HDR tandems. Other indications for an ultrasound include discrepancies in the uterine length from one insertion to the next, radiographic evidence of a perforation (i.e., tandem too high in the pelvis), and an inability to sound the uterus. The last indication is rare, but has occurred in two patients. Because of the large single fractions that are used in HDR brachytherapy, an ultrasound is strongly recommended to verify tandem placement if any concern exists over a perforation. The likelihood of creating a fistula in the bowel or rectum greatly increases if the tandem is abutting either of these structures. In fact, one patient fistulized 6 weeks after completing five HDR treatments. In reviewing the films and details of the insertion, the tandem had perforated the uterus and was abutting the bowel in at least two of the five insertions. We therefore use ultrasound more liberally if clinically indicated.

In summary, ultrasound is a useful imaging modality in HDR brachytherapy. Its judicious use facilitates accurate tumor assessment (uterine cancer) and minimizes the chance of overdosing normal tissues.

Conclusions

Imaging plays an extremely important role in brachytherapy. Irrespective of the radiation source, applicator used and dose rates employed, the precise and accurate delivery of treatment is essential. Errors of only a few millimeters in the spatial position of the source(s) can easily result in the delivery of errors >10 mm. The localization errors can be minimized by using imaging systems with good spatial resolution, reproducible positioning capability, isocentric mount, and not requiring patient movement and repositioning between different images. Ideally, it would be excellent to have two biplanar mounted (orthogonal and lateral) fluoroscopic and radiographic systems capable of operating simultaneously or at least sequentially.

References

1. Granai CG, Doherty F, Allee P, et al. Ultrasound for diagnosing and preventing misplacement of intrauterine tandems. Obstet Gynecol 1990;75:110–113.
2. Wong F, Bhimgi S. The usefulness of ultrasonography in intracavitary radiotherapy using Selectron applicators. Int J Radiat Oncol Biol Phys 1990;19:477–482.
3. McGinn CJ, Stitt JA, Buchler DA, et al. Intraoperative ultrasound guidance during high dose rate intracavitary brachytherapy of the uterine cervix and corpus. Endocuriether Hyperthermia Oncol 1992;8:101–104.
4. Fletcher GH. Textbook of Radiotherapy. Lea and Febiger, Philadelphia, 1980.
5. International Commission on Radiation Units and Measurements (ICRU). Dose and Volume Specification for Reporting Intracavitary Therapy in Gynecology. ICRU, Bethesda, MD, 1985.
6. Hughes HA. Accuracy of foreign body localization for "Tube Shift" radiographs. Br J Radiol 1956;29:116–118.
7. Fitzgerald LT, Mauderli W. Analysis of errors in three-dimensional reconstruction of radium implants from stereo radiographs. Radiology 1975;115:455–458.
8. Sharma SC, Williamson JF, Cytacki E. Dosimet-

ric analysis of stereo and orthogonal reconstruction of interstitial implants. Int J Radiat Oncol Biol Phys 1982;8:1801–1805.

9. Niroomand-Rad A, Thomadsen B, Vainio P. Evaluation of the reconstruction of brachytherapy implants in three-dimensions from stereo radiographs. Radiother Oncol 1987;8:337–342.

10. Amols HI, Rosen II. A three-film technique for reconstruction of radioactive seed implants. Med Phys 1981;8:210–214.

11. Rosenthal MS, Nath R. An automatic seed identification technique for interstitial implants using three isocentric radiographs. Med Phys 1983;10:475–479.

12. Altschuler MD, Findlay PA, Epperson RD. Rapid, accurate, three-dimensional location of multiple seeds in implant radiotherapy treatment planning. Phys Med Biol 1983;28:1305–1318.

13. Siddon RL, Chin LM. Two-film brachytherapy reconstruction algorithm. Med Phys 1985;12:77–83.

14. Thomadsen BR, Shahabi S. Video tape recording assistance in radiotherapy seed identification. Abstract. Med Phys 1987;14:476.

15. King CG, Stockstill TF, Bloomer WD, et al. Point dose variations with time in brachytherapy for cervical carcinoma. Abstract. Med Phys 1993;19:777.

16. Thomadsen BR, Shahabi S, Stitt JA, et al. High dose rate intracavitary brachytherapy for carcinoma of the cervix: The Madison System: II. Procedural and physical considerations. Int J Radiat Oncol Biol Phys 1992;24:349–357.

17. Adams G. Errors in brachytherapy. In: Wright A, Boyer A (eds). Advances in Radiation Therapy Treatment Planning. American Institute of Physics, New York, 1983, pp. 575–600.

Chapter 10

Radiation Protection

Nina Samsami, Ph.D.,
Robert Peterson, B.S.,
Subir Nag, M.D.

Introduction

The term brachytherapy means treatment with radioactive sources at short distances. In brachytherapy, the radioactive sources may be inserted into the malignant tissue so that a very high dose of radiation can be delivered just where it is needed. This must be achieved while protecting the general public and health care workers from the adverse effects of radiation. In 1954 the National Committee on Radiation Protection put forth the principle that radiation exposures should be kept "As Low As Reasonably Achievable" (ALARA).[1] The ALARA philosophy is based on adopting a conservative assumption that any radiation exposure may carry some risks. This philosophy applies to occupational workers and the members of the general public. The quantity of radiation dose that personnel working with brachytherapy sources, i.e., occupational radiation workers, may be exposed to is regulated by either state or federal agencies. Dose limits for radiation workers, the general public, pregnant women, and embryo/fetuses, according to Subparts C and D of Title 10 CFR, Part 20, are listed in Table 1.[2]

The US Nuclear Regulatory Commission (NRC) requires all medical licensees to establish an ALARA Program. This can usually be achieved through the use of proper safety procedures and training. The required contents of an ALARA Program are given in 10 CFR Part 35.20.

In brief, distance, shielding, and time are the three basic variables involved in radiation protection. By manipulation of one or a combination of these three variables, radiation exposure can be reduced considerably. Detailed recommendations for reducing radiation exposure in handling radioisotope sources are given in NCRP No 40 and 48.[3,4]

Distance

Radiation exposure is inversely proportional to the square of the distance from the source. This relationship between distance and radiation exposure is called the Inverse Square Law. Increasing the distance from a radiation source reduces the radiation exposure of an individual. For instance, doubling the distance quarters the radiation exposure. Hence, it is clear that it is important to stay as far as possible from the radiation source. Long handled tools should be used to handle brachytherapy sources, and a protective distance (preferably >6 feet) between the radioactive patient and health care workers should be maintained whenever possible. For instance, one should stand at either the head or foot of the bed of patients with intracavitary

From Nag S (ed): *Principles and Practice of Brachytherapy.* © Futura Publishing Co., Inc., Armonk, NY, 1997.

Table 1.
Yearly Dose Limits for Radiation Workers, General Public, Pregnant Women,
and Embryo/Fetuses

For Radiation Workers:	
Whole body dose equivalent	50 mSv (5 Rem)
Eye dose equivalent	150 mSv (15 Rem)
Shallow dose equivalent (to skin or extremity)	500 mSv (50 Rem)
Dose to embryo/fetus for pregnant workers during the entire pregnancy	5 mSv (0.5 Rem)*
Minors (age < 18 years)	10% of the limits for adults
For the General Public:	
Total effective dose equivalent (TEDE)	1 mSv (0.1 Rem)**

* Summation of deep dose equivalent to the declared pregnant woman and dose to the embryo/fetus.
** The dose at unrestricted area from external source should not exceed 0.002 rem (0.02 mSev) in any one hour.

implants or at the side of the bed farthest from the implant for patients with head-and-neck implants. Persons not providing direct care should stop at the doorway when visiting or providing patient education.

Shielding

The use of various high density materials as shielding will reduce radiation exposure. The most commonly used materials are lead and concrete. In choosing the type of material for shielding, one must consider the type and energy of radiation. For instance, low energy emissions such as those from I-125 or those used for fluoroscopy can be easily shielded by a thin layer of lead, such as a lead apron. However, for brachytherapy patients with high energy removable implants, lead aprons provide little protection since they only minimally absorb high energy radiation. With these implants, a lead bedside shield could be used to reduce radiation exposure. When properly used, this shielding can provide additional protection from radiation exposure; however, shielding equipment is cumbersome, and often its use causes nursing staff to spend additional time in the patients' rooms maneuvering the shields. If nurses follow the guidelines for limiting time spent in patients' rooms and maintain the maximum possible distance from the radioactive source, they can minimize their exposure regardless of the presence or absence of shielding.

Time

The quantity of radiation exposure is directly related to time. Simply put, the longer an individual remains within a radiation field, the more radiation exposure that person will receive. Guidelines for the length of time that one can spend with the radioactive patient must be posted on the patient's chart and door. Although nursing personnel can exceed these guidelines in cases in which extra medical care is required, radiation exposure should always be minimized by using time efficiently. After the patient has been returned to the room and before radioactive sources are loaded, the maximum amount of direct nursing care should be provided. Vital signs and the applicator site should be checked, comfort measures should be provided, and call button and personal objects should be placed within the patient's reach. The patient should be encouraged to care for himself/herself, and nursing staff should be rotated. The necessity of limiting staff exposure should be explained to the patient and the patient should be reassured that adequate nursing care will be maintained. With the application of measures such as these, time spent with the radioactive patient can be minimized without compromising patient care.

Starting a New Brachytherapy Program

The important factors to be kept in mind when designing a new brachytherapy program is the need to protect the general public and the health care workers from the adverse effects of radiation, to comply with regulatory guidelines, and to have personnel well-trained in and familiar with brachytherapy safety procedures.

Licensing

In the US institutions establishing a program to work with radioisotopes need an appropriate license from either the NRC or, in the "agreement states," from the state health department. This authorization involves completion of a special material license form, NRC Form 313, which requires information on the type of radioisotopes to be purchased, their purpose and intended use, the maximum amount to be possessed at any one time, the training and experience of the individual responsible for radiation safety program, the radiation detection instruments available, personnel monitoring devices, laboratory facilities, handling equipment, waste disposal procedures, and the quality management program. The institution is responsible for providing a radiation safety program that ensures ALARA doses to radiation workers and members of the public.

A broad scope license[4] is issued to institutions involved in research and medical use of radioisotopes. The NRC authorizes the Radiation Safety Committee (RSC) of the institution to oversee the safe use of radioisotopes. The RSC consists of a radiation safety officer, a representative of management, and persons trained and experienced in the safety handling of radioactive materials. RSC is responsible for development of documentation procedures and implementation of a radiation protection program in accordance with the scope and extent of licensed activities and sufficient to ensure compliance with the NRC regulations. It is essential that individuals working with radioisotopes receive proper training and continuing education in radiation safety and in ALARA concepts.

The license for the medical use of radioactive materials may also be issued to individual physicians properly trained in the handling and use of medical radioisotopes. It is essential that all licensing requirements have been met before starting a brachytherapy program.

Training Requirements

It is important that each individual dealing with brachytherapy sources receives appro-

priate radiation safety training related to his/her duties. The basic training program for radioisotope user must cover safety, radioactivity measurements, monitoring techniques, radiation calculation, and biological effects. In addition, radiation workers should know their rights to access personnel exposure data, regulations, amendments, and inspection reports. They should not proceed with a treatment unless they are familiar with all aspects of the treatment. All training should be documented and kept on file for inspection.

Receipt and Assay of Radionuclides

A package containing radionuclide must be monitored immediately after receipt for any damage, contamination, or leakage. This monitoring must be completed no later than 3 hours after the package is received during the normal working hours or not later than 3 hours from the beginning of the next working day if it is received after working hours (10 CFR 20.1906). If the contamination in excess of 22,000 dis/min per cm^2 is found at the package surface or if the radiation level exceeds 200 mrem/hr at the surface or 10 mrem/hr at one meter from the surface, the licensee must notify the final delivery carrier immediately and the appropriate NRC Inspection Office by telephone, mailgram, or facsimile (10 CFR 71.87, 10 CFR 71.47). Each licensee must establish and maintain written procedures for safely opening packages containing radioactive materials.

Brachytherapy sources should be assayed upon opening of the package or container. The seeds are assayed in a well-type ionization chamber. The measured values are compared with the activity of the seeds recorded in shipper's certificate and documented in the assay book.

Storage and Control of Brachytherapy Sources

For a brachytherapy program, it is necessary to provide a special storage room "hot lab" designed for the storage of the anticipated types and quantities of brachytherapy sources. This room should be secured and be accessible only to designated workers and should preferably be close to the area where the sources are calibrated and will be ultimately used (CFR 20.1801). Usually cesium-137 and radium-226 sources are stored in a locked lead safe. Other brachytherapy sources such as palladium-103, iodine-125, gold-198, and iridium-192 are stored in their shipping containers. The radioisotopes should be adequately shielded such that the surface exposure rate is <10 mR/hr. Access to the brachytherapy storage area must be controlled at all times. The room must be posted with appropriate signs in accordance with applicable regulations (CFR 20.1902). Proper inventory of brachytherapy sources must be maintained in a log book, and is mandated by regulators. Inventory of brachytherapy sources is performed at least on a quarterly basis and contains the following information:

1. Model number of each source,
2. Serial number,
3. Location of each source,
4. Radionuclide,
5. Nominal activity of each source.

To insure that all sources that were used for a patient have been removed and returned to the storage room, an inventory of the brachytherapy sources should be conducted at the conclusion of each treatment.

The areas adjacent to the brachytherapy storage sites must be surveyed to ensure that radiation levels are at acceptable levels. These records must be retained for a minimum of 3 years.

Transportation of Brachytherapy Sources

Proper procedures must be followed to insure safety and efficiency when brachytherapy sources are transported within a medical institution (e.g., from the "hot lab" to the patient's room). Brachytherapy sources must be transported in shielded carriers, preferably on a cart. To ensure stability, the carriers should not be cumbersome or top-heavy. The shielding should be thick enough to reduce external radiation levels at contact to 200 mR/hr (10CFR 70.47), (the thickness of lead for providing additional shielding may be found in NCRP report #37).[5] Radioisotopes with high energy emissions (cesium-137, iridium-192)

will require thick lead shielding as opposed to iodine-125 or palladium-103, which require only minimal shielding. The transporter should be equipped with a portable radiation survey meter and remote handling tools in case of an accident.

Patient Surveys

Promptly after brachytherapy sources have been implanted in a patient, a radiation survey must be performed in areas in and around the patient's room. The survey must include patient's name, total activity of the sources at that day, and the date and time of insertion. Before release of the patient from the hospital, the patient and the patient's room must be surveyed again. In case of temporary implants, the survey must be performed upon removal of brachytherapy sources from the patient to insure that all sources have been removed from the patient and the room. The survey must include the date of the survey, patient's name, radiation levels from the patient and locations within the room and the surveyor's signature. This record must be retained for 3 years.

Storage for Decay or Disposal

Cesium-137 and radium-226 have long half-lives and hence are used repeatedly over a number of years. When these sources lose their effectiveness they must be disposed of, and their disposal can become a problem because of the lack of disposal sites and the reluctance of other companies to take these sources. As a result, the department often must keep these sources for an indefinite period of time.

Iridium-192 sources, which have an intermediate half-life, are usually used only once and are returned to the supplier for disposal. Alternatively, iridium-192 wires can be used repeatedly over a period of a few months and then returned to the supplier for disposal. Before the sources are returned to the supplier, a smear wipe of the inner container must be taken to ensure that there is no contamination. A complete shipper's certification form must accompany the shipment to the supplier. Records of such transactions must be kept. Shipping of these sources must meet applicable Department of Transportation regulations. Usually the supplier of the brachytherapy sources will send instructions about the proper return of the sources.

Low energy brachytherapy sources (iodine-125, and palladium-103) are easily shielded and are disposed of more easily. These sources have half-lives of 60 days or less and must be stored for decay for a minimum of 10 half-lives (10 CFR 35.92). Short half-life radioisotopes like gold-198 are also stored for 10 half-lives for decay. Before radioisotopes can be disposed, their radiation level must be indistinguishable from background radiation level with a radiation detection survey meter set on its most sensitive scale and no shielding must exist between detector and radioisotope (10 CFR 35.92). Records for this type of disposal must include the date at which the sources were put into storage, radionuclide, activity, date of disposal, survey meter used, background dose rate, dose rate of the brachytherapy source, and the name of the individual who performed the disposal. In all cases, brachytherapy sources must be disposed of in accordance with applicable regulations.

Posting Notice to Employees

The licensee must post current copies of NRC-3 form, "NOTICE TO EMPLOYEES" in a sufficient number of places to permit individuals involved in licensed activities to observe them. A copy of radiation protection rules and all of the operating procedures or restrictions that apply to the individual's work and the provisions related to them must be available to them. The employee is responsible for becoming familiar with these rules and operating procedures. A licensee must provide a written report of an individual's exposure to him/her if the individual's exposure exceeds any applicable limits as set forth in the rules.

Posting of Areas

The licensee is required to post radiation signs in the areas where levels of radiation or radioactivity are present. The common types of signs and the circumstances requiring their use follow:

1. A **"Caution Radiation Area"** sign is required in the areas where individuals may receive a dose equivalent in excess of 0.005 rem (0.05 mSv) in 1 hour at 30 centimeters from the radiation source.

2. A **"Caution Radioactive Material"** sign is required where radioactive materials are used in an amount exceeding quantities listed in appendix C of 10 CFR part 20.

3. An **"Airborne Radioactivity Area"** or "**Danger Radioactivity Area**" sign is required if the concentration of airborne materials present exceeds the derived air concentration (DAC) specified in appendix B, CFR 20, or if an individual could receive in 1 week a total intake of 0.6 percent of annual limit on intake (ALI) or 12 DAC.

4. A **"High Radiation Area"** sign is required where the radiation level could result in an individual receiving a dose equivalent in excess of 0.1 rem (1 mSv) in 1 hour at 30 centimeters from the radiation source.

5. A **"Very High Radiation Area"** sign is required in the areas in which an individual could receive an absorbed dose in excess of 500 rads (5 Gy) in 1 hour at one meter from the radiation source.

Radiation Detectors

Survey Meters

Two types of radiation monitoring devices are useful for survey of medical radiation facilities. First, survey meters, such as Geiger-Muller counters or scintillation detectors, are useful for detection of radiation in the medical facility or in the vicinity of the patient undergoing brachytherapy procedure. These devices are useful only for detection of radiation and should not be used to measure exposure rates despite the fact that some survey meters are calibrated to read in mR/hr. Another type of monitoring device, the ion chambers (by Keithley or Victoreen), can be used to measure gamma rays with energies from 7 keV to 2 MeV. There are some problems associated with ion chambers. Their response to γ and x-rays change with incident photon energy since photon absorbtion and penetration through the chamber walls and gas volume is an energy-dependent process. As with any survey meter, these devices must not be used for calibration of radioisotopes.

Personal Monitoring Devices

Personal monitoring devices must be worn on the chest or abdomen in all controlled areas where there is a possibility of receiving a dose exceeding one tenth of applicable maximal permissable dose. These devices must be left at the work site in the specific location at the end of each day. Personal monitoring is valuable for checking the adequacy of a radiation protection program; therefore, any accidental mishandling of these devices should be reported to the radiation safety officer. Different types of personal monitoring devices are discussed below.

Film Badge

The most common device used to monitor individual whole-body exposure to x- and gamma radiation and charged particles is the film badge. This dosimeter must be worn on chest or abdomen. A film badge is made of a dental film covered by a thin copper, stepped wedge filter to detect various quality of radiation. The film is backed by the lead foil to absorb backscattered radiation. Commercial laboratories provide fresh film badges monthly and process the previous film badges, comparing them with standard film exposed to known quantities of radiation. The amount of exposure of each film badge is reported to the corresponding institution.

Pocket Ionization Chamber

The pocket ionization chamber is another personal monitoring device that consists of an ionization chamber and a built-in electrometer for reading the radiation dosage. The pocket ionization chamber must be handled carefully. Leakage across the insulator may result from exposure to excessive moisture. Although, this device does not provide a permanent record, it is the best available personal monitor for reading exposure level directly.

Thermoluminescence Dosimeter

Thermoluminescence Dosimeter (TLD) detectors consist of crystals that have a unique ability to store energy when they are exposed to radiation. The radiation raises the electrons of the crystal to the metastable state. They remain in excited states until they are heated to a temperature high enough to cause electrons to return to their normal state by emission of light. The energy absorbed is proportional to the amount of light emitted, which can be measured by a photomultiplier tube. Lithium fluoride activated with magnesium and titanium is most suited for TLD. TLD materials have some advantages over other personal monitors in that they are less affected by environmental changes. Although photographic emulsions (film) holds information permanently if it is developed, they are not reusable. TLD monitors can be annealed and used over again.

Radiation Safety Issues Involved in Permanent Brachytherapy

There are many radiation safety issues involved in permanent brachytherapy including source handling and transportation, loss or rupture of seeds, room and patient surveys, and procedures to follow in the event of the death of permanently implanted patients.

The common radioisotopes used for permanent brachytherapy, i.e., Pd-103 and I-125, have low energy and short half-lives and hence require minimal precautions. The sources are loaded in shielded cartridges by long forceps and transported to the operating room in shielded, metal containers. The seeds are autoclaved for 3 minutes; longer autoclaving is inadvisable as the integrity of the seeds may be breached. After the patient has been implanted, but before he/she leaves the operating room, radiation measurements are taken at bedside 3 feet and 6 feet from the patient. The operating room floor, blood suction bottles, garbage bags, needles, and autoclave are surveyed after the patient leaves the operating room. Any seeds found in the operating room must be stored in a lead shielded container and picked up by the radiation safety officer for proper radioactive disposal. Patients with

**GUIDELINES FOR INDIVIDUALS COMING IN CONTACT
WITH PERMANENTLY IMPLANTED PATIENTS**

The Arthur G. James Cancer Hospital and Research Institute
Department of Radiation Oncology

_____ (name) was implanted on _____ , 19___ with _____

millicuries of Iodine-125/Palladium-103 in the form of _____ (number) seeds into

_____ (organ).

There is minimum radiation exposure at the implanted area.
NO RADIATION SAFETY PRECAUTIONS ARE NECESSARY AFTER _____ .
The bracelet may be removed at the above date.

UNTIL THEN, IT IS SUGGESTED THAT:

1.   Children or pregnant women not come in contact with the implanted area of patient more than 1 hour per day. (There is no restriction to the time spent at a distance of 3 feet from the patient.)
2.   Pregnant staff are to contact Radiation Oncology if they have concerns about caring for permanently implanted patients.
3.   Every physician consulted concerning this patient must be shown this form.
4.   In the unlikely event that a seed becomes dislodged, please put in metal container, and inform Radiation Oncology (293-8415), who will inform you on proper disposal.
5.   If the patient is to be hospitalized, have surgery at the implanted site, or if death should occur, **you must immediately notify RADIATION ONCOLOGY, at the Ohio State University Hospitals at 614-293-8415 during working hours or after hours Radiation Oncology On-Call Physician through hospital operator at 614-293-8000 for details of radiation precautions.**

_____

_____

My signature below constitutes my acknowledgement (1) that I have read, (or it has been read to me), and agree to the foregoing, (2) that the guidelines for individuals coming in contact with permanently implantable patients have been explained to my satisfaction by the staff or physicians and that I have all the information that I desire, and (3) that I will wear the identification bracelet until the stated removal date.

X_____ Date_____
    (patient)

X_____ Date_____
    (witness)

Patient Copy

Figure 1. Written instructions given to patients with permanent implants. This form is printed in triplicate such that a copy can be posted in the patient's room and another copy placed in the patient's chart.

I-125 or Pd-103 implants can be discharged home after they have recovered from surgery. The patient should be provided with written instructions regarding radiation precautions (Figure 1) and should wear a "medical alert" bracelet at all times for the duration of radiation precautions. This bracelet indicates the radioisotope implanted, the duration that the radiation precautions should be observed, and the names and phone numbers of per-sons to be notified in the event of an emergency.

Permanently Implanted Patients Undergoing Emergency Surgery

The guidelines for permanently implanted patients undergoing emergency surgery are given in NCRP report #37 and are summarized below. The radiation oncology physician is to identify the area of the implantation. If the surgery involves the area of the previous implant, suction is to be avoided if at all possible. If necessary, the area of the tumor containing the implant is to be removed by the surgeon. The seeds are to be retrieved by the radiation oncology physician, taking care not to damage any seeds; and all must be accounted for if possible. If it is not possible to retrieve the seeds, a radiograph of the specimen should be obtained so that the seeds can be accounted for. Any loose seeds in the body cavity are to be retrieved. The surgeon then continues with the surgery. The seeds are to be stored for radioactive decay in a shielded container. If the seeds were not individually re-

trieved, the entire organ should be frozen and picked up by the radiation safety officer for radioactive disposal.

Death of Patients with Permanent Implants

The procedure to follow when a permanently implanted patient expires is summarized here and detailed in NCRP Report #37. At the time of the implantation, the patients are given a "medical alert" bracelet noting the radioisotope implanted, the duration that the radiation precautions are to be observed, and the names and phone numbers of persons to be notified in the event of an emergency. Such

Form for Radioactivity Report Accompanying a Body

_____Hospital

Report to Funeral Director from Radiation Safety Officer (or delegate) on radioactivity.

☐   This body does not contain significant amount of radioactive materials. No special precautions are required if standard embalming procedures are employed.

☐   This body contains a significant amount of radioactive material:

Radioisotope   _____

Amount   _____ mCi

The following precautions are to be observed:

_____

_____

_____

Signed _____
              Radiation Safety Officer (or Delegate)

Date _____

Figure 2. An acceptable form for radioactivity report to accompany the body after death of a person with permanent implant.

a bracelet warns hospital personnel in the event that the patient is rehospitalized; upon the patient's death, this bracelet facilitates notification of the radiation oncologist who performed the implant and who is then responsible for determining whether the body is to be autopsied, cremated, or buried without an autopsy. The physician should also notify the radiation safety officer at the hospital where the death occurred. A form (Figure 2) that indicates which isotope is present in the body and gives any necessary instructions or precautions that the funeral director should observe when handling the body should accompany the body to the funeral home.

If the body is to be autopsied, the pathology department should be notified that the body is radioactive and that the radiation precautions need to be observed. If at all possible, the organ containing the radioactive seeds should be removed first. The entire body should then be checked to confirm that there is no residual radioactivity. If there is residual radioactivity, the seeds remaining in the body must be detected, removed, and placed in a shielded container.

If the body is to be cremated, the radioactive seeds in the implanted organ should be carefully retrieved and placed in a shielded container for decay. If this cannot be easily done, the organ (or part of it) can be frozen and sent to radiation safety for disposal.

If the body is to be buried without autopsy and if the implanted organ can be replaced in the body cavity, the funeral home can be notified that they may proceed with standard embalming procedures.

Radiation Safety Issues Involved in Removable Implants

The radioisotopes most often used for temporary implants are Ir-192, Cs-137, and occasionally, I-125. Ir-192 seeds come from the manufacturer encased in nylon ribbons to facilitate loading into preplaced catheters. Ir-192 is generally returned to the manufacturer after each use, although it can be reused, if required. Cs-137 sources have a long half-life of 30 years and are reused; they are kept in specially designed vaults at the therapy centers. These sources are encased in 2 cm tubes and are used primarily for gynecological implants. I-125 sources, which are also used for permanent implants, come from the manufacturer as individual seeds. I-125 temporary implants are most frequently used in eye plaques; they are occasionally used for brain and breast implants. The radiation safety issues relating to removable implants include the preparation and transportation of the sources prior to implant, the procedures to be followed after the seeds have been implanted, procedures to be followed in the event a source becomes dislodged or lost, and procedures to be followed after source removal.

Source Preparation

Considerable care must be given to source preparation and especially to the cutting of Ir-192 ribbons. Utmost care must be taken to ensure that a radioactive seed is not cut during this procedure and that the cut fragment of the iridium ribbon is not lost. For these reasons, it is recommended that ribbons containing Ir-192 seeds not be cut unless absolutely necessary. These sources must be prepared behind lead blocks to minimize the radiation exposure involved.

Patient Care

Private rooms should be provided for patients with removable implants. Radiation precaution signs and time restrictions should be posted on the patient's door. Because the sources are sealed there is minimal risk of contamination. However, a possible risk arises if the sources are damaged or lost. Therefore, the linen and food trays should be inspected before they are removed from the room to make certain that no sources have been inadvertently lost. Any dressings over the implanted area should be changed only by the radiation oncology staff to ensure that there are no displacement of the radioactive sources. Before the patient's discharge, the patient and the room should be surveyed by Radiation Safety to confirm that there is no residual radioactivity.

Radiation Emergencies

Lost Source(s)

If any radioactive sources are lost or misplaced, the Office of Radiation Safety should be notified immediately. The path of the source should be retraced and areas where the source was used should be surveyed using an appropriate survey meter. The missing source should be recovered and placed in a shielded container. Any sources not recovered should be reported to the Radiation Safety Office.

Dislodged Source

If a source becomes dislodged, spilled, or discharged during patient treatment, it should be picked up using long-handled tools and placed into the lead carrier. The radiation oncologist and radiation safety officer should be notified immediately.

Delirious Patient

Patients becoming delirious during treatment may require restraint or medication so as not to pose a threat to themselves or to the staff. The radiation oncologist must be notified of the patient's condition, and a decision to terminate the brachytherapy treatment may be required.

Radiation Safety Issues Involved in HDR Brachytherapy

Remote controlled afterloading systems offer important radiation safety advantages by eliminating the radiation exposure to medical caregivers. However, the very high activity of the Ir-192 sources used in HDR remote afterloading units necessitates a rigorous radiation safety and emergency program to ensure the safety of the patient and to minimize the radiation exposure to the support personnel in the event of an emergency. The primary radiation safety concerns are room security, radiation monitoring during treatment, and emergencies such as failure of the source to retract after completion of treatment.

Room Security

Access to the room in which the HDR unit is located must be limited to authorized personnel, and the room must be locked when the unit is not in use. This is easily done if the

room is dedicated specifically for HDR and no other types of treatments are performed there. Frequently, however, the HDR unit shares the room with another treatment unit such as a linear accelerator. In this case, the room door remains unlocked during external beam treatments. It is essential that access to this room be monitored continually during external beam treatments and that the room be locked after working hours.

Radiation Monitoring During Treatment

Radiation exposure in the treatment room is monitored by wall-mounted radiation monitors. These monitors typically have both an audible alarm (beeping sounds) and visual display (flashing lights) as warning signals to indicate that the source is out of the safe. The visual mode is the most convenient for actual treatments and is most often used. The monitors should be positioned so that the warning light is visible through the treatment room door or on a remote video monitor. A backup battery pack should be used so that the monitor will continue to function in the event of a power failure. After each treatment, the patient should be checked with a survey meter to ensure that no radioactive material remains in the patient.

Emergency Situations

Emergency situations include but are not limited to the following situations:

1. Failure of the source to retract into the leaded safe within the treatment unit at the end of treatment;
2. The source becoming stuck at one dwell position;
3. Compromise of the integrity of the connection between the source and the cable.

The procedures to be followed in the event of an emergency during the use of HDR units are found in the user's manual of the specific HDR unit. All those involved in the brachytherapy treatments should be familiar with the procedures and should be aware of their responsibility in the event of an emergency before embarking on any treatments. This policy should be clearly spelled out in a written procedural manual accessible to all in the department. In-service training should be held regularly to update all members of the team.

Hazards To Nursing Personnel In Brachytherapy

Because radiation is emitted from these patients, nursing personnel must be trained in proper radiation safety techniques to minimize their radiation exposure. The following should be included in the radiation safety training:

1. Size and appearance of the brachytherapy sources;
2. Instructions for handling a dislodged source;
3. Basic radiation safety concepts;
4. Nursing care instructions;
5. Patient control procedures;
6. Visitor control procedures;
7. Risks of radiation exposure; and
8. Procedures for notification of the authorities if the patient dies or has a medical emergency.

Details of radiation precautions to be followed by nurses caring for patients with radioactive implants are detailed in Chapter 32.

References

1. International Commission on Radiological Protection : Recommendation of the International Commission on Radiological Protection. ICRP Publication, 26. Pergamon Press Ed., Oxford, 1977.
2. United States Nuclear Regulatory Commission, Title 10, Chapter 1, Code of Federal Regulations—Energy, Part 20.
3. NCRP 1972. Protection Against Radiation from Brachytherapy Sources. National Council on Radiation Protection and Measurement. Bethesda, MD, Report 40.
4. NCRP 1976. Radiation protection for Medical and Allied Health Personnel. National Council on Radiation Protection and Measuremen. Bethesda, MD, Report 48.
5. NCRP 1970. Precautions in the Management of Patients Who Have Received Therapeutic Amount of Radionuclides. Bethesda, MD, Report 37.

PART II

Clinical Body Sites

Brachytherapy for Skin Cancer

Juanita M. Crook, M.D., FRCP(C),
Peter J. Fitzpatrick, M.B., B.S., FRCP(C), FRCR

Introduction

Following the discovery of x-rays in 1895, skin changes from the new rays were soon noted. This was the beginning of radiotherapy; "the x-rays" were used to treat basal cell carcinomas of the skin, in both Europe and North America, before the turn of the century.[1] The first written paper was probably that published in the British Medical Journal by Sequeira in 1901 when he reported on the responses of 12 patients with rodent ulcers treated by x-rays. In 1898 radium was made from pitchblende by Marie Curie, and Henri Becquerel reported the first case of radiation dermatitis caused by this new substance. A rash developed on his body adjacent to where he had placed a radium tube in his waistcoat for several hours. This radium was used by Danlos of the Hospital St. Louis in Paris to treat skin diseases in 1902 and was the start of brachytherapy. In the first two decades of the century, both x-rays and radium were used extensively to treat skin cancer with radium use peaking in the 1920s and 1930s. Radium was used both in the form of plaques for surface application and in needles for interstitial treatment. Radon gas, a by-product of radium, was put into glass seeds and also used for both interstitial and surface application. Over the years, radium and radon have been replaced in turn by radioactive cobalt needles,

tantalum wire, gold grains, iridium wire or seeds, and iodine seeds. Today, the most commonly used isotope for interstitial implantation of skin cancers is iridium-192.

Nonmelanoma skin cancer is a highly curable malignancy with a wide variety of effective treatment options. As over 80% occur on sun-exposed skin, particularly the face, cosmesis is an important factor in treatment selection. Tumors occurring in relatively flat anatomical areas can be readily and simply treated by external radiotherapy (either orthovoltage[2,3] or electron beam). Brachytherapy, using interstitial techniques or surface applicators, tends to be reserved for sharply curved surfaces, such as the nose, inner canthus, ears, and lips.

Interstitial Low-Dose-Rate Brachytherapy

Dosimetry

Adherence to the rules of an established system of dosimetry is necessary for optimal results. Since much of the world experience in skin brachytherapy has been obtained using the Paris system of dosimetry, the key components of that system will be reviewed.

The Paris system specifies a simple and straightforward set of rules concerning implant geometry, dose calculation, and pre-

From Nag S (ed): *Principles and Practice of Brachytherapy*. © Futura Publishing Co., Inc., Armonk, NY, 1997.

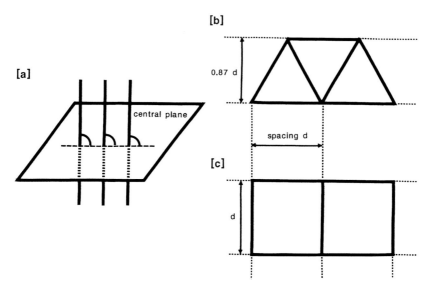

Figure 1. a) For implants containing more than one plane, equidistant radioactive lines intersect the central plane in a triangular or square pattern. b) The separation between planes is equal to 0.87 × spacing between the lines for patterns "in triangles" and c) equal to the spacing for patterns "in squares."

scription, and is readily applicable to implantation of most cutaneous sites. Although the Paris system was developed for iridium wire, it is also applicable to seed ribbons, provided that the spacing between the centers of consecutive seeds are <1.5 times the active length of the individual seeds.[4]

1. Radioactive lines must be rectilinear, parallel, and arranged so that their centers are located in the same plane, perpendicular to the direction of the lines (called the central plane, see Figure 1).
2. The linear activity must be uniform along each line and identical for all lines.
3. Adjacent radioactive lines must be equidistant from each other. In volume implants involving more than one plane, the separation between the planes must be such that the principle of equidistant lines is still observed. The intersection of the lines with the central plane of the implant should form a pattern of either squares or equilateral triangles (Figure 1).

The spacing, length, and number of lines depend on the situation and can be readily calculated when the dimensions of the volume to be implanted have been determined. By convention in the Paris system, the isodose enclosing the target volume is called the reference isodose and is calculated in the central plane of the implant. The reference isodose is 85% of the basal-dose-rate, which is the average of the dose-rate minima in the central plane.

The dose is prescribed at the reference isodose, the shape and dimensions of which depend on the geometry of the source placement and can be predetermined. For single plane implants, the length of the volume enclosed by the reference isodose is 0.7 times the active length of the iridium wire sources (Figure 2). The width is greater than the distance between the two outermost lines by the addition of the "lateral margin" on each side (0.37 times the spacing between the lines). The treated thickness is 0.5 times the spacing for a two line implant, and 0.6 times the spacing for three or more lines. The ideal spacing is 10–15 mm. The sources should be placed 2–3 mm under the skin surface so that they

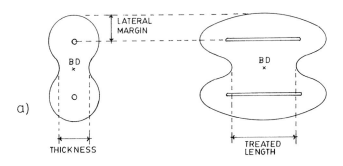

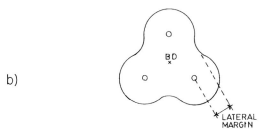

Figure 2. Shows the reference isodose for a) single plane two line implant and b) three line implant in a triangular array.

are midway in the treated thickness. This avoids linear overdosing of the skin surface and ensures optimal dose penetration.

Dosimetric calculations are generally based on orthogonal films. The dose-rate minima in the central plane are calculated and averaged to give the basal-dose-rate. The isodoses can then be expressed as a percentage of the basal-dose-rate or as actual dose rates in cGy/hr.

Optimal linear activity ranges from 1.3–1.8 mCi/cm (linear Kerma rate of 5.6-7.7 uGy/hr in air at 1 m). A prescribed dose of 60 Gy at the 85% reference isodose will take 4–6 days to deliver at a dose rate of 0.45–0.7 Gy/hr. Dose rates of 0.3–0.9 Gy/hr are acceptable,[5] but for skin implants dose rates in the upper end of this range are often preferable.

Once the target volume has been determined, the geometry of the implant is planned according to the principles of the Paris system. The required number of radioactive lines and their lengths are specified. The minimum spacing between the lines should never be <8 mm for short lines, or 12–15 mm for the longest lines (>10 cm). Slight errors in parallelism become very significant when the spacing is too narrow relative to the source length. Spacing should never be >15 mm for short lines, or 22 mm for very long lines. If these limits are exceeded, the relative dose in the immediate vicinity of the source is too high, increasing the risk of tissue necrosis. The hyperdose sleeve, the volume of tissue surrounding a radioactive line that receives a dose equal to or greater than twice the prescribed dose (2x the reference dose or 170% of the basal dose), should be kept under 8 mm.[5]

Techniques

All implants are performed in an operating room under sterile conditions, usually under local anesthesia but often with sedation. The choice of implant technique depends on the anatomical site, the morphology and dimensions of the tumor, and on personal preference. A nonrigid guide system is preferred for superficial tumors in sites of rapidly changing contour, while a rigid system would be chosen for more extensive infiltrating or ulcerating carcinomas especially if more than one plane is required. For a full description of techniques see reference 6.

Small Nylon Tube Technique

Either a straight or three eigths curved 5-cm suture needle is used to position a 2–0 silk or nylon suture subcutaneously along the desired track of each source. Each iridium wire source is loaded into one end of a 50-cm length of fine nylon tubing (external diameter 0.85 mm). With the loaded end in a lead safe beside the patient, the free end is threaded over the appropriate suture for 10 cm and clamped such that traction on the suture will pull the tube along its course. When the end of the tube reemerges from the skin, the clamp is removed and the tube advanced until the iridium wire is correctly positioned. When all sources have been placed satisfactorily, excess tubing is trimmed off and light plastic transverse spacers are threaded over the cut ends and held in place with metal buttons.

Double Plastic Tube Technique

This is also a nonrigid system but instead of suture threads, 1.6-mm diameter, 10-cm hollow steel needles (17 gauge) are positioned subcutaneously along the track of each source. A 20-cm steel obturator is inserted into each needle and 1.6-mm diameter nylon tubing is threaded over the obturator until it abuts the blunt end of the needle. It is then advanced through the tissues, pushing the needle out ahead of it.[7] When each needle has been replaced by a length of plastic tubing, transverse plastic spacers are threaded over the ends. The Iridium-192 sources, encased in short lengths of fine plastic carrier tubing (diameter: 0.85 mm) are then loaded and held in place with metal buttons.

Hypodermic Needle Technique

This rigid system is ideal for two plane implants, or when three needles are required in a triangular configuration as for carcinoma of the lip. Needles that are 19.5 gauge (external diameter 0.8 mm, internal diameter 0.5 mm) 6, 8, or 10 cm long, are positioned using a predrilled template and remain in place for the duration of the implant. Lead caps are crimped over one end, both closing the needle and holding the template in place. The required length of iridium wire is loaded into each needle and pushed into place with a stylet. A nylon "fishing line" spacer keeps the source in position and can be held with a friction-fit plastic cap.

If 17-gauge (1.6-mm diameter) steel needles are required for greater strength or rigidity in larger volume implants, 10-cm needles are usually chosen. The ends are left protruding and are secured with retaining templates and lead caps.

Dose and Dose Rate

A tumor dose of 60 Gy prescribed at the 85% reference isodose is recommended. Dose rates of 0.3–0.9 Gy/hr are acceptable, but for convenience and to minimize the length of hospital stay, 0.7–0.9 Gy/hr is suggested. No correction in prescribed dose is made for dose rates within this range. For larger volume implants, a lower dose rate is preferable.

Loading, Monitoring, and Reactions

In all cases, the sources are cut and prepared by source-handling personnel applying the principles of radiation protection. The implant is performed using the nonradioactive guide systems described above, with no exposure to the brachytherapist or operating room assistants. When the geometry is considered optimal, the prepared sources are brought to the implant suite in a mobile lead safe and can be rapidly loaded into position. The use of individual mobile lead shields and long-handled forceps reduces exposure to well within radiation safety standards.

The patient is transported to a shielded room for the duration of the implant. Patients are usually self-sufficient, have minimal discomfort, and require very little nursing care. Visitors must maintain a safe distance from the patient and are limited to half an hour per day. The implant position is verified twice daily.

Localized moist desquamation develops

10–12 days after removal of the implant, reaches a peak at 3 weeks, and heals in about 6 weeks. Gentle cleansing and application of a topical antiseptic are required until reepithelialization is complete. The patient should be reviewed 6-weeks postimplant to assess healing. The eventual scar will correspond to the area of skin disruption by the tumor. Late radiation skin changes such as telangiectasia and hypo- or hyperpigmentation are in proportion to the dose over 60 Gy.

Specific Sites

External Ear

Although carcinomas of the external ear would most often be managed by external radiotherapy using either orthovoltage photons or electron beams, interstitial implantation performed under local anesthesia yields excellent results. Mazeron et al.[8] reported only one local failure in a series of 70 patients implanted using either the hypodermic needle technique or the fine plastic tube technique. Good to excellent cosmesis was obtained in 78% of patients with tumors <4 cm, but was generally poor for tumors >4 cm. Cartilage necrosis occurred in three patients, but only

in tumors >4 cm. Amputation of the pinna was required in each case. Superficial epidermal ulcers (0.5–1.5 cm) occurred in nine patients and healed spontaneously within 3–9 months. The risk of late skin ulceration was 25% for tumors >3 cm, but only 10% for those <3 cm.

Nose

Carcinomas of the skin of the external nose present special management problems. The rapidly changing contour makes delivery of a uniform dose from external irradiation difficult but poses no problem for the brachytherapist. Nonrigid techniques adapt themselves very well to the anatomical contours for superficial tumors, while a rigid technique can be used for deeply infiltrating tumors or those involving the columella. To assist in the selection of implant technique, guidelines have been developed for the different regions of the nose.[6]

Ala Nasae

Sources are usually oriented parallel to the border of the nostril, extending across the nasolabial sulcus if necessary. The most inferior

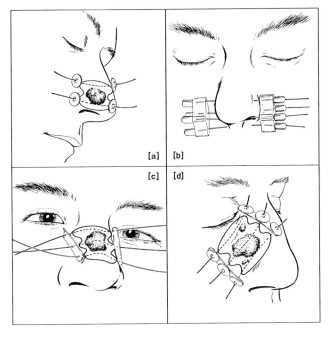

Figure 3. Clinical applications. a) Ala nasae: two line implant using small plastic tube technique. Reference isodose shown; b) Columella: two plane, four line implant using hypodermic needle technique with plastic templates; c) Bridge of nose: three line implant using small plastic tube technique. Metal buttons not shown. Reference isodose superimposed; d) Upper lateral surface: three line implant for multifocal tumor using small plastic tube technique. Reference isodose shown.

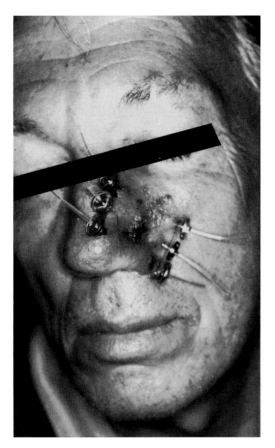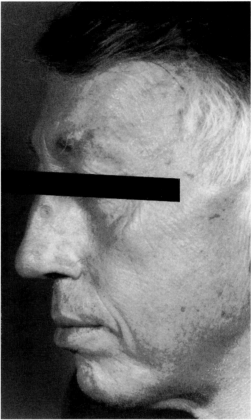

Figure 4. A) Ala nasae implant showing plastic tube technique using three lines held by spacers and metal buttons. B) Result 3-years posttreatment (60 Gy).

source should be several mm from the free edge of the nostril to avoid overdosage (Figures 3a and 4).

Columella

A transversely oriented, two plane implant using a hypodermic needle technique with 4–6 needles piercing the nasal cartilage is usually best. This can easily be adapted to include tumor extension to the nasal septum, tip of the nose, or upper lip. Predrilled plastic templates guide placement and maintain spacing. Needles are held in position with lead caps (Figures 3b and 5).

Tip of the Nose

For small to medium sized lesions, the small plastic tube technique is ideal. The coplanar

sources follow the curvature of the tip. More extensive lesions may require a hypodermic needle technique using a triangular or square array.

Bridge of the Nose

For lesions that straddle the bridge of the nose, the radioactive lines should be oriented obliquely relative to the dorsal ridge, forming a plane that is spiralled (Figure 3c). Either the small plastic tube or double plastic tube technique can be used.

Upper Lateral Surface and Nasolabial Sulcus

Orientation of the wires parallel to the nasolabial sulcus is best, including the lower eyelid or medial canthus if necessary (Figure 3d).

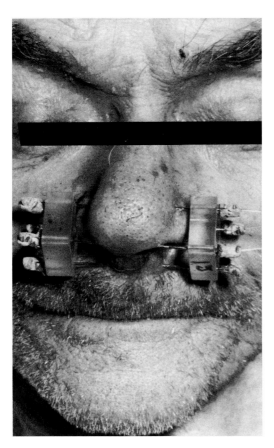

Figure 5. Columella implant using four 19.5-gauge needles in a square array, held by pre-drilled templates and lead caps.

Either the small plastic tube or double plastic tube technique can be used. Care should be taken to avoid the lacrimal punctum and lacrimal duct. Placement of a lacrimal duct stent prior to implantation will facilitate this.

Results of Interstitial Brachytherapy for Carcinoma of the Skin of the Nose

The European Curietherapy Group reported a retrospective review of the results of radical radiation of carcinoma of the skin of the nose in 1676 patients at 22 centers.[9] Fourteen of the 22 centers used interstitial iridium to treat 468 patients. There were 407 basal cell carcinomas and 61 squamous cell carcinomas with a median follow-up of 4.5 years. Local recurrence rate was 2.5% for tumors <2 cm (9/362) and 3% for those 2–3.9 cm (3/94).

Only ten tumors >4 cm were implanted and none recurred. No improvement in local control was seen with doses above 62 Gy.

Cosmesis was judged according to the extent of scarring, color change, and nasal deformity, and was found to be good in 50%, fair in 32%, and poor in 6%. Necrosis rates were 1.5% for tumors <2 cm and 5.5% for those >2 cm. For doses of 58–62 Gy, the necrosis rate was 1% but rose to 4% for doses over 62 Gy.

Eyelids

Carcinomas of the lower eyelid and inner canthus are easily managed by interstitial implantation. In most cases a single plane implant using either a single line or two parallel lines is sufficient. The small plastic tube technique is generally preferred. To avoid ocular complications, the radioactive lines should not traverse more than one half the length of the lid margin.[5] For carcinomas of the upper eyelid, brachytherapy is not the treatment of choice and is considered to be contraindicated by some authors.[5]

Daly et al.[10,11] have reported on brachytherapy of 192 eyelid tumors. Eighty-five were on the lower lid, 87 involved the inner canthus, 11 were on the upper lid, and 9 at the lateral canthus. With a median follow-up of 4 years, the local control achieved for previously untreated tumors was 98% (133/136). The dose prescribed ranged from 60–70 Gy. In 80% of cases cosmesis was excellent and no late cutaneous sequellae were detectable. Late side effects consisted of eyelid aperture reduction (5%), epiphora (6%), ectropion (4%), and loss of substance (4%). One patient developed an ulcerated cornea, one had hypertrophic conjunctivitis, and two developed cataracts. The authors suggest the use of lead contact lenses during the duration of the implant. Thermoluminescent measurements performed on the center of the closed upper eyelid during an inner canthus or lower eyelid implant show dose rates ranging from 5–15 cGy/hr for total doses of up to 1250 cGy (Crook, personal communication).

Lip

Over 90% of squamous carcinomas of the lip occur on the lower lip with the remainder equally divided between the upper lip and

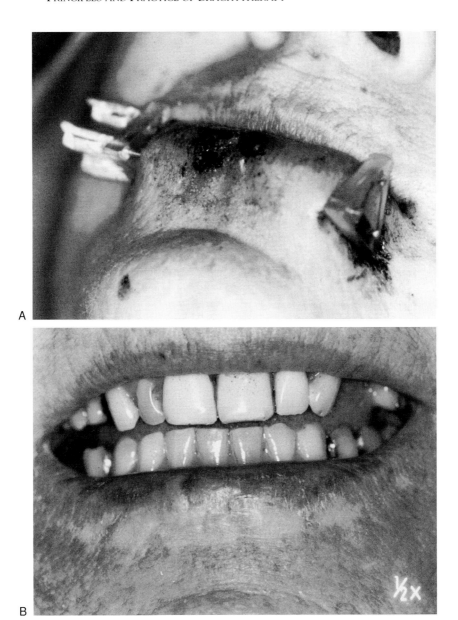

Figure 6. A) Lower lip implant using three 19.5-gauge needles in a triangular array, held by predrilled templates and lead caps. B) Result 3-years posttreatment (60 Gy).

the commissure.[12] Carcinoma of the lip can be simply and effectively managed by brachytherapy making it the treatment of choice in many European centers.[13–15] The hypodermic needle technique is generally preferred and can be performed under either neuroleptic or general anesthesia. As for any other oral cancer, patients should have a dental assess-

ment prior to radiotherapy. A mandibular shield can be constructed to distance the implant from the mandibular gingiva and from the upper lip.[16]

For small superficial lesions up to 5-mm thick, a single plane implant consisting of two horizontally oriented lines bracketing the lesion is adequate. For thicker or more exo-

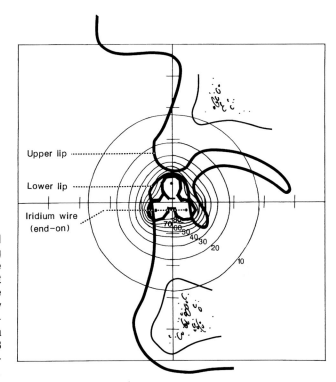

Figure 7. Line drawing of sagittal section through lip implant using three needles in triangular array. The superimposed isodoses show that without protective prosthesis the dose to the upper lip is approximately 75 cGy/hr and to the gingiva approximately 60 cGy/hr. The addition of a prosthesis pushing the sources 3 mm further away from the healthy tissues will reduce this by about 35%.

phytic tumors, three lines should be oriented in a horizontal triangular array maintained with predilled lucite templates (Figure 6). The first needle is placed submucosally at the junction of the moist mucosa with the vermillion of the lip, the second is just inferior to the junction of the vermillion with the labial skin, and the third submucosally just above the labiogingival sulcus (Figure 7).[5]

Lesions with more extensive involvement of the surface of the lip (<4 cm) can be managed by either the rigid hypodermic needle technique, which maintains optimal geometry, or a flexible double plastic tube technique, which is more comfortable for the patient. A triangular array can be used with either technique.

When the tumor involves the commissure, a double plastic tube technique is preferred. The needles are inserted through the skin of the cheek lateral to the lesion and advanced medially to exit through the skin or mucosa of the upper and lower lips. Good parallelism can usually be achieved with the mouth closed, and can be maintained by using predrilled plastic spacers.[5]

The European Curietherapy Group reported on 2747 lip cancers treated at 23 different centers.[17] The majority using iridium, 1870 were treated with brachytherapy. The median dose prescribed (according to the Paris system) was 65 Gy. The local failure rate was 2.5% for tumors <2 cm (T1), 5% for those 2–4 cm (T2), and 11% for those >4 cm (T3). Eighty-two percent of T1 tumors and 51% of T2 tumors had no detectable cosmetic or functional sequelae. Cosmetic sequellae, but no functional impairment, were observed in 17% of T1 and 44% of T2.

Resource Considerations

Most skin brachytherapy procedures can be completed in 30–45 minutes. This includes the sterile preparation of the patient, planning of the treatment volume and implant geometry, injection of local anesthesia, insertion of nonradioactive needles or tubes, orthogonal x-ray verification, and loading and securing of radioactive sources. A nurse is required to assist, and a dosimetrist cuts and prepares the required sources. Computer dosimetry is performed using the orthogonal films and generally takes

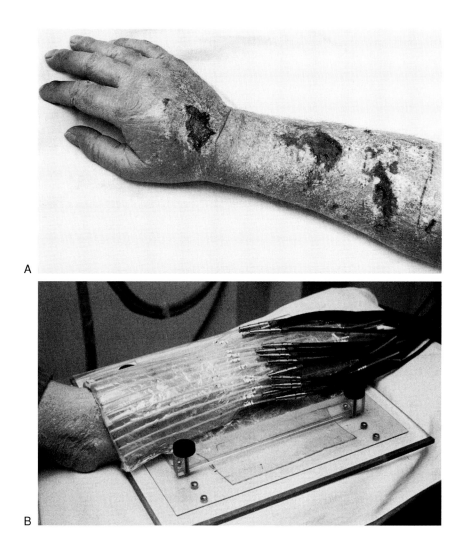

Figure 8. A) Right forearm showing widespread actinic change with multiple squamous and basal cell carcinomas in a patient with xeroderma pigmentosa. B) Forearm treated to 4000 cGy in 14 fractions using HDR brachytherapy.

about 30–45 minutes. For a dose of 60 Gy, 4–6 days of hospitalization are required.

Surface Applicators—High-Dose-Rate Brachytherapy

In the past, radioactive moulds have been applied to skin tumors and worn either continuously or, more commonly, for several hours a day for 1–2 weeks. The major disadvantages of this technique are the radiation exposure to the members of the health care team and the time taken to deliver treatment.[18,19] The development of high-dose-rate (HDR) remote afterloading brachytherapy units has enabled radiation oncologists to review the use of surface moulds in cases where surface irregularity, proximity to bone, or poor intrinsic tolerance of tissues do not allow for satisfactory treatment by an external beam.[20] HDR remote afterloaders provide an alternative method of treatment with good radiation dosimetry, patient convenience, and operator safety. An accurate and cancericidal dose of radiation at any depth below the sur-

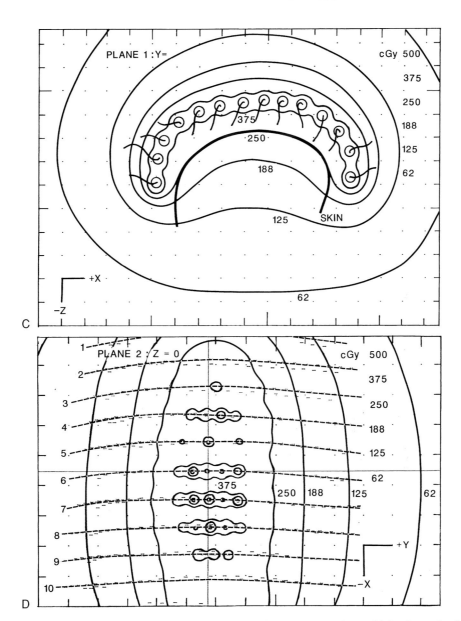

Figure 8. *(continued).* C) *Isodose distribution through transverse plane.* D) *Isodose distribution through longitudinal plane.*

face is achieved by varying the source to skin distance (SSD) to fit the clinical situation.

Treatment Planning

The Nova Scotia Cancer Center has applied the Nucletron HDR brachytherapy unit to the treatment of skin cancers using single plane surface applicators. The principles for treatment with surface applicators that were firmly established in the 1930s remain unchanged. In the past, the dosimetry was based on either the Manchester system[21] developed by Patterson and Parker in the 1930s, or the Paris system[5] developed in the 1970s by Pierquin and Dutreix.

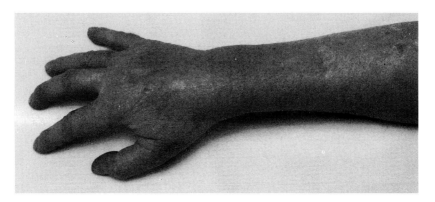

Figure 8. *(continued). E) Appearance 18 months posttreatment.*

The HDR brachytherapy system has a dedicated computer program that is used to individualize treatment for each patient. Special applicators with built-in shielding are available but individual moulds can be constructed if preferred.[22,23] The dose is prescribed at the normal skin surface and is measured at the apex of the tumor and at depths of 2 and 5 mm below the surface. Treatment planning begins with a careful assessment of the tumor in three dimensions. Areas of potential spread must be included in the irradiated volume to avoid geographic miss. The area to be irradiated is marked on the skin. The target volume is then determined and, from the depth of tissue to be irradiated, the optimum SSD is calculated. For most cases, a satisfactory mould can be made from 5-mm thick sheets of wax. The HDR catheters are spaced 1 cm apart and are placed on or between the layers of wax to achieve the necessary SSD. The wax is warmed and moulded to the surface contour and then allowed to harden. For some tumors, a plastic shell is required for fixation and accurate apposition of the radioactive sources to the tumor.

The area to be irradiated is outlined with lead pellets placed on the skin. The mould is then reapplied and orthogonal simulation films are obtained using dummy sources. The information is digitalized in the Nucletron Planning Computer and isodose distributions are obtained in three planes. The tumor dose is prescribed at the normal skin surface, which is made to coincide with the 100% isodose line.

There is a wide range of recommended doses and fractionation schemes for treating skin cancer. We elected to use the same tumor dose that would have been used for a discontinuous, single plane, cobalt-60 mould or for external beam therapy in a similar situation, without allowance for the different dose rate. Doses in the range of 3500 cGy in 5 fractions to 5000 cGy in 10 fractions have been used with success in HDR moulds (Figure 8). The skin cancer literature for external irradiation provides data bases for control and complication rates and for comparison with our increasing HDR experience.

Conclusion

With almost a century of experience to draw on, radiation therapy continues to play an important role in the management of nonmelanoma skin cancer. Selection of cases for brachytherapy depends on the anatomical tumor site and tumor configuration, the available expertise, financial resources, patient acceptance, and desired cosmesis.

References

1. Mould RF. A Century of X-rays and Radioactivity in Medicine. Institute of Physics Publishing, Bristol and Philadelphia, 1993, pp. 126–131.
2. Fitzpatrick PJ. Cancer of the lip. J Otolaryngol 1984;13:32–36.
3. Fitzpatrick P, Thompson GA, Easterbrook WM, et al. Basal and squamous cell carcinoma of the eyelids and their treatment by radiotherapy. Int J Radiat Oncol Biol Phys 1984;10:449–454.

4. Marinello G, Valero M, Leng S, et al. Comparative dosimetry between iridium wires and seed ribbons. Int J Radiat Oncol Biol Phys 1985;11: 1733–1739.

5. Pierquin B, Wilson JF, Chassagne D, et al. Skin: Modern Brachytherapy. Masson Publishing Inc., New York, 1987, pp. 273–285.

6. Crook JM, Mazeron JJ, Marinello G, et al. Interstitial iridium 192 for cutaneous carcinoma of the external nose. Int J Radiat Oncol Biol Phys 1990;18:243–248.

7. Raynal M. Endocuriethérapie des cancers cutanés par mise en place direction des gaines plastiques porte-fils d'iridium-192. J Radiol Electrol 1977;58(11):713–714.

8. Mazeron JJ, Ghalie R, Zeller J, et al. Radiation therapy for carcinoma of the pinna using iridium 192 wires: A series of 70 patients. Int J Radiat Oncol Biol Phys 1986;12(10):1757–176.

9. Mazeron JJ, Chassagne D, Crook J, et al. Radiation therapy of carcinomas of the skin of the nose and nasal vestibule: A report of 1676 cases by the "Groupe European de Curiethérapie" (RTO 00509). Radiother Oncol 1988;13: 165–173.

10. Daly NJ, De Lafontan B, Combes PF. Results of the treatment of 165 lid carcinomas by iridium wire implant. Int J Radiat Oncol Biol Phys 1984; 10:455–459.

11. De Lafontan B, Daly N, Bachaud JM, et al. La curiethérapie des épithéliomas palpébraux par iridium 192. J Fr Ophtalmol 1986;9(6–7): 471–479.

12. Daly NJ, Combes D, Combes PF. Results of the radiotherapeutic management of 323 patients with squamous cell carcinoma of the lip. J Eur Radiother 1981;3:205–213.

13. Gerbaulet A, Chassagne D, Hayem M, et al. Thérapie: L'épithélioma de la lèvre. J Radiol Electrol 1978;59:603–610.

14. Pierquin B, Chassagne D, Pieter E, et al. L'endocuriethérapie par iridium 192 des carcinomes épidermoides de la lèvre inférieure. J Radiol Electrol 1972;53:207–212.

15. Pigneux J, Richaud PM, Lagarde C. The place of interstitial therapy using 192 iridium in the management of carcinoma of the lip. Cancer 1979;43:1073–1077.

16. Hardie J, Ringland TC, Esche BA, et al. Oral malignancies: Interstitial irradiation and protective prostheses. Oral Health 1990;80:3, 51–60.

17. Mazeron JJ, Richaud P. Compte rendu de la XVIII réunion du groupe européen de curiéthérapie. J Eur Radiother 1984;1:50–56.

18. Ashby MA, Pacella JA, DeGroot R, et al. Use of radon mould technique for skin cancer: Results from the Peter MacCallum Cancer Institute (1975–1984). Br J Radiol 1989;62:608–612.

19. Michael AA, Pacella JA, de Groot R, et al. Use of a radon mould technique for skin cancer: Results for the Peter MacCallum Cancer Institute (1975–1984). Br J Radiol 1989;62:608–612.

20. Pirrazzo M, Stablle BS, Shih L, et al. HDR remote afterloading as an alternative to electrons for therapy of superficial tumors. Select Brachytherapy J 1992;6(1):11–13.

21. Merredith WJ (ed). Radium Dosage. The Manchester System. Livingstone, Ltd, Edinburgh, 1967.

22. Brock A, Pohlmann S, Prager W. Surface applicators for HDR brachytherapy in the head and neck region. Act Selectron Brachytherapy J 1992;3(Suppl):22–25.

23. Kitchen CL, Dalton AE, Pope BP, et al. Surface applicator for basal cell carcinoma of the right pinna: A case report. Act Selectron Brachytherapy J 1991;5:140.

Chapter 12

Interstitial Radiation Therapy for Brain Tumors

Minesh P. Mehta, M.D., Penny K. Sneed, M.D.

Introduction

Although malignant gliomas (MGs) are relatively uncommon neoplasms, accounting for only about 40% of the approximately 17,000 new annual cases of central nervous system (CNS) malignancies diagnosed in the United States every year, their clinical impact continues to far outweigh their incidence because of their high fatality rate.[1] Glioblastoma multiforme (GBM), which accounts for about 80% of all MGs, has an annual United States incidence in excess of 5000 cases and the median and 5-year survival is typically 9–10 months and 5%, respectively[2]; 5-year survival for anaplastic astrocytoma is typically under 20%.

MG rarely metastasize and mortality is primarily attributed to near-universal local failure. Hochberg and Pruitt[3] demonstrated that over 80% of failures occur within 2 cm of the primary tumor, with only 1/35 (3%) patients in their series having recurrence outside this 2-cm "risk zone." Similarly, in a trial of radiotherapy plus a nitroimidazole radiosensitizer, Urtasun et al. reported all recurrences within the initial target volume.[4] Autopsy studies[5] as well as stereotactic localization biopsy studies[6] have demonstrated that microscopic spread of tumor is present at the time of diagnosis beyond the zone of enhancement. Additionally, local control in these tumors is com-

promised by significant regions of hypoxia[7] as well as the relative inability of chemotherapeutic drugs to perfuse through the blood brain barrier into the tumor.[8] These biological observations provide strong rationale for the investigation of aggressive modalities of local control in an attempt to improve the overall outcome in patients with malignant glioma.

Rationale for Dose Escalation in Malignant Glioma

There is compelling evidence from in vitro studies[9] that a dose-response relationship exists above 60 Gy. Clinical trials conducted by the Brain Tumor Cooperative Study Group in the 1970s established improvement in local control and survival in patients with MGs treated with postoperative radiotherapy compared to patients undergoing surgical resection only. In addition, subsequent analysis of their serial trials demonstrated a possible dose response survival relationship over a range from 45–62 Gy.[10] The median survival improved from 14 weeks at <45 Gy to 42 weeks at 60 Gy; these data are presented in Table 1. Further confirmatory data have recently become available from a Medical Research Council trial of two radiotherapy doses in the treatment of malignant glioma.[11] These trials form the basic rationale for supporting first,

From Nag S (ed): *Principles and Practice of Brachytherapy.* © Futura Publishing Co., Inc., Armonk, NY, 1997.

Table 1.
Local Control is a Function of Dose

Dose (Gy)	MS (Weeks)	25% Survival	p
0	18	N/A	N/A
<45	14	N/A	ns
50	28	52	<0.001
55	36	57	<0.001
60	42	68	<0.001

Local control is a function of dose; median survival increases from 14 weeks at <45 Gy to 42 weeks at 60 Gy; MS = median survival; 25% survival = 25th percentile survival (Data from Walker et al. ref 10).

the use of postoperative radiotherapy, and second, for considering dose escalation.

Unfortunately, our ability to escalate the external beam radiotherapy dose is severely limited by the accompanying increase in neurotoxicity. For example, Marks et al.[12] have demonstrated that the risk of brain necrosis increases substantially with doses above 60–70 Gy. In addition, substantial clinical evidence indicating improved local control beyond 60 Gy is lacking. In an analyses of more than 600 patients treated on an intergroup Radiation Therapy Oncology Group/Eastern Cooperative Oncology Group (RTOG/ECOG) study, 70 Gy did not result in increased survival compared to 60 Gy.[13] RTOG 83–02, a randomized phase I dose-escalation trial of XRT twice a day accrued over 700 cases from a dose range of 64.8–81 Gy and although the 72 Gy arm had the best survival, toxicity beyond this dose resulted in worse survival.[14] In the prospective phase I/II dose escalation study by Fulton and colleagues,[15] external beam doses up to 80 Gy using a hyperfractionated regimen of 1 Gy three times a day were achieved without substantial toxicity or evidence of improved local control or survival.

These clinical studies may be interpreted as representing a response ceiling at 60 Gy without substantial increase in local control or survival improvement up to 80 Gy. This does not necessarily rule out the possibility of improved local control at doses beyond these levels. It is the latter argument that forms the primary rationale for delivering brachytherapy for malignant tumors of the brain. As will be shown from the clinical trials described later in this chapter, the total cumulative doses with the use of brachytherapy and external beam radiation typically exceed 100 Gy and it may well be possible that such high radiation doses are necessary to achieve adequate tumor control for this highly malignant disease process.

Historical Considerations

One of the earliest reports of the use of brachytherapy in brain tumors dates back to 1912 when Hirsch[16] treated a pituitary adenoma with radium insertion in the sella turcica. As early as 1914, Frazier[17] reported the effects of radium implants on parenchymal brain tumors. Up to the 1950s, several publications outlining anecdotal reports of the use of brachytherapy for malignant brain tumors appeared in the literature and have been summarized in a historical review article by Bernstein and Gutin.[18] The vast majority of these implants were performed at the time of open craniotomy without the use of any fixation or guiding devices. The advent of the principles of stereotaxis led to the development of externally fixated frames that permitted stereotaxic biopsies as well as implantation of brain tumors without resorting to a craniotomy. The early pioneers of the stereotactic technique were Talairach[19] in Paris who performed stereotaxic implantation of radioactive gold seeds into inoperable brain tumors and Mundinger and Weigel[20] in Freiburg, Germany who performed almost 500 implants using iridium-192 as well as iodine-125.

The recent history of interstitial implantation for brain tumors has been characterized by the enormous advances in imaging technology, particularly CT and MR as well as the availability of sophisticated computerized treatment planning systems that permit refined and relatively rapid treatment planning. More recently, the availability of newer isotopes such as Ir-192, the development of remote afterloaders, the availability of high-dose-rate (HDR) techniques, and the recent integration of hyperthermia with brachytherapy techniques for malignant brain tumors have led to further advances in this field.

Radiobiological Considerations

Brachytherapy for malignant brain tumors offers several potential radiobiological advantages. The typical implant delivers a dose of approximately 0.3–1.0 Gy/hr over a 50- to 150-hour period of time. This continuous low-dose radiation produces a G_2/S block, resulting in accumulation of proliferating tumor cells in the relatively radiosensitive G_2 phase.[21] This accumulation in a relatively radiosensitive phase has also been demonstrated in vitro using malignant glial cell lines.[22] A second major radiobiological benefit of continuous low-dose-rate (LDR) radiation is the minimization of the oxygen effect. Ling and colleagues[23] have demonstrated that the oxygen enhancement ratio is lowered for low dose-rate radiation, possibly because continuous delivery of radiation impairs the ability to repair sublethal damage. A secondary effect may well be the occurrence of reoxygenation during the course of continuous LDR radiotherapy. The third major radiobiological advantage of brachytherapy is prevention of tumor repopulation. Hall[24] has described inhibition of tumor cell repopulation when radiation is given continuously at 0.4–0.6 Gy/hr. These three radiobiological advantages would lend theoretical support to a possible benefit from brachytherapy.

Physics Considerations

These issues have been discussed in greater detail in other chapters in this book. A full description of the radiation physics issues will, therefore, not be repeated. The major isotopes used for brachytherapy for parenchymal brain lesions include high activity iodine-125 and iridium-192. Both of these isotopes are typically used in temporary implants delivering between 0.3–0.6 Gy/hr. Iodine-125 has certain shielding advantages over iridium-192 because of its relatively low energy. In addition, iridium-192 is also used in the form of a high activity source within HDR remote afterloaders. Other isotopes that have been used for CNS brachytherapy include gold, cobalt, cesium, phosphorous, and yttrium.

In general, these isotopes are placed in plastic catheters that have been implanted into the tumor using standard principles of volume implants. After delivering the appropriate dose, the radioactive sources as well as plastic catheters are removed. Permanent implants are generally not performed for parenchymal brain tumors. With remote afterloading, multiple fractions given daily or twice daily over several days are utilized.

Technical Description

The two institutions with the largest experience with CNS brachytherapy in the United States are the University of California at San Francisco (UCSF) and The Joint Center for Radiation Therapy (JCRT) in Boston. Both of these institutions utilize temporary, removable high activity iodine-125 sources.

The Iodine-125 Technique (UCSF)

After initial tissue diagnosis and maximal possible tumor debulking, patients with newly diagnosed MG receive a course of external beam radiation to a median dose of 60 Gy using standard fractionation. In several serial in-house studies, this dose of external beam radiotherapy has been combined with either oral hydroxyurea as a radiosensitizer or chemotherapy. The brachytherapy boost is typically performed 3 weeks after completion of external beam radiation. The implant is performed with a stereotactic base ring that is affixed under local anesthesia to the patient's skull. After mounting an image localization fiducial system, a stereotactic localization CT scan is performed (Figure 1). These axial imaging data are transferred to a treatment planning computer and the target volume as defined by contrast enhancement is outlined on each image without additional margin. Using in-house software,[25] a "simulation implant" is performed by placing between 2–6 catheters perpendicular to the skull surface and penetrating the tumor. Two or three iodine-125 sources are placed within each of the simulated catheters typically separated by 3–4 mm. The treatment planning program allows differential spacing as well as the use of differential activity. The aim is to produce a median isodose contour of 0.5 Gy/hr covering most of the target volume as evaluated on a dose volume histogram. Intratumor heterogeneity is not considered a major limitation. Once an

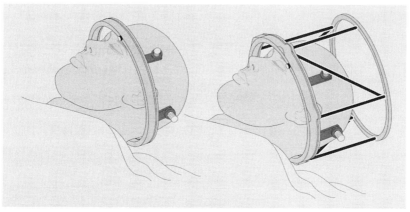

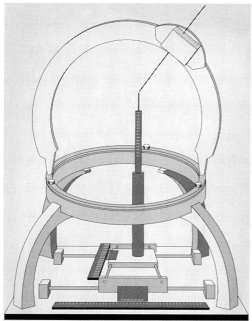

Figure 1. The technique for interstitial implantation. After placement of a stereotactic headframe under local anesthesia (A), a treatment planning CT scan is obtained and the tumor volume is identified. Intraoperatively, verification of the coordinates is carried out using a phantom base (B).

approved plan is generated, the stereotactic coordinates and frame angles for the target points are printed out. The actual implant procedure is performed under local anesthesia using prophylactic antibiotics. For each of the catheters, the target point coordinates are set on the stereotactic phantom base and the frame angles are set on the arc ring assembly to confirm the catheter trajectory. This arc ring system is then transferred to the base frame that had previously been attached to the patient's head. After anesthetizing and incising the skin, a small hole is drilled through the skull with a twist drill. The dura is perforated

with K-wires, and closed end silastic catheters are implanted. The catheter is fixed to the skull surface using a purse string suture and also a collar that is glued to the catheter with cyanoacrylate. After all the brain implant catheters have been inserted, the iodine-125 sources, which are housed in individual catheters corresponding to the implant catheters, are loaded and secured in place with a surgical clip. Orthogonal radiographs using a fiducial marker box are obtained in the operating room so that the exact placement of each of the iodine-125 seeds can be verified and reentered into the treatment planning program to

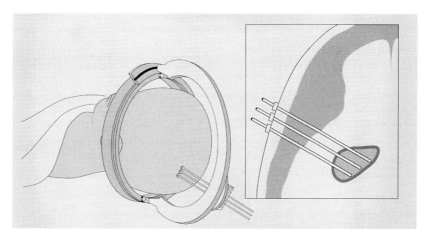

Figure 1. *(continued). Single or multiple, closed-end catheter trajectories are then planned, either with or without a template. The catheters are usually inserted under local sedation by making twist drill holes in the skull. They are affixed to the skin with collar buttons (C).*

generate actual isodose contours. At UCSF, the dose volume histogram is utilized for final dose prescription. The isodose contour that encompasses 95%–98% of the target at a dose range of 0.4–0.6 Gy/hr is utilized.

Template-Based Techniques

At several centers,[26,27] a rigid template, affixed to the arc system of the stereotactic frame, is utilized for catheter placement. These prefabricated templates have predrilled openings with fixed separation ranging from 7–12 mm (Figure 1). The template affixes to the stereotactic frame arc and the parallel openings within it allow placement of catheters that are, therefore, more or less parallel to each other. In the UCSF technique, no specific attempt is made to ensure parallelism. The template-based techniques not only allow for placement of parallel catheters, but also typically result in placement of a larger number of catheters, usually ranging from 6–15. As a consequence, the distribution of the radioisotope seeds within the tumor tends to be more uniform, resulting in less heterogeneity of dose within the target volume. The procedure for placing catheters with the template technique is similar to that without the template. At some institutions,[28] to provide further catheter stability, a piece of silastic is sewed to the scalp. This piece of silastic tends to constrict

the catheter from all directions, thereby providing a better fit and reducing the possibility of catheter displacement.

Several variations on this theme have been utilized. For example, at The Joint Center,[29] the volume implanted is defined as the enhancing region on CT plus a 5-mm margin in all three dimensions. The Boston Group also uses coaxial silicone catheters and delivers a total of 50 Gy at 0.4 Gy/hr using iodine-125 sources ranging from 20–50 milliCuries in activity. They have typically used between 3 and 11 catheters.

High-Dose-Rate Techniques

The basic principles underlying an HDR implant do not differ from those for LDR implants. The techniques revolve around using single or multiple catheters that are then attached to the remote afterloader. The brachytherapy dose is usually delivered in multiple fractions given either once or twice a day, usually over 3–5 days. Occasionally, a single fraction is used. Modern remote afterloaders are typically equipped with advanced treatment planning programs that allow variation in dwell time in order to produce a distribution of dose, configured to the tumor shape. The details of individual techniques are addressed in the section below.

Clinical Indications

Brachytherapy has been utilized for the management of a variety of different neoplasms including primary and recurrent malignant glioma, metastases, skull base tumors, craniopharyngioma, and several pediatric tumors. The largest body of experience is with malignant glioma.

Brachytherapy for Primary Malignant Glioma

The Joint Center for Radiation Therapy Experience

In one of the largest clinical trials reported to date, Loeffler and colleagues,[29] reported on 35 patients with glioblastoma that were treated with stereotactic brachytherapy as part of an initial treatment plan between 1987 and 1990. In order to qualify for the study, patients had to have a Karnofsky performance status of at least 70%, a unifocal and radiographically well defined supratentorial tumor measuring 5 cm or less in greatest diameter; patients were ineligible if the tumor involved the corpus collosum or ependymal surfaces of the brain. Thirty-three of the 35 patients underwent surgical debulking initially, and two patients had stereotactic biopsies. Two weeks after surgery, external beam radiotherapy was initiated. The enhancing mass with a 3- to 4-cm margin was treated with 1.8 Gy daily fractions to a total dose of 59.4 Gy. Two weeks after completion of external beam therapy, brachytherapy was performed using the Brown-Roberts-Wells head frame and high activity iodine-125 sources (20–50 mCi) to deliver a minimum tumor dose rate of 0.4 Gy/hr for a total of 50 Gy. Typically, 3–11 catheters were utilized. The median treatment volume was 25 cc with a range of 3–75 cc.

This group of 35 patients was compared retrospectively with a cohort of 40 patients (Table 2) with GBM fulfilling all of the clinical and radiographic criteria that would have made them eligible for the brachytherapy protocol, but who were not treated with brachytherapy. This cohort was derived from a prior group of historic controls from The Joint Center. Survival at 1 year after diagnosis was 87% for the brachytherapy group and 40% for the

Table 2.
JCRT Case Comparison Study of Brachytherapy (Glioblastoma Multiforme)

	Brachy	Control	p
n	35	40	N/A
MS (months)	27	11	<0.004
% 1 year surv	87	40	<0.001
% 2 year surv	57	12.5	<0.001

Brachy = brachytherapy group; n = patient numbers; MS = median survival; surv = survival; JCRT = The Joint Center for Radiation Therapy. (Data from Wen, ref 30).

control group, which was statistically significant with a P<0.001. At 2 years, the survival in the control group was 12.5%; whereas, the brachytherapy group had a survival of 57%. This was also statistically significant. The median survival time for the brachytherapy group was 27 months, versus 11 months for the control group (P<0.004). This matched analysis with historic controls is suggestive of a significant advantage not only in median survival, but also in long-term survival for GBM.

Forty percent of the patients (14) in the brachytherapy group required reoperation at a median of 6 months after implantation. Typically, reoperation was performed more commonly in patients with larger tumors. The surgical intervention was prompted by increasing mass effect on radiographic studies as well as by neurological deterioration. The authors described that the resected tissue was generally firm, avascular, and well demarcated from the surrounding brain, suggesting the probable occurrence of necrosis within the high-dose region. Microscopic examination revealed residual neoplastic cells in most of the resected specimens. The significance of malignant cells centrally is unclear. The most common site of failure was outside the implanted volume.

The toxicities encountered with brachytherapy included four scalp infections, one brain abscess necessitating surgical intervention, and one intracranial hemorrhage requiring surgical evacuation for a major acute toxicity rate of 6 of 35 (18%). In addition, patients undergoing brachytherapy experienced a decline in median performance status up to 12 months after completion of implantation. The median Karnofsky Performance Status (KPS) declined from 80% at implantation to 70% at 6 months to 60% at 12 months. Interestingly, a further decline in KPS beyond 12 months was not noted.

In a recent update of their data,[30] the group from The Joint Center has reported on an updated series of 56 patients with glioblastoma treated with stereotactic brachytherapy as part of their initial therapy. The median survival for patients undergoing brachytherapy was 18 months compared with 11 months for a matched brachytherapy control group with similar clinical and radiological features (P<0.0007). In the brachytherapy group, the 1-, 2-, and 3-year survival rates were 83%, 34%, and 27% compared to rates of 40%, 12.5%, and 9% for the control group. The reoperation rate was 64%. The median survival of the 36 patients undergoing reoperation was 22 months compared to 13 months for the group not undergoing reoperation. This observation of improved survival in the reoperated group has led to the speculation that reoperation is contributing to improved survival in patients undergoing brachytherapy because of further tumor debulking. An alternative hypothesis explaining this improved survival is based on the fact that patients undergoing re-resection typically have substantially more necrosis and that the therapeutic window for this tumor may be so narrow that it may almost be necessary to produce necrosis in order to achieve long-term tumor control.

The UCSF Experience

The first temporary high activity iodine-125 brain implant boost for primary GBM was performed at UCSF in 1981. From February 1981 to December 1992, 159 consecutive adults with primary GBM were treated with an implant boost in addition to surgery, external beam radiotherapy (59.4–61.2 Gy), and implant boost with a median of 55 Gy at 0.43 Gy/hr using a median of seven sources and a median of three catheters with or without hydroxyurea sensitization.[31] The median survival of this group of patients exceeded 19 months with 1-, 2-, and 3-year actuarial survival rates of 85%, 36%, and 20%. The reoper-

ation rate exceeded 50%, and patients with GBM who underwent reoperation showed significantly longer survival than those who did not with a median survival of 110 versus 77 weeks.

Literature Review

Several authors[30–40] have described their experience in a number of reviews. A comprehensive summary illustrating the experience in over 500 cases is presented in Table 3. Unfortunately, some authors have reported their experience without providing a breakdown of the histologic type or the number of patients treated upfront versus those treated at recurrence. These data are very difficult to interpret and, other than providing baseline information in terms of pilot feasibility experience, serve little purpose.

Chun and colleagues[38] have reported the treatment results in 37 patients with malignant brain neoplasms treated with iridium-192 implantation. Twenty-nine of these patients had high-grade gliomas with 20 carrying a diagnosis of GBM. These 20 patients received an interstitial implant together with external beam radiotherapy as part of their initial management. The external beam dose was 60 Gy followed by an interstitial implant within 2–3 weeks. The implant dose was escalated from 60–100 Gy resulting in a total tumor dose ranging from 120–160 Gy. In general, 3–8 catheters spaced 1–1.5 cm apart were utilized with seed activity sufficient to yield an 80–100 cGy/hr isodose surface covering the tumor. The overall survival in the 20 patients with primary GBM was 14 1/2 months. Interestingly, in this series, escalation in dose did not yield improvement in either local tumor control or overall survival. Also, unlike the experience from UCSF and JCRT, reoperation did not provide a significant survival benefit to patients in this series.

Kumar and colleagues[37] have described an intraoperative remote afterloading endocurietherapy technique with high activity cobalt-60 for the treatment of GBM. Unlike the catheter-based systems, in this technique a specially adapted intracranial probe, the Kumar flange, is utilized. This stainless steel, blunt-ended 5-mm diameter probe is inserted without a stereotactic frame and can be angled 15°

Table 3.
Clinical Studies of Brachytherapy Boost for Glioblastoma Multiforme

Author	Isotope	Dose in Gy		Pt	Survival Parameters: Months & %			
		Implant	Ext		Median	1 Year	2 Years	3 Years
Sneed	I 125	55	59.4	159	19	85	36	20
Wen	I 125	50	59.4	56	22	83	34	27
Mundinger	Ir 192[a]	40–45	[a]	62	<10	—	—	—
Patchell	Cf 252[b]	21–31	60	48	10	—	19	—
Selker	Ir 192	—	—	47	16	—	—	—
Stea	Ir 192	40	45	37[c]	14	60	18	10
Ostertag	I 125[d]			34	6			
Kumar	Co 60	20	60	30	7	42	—	
Stea	Ir 192[e]	32	50	25[e]	24	80	50	38
Chun	Ir 192	60–100	60	20	15	—	—	—
Yakar	I 125	55	55	17	12	—	—	—
Garcia	Ir 192[f]	15	46	7	20	60	—	—
Total				542	6–24	42–85	18–50	10–38

Gy = Gray; Ext = external beam dose; Pt = patient numbers.
[a] High dose rate one fraction remote afterloading; variable ext dose (some received none).
[b] The implant dose is photon-equivalent Gy.
[c] 28 glioblastoma and 9 anaplastic astrocytoma.
[d] Low activity Iodine 125.
[e] Hyperthermia used; 17 glioblastoma and 8 anaplastic astrocytoma.
[f] High dose rate remote afterloading multifraction schema.

in any direction because of the presence of a ball-valve. This probe permits insertion of a 3-mm diameter nylon tube that is connected to a high activity cobalt-60 remote afterloader. In essence, this results in a single line source implant delivering 20 Gy to the tumor edge. Because of the utilization of only a single line source, substantial intratumoral heterogeneity of dose is encountered. A total of 60 Gy additional external beam therapy is delivered following brachytherapy. In a series of 30 patients with GBM, the median survival was only 7 months. The reason the median survival in this series is substantially worse than in other trials is unclear, but it could represent patient selection factors. Another possible explanation could be that the significant intratumoral dose heterogeneity results in unacceptably high levels of necrosis that could contribute to early patient demise.

Yakar and colleagues[39] have reported a series of 17 patients with newly diagnosed GBM treated with high activity iodine-125 sources. These patients received 50–60 Gy external beam radiotherapy with Carmustine (BCNU) followed by iodine-125 implantation to a total of 55–60 Gy at 40 cGy/hr. The median survival was 12 months. This group of investigators felt that the risk of injury to the surrounding normal tissue was unacceptably high with the high doses of brachytherapy delivered with temporary iodine-125 implant. Therefore, in order to reduce this risk, they initiated a new approach using permanent implants with a lower dose rate. In a group of 50 patients, permanent implantation of iodine-125 seeds at a dose rate of 4–7 cGy/hr to a total dose of 100–120 Gy with concurrent external beam radiotherapy of 50 Gy was delivered following surgical resection. The authors hypothesized that the biological rationale of this protocol was to increase the effectiveness of the LDR implant by a concurrent daily boost of external radiation, thus inhibiting the proliferation of tumor cells during the protracted low-dose radiation treatment. In a preliminary analysis[41,42] of survival between the groups treated with permanent versus temporary implants in terms of effectiveness in tumor control, they concluded that the LDR implant with concurrent external beam radiotherapy seemed to offer the best chance for long-term survival without deterioration in the patient's clinical condition.

Unlike the results with high activity iodine-125 sources, the clinical results of low activity iodine-125 sources have not been favorable. Ostertag and Kreth[36] reported a median survival of only 6 months in 34 patients with GBM treated with low activity iodine-125 brachytherapy at a dose rate of 0.1 Gy/hr.

Although most groups have focused on using either high activity iodine-125 or iridium-192 seeds for interstitial brachytherapy for malignant glioma, the group from the University of Kentucky[33] has utilized californium-252 primarily because of its mixed photon/neutron emission with the assumption that the neutron component may improve the efficacy of tumor kill. Previous studies of external neutron radiation have suggested a high incidence of tumor clearance. In their first study, 56 patients with MG were treated with surgical debulking followed by implantation of californium-252 sources within afterloading catheters. Approximately 300 neutron rads (21–31 Gy photon equivalent dose) were delivered with the implant, and subsequently an external conventional photon dose of 60–70 Gy was added for a total photon equivalent dose of 81–91 Gy. In the 48 patients with GBM, the median survival time was 10 months, and the 2-year survival rate was 19%.

In a subsequent phase I study, 31 patients with MG (27 patients had glioblastoma) were treated with californium implant only to a total dose of 9–14 neutron Gy (54–85 Gy photon-equivalent dose, assuming a relative biological effectiveness of 6 for californium-252).[43] Interestingly, in this phase I study, scalp necrosis occurred in six patients, and both necrosis and infection occurred in four others, for an overall significant scalp toxicity rate of 33%. In addition, five patients died within 1 month of the procedure and, therefore, did not live long enough to demonstrate potential scalp necrosis. A reevaluation of the dosimetry showed that patients developing scalp necrosis had scalp doses ranging from 10–33 neutron Gy with a median dose of 13 neutron Gy as contrasted to a dose of <7 neutron Gy in those patients not developing scalp necrosis.

More recently, remote afterloading techniques have been introduced in the management of these tumors. Garcia et al.[40] have performed several implants using multiple nylon catheters that are then attached to a remote afterloading high activity iridium-192 source (Nucletron MicroSelectron HDR unit [Nucletron Corporation, Columbia, MD, USA]). Typically, the patients are treated with external beam radiation therapy to 46 Gy in 23 fractions. Multiple parallel catheters are implanted using a rigid acrylic template. In their current protocol, a total dose of 15 Gy is delivered at 1 cm from the periphery of the outer most catheters, administered in three equal fractions given over 3 consecutive days. In addition, the treatment is combined with hyperthermia using a commercially available computer controlled conductive heating system. The protocol specification is 48 hours of moderate temperature hyperthermia with a minimum tissue temperature of 41.5°C to be delivered over a 64-hour period in 3-hour fractions every 4 hours. They have reported median survival of 19.5 months for the first seven glioblastoma patients.

Mundinger and Sauerwein designed the Gammamed remote afterloading device and have treated several patients with intracranial neoplasms with a single catheter technique. In this particular technique, a metallic tube or catheter 3 mm in diameter is stereotactically implanted into the tumor and a single dose (typically 40–45 Gy) of HDR remote afterloading brachytherapy is delivered. In a group of 62 patients with glioblastoma, median survival of just under 10 months was noted.[40] Not all patients in Mundinger's series received external beam radiotherapy.

Ashpole and colleagues[44] have described a new method of using intracranial radiation utilizing a remotely controlled afterloading system with a modified endotracheal tube as the applicator. This system uses the Selectron LDR/MDR (Nucletron) using cesium-137 in spherical pellets in a linear source train within a sealed system. This applicator is implanted at the time of surgical resection and an inflated balloon stabilizes the applicator. No significant clinical data are available at this time.

The group at the Baylor College of Medicine[45] has developed a catheter system for fractionated HDR brachytherapy for intracranial gliomas, and a phase I dose escalation study has been initiated. Clinical results are awaited.

In a modification of Mundinger's technique, Sparenberg and Ernst[46] have designed a screw that fits on Mundinger's metal tube to allow insertion of the tube for up to 8 days, permitting fractionated remote afterloading. They have delivered a marginal tumor dose of 30 Gy at a daily fractionation of 2 Gy twice daily using an iridium afterloading technique followed by 30–40 Gy external beam radiation. In 16 previously untreated patients with MG, the 1-year survival was 41%. Unfortunately, the breakdown between GBM and anaplastic astrocytoma was not reported. It would appear therefore, that in large measure, the experience with HDR remote afterloading brachytherapy for MG is anecdotal at best, and prospective clinical studies have only recently been initiated.

Thermoradiotherapy for Newly Diagnosed Glioblastoma Multiforme

Stea and colleagues[35] have recently reported on a retrospective comparison of interstitial irradiation versus interstitial thermoradiotherapy for supratentorial MG. In this study, 25 patients received external beam radiotherapy and interstitial boost with hyperthermia, and another 37 patients received the same therapy without the adjuvant hyperthermia. The median survival was 23.5 months in the thermoradiotherapy group versus 13.3 months in the nonhyperthermia group.

The groups from Dartmouth[47] and UCSF[31] have also initiated preliminary clinical trials investigating thermoradiotherapy for newly diagnosed GBM. In the UCSF trial, patients with newly diagnosed GBM undergo surgery and external beam radiotherapy to 59.4 Gy at 1.8 Gy per fraction with oral hydroxyurea utilized as a radiosensitizer. At completion of external beam radiotherapy, patients are reevaluated for suitability for implantation and randomized to brachytherapy boost alone or interstitial microwave hyperthermia in conjunction with brachytherapy. As of mid-1994, a total of 50 patients had been enrolled on this randomized study, results of which are eagerly awaited.

Controversies and Randomized Trials

Although brachytherapy for MG is based on sound biological principles, the divergent clinical results with median survival ranging from 6–24 months have left doubt regarding the efficacy of this technique. The improvement in the median survival documented in the larger studies reported from JCRT and UCSF has been compared with matched controls. A major criticism of several of these clinical trials is the inherent selection bias. Only about 20%–30% of all patients with newly diagnosed GBM are eligible for brachytherapy based on size and location criteria. Critics of brachytherapy have, therefore, challenged the validity of the claims of improved survival by suggesting that similar patients treated with external beam radiotherapy alone also achieve improved survival.[48] In fact, in the study by Wen and colleagues[30] from JCRT, patients treated with brachytherapy were matched with controls that would be eligible for brachytherapy and a statistically significant improvement in survival was noted. Similar results were also noted by Florell and colleagues,[49] with brachytherapy eligible patients treated with external beam radiation only having a median survival of 14 months compared to 6 months for those ineligible for implantation.

In addition, a further criticism levied against some of these studies is the utilization of additional chemotherapy as well as re-resection at the time of clinical and radiographic deterioration with the suggestion that repeat resection may in fact be responsible for improving survival in some of these clinical trials. The high reoperation rate, in excess of 50%, imposes a substantial clinical burden on physicians managing these patients, once again raising several questions regarding the utility of this technology. To determine the value of reoperation alone without further therapy, Dirks and colleagues[50] performed a second resection in 43 patients with recurrent supratentorial glioblastoma at the time of tumor progression. Median survival after reoperation was 19 weeks, which is substantially shorter than the median survival of patients undergoing brachytherapy at recurrence. Reoperation, therefore, confers a modest, but very small increase in survival.

The only logical way to address such concerns and criticisms is through the mechanism of well designed prospective randomized trials. The Brain Tumor Cooperation Group (BTCG) randomized trial[51] of conventional external beam radiotherapy with or without a preceding brachytherapy boost has recently been completed. A full analysis with detailed long-term follow-up is expected in mid-1995. In this multicenter randomized trial that was initiated in 1987, all patients received external beam radiotherapy and BCNU. In the experimental arm, interstitial radiotherapy using temporary iodine-125 implants was carried out. The study eligibility criteria required an implantable target in a patient (>15 years of age) with supratentorial MG with a Karnofsky performance >50%. The Karnofsky performance status is an important factor to bear in mind when comparing the results of this randomized trial with single institution data. Because KPS represents a major prognostic factor in MG, results of clinical studies are highly dependent on the proportion of patients with lower KPS values. Initially, the external beam radiotherapy dose was 43 Gy whole brain plus 17.2 Gy boost, but subsequently the whole brain radiotherapy was deleted and patients were treated with partial brain radiotherapy to a total of 60.2 Gy to the tumor plus 3-cm margin. BCNU was given at 200 mg/m^2 intravenously at 8-week intervals. The brachytherapy dose was 60 Gy at 40 cGy/hr at the tumor periphery. Preliminary evaluation revealed that the reoperation rate in both arms was comparable. Once again, this is an important fact to bear in mind because previous nonrandomized studies have been criticized for the high incidence of reoperation in the brachytherapy group. A statistically significant survival advantage was noted for the brachytherapy arm of the study. These preliminary results are very encouraging, not only because the study is positive and, therefore, puts to rest a number of controversies regarding the role of brachytherapy in MG, but also because there are very few prospective randomized trials of brachytherapy that exist in the literature and this study will be regarded as a landmark trial. In addition, two other randomized trials of brachytherapy in MG are currently under way.[52,53] It is expected that these trials will be completed and

some results will be available by mid-1997. It is, therefore, very likely that primary MGs may serve as one of the first clinical sites where randomized trials define the role of brachytherapy.

The recent emergence of radiosurgery as a potential modality to provide a noninvasive boost is an exciting, new, and potentially challenging development for brachytherapy. In the largest nonrandomized retrospective evaluation of 115 patients with GBM, compared to 1500 patients from sequential Radiation Therapy Oncology Group (RTOG) studies not undergoing radiosurgery, Sarkaria et al.[54] utilized the nonrecursive partitioning analysis model described by Curran and colleagues.[55] This statistical model allows for categorization of patients with MG into six prognostic classes, thereby balancing for various prognostic factors. The authors suggest a probable survival advantage (Table 4) in some groups of patients with MG using radiosurgery boost. The survival figures appear comparable to the brachytherapy series. The RTOG has recently initiated a prospective randomized trial to assess the benefit of a radiosurgery boost in patients with GBM.

Brachytherapy for Primary Anaplastic Astrocytoma

Because anaplastic astrocytoma are relatively uncommon compared to GBM, limited clinical data are available. In addition, the recent recognition that anaplastic astrocytoma have a more favorable outcome in GBM necessitates that the brachytherapy data be looked at in light of the best results available from the nonbrachytherapy studies. In a series of clinical trials using external beam radiotherapy with hydroxyurea sensitization and either single agent BCNU or procarbazne and vincristine (PCV) chemotherapy, the UCSF/NCOG (Northern California Oncology Group) group has demonstrated a survival advantage with PCV. In a subsequent trial utilizing bromodeoxyuridine radiosensitization[56] in place of hydroxyurea, the median survival for patients with anaplastic astrocytoma was noted to be 5 years. In addition, a recent single arm study from the National Cancer Institute (NCI)[57] using iododeoxyuridine also shows median survival in excess of 5 years

Table 4.
Radiosurgery Survival Stratified by Prognostic Class

Class	Radiosurgery Study			RTOG Study		
	MS (Months)	2 Year % S	n	MS	2 Year % S	n
1	N/A[a]	81[b]	17[b]	58.6	76	139
2	N/A[a]	N/A[b]	N/A[b]	37.4	68	34
3	38.1	75	24	17.9	35	175
4	19.6	34	35	11.1	15	457
5	13.1[c]	21[c]	43[c]	8.9	6	395
6	N/A[c]	N/A[c]	N/A[c]	4.6	4	263

When stratified by prognostic class, radiosurgery appears to produce a survival benefit compared to the RTOG patients who did not receive a radiosurgery boost. (Reproduced with permission from Sarkaria, et al. ref 54). MS = median survival; % S = percent survival; n = patient numbers.
[a] Median survival not reached.
[b] Groups 1 and 2 combined.
[c] Groups 5 and 6 combined.

for 22 patients. A summary of the various trials of radiosensitization in anaplastic astrocytoma is provided in Tables 5 and 6, and these show consistently high survival rates. These favorable results, therefore, form a baseline to compare the results of brachytherapy to.

In the series reported by Mundinger et al.[58] in 1980, 34 patients with anaplastic astrocytoma underwent brachytherapy with iridium-192 or iodine-125. The 3- and 5-year survival rates were 66% and 45%.

In the UCSF experience,[31] 52 patients with high grade nonglioblastoma gliomas underwent high activity iodine-125 interstitial brachytherapy to 52.6 Gy with a median ex-ternal beam dose of 59.4 Gy. The median survival of this group of patients was 36 months with 1- and 3-year survivals of 84% and 51%. However, the authors noted that when compared to the overall results for 357 patients with highly anaplastic astrocytoma treated from 1979–1989 on a variety of UCSF and NCOG protocols, the median survival was 39.4 months and it, therefore, appeared that interstitial brachytherapy did not afford survival advantage. Therefore, the group at UCSF does not recommend brachytherapy for anaplastic gliomas.[59]

The results of LDR iodine-125 sources have also not demonstrated any significant survival advantage. In fact, in the study reported by Ostertag and Kreth,[36] a median survival of only 8 months was noted for 75 patients with grade 3 anaplastic astrocytoma. The results of brachytherapy from several clinical trials are summarized in Table 7.

Table 5.
UCSF/NCOG Results for Anaplastic Astrocytoma

Protocol	Median Survival (Weeks)	
	AA	GBM
RT/OHU/BCNU	82	57
RT/OHU/PCV	157	50
RT/BUdR/PCV	252	64

Results from sequential trials show improved survival for anaplastic astrocytoma (AA) compared to glioblastoma multiforme (GBM), with external beam radiotherapy (RT) combined with bromodeoxyuridine (BUdR) and PCV (Procarbazine; CCNU (Lomustine), Vincristine) chemotherapy compared to hydroxyurea (OHU). (Data from Levin, et al. ref 56). BCNU = Carmustine; UCSF/NCOG = University of California at San Francisco/Northern California Oncology Group.

Brachytherapy for Low Grade Glioma

The role of brachytherapy in the management of patients with low grade glial neoplasms is controversial, primarily because of the long natural history of these tumors and secondarily because the exact roles of surgery and external beam radiotherapy remain poorly defined. A few anecdotal series have been reported in the literature and are summarized here.

In a series of 45 patients[60] with inoperable

Table 6.
Radiosensitization Studies: Anaplastic Astrocytoma

Study	Sensitizer	MS (Months)	1 Year % S	2 Year % S
Hegarty	IA BUdR	N/A	200	65
Levin	IV BUdR	63	80	65
Urtasun	IV IUdR	N/A	74	68
Sullivan	IV IUdR	N/A	71	57

Data from ref. 57 demonstrating consistently good survival for anaplastic astrocytoma treated with halogenated pyrimidines, either iododeoxyuridine (IUdR) or bromodeoxyuridine (BUdR), given intra-arterialy or intravenously. MS = median survival (in months); N/A = not yet reached; S = survival.

low grade cerebral neoplasms, iodine-125 stereotactic brachytherapy was used. The majority of these tumors were either grade 1 or grade 2 astrocytoma or oligodendroglioma. With follow-up ranging from 2½–6 years, the authors reported a 66% tumor control rate on follow-up radiographic studies and functional status determination. In this series, age <40 appeared to be an important prognostic factor. The authors also noted that diffuse infiltrating cortical/subcortical tumors, optochiasmatic gliomas, hypothalamic, and lower brain stem neoplasms did not respond satisfactorily to iodine-125 radioisotope implantation. Ostertag,[61] using both low activity permanent and high activity temporary iodine-125 implants, has treated 136 patients with low grade glioma or ependymoma. Although a full statistical analysis is not available, it was the author's opinion that brachytherapy was utilized in these situations primarily to enhance and complement the role of surgery. In other words, patients underwent maximal possible surgery and subsequently brachytherapy was used principally for the slowly proliferating, differentiated, minimally resectable tumors in functional and critical areas in order to avoid operative damage to healthy brain.

In the UCSF experience,[62] 16 patients with primary low grade gliomas received an implant dose ranging from 38.7–86.2 Gy with a median survival of 226 weeks and 1- and 3-year survival of 94% and 74%. In addition, the median survival duration for 22 patients with recurrent low grade glioma receiving between 37–150 Gy brachytherapy dose was 81 weeks with 1- and 3-year survival figures of 64% and 32%. These latter data would indicate that in patients with low grade glioma who have undergone prior therapy and for whom no further options are available, brachytherapy may still afford reasonable survival.

Table 7.
Brachytherapy Boost for Anaplastic Astrocytoma

Author	Isotope	Dose in Gy Implant	Ext	Pt Nos	Survival: Months & % Median	1 Year	3 Years	5 Years
Ostertag	I 125[a]	—	—	75	8	—	—	—
Sneed	I 125	52.5	59.4	52[b]	36	84	51	—
Mundinger	[b]	40–45	[b]	34	—	—	66	45
Patchell	Cf 252	21–31[d]	60	8	17	—	—	—
Total				169	8–36			

[a] Low activity iodine seeds.

[b] This group includes all high-grade nonglioblastoma gliomas.

[c] Iodine 125 in some and iridium 192 in others; variable ext dose (some not receiving any).

[d] Photon-equivalent dose.

(From refs 31, 33, 36, 58).

Brachytherapy for Recurrent Malignant Glioma

A considerable amount of experience in managing patients with recurrent MG with brachytherapy has been accumulated, primarily because several institutions embarking upon CNS brachytherapy programs have elected to select this group of patients as a preliminary target. As a consequence, institutions, typically on the early phase of the learning curve, tend to treat substantial numbers of patients with recurrent MG. This factor must be borne in mind when interpreting results of these trials. In addition, these patients have limited further therapeutic options, and interstitial brachytherapy is frequently performed with a purely palliative intent. As a result, the selection criteria and the implant specifications may not necessarily be of the same level of stringency as those for newly diagnosed MG.

In one of the largest experiences reported to date, the UCSF[31] group reported median survival of just about 1 year for 111 adults with recurrent MG. In this series, there were 66 patients with recurrent GBM and 45 with recurrent high grade nonglioblastoma tumors. No significant differences in outcome were noted between these two groups. Subsequently, UCSF reported their experience with thermoradiotherapy for recurrent MG. Twenty-five patients with recurrent glioblastoma and 16 with recurrent nonglioblastoma were treated to a median implant dose of 59 Gy at 0.44 Gy/hr with concomitant hyperthermia to a minimum of 41.2°C with a median survival of 49 weeks in the glioblastoma group and 140 weeks in the nonglioblastoma group.

Selker et al.[34] have reported another large series of 61 patients with recurrent GBM undergoing iridium-192 interstitial implantation, with a median survival of 13 months.

Shrieve and colleagues[63] recently reported the results from JCRT on 118 patients with recurrent GBM treated either with interstitial brachytherapy or stereotactic radiosurgery. The patient characteristics were similar in the two groups. The median brachytherapy dose was 50 Gy, using high activity iodine-125 seeds. The median survival of the 32 patients treated with interstitial brachytherapy was 10.9 months, comparable to the median survival of 10.2 months for the 86 patients treated with stereotactic radiosurgery. The 12- and 24-month survivals for the brachytherapy and the radiosurgery groups were 38% and 14% and 45% and 19%, respectively. These data are very provoking because they suggest that radiosurgery may produce results comparable to brachytherapy for recurrent MG, especially glioblastoma; and because this therapeutic modality is noninvasive, it may therefore challenge brachytherapy as a management option in the future. Table 8 is a comparison of selected institution[63,64] data illustrating the similarity in outcome between patients managed with radiosurgery and brachytherapy for recurrent MG.

In Table 9, a comprehensive review of the literature for brachytherapy results for recurrent MG is provided. Results from over 450 patients are available, and median survival ranges from 6–35 months, with most studies reporting a narrow range of 8- to 12-month survival at the time of recurrence. It must, therefore, be concluded that for most patients with recurrent MG, brachytherapy probably provides palliation and results in a median survival of 8–12 months. Newer modalities such as stereotactic radiosurgery may well provide equal results.

Brachytherapy for Brain Metastases

The standard management for most patients with brain metastases remains whole brain radiotherapy. In a recent randomized trial,[65] a statistically significant survival advantage was noted for patients with single brain metastasis undergoing surgical resection followed by whole brain radiotherapy compared to those receiving whole brain radiotherapy only. Such data would imply that improved local control in selected patients with brain metastases may impart survival advantage. Based on such considerations, selected patients with brain metastases have undergone brachytherapy. For example, in the UCSF series,[66] 14 patients with progressive metastatic brain lesions have been treated with temporary implantation of high activity iodine-125 sources. Four of these patients had undergone prior surgery and 13 had received prior external beam whole brain radiotherapy. Whereas four of the patients re-

Table 8.
Radiosurgery vs Brachytherapy for Recurrent Glioma

Institution	Boost	Dose (Gy)	#	MS (Months)	REOP%
JCRT	I 125	50	32	11.5	44
UCSF	I 125	64.4	66	12	38
JCRT	RS	13	86	10	22
Mayo	RS	15	14	9	—
UCLA	RS	24.4	17	10	29

Comparison of stereotactic radiosurgery and brachytherapy for recurrent malignant glioma (from refs 63 & 64). # = patient numbers; MS = median survival; REOP = reoperation rate; JCRT = The Joint Center for Radiation Therapy; UCSF = University of California at San Francisco; UCLA = University of California at Los Angeles; Mayo = Mayo Clinic at Rochester.

ceived brachytherapy as a boost, ten underwent the procedure at recurrence following conventional radiation therapy. The median survival for the entire group was 80 weeks, with 10 of the 14 patients surviving more than 12 months. Radiographic improvement was seen in 6 of 40 lesions, with the rest demonstrating stable disease. These results are certainly encouraging and would suggest the need for further evaluation of this modality in the management of selected patients with brain metastases. Once again, however, it must be noted that radiosurgery is now being frequently used in the management of these patients, and in a recent review of the world literature, Mehta[67] has described local control rates in excess of 80% in over 1000 patients (Table 10).

The Role of Brachytherapy for Pediatric Brain Tumors

Unlike the situation in adults, there has been very limited experience with brachy-

Table 9.
Brachytherapy for Recurrent Malignant Glioma

Author	Isotope	Dose	Pt Nos	Survival Parameters: Months & %	
				Median	1 Year
Sneed	I 125	64.4	111	12	50
Selker	Ir 192	—	61	13	—
Sneed	I 125	59	41	12/35[a]	—
Larson	Au 198	—	33	9/17[b]	—
Shrieve	I 125	50	32	10	38
Fass	I 125	—	29	15	—
Matsumoto	Ir 192	—	23	18	—
Zamorano	I 125	—	23	10	—
Stea	Ir 192	40/50[c]	21[c]	8	24
Lucas	Ir 192	—	20	10	—
Kumar	Co 60	20	19	6	19
Bernstein	I 125	70	18	10	—
Shehata	[d]	60	16	9	—
Hitchon	I 125[e]	55–270	11	6	—
Total			458	6–35	19–50

[a] Median survival 12 months for 25 rec GBM and 35 months for 16 rec non-GBM.

[b] Median survival 9 months for 13 rec GBM and 17 months for 20 rec AA.

[c] 13 patients received 50 Gy implant, 8 had 40 Gy implant and hyperthermia.

[d] Various isotopes used.

[e] Low activity seeds in 7 and high in 4.

Table 10.
Brain Metastases: Local Control with Radiosurgery

Institute	Unit	# Lesions	Dose (Gy)	% Control
Wisconsin	Linac	58	18.3	82
Cologne	Linac	66	18.0	83
Heidelberg	Linac	102	17.2	95
Karolinska	Gamma	300	29.0	94
Sapporo	Gamma	132	27.0	95
Sendai	Gamma	77	26.0	99
GK Users	Gamma	116	18.0	83
Pittsburgh	Gamma	53	16.0	85
Harvard	Linac	330	16.0	88
Stanford	Linac	47	24.6	88
Total		1281	16–29	82–99

Data from ref 67.

therapy in childhood CNS tumors. This is primarily due to the relatively low incidence of brain tumors in children and also because of the occurrence of primitive undifferentiated tumors in this age group, which tend to have a substantially wider spectrum of failure than the very localized failures seen in adult brain tumors. Interstitial brachytherapy is, therefore, limited to the glial neoplasms that occur at a low frequency in this age group. In addition, colloidal isotope therapy has also been utilized for cystic tumors, primarily craniopharyngiomas, and a few cystic gliomas in this age group.

Interstitial Implants for Pediatric Gliomas

Perhaps the largest experience comes from Mundinger's group[68] who have reported their experience with 111 permanent implants in a series of 204 patients with diencephalic gliomas. This series included 117 patients with grade 1 astrocytoma, 58 patients with grade 2 astrocytoma, 23 patients with grade 3 astrocytoma, and 6 patients with GBM. The 5-year survival rates were substantially different depending on whether an iridium-192 or an iodine-125 implant was performed. For example, in grade 1 astrocytoma, the 5-year survival rates were 54.6% for iridium-192 and 22.2% for iodine-125. A slight difference in survival between the two implant techniques was also noted for grade 2 astrocytoma, with the iridium-192 group experiencing 31% 5-year survival compared to 21% for the iodine-125 group. The iridium-192 group received

120 Gy compared to a slightly lower dose range of 90–110 Gy for the iodine-125 group.

Gutin and colleagues[69] have utilized both high activity temporary iodine-125 and permanent low activity iodine-125 implants in children. They have reported a total of nine patients treated by their group. Because this group was quite heterogeneous in terms of prior therapy, this experience served primarily to illustrate the feasibility of performing brachytherapy in this age group.

Other smaller experiences have been reported by Godano et al.,[70] who used permanent iodine-125 seeds in 15 patients with low grade glioma without external beam radiation. A total dose of 80–120 Gy was delivered at the tumor edge. Unfortunately, no substantial survival or response data were presented.

Laperiere[71] have performed iodine-125 implants in five recurrent posterior fossa childhood tumors. A peripheral dose of 100 Gy was delivered with permanently implanted low activity iodine-125 seeds. Two of the five patients died postoperatively, and three patients with medulloblastoma were functional following the implant, but subsequently developed cerebral spinal fluid (CSF) seeding.

Voges and colleagues[72] have treated six children with high grade gliomas of the brain stem with brachytherapy and external beam radiotherapy and an additional 13 children with low grade gliomas with brachytherapy alone. A dose of 50–65 Gy was delivered using low activity iodine-125 seeds for the children with high grade lesions whereas the

in three Radiation Therapy Oncology Group malignant glioma trials. J Natl Cancer Inst 1993; 85:704–710.

56. Levin VA, Wara WM, Gutin PH, et al. Initial analysis of NCOG 6G82–1: Bromodeoxyuridine (BUdR) during irradiation followed by CCNU, procarbazne and vincristine (PCV) chemotherapy for malignant gliomas. Proc Am Soc Clin Oncol 1990;9:91.

57. Sullivan FJ, Herscher LL, Cook JA, et al. National Cancer Institute (Phase II) study of highgrade glioma treated with accelerated hyperfractionated radiation and iododeoxyuridine: Results in anaplastic astrocytoma. Int J Radiat Oncol Biol Phys 1994;30:583–590.

58. Mundinger F, Ostertag CB, Birg W, et al. Stereotactic treatment of brain lesions. Appl Neurophysiol 1980;43:198–204.

59. Prados MD, Gutin PH, Phillips TL, et al. Highly anaplastic astrocytoma: A review of 357 patients treated between 1977 and 1989. Int J Radiat Oncol Biol Phys 1992;23:3–8.

60. Frank F, Fabrizi AP, Gaist G, et al. Late considerations in the treatment of low-grade malignancy cerebral tumors with iodine-125 brachytherapy. Applied Neurophysiol 1987;50:302–309.

61. Ostertag CB. Stereotactic interstitial radiotherapy for brain tumors. J Neurol Sci 1989;33:83–89.

62. Sneed PK, Larson DA, Gutin PH. Brachytherapy and hyperthermia for malignant astrocytomas. Sem Oncol 1994;21:186–197.

63. Shrieve DC, Alexander E, Wen PY, et al. Comparison of stereotactic radiosurgery and brachytherapy in the treatment of recurrent glioblastoma multiforme. Int J Radiat Oncol Biol Phys 1994;30(Suppl 1):165.

64. Selch MT, Ciacci JD, DeSalles AA, et al. Radiosurgery for primary malignant brain tumors. In: DeSalles AA, Goetsch S (eds). Stereotactic Surgery and Radiosurgery. Medical Physics Publishing, Madison, WI, 1993, pp. 335–352.

65. Patchell RA, Tibbs PA, Walsh JW, et al. A randomized trial of surgery in the treatment of single metastases to the brain. N Engl J Med 1990;322:494–500.

66. Prados M, Leibel S, Barnett CM, et al. Interstitial brachytherapy for metastatic brain tumors. Cancer 1989;63:657–660.

67. Mehta MP. Radiosurgery for brain metastases. In: DeSalles AA, Goetsch S (eds). Stereotactic Surgery and Radiosurgery. Medical Physics Publishing, Madison, WI, 1993, pp. 353–368.

68. Etou A, Mundinger F, Mohadjer M, et al. Stereotactic interstitial irradiation of diencephalic tumors with iridium-192 and iodine-125: 10 years follow-up and comparison with other treatments. Child's Nerv Syst 1989;5:140–143.

69. Gutin PH, Edwards MSB, Wara WM, et al. Preliminary experience with iodine-125 brachytherapy of pediatric brain tumors. Concepts Pediatr Neurosurg 1985;5:187–206.

70. Godano U, Frank F, Fabrizi AP, et al. Stereotactic surgery in the management of deep intracranial lesions in infants and adolescents. Child's Nerv Syst 1987;3:85–88.

71. Laperiere NJ. A critical analysis of experimental radiation modalities in malignant astrocytoma. Can J Neurol Sci 1989;17:199–208.

72. Voges J, Sturm V, Berthold F, et al. Interstitial irradiation of cerebral gliomas in childhood by permanently implanted 125 iodine: Preliminary results. Klin Padiatr 1990;202:270–274.

73. Thompson ES, Afshar F, Plowman PN. Pediatric brachytherapy. II. Brain implantation. Br J Radiol 1989;62:223–229.

74. Berg E, van den Berge JH, Blaauw G, et al. Intra-cavitary brachytherapy of cystic craniopharyngiomas. J Neurosurg 1992;77:545–550.

75. Kumar PP, Good RR, Jones EO, et al. Choice of isotope in the treatment of recurrent cystic craniopharyngioma, a case report. Endocuriether/Hypertherm Oncol 1985;1:201–206.

76. Saaf M, Thoren M, Bergstrand CG, et al. Treatment of craniopharyngiomas—the stereotactic approach in a ten to twenty-three years' perspective. II. Psychosocial situation and pituitary function. Acta Neurochir 1989;99:97–103.

77. van den Berge JH, Blaauw G, Breeman WA, et al. Intracavitary brachytherapy of cystic craniopharyngiomas. J Neurosurg 1992;77:545–550.

78. Pollack IF, Lunsford LD, Slamovits TL, et al. Stereotactic intracavitary irradiation for cystic craniopharyngiomas. J Neurosurg 1988;68:227–233.

79. Backlund EO. Colloidal radioisotopes as part of a multimodality treatment of craniopharyngiomas. J Neurosurg Sci 1989;33:95–97.

80. Julow J, Lanyi F, Hajda M, et al. Further experiences in the treatment of cystic craniopharyngiomas with yttrium-90 silicate colloid. Acta Neurochir 1988;42:113–119.

Chapter 13

Brachytherapy for Cancer of the Head and Neck

Jonathan J. Beitler, M.D., M.B.A.,
Bhadrasain Vikram, M.D.,
Peter C. Levendag, M.D., Ph.D.

General Principles

Patient selection is based on patient factors and tumor factors. Patient factors include coexistent disease, age, motivation, and performance status of the patient. Tumor factors include tumor location, extension, and previous therapy. Once the decision has been made to perform brachytherapy, the clinician must decide on the clinical target volume to be treated and determine the safest technique to deliver the tumoricidal dose and dose rate. Optimal definition of the target volume and realistic pre- and postprocedure planning are the steps that the experienced brachytherapist has mastered.

Patient Factors

An ideal patient is intelligent, well motivated, and has no medical or social difficulties. Such patients are the exception rather than the rule, and each criterion for patient selection deserves due consideration.

The patient who understands the rationale and technique of the implant is the one who will be cooperative and most satisfied with the result. The patient should understand and accept the necessity for radiation precautions without becoming irrational. The patient should also be realistically informed about the indignities and discomfort of the implant and the brachytherapy treatment. The need for self-care (i.e., suctioning, cleaning, and bathroom needs) should be explained. Particularly when the procedure involves a concomitant tracheostomy, the more teaching performed preoperatively, the better.

The team needs to discuss methods of communication appropriate to the patient and the implant. A child's erasable drawing tablet for writing is inexpensive and very useful for those patients who are literate. The plan for nutrition should be discussed with the patient, and any feeding tube insertion should be done under general anesthesia.

Age alone is not a contraindication to brachytherapy. Disorientation, however, is a contraindication to afterloaded brachytherapy when the ability to deliver the treatment is compromised. Disoriented patients can pull either catheters or low-dose-rate (LDR) sources and, thereby, compromise both their own care and the safety of hospital employees and visitors. A perfectly oriented patient in an out-patient setting may suffer disorientation as an in-patient. The "sundowner syndrome,"

From Nag S (ed): *Principles and Practice of Brachytherapy.* © Futura Publishing Co., Inc., Armonk, NY, 1997.

disorientation at sunset, is particularly difficult to predict and the clinician should inquire of the family about episodic generalized confusion and specific inquiry should be made about disorientation during any recent hospitalization. Potential problems of alcohol or narcotic withdrawal demand early consultation with appropriate specialists.

It is well known that dental disease increases the risk of osteonecrosis for patients undergoing external radiation therapy[1] (ERT) and/or implant.[2] Whether or not the patient will also undergo external radiation treatment, a dental evaluation, including Panorex films, before implant is highly desirable. Early dental extractions (allowing up to 21 days for wound healing[2]) and early repair of compromised dentition should be the rule. Sodium fluoride gel treatments have been shown to decrease dental caries[3] and considering the shift of oral microflora to acidogenic strains,[4] the neutral rather than the acidic sodium fluoride gel is recommended. The role of pilocarpine in preventing cavities and subsequent osteonecrosis has yet to be demonstrated.

Tumor Factors

Much of the failure pattern in head and neck cancer treatment is local and regional rather than systemic. Distinct from most other sites, lymph node treatment in the head and neck cancer patient affects not only regional control but may also affect survival. If local and regional control are important and brachytherapy represents a better method of delivering effective therapy to a biologically significant target, then brachytherapy should be important. We believe there are roles for brachytherapy throughout the head and neck region, but we acknowledge that there is a

pressing need for phase III studies to support this belief.

Table 1 summarizes the indications for brachytherapy. Definitive brachytherapy is well established for treatment of the lip, oral tongue, floor of mouth, and to a lesser extent for the base of tongue and the tonsil. Brachytherapy as a method for delivering a localized boost is appropriate for most sites in the oral cavity, oropharynx, and nasopharynx. We use brachytherapy postoperatively after external beam therapy for patients with positive surgical margins. Brachytherapy is also useful intraoperatively for gross residual disease at the primary site or for extensive neck disease.

Recurrences of most sites of the head and neck have been treated with brachytherapy because of the need to deliver a high dose to tumor and to maximally spare surrounding normal tissues. Particularly in the patient who has received previous ERT, the density of critical structures in the head and neck region limits which structures the radiation oncologist can deliberately "over-treat." Though treatment of recurrences includes a higher risk of complications, brachytherapy may be the only method of delivering what might be a curative dose to a recurrent tumor. If the recurrence can be covered by an appropriate isodose, the risk benefit considerations often support subjecting involved normal structures to higher doses than can be "safely" tolerated. Consider the recurrent larynx cancer patient faced with a total laryngectomy; for a patient who depends on his voice, even a relatively high risk of laryngeal necrosis due to brachytherapy salvage may be quite acceptable. We have successfully used brachytherapy to salvage the archetypal Philadelphia lawyer seeking to preserve his voice. In highly selected patients, we have implanted sites from the base of skull to the hypopharynx.

Table 1.
Role of Brachytherapy

Definitive Brachytherapy Well Established	Definitive Brachytherapy Used	Brachytherapy as a Boost	Brachytherapy for Positive or Close Margins	Gross Residual Disease after Surgery
Oral tongue Floor of mouth Lip	Base of tongue Tonsil	Tongue Floor of mouth Tonsil Nasopharynx	Anywhere	Anywhere

Contraindications for brachytherapy include lesions invading bone, with lesions overlying bone being a relative contraindication. Relative contraindications also include a high risk of fistulization, radionecrosis of either bone or soft tissue, a high risk of injuring some critical structure at the time of catheter insertion, or advanced disease that has not responded to external radiation.

In the head and neck region it is difficult to achieve adequate margins for sarcomas. Because postoperative external therapy necessitates treating a large area to a relatively high dose, it is particularly morbid. Just as the density of crucial structures limits the surgeon, the radiation oncologist is also limited by surrounding normal tissues. We believe with brachytherapy the target volume might be more precisely covered and is well suited not only to treatment of high grade lesions, but also to low grade lesions with close or positive margins.

Second primaries in previously irradiated fields may also be considered for brachytherapy, especially if surgery is not possible, or is particularly morbid.

Defining the Clinical Target Volume

Preplanning of the implant is accomplished through a physical exam, CT and/or MRI, and a knowledge of the natural history of the disease. Once the target volume is delineated, the target volume is measured and then the technique of implantation is decided. Critical normal structures and obstructing bony features determine the tactics of access. Close cooperation with surgical colleagues is often an important part of the preimplant planning.

Under anesthesia in the operating room, the patient is reexamined, exposure optimized, and the preplanned implant is accomplished. Fine tuning of the preplanned technique is frequently necessary. Postimplant localization using orthogonal films and, increasingly, CT scans, allows the physician to evaluate and optimize the isodose distribution to best encompass the target volume while sparing normal tissue. In the future, improved technology will allow the clinician to better decide if the target volume was adequately covered in three dimensions.[5]

Temporary Versus Permanent Implants

Our preferred radionuclides are Iridium-192(Ir-192)and Iodine-125 (I-125). Temporary implantations have a higher dose rate and are loaded after localization and plan optimization. Temporary implantation exacerbates the acute response and must be temporally separated from a course of external radiation to the head and neck. Permanent implantation of I-125 has the advantages of a same day admission and discharge, and due to the low dose rate, mucosal reactions are much more limited. However, because of its extremely low energy, geographic misplacement of I-125 will lead to misadministration of brachytherapy. I-125 can be inserted as radioactive pellets via a Mick Applicator (Mick Radio-nuclear Instruments, Bronx, NY, USA) as seeds embedded on absorbable suture or on a plastic mold applied to a target surface.

Required activity for I-125 implantations is based on the preimplant target volume.[6] For an average dimension of 3 cm or less, we multiply the average dimension by five to obtain the activity necessary to administer a minimum target dose of 160 Gy. For target volumes of >3 cm average dimension, we use the nomograph of Anderson[7] to calculate I-125 requirements.

Intersource spacing for temporary implants should be <15 mm (we use 10 mm for LDR and 5 mm for high-dose-rate [HDR]).[8] Generally, planes should be 10–15 mm apart.

Special Considerations in the Operating Theater

In the operating room, the anesthesia team must be made aware of the operative goals of the brachytherapist. Any temporary implant of the oropharynx, hypopharynx, and larynx should be preceded by a tracheostomy to maintain an adequate airway. The tracheostomy tube should be of the cuffed category and during the procedure the cuff should be inflated. Permanent implantation of the oropharynx, hypopharynx, and larynx causes less edema and mucosal reaction and nasotracheal intubation can be contemplated.

Head and neck patients often suffer severe trismus, and if a nasal intubation is impossible either conventionally or fiberoptically, an elective tracheostomy is preferable to a fractured mandible. Particular caution is advised if the patient has undergone prior mandibular reconstruction—we have witnessed a mandibular fracture caused by an anesthesiologist's failure to respect the fragility of a mandibular reconstruction that had received external therapy prior to a planned implant.

Both permanent and temporary oral cavity implantations can be carried out with nasotracheal intubation. Reintubation can be difficult and when in doubt, the anesthesiologist should be encouraged to be cautious with extubation. A nasal trumpet has occasionally been useful to overcome postanesthesia upper airway occlusion.

A wide selection of appropriately sized mouth gags is important for optimizing exposure to the oral cavity and oropharynx. Storz© (Culver City, CA, USA) stocks eight sizes of Davis Blades for tongue retraction and are used with either the Davis type, the Palate type, the Davis-Boyle, or the Leivers type mouth gags. Jennings mouth gags come in small, medium, and large, and the Whitehead-Jennings retractor comes in four sizes. Side gags are somewhat easier to apply but the conventional mouth gags tend to open the full mouth wider and have more attachments for manipulation of the tongue.

Yankauer suction tips may be too bulky for head and neck work and finer suction tips are available and valuable. We recommend adequate surgical sponges or sterile gauzes be readily available in the operating room for unexpected bleeding. If throat packing is used, the end of the packing should come out of the mouth to ensure that the packing is not forgotten.

Applicators

Afterloading can be done through any sterile catheters including conventional angiocatheters, but we find Flexiguides (Best Industries, Inc., Springfield, VA, USA) to be optimal. These flexible 16-gauge catheters come in 20-, 30-, and 40-cm sizes and have appropriate trochars for each length catheter. The catheters can be used with either HDR or LDR afterloading treatments. Though the tips are pointed, a small skin incision will allow for easier catheter introduction. Allowance

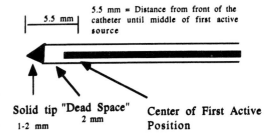

Figure 1. Relationship of catheter tip to position of the first active source.

should be made for the "front" of the catheter. The solid tip is 1–2 mm. The very front of the channel is not loadable and is 2 mm. The source itself is 4.5 mm and thus the center of the source is roughly 5.5 mm from the front of the solid tip of the catheter (Figure 1). More specific information concerning the source and its characteristics is available from Nucleotron Microselectron System© (Nucleotron Corporation, Columbia, MD, USA) and other venders.

Interstitial implantation of I-125 sources can be readily accomplished using the Mick Applicator. The 17-gauge metal needles allow for intraoperative imaging, and with practice, seeds are easily implantable at 5-mm intervals. In the head and neck, seed loss can occur due to insufficient depth of the implant (i.e., <5 mm beneath the surface) as well as due to a seed remaining in the needle; thus, to account for seed loss, we routinely implant 10% more activity than either our formulas or nomograms recommend.

In the head and neck, particular attention should be made to securing the needle with Mixter or another right angle clamp so that the needle is not inadvertently pushed in during attachment of the Mick Applicator. Generally I-125 insertion is a two person procedure.

Optimization of Dose Distribution and Dose Rate

Interstitial implants are rarely perfect and afterloading allows either HDR or LDR Iridium-192 treatments to be optimized via differential loading. Using HDR brachytherapy, we have described a method of CT-assisted dosimetry[9] for optimization, which we hope to see improved upon. Experience is growing with the use of the postimplant CT scan as an aid in treatment planning[9]; but unconquered problems include tissue inhomogeneity, tissue air-interface, software compatibility problems, and unsatisfactory graphics.

The Creteil Group[10] believes that the dose rate should be at least 50 cGy/hr even for LDR temporary implantation. The Creteil reference isodose is 85% of the basal dose (basal dose being the arithmetic mean of the dose-rate minima). The Paris system prescribes to the basal dose in an attempt to achieve dose homogeneity. Our custom is to prescribe to the highest isodose that covers the target volume, just as in external beam radiothrapy. We acknowledge that our method does not address the dose inhomogeneity problem but there are also little data to indicate if there is a critical volume that when "overdosed" is likely to cause an increased complication risk clinically. We do attempt to record the D_{max} to an arbitrary volume of 1 cm^3, but further software development is needed for these purposes.

At this time, we recommend that isodose plans with the same orientation and magnification as the orthogonal localization films be prepared. With this method, the appropriate isodose distribution can be placed behind the localization film and not only is seed placement checked, but the clinician may have the opportunity to correlate the isodose curves with the radiological anatomy. Orthogonal distributions alone may mislead the clinician, and a true understanding of the isodose distribution requires multiple distributions along different planes. The larger the target volume or the more the topography changes, the more isodose distributions are generated. At a minimum, we obtain distributions every 3 cm in plane perpendicular to the implant. The Brachytherapy Subcommittee of the Radiation Therapy Oncology Group (RTOG) recommends evaluating implants based on at least three CT scans (if possible, obtained perpendicular to the long axis of the implant) to evaluate how the prescription isodose address the outlined target volume on each CT slice. Obviously if the target volume is "ad-

justed" to the isodose curves, we are defeating the purpose of our optimization process.

Inhomogeneity within the target volume is an unavoidable problem and it is crucial to know the combination of dose and volume that increases the probability of a treatment related complication. A goal of every brachytherapist should be to gather data to aid in this analysis. Despite signigicant technical advances in software in general and dose-volume histograms in particular, Dmax to a contiguous 1 cm^3 volume is not reported by any of the current treatment planning systems. Some brachytherapists obtain treatment planning CT scans after implant and it certainly is possible to draw the highest isodose curve on each transverse plane that covers a contiguous area of 1 cm^2. By doing this every 1 cm throughout the volume treated, one approaches a rough approximation of the Dmax to a contiguous 1 cm^3 volume and we could correlate later complications with the region of the maximum dose. Performing the process every centimeter in the long axis of the implant (with sagital cuts) may eventually become more accurate, especcially if the software handles each dwell position as a short line of radiation rather than a point source. Idealy, in a multiinstitutional trial, implants should be evaluated using the minimum dose to the target volume, and the Dmax to a contiguous volume. Like our experience with external radiation we need to balance the probability and utility of local control with the normal tissue complication probability for each structure within the body.

Integrated Brachytherapy Units

Recently, in several institutions around the world, so-called integrated brachytherapy units (IBUs), have been established. The IBU basically consists of a dedicated, shielded operating suite that is fully equipped to perform any type of head and neck surgery in conjunction with a HDR remote controlled afterloading machine. Integrated in the operating room is a dedicated simulator in combination with a specifically designed operating table. On-line dosimetry is under development. The IBU can ultimately provide the basis for a geometrically perfect source configuration and optimized dose distribution by perioperative

TEMPLATE

micro Selectron HDR

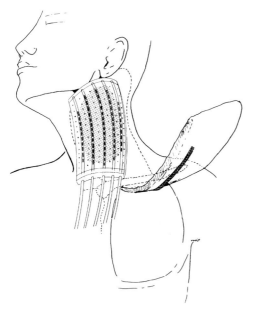

Figure 2. Single plane implant using a flexible silicone template in the dissected N3 neck.

filmless simulation, on-line treatment planning, and immediate catheter repositioning.[11] The IBU will allow either a single large fraction or the first of many fractions with smaller fraction sizes. A typical example for the implementation of a single high dose, single plane implant in the IBU is the use of a flexible silicone template in the dissected N3 neck (Figure 2).

Specific Sites

Lips

Squamous cell cancers of the lip that are 2 cm or smaller have a high probability of cure and a low rate of regional node metastases. Regional failure for primary stage I or II lip cancer is 4%–7%.[12–14] We believe that regional treatment is therefore, unwarranted for tumors 2 cm or less and probably unnecessary for tumors 4 cm or less in size. Fortunately, most lesions are small in presentation and can be successfully controlled with either surgery or radiation therapy.[15,16] When surgery will

Table 2.
T1/T2 Lip Cancer: Implant Alone

Author	Local Control	Number of Patients
Orecchia (1991)	94%	47
Cowen (1990)	96%	248

produce a cosmetic deformity, brachytherapy becomes the treatment of choice.

Recurrent lip carcinomas, particularly those whose initial size were >1 cm have a 30%–35% rate of subsequent cervical metastases[15] and treatment should include regional therapy.

Technique

Angiocatheters happen to be a convenient length for most lip cancers. Angiocatheters are inserted perpendicular to the lips for tumors involving the commissural area and in the plane of the lips for other tumors. Catheters are inserted *beyond* the lateral limit of the area of gross disease. The planning target volume includes the gross target volume plus at least 1 cm of margin. Based on the experience of Cowen et al.[17] and Orecchia et al.,[14] 60–80 Gy via LDR Ir-192 is adequate treatment. We are not aware of a published experience with the HDR approach.

Results

Results[14,17] are shown in Table 2.

Oral Tongue

Small squamous cell carcinomas of the lateral oral tongue, without clinically apparent adenopathy, can be managed by surgical excision and bilateral selective neck dissections. Postoperative ERT is dictated by the pathological findings. Definitive surgery may well be appropriate if there are no functional consequences to the partial glossectomy.

Brachytherapy, with or without external irradiation, has long been used for treating oral tongue cancers. Fu et al.[18] and Mendenhall et al.[19] suggest greater efficacy of radiation therapy for local control of oral tongue lesions as the proportion of treatment delivered by implant is increased. We and others[20,21] believe that optimal radiation treatment of the tongue is not a combination of brachytherapy and external therapy for the primary, but brachytherapy alone for the primary tongue tumor and either elective external radiation to a dose of 50 Gy to both sides of the clinically negative neck or bilateral neck dissections. When the tumor is ≤1 cm in greatest dimension[22] or <2 mm in depth,[23] an argument can be made against elective regional treatment.

Technique

The tongue lesion is carefully measured in the clinic and again under anesthesia. Because clinical understaging is so common, the implantation is planned to cover a planning target volume at least 2 cm beyond the gross tumor volume. Prior to treatment we insert permanent metal markers to radiographically delineate the original borders of the tongue tumor and we draw detailed tumor diagrams and photograph the area. Marker insertion can be performed in the clinic or in the operating room.

With a heavy silk suture, the tongue is retracted so that the target volume does not overlie the patient's mandible. We insert the catheters submentally in parallel rows and find that a number fifteen surgical scalpel is useful in penetrating the skin prior to catheter insertion. Prior to irradiation, the dose distribution and clinical situation may warrant the use of intraoral wax-covered lead stents to limit the dose to the mandible.

We chose a separation between planes of between 1 and 1.5 cm. Rather than differentially load the source closest to the surface,[24] we prefer to extend the catheter 1 cm beyond the dorsum of the tongue. To protect the palate from mechanical trauma as well as to ensure that our implant covers any exophytic disease above the surface of the tongue, we use two "half moon" spacers and a metal button. The metal button is inserted so that the top button is facing flat side superiority. Buttons and spacers are secured with long (15 inch) 00 silk sutures and brought out through the mouth. The implant is designed to be treated 1 cm above the surface of the tongue. The inferior portion of the catheter is secured using metal buttons crimped (gently) around the catheter and sutured to the skin (Figures 3A-3D).

After irradiation is complete the catheters are removed by gentle traction on the oral end of the catheter, then the exposed catheter is amputated flush with the submental skin. Then, using the sutures already coming out of the oral cavity the catheters are pulled out of the mouth. The mouth is irrigated after the catheters have been removed.

Using LDR Ir-192, 60–70 Gy is an appropriate dose for definitive treatment.

Results

Results[20,21,25] are shown in Table 3.

Floor of Mouth

Floor of mouth cancers treated with definitive implantation have good local regional control and brachytherapy represents appropriate treatment for lesions 3 cm or less, providing there is no gingival involvement.[26] Just as in oral tongue cancers, neck dissection or elective neck treatment should be the rule except for the very smallest primary cancers (depth <1.5 mm[27]). We do not feel that implant, ERT, or a combination thereof is the treatment of choice for floor of mouth lesions >3 cm.[28]

Technique

Floor of mouth cancer is treated much like oral tongue cancer. However, instead of being able to retract the tongue from the region of overlying bone, either spacers or intraoral shields are used to protect nearby bone.[29] Mazeron et al.[26] recommend a dose of 65 Gy (Paris system) for floor of mouth tumors confined to the floor of mouth, and 65–70 Gy if there is lingual involvement.

Results

Mazeron et al.[21,26] found that within the T2 stage, local control rate varied by size of primary (Table 4). T2a tumors (≤3 cm) had an 80% local control versus a 50% local control for T2b (>3 cm) tumors. Gingival extension also decreased local control[21] (53% vs 20%, P<0.04). Primary tumor control was similar for those tumors treated exclusively with im-

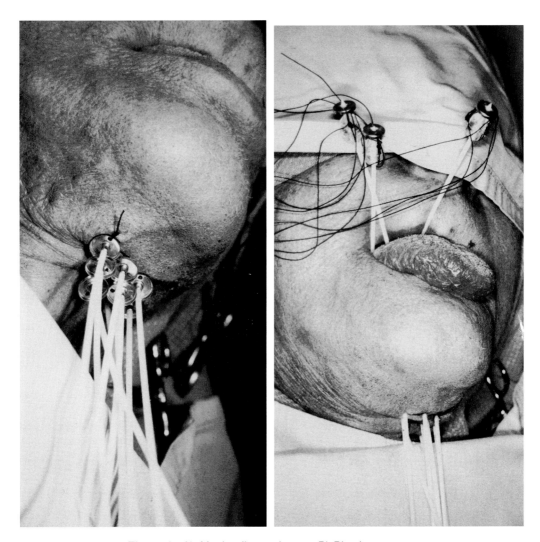

Figure 3. A) Afterloading catheters; B) Plastic spacers;

Table 3.
Oral Tongue Cancer*

Author	Local Control	Stage	Number of Patients
Implant Alone:			
Shibuya (1993)	85%	T1/T2	226
Pernot (1992)	90%	T2	70
Mazeron (1994)	88%	T2	85
Implant & XRT:			
Shibuya (1993)	87%	T1/T2	62
Pernot (1992)	51%	T2	77
Mazeron (1994)	46%	T2	33

* Minimum follow-up = 2 years.

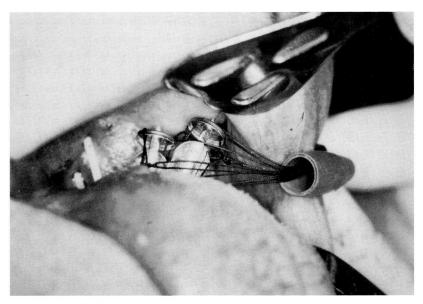

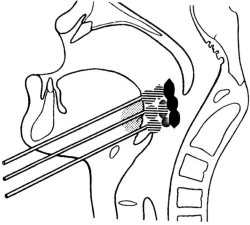

Figure 3. *(continued).* C) Metal buttons (crimped). The spacers and the intraoral metal buttons are secured with two heavy ties that exit orally. The ties are kept together by enclosing them within a large Penrose drain. D) Schematic drawing of the base of tongue implantation. Using spacers and buttons, the implant is designed to treat 1 cm beyond the surface of the tongue—New York Technique.

plant compared to those treated with external radiation and implantation (74% vs 70%).

Base of Tongue

Base of tongue cancer has a greater propensity for lymphatic spread then oral tongue cancer, and once again is frequently understaged by clinical exam. Experts disagree[30–34] about the role of brachytherapy, external radiation, and surgery. The Gainesville group[35] reports results similar to interstitial implant with ERT alone for T1 and T2 base of tongue lesions and implants only those tumors that are small, discrete, and located in the anterolateral base of tongue.

An implant is used by us as a boost for most patients treated with external therapy. For T3 lesions, the strategy of downsizing the lesion by ERT and then boosting with interstitial irradiation is an attractive alternative to total glossectomy and laryngectomy. In selected T4 lesions the combination of ERT and chemotherapy is under active investigation by us and others.

Technique

New York Group. Implantation of the base of tongue requires a tracheostomy with a cuffed tracheostomy tube. As in the oral

Table 4.
Floor of Mouth: Implant Alone
(Mazeron, 1990)

Local Control	Stage	Number of Patients
94%	T1	46
80%	T2a*	44
58%	T2b*	26

* T2a ≤ 3 cm, T2b > 3 cm.

tongue and the floor of mouth, our preferred approach is submental. In the base of tongue, however, the flexi-guide catheters are directed posteriorly as well as superiorly.

Since our methodology was originally described[29] in 1981 we have modified our method of fixation on the tongue surface. As described in the section on oral tongue, we use two spacers in addition to our metal button to treat 1 cm superior to the surface of the tongue (Figure 3). The currently used flexi-guides also allow for HDR afterloading.

Insertion of Afterloading Catheters

After the catheter position has been verified by clinical palpation and/or intraoperative localization x-rays, the catheter is fixed in the tongue base. Just as in the floor of mouth and oral tongue, we use two half moon plastic spacers and a metal button to be sure that the catheter tip extends at least 1 cm beyond the dorsal surface of the tongue and the reference isodose would, therefore, encompass all exophytic surface disease.

We caution that though removal of the catheters is relatively painless, in roughly 5%–10% of the base of tongue cases we, and others,[32] have experienced significant bleeding at the time of atraumatic catheter removal. This risk seems to be elevated in patients implanted for recurrent cancers. Because of this possibility we usually remove the catheters in the operating theater, using the protection of an inflated, cuffed tracheostomy.

Rotterdam Group. Prior to 1985, at the Dr. Daniel den Hoeb Cancer Center-Rotterdam (DDHCC), surgery for either early or late stage base of tongue cancer was considered too mutilating and patients were treated by external radiation alone. In 1986, the combined treatment of ERT and LDR interstitial implant (LDR-IRT), with or without a neck dissection, was initiated and with encouraging results (Table 5) became the standard treatment policy. In more recent years either pulsed-dose-rate (PDR) brachytherapy regimes (1 Gy per fraction, 3-hour intervals, 8 fractions per day) or hyperfractionated HDR (two daily fractions of 3 Gy per fraction with 6-hour intervals) has been the DDHCC standard of care.[36,37] Both the PDR and HDR systems take advantage of the single stepping source and optimization software to provide better distributions for interstitial implants.[11] A single plane of a soft palate and base of tongue implant is shown (Figures 4 and 5).

Results

The results of treatment by external beam irradiation plus local boost brachytherapy for T1 and T2 primary tumors of the base of tongue are shown in Table 6.[32,33,38]

Table 5.
Evolution of Treatment Protocol for Advanced Base of Tongue Cancer*

Modalities	Evolution Protocol	Year Protocol	Local Control	Survival Local Relapse Free	Survival Overall
ERT	Standard	1974–1985	33% (11/33)	25% (5 years)	20% (5 years)
ERT	Optional	1986–1987	33% (2/6)		
ERT + IRT**	Optional	1986–1987	75% (6/8)		
ERT + IRT**	Standard	1988–1991	73% (11/15)	73% (3 years)	55% (5 years)

* Head and neck surgery DDHCC/AZR; Levendag, et al., 199.

** Low-dose-rate brachytherapy.

ERT = external beam radiotherapy; IRT = interstitial radiotherapy.

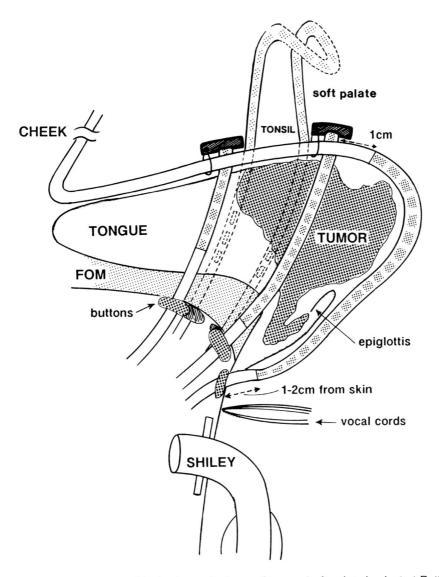

Figure 4. Single plane of a base of tongue/soft palate implant at Rotterdam.

Tonsil

Early stage squamous cell cancer of the tonsil can be cured by surgery,[39] external radiation,[40–42] or external radiation combined with brachytherapy.[43–45] We believe that radiation therapy is the treatment of choice for most early tonsil cancers. When the patient has either ipsilateral N2 neck disease or tongue extension, bilateral external radiation to 45–50 Gy following interstitial implantation of the primary tumor and/or the cervical dis-

ease may preserve some parotid salivary response to gustatory stimulation.[46]

Advanced tonsil cancer is conventionally treated with surgery and postoperative ERT. We prefer definitive surgery, adjuvant external radiation with I-125 implant reserved for positive[47] or close[48] margins for advanced tonsil cancer.

Technique

After reviewing the pretherapy diagrams and imaging studies, the clinical target vol-

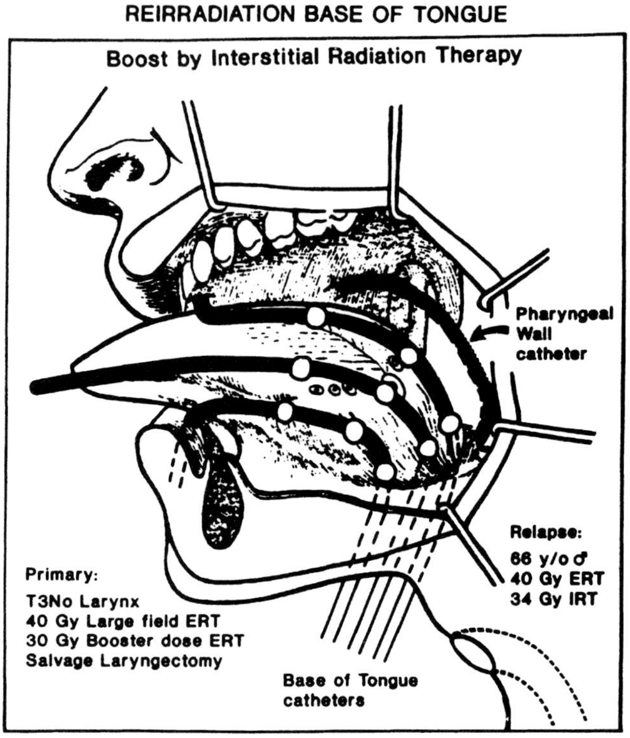

REIRRADIATION BASE OF TONGUE

Boost by Interstitial Radiation Therapy

Pharyngeal Wall catheter

Primary:

T3No Larynx
40 Gy Large field ERT
30 Gy Booster dose ERT
Salvage Laryngectomy

Relapse:
66 y/o ♂
40 Gy ERT
34 Gy IRT

Base of Tongue catheters

Figure 5. Base of tongue irradiation—Rotterdam Technique.

ume is defined under general anesthesia. A flexi-guide catheter is introduced through the skin, just anterior and medial to the angle of the mandible. Under bimanual palpation, the catheter is gently guided superiorly and submucosally along the anterior tonsillar pillar until its tip reaches the base of the skull. A second catheter is passed posterior to the first catheter, along the posterior tonsillar pillar. The catheters are secured on the skin with metal snaps and nonabsorbable sutures.

For tonsillar lesions that encroach onto the base of the tongue or soft palate, a medial plane of catheters is created parallel to the first plane. These catheters enter through the submental skin, pierce the dorsum of the base of the tongue, and then penetrate the soft palate so the tips are resting in the nasopharynx. To protect the airway, a preliminary tracheostomy is indicated.

Results

Results are shown in Table 7.[43–45]

Soft Palate

In patients with squamous cell cancers of the soft palate there is a high risk of nodal involvement[49] and both sides of the neck should be addressed. In patients with T1–3 primary lesions and clinically negative necks, excellent functional and curative results are achieved with Ir-192, and 45–50 Gy of ERT. Contraindi-

Table 6.
Base of Tongue: XRT + Implant

Author	Initial Local Control	Stage (Minimum Follow-Up)	Number of Patients
Crook (1988)	85%	T1 (5 years)	13
Crook (1988)	71%	T2 (5 years)	35
Harrison (1992)	92%	T1/T2 (22 months)	25

Table 7.
Tonsil: XRT and Implant

Author	Local Control	Stage*	Number of Patients
Pernot (1992)	89%	T1-2/N0	120
Pernot (1992)	83%	T1-2/N+	48
Pernot (1992)	65%	T3 N0	52
Pernot (1992)	70%	T3 N+	49
Puthawala (1985)	84%	III/IV	80
Mazeron (1994)	100%	T1/T2	33

* Two year minimum follow-up.
XRT = external radiation therapy.

cations[45] include extension to the retromolar trigone, the pterygomandibular space, nasopharynx, and intermaillar commissure.

Technique

Depending on the original size of the gross tumor volume, catheters are implanted via a submental approach, similar to the tonsil. In Rotterdam, the catheters are sutured onto the soft palate (Figures 6 and 7). The New York group prefers to extend these catheters superiorly toward the base of the skull. Multiple parallel, sagittal planes, 10–15 mm apart, are created in order to encompass the entire lesion with a 1- to 2-cm margin. All catheters are secured on the submental skin with metal buttons and nonabsorbable sutures.

Results

Results are shown in Table 8.[45,50,51]

Larynx and Hypopharynx

The technique[52] for interstitial implantation of tumors in the hypopharynx and larynx in-

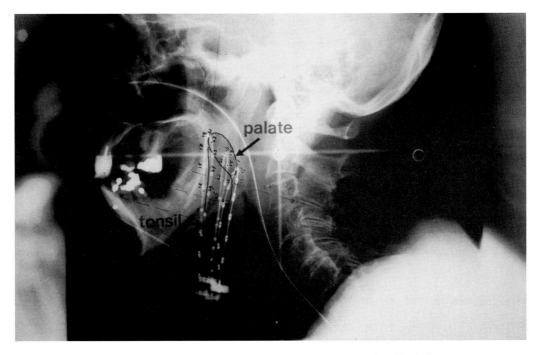

Figure 6. Anterior simulation film, soft palate—Rotterdam Technique.

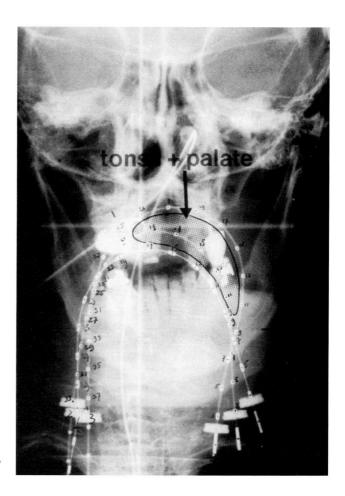

Figure 7. Lateral simulation film, soft palate—Rotterdam Technique.

volves the placement of flexi-guides in a posterior direction through the midline of the neck at intervals of 1–1.5 cm, in sagittal planes. A preliminary tracheostomy is performed. The most superior catheter is introduced just superior to the level of the hyoid bone and additional catheters are introduced through the thyroid notch, through the cricothyroid membrane, and between the tracheal rings. The needles extend posteriorly into the prevertebral fascia. As many additional sagittal planes, 10–15 mm apart, are created parallel to this midline plane as is necessary. The second plane is medial to the major blood vessels and the catheter tip extends posteriorly to the level of the vertebral bodies. The third plane is lateral to the major vessels and the catheter tip extends posteriorly as far back

as the transverse processes. Finally, a coronal plane is created to "cross" the distal end of the implant. This is accomplished by introducing the flexi-guide catheters through the lateral neck, posterior to the major vessels, such that the needles traverse the prevertebral fascia and are perpendicular to the previously described planes of catheters. To date, experience with this procedure is anecdotal, and few results are available.

Nasopharynx

New York Group. Radiotherapeutic salvage of local failures after ERT can be achieved with intracavitary irradiation of the nasopharynx.[53–55] However, intracavitary techniques must overcome positional uncertainty. Intra-

Table 8.
Soft Palate External RT + Implant and <u>Implant Alone</u>

Author	Initial Local Control	Stage (Minimum Follow-Up)	Number of Patients
Esche (1988)	100% & <u>100%</u>	T1	24 & <u>10</u>
Esche (1988)	2/5 & <u>2/2</u>	T2	5 & <u>2</u>
Mazeron (1987)	81% & <u>100%</u>	T1 (2 years)	16 & <u>10</u>
Mazeron (1987)	85% & <u>4/4</u>	T2 (2 years)	13 & <u>4</u>
Pernot (1992)	95%	T1/T2 (3 years)	96

cavitary irradiation of a region at risk that may be <1 cm³ relies heavily on a source that if not "flopping in the breeze" can be disturbed by any inadvertent movement of the afterloading catheters. While positional uncertainties can be reduced by the use of mold applications,[54] or the use of intranasopharyngeal endotracheal tubes,[55] the New York group prefers interstitial techniques.[56] The area at risk can be directly visualized and the sources are placed securely submucosally (i.e., within the target volume). Because the source position is fixed, the dosimetry for interstitial brachytherapy is more certain.

Local control of cancers of the nasopharynx has long been recognized to exhibit a dose response to ERT.[57–60] Our encouraging experience with interstitial implants for recurrent cancer of the nasopharynx,[61] and the evidence for improved local control with increasing doses of radiation led us to use interstitial boosts after ERT (Figure 8).

The technique of interstitial implantation is dependent on accurate estimation of the site and size of the target volume. This is determined by endoscopy, and CT or MRI scans. The patient is examined fiberoptically every week during ERT and tumor response is recorded on lesion diagrams. Though the tumor may initially fill the nasopharynx and bulge into the nasal cavity, our experience is that external radiation usually is successful in obtaining a complete or near-complete response. The radiation oncologist must observe the responding tumor to decide on the site of the tumor within the nasopharynx to be implanted. We believe the tumor disappears last from the site of origin. At CT scan is repeated 2–4 weeks after ERT to compare to the pretherapy scan in order to help determine the residual volume. Residual retropharyngeal fullness as shown by the postexternal therapy CT scan may be implanted.

The size of the area is estimated, and the target volume in a complete responder is deemed to be 1×1×0.5 cm. With our preexternal and postexternal CT scans, the patient is brought to the operating room 3–4 weeks after ERT. Using oropharyngeal intubation, we first examine and palpate the nasopharynx and neck under anesthesia. We find that both the rigid and flexible endoscopes are useful in visualizing the target volume but prefer the rigid endoscope with suction and irrigation attachments for the actual implant. Primary sites in the vault, fossa of Rosenmuller, and torus tubaris are implanted through a needle inserted in the nose. Lesions of the posterior wall or retropharyngeal disease are sometimes more easily implanted transorally. The endoscopy equipment and the needle insertion need not be through the same orifice (Figure 8).

Despite suction and irrigation, once the first needle has been inserted sometimes even a small amount of bleeding impairs visualization. Subsequent needles are inserted with reference to the first needle. Needle position is confirmed with lateral x-rays in the operating room, and 3–4 seeds are inserted per needle. Because the depth of the submucosa in a complete responder is particularly shallow, the seeds are not spaced but are deposited end to end. Extreme care should be exercised in posterior implants when there has been bone destruction in the clivus so as not to impale the brain stem.

After the implant, the area is reinspected for bleeding and packed if necessary. The patient is discharged a few hours later, after formal localization films.

Rotterdam Group. In the DDHCC, intracavi-

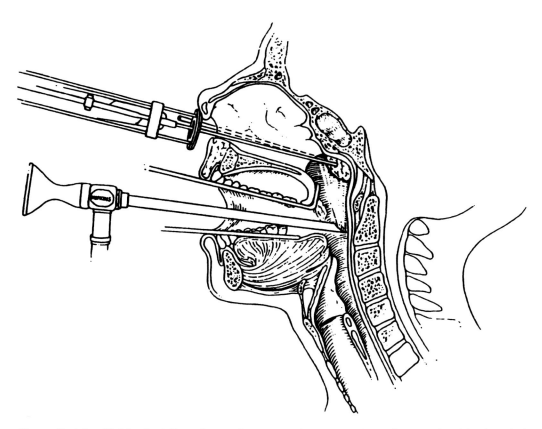

Figure 8. Interstitial implantation of nasopharynx; endoscope and needles need not be inserted through the same orifice.

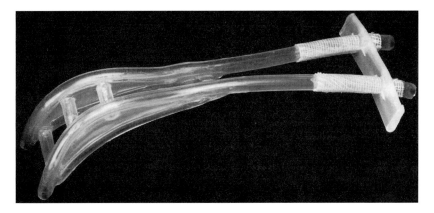

Figure 9. Intracavitary irradiation of nasopharynx—mold applicator used in Rotterdam.

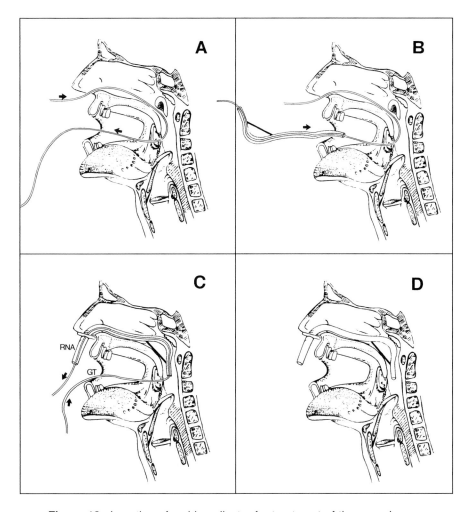

Figure 10. Insertion of mold applicator for treatment of the nasopharynx.

tary irradiation has been the method of choice for boosting the nasopharynx.[62] For this purpose a flexible silicone mold was developed, which is introduced into the nasopharynx after a dose of 60 Gy ERT-conventional fractionation (T1–3N0 tumors) or after a dose of 70 Gy ERT (T1–3N+ or T4N0,+ tumors) (Figures 9 and 10). This mold will remain in situ for the duration of the HDR brachytherapy boost treatment, i.e., 2–4 days. After a treatment planning procedure with optimization of specific normal tissue dose points (that is, if the nasopharynx receives 100% of the prescribed dose specified, normal tissues are to receive as low a dose as possible, see Table 9), 3 Gy per fraction is prescribed to the naso-

pharynx at the level of the base of the skull. For patients having received 60 Gy ERT, two fractions of 3 Gy (six fractions in total) are given as a booster dose by means of intracavitary irradiation (cumulative dose nasopharynx 78 Gy). Those who received 70 Gy previously are boosted by four fractions of 3 Gy (two fractions per day), which is a cumulative dose of 82 Gy to the nasopharynx.

Results

Twenty consecutive New York patients were treated using the technique described below. They received 50–70 Gy of external radiation, which was then electively boosted

Table 9.
DDHCC—Intracavitary Brachytherapy for the Nasopharynx

Dose Points	Before Optimization	After Optimization
Nasopharynx	100%	104%
Node Rouviere	158	116
Retina	29	21
Optic Chiasm	38	25
Pituitary Gland	28	22
Nose	169	92
Foramen Ovale	37	47
Foramen Lacerum	56	68
Palate	204	110
Cord	87	47

Table 10.
Rotterdam–Nasopharynx: Local Relapse Free Survival (LRFS) and Overall Survival (OS)

		Brachytherapy 1990–1992	External Beam 1965–1985, >50 Gy
T 1–3	LRFS	96%, 2 years	68%, 5 years
T 1–4	LRFS	92%, 2 years	52%, 5 years
	OS	78%, 2 years	30%, 5 years

to 160 Gy (permanent dose).[63] At a median follow-up of 2 years, there have been no local recurrences and, probably because of the lower activity used in the latter series (7.5 mCi versus 11 mCi in the earlier series for recurrent disease), there have been no instances of radionecrosis.

The results at DDHCC were recently compared to the previous DDHCC experience using ERT only. A summary of the tumor control rates (local relapse-free survival) and overall survival can be depicted from Table 10.

Special Situations

Boost Implants as Postoperative Radiation Therapy

We have recently reviewed our experience using postoperative and postexternal radiation therapy, I-125 implants for 32 consecutive patients who were at high risk of recurrence due to positive margins. Our goal was to treat the region at risk to a permanent dose of 120 Gy and we usually used 10–12 I-125 seeds (activity 0.60–0.67 mCi per seed) to the region of the microscopically positive margin. The size of the area we estimated to be at risk influenced the activity implanted. The brachytherapists' deductive skills were used to ascertain the exact location of the region at high risk by studying the operative report, the pathology report, the preoperative CT or MRI

scans, and also by visiting the pathologist and examining and orienting the actual surgical specimen. With a median follow-up of 24 months, the local control rate is 94%.[47]

Salvage Irradiation

Radiation of second malignancies in previously irradiated fields can be accomplished through brachytherapy[64] or external therapy.

Reirradiation of recurrent primary cancers has been performed for the wide range of head and neck tumors[64–72] (Table 11). For salvage, meaningful reirradiation generally means retreatment to a dose of 50 Gy, therefore, after radiation failures, first consideration should go to salvage surgery. Often surgery is not possible and reirradiation can offer a moderate chance of local control, particularly in the nasopharynx, oropharynx, and larynx. Despite respectable local control, overall survival remains unacceptably low. We are currently investigating the use of chemotherapy to downsize disease prior to implantation. To date, it remains unclear if tumor control is significantly improved, but the downsizing by systemic therapy may reduce the acute and chronic complications. Another strategy to reduce the risk of complications is to perform the implant in two separate sittings a few weeks apart rather than give the entire retreatment dose at once.

Conclusion

In 1971,[73] Pierquin et al. described a local control rate of 95% with Iridium treatment for

Table 11.
Reirradiation

Author	Site	Local Control	Overall Survival	Complications
Wang (1987)	Nasopharynx		45%	4%
Pryzant (1992)	Nasopharynx	35%	21%	15%
Wang (1993)	Larynx	61%	93%	0%
Levendag (1992)	All sites	50%	20%	28%
Mazeron (1987)	Oropharynx	69%	14%	27%
Housset (1992)	Neck	57%	13%	37%
Langlois (1988)	Tongue/oropharynx	59%	48%	23%
Stevens (1994)	All sites	60%	37%	13%
Pieffert (1994)	Tonsil/palate	78%	30%	13%

oral tongue and floor of mouth tumors <4 cm in size. Despite these results, there was little doubt that most such tumors were treated by surgical resection. Today, as in the past, "the proposition that surgery is the best method or preferred method of treatment of these lesions merits serious debate."

References

1. Murray CG, Daly TE, Zimmerman SO. The relationship between dental disease and radiation necrosis of the mandible. Oral Surg Oral Med Oral Pathol 1980;49:99–104.
2. Marx RE, Johnson RP. Studies in the radiobiology of osteonecrosis and their clinical significance. Oral Surg Oral Med Oral Pathol 1987; 64:379–390.
3. Dreizen S, Brown LR, Daly TE, et al. Prevention of xerostomia-related dental caries in irradiated cancer patients. J Dent Res 1977;56: 99–104.
4. Brown LR, Dreizen S, Handler S, et al. Effect of radiation-induced xerostomia on human oral microflora. J Dent Res 1975;54:740–750.
5. Roy JN, Wallner KE, Chiu-Tsao S, et al. CT-based optimized planning for transperineal prostate implant with customized template. Int J Radiat Oncol Biol Phys 1991;21:483–489.
6. Anderson LL, Moni JV, Harrison LB. A nomograph for permanent implants of palladium-103 seeds. Int J Radiat Oncol Biol Phys 1993; 27:129–135.
7. Anderson LL. Spacing nomograph for interstitial implants of I-125 seeds. Med Phys 1976;3: 48–51.
8. Simon JM, Mazeron JJ, Pohar S, et al. Effect of intersource spacing on local control and complications in brachytherapy of mobile tongue and floor of mouth. Radiother Oncol 1993;26: 19–25.
9. Mishra S, Chadha M, Panigrahi N, et al. Computed tomography-assisted three-dimensional dosimetry in high dose rate brachytherapy. Endocurie Hyperther Oncol 1994;10:71–77.
10. Mazeron JJ, Simon JM, LePechoux C, et al. Effect of dose rate on local control and complications in definitive irradiation of T1–2 squamous cell carcinomas of the mobile tongue and floor of mouth with interstitial iridium 192. Radiother Oncol 1991;21:39–47.
11. Kolkman-Deurloo IKK, Visser AG, Niel CGJH, et al. Optimization of interstitial volume implants. Radiother Oncol 1994;31:229–239.
12. Cerezo L, Liu FF, Tsang R, et al. Squamous cell carcinoma of the lip: Analysis of the Princess Margaret experience. Radiother Oncol 1993; 28:142–147.
13. Petrovich Z, Parker RC, Luxton G, et al. Carcinoma of the lip and selected sites of the head and neck skin. A clinical study of 896 patients. Radiother Oncol 1987;8:11–17.
14. Orecchia R, Rampino M, Gribaudo S, et al. Interstitial brachytherapy for carcinomas of the lower lip. Results of treatment. Tumori 1991; 77:336–338.
15. Baker SR, Krause CJ. Carcinoma of the lip. Laryngoscope 1980;90:19–27.
16. Million RR, Cassisi NJ, Mancuso AA. Oral cavity. In: Million RR, Cassisi NJ (eds). Management of Head and Neck Cancer: A Multi-Disciplinary Approach. Second Edition. J.B. Lippincott, Philadelphia, PA, 1994, p. 391.
17. Cowen D, Thomas L, Richaud P, et al. Cancers des levres: Resultats du traitment de 299 patients. Ann Oto-Laryng (Paris) 1990;107: 121–126.

18. Fu KK, Chan EK, Phillips TL, et al. Time, dose and volume factors in interstitial radium implants of carcinoma of the oral tongue. Radiology 1976;119:209–213.

19. Mendenhall WM, Van-Cise S, Bova FJ, et al. Analysis of time-dose factors in squamous cell carcinoma of the oral tongue and floor of mouth treated with radiation therapy alone. Int J Radiat Oncol Biol Phys 1981;7:1005–1011.

20. Pernot M, Malissard L, Aletti P, et al. Iridium-192 brachytherapy in the management of 147 T2N0 oral tongue carcinomas treated with irradiation alone: Comparison of two treatment techniques. Radiother Oncol 1992;23:223–228.

21. Mazeron JJ, Grimard L, Benk V. Curietherapy versus external irradiation combined with curietherapy in stage II squamous cell carcinomas of the mobile tongue and floor of mouth. Recent Results Cancer Res 1994;134:101–110.

22. Bradfield JD, Scruggs RP. Carcinoma of the mobile tongue: Incidence of cervical metastases in early lesions related to the method of primary treatment. Laryngoscope 1983;93:1332–1336.

23. Spiro RH, Huvos AG, Wong GY, et al. Predictive value of tumor thickness in squamous cell carcinoma confined to the tongue and floor of the mouth. Am J Surg 1986;152:345–350.

24. Schmidt-Ullrich R, Zwicker RD, Wu A, et al. Interstitial Ir-192 implants of the oral cavity: The planning and construction of volume implants. Int J Radiat Oncol Biol Phys 1991;20:1079–1085.

25. Shibuya H, Hoshina M, Takeda M, et al. Brachytherapy for stage I & II oral tongue cancer: An analysis of past cases focusing on control and complications. Int J Radiat Oncol Biol Phys 1993;26:51–58.

26. Mazeron JJ, Grimard L, Raynal M, et al. Irridium-192 curietherapy for T1 and T2 epidermoid carcinomas of the floor of mouth. Int J Radiat Oncol Biol Phys 1990;18:1299–1306.

27. Mohit-Tabatabai MA, Sobel HJ, Rush BF, et al. Relation of thickness of floor of mouth stage I and II cancers to regional metastases. Am J Surg 1986;152:351–353.

28. Marks JE, Lee F, Smith PG, et al. Floor of mouth cancer: Patient selection and treatment results. Laryngoscope 1983;93:475–480.

29. Levendag PC, Visch LL, Driver N. A simple device to protect against osteoradionecrosis induced by interstitial irradiation. J Prosthet Dent 1990;63:665–670.

30. Foote RL, Parsons JT, Mendenhall WM, et al. Is interstitial implantation essential for successful radiotherapeutic treatment of base of tongue carcinoma? Int J Radiat Oncol Biol Phys 1990;18:1293–1298.

31. Foote RL, Parsons JT, Mendenhall WM, et al. Response to Goffinet, Harrison, Puthawala, and Syed. Int J Radiat Oncol Biol Phys 1991;21:868–869.

32. Goffinet DR, Harrison LB. 192 irridium implantation of the base of tongue. Int J Radiat Oncol Biol Phys 1991;21:867.

33. Puthawala A, Siyed MN. Response to article by Foote et al. Int J Radiat Oncol Biol Phys 1991;21:868.

34. Gardner KE, Parsons JT, Mendenhall WM, et al. Time-dose relationships for local tumor control and complications following irradiation of squamous cell carcinoma of the base of tongue. Int J Radiat Oncol Biol Phys 1987;13:507–510.

35. Million RR, Cassisi NJ, Mancuso AA. Oropharynx. In: Million RR, Cassisi NJ (eds). Management of Head and Neck Cancer. Second Edition. J.B. Lippincott, Philadelphia, PA, 1994, p. 414.

36. Levendag PC, Vikram B, Yin W, et al. High dose rate brachytherapy for cancer in the head and neck. In: Nag S (ed). High Dose Rate Brachytherapy: A Textbook. 1994, p. 237–273.

37. Levendag PC, Visser AG, Kolkmas-Deurloo IK. HDR & PDR brachytherapy with special reference to base of tongue cancer. In: Mould RF, Batterman JJ, Martinez AA, et al. (eds). Brachytherapy from Radium to Optimization, 1994, pp. 132–148.

38. Harrison LB, Zelefsky MJ, Sessions RB, et al. Base-of-tongue cancer treated with external beam irradiation plus brachytherapy: Oncologic and functional outcome. Radiology 1992;184:267–270.

39. Remmler D, Medina JE, Byers RM, et al. Treatment of choice for squamous cell carcinoma of the tonsillar fossa. Head Neck Surg 1985;7:206.

40. Bataini JP, Asselain B, Jaulerry C, et al. A multivariate primary tumour control analysis in 465 patients treated by radical radiotherapy for cancer of the tonsillar region: Clinical and treatment parameters as prognostic factors. Radiother Oncol 1989;14:265–277.

41. Lee WR, Mendenhall WM, Parsons JT, et al. Carcinoma of the tonsillar region: A multivariate analysis of 243 patients treated with radical radiotherapy. Head & Neck 1993;15:283–288.

42. Wong CS, Ang KK, Fletcher GH, et al. Definitive therapy for squamous cell carcinoma of the tonsillar fossa. Int J Radiat Oncol Biol Phys 1989;16:657–662.

43. Mazeron JJ, Lusinchi A, Marinello G, et al. Interstitial radiation therapy for squamous cell carcinoma of the tonsillar region: The Creteil

experience (1971–1981). Int J Radiat Oncol Biol Phys 1986;12:895–900.

44. Puthawala AA, Syed AMN, Eads DL, et al. Limited external irradiation and interstitial iridium implant in the treatment of squamous cell carcinoma of the tonsillar region. Int J Radiat Oncol Biol Phys 1985;11:1595–1602.

45. Pernot M, Malissard L, Taghian A, et al. Velotonsillar squamous cell carcinoma: 277 cases treated by combined external irradiation and brachytherapy—results according to extension, localization and dose rate. Int J Radiat Oncol Biol Phys 1992;23:715–723.

46. Tsujii H. Quantitative dose-response analysis of salivary function following radiotherapy using sequential ri-sialography. Int J Radiat Oncol Biol Phys 1985;11:1603–1612.

47. Beitler JJ, Smith RV, Silver CE, et al. Close or positive margins after surgical resection for the head and neck cancer patient: the addition of brachytherapy improves local control. Submitted for publication. 1997.

48. Looser KG, Shah JP, Strong EW. The significance of "positive" margins in surgically resected epidermoid carcinoma. Head Neck Surg 1978;1:107–111.

49. Lindberg R. Distribution of cervical lymph node metastases from squamous cell carcinoma of the upper respiratory and digestive tracts. Cancer 1972;29:1446–1449.

50. Mazeron JJ, Marinello G, Crook J, et al. Definitive radiation treatment for early stage carcinoma of the soft palate and uvula: The indications for iridium 192 implantation. Int J Radiat Oncol Biol Phys 1987;13:1829–1837.

51. Esche BA, Haie CM, Gerbaulet AP, et al. Interstitial and external radiotherapy in carcinoma of the soft palate and uvula. Int J Radiat Oncol Biol Phys 1988;15:619–625.

52. Vikram B, Bosl GJ, Pfister D, et al. New strategies for avoiding total laryngectomy in patients with head and neck cancer. NCI Monograph 1988;6:361–364.

53. Henschke UK, Hilaris BS, Mohan GD. Therapy of recurrent cancer of the nasopharynx. Am J Roentgenol 1963;90:386–395.

54. Suit HD, Lloyd RS, Andrews JR, et al. Technique for intracavitary irradiation of the nasopharynx. Am J Roentgenol 1960;84:629–631.

55. Wang CC, Busse J, Gitterman M. A simple afterloading applicator for intracavitary irradiation of carcinoma of the nasopharynx. Radiology 1975;115:737–738.

56. Vikram B, Hilaris BS. Transnasal permanent interstitial implantation for carcinoma of the nasopharynx. Int J Radiat Oncol Biol Phys 1984;10:153–155.

57. Bedwinek JM, Perez CA, Keys DJ. Analysis of failures after definitive radiation for carcinoma

of the nasopharynx. Cancer 1980;45:2725–2729.

58. Moench HC, Phillips TL. Carcinoma of the nasopharynx—review of 146 patients with emphasis on radiation dose and time factors. Am J Surg 1972;124:515–518.

59. Vikram B, Mishra UB, Strong EW, et al. Patterns of failure in carcinoma of the nasopharynx: I. Failure at the primary site. Int J Radiat Oncol Biol Phys 1985;11:1455–1459.

60. Wang CC, Meyer JE. Radiotherapeutic management of carcinoma of the nasopharynx—An analysis of 170 patients. Cancer 1971;28:566–570.

61. Vikram B. Permanent iodine-125 implants for recurrent carcinoma of the nasopharynx. Endocurie Hypertherm Oncol 1986;2:83–85.

62. Levendag PC, Visser AG, Kolkman-Deurloo IKK, et al. HDR brachytherapy with special reference to cancer of the nasopharynx. In: Mould RF, Battermann JJ, Martinez AA, et al. (eds). Brachytherapy from Radium to Optimization, Nucletron International B.V. Veendendaal, The Netherlands, 1994, pp. 121–131.

63. Vikram B, Mishra S. Permanent iodine-125 boost implants after external radiation therapy in nasopharyngeal cancer. Int J Radiat Oncol Biol Phys 1994;28(3):699–701.

64. Peiffert D, Pernot M, Malissard L, et al. Salvage irradiation by brachytherapy of velotonsillar squamous cell carcinoma in a previously irradiated field: Results in 73 cases. Int J Radiat Oncol Biol Phys 1994;29:681–686.

65. Stevens KR, Britsch A, Moss WT. High-dose reirradiation of head and neck cancer with curative intent. Int J Radiat Oncol Biol Phys 1994;29:687–689.

66. Levendag PC, Meeuwis C, Visser AG. Reirradiation of recurrent head and neck cancers: External and/or interstitial radiation therapy. Radiother Oncol 1992;23:6–14.

67. Wang CC. Reirradiation of recurrent nasopharyngeal carcinoma. Treatment, techniques and results. Int J Radiat Oncol Biol Phys 1987;13:953–956.

68. Wang CC, McIntyre J. Reirradiation of laryngeal carcinoma. Techniques and results. Int J Radiat Oncol Biol Phys 1993;26:783–785.

69. Housset M, Barret JM, Brunel P, et al. Split course interstitial brachytherapy with a source shift: The results of a new technique for salvage irradiation in recurrent inoperable cervical lymphadenopathy greater than or equal to 4 cm in diameter in 23 patients. Int J Radiat Oncol Biol Phys 1992;14:1071–1074.

70. Langlois D, Hoffstetter S, Malissard L, et al. Salvage irradiation of oropharynx and mobile tongue about 192 iridium brachytherapy in

Centre Alexis Vautrin (published erratum appears in 16:A1,1989). Int J Radiat Oncol Biol Phys 1988;14:849–853.

71. Mazeron JJ, Langlois D, Glaubiger D, et al. Salvage irradiation of oropharyngeal cancers using Iridium 192 wire implants. Int J Radiat Oncol Biol Phys 1987;13:957–962.

72. Pryzant RM, Wendt CD, Delcos L, et al. Retreatment of nasopharyngeal carcinoma in 53 patients. Int J Radiat Oncol Biol Phys 1992;22: 941–947.

73. Pierquin B, Chassagne D, Baillet F, et al. The place of implantation in tongue and floor of mouth cancer. JAMA 1971;215:961–963.

Chapter 14

Brachytherapy for Ocular Disease

James Fontanesi, M.D., Subir Nag, M.D.

Editor's note: All iodine-125 doses are to be reduced by 15% when using the new I-125 calibration standards established by the National Institute of Standards and Technology (NIST) after November 1, 1996. Subir Nag, M.D.

Introduction

The efficacy of brachytherapy in the management of malignant and benign ocular diseases has been well documented.[1–3] In fact, the use of brachytherapy has a long record of use, with documentation of clinical use as early as 1931.[4] This chapter will describe the historical use, present day application, and possible future use of brachytherapy to treat ocular diseases.

Uveal Melanoma

Uveal melanomas are a relatively rare malignancy with approximately 1500 new cases in the United States each year.[5] The peak incidence occurs in the sixth decade, with male to female ratio estimated at 1.06. Histologic classification of ocular melanomas was initially proposed by Callender et al. in 1942[6] and modified by McLean et al. in 1970.[7] There was excellent correlation between histologic subgroups, with spindle A type lesions, those with heavy argyrophic fiber content, and tumors with light pigment content having improved 5-year survival. In addition to these histologic characteristics, several important clinical features have also been reported. Factors suggestive of poorer prognosis include location anterior to equator, tumor diameter >14 mm, and age >60 years.

These tumors grow very slowly; therefore, small tumors (<2.5 mm in height) can be followed and treated when there is documented rapid growth. Until recently, the standard treatment has been enucleation. Alternative management includes local eye wall resection,[8] laser photocoagulation,[9–11] cryotherapy,[12] external beam irradiation (EBI) with x-rays,[13] proton beam,[14] or helium ions,[15] and the implantation of radioactive plaques using radon-222,[9,16–18] cobalt-60,[2,19–22] gold-198,[23] iodine-125,[24–30] Ru-106/Rh-106,[31,32] iridium-192,[33] and recently, palladium-103.[34]

Of these alternatives, brachytherapy is the most commonly used approach. Moore and Scott[35] have reported implantation of radon seeds as early as 1929. Until this decade, the most commonly used isotope was cobalt-60, popularized by Stallard.[2] Although there was good control of tumor, long-term visual acuity was poor due to the high energy radiation of the cobalt.[20–22] Iodine-125 eye plaques were introduced in the 1980s because the lower energy emission of I-125 offered two advantages: first, the seeds could be easily shielded by a thin layer of gold, thereby reducing the radiation hazard to caregivers and visitors to a minimum; and second, because of the lower penetration of I-125 rays, the dose received by

From Nag S (ed): *Principles and Practice of Brachytherapy*. © Futura Publishing Co., Inc., Armonk, NY, 1997.

normal structures of the eye (lens, opposite retina, etc.) was much lower than that delivered with cobalt-60.[26] Hence, I-125 is currently the radioisotope most commonly used in ocular brachytherapy.

Among the available treatment alternatives, the ideal treatment for choroidal melanoma should destroy the tumor while maintaining useful vision, have few adverse effects, and provide the patient with the best prognosis for life.[20] There is intense debate as to the best management. Those individuals who support the use of enucleation point out that after irradiation, regardless of technique, there will be a number of patients who will harbor not only viable tumor capable of local growth but also metastatic disease.[36,37] Those who advocate the use of radioactive episcleral plaque therapy (REPT) point out the reported increase in death due to metastatic disease in the immediate postoperative time frame (8% at 2 years) and the fact that in large single institutional data there is preservation of vision with a low overall metastatic rate.[38,39] In an effort to answer these questions, a national study that allows for a randomization between REPT and enucleation in patients with medium sized lesions, the Collaborative Ocular Melanoma Study (COMS), has been designed and implemented.[40,41]

Indications for I-125 Plaque Therapy

1. There should be potential for good vision after therapy, as determined by tumor size and location: a) the tumors should be of medium size, i.e., <16 mm at greatest diameter and <10 mm in height; and b) the tumors should be at least 1–2 mm from the optic nerve or macula.
2. Patients who do not meet the above criteria can be treated with an eye plaque if: a) the patients have no useful vision in the contralateral eye; or b) the patent refuses enucleation.

Construction of the I-125 Eye Plaque

The dimensions and location of the tumor is determined from direct fundoscopy, A and B scan ultrasound by the opthalmologist. Various types of plaques can be used. At the Ohio State University, custom made "Nag" eye plaques are made from 0.6-mm thick, 18k gold, in various sizes and shapes (Dental Ceramics, Inc., Reynoldsburg, OH, USA) to conform to the size and shape of the tumor (Figure 1). The radius of curvature of the plaques is 12 mm to conform to the curvature of the eyeball. The plaques have apertures on the lateral wings to allow sutures to be placed to hold the plaque onto the sclera. Elongated anterior wings (rabbit ears) have been designed to reach posteriorly located tumors (close to the macula). The inner surface of the plaques is raised 2 mm from the surface of the sclera to reduce the radiation dose to the

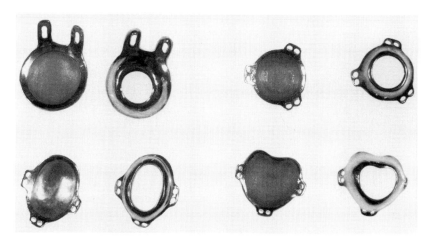

Figure 1. Various shapes and sizes of custom made "Nag" eye plaques being used at the Ohio State University.

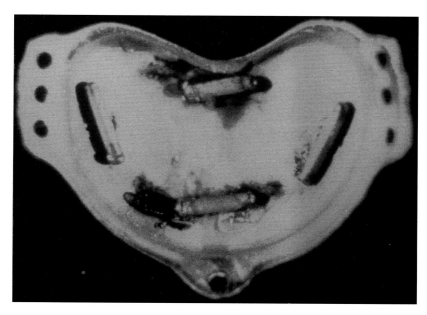

Figure 2. Four I-125 seeds attached to the concave surface of a kidney shaped eye plaque.

sclera. The required number of radioactive I-125 seeds (Medi-Physics, Inc., Arlington Heights, IL, USA) of 370–740 mBq (10–20 mCi) are attached to the inner surface of the plaque using commercially available super glue (Figure 2). The seeds can be removed, if necessary, by dissolving the glue with acetone. We prescribe 100 Gy minimum peripheral dose to the apex of the tumor in 3–5 days. Generally, the sclera receives 200–500 Gy during that time.

Placement of the Eye Plaque

The patient is examined under general or local anesthesia by the ophthalmologist and the radiotherapist using direct and indirect ophthalmoscopy. A peritomy is performed, and the area of the sclera overlying the tumor is exposed. If necessary, the overlying rectus muscle can be divided. The margins of the tumor are marked on the overlying sclera. A dummy (nonradioactive) plaque identical in shape and size to the radioactive plaque to be used is then placed on the sclera over the tumor to confirm accurate localization. Scleral sutures are positioned to ensure that the tumor and a 1- to 2-mm margin will be ade-

quately covered by the plaque (Figure 3). The dummy plaque is then removed and replaced with the presterilized radioactive plaque. If the rectus muscle has been divided, it is temporarily resutured over the plaque. A lead rubber patch is placed over the orbit (Figure 4). When the desired radiation dose has been delivered, the plaque is removed under local or general anesthesia. The rectus muscle is returned to its insertion, and the conjunctival flap is closed.

Collaborative Ocular Melanoma Study

COMS has two ongoing randomized controlled trials:

1. medium sized choroidal melanomas between 2.5–10.0 mm in height and <16 mm in basal diameter are randomized to receive I-125 plaque therapy versus enucleation;
2. large choroidal melanomas >10 mm in height or >16 mm in basal diameter are randomized to receive standard enucleation versus preoperative external beam radiation of 20 Gy followed by enucleation.

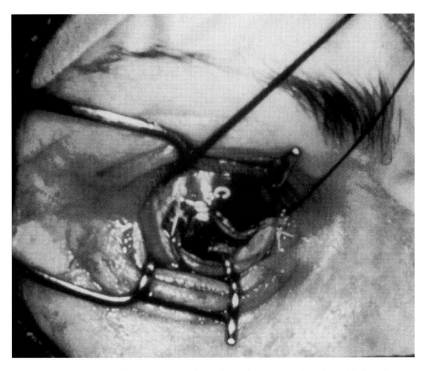

Figure 3. The radioactive eye plaque sutured on the sclera over the choroidal melanoma.

Since large melanomas are not treated by brachytherapy, this chapter will discuss only the medium sized melanomas that are treated by brachytherapy.

The idea of initiating a prospective randomized trial of enucleation versus radiation plaque for ocular melanomas was suggested at the meeting COMS held in Sun Valley, Idaho, in 1980. The COMS was funded in September 1985, and included 19 clinical centers. There are currently 42 centers in COMS. About 2400 patients must be enrolled for this study to be able to detect a 25% relative difference in cumulative 5-year modality with reasonable confidence.

The COMS plaques (seed carrier inserts), manufactured by Trachsell Dental Studio, Inc. (Rochester, MN, USA) consist of a gold outer plaque and a flexible inner plastic plaque that are available in five standard sizes of various diameters from 12–20 mm (Figure 5). The outer plaques are made of gold and have a lip. The plaques are designed so that the surface of the seeds and the sterile surface of the outer plaque are separated by 1 mm of plastic.

The inner plaques have grooves to accommodate the I-125 seeds. The I-125 seeds are placed in the seed carrier insert and attached to the gold plaque using small amounts of silicone adhesive. The plaque size is chosen to include the entire tumor base and a 2- to 3-mm margin on all sides. A 100 Gy dose is delivered at the apex or at 5 mm (whichever is greater) at a rate of 0.5–1.25 Gy/hr. Hence, the entire treatment is generally completed in $3\frac{1}{2}$–8 days.

The I-125 seeds, arranged in concentric rings throughout the inner plaque and coming to within 1 mm of the edge of the plaque, are loaded so that the 100 Gy isodose surface passes through the prescription point, encompasses the tumor, and extends to or beyond the edge of the plaque (Figure 6). The plaques are sterilized by gas sterilization.

Institutional Experience

The treatment of uveal melanoma with REPT is no longer limited to a few institutions. In fact its use has been reported worldwide,

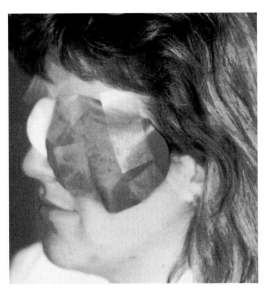

Figure 4. A lead rubber patch placed over the eye to reduce radiation exposure to visitors and caregivers.

node status, and distant metastasis, has been the most replicable system and should be used in further communications regarding tumor description (Table 1).

The most extensive experience with REPT has been reported by the Wills Eye Institute.[21] This experience included 178 patients treated with Co-60 and an additional 232 who had enucleation in a nonrandomized comparison in which there was minimum 5-year follow-up. Despite the fact that the Co-60 patients had a statistically increased number of patients with known poor prognostic factors such as large basal diameter, increased tumor height, and anterior location, no statistical difference in survival was noted between the two groups. Fifty percent of these patients retained useful vision at 5-year follow-up, although a steady decline in the vision was noted.

with various criteria for treatment and the dose and/or isotope used. However, despite the fact that REPT is being used in numerous centers, there has been little agreement as to the actual description of tumors. The American Joint Committee on Cancer criteria, which is based on both tumor diameter and height,

Two recent large institutional series also document the efficacy of REPT. Fontanesi et al.[27] reported on 144 patients treated with I-125 and documented 130/144 with ocular survival (median follow-up of 49 months). The interesting aspect of this series was the standardization of apical dose to 75 Gy over 5 days, which represented a decrease of approximately 25% over most other reported series using I-125. The other recent retrospective study from the University of California at San

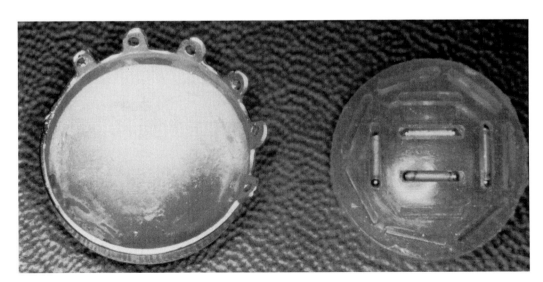

Figure 5. COMS outer gold plaque and the inner plastic insert containing I-125 seeds.

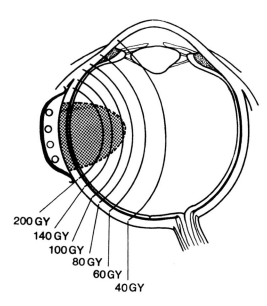

200 GY
140 GY
100 GY
80 GY
60 GY
40 GY

Figure 6. Cross-section of the globe showing the 100 Gy isodose passing through the apex of the tumor.

Francisco demonstrated local tumor control of 91.7%, with a mean follow-up of 35+ months.[28] Actuarial local control at 5 years was 82%, and reported visual acuity was 20/200 or better in 58%.

It thus is evident from these and other single institution studies that the use of REPT for the treatment of small and medium size lesions appears to provide good local control rates and metastatic rates similar to other irradiation series or surgical series.[22,29,42] However, there is little information that deals with treatment of large tumors with REPT. There has been concern that the physical parameters of delivering dose with a single plane implant for a volume of tumor would lead to unacceptably high rates of local failure and complications. This reasoning was based in part on the physical aspects of the inverse square law and its relationship to radiation. Recently there has been renewed interest in the treatment of these large lesions by several groups. Fontanesi et al. reported on 64 patients who were treated with REPT for lesions >1000 mm³ and/or >10 mm in height. Fifty-six of 64 patients maintained ocular control 12–96 months post-REPT (median = 50), and 30 of the 56 patients had useful binocular vision at last follow-up. In addition, a metastatic

rate of 7% was noted.[43] The findings of this series prompted the authors to reexamine the mechanism of action of REPT on ocular melanomas. In their research, which was largely based on review of enucleated globes and posttreatment fluorescein angiography, it was noted that the blood supply to the tumor (which is unique in that it can originate only through the base of the tumor) was dramatically altered. The authors then retrospectively reviewed a series of small and medium sized lesions and calculated that scleral doses of 200–400 Gy had been delivered. It was not surprising to find that some of the large lesions received as high as 1200 Gy to the sclera. Hence, it is postulated that the mechanism of action of REPT on ocular melanoma is at least partially due to reduction of blood supply to the tumor by the vascular sclerosing effect of irradiation. These findings led to the development of a pilot trial that now prescribes the dose to a 3-mm region above the plaque while recording the apical doses. Initially this trial was designed for large lesions, but has subsequently been modified to include small and medium lesions. The initial series of patients treated in this pilot study had "large lesions" and have shown very promising results, although longer follow-up is required.[44]

There can be no question that the use of REPT plays an important role in the management of ocular melanomas. However, there are still questions as to which patients will benefit most from the various therapeutic options.

Although most series to date have reported on the experience using Co-60 and iodine-125 REPT, several other isotopes are presently being evaluated. Lommatzsch[45] reported on an ongoing series of 309 patients treated between 1964 and 1984 with the beta emitting Ru-106/Rh-106 isotope. Of 188 patients having at least 5-year follow-up, 130 (69.1%) were regarded as having successful therapy, while 40 required enucleation for tumor regrowth. Dose to the tumor apex was "at least 100 Gy." Only 64 tumors (20.7%) exceeded basal diameter of 15 mm or height of 5 mm. Since the beta rays have limited penetration, the Ru-106/Rh-106 plaques are generally reserved for tumors of <5 mm in height.

Another more recent addition to the isotopes used to treat ocular melanomas is palladium-103 (Pd-103). Because it has a lower

Table 1.
AJCC Staging Criteria for Uveal Melanoma

		Primary Tumor (T)	Lymph Node (N)	Distant Metastasis (M)
Iris	Tx	Primary tumor cannot be assessed	NX Regional lymph nodes cannot be assessed	MX Presence of distant metastasis
	T0	No evidence of primary tumor		
	T1	Tumor limited to the iris	N0 No regional lymph node metastasis	M0 No distant metastasis
	T2	Tumor involves one quadrant or less, with invasion into the anterior chamber angle	N1 Regional lymph node metastasis	M1 Distant metastasis
	T3	Tumor involves more than one quadrant, with invasion into the anterior chamber angle		
	T4	Tumor with extraocular extension		
Ciliary body	Tx	Primary tumor cannot be assessed	NX Regional lymph nodes cannot be assessed	MX Presence of distant metastasis
	T0	No evidence of primary tumor		
	T1	Tumor limited to cilliary body	N0 No regional lymph node metastasis	M0 No distant metastasis
	T2	Tumor invades into anterior chamber and/or iris	N1 Regional lymph node metastasis	M1 Distant metastasis
	T3	Tumor invades choroid		
	T4	Tumor with extraocular extension		
Choroid	Tx	Primary tumor cannot be assessed	NX Regional lymph nodes cannot be assessed	MX Presence of distant metastasis
	T0	No evidence of primary tumor		
	T1	Tumor 10 mm or less in greatest dimension with an elevation 3 mm or less	N0 No regional lymph node metastasis	M0 No distant metastasis
	T1a	Tumor 7 mm or less in greatest dimension with an elevation 2 mm or less	N1 Regional lymph node metastasis	M1 Distant metastasis
	T1b	Tumor more than 7 mm but not more than 20 mm in greatest dimension with an elevation of more than 3 mm but not more than 5 mm		
	T2	Tumor more than 10 mm but not more than 15 mm in greatest dimension with an elevation of more than 3 mm but not more than 5 mm		
	T3	Tumor more than 15 mm in greatest dimension or with an elevation more than 5 mm		
	T4	Tumor with extraocular extension		

Staging Grouping							
Iris and Ciliary Body				Choroid			
I	T1	N0	M0	IA	T1a	N0	M0
II	T2	N0	M0	IB	T1b	N0	M0
III	T3	N0	M0	II	T2	N0	M0
IVA	T4	N0	M0	III	T3	N0	M0
IVB	Any T	N1	M0	IVA	T4	N0	M0
	Any T	Any N	M1	IVB	Any T	N1	M0
					Any T	Any N	M1

AJCC = American Joint Commission on Cancer.

energy emission (21 keV) than I-125, Pd-103 gives a lower dose to the other normal structures of the eye. However, it is more expensive and its lower penetration may make it less suitable for treating very large tumors. A recent report by Finger et al.[34] reported encouraging early results in 23 patients who received 80–100 Gy at the apex or 40–50 Gy at the apex with adjunct microwave hyperthermia; one of the 23 had enucleation for tumor progression. The major drawback to this report was the short follow-up (median = 13.5 months).

For selected patients with ocular melanoma, REPT appears to be a viable alternative therapy to enucleations. Most institutions report >80% local control and 5-year survival.

The completion of the COMS study will provide further information regarding local control and survival. The present recommendation for apical dose is between 75–100 Gy of I-125 brachytherapy to the tumor apex although there is ongoing clinical trials to determine if calculation of dose to the apex or base of the tumor is more appropriate.

Retinoblastoma

Retinoblastoma (RB) is a malignant process that arises from the neural retina.[46] Primarily a disease of children, it has no racial or sexual predilection, and it will account for 300–350 cases annually in the United States.[47] Approximately 20%–30% of these cases will have germ line mutations, which are inheritable, with the remaining children having sporadic RB development. However, it has been estimated that up to 10% of the "sporadic" cases will also have a germ line mutation. While overall, the majority of the RB cases will have been diagnosed by the age of 6, a majority of those who present with the hereditary form of RB will be diagnosed by age 2.[48] These are the children who are at highest risk for development of second malignant neoplasms, with incidence of 90% at 30 years postdiagnosis reported.[43] It is with this knowledge that we review the use of brachytherapy in the treatment of RB.

Recurrent Retinoblastoma

The treatment of primary RB continues to undergo reevaluation as to the optimal radiation dose required for tumor sterilization. In addition, the advantages of various lens-sparing techniques when compared to enfosse treatment are being explored, and new therapies such as cryotherapy, photocoagulation, laser therapy, or chemotherapy in an effort to delay or to eliminate the use of irradiation are being evaluated. These and other questions are the reasons why multimodality therapy is vitally important in treatment decisions regarding RB. However, despite all these questions that are being evaluated, enucleation and EBI remain the most common forms of therapy. Those children who receive irradiation can expect about a 30%–50% incidence of failure (Table 2).[49–56] A majority of these failures can, however, be retreated with the most common forms of retreatment including enucleation, cryotherapy, and REPT.

Stallard's[1] series, the largest reporting the use of REPT in the treatment of recurrent RB, reported excellent results with the use of Co-60 REPT. The descriptions of the technique of placement and the criteria for treatment have been accepted as the standard by which other REPT is judged. These criteria include an eye with one or two lesions each <10 mm in diameter with <$\frac{1}{4}$ of the retina involved. The availability of Co-60, with its well known energy profile and radioactive properties, made its use logical (Table 3). Stallard's results were soon replicated by other groups (Table 4). However, concerns about radiation safety and the desire to limit dose to the affected sites

promoted investigation of new radioactive isotopes that have been evaluated in various institutional clinical trials. These sources include iodine-125, ruthenium-106, and iridium-192 (Table 3). To date, use of these newer sources has produced promising early results similar to those reported with Co-60 plaques. However, there has been no randomized trial to evaluate possible differences. There have, however, been attempts to use the various isotopes for specific lesion criteria. Shields et al.[57] in reporting on the Wills Eye Institute experience, described the use of various isotopes based on tumor dimensions. In addition, early results with Ru-106 (similar to those reported by Lommatzch for this beta emitter) produced a favorable early impression. However, it is best used for tumors of shallow height (≤5 mm).[58] The Wills Eye Institute has also pioneered the use of "rotating" plaques with large lesions and/or vitreous seeds.[59] This technique is in direct opposition to the original use proposed by Stallard, yet early results are encouraging. It is interesting that most series, regardless of isotope, have reported salvage rates of 60%–80% with vision when doses of 35–45 Gy to the apex of the tumor are delivered.

The technical aspects of placement of the actual plaque have many variations. However, in general, tumors are first evaluated by ultrasound to give information relating to geometry, basal diameter, and height. After evaluation and dose planning, an isotope and seed activity based on the dosimetry plan are selected. At the time of placement, the tumor is identified; and, after the localization process (usually with diathermy) to mark basal diameter, a dummy plaque made of clear material and identical to the planned plaque is used to determine that the plaque will be large enough to cover the tumor base. Then the radioactive plaque is sutured into place and remains in place for 3–5 days depending on selected dose rates. Dose rates at the sclera and apex and total apical doses reported in published series are found in Table 4.

Primary Irradiation for Retinoblastoma

The use of brachytherapy in the initial radiotherapeutic management of RB was initially described by Moore et al.[4] In that report, it was shown that RB could effectively be ster-

Table 2.
Local Control of Retinoblastoma with Irradiation Alone

Author (Ref No.)	Date	Age	RE Group	No. Eyes Irradiated	Total Dose (Gy)	Dose Daily (cGy)	Technique	Local Control	Follow-Up
Schipper[49]	1985	2 week–91 months (median = 6.5 months)	I–III IV–V	35 19	45	300	Lens Sparing	16/35 (45.7%) 6.19 (31.5%)	2–12 years (median = 6 years)
Cassady[51]	1969	N/A	I–III IV–V	120 103	35–60 Gy 32.5–45	333–400[1]	Lens Sparing	RE-I-III <40 Gy 22/30 (73.3%) >40 Gy 66/90 (73.3%) <40 Gy 8/43 (18.6%) RE-IV-V >40 Gy 13/60 (21.6%)	5–14 years
McCormick[52]		1–60 months (median = 10.4)	I–III IV–V	66 37	38.5–50 42–44	200–250	Anterior Lens Sparing (n = 67) Modified Lateral Beam (n = 53)	RE-I-III ALS 35[2]% MLB 75% (P = .0009) RE-IV-V ALS 38% MLB 50% (P = .7)	Mean = 36 months
Bedford[53]	1971	1 month–5 years (avg 1 year)	N/A	58	40	N/A	Anterior	30/58	66% ≥2 years 81% > year
Gagnon[54]	1980	Newborn–6½ years	I–III IV–V	18 10	45–50	200	Ipsilateral Horizontal	20/28	2–36 years
Foote[55]	1989	0.5–39.2 months (median = 4.6)	I–III IV–V	15 10	39–51	180–300	Anterior (n = 11) Lens Sparing (n = 14)	7/11 4/14 (median = 31.5)	6.5–112.5 months
Abramson[56]	1983	0–6 months (median = 3.6)	I–III V	132	180–300	N/A	N/A	85/132	
SJ Series[50]	1993	13–70 months (median = 16)	I–V	19	25–45	170–225 (n = 13) 225 (n = 8)	Anterior (n = 11) Lens Sparing	12/19	13–301 months (median = 130 months)

[1] Given three times per week.
[2] Estimate from relapse free data.

299

Table 3.
Commonly Used Radionuclides for Ocular Brachytherapy

Symbol	Half-Life	Average Gamma Ray (MeV)	HVL in Lead (cm)
Co-60	5–6 Years	1.25	1.2
I-125	60–25 Days	0.028	0.002
Ir-192	74.2 Days	0.38	0.3
Ru/Rh-106	367 Days	3.5 (Beta)	Range Max E $=$ 1800 mg/cm^2
Pd-103	17 Days	0.021	0.004

ilized with modest doses of irradiation delivered with a Co-60 plaque. Criteria for use was based on size (1 or 2 sites; <10-mm diameter) and location. It has since been noted that the precision of the dose that can be obtained with the use of REPT also may have several other benefits, including limiting the amount of irradiation delivered to normal tissues in patients who may already have a genetic predisposition to second malignant tumors, especially in treated areas. This dose limitation may also result in improved visual acuity when compared to that in those who receive EBI, and it allows the further use of irradiation via external beam techniques or replaque. Although REPT was not used as frequently in the earlier reports, there are an increasing number of institutions that are reporting its use in the primary management of RB (Table 5).[57,60,61]

The primary indications for the use of REPT in the primary radiotherapeutic management of RB include solitary, unilateral, nonfamilial cases not amenable to nonirradiated techniques (i.e., cryotherapy), and small tumors in the remaining eye after enucleation of the worst vision eye in bilateral RB. The success that has been noted in some groups has led to the use of the Wills Eye Institute "rotating plaques." In this technique, the plaques (usually two with larger tumors) are rotated through the four quadrants of the eye in an attempt to treat large tumors and/or tumors with vitreous seeding.[59] However, despite early high expectations, the Wills Eye Institute has justifiably voiced concern in publications that this experimental technique might result in a decrease in local control rate when compared to the use of EBI in these advanced cases.

Thus, from the various institutional experience, we can develop a consensus as to the role of REPT in the treatment of RB. For primary irradiation of RB, REPT is best used for small peripheral lesions in those patients with sporadic unilateral disease or in the treatment of the remaining eye after enucleation of bilateral RB worst vision eye. Those patients who present with small isolated foci of recurrent RB after previous EBI and in whom other forms of salvage therapy are not an option (i.e., cryotherapy, photocoagulation) and in whom there is a reasonable expectation for vision are also candidates for REPT. The review of literature suggests that 40 Gy (prescribed to the apex of the lesion as identified

Table 4.
REPT for Recurrent Retinoblastoma

Author (Ref)	Year	No. Eyes	Source	Apical Dose (Total)	Scleral Dose (Total)	Previous Dose	Local Control	Follow-Up (Months)
Kock[60]	1986	5	Co-60	33–64 Gy	49–60 Gy	4/5	3–20	
Shields[57]	1989	36	Co-60 I-125 Ir-192 Ru-106	35–40 Gy	30–160 Gy	N/A	22/36	13–144
Fass[74]	1991	75	Co-60	30–50 Gy	30–500 Gy	30–60 Gy	45/75	2–252
Fontanesi[75]	1992	9	I-125	40 Gy	30–120 Gy	21–40 Gy	8/9	12–48

REPT = radioactive episceral plaque therapy.

Table 5.
REPT for Primary Retinoblastoma Therapy

Author (Ref)	Year	No. Eyes	Source	Apical Dose (Total)	Scleral Dose (Total)	Local Control	Follow-Up (Months)
Shields[57]	1989	5	Co-60 I-125 Ir-192 Ru-106	40 Gy	Up to 160 Gy	13/15	13–144
Kock[60]	1986	28	Co-60	N/A	33–64 @ 2 mm	15/28	2–21
Stallard[61]	1966	69	Co-60	35 Gy	N/A	63/69	N/A

REPT = radioactive episceral plaque therapy.

on ultrasound) given over 3–4 days has resulted in up to 80% long-term local control.

Pterygia

The use of postoperative beta irradiation for pterygium has been shown to be effective in the reduction of recurrence.[62–64] Despite this widely held knowledge, there is no agreement as to the total dose, fraction size, or time to initiation of therapy.[65,66] In addition, a wide range of complications has been described. This section will endeavor to clarify and review the literature and develop recommendations for therapy.

Pterygia is a triangular shaped proliferative fibrovascular tissue that originates from the canthus and grows toward the limbus and cornea; most commonly, it is nasally located. Treatment, which is recommended for visual loss, is more often sought for cosmetic reasons. The most common form of therapy is total resection; however, in approximately one third of patients, resection cannot be completed.

Beta irradiation has had a long-standing role in the postoperative treatment of pterygium, and various series report large numbers of patients (Table 6).[67,68] The indications for therapy include incomplete resection and regrowth following resection. Although various sources have been described, strontium-90 is clearly the preferred source. A beta emitter with maximum energy of 0.554 MeV and an average of 0.21 MeV, strontium-90 decays to yttrium-90, which emits a maximum energy of 2.27 MeV and average energy of 0.89 MeV.

The results that have been published are remarkable in their similarity. Most series report on treatment with application in the immediate postoperative setting, although there has been suggestion to the contrary. There has also been a clinical trial evaluating "sandwich" therapy pre- and postoperatively. The normal fractionation scheme has used 600–800 cGy per fraction to a total dose of

Table 6.
Brachytherapy for Pterygium

Author (Ref)	Year	No. Eyes	Pre-Tx Surgery	Source	Dose	Follow-Up
Duggan[71]	1966	25	Y	SR-90	1000–12000 cGy	24/25 Good results
		3	N	SR-90	1000–10104 cGy	3/3 Good results
Haik[72]	1966	314	Y	SR-90	900 cGy	2/314 Recurrence
		131	Y	Ra-226	900 cGy	2/131 Recurrence
Bahrassa[67]	1983	83	Y	SR-90	18–22 Gy	5% Recurrence 5% Cataract
Pinkerton[68]	1979	975	Y	SR-90	<30 Gy	6% Recurrence 20 year follow-up

1800–2100 cGy surface dose. It is important to take care to include all cut surfaces in the operative bed, especially in the bulbar conjunctiva. Several authors have stressed the importance of entirety of coverage and have recommended multiple placements per fraction, realizing potential overlap regions.[69,70] Local control rates in high risk patients or those with a history of recurrence after surgery have ranged between 61%–98%.[71–73]

Conclusions

Although relatively infrequent in number, primary tumors of the eye present special challenges to the radiation oncologist. It is vital that a multimodality team evaluate all patients in an effort to determine the ideal patient for consideration of brachytherapy application. Because of the eye's unique role as a sensory organ and its small size, especially careful planning for the use of REPT is necessary, since complications of therapy can be as devastating as initial management with enucleation. Although other forms of irradiation (protons, stereotactically delivered irradiation, and heavy particles) are being investigated, their dependence on technology and eye fixation can be problematic when compared to REPT. The use of REPT is also justified in salvage attempts for selective recurrent RB. In addition, beta emitters such as strontium-90 are effective in the treatment of a benign condition, pterygium. The future of the therapy of ocular tumors is exciting, with the development of an increasing array of radioisotopes to be investigated and possible dose reduction to reduce morbidity in selected patients.

References

1. Stallard HB. The treatment of retinoblastoma. Second Cong Eur Soc Ophthal, Vienna 1964. Ophthalmodlogica 1966;151:214–230.
2. Stallard HB. Radiotherapy for malignant melanoma of the choroid. Br J Ophthal 1966;50:147.
3. Haik GM, Ellis GS, Nowell JF. The management of pterygia with special reference to surgery combined with beta irradiation. Tran Am Acad Ophthalmol Otolaryngol 1962;66:776–784.
4. Moore RT, Stallard MD, Milner JG. Retinal glio-mata treated by radon seeds. Br J Ophthalmol 1931;15:673.
5. Petrovich A, Liggett P, Luxton G, et al. Radioactive plaque therapy in the management of primary malignant ocular melanoma: An overview. Endocurie/Hypertherm Oncol 1990;6:131–141.
6. Callander GR, Wilder HC, Ash JE. Five hundred melanomas of the choroid and ciliary body followed five years or longer. Am J Ophthalmol 1942;25:962–967.
7. McLean IW, Foster WD, Zimmerman LE, et al. Modifications of Callander's classification of uveal melanoma at the Armed Forces Institute of Pathology. Am J Ophthalmol 1983;96:507–252.
8. Peyman GA, Axelrod AJ, Graham RO. Full-thickness eye wall resection. An experimental approach for treatment of choroidal melanoma: Evaluation of cryotherapy, diathermy, and photocoagulation. Arch Ophthalmol 1974;91:219–222.
9. Boniuk M, Girard LJ. Malignant melanoma of the choroid. Treated with photocoagulation, transscleral diathermy, and implanted radon seeds. Am J Ophthalmol 1965;59:212–216.
10. Vogel MH. Treatment of malignant choroidal melanomas with photocoagulation. Evaluation of 10-year follow-up data. Am J Ophthalmol 1972;74:1–11.
11. Meyer-Schwickerath G. The preservation of vision by treatment of intraocular tumors with light coagulation. Arch Ophthalmol 1961;66:458–466.
12. Lincoff H, McLean J, Long R. The cryosurgical treatment of intraocular tumors. Am J Ophthalmol 1967;63:389–399.
13. Bornfield N, Alberti W, Foerster MH, et al. External beam therapy of choroidal melanoma preliminary report. Trans Ophthal Soc UK 1983;103:68–71.
14. Gragoudas ES, Goitein M, Koehler AM, et al. Proton irradiation of small choroidal malignant melanomas. Am J Ophthalmol 1977;83:665–673.
15. Char DH, Saunders W, Castro JR, et al. Helium ion therapy for choroidal melanoma. Ophthalmology 1983;90:1215–1225.
16. Davidorf FH, Makley TA, Lang JR. Radiotherapy of malignant melanoma of the choroid. Trans Am Acad Ophthalmol Otolaryngol 1976;81:849–861.
17. Fingerhut AG, Collins VP. Local treatment of retinal tumors with radon. Radiology 1963;81:1003–1007.
18. Moore RF. Choroidal sarcoma treated by the intraocular insertion of radon seeds. Br J Ophthalmol 1930;14:140–152.

19. Migdal C. Choroidal melanoma: The role of conservative therapy. Trans Ophthal Soc UK 1983;103:54–58.

20. Shields JA, Augsburger JJ, Brady LW, et al. Cobalt plaque therapy of posterior uveal melanomas. Ophthalmology 1982;89:1201–1207.

21. Markow AM, Brady LW, Shields JA, et al. Malignant melanoma of the eye: Treatment of posterior uveal lesion by Co-60 plaque radiotherapy versus enucleation. Radiology 1985;156:801–803.

22. Beitler J, McCormick B, Ellsworth R, et al. Ocular melanoma: Total dose and dose rate effects with Co-60 plaque therapy. Radiology 1990;176:275–278.

23. Chenery SGA, Japp B, Fitzpatrick PJ. Dosimetry of radioactive gold grains for the treatment of choroidal melanoma. Br J Radiol 1983;56:415–420.

24. Robertson DM, Earle J, Anderson JA. Preliminary observations regarding the use of iodine-125 in the management of choroidal melanomas. Trans Ophthal Soc UK 1983;103:155–160.

25. Sealy R, Buret E, Cleminshaw H, et al. Progress in the use of iodine therapy for tumors of the eye. Br J Radiol 1980;53:1052–1060.

26. Packer S, Rotman M, Salanitro P. Iodine-125 irradiation of choroidal melanoma. Clinical experience. Ophthalmology 1984;91:1700–1708.

27. Fontanesi J, Meyer D, Shizhao X, et al. Treatment of choroidal melanoma with I-125 plaque. Int J Radiat Oncol Biol Phys 1993;26:619–623.

28. Quivey JM, Char DH, Phillips TL, et al. High intensity 125-iodine (^{125}I) plaque treatment of uveal melanoma. Int J Radiat Oncol Biol Phys 1993;26:613–618.

29. Bosworth J, Packer S, Rotman M, et al. Choroidal melanoma: I-125 plaque therapy. Radiology 1988;169:249–251.

30. Fontanesi J, Meyer D, Shizhao Z, et al. High-activity iodine-125 episcleral plaque therapy for large choroidal melanoma. Endocurie Hyphertherm Oncol 1994;10:105–109.

31. Busse H, Muller R. Techniques and results of ^{106}Ru/^{106}Rh radiation of choroidal tumors. Trans Ophthal Soc UK 1983;103:72–77.

32. Foerster MH, Wessing A, Meyer-Schwickerath G. The treatment of ciliary body melanoma by beta radiation. Trans Ophthal Soc UK 1983;103:64–67.

33. Japp B, Payen D, Gallie BL, et al. Individualized iridium-192 wire moulds for treatment of large accessible malignant melanomas of the choloid. Int J Radiat Oncol Biol Phys 1982;8:113.

34. Finger PT, Buffa A, Mishra S, et al. Palladium-103 plaque radiotherapy for uveal melanoma. Ophthalmology 1994;101:256–263.

35. Moore F, Scott PS. Clinical and pathological report of bilateral glioma retinae. Proc P Soc Med (Ophthalmol Sect) 1929;22:39–50.

36. Donoso LA, Berd D, Augsburger JJ, et al. Metastatic uveal melanoma. Pretherapy serum liver enzyme and liver scan abnormalities. Arch Ophthalmol 1985;103:796–798.

37. Kleineidam M, Guthoff M, Bentzen S. Rates of local control, metastasis, and overall survival in patients with posterior uveal melanomas treated with ruthenium-106 plaques. Radiother Oncol 1993;28:148–156.

38. Zimmerman LE, McLean IW. An evaluation of enucleation in the management of uveal melanomas. Am J Ophthalmol 1979;87:741–760.39. Maumenee AE. An evaluation of enucleation in the management of uveal melanomas. Am J Ophthalmol 1979;87:846–847.

40. Straatsma BR, Fine SL, Earle JD, et al. The collaborative ocular study research group: Enucleation versus plaque irradiation for choroidal melanoma. Ophthalmology 1988;95:1000–1004.

41. Collaborative Ocular Study Research Group. Design and methods of a clinical trial for a rare condition: The collaborative ocular melanoma study. COMS Report No. 3, Controlled Clinical Trials 1993;14:362–391.

42. Lean E, Cohen D, Liggett P, et al. Episcleral radioactive plaque therapy: Initial clinical experience with 56 patients. Am J Clin Oncol (CCT) 1990;13(3):185–190.

43. Abramson DH, Ellsworth RM, Kitchin FD, et al. Second non-ocular tumors in retinoblastoma: Are they radiation induced? Ophthalmology 1984;91:1352–1355.

44. Fontanesi J, Pratt CB, Meyer D, et al. Radiation therapy for retinoblastoma patients less than one year of age. IXth Meeting of International Society for Genetic Eye Diseases, VIth International Symposium on Retinoblastoma. Siena, Italy, June 1–3, 1992. Ophthalmic Paediatr Genet.

45. Lommatzsch PK. Results after B-Irradiation (^{106}Ru/^{106}Rh) of choroidal melanoma. Am J Clin Oncol 1987;10:146–151.

46. Lemieux N, Leung T, Michaud J, et al. Neuronal and photorecptor differentiation of retinoblastoma in culture. Ophthalmic Pediatr 1990;11:109–120.

47. Devesa SS. The incidence of retinoblastoma. Am J Ophthalmol 1975;80:263–265.

48. Ellsworth RM. The practical management of retinoblastoma. Trans Am Ophthalmol Soc 1969;67:462–534.

49. Schipper J, Tan KEWP, Peperzeel HA: Treat-

ment of retinoblastoma by precision megavoltage radiation therapy. Radiother Oncol 1985; 3:117–132.

50. Fontanesi J, Pratt CB, Kun LE, et al. Treatment outcome and dose response relationship in infants younger than one year treated for retinoblastoma with primary irradiation. Med Pediatr Oncol 1996;26:297–304.

51. Cassady JR, Sagerman RH, Tretter P, et al. Radiation therapy in retinoblastoma. Radiology 1969;93:405–409.

52. McCormick B, Ellsworth R, Abramson D, et al. Results of external beam radiation for children with retinoblastoma: A comparison of two techniques. J Pediatr Ophthalmol Strab 1989; 26:239–243.

53. Bedford MA, Bedotto C, Macfaul PA. Retinoblastoma: A study of 139 cases. Br J Ophthalmol 1971;55:17–27.

54. Gagnon JD, Ware CM, Moss WT, et al. Radiation management of bilateral retinoblastoma: The need to preserve vision. Int J Radiat Oncol Biol Phys 1980;6:669–673.

55. Foote RL, Garretson BR, Schomber PJ, et al. External beam irradiation for retinoblastoma: Patterns of failure and dose-response analysis. Int J Radiat Oncol Biol Phys 1989;16:823–830.

56. Abramson PH, Ellsworth R, Rosenblatt M. Retreatment of retinoblastoma with external beam irradiation. Arch Ophthalmol 1982;100: 1257–1260.

57. Shields J, Giblin M, Shields C, et al. Episcleral plaque radiotherapy for retinoblastoma. Ophthalmology 1989;96:530–537.

58. Lommatzsch P. Die anwendung von betastrahlen mit ^{106}Ru/^{106}Rh: Applikatoren bei der behandlung des retinoblastoms. Klin Montsbl Augenheilkd 1970;156:662–669.

59. Brady L, Markoe A, Amendola B, et al. The treatment of primary intraocular malignancy. Int J Radiat Oncol Biol Phys 1988;15: 1355–1361.

60. Kock E, Rosengren B, Tengroth B, et al. Retinoblastoma treated with a ^{60}Co applicator. Radiother Oncol 1986;7:19–26.

61. Stannard C, Sealy R, Shackelton D, et al. The use of iodine-125 plaques in the treatment of retinoblastoma. Ophthal Pediat Gene 1987; 8(2):89–93.

62. Dusenbery KE, Alul I, Holland E, et al. β irradiation of recurrent pterygia: Results and complications. Int J Radiat Oncol Biol Phys 1992; 24:315–320.

63. Ozarda AT. Evaluation of post excisional strontium-90 beta ray therapy for pterygium. South Med J 1977;70:1304.

64. Van den Brenk HAS. Results of prophylactic postoperative irradiation in 1,300 cases of pterygium. Am J Roentgenol Rad Ther Nucl Med 1968;103:723–733.

65. Bernstein M, Unger SM. Experiences with surgery and strontium-90 in the treatment of pterygium. Am J Ophthalmol 1960;49:1024–1029.

66. Lentino W, Zaret MM, Rossignol B, et al. Treatment of pterygium by surgery followed by beta radiation. Am J Roentgenol Rad Ther Nucl Med 1959;81:93–98.

67. Bahrassa F, Datta R. Postoperative beta radiation treatment of pterygium. Int J Radiat Oncol Biol Phys 1983;9:679–684.

68. Pinkerton OD. Surgical and strontium treatment of pterygium: Recurrence and lens changes. Age statistics. Ophthalmic Surg 1979; 10:45–47.

69. Rahman SM, Chung CK, Constable WC. Postoperative beta irradiation in the treatment of pterygium. South Med J 1979;72:823–826.

70. Cooper JS. Postoperative irradiation of pterygia: Ten more years of experience. Radiology 1978;128:753–756.

71. Duggan HE. Results using the strontium-90 beta-ray applicator on eye lesions. J Can Assoc Radiol 1966;17:132–137.

72. Haik GM. The management of pterygia. Am J Ophthalmol 1966;61:1128–1134.

73. Cooper JS, Lerch IA. Post-operative irradiation of pterygium: An unexpected effect of the time/dose relationship. Radiology 1980;135: 743–745.

74. Fass D, McCormick B, Abramson D, et al. Cobalt-60 plaques in recurrent retinoblastoma. Int J Radiat Oncol Biol Phys 1991;21:625–267.

75. Fontanesi J, Sutphen E, Pratt CB, et al. Treatment of recurrent retinoblastoma. IXth Meeting of International Society for Genetic Eye Disease/VI International Symposium on Retinoblastoma. Siena, Italy, 1992, p. 17.

Chapter 15

Esophageal Brachytherapy

Laurie E. Gaspar, M.D., Subir Nag, M.D.

Introduction

Despite the continued availability of brachytherapy, external beam radiation therapy (EBRT) or surgery have formed the backbone of therapy of esophageal cancer for years. Unfortunately, the 5-year survival or cure rates have been notoriously poor following either radiation or surgery as a single modality.[1–4] In a Radiation Therapy Oncology Group (RTOG) study, radiation alone to 64 Gy was associated with a 62% incidence of locoregional recurrence; there were no 3-year survivors.[7] The high failure rate observed clinically following EBRT is supported by autopsy studies demonstrating persistent tumor in the esophagus at the time of death in 78% of patients.[6] Mantravadi[6] found that local and regional tumor caused the death of 111/148 (74%) patients, whereas distant metastases led to death in only 27/148 (18%). Fifteen percent of patients developed fistulae between the esophagus and trachea or bronchus due to direct extension of the primary tumor.

The low survival associated with radiation or surgery alone have inspired studies of combined modality therapy. A phase III prospective, randomized study by the RTOG evaluated the efficacy of four courses of combined 5-fluorouracil (5-FU) (1000 mg per square meter of body-surface area daily for 4 days) and cisplatin (75 mg per square meter on the first day) concurrent with 50 Gy EBRT, as compared with 64 Gy of radiation therapy alone.[5] The median survival following radiation alone was 8.9 months, as compared with 12.5 months following combined modality (P<0.001). At 3 years there were no survivors with radiation alone while the estimated 3-year survival is 31% with chemoradiation.[7] Severe and life-threatening acute side effects occurred in 44% and 20%, respectively, of the patients who received combined modality therapy, as compared with 25% and 3% of those treated with radiation alone. The increased side effects in the chemoradiation group were attributable to hematological side effects as well as mucositis of the oral cavity, pharynx, and esophagus. The combined modality group experienced a 3% incidence of severe or life-threatening pneumonitis and a 2% incidence of severe nervous system complications. Neither of these complications occurred in the radiation alone group. Despite the increased toxicity observed in the chemoradiation group, persistent or recurrent disease at the primary site was a major problem, occurring by 12 months in 62% and 44% of the radiation only and chemoradiation group, respectively. Compared to the radiation alone arm, both local and distant recurrences were reduced in the chemoradiation arm. Only 7% of patients in the chemoradiation arm developed distant metastases without simultaneous local recurrence.

A nonrandomized study from Fox Chase Cancer Center, Philadelphia, PA, utilizing

From Nag S (ed): *Principles and Practice of Brachytherapy*. © Futura Publishing Co., Inc., Armonk, NY, 1997.

chemoradiation (5-FU and mitomycin-C concurrent with 60 Gy EBRT) resulted in local control and 3-year survival rates comparable to the RTOG randomized trial.[8] Late toxicity was described as "moderate" since esophageal strictures requiring one or two dilatations occurred in only 10 of 90 treated patients (11%). No patients required more than two dilatations. One patient (1%) developed transient radiation pneumonitis, and one (1%) died secondary to pneumonitis and mediastinitis.

Although recent advances in chemoradiation have prompted renewed enthusiasm for the nonsurgical management of cancer of the esophagus, the long-term survival remains modest and is associated with acute and late side effects. The incidence of acute esophageal toxicity and pneumonitis in the above studies, while acceptable, suggests that the current accepted doses of chemotherapy and conventional EBRT are approaching the tolerance of the surrounding normal tissues. Despite the impressive 3-year survival rate of >30% obtained with chemoradiation, the locoregional recurrence/progression rates of approximately 40% are unacceptably high. Brachytherapy is one of the several radiotherapeutic techniques available for escalation of the dose to the primary tumor site.[9,10] Esophageal brachytherapy offers several potential advantages when compared to dose escalation studies utilizing EBRT. The most obvious advantage is in terms of dose distribution; irradiating the tumor to a high dose with relative sparing of the surrounding normal tissues. Secondary advantages may be rapid relief of dysphagia, shortening of treatment time, and patient convenience.

Esophageal brachytherapy has been described in early radiation oncology literature. Barcat and Guisez[11] in 1909 were among the first to observe the results of local application of radium in esophageal cancer. In 1925, Guisez[12] reported his experience using radium bougie application. In the latter part of the century Dickson[13] reviewed the use of radon seeds, radium bougie, and tantalum wire for brachytherapy treatment of esophageal cancer. Rider and Mendoza[14] reported a 37% 3-year survival with a median survival of 24 months for patients treated with radium bougie and external radiation therapy. Bottrill

Table 1.
Indications for Brachytherapy

1. Unifocal disease
2. Primary tumor <10 cm long
4. Thoracic location
5. No evidence of intra-abdominal disease
6. No evidence of distant metastasis
3. Adenocarcinoma or squamous cell Ca

et al.[15] proposed an iridium afterloading technique for irradiation of the esophagus using a special esophageal catheter having an inner and outer balloon. Clinical studies in Japan with high-dose-rate (HDR) afterloading cobalt sources following external beam irradiation supported the use of this modality in the potentially curative setting.[16]

Methods

Patient Selection

Radiation therapy, particularly with brachytherapy, is potentially curative in the select group of patients with unifocal, nonmetastatic adenocarcinoma or squamous cancers of the thoracic esophagus <10 cm in length (Table 1). Extraesophageal spread (without fistula), primary >10 cm in length, macroscopic regional lymphadenopathy or tumor extension to the cardia are not clear contraindications to brachytherapy, but are factors associated with a poorer outcome (Table 2).[17,18] Esophageal tumors are notorious for the presence of skip lesions, which can be located up to 8 cm away and may represent either synchronous tumors or lymphatic spread that has extended into the mucosa. Patients with skip lesions are poor candidates for brachytherapy given the intervening normal esophageal mucosa that

Table 2.
Poor Candidates for Brachytherapy: Relative Contraindications

1. Extra-esophageal spread (wihtout fistula)
2. Primary tumor >10 cm long
3. Macroscopic regional lymphadenopathy
4. Extension to cardia
5. Patients with skip lesions
6. Cervical location

Table 3.
Contraindications for Brachytherapy

1. Severe stenosis that cannot be bypassed
2. Tracheo-bronchial involvement
3. Tracheo-esophageal fistula
4. Deep mucosal ulceration

would be subjected to an unnecessarily high dose of radiation.

Contraindications to esophageal brachytherapy include stenosis that cannot be bypassed, fistula, or patient refusal (Table 3). Bronchoscopy is required for patients with tumors extending from 18–32 cm from the incisors in order to detect tracheal or bronchial wall invasion. Bronchoscopic evidence of airway involvement has been an accepted contraindication to brachytherapy because of the potential for development of brachytherapy-induced fistulae. Among the sparse reports of brachytherapy in the management of cervical esophagus cancers, Gaspar et al.[19] have reported development of tracheo-esophageal fistulae in two of two cervical esophageal cancer patients after treatment with 50 Gy external beam, 14 Gy brachytherapy in two fractions, 1 week apart and concurrent chemotherapy.

Although clinical experience with esophageal brachytherapy has dealt mostly with squamous cell cancers of the midthoracic region, there is no clear evidence that brachytherapy is less effective for adenocarcinoma pathology.[19–21] The observation of an increasing incidence of adenocarcinoma of the distal esophagus has been noted in several studies.[22–24] The location of adenocarcinomas in the distal esophagus involving the gastro-esophageal junction raises concerns that brachytherapy may inadequately cover the distal tumor extension, particularly if there is gastric involvement. The literature suggests that compared with squamous cancers, adenocarcinomas respond as well but have a higher incidence of distant metastases as the site of first relapse.[19,25]

The esophagus is drained by a rich supply of lymphatics with multiple interconnecting channels allowing for early lymphatic metastases. The esophagus is the only portion of the gastrointestinal tract that lacks a serosa,

thereby allowing early direct spread of the tumor. Because the esophagus is a distensible organ, dysphagia is infrequent until obstruction occurs secondary to circumferential involvement of the esophageal wall. Cancer of the esophagus is usually diagnosed late, after symptoms have developed due to extensive locoregional disease.

Clinical staging of esophageal cancer is very relevant to the radiation oncologist considering esophageal brachytherapy in order to appropriately identify patients for this procedure, as well as for accurate tumor localization and treatment prescription. Prior to 1987 the TNM clinical staging classification was based on tumor length, degree of obstruction, and circumferential involvement. These tumor features were usually assessed by esophagoscopy and barium swallow examination. The 1987 UICC/TNM staging classification is more surgically oriented; requiring the esophagectomy specimen in order to accurately determine depth of esophageal wall involvement.[26] The recent availability of CT, MRI, and endoscopic ultrasound have led to proposals for noninvasive staging systems.

Based on normal measurements of the esophageal wall and lumen, CT staging criteria according to the wall thickness have been proposed (Table 4).[27] The normal esophageal wall thickness in the upper thoracic esophagus averages approximately 3 mm by CT scan.[28] The mean diameter of the upper thoracic esophagus (apposed walls) averages 14 mm in the anteroposterior dimension (range 11–20 mm) and 18 mm in the transverse dimension (range 11–28 mm). Specific CT criteria predictive of a poor prognosis include evidence of tracheal, aortic, or pericardial

Table 4.
Computerized Tomography
Staging Criteria[27]

CT-T0	No thickening of wall, <5 mm
CT-T1, T2	Thickening of the wall >5 mm, <10 mm
CT-T3	Thickening of the wall >10 mm with mediastinal involvement
CT-T4	Thickening of the wall with mediastinal involvement and invasion into adjacent structures

invasion.[27,29] In the normal patient, the esophagus is usually in direct contact with the posterolateral wall of the trachea and left mainstem bronchus.

CT criteria for tracheal or bronchial invasion are described as displacement of the entire trachea by an esophageal mass or indentation of the posterior wall of the trachea by the esophageal tumor without an intervening fat plane. One cannot always rely on the absence of a fat plane as evidence of invasion into adjacent organs, for the normal esophagus lacks fat planes at some levels. Also, patients with cachexia can be expected to have less fat. Invasion of the pericardium or aorta is based on the focal absence of a fat plane between the esophageal mass and the adjacent organ, assuming fat planes are present above and below the tumor. The middle third of the esophagus lies in direct contact with the descending aorta, often without a visible intervening fat plane. Aortic invasion is rare, occurring in approximately 2%. Invasion of the aorta is predicted with 80% accuracy by CT if there is no intervening fat plane between the tumor and aorta and the region of contact between vessel and esophageal tumor is >90° of the aortic circumference.

Using the CT criteria summarized above, it is estimated that over 70% of patients have some degree of extraesophageal mediastinal involvement at initial presentation. Currently, the CT appears superior to MRI for the detection of mediastinal invasion.[28] With future technological advances, including development of respiratory gating techniques that can be used routinely, MRI may become more accurate in assessing the extent of mediastinal disease.

Interest has been increasing in the use of endoscopic ultrasound; a new technique in which high-frequency, high-resolution real-time ultrasound images are obtained from within the esophageal lumen by use of an ultrasound probe incorporated into the tip of a fiber optic endoscope.[30] With this technique the esophageal mucosa, submucosa, and muscularis propria layers can be identified and the depth of tumor invasion can be assessed. In experienced hands, the ultrasound is superior to CT in evaluating tumor involvement of the esophageal wall. However, problems have been identified. The large 13-mm

transducers used by some investigators have been found to be "noisy" due to the motor in the mechanical sector of the scanner. The blunt end of the transducer makes it difficult to pass through the esophageal lumen at times. Apart from the technical difficulty of passing transducers through tight esophageal strictures, there is a lower accuracy in staging tumors with tight stenoses.[31] With newer technology, increased availability, and experience endoscopic ultrasound will be more valuable in the future.

In summary, CT appears to be superior to barium swallow and MRI in defining the superior, inferior, and lateral margins of esophageal cancers. Endoscopic ultrasonography may be of benefit in the future as transducers become smaller and experience with this technique evolves. Radiological evidence of involvement of the trachea, bronchus, and/or aorta is a contraindication to radical radiation with brachytherapy, given the potentially hazardous outcome of fistulae formation. However, brachytherapy is otherwise suitable to treat minimal mediastinal invasion, since this presumably had been present, though unsuspected, in many patients treated with brachytherapy in the past and only a small percentage of these patients later developed fistulae.

Catheter Insertion

While techniques of endo-esophageal radiation vary, one technique that can be applied to HDR, medium-dose-rate (MDR), or low-dose-rate (LDR) will be described in detail. A well lubricated, 18Fr nasogastric tube is inserted transorally (or transnasally) into the esophagus, past the distal aspect of the esophageal cancer. A tube of this diameter must ordinarily be passed under fluoroscopic or direct visual control. We do not recommend blindly inserting large semirigid nasogastric tubes or commercially available brachytherapy applicators, i.e., >4 mm, due to the risk of esophageal perforation.[32] A hollow needle is used to pierce the lumen of the nasogastric tube close to the mouth (or nostril). A 14-gauge needle is used to insert LDR or 5Fr HDR catheters. A 12- or 13-gauge needle is required to insert 6Fr HDR catheters. The blind-ended nylon afterloading catheter is then passed through the needle into the

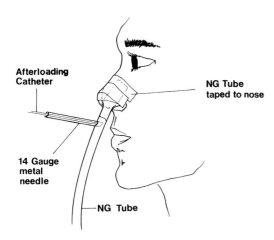

Figure 1. Placement of nasogastric tube and afterloading brachytherapy catheter.

lumen of the nasogastric tube (Figure 1). The afterloading catheter is then advanced under fluoroscopic control such that its tip is placed approximately 3 cm distal to the tumor site; assuming that the brachytherapy is to encompass the primary tumor length with a 3-cm margin proximally and distally, as in Figure 2. The metal needle is then removed. A metal

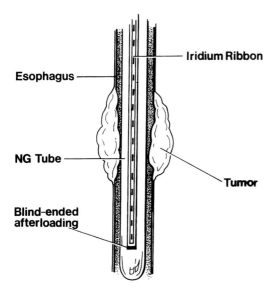

Figure 2. Nasogastric tube with afterloading catheter containing low-dose-rate iridium ribbon (or showing the HDR dwell positions). Active length encompassing the esophageal cancer with a 3-cm margin superiorly and inferiorly.

button is threaded over the nylon catheter until it reaches the nasogastric tube, then secured to the wall of the nasogastric tube with a suture in order to keep the afterloading catheter and the nasogastric tube in a secure position. The nasogastric tube is then taped to the mouth (or nostril) to prevent further movement. Dummy sources are then inserted into the afterloading catheter until it reaches the blind end. Anteroposterior and lateral orthogonal radiographs are obtained and computerized dosimetry performed. Optimized dose distributions can be achieved by varying the source activity and/or dwell time. Dummy sources are then removed and replaced by the HDR or MDR transfer cable or the LDR radioactive sources. When the treatment is completed, the catheters and nasogastric tubes are removed, and the patient may resume oral feeds as soon as the gag reflex has returned. Temporary absence of the gag reflex will only be a problem if topical anesthetics were used during placement of the nasogastric tube.

Esophageal brachytherapy can be accomplished with smaller diameter applicators, i.e., 3- to 4-mm diameter, if fluoroscopy or direct visualization with esophagoscopy is not available. A 12Fr or 14Fr nasogastric tube containing the afterloading catheter and dummy seeds can often be inserted blindly transorally or transnasally without much difficulty in a patient who is able to swallow at least liquids. The afterloading catheter and dummy seeds stiffen the nasogastric tube and must extend to the tip of the nasogastric tube. This may require cutting the proximal aspect of the nasogastric tube. The position of the nasogastric tube should be confirmed radiographically to ensure that it is not lodged in a bronchus. The nasogastric tube should be secured to the side of the mouth (or nostril) with tape or specially designed oral stents. Detection of subsequent movement of the nasogastric tube or afterloading catheter is easier if it is marked or if tape is placed at specific points (e.g., on the nasogastric tube at the mouth or nostril and on the afterloading catheter at the end of the nasogastric tube, etc.). Alternatively, the length of the protruding catheter can be measured and recorded.

Radionuclides

LDR brachytherapy (i.e., <200 cGy/hr) has generally been performed with iridium seeds placed in ribbons. The seeds are spaced no more than 1 cm apart (measured from center to center) and are frequently 0.3 or 0.5 cm apart. LDR brachytherapy is an in-patient procedure conducted over 24–48 hours. Adaptations of LDR esophageal brachytherapy catheters have been suggested to enable gastric suction during these prolonged sessions, reducing the possibility of aspiration of saliva or gastric contents.[33] MDR brachytherapy (i.e., 200–1200 cGy/hr) has been performed with cesium, cobalt, or radium.[17,34] Remote afterloading machines containing cesium have been adapted for MDR esophageal brachytherapy making cesium the currently preferred MDR source. HDR brachytherapy (i.e., >1200 cGy/hr) can be accomplished with cobalt or iridium. Concerns regarding radiation exposure to medical personnel have prompted many investigators to acquire remote afterloading machines containing small iridium sources. The treatment planning systems allow the dwell positions to be as close as 0.25 cm apart, but 0.5 cm between source steps provides a satisfactory dose distribution.

No single source or dose rate has proven itself superior to another in clinical studies (Table 5). The choice of source and dose rate varies with personal preference, availability of shielded rooms, and equipment. Iridium is currently the source used most frequently in esophageal brachytherapy; often in combination with remote afterloading machines.

Applicators

Applicators used in esophageal brachytherapy vary in size but often range from 4–10 mm in diameter (Table 5). Proponents of larger lumen endoluminal catheters point out the well known physical fact that small caliber catheters deliver a high dose to the esophageal mucosa, relative to the prescription depth (usually 1 cm). Attempts to match the caliber of the esophageal applicator to the diameter of the lumen have been described but such customized treatment will make interpretation of clinical results difficult.[35] The variation in dose to esophageal mucosa with increasing diameter of the applicator is demonstrated in Figure 3 and Table 6. Another possible drawback of a small esophageal applicator is that it may occupy an eccentric position within a patent esophagus.[36] Dosimetry in such a situation would be extremely difficult to predict. Bougie-type afterloading applicators of up to 16Fr in external diameter are now commercially available. These applicators may allow exact positioning of the applicator within the region of stenosis, allowing a homogeneous dose to the esophageal mucosa with a simultaneous dilatory effect.

Timing or Sequencing

While most reports have used esophageal brachytherapy as a boost following EBRT there are several reasons to use brachytherapy first. In patients with severe obstruction the esophageal applicator acts as a mild dilator and on this basis dysphagia can immediately improve after brachytherapy. The high single doses associated with brachytherapy may alleviate dysphagia within a few days. Others advocate EBRT prior to brachytherapy due to the possible shrinkage of the tumor during EBRT, theoretically allowing an improved dose distribution with brachytherapy. In an effort to resolve the question of optimal sequencing of brachytherapy and EBRT, a prospective, randomized study was initiated in a Canadian institution.[37] Two hundred patients were randomized to receive brachytherapy 1500 cGy at 1 cm from the central source position (MDR or HDR) either preceding or following EBRT 40 Gy in 15 fractions in 3 weeks. Preliminary results suggest that brachytherapy following external beam may yield a higher rate of pathologically negative specimens (51% vs 38.2%) than brachytherapy preceding external beam.[37]

Dose Prescription and Sequencing

The maximum tolerated dose of brachytherapy will be determined by many treatment related factors, such as sequencing, timing, and dose of chemotherapy or EBRT, and by brachytherapy parameters such as applicator diameter, dose rate, active length, interval, and fractionation of brachytherapy treatments.

Table 5.
Selected Clinical Trials of Brachytherapy and EBRT in Cancer of the Esophagus

Author/Study (ref)	HDR				MDR		LDR	
	Gaspar (41)	Mantravadi (20)	Hishikawa (46)	Sur (48)	Kumar (42)	Hyden (43)	Caspers (49)	Hareyama (17)
Number of patients	50	40	148	25	75	46	35	101
Pathology	Sq 46, Adeno 4	Sq 29, Adeno 11	Sq 148	Sq 25	Sq 75	Sq 45, Adeno 1	Sq 21, Adeno 14	Sq
Stage 1978 UICC	Stg II 84%, Stg III 16%	Stg I 7.5%, Stg II 32.5%, Stg III 47.5%, Stg IV 12.5%	LD 45%, ED 55%	All M0	All M0	Stg I–II 61%, Stg III–IV 39%	All M0	Stg I 30%, Stg II 71%
Chemotherapy	5FU, DDP	5 FU, Mito-C	—	—	—	—	—	—
EBRT (Gy/weeks)	50/5	45–55/5–6	60/6	35/3	40–55/4–6	50/6	50–60/5–6	50–60/5.5–6
Brachytherapy Gy per fraction at 1 cm	5	5	6	6	8–15	20	15–20[b]	4–10 Gy
No. of fractions	2–3	2	2	2	1	1–3	1	1–3
Fraction Interval	1 week	2 weeks	3–4 days	1 week	—	2 weeks	—	1 week
Applicator Diameter	6 mm	6 mm	10 mm	8 mm	NS	11 mm	3 mm	10 mm
Late Complications: Stricture	4%	22%	4%	25%	10/75	2/46	9%	3%
Ulcer	—	—	28%	—	—	—	14%	3%
Fistula	12%	—	10%	—	4/75	1/46	6%	—
Local Control	76%	77%	2 year, LD 64%, 2 year, ED 45%	NS	33/75	65%	43%	5 year–31%
Survival	1 yr 48%	3 yr, Stg II 44%, Stg III 31%	5 year, LD 18%*, 2 year, ED 7%*	1 yr 69%*	1 yr 39%	5 yr, Stg I–II 12%*, Stg III–IV 0%*	2 yr 10%	5 yr, Stg I 43%*, Stg II 21%*

* = actuarial; Adeno = adenocarcinoma; b = Dose calculated at 11.5 mm from mid-source; EBRT = external beam radiation therapy; ED = extensive disease; HDR = high-dose-rate; LD = limited disease; LDR = low-dose-rate; MDR = medium-dose-rate; NS = not stated; Sq = squamous; Stg = stage; MitoC = Mitomycin-C; 5-FU = 5-Fluorouracil; DDP = Cisplatinum.

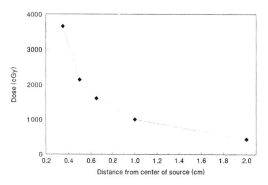

Figure 3. Dose (cGy) with increasing distance from midsource or midposition of radionuclide.

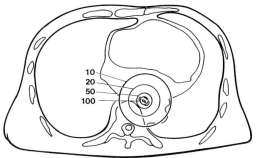

Figure 4. Schematic dose-distribution on chest computerized tomography scan. The spinal cord receives about 10% of dose at 1 cm from the midsource.

The normal tissue of most concern with esophageal brachytherapy, both in terms of acute and chronic side effects, is the normal esophageal mucosa and underlying fibromuscular wall. Relative to EBRT, brachytherapy offers the potential advantage of increasing the dose to the esophageal tumor while delivering a relatively low dose to the surrounding normal tissues, particularly the lung, spinal cord, and adjacent normal esophageal mucosa. Figure 4 is a schematic presentation of the dose fall-off using a 1-cm applicator. If the dose is prescribed at a 1 cm depth from the source axis, the spinal cord receives approximately 10% of the prescribed dose.

Acute esophagitis occurring within 3 months of brachytherapy treatment has not been well quantified in the literature. If combined with chemoradiation to 50 Gy external beam, it is likely that severe or life-threatening esophagitis will occur in >5% given the experience with chemoradiation alone.[5] Supportive measures such as intravenous hydration and gastro- or jejunostomy feedings must be made available.

Chronic esophageal ulcers, fistula, or stricture formation have been more thoroughly reported. Few of these studies involve concurrent chemotherapy, prompting caution in applying these dose/fractionation schemes in the multi-modality setting. In the series reported by Hishikawa et al.[38] in which patients received 1–4 fractions, twice weekly, of 6 Gy HDR with a 1-cm esophageal applicator, 90% (15/17) of patients with tumor control developed ulcerations and 20% developed fistulae.[38] Ulcers developed within 1–12 months following completion of therapy with a median of 5 months. Disease stage and tumor morphology were not significantly different between the patients with or without ulceration. Based on this experience, the maximum tolerated brachytherapy dose was estimated to be 12 Gy in two fractions within 1 week, starting 2 weeks after 60 Gy external beam over 6 weeks. With this dose reduction the incidence of esophageal ulcers decreased to 50%.[39]

The High Dose Rate Brachytherapy Group (HIBWOG) had proposed the following dose schedules for treatment of carcinoma of the esophagus.[40] Patients not receiving chemotherapy would receive EBRT of 60 Gy in 30–33 fractions over 6–7 weeks, reducing field after 40 Gy. HDR brachytherapy of 5 Gy at 1 cm was to be given once a week on weeks 4, 5, and 6. For patients treated with chemotherapy (Cis-Platinum at 100 mg/m² on day 1 and 23 with continuous infusion 5 FU at 1000 mg/m² on days 1–4), the EBRT dose was re-

Table 6.
Dose (cGy) at Selected Distances from Midsource or Midposition of Radionuclide

Catheter (cm)	Dose (cGy)		
	Surface	1.0 cm	2.0 cm
0.6	3661	1000	433
1.0	2140	1000	433
1.3	1614	1000	433

stricted to 50 Gy in 25–28 fractions. The HDR dose schedule was not altered.

In the recently completed RTOG clinical trial (RTOG 92–07), chemotherapy with cisplatinum at 75 mg/m^2 and 4-day infusion of 5–FU 1000 mg/m^2/day was given on weeks 1, 5, 8, and 11.[41] EBRT of 50 Gy in 25 fractions was given starting on day 1 and reducing fields after 30 Gy. HDR brachytherapy of 15 Gy at 1 cm from the midsource was given in 5 Gy fractions once a week on weeks 8, 9, and 10. HDR brachytherapy was later reduced to 10 Gy at weeks 8 and 9 after reports of esophageal fistulae. The LDR arm of this study was conducted with the same chemotherapy and EBRT and delivered 20 Gy of LDR brachytherapy with Ir-192 at a dose rate of 0.5–1.0 Gy/hr during week 8. Low accrual in the LDR group precludes analysis of toxicity or efficacy with this dose rate. Treatment related esophageal fistulae developed in 12% of the HDR group. Median survival was 11.5 months. The toxicity observed in this study suggests that the tolerance of the esophagus to HDR brachytherapy may be in the range of 10 Gy given in two fractions when given with simultaneous chemotherapy and EBRT.

A study of MDR in which the incidence of ulcerations or strictures was only 3% in long-term survivors suggests that 5500–6000 cGy external beam followed by 1500–2000 cGy MDR in 2–3 weekly fractions may be the maximally tolerated dose.[17] Acute reactions were limited to mild esophagitis. Based on the late complications observed with this dose/fractionation scheme, the authors felt that they were approaching maximally tolerated doses. Clinical experience from India concluded that 50–55 Gy EBRT followed by a single fraction of 10–12 Gy MDR brachytherapy may be the optimal dose with respect to complications and local control.[42] This was based on the observation of a 45% incidence of local control with a 25% complication rate, consisting of fistulae or strictures. Higher intraluminal doses were associated with an unacceptable complication rate of 70%.

The tolerance of the esophagus to LDR brachytherapy is more difficult to determine from the literature. Following 5000 cGy EBRT patients appear to tolerate 4000 cGy delivered with an 11-mm applicator, given in two fractions separated by 2 weeks.[43]

Various attempts have been made to decrease the incidence or severity of esophagitis with mucosal protective agents. Antiulcer prophylaxis was introduced in Japan using geranylgeranylacetone (teprenone, Eisai Co., Tokyo, Japan) which stimulates gastrointestinal mucous production.[39] Ulcers developed in 39% of 23 patients treated with the ulcer prophylaxis regimen, a significant decrease compared to the incidence observed without prophylaxis (P<0.01). A randomized prospective study has yet to be done in esophageal cancer to confirm these findings but a similar mucosal protective agent failed to decrease oral mucositis in a double blind, placebo controlled, randomized study of head and neck cancers.[44]

The length of adjacent "normal" esophagus treated with the brachytherapy boost is usually 1–2 cm proximal and distal to the primary, although the literature is seldom clear as to how the length of esophagus to be boosted with brachytherapy is determined. Some described techniques simply use a fixed active length such as 12 cm.[45] The drawbacks of larger margins will be more pronounced with small caliber esophageal applicators delivering relatively large doses of radiation to normal mucosa. This issue of appropriate margin may never be satisfactorily resolved in clinical trials.

We presently recommend EBRT doses of 50 Gy in 25 treatments (reducing fields after 30 Gy) with chemotherapy or 60 Gy in 30–33 treatments (reducing fields after 40 Gy) if chemotherapy is not added. This is followed by HDR brachytherapy of 10 Gy in 2 weekly fractions or single 20 Gy LDR brachytherapy over 2 days. We have the most experience with initiating the brachytherapy 2–3 weeks from completion of EBRT. Brachytherapy should not be given simultaneously with chemotherapy. Our current preference is to treat the posttherapy length, determined by esophagoscopy, with a 1- to 2-cm margin.

Results

Treatment with Curative Intent

Brachytherapy Alone

With the exception of a few reports of brachytherapy alone in the treatment of locally advanced or metastatic esophageal cancer, most North American investigators have utilized brachytherapy as a boost following EBRT. The largest experience with brachytherapy alone is from a rural area of Linxian County in China in which external beam facilities were not available.[45] Over 200 patients with cancer of the esophagus found during a mass screening program were treated by brachytherapy alone (cobalt-60 at 750–786 cGy/hr). Each patient received a series of 8–hour applications at 1-week intervals, with the dose specified at a depth of 0.5 cm, to a 12 cm length of esophagus. Between 2–4 brachytherapy applications were used. As expected from a screening program, tumors often were small at the time of diagnosis; 67% were 5 cm or less in length. Acute esophagitis was observed from the third day to 1-month posttreatment. Severe odynophagia or chest and back pain was experienced by 66% and 49%, respectively. Erythema, ulceration, and pseudomembrane formation was observed within the irradiated area in the minority (9%) of patients reendoscoped following radiation. Treatment related strictures developed in 11% of patients. Seventy percent of deaths were attributed to local failure and survival rates at 1, 3, and 5 years were 34.5%, 13.8%, and 8.4%, respectively. These survival rates rival the historical results after EBRT alone, but because the patients entered into this study through a screening program that clearly helped to identify those with early, superficial disease, the results cannot be easily compared.

Other smaller series exist in which brachytherapy alone was used. Hishikawa et al.[46] described six medically inoperable patients with small, superficial esophageal cancer treated in Japan with HDR brachytherapy alone. These patients were treated to a total dose of 24 Gy, 6 Gy/fraction, two fractions a week, to a field encompassing the tumor with a 2.5- to 4-cm margin superiorly and inferiorly. Although a complete response was documented endoscopically within 1 month in all patients, locoregional failure occurred in 3 patients at 7, 13, and 16 months after HDR brachytherapy; one failing in the esophagus, two failing in the mediastinal lymph nodes. Three of the six patients developed late temporary esophageal ulcers.

The low survival and local control documented in the larger Chinese experience suggests that brachytherapy alone is not appropriate curative treatment for more advanced lesions. However, brachytherapy alone may play a role in the treatment of superficial, small lesions, especially if EBRT is unavailable or contraindicated.

External Beam Radiation Therapy and Brachytherapy Boost

There are two prospective randomized studies comparing brachytherapy and EBRT with external beam alone for the treatment of cancer of the esophagus.[45,47,48] In a study in China, 200 patients with tumors mainly in the upper or middle third of the esophagus were treated.[44,47] Only 14 patients (7%) had tumors measuring >7 cm in length. The group randomized to external beam alone were treated to 70 Gy in 35 fractions over 7 weeks. The combined group received 50 Gy external beam followed by MDR brachytherapy, one application per week with a total of 3–4 applications, delivering a dose of 19.6 Gy or 26.16 Gy. A statistically significant difference in 5–year survival (17% vs 10%, P<0.05) was found favoring the combined group. Local recurrences were more frequent in the external beam group than in the combined group (61.3% and 43%, respectively). Perforation or hemorrhage occurred in 12.6% of each treatment group.

The other randomized trial, from India, included 50 patients: 25 who received 55 Gy EBRT and 25 who received 35 Gy EBRT supplemented by 12 Gy HDR brachytherapy (in two HDR treatments, 1 week apart). The doses were designed to be biologically equivalent. The group receiving brachytherapy had better relief of dysphagia (70.6% vs 37.5%) than the EBRT only arm), improved local control (70.6% vs 25%), and improved 1-year actuarial survival (78% vs 47%). However, the incidence of strictures was higher in the brachytherapy arm as compared to the EBRT arm (8% vs 4%, respectively).

Several retrospective studies comparing external beam with or without a brachytherapy boost claim improved survival, local control and swallowing ability favoring patients treated with brachytherapy.[18,49–51] For example, Petrovich[52] found that the 5-year actuarial survival with 50 Gy external beam and 40 Gy LDR brachytherapy boost was 11%, as compared to only 2% for patients treated with 55 Gy external beam only (P<0.001).[52] Caspers et al.[49] retrospectively examined actuarial survival following external beam alone to 50–60 Gy and the same external beam with a 15–20 Gy LDR boost.[49] Local control and survival were found to be strongly correlated. Although the 6-month survival and local control were improved in the brachytherapy group, the 1- and 2-year survival of 42% and 10%, was not significantly better than the experience with external beam alone. Late complications were seen in 17% (6/35) of patients, of which there was one case of fatal massive bleeding and two fatalities due to esophagopleural fistulae.

The largest experience with esophageal brachytherapy probably comes from Japan where the histology is almost always squamous. Hishikawa et al.[18,38] reported no improvement in survival but reported a significant improvement in 2-year local control with external radiation (median of 50 Gy) and 12 Gy HDR brachytherapy in two fractions when compared to 50 Gy or more external beam only. The 5–year survival rate in 66 patients without distant metastases, treated with the combination of external beam and HDR brachytherapy, was 18% and the 1- and 2-year actuarial local control rate were 66% and 64%, respectively. Cause of death was attributed to local failure in 28% of patients, local failure with distant metastases in 12%, distant metastasis in 29%, and intercurrent disease in 31%.

Other retrospective reports have found that the esophageal brachytherapy boost is unnecessary if a high dose of EBRT is delivered. Chatani et al.[52] retrospectively examined the outcome in patients who received either 70 Gy external beam or 60 Gy external beam with an HDR brachytherapy boost of 10 Gy given in two fractions, 1 week apart. They found that local control with EBRT alone was significantly higher than with external beam and brachytherapy boost (79% and 55%, respectively). Toxicity and disease-free survival were similar between the two groups.

Interpretation of retrospective studies is always difficult. One interesting study conducted in Japan concluded that patient selection may account for the improved survival observed following esophageal brachytherapy.[53] Barium swallows were used to retrospectively assess the feasibility of inserting a 1-cm tube for intraluminal irradiation. The

survival in patients receiving and not receiving brachytherapy was not statistically different once the extent of obstruction was taken into consideration.

Selected clinical results of esophageal brachytherapy boost are summarized in Table 5. The variation in local control and toxicity in these retrospective reviews indicate the need for prospective clinical trials with clearly defined local control and toxicity definitions.

Concurrent Chemoradiation and Brachytherapy Boost

Few studies have used state-of-the-art concurrent chemoradiation with an intraluminal boost. Chemotherapy is clearly an important modality in terms of local control, toxicity, and survival outcome and should be incorporated into future esophageal cancer brachytherapy trials.[5,7,8] Mantravadi et al.[20] have the largest reported series (40 patients) treated with 45–55 Gy external beam concurrent with two courses of 5-FU and mitomycin-C, followed 2 and 4 weeks later by 5 Gy intraluminal boost. Results of this study are summarized in Table 5. Three-year survival figures of 44% for stage II and 31% for stage III are in the same range as those reported with chemotherapy-external beam alone. Local control was excellent with only 23% of patients developing recurrent local disease. Distant metastases without local recurrence developed in another 23% of patients; an unusually high percentage for most radiation series. The most common late effect encountered was stricture formation, defined as narrowing requiring one or more dilatations. This occurred in 23% of patients. Factors determined to be predictive of stricture formation were circumferential tumor involvement, tumor length >6 cm, and external radiation dose of 54 Gy or more.

The RTOG recently completed accrual to a phase I/II study to further evaluate EBRT and brachytherapy with concurrent chemotherapy.[41] Brachytherapy was given concurrent with the third cycle of chemotherapy 2 weeks following 50 Gy EBRT concurrent with two cycles of 5-FU and cisplatin. Depending on institutional preference, the brachytherapy could be either HDR or LDR. The HDR was initially given as 15 Gy at 1 cm from the mid-source position in three fractions. After reports of esophageal toxicity (fistulae), the HDR brachytherapy dose was revised to 10 Gy in two fractions in week 8 and week 9. The LDR dose was a single fraction of 20 Gy. Cervical esophageal lesions were excluded due to concerns about brachytherapy-induced tracheo-esophageal fistulae. To obtain an adequate distal margin, tumors of the distal esophagus that are within 1 cm of the gastro-esophageal margin were not eligible. The study required that the active treatment length encompassed the primary tumor with a 1-cm margin proximally and distally. Tumor length was defined as the longest tumor measurement on the pretreatment CT scan, esophagoscopy, or barium swallow. Slow accrual to the LDR group led to discontinuation of this dose rate prior to the accumulation of sufficient patient numbers to allow statistical analysis. Preliminary results within the HDR group suggest that the efficacy of the regimen did not justify the 12% incidence of treatment related esophageal fistulae. This regimen will not be tested further within the RTOG.

Neoadjuvant Esophageal Brachytherapy

Surgery alone is associated with median survival times of 12–24 months.[2,3,24] Few studies have analyzed the added benefit of brachytherapy, with or without EBRT or chemotherapy. One study from Canada gave patients with esophageal cancers arising below the carina preoperative brachytherapy, 15 Gy HDR or MDR, either before or after 40 Gy external beam in 15 fractions in 3 weeks.[25,37] Transhiatal esophagectomy was done 4–6 weeks later in resectable patients. Postoperative mortality was only 1%. In 73 patients resected with curative intent, 4-year actuarial disease specific survival rate was 25% for squamous cell cancers and 22% for adenocarcinomas. No difference was observed in the pathological response or survival for those patients with squamous cancer as compared to adenocarcinoma. In 104 resected patients the esophagectomy specimen was free of tumor in 43%. Since both external beam and brachytherapy were used, it is not possible to detect the benefit from any one of these radiation modalities alone.

In an effort to reduce possible complications associated with preoperative EBRT,

brachytherapy has been combined with 5-FU and mitomycin-C preoperatively. In a small group of 11 patients postoperative morbidity and mortality due to adult respiratory distress syndrome was 55%.[54] The explanation for this high complication rate is not clear, particularly in light of other small series in which complications attributable to preoperative chemotherapy and brachytherapy were not noted.[55]

Surgical Salvage Following Radiation

Prior external beam and brachytherapy is not an absolute contraindication to surgical salvage. In one report, surgery as attempted salvage following 55–60 Gy external beam and 15–20 Gy MDR brachytherapy surgery was performed in 23 patients with local recurrence or tumor persistence.[17] Five (21.7%) of these patients survived 5 years, indicating that consideration of salvage surgery is warranted.

Treatment with Palliative Intent

The decision to treat cancer of the esophagus with palliative or curative intent is not always an easy one. Although most oncologists would agree that palliative treatment is appropriate for patients with systemic metastases, the curability of patients with evidence of regional lymph node metastases or bulky disease or of patients who are in poor medical condition is more controversial. Some form of treatment for dysphagia is invariably required, since locally recurrent or persistent disease and aspiration pneumonia is responsible for most deaths (more than 80% in some series).[34] Although some reviews have concluded that esophagectomy or gastric interposition provides the best relief of dysphagia, most clinicians agree that the associated morbidity and mortality are too high to recommend surgery purely for palliation.[56]

Once the patient has been deemed incurable, there is still controversy regarding the most effective method of palliation. Is brachytherapy able to provide quicker or more prolonged relief of dysphagia than other modalities available such as surgery, laser treatment, or endo-esophageal tubes? Few prospective studies have been done to compare brachytherapy with other methods of palliation such as dilatation, laser therapy, EBRT, chemoradiation, etc.

EBRT alone provides effective relief of dysphagia but the benefit is often short lived. In a retrospective study from the University of California, San Francisco, significant relief of dysphagia lasting for 2 months was experienced by 66% of patients with squamous cell cancer following 50–60 Gy external beam.[57] However, 20% of patients were unable to complete the prescribed course of radiation, usually due to rapidly progressive disease. Symptomatic local progression occurred by 3 months in over half of the patients completing therapy and 23% of the patients eventually required endo-esophageal intubation with celestin tube placement due to progressive dysphagia. The addition of concurrent chemotherapy with dose/fractionation schedules similar to those used during curative treatment has been found to provide more lasting palliation in the majority of patients with locally-advanced or metastatic disease.[8] However, the median survival was still only 7–9 months with approximately 2 of these months spent in treatment.

Brachytherapy Alone

Palliation of dysphagia can be achieved with brachytherapy alone. Fontanesi et al.[58] reported relief of dysphagia and objective tumor response endoscopically by 2 weeks in five of five patients given one course of 50–53 Gy LDR brachytherapy, with the dose specified at 0.5 cm. In another small series of ten patients, relief of dysphagia was achieved in nine patients for an average duration of 5 months after 2000 cGy LDR (dose specified 1 cm from source), given in three fractions over 5 days.[59] Jager and colleagues[60] claimed relief of dysphagia in 69% of 36 patients who received 15 Gy MDR. The median survival for the whole group of 36 patients was only 4 months despite the fact that 61% (22/36) had no distant metastases at the time of treatment. The median dysphagia-free duration was 4.5 months. Brachytherapy was found to provide equivalent palliation for both squamous and adenocarcinomas.

In an effort to compare brachytherapy with laser therapy, Low and Pagliero[61] randomized 23 consecutive patients with advanced esophageal cancer to either endoluminal brachytherapy or laser treatment. The treatment was considered palliative because of the presence of distant metastases, serious medical conditions, or locoregional spread involving the bronchus, aorta, or vertebral column. Brachytherapy consisted of 1500 cGy HDR at a distance 1 cm from the catheter, with an 8-mm catheter to a length of 13 cm. Initial improvement in dysphagia scores was observed in 83% and 91% of the brachytherapy and laser groups, respectively (P>0.05) This improvement in dysphagia was maintained for more than 2 months in at least 75% of patients. Retreatments were required three times more often following laser therapy, but the frequency of eventual treatment failures was equal between the laser and brachytherapy group. Minor complications, particularly transient early dysphagia, were more common in the brachytherapy group. Thirty-three percent of patients experienced dysphagia lasting 3–7 days, although the only major late complication, a fistula, occurred in the laser group. Based on this experience, the authors concluded that brachytherapy was associated with a shorter hospital stay and less need for further therapy. Interestingly, luminal patency did not always correlate with the degree of dysphagia, supporting the existence of tumor related anorexia as a contributing factor to weight loss.

In another study, 39 patients (adenocarcinoma, 22; squamous, 17) were randomized to either Nd:YAG laser recanalization alone or laser recanalization with subsequent endoluminal afterloading irradiation.[62] A 3-day time interval between laser treatment and endoluminal irradiation was felt to be necessary to reduce the risk of excessive esophagitis. The brachytherapy group received 3 weekly fractions of 7 Gy HDR. If dysphagia recurred in the brachytherapy group, a further three fractions was given, i.e., 42 Gy in six fractions. Twenty-one percent of patients developed esophagitis following brachytherapy. Restenosis occurred eventually in all patients in both treatment groups. Although not statistically significant, squamous cell carcinoma patients in the brachytherapy group showed a prolonged dysphagia-free first interval as compared to the squamous cancers in the laser only group (65 vs 30 days, P<0.03). This prolonged dysphagia-free interval with brachytherapy was not seen in patients with adenocarcinoma. There was a more frequent need for subsequent intervention in patients with adenocarcinoma as compared to squamous cell cancer. The conclusion reached from this study was that brachytherapy may provide palliation superior to that obtained with laser alone in patients with squamous cell cancer. It may also be concluded from this study that neither laser alone nor laser with brachytherapy provides effective palliation in patients expected to live more than 4–8 weeks.

Brachytherapy as a Palliation Boost

Brachytherapy combined with a short course of external beam is an attractive alternative to achieve equivalent or superior palliation in less total treatment time. Brachytherapy may also be cost effective when compared to other palliative options although the economic benefits have not been analyzed extensively. In Britain, palliative intubation is estimated to cost five to six times that of brachytherapy.[21] Gaspar et al.[19] treated 30 patients with cancer of the esophagus palliatively with 30 Gy external beam in ten fractions and a single fraction of 10–15 Gy HDR brachytherapy. Relief of dysphagia was evident in most patients within 2–3 weeks of completing therapy. Although the ability to swallow at least liquids was maintained for 6 months in approximately 40% of surviving patients, recurrent dysphagia was a major problem in the majority, particularly those surviving beyond 6 months. In view of these observations, the authors recommended longer courses of EBRT, i.e., 50 Gy in 25 fractions over 5–6 weeks, with a brachytherapy boost for patients without distant metastases in whom the anticipated survival is more than 6 months.

A preliminary report suggests the potential benefit of chemoradiation with brachytherapy boost.[63] Thirty-two patients with locally advanced or metastatic esophageal cancer were treated with 55.8 Gy external beam in 1.8 Gy daily fractions concurrent with 5–FU and mitomycin-C, with two fractions of HDR brachytherapy given 1 and 3 weeks following completion of chemoradiation. Each intraluminal brachytherapy treatment delivered 7 Gy, specified at a 1 cm depth. Actuarial median survival was 15 months. Treatment was well tolerated, although mucositis developed in all patients. This treatment regimen merits further investigation.

Summary

Results of recent chemo-external beam studies (3-year survival rates of >30%, but associated locoregional recurrence/progression rates of approximately 40%) suggest a need for dose escalation for esophageal cancer.[5,7,8] Brachytherapy is one of the several radiotherapeutic techniques available for escalation of the dose to the primary tumor site. Compared to EBRT, esophageal brachytherapy offers several potential advantages in providing dose escalation, including delivery of a high tumor dose with relative sparing of the surrounding normal tissues, rapid relief of dysphagia, shortening of treatment time, and patient convenience.

With the exception of a few reports of brachytherapy alone in the treatment of locally advanced or metastatic esophageal cancer, most North American investigators have used brachytherapy as a boost after EBRT. The choice of radioactive source and dose rate varies with personal preference and with availability of shielded rooms and equipment. Iridium is currently the source used most frequently in esophageal brachytherapy, usually as remote HDR brachytherapy.

While results of further studies are pending, for primary esophageal carcinoma, we currently recommend cisplatinum and 5-FU chemotherapy concurrent with 45–50 Gy EBRT (reducing fields after 30–40 Gy), followed by a brachytherapy boost of 10 Gy HDR in 2 weekly fractions of 5 Gy each or 20 Gy LDR in a single application, prescribed at 1 cm from the source. The active treatment length should encompass the pretreatment primary tumor with a 1–2 cm proximal and distal margin. Endoscopic ultrasonography may be of benefit in target definition. Consideration of salvage surgery is warranted.

For palliative management of esophageal cancer in patients with distant metastases, we recommend a 2- to 3-week course of EBRT and a brachytherapy boost of 10–15 Gy HDR or 15–20 LDR given in a single fraction. Concurrent chemotherapy should be considered, if tolerated.

Absolute contraindications to brachytherapy include broncho-esophageal, aortic-esophageal, or tracheo-esophageal fistula, deep mucosal ulceration, and cervical esophageal involvement. Prospective clinical studies with objective end points are necessary to rigorously assess the role of esophageal brachytherapy.

Editor's note: The American Brachytherapy Society (ABS) issued guidelines for brachytherapy of esophageal cancer after this chapter was written. The ABS recommendations parallels those given in this chapter. (Gaspar LE, Nag S, Herskovic A, Mantravadi P, Speiser B. American Brachytherapy Society (ABS) Consensus Guidelines for Brachytherapy of Esophageal Cancer. Int J Radiat Oncol Biol Phys. In press, 1997.) Subir Nag, M.D.

References

1. Beatty JD, DeBoer G, Rider WD. Carcinoma of the esophagus—pretreatment assessment, correlation of radiation treatment parameters with survival, and identification and management of radiation treatment failure. Cancer 1979;43:2254–2267.
2. Mannell A, Becker PJ. Evaluation of the results of oesophagectomy for oesophageal cancer. Br J Surg 1991;78:36–40.
3. Kasai M, Mori S, Watanabe T. Follow-up results after resection of thoracic esophageal carcinoma. World J Surg 1978;2:543–551.
4. Newaishy GA, Read GA, Duncan W, et al. Results of radiotherapy of squamous cell carcinoma of the esophagus. Clin Radiol 1982;33:347–352.
5. Herskovic A, Martz K, Al-Sarraf M, et al. Combined chemotherapy and radiotherapy compared with radiotherapy alone in patients with cancer of the esophagus. N Engl J Med 1992;326:1593–1598.
6. Mantravadi R, Lad T, Briele H, et al. Carcinoma of the esophagus: Sites of failure. Int J Radiat Oncol Biol Phys 1982;8:1897–1901.
7. Al-Sarraf M, Pajak T, Herskovic A, et al. Progress report of combined chemo-radiotherapy (CT-RT) versus radiotherapy (RT) alone in patients with esophageal cancer, an intergroup study (Abstract). Proceedings of ASCO 1993;12:197.
8. Coia LR, Engstron PF, Paul AR, et al. Long-term results of infusional 5-FU, mitomycin-C and radiation as primary management of esophageal carcinoma. Int J Rad Oncol Biol Phys 1991;20:29–36.
9. Gaspar L. Radiation therapy of esophageal cancer: Improving the therapeutic ratio. Semin Radiat Oncol 1994;4(3):192–201.
10. Nori D, Allison R. Prospects for improved treatment results with radiation dose escalation in esophageal cancer. Endocurie/Hyperthermia Oncol 1993;9:63–67.
11. Barcat, Guisez. Essais de traitement de quelques cas d'epithelioma de l'oesophage par les applications locales directes de radium. Bul Mem Soc Med Hop Par 1909;26:717–712.
12. Guisez J. Malignant tumors of the esophagus. J Laryngol Otol 1925;40:213–232.
13. Dickson RJ. Radiation therapy in carcinoma of the esophagus—a review. Am J Med Sci 1971;241:662–677.
14. Rider WD, Mendoza RD. Some opinions on the treatment of cancer of the esophagus. Am J Roentgenol 1969;105:514–517.
15. Bottrill DO, Plane JH, Newaishy GA. A proposed afterloading technique for irradiation of the oesophagus. Br J Radiol 1979;52:573–574.
16. Abe M, Kitagawa T. Treatment of esophageal cancer with high dose rate intracavitary irradiation. Tohuku J Exp Med 1981;134:159–167.
17. Hareyama M, Nishio M, Kagami Y, et al. Intracavitary brachytherapy combined with external beam irradiation for squamous cell carcinoma of the thoracic esophagus. Int J Rad Oncol Biol Phys 1992;24:235–240.
18. Hishikawa Y, Kurisu K, Taniguchi M, et al. High-dose-rate intraluminal brachytherapy for esophageal cancer: 10 years experience in Hyogo College of Medicine. Radiother Oncol 1991;21:107–114.
19. Gaspar LE, Kocha WI, Barnett R, et al. Cancer of the esophagus: Brachytherapy, EBRT and chemotherapy. Cancer J 1993;6(4):196–200.
20. Mantravadi RVP, Crawford JN, Gates JO, et al. Combined Chemotherapy and External Radiation Therapy Plus Intraluminal Boost with High Dose Rate Brachytherapy for Carcinoma of the Esophagus. Proc. 76th Annual Meeting of the American Radium Society, Bermuda, April 22–26, 1994, p. 18.
21. Flores AD, Rowland CG, Yin W. High dose rate brachytherapy for carcinoma of the esophagus. In: Nag S (ed). High Dose Rate Brachytherapy: A Textbook. Futura Publishing Co., Inc., Armonk, NY, 1994, pp. 275–294.
22. Harvey JC, Kagan AR, Ahn C, et al. Adenocarcinoma of the esophagus: A survival study. J Surg Oncol 1990;45:29–32.
23. Whittington R, Coia LR, Haller DG, et al. Adenocarcinoma of the esophagus and esophago-

gastric junction: The effects of single and combined modalities on the survival and patterns of failure following treatment. Int J Radiat Oncol Biol Phys 1990;19:593–603.

24. Finley RJ, Inculet RI. The results of esophagogastrectomy without thoracotomy for adenocarcinoma of the esophagogastric junction. Ann Surg 1989;210(4):535–543.

25. Hay JH, Haylock BJ, Flores AD, et al. Influence of histology on results of pre-op radiotherapy for carcinoma of the lower esophagus and cardia. Proc Royal College of Physicians and Surgeons, 736, 1993.

26. International Union Against Cancer TMN Classification of Malignant Tumors, Fourth Edition. Springer-Verlag, 1987.

27. Halvorsen RA, Magruder-Habib K, Foster WL, et al. Esophageal cancer staging by CT: Long-term follow-up study. Radiology 1986;161:147–151.

28. Quint LE, Glazer GM, Orringer MB. Esophageal imaging by MR and CT: Study of normal anatomy and neoplasms. Radiology 1985;156:727–731.

29. Halvorsen RA, Thompson WM. Computed tomographic staging of gastrointestinal tract malignancies part I. Esoph Stomach Invest Radiol 1987;22(1):2–16.

30. Shorvon PJ. Upper gastrointestinal endoscopic ultrasonography in gastroenterology. Br J Radiol 1987;60:429–438.

31. Hordijk ML, et al. Influence of tumor stenosis on the accuracy of endosonography in preoperative tumor staging of esophageal cancer. Endoscopy 1993;25:171–175.

32. Hay JH, Flores AD. Letter to editor. Br J Radiol 1990;63:583–584.

33. Pizzi GB, Beorchia A, Cereghini ME, et al. A new technique for endocavitary irradiation of the esophagus. Int J Rad Oncol Biol Phys 1989;16:261–262.

34. Flores AD, Nelems B, Evans K. Impact of new radiotherapy modalities on the surgical management of cancer of the esophagus and cardia. Int J Rad Oncol Biol Phys 1989;17:937–944.

35. Fietkau R, Ell Ch, Hochberger J, et al. New applicator system for the intraluminal high dose rate irradiation of the esophageal carcinoma. Strahlenther Onkol 1991;167:301–304.

36. Ell C, Hochberger J, Fietkau R, et al. New bougie applicator system for intraluminal high dose rate afterloading radiotherapy of esophageal carcinoma. Endoscopy 1993;25(3):236–239.

37. Keyes M, Haylock B, Hay JH. An evaluation of pathological effect of pre or post external beam brachytherapy in radical radiotherapy of

carcinoma of esophagus. Proc Roy Coll Phys Surg, 1994.

38. Hishikawa Y, Kamikonya N, Tanaka S, et al. Radiotherapy of esophageal carcinoma: Role of high-dose-rate intracavitary irradiation. Radiother Oncol 1987;9:13–20.

39. Hishikawa Y, Izumi M, Kurisu K, et al. Esophageal ulceration following high-dose-rate intraluminal brachytherapy for esophageal cancer. Radiother Oncol 1993;28(3):252–254.

40. Nag S, Abitbol A, Clark D, et al. Clinical guidelines for HDR brachytherapy: A report of the High Dose Rate Brachytherapy Working Group (HIBWOG). 15th Annual Meeting of the American Endocurietherapy Society, Beavercreek, CO, December 9–12, 1992.

41. Gaspar LE, Chunlin Q, Kocha WI, et al. A phase I-II study of external beam radiation, brachytherapy and concurrent chemotherapy in localized cancer of the esophagus (RTOG 9207): Preliminary toxicity report. Int J Radiat Oncol Biol Phys 1995;32(S1):207(132).

42. Kumar MU, Swamy K, Supe SS, et al. Influence of intraluminal brachytherapy dose on complications in the treatment of esophageal cancer. Int J Radiat Oncol Biol Phys 1993;27:1069–1072.

43. Hyden EC, Langholz B, Tilden T, et al. External beam and intraluminal radiotherapy in the treatment of carcinoma of the esophagus. J Thorac Cardiovasc Surg 1988;96:237–241.

44. Epstein JB, Wong FLW. The efficacy of sucralfate suspension in the prevention of oral mucositis due to radiation therapy. Int J Radiat Oncol Biol Phys 1994;28(3):693–698.

45. Yin WB. Brachytherapy of carcinoma of the esophagus in China, 1970–1974 and 1982–1984. In: Martinez AA, Orton CG, Mould RF (eds). Brachytherapy: HDR and LDR. Nucletron Corp., Columbia, MD, 1990, pp. 52–56.

46. Hishikawa Y, Kurisu K, Taniguchi M, et al. High-dose-rate intraluminal brachytherapy (HDRIBT) for esophageal cancer. Int J Radiat Oncol Biol Phys 1991;21:1133–1135.

47. Wang RZ, Zhao RO. Combined intracavitary and external radiotherapy for esophageal carcinoma: A prospective randomized clinical trial on 128 patients. Chin J Radiat Oncol 1987;1:41–43.

48. Sur RK, Singh DP, Sharma SC, et al. Radiation therapy of esophageal cancer: Role of high dose rate brachytherapy. Int J Radiat Oncol Biol Phys 1992;22(5):1043–1046.

49. Caspers RJL, Zwinderman AH, Griffioen G, et al. Combined external beam and low dose rate intraluminal radiotherapy in oesophageal cancer. Radiother Oncol 1993;27:7–12.

50. Petrovich Z, Langholz B, Formenti S, et al. Management of carcinoma of the esophagus: The role of radiotherapy. Am J Clin Oncol (CCT) 1991;14(1):80–86.

51. Petrovich Z, Langholz B, Formenti S, et al. The importance of brachytherapy in the treatment of unresectable carcinoma of the esophagus. Endocurie/Hypertherm Oncol 1989;5: 201–208.

52. Chatani M, Matayoshi Y, Masaki N. Radiation therapy for the esophageal carcinoma: External irradiation versus high-dose rate intraluminal irradiation. Strahlenther Onkol 1992;168: 328–332.

53. Nakajima T, Fukuda H, Hosono M, et al. Intraluminal irradiation for T2MO esophageal cancer: Effect of patient selection on prognosis. Radiat Med 1992;10(3):123–128.

54. Scholz J, Steinhofel U, Durig M, et al. Postoperative pulmonary complications in patients with esophageal cancer. Clin Investig 1993;71(4): 294–298.

55. Peddada AV, Harvey JC, Anderson PJ, et al. High dose rate intraluminal radiation in a combined modalit treatment plan for carcinoma of the esophagus. J Surg Oncol0 1993;52: 160–163.

56. Brown SG. Palliation of malignant dysphagia: Surgery, radiotherapy, laser, intubation alone or in combination? Gut 1991;32(8):841–844.

57. Wara WM, Mauch PM, Thomas AN, et al. Palliation for carcinoma of the esophagus. Radiology 1976;121:717–720.

58. Fontanesi J, Rodriguez RR, Robison JC. Intracavitary irradiation as a primary treatment for unresectable esophageal carcinoma. Endocurie/Hypertherm Oncol 1989;5:231–234.

59. Fleischman EH, Kagan AR, Bellotti JE. Effective palliation for inoperable esophageal cancer using intensive intracavitary radiation. J Surg Oncol 1990;44:234–237.

60. Jager JJ, Pannebakker M, Rijken J, et al. Palliation in esophageal cancer with a single session of intraluminal irradiation. Radiother Oncol 1992;25(2):134–136.

61. Low DEJ, Pagliero KM. Prospective randomized clinical trial comparing brachytherapy and laser photoablation for palliation of esophageal cancer. J Thorac Cardiovasc Surg 1992; 104(1):173–178.

62. Sander R, Hagenmueller F, Sander C, et al. Laser versus laser plus afterloading with iridium-192 in the palliative treatment of malignant stenosis of the esophagus: A prospective, randomized, controlled study. Gastrointest Endosc 1991;37(4):433–440.

63. Staar S, Mueller RP, Achterrath W. Intensified treatment for inoperable esophagus cancer: Simultaneous radiochemotherapy combined with HDR intraluminal brachytherapy. Results of a phase II trial (Abstract). Proceedings of ASCO 1993;12:223.

Chapter 16

Brachytherapy for Lung Cancer

Minesh P. Mehta, M.D., John P. Lamond, M.D.,
Dattatreyudu Nori, M.D., Burton L. Speiser, M.D.

Introduction

With an annual incidence of more than 160,000 in the United States and a mortality rate of over 80%, lung cancer represents our greatest oncologic challenge.[1] Although surgery has been demonstrated to be an effective single treatment modality for localized early stage non-small lung cancer, only a minority (approximately 20%) of patients are currently diagnosed with localized disease amenable to complete surgical resection. Of those patients with more advanced local disease, most will receive external beam irradiation with or without chemotherapy, with <10% 5-year survival.

The majority of lung cancer patients eventually have symptoms related to local progression and subsequently die from local regional failure. Local failure rates between 31%–51% have been reported in several Radiation Therapy Oncology Group (RTOG) studies that had utilized external beam irradiation alone.[2] Commonly reported symptoms from failure of local control include cough, dyspnea, pain, and hemoptysis, with the majority of symptoms related to endobronchial disease.[3] Therefore, management of the endobronchial and peribronchial component of lung cancer is quite important, even in some patients with metastatic disease. In 300 consecutive autopsies from the Veterans' Administration Lung Group (VALG) protocols, residual intrathoracic tumor was responsible for death in 75% of the patients with squamous cell carcinoma and 50% of the patients with adenocarcinoma and large cell carcinoma of the lung.[4]

Increasing the total dose of external beam radiation has been attempted to help improve local control rates. Data from two randomized RTOG lung cancer trials demonstrated that the local regional failure rate was dose dependent, with a failure rate of 48% with 40 Gy continuous radiation, 38% with 40 Gy split course or 50 Gy continuous regimen, and 27% for the 60 Gy continuous regimen.[5] The RTOG then conducted phase II studies utilizing escalating total doses of hyperfractionated radiation (60, 64.8, 69.6, 74.4, and 79.2 Gy in 1.2 Gy bid fractions). There was statistically significant improvement in patients with favorable prognostic signs who received 69.6 Gy in comparison to previous RTOG trials that used the standard 60 Gy in daily 2 Gy fractions.[6] No additional benefit was obtained in those patients who received higher radiation doses. Although there appeared to be no significant differences in the risks of acute or late effects in normal tissues among the five treatment arms, it is possible that more rigorous methods of measurement may have unmasked differences among the treatment groups. Recently, there has been great interest in better quantitating pulmonary, cardiac, and

From Nag S (ed): *Principles and Practice of Brachytherapy.* © Futura Publishing Co., Inc., Armonk, NY, 1997.

Table 1.
Lung Brachytherapy General Guidelines

Treatment	Indication	Potential Brachytherapy Techniques
Brachytherapy alone	Very early stage endobronchial disease	Temporary endobronchial or permanent interstitial
	Localized disease where resection requires removal of lung tissue beyond patient tolerance	Temporary or permanent interstitial
Surgery, external beam radiation with brachytherapy as boost	Locally advanced disease with subtotal surgical resection, typically secondary to invasion of major structures or mediastinal lymph nodes	Permanent vicryl suture or gel foam; temporary interstitial; temporary endobronchial
External beam radiation with brachytherapy as boost	Locally regionally advanced inoperable disease	Temporary or permanent interstitial; temporary endobronchial

other effects in patients who receive thoracic radiation.[7,8] Many studies have shown that normal tissue toxicity is a function of the dose and volume of the tissue irradiated, lending credence to the suspicion that the toxicities may be higher in those patients treated to higher total doses.

Thus, as far as local control is concerned, a dose response relationship in lung cancer exists, but the response appears limited when using standard external beam radiation. Based on experience in other disease sites, where radiation alone is used to treat gross disease and doses of 70–80 Gy or greater are usually required for local control, it is quite understandable that the local control is poor when using only 60 Gy. Brachytherapy is effectively used in other disease sites, including its frequent use in gynecological and head and neck cancer, to boost a region to a higher

dose than can be safely achieved with external beam radiation alone.

Brachytherapy for lung malignancies has been used for a variety of clinical indications, with a number of radiation sources and techniques, as summarized in Tables 1 and 2. Brachytherapy may be used alone, with surgery, or with external beam radiation. The intent of treatment may be for cure or for palliation of symptoms.

This chapter will initially review the techniques and results of intraoperative interstitial brachytherapy, including the substantial Sloan-Kettering experience. Next, the various techniques and results of endobronchial brachytherapy will be reviewed. Other nonbrachytherapy treatment techniques are discussed, but direct comparisons from prospective controlled randomized trials are lacking.

Table 2.
Commonly used Radionuclides for Lung Brachytherapy

Nuclide	Average Photon Energy (MeV)	Half-Life (Days)	Application
I-125	0.028	59.6	Interstitial implant (volume planar); interstitial temporary implant; transbronchial implant
Ir-192	0.350	74.0	Interstitial temporary planar or intraluminal; remote afterloading temporary or intraluminal
Pd-103	0.021	17.0	Interstitial implant (volume or planar)

Interstitial Brachytherapy

History

Interstitial implantation of the lung combined with resection was first performed by Graham and Singer[9] in the United States in 1933. After completion of a left pneumonectomy for bronchogenic carcinoma, they inserted seven radon seeds into the bronchovascular stump. During the 1960s, Henschke[10] reported on the first major study using intraoperative brachytherapy in 117 patients with early encouraging results.

Although the initial results with interstitial brachytherapy used at thoracotomy had been encouraging, this form of treatment was restricted to a few institutions for two reasons: 1) the technique of interstitial implantation was more difficult to learn than external beam therapy since it required both knowledge of radiotherapy and surgical skills; and 2) interstitial implantation with high energy radionuclides, such as Rn-222, Au-198, and Ir-192, posed problems of radiation exposure to the operator and to the personnel caring for the patient. During the mid-1960s, Henschke et al.[11] introduced the modern afterloading techniques for brachytherapy to minimize radiation exposure to the operating personnel.

The introduction of low energy Iodine-125 gamma ray encapsulated sources in 1965 by Hilaris and Holt[12] removed some of the obstacles to interstitial irradiation. Iodine-125 has a low energy gamma emission (30 Kv) and a long half-life (60 days). The long half-life allows these sources to be stored in the hospital and makes interstitial implantation available on short notice, simplifying the problem of source availability. The low gamma energy has also resulted in a substantial reduction in radiation exposure. The introduction of Palladium-103, a low energy isotope in thoracic tumors by Nori[13] has added a new dimension to intraoperative brachytherapy. Its short half-life and higher initial dose rate have greatly expanded the applications of brachytherapy for rapidly growing and anaplastic non-small cell lung cancers. In addition, the introduction of new technologies such as computerized dosimetry has improved our ability to accurately determine the radiation dose distribution within the implanted volume.[14] The radiation dose distribution is readily adaptable to the tumor shape and falls rapidly outside the implanted tumor, thereby sparing surrounding normal lung that would be damaged with external irradiation.

A number of interstitial brachytherapy techniques can be applied in the treatment of non-small cell lung cancer. The brachytherapy technique used depends on tumor location and the amount of gross disease left after surgery. Discrete lung masses are permanently implanted with I-125 or Palladium-103 seeds. Chest wall, small mediastinal lesions, and positive margins of resection are treated by temporary Ir-192 implantation (low-dose-rate [LDR] or remote afterloading high-dose-rate [HDR]). These areas when appropriate can also be treated by I-125 or Pd-103 in suture seeds using specialized techniques described in the text. Since the suture and gel techniques do not involve the placement of sources within the tumor bed, but against it, the term intraoperative brachytherapy has been used by some authors.[15]

Indications

Intraoperative brachytherapy has good curative potential in patients with small to medium size lung tumors that are well defined and have not metastasized to lymph nodes.[16] In general, the indications include:

1. Patients with limited pulmonary reserve and in whom adequate resection requires the removal of lung tissue beyond patient tolerance.
2. Patients with hilar tumors adherent to the major vessels with no clearance for safe dissection.
3. Patients with tumors extending to the mediastinum and attached to trachea, esophagus, aorta, superior vena cava, or pericardium.
4. Patients with extensive involvement of chest wall or spine in whom complete excision is not possible.

Techniques

Permanent Implantation Technique for Palpable Masses

The techniques of interstitial implantation of encapsulated radioactive sources vary depending on the type of implantation used. Permanent implants are interstitial implants in which the radioactive sources are permanently left in the tissue. Temporary implants, sometimes called "removable" implants, are interstitial implants in which the radioactive sources are removed after the desired dose has been delivered.[17]

Most interstitial implants for carcinoma of the lung are done through a posterolateral thoracotomy approach. The first step of the procedure consists of delineating the area to be treated and measuring it. The second step consists of determining the number of sources required using the nomogram. This is based on the average dimension of the tumor and the strength of the radioactive sources. The dimensions of the target volume includes the measured three dimensions of the tumor, with a 1-cm margin around it. The nomogram, in addition, gives the spacing to be used between needles. The cumulative dose with this system is 13,000–16,000 cGy with I-125 and 10,000–12,000 cGy with Palladium-103. Typically it is preferred to insert the hollow needles first in the periphery of the tumor mass. The third step is the afterloading with radioactive sources. Several commercially available implantation instruments have been used during the past few years. After insertion of the radioactive sources, each needle is retracted and detached from the applicator (Figure 1). The process is repeated with each needle until all needles have been implanted. On the average, the procedure adds 30–45 minutes to the operating time and has not increased hospital stay. During the implantation a careful record should be kept of the number of implanted Iodine-125 or Palladium-103 sources, the activity per source, and the spacing between sources inserted along each needle. Figure 2 shows a radiograph of a permanent implant in a patient with stage I lung cancer. A 4-year follow-up radiograph is also shown, demonstrating complete shrinkage of the implanted tumor.[15]

Permanent Vicryl Suture or Gelfoam Impregnated with I-125 or Pd-103 Seed

In the surgical treatment of large mediastinal or chest wall tumors, negative margins of surgical resection are often unattainable. Tumors often adhere to critical vessels or bone or other visceral structures and resection is often incomplete. The usual method of sterilizing a tumor bed in this situation is with external beam radiation; however, local control is often unsatisfactory because of risk of toxicity with higher doses of external radiation. In addition, treatment with external beam radiation must be delayed until there is adequate wound healing, potentially allowing time for tumor growth and dissemination.

The suture technique includes a curved needle attached to the Vicryl suture, which facilitates anchoring of the suture on the tissue. The number of sutures to be applied for a given target area can be obtained from the planar implant guide. The target area includes all visible or suspected tumor extension with a minimum 1-cm margin.

Previously, a versatile permanent planar implant technique using I-125 seeds embedded in Gelfoam was reported.[18–20] This technique is extremely useful in situations when there is inadequate stroma available for suturing. Areas that were previously unimplantable because of the proximity of critical structures are now readily implanted without the risk of intraoperative or perioperative complications. The Gelfoam plaques can be prepared with I-125 or Palladium-103 isotopes. The target region is measured in its length and width and then a planar implant nomograph is used to estimate the number of radioactive seeds or ribbons required to deliver a minimal peripheral dose of 16,000 cGy or 10-12,000 cGy for palladium. Loose I-125 or palladium seeds can also be implanted in the Gelfoam plaque. Based on nomograph calculation, a matrix is drawn on the Gelfoam with mesh points corresponding to where each seed should be placed. The radioactive seeds can be placed into the Gelfoam matrix by using either long forceps or a standard Mick applicator (Mick Radio-Nuclear Instruments, Bronx, NY, USA) (Figure 3). After the seed placement is completed, a layer of Surgilube is applied to the entry points on the Gelfoam. At this point, another piece of Gelfoam of equal dimensions is sandwiched to the radioactive Gelfoam plaque, using large hemoclips. This completed Gelfoam plaque can then be secured onto the tumor bed either by clips or by using an absorbable suture placed across

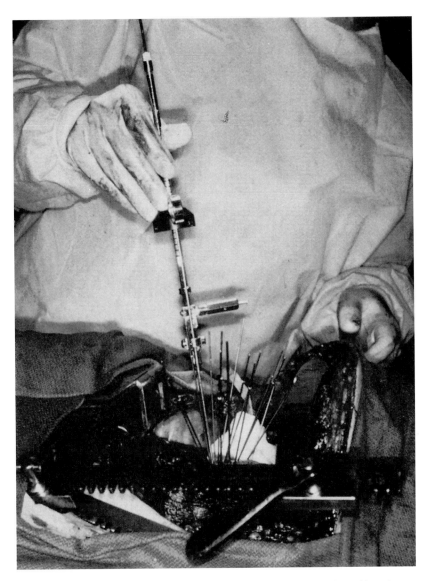

Figure 1. Intraoperative interstitial implant. The afterloading needles are placed into the unresectable tumor. Mick applicator is attached to the needle to deposit the radioactive seeds at prescribed depths.

the plaque from one end of the tumor bed to the other end. When warranted, the Gelfoam plaque may be fixed in place by using a Dexon/Vicryl mesh, which may be sutured or clipped to the tumor bed to prevent slippage. Various steps of this procedure are shown in Figure 3.

The low average photon energy of I-125 or Pd-103 limits radiation exposure, requires little or no postoperative radiation precau-

tions, and thus also reduces hospital costs by eliminating the need for a shielded room. The rapid attenuation of dose beyond the implanted site also reduces the normal tissue damage by limiting the integral dose. The technique described here (Nori/Hilaris technique) has been applied in a variety of clinical sites in thoracic malignancies without untoward complications or any undue prolongation of hospitalization stay. Figure 4 shows

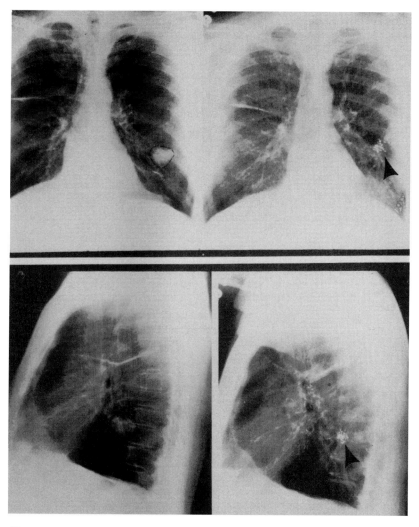

Figure 2. Unresectable tumor in the left lower lobe implanted with I-125 pellets. Also seen is a 4-year follow-up radiograph showing complete shrinkage of the implanted mass with no evidence of radiation changes in the normal lung.

the axial chest CT in a 54-year-old patient who presented with non-small cell lung cancer who underwent an intraoperative I-125 plaque implant for minimal residual disease after resection near the arch of the aorta.[15]

The Gelfoam plaque is extremely useful for treating close or positive microscopic margins in such sites as the mediastinum and paraspinal area. In these sites, the close or positive surgical margins are generally in proximity to vital structures. Further attempts at resection may involve a major surgical extirpation, and

a standard afterloading removable implant technique may not be technically feasible following such a procedure.

The preparation of the Gelfoam plaque with Vicryl mesh (corresponding to the required surgical tumor bed) is performed outside the patient; hence seed placement and measurements can be done with a relatively high degree of accuracy and reproducibility. The flexibility of the Gelfoam Vicryl plaque enables the implant to be used on highly irregular tumor bed defects. The placement of

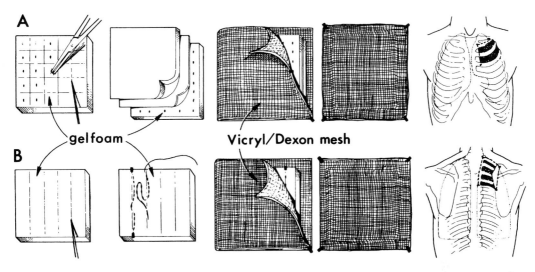

Figure 3. Step by step diagrams for Gelfoam plaque implants. A) Gelfoam plaque implant using individual I-125 or Pd-103 seeds. B) Gelfoam plaque implant using vicryl sutures.

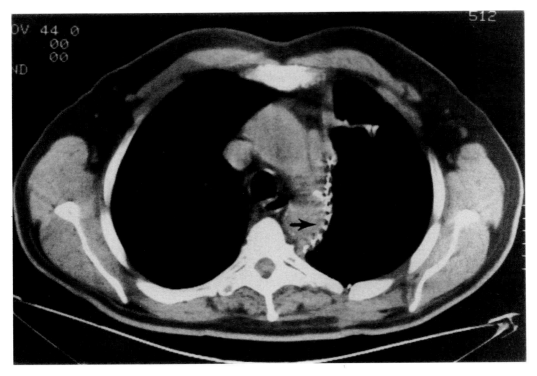

Figure 4. Placement of a Gelfoam plaque implant in the mediastinum after complete resection of a tumor with positive margins.

the Gelfoam plaque between two layers of absorbable Vicryl-Dexon mesh decreases the likelihood of displacement of the sources or seeds and an additional single Dexon suture across the plaque after its placement in the tumor bed further assures accurate positioning of the plaque.

Temporary Interstitial Implantation Technique

Temporary implants with Ir-192 (LDR or remote afterloading HDR) or high activity I-125 are useful in the treatment of mediastinal, paravertebral, or chest wall tumors.

The technique of temporary interstitial brachytherapy is as follows: the skin of the anterior chest wall between the nipple and anterior axillary line is marked with a sterile pen to indicate the points through which the catheters will be passed into the chest. A hollow, straight stainless steel needle (17 gauge, 15 cm long) is inserted into the chest through the planned mark on the skin. The closed end of a plastic catheter is threaded through the stainless steel needle until it emerges from the opposite end of the needle. The needle is then removed while the plastic catheter is held in the chest and the needle is pulled out through the chest wall. In this manner, the process is repeated for the planned number of afterloading catheters determined using the "planar implant guide."[21] Each catheter (with an inner steel cable) is placed in the desired position in the mediastinum and secured with number 2 or 3 chromic or Dexon suture material. Metallic clips are placed near each closed end of the catheter for later identification of this end on the localization radiographs. The afterloading catheters are then fixed to the skin by threading a plastic hemisphere through the projecting end of the catheter, followed by a stainless steel button. The stainless steel button is then secured to the skin with silk sutures.

The radioactive sources are afterloaded into the catheters 3–5 days after surgery in order to facilitate the nursing care in the first postoperative days and to allow some time for tissue healing that will decrease the risk of complications. This technique is used to deliver additional radiation doses to the mediastinum, chest wall, and paravertebral resection sites. In LDR Ir-192 temporary implants, a minimal peripheral dose of 3000 cGy is prescribed and is supplemented with 4500–5000 cGy of external beam radiation. The evaluation of the dosimetric calculations and the determination of the implanted time is done according to the guidelines previously described.[22]

In HDR Ir-192 intraoperative temporary remote afterloading implants, a minimal peripheral dose of 1000 cGy is delivered in 3–4 minutes and the afterloading catheters are removed following the treatment. Figure 5 shows the placement of three remote afterloading catheters used to treat positive surgical margins with intraoperative radiation after chest wall resection. It also shows the three-dimensional dose reconstruction encompassing the target volume.[15]

Results

The results of treatment with interstitial brachytherapy is presented in Table 3.[15]

Results in Early Non-Small Cell Lung Cancer

Very few reports in the literature refer to the results of curative radiation therapy in early lung cancer. From 1958–1984, 55 patients with stage I and II non-small cell lung cancer were surgically explored and treated with intraoperative brachytherapy without surgical resection. Locoregional control was 100% in small T1 lesions and 70% in large T2 lesions. The overall 5-year survival rate was 32% and the disease-free survival rate was 63%.[22]

Results in Locally Advanced Non-Small Cell Lung Cancer

From 1977–1980 an additional 88 patients with stage III non-small lung cancer with involved mediastinal nodes were treated with a combination of surgery, brachytherapy, and postoperative external radiation. This combined approach has improved the local control rate from 63% in the earlier period to 75%. The median survival was 26 months and 2-year survival was 51%.[23] In patients who sur-

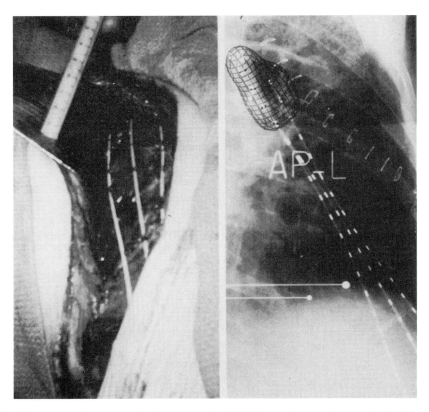

Figure 5. Placement of catheters for intraoperative HDR brachytherapy in a patient with a resected chest wall tumor with positive margins. A dose of 1000 cGy was delivered and the catheters were removed. A three-dimensional isodose is also shown.

vived more than 2 years and in whom the lung cancer was locally controlled, no significant pulmonary toxicity was appreciated.[24]

Results in Unresectable Tumors with Negative Nodes (T3NO)

From 1986–1987, 225 patients underwent exploration, resection, and/or brachytherapy. Forty-nine patients underwent complete resection with a reported 2-year survival of 29%. Patients in whom only a partial resection was possible and who underwent brachytherapy in addition had a 2-year survival of 30%.

Patients who received brachytherapy without resection had a 21% 2-year survival and the biopsy only group had a 9% 2-year survival. Patients with incomplete resection and brachytherapy had similar 2-year survival compared with patients who underwent complete resection.[25] Figure 6 shows pre- and 10-

year posttreatment radiographs in a patient with unresectable tumor who underwent intraoperative brachytherapy.

Results in Superior Sulcus Tumors

Intraoperative brachytherapy has been particularly useful in superior sulcus tumors.[26,27] The majority of these patients are unresectable because of extension to the brachial plexus and to the spine. Treatment by external radiation therapy alone or surgery alone has usually been inadequate. Hilaris et al.[27] reported 127 patients treated by surgery combined with interstitial brachytherapy or external beam irradiation or both. Sixty-six patients received preoperative external irradiation and 61 patients did not. Patients who had either a partial resection or no resection were treated by brachytherapy.

In the absence of regional or distant metas-

Table 3.
Results of Interstitial Brachytherapy in Non-Small Cell Lung Carcinoma

Author	Patient Category	No. of Patients	Brachytherapy Technique	Results of Treatment %	
				Local Control	Survival (Years)
Hilaris[22]	Early stage Stage I	55	Permanent interstitial	85	33 (5 year)
Hilaris[24]	Locally advanced Unresectable tumors with negative nodes	322	Permanent interstitial	71	20 (2 year)
Hilaris[24]	Locally advanced Unresectable tumors with positive nodes	152	Permanent interstitial	63	9 (2 year)
Hilaris[23]	Locally advanced Unresectable tumors with positive nodes	88	Permanent implant of primary + temporary implant (Ir-192) of mediastinum (3000 cGy/3 days)	76	51 (2 year)
Burt[25]	Locally advanced Chest wall tumors (T3N0)	225	Permanent interstitial and/or temporary implants	70	29 (2 year) Complete resection only 30 (2 year) Incomplete resection + brachytherapy 21 (2 year) brachytherapy 9 (2 year) Biopsy only
Hilaris[27]	Locally advanced Superior sulcus tumors	127	Pre-op RT, partial resection + permanent and/or temporary implant	70	20 (10 year)

RT = radiotherapy.

tases, better survival was observed. Survival was best when the tumor was completely resected. However, the majority had unresectable tumors and were treated primarily by interstitial brachytherapy. The 5- and 10-year survival of this group of patients was 20%.[27]

Endobronchial Brachytherapy

Endobronchial tumor may be controlled by a variety of different methods, either used singly, or in combination. The commonly reported methods are biopsy recanalization, electrocoagulation, cryosurgery, laser resection, photodynamic therapy, endobronchial prosthesis, external beam radiotherapy, and endobronchial brachytherapy (both HDR and

LDR). These methods are tabulated in Table 4. In this section, the historical evolution of endobronchial radiation, current techniques, results, and side effects will be reviewed. A summary of complimentary and competing treatment modalities is provided at the end of this section.

History

The earliest reported use of endobronchial brachytherapy is credited to Sidney Yankauer[28] from New York who in 1922 reported on implantation of radon capsules (via a rigid bronchoscope under local anesthesia) in two patients with bronchial carcinoma with good response. Soon thereafter, Kernan[29] and later

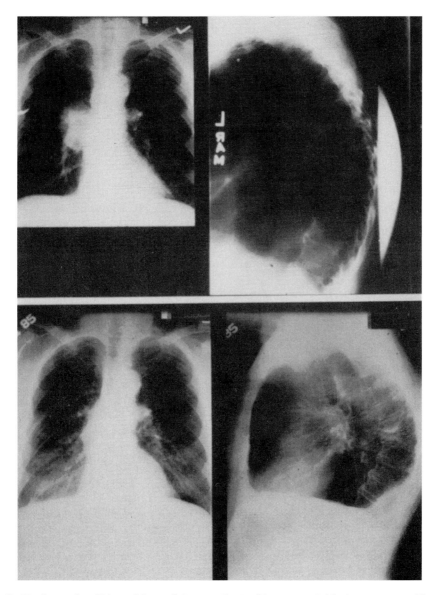

Figure 6. Radiographs (PA and lateral) in a patient with unresectable lung cancer. The patient underwent intraoperative brachytherapy with permanent as well as temporary implant. A 5-year follow-up radiograph showing complete resolution of the masses is shown. The patient is currently free of disease at 11 years following the procedure.

Pancoast[30] also reported their experiences with endobronchial brachytherapy. Unfortunately, this technique suffered from two main disadvantages, i.e., the relatively large size of the radon capsules and the low specific activity requiring long residence times up to 5 days. Consequently, no major clinical series were reported until the 1940s when Ormerod[31] presented his experience in 100 patients, focusing principally on the considerable limitations of radon seed implantation. This led to the abandonment of any major activity in the field of endobronchial brachytherapy for almost two decades.

Table 4.
Techniques for the Management of
Endobronchial Disease

1. Biopsy recanalization
2. Electrocoagulation
3. Cryosurgery
4. Laser therapy
5. Photodynamic therapy
6. Endobronchial prosthesis
7. External beam radiotherapy
8. Brachytherapy

In the 1960s, endobronchial brachytherapy enjoyed a brief resurgence and sudden demise due to the introduction of cobalt-60 beads.[32] These beads, with a diameter of 6–8 mm, could be attached to an iron wire that could be implanted into the bronchial tree. Compared to the relatively low activity of radon of 30 millicurie, these beads were more than twice as active at 80 millicurie, permitting a relatively short residence time of 3–5 hours. Unfortunately, the lack of afterloading led to considerable personnel exposure, resulting in the abandonment of the technique by the late 1960s.[33]

By 1964, Henschke et al.[34] had already introduced a hand-cranked, remote afterloading device with a Co-60 source for use in cervical carcinoma. Within a few years, the hand-crank was replaced by a motor and the stepwise motion of the source permitted the delivery of tailored brachytherapy. Sauerwein developed computerized control for the device, which was named Gammamed I, and this became available for endobronchial treatment in 1979.[35] During this period, experience was being reported not only with this new device,[36,37] but also with cesium-137[38,39] and with interstitial implantation of gold[40] and iodine. Although this technique reportedly produced excellent palliation in a series of 27 patients,[40] the risks of permanent interstitial implantation included hemorrhage, edema, and the potential for seed loss into the pleural space and, as a consequence, this technique did not become widespread.

Two developments in the 1980s led to a significant increase in the utilization of endobronchial brachytherapy. First, the advent of fiberoptic bronchoscopy and its widespread dissemination as well as the simultaneous use of effective local anesthesia, antitussive agents, and intravenous sedation allowed the insertion of small caliber afterloading catheters in every major branch of the tracheobronchial tree, even in critically ill patients. These flexible catheters could be inserted under direct visual guidance and subsequently afterloaded either manually or with remote afterloaders. The second major development was the availability of high activity iridium-192 that could either be obtained as multiple end-to-end seeds simulating a line source or as high activity seeds driven by a remote afterloader.[41]

The 1980s were characterized by the parallel development of several of these techniques. In 1985, Schray et al.[42] reported on the use of a 2-mm diameter, 125-cm long blind-end nylon catheter manually afterloaded with iridium seeds and left in situ for 30–60 hours. The dose rate at 1 cm was usually 50–100 cGy/hr. In 1986, Joyner and Hauskins[43] manually placed iridium seeds into an angio-catheter with an anchoring balloon. The large size precluded the use of the accessory channel on the bronchoscope, and therefore, this angio-catheter was slid over a guide wire that was inserted first at the time of bronchoscopy. Seagren et al.,[37] in 1985, used a 3-mm cobalt-60 seed for HDR treatment with a 4-mm diameter and 46-cm long catheter, which could not be used in the distal airways because of width considerations. In the same year, Korba et al.[44] reported on the use of a 10 curie, 1.2-mm diameter, and 1-cm long iridium-192 source attached to a 2-mm thick cable that was driven by a remote afterloader. The microSelectron-HDR was developed in the late 1980s. It uses a 1.1-mm diameter, 6-mm long high activity iridium-192 source attached to a 1.1-mm diameter cable that can be inserted into a 5Fr (1.7 mm) catheter. The source position can be programmed in 1–48 dwell positions, either in 2.5- or 5-mm increments, thereby allowing coverage of up to 12 or 24 cm length.

Techniques

Program Prerequisites

The prerequisites for an effective endobronchial brachytherapy program are:

1. A reliable remote afterloading machine characterized by excellent shielding, small source diameter, high specific activity, availability of multiple channels and computer control, which allows modulation of source position, dwell spaces, and dwell times for HDR or readily available iridium seeds for LDR brachytherapy.
2. A good treatment planning program that allows rapid and accurate calculation of the dose distribution.
3. Suitable endobronchial catheters.
4. A dedicated team of pulmonologists, radiation oncologists, radiation physicists, and support personnel functioning within a short distance of both the radiation therapy facility as well as the endoscopy suite.

Catheter Placement

Prior to the procedure, thorough evaluation of the patient including a full history and physical examination as well as all pertinent laboratory parameters is essential. It is critical to be aware of the patient's cardiac and pulmonary status. Pretreatment CT sometimes aids in localizing the obstruction. At the University of Wisconsin, coagulation studies are not routinely obtained unless a biopsy is also planned.

The procedure is performed in a fully equipped endoscopy suite. Patients are continually monitored in terms of pulse, blood pressure, pulse oximetry, and ECG at 3- to 5-minute intervals. Continuous oxygen at 3–4 liters per minute is provided per nasal cannula. The nasal passages are anesthetized using 10% lidocaine jelly. Demerol, 50–100 mg, intravenous or intramuscular is used for sedation. Either atropine (0.4–0.6 mg intravenous) or glycopyrolate (200–400 μg) is used to minimize secretions. If necessary, codeine, 30–60 mg intramuscular may be used as an antitussive. To provide adequate sedation, midazolam 0.5–1 mg intravenous is used and repeated as necessary. Usually a total dose of 1–3 mg is needed, but age is a very important factor in determining total dose. Airway anesthesia is attained with 1% lidocaine in 2- to 3-mL aliquots. In order to ensure adequate anesthesia of the vocal cords, 4–5 squirts of

2–3 mL each are usually necessary. Further lidocaine, as necessary, is used once the bronchoscope has been negotiated past the vocal cords. As a matter of routine practice at the University of Wisconsin, a video camera head with photographic documentation of the lesion is used. It is extremely useful to measure the distance between the proximal and, if possible, the distal end of the tumor from a fixed internal landmark such as the tracheal carina. This allows determination of the longitudinal tumor dimension, which can be correlated to a reference point on the simulator radiographs, i.e., the carina. After inspection of both sides and determination of the number of catheters required, placement is carried out through the accessory port. A radioopaque internal stiffening cable assists in placing the catheter without kinking, dislodgment, or getting stuck at the obstruction. The goal is to place the catheter at some distance past the obstruction. The distal airways actually hold the catheter in place without the need for fixating devices. The placement is confirmed visually and fluoroscopically, and the bronchoscope is withdrawn under continuous fluoroscopy to maintain catheter position. The catheter is then secured at the nose, marked with indelible ink to provide a visual alert in case of displacement, and as an additional precautionary measure, the external length from the tip of the nostril is documented and verified again prior to actual treatment.

Endobronchial Applicators

A variety of different applicators are available for HDR brachytherapy. The major differences between various applicators usually affect the caliber, the length (100 vs 150 cm), the composition, the presence of a radio-opaque tip, the presence of an inflatable balloon, and the presence of distance markers. Although various systems including outer sheaths, balloons, and cages have been designed to hold the catheter in a central location in the airway, in order to avoid localized hot spots on the bronchial mucosa, these have generally not been found to be necessary in the vast majority of patients. The simple procedure of lodging the catheter distal to the obstructed airway is sufficient to hold it in place. Metal-tipped catheters should obviously be avoided if concomitant hyperthermia is contemplated. The most common calibers used are either 5Fr (1.7 mm) or 6Fr (2 mm). If a 6Fr catheter is used, a bronchoscope with a 2.2-mm diameter port hole is required. In contrast, if a 5Fr catheter is used, a bronchoscope with a 2.0-mm diameter port hole is sufficient. When starting out, it is advisable to ensure that the bronchoscope will accommodate the catheter to be used. The 6Fr catheter is better at negotiating acute curvature such as the right upper lobe. These catheters are usually quite flexible, but the larger 4-mm catheter is not as flexible. This semirigid catheter has the advantage of keeping its shape during treatment, and dislocation is extremely uncommon. Its introduction requires a ventilation tube, which mandates the use of the oral instead of the nasal route. Although extensively used in Europe, it is not commonly utilized in the United States.

Remote Afterloaders

The Gammamed II (Frank Baker Associates, Pequannock, NJ, USA) and the microSelectron (Nucleotron Corporation, Columbia, MD, USA) HDR are the leading afterloading machines currently on the market. Recently, the Omnitron (Omnitron International, Houston, TX, USA) with its ultra small source has also become available. Currently, the manufacturers provide the software for dosimetry.

Treatment Planning

The routine at the University of Wisconsin involves using the microSelectron HDR (10 Curie initial activity, changed approximately every 3 months at 4.3 Ci) with 6Fr catheters, and obtaining orthogonal radiographs with dummy seeds in place at the "best" angles as determined at the simulator. The seed positions are then digitized from dwell position 1. Although a spacing of 2.5 mm is used to provide 48 dwell positions, this can be varied. In general, the first dummy seed is labeled as the first dwell unless the implant length is expected to exceed 48 dwell positions. Optimization points are then placed at target radii in four cardinal directions, starting from the first active dwell position. As a rough guide, the first active dwell position is usually placed at

approximately half the radial treatment distance from the catheter. When using multiple catheters, it is crucial not to put optimization points closer than the prescription distance. The spinal cord, at several levels, is always entered in. The current treatment planning system, Nucletron Planning System (NPS), runs on a Silicon Graphics Iris Indigo workstation and is compatible with other UNIX workstations, but not DOS.

Various dose calculation techniques have been described, including the semiorthogonal reconstruction, the isocentric method, and the variable angle reconstruction. They are explained in detail in the treatment planning chapter.[45–47]

The Prescription Point

Because various authors have used different prescription points, total doses, and number of fractions, meaningful comparison between different studies is not always possible. Some authors[48] have suggested adopting 1 cm as the standard, but this is not universally accepted.[49] In fact, prescription depths ranging from 0.5–2 cm have been used, and these differences reflect the changing caliber of the tracheo-bronchial tree, the eccentric location of some catheters that are pushed to one side by the endoluminal tumor, as well as the desire to treat some of the peribronchial tumor in order to achieve a sustained response. Of course, toxicity concerns also affect the choice of the prescription point. With improvements in technology, three-dimensional brachytherapy planning may become feasible and cost effective and may then permit tailoring of the dose distribution to the three-dimensional shape of the tumor. The longitudinal margin is usually 1–2 cm and is not the subject of much debate.

Dose and Fractionation

The dose and fractionation for HDR brachytherapy varies widely, ranging from 15 Gy in one fraction to 4–5 fractions of 4 Gy each. The prescribed dose is, of course, highly dependent on the depth prescribed. A 1-week interval between fractions is most commonly used. At the University of Wisconsin, however, we typically prescribe four fractions of

4 Gy each, prescribed to 1 cm depth, given twice daily over 2 days. Depending on the previous total irradiated dose or location (for example, the left upper lobe bronchus), the prescribed depth or number of fractions may be reduced. The endobronchial catheter remains in place between fractions, thus eliminating the need for multiple bronchoscopies. The majority of patients treated with this regimen have been treated on an out-patient basis.

The routine previously used at the University of Wisconsin for LDR brachytherapy involved a similar bronchoscopic procedure as that described for HDR. A 1.6-mm polyethylene catheter was typically placed 2 cm distal to the tumor. Different sized diameter catheters have been used in other institutions.[42] Iridium-192 with activities of 37–48 MBq per seed were used, with a dose rate of 35–40 cGy/hr at 2 cm from the center of the source. Patients were typically prescribed 20–30 Gy, at a depth of 2 cm, with 2 cm proximal and distal tumor margins. CT scanning was used in treatment planning to better assess the dose distribution prior to the placement of the radioactive seeds. All patients required hospitalization in a lead-lined room during treatment (usually 2 days).

Results

Endobronchial brachytherapy is most often used for palliative purposes, but is slowly being explored in selected patients as a form of boost with curative intent. No major prospective randomized multi-institution studies of this modality have been reported, and the lack of uniformity and standardization has remained a major obstacle.

The following are the major clinical questions:

1. Should brachytherapy be used alone or in combination with laser debulking?
2. Is LDR or HDR brachytherapy more clinically advantageous?
3. What is the appropriate dose, fractionation, and prescription point?
4. How should palliation be measured?
5. Which patients might benefit from the integration of an up-front endobronchial boost as curative therapy?
6. What is the toxicity profile?

Palliative Endobronchial Brachytherapy

This is perhaps the single most common indication of endobronchial brachytherapy. Both LDR and HDR techniques have been used. Several single institution results of LDR have now been published and are summarized in Table 5. Symptomatic improvement is reported in 50%–100% of these patients, radiographic improvement in 17%–78%, and bronchoscopic improvement in 60%–93%.[42,50–58]

Similar results have been reported in almost 1000 patients treated with HDR brachytherapy.[35,37,51,57–66] A number of different treatment schema have been reported and are summarized in Table 6. The functional, radiographic, and endoscopic improvement following HDR endobronchial brachytherapy is summarized in Table 7, and it ranges from 50%–100% for clinical improvement, 46%–88% for radiographic reaeration, and 59%–100% for bronchoscopic response. This variability is explained by several factors, including inhomogenous groups of patients and tumors, variable additional treatments including laser and external radiation, as well as the use of different treatment schema. Therefore, the exact contribution of each of these variables is impossible to tease out.

Although some authors[63] have suggested that the addition of laser improves outcome significantly, this is not borne out in some of the larger series.[59] Similarly, it is difficult to make a case for higher doses because a clear cut, dose-response relationship does not seem to be apparent. In fact, the only relatively strong data supporting a dose-response relationship come from an LDR study reported by Lo et al.[53] and illustrated in Figure 7.

Speiser has described a concise and user-friendly symptom index wherein the four major problems associated with airway occlusion, hemoptysis, pneumonia, dyspnea, and cough are graded on a subjective scale from 0–4 (Table 8). He has also described an "obstruction" score for assessment of the degree of endoluminal blockage at the time of endoscopy. At the University of Wisconsin, a "symptom resolution" data sheet has been

Table 5.
Results of Low-Dose-Rate Trials

Author	Patients	Symptoms Improved	X-Ray Improved	Bronch Improved
Allen[50]	15	100%	38%	NA
Lo[53]	87	59%	NA	76%
Locken[54]	18	83%	NA	70%
Mehta[51]	66	78%	78%	93%
Paradelo[55]	32	66%	21%	85%
Roach[52]	17	53%	17%	60%
Schray[42]	65	NA	NA	60%
Susnerwala[56]	14	50%	75%	NA

utilized for determination of response (Table 9). The use of such tools is highly encouraged as it allows for some standardization in this field. Since the palliative response from endobronchial brachytherapy is usually good to excellent, the modality has now become almost routine in patients with an endobronchial recurrence. An important aspect of this palliation is its durability. It appears from most studies that almost $\frac{2}{3}$ to $\frac{3}{4}$ of the remainder of the patients' lifetime is rendered symptom-improved or symptom-free.[51]

Table 6.
Literature Review of
Endobronchial Schema

Author	Patients	Dose (Gy)*	Fractions
Bedwinek[62]	38	18	3
Burt[60]	50	15–20	1
Fass[61]	15	3–36	1–6
Gauwitz[58]	24	18	2
Kohek[64]	81	10–21	2–3
Macha[35]	56	22.5	3
Mehta[51]	66	32	4
Miller[63]	88	30	3
Nori[57]	15	60	3
Seagren[37]	20	10	1
Speiser[59]	144	30	3
Speiser[59]	151	22.5	3
Speiser[59]**	47	15	3
Stout[65]	100	15–20	1
Sutedja[66]	31	30	3
Total	926		

* Dose at 1 cm.

** Intermediate dose rate.

Curative Endobronchial Brachytherapy

The logical patient group that could ideally be treated with endobronchial radiation for cure would be patients with in situ disease picked up on screening bronchoscopy. Such patients are not frequently encountered and, in the few small series reported, they have generally been treated with phototherapy.[67]

There is a small but increasing body of data that would suggest that, in selected patients with more advanced disease, endobronchial brachytherapy as an additional boost to external beam radiotherapy is useful. Reddi and Marbach[68] reported on a small study of 32 patients with newly diagnosed advanced non-small cell lung cancer treated with initial 60 Gy in 30 fractions followed by HDR boost endobronchial radiation of 7.5 Gy at 1 cm with an optional second and third brachytherapy boost 2 and 4 weeks later if residual tumor was found at repeat bronchoscopy.[68] The re-aeration response was 100%. In the eight patients in whom 3-month biopsies were available, none demonstrated residual tumor. The median survival, however, was only 8 months. Aygun and colleagues[69] reported on 62 patients with medically inoperable or surgically unresectable disease treated with both external beam radiotherapy to 50–60 Gy and HDR brachytherapy in three to five fractions of 5 Gy at 1 cm. The median survival was slightly better at 13 months but probably reflected the fact that some patients had stage I disease. They noted that median survival for N_o patients was 20 months compared to 9 months for N_+ patients. Bastin et al.[70] have previously reported on a group of 22 patients

Table 7.
Outcome Data for HDR Endobronchial Brachytherapy

Author	Clinical Response	Radiographic Response	Bronch Response
Bedwinek[62]	76%	64%	82%
Burt[60]	50%–86%	46%	88%
Fass[61]	75%	NA	NA
Gauwitz[58]	88%	83%	100%
Kohek[64]	65%–77%	26%	61%
Macha[35]	74%	88%	75%
Mehta[51]	71%–100%	85%	NA
Miller[63]	NA	NA	80%
Nori[57]	80%	88%	NA
Seagren[37]	94%	NA	100%
Speiser[59]	85%–99%	NA	80%
Stout[65]	51%–86%	46%	NA
Sutedja[66]	NA	NA	72%

with newly diagnosed stage IIIA or B non-small cell lung cancer who were ineligible for other protocols because of poor KPS, weight loss, significant atelectasis/collapse, or other factors and were, therefore, treated with up-front brachytherapy followed by 60 Gy external radiation. A 67% reaeration rate was noted and, using sequential volume integration, it was demonstrated that 47% and 25% of the lung volume was spared external radiation in patients achieving complete and partial reaeration, respectively. Although there was a trend toward improved survival among reaerators, the overall median survival was only

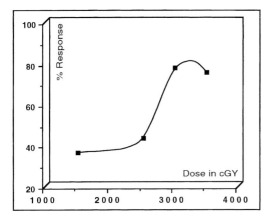

Figure 7. Dose-response relationship (clinical improvement). Data from Lo et al.[53] based on LDR dose at 2 cm.

34 weeks. In a case report from Sutedja,[71] a patient with unresectable cancer because of disease extending to the main carina was rendered resectable following brachytherapy.

Such data suggest that, in selected patients, endobronchial boost therapy is likely to produce significant reaeration and hence sparing of lung volume from subsequent external radiation. A few cases may even become resectable. Demonstration of a considerable survival advantage will, however, require a larger clinical trial with adequate controls.

Another innovative curative application of this modality is in an adjuvant setting following surgical resection, which leaves behind minimal disease at the bronchial stump, either as a positive margin or as positive washings following resection. Macha and Wahlers[72] have recently reported on a series of 17 such patients treated on a pilot study with tumor-free survival times of up to 4 years.

Complications

Fatal Hemoptysis

Relatively little has been reported on the long-term tolerance of the tracheo-bronchial tree to HDR endobronchial brachytherapy. However, more detailed follow-up of patients treated with this modality is beginning to demonstrate that a certain proportion of patients experience fatal hemoptysis. The estimates of the occurrence of this complication

Table 8.
Sympton Index

Score	Definition
	Hemoptysis
0	None
1	<2 times/week
2	<daily but >2 times/week
3	Daily, bright red blood or clots
4	Decrease of Hb/Hct. >10%, >150 cc, requiring hospitalization or leading to respiratory distress
	Pneumonia/Elevated Temperature
0	Normal temperature, no infiltrates, WBC <10,000
1	Temperature >38.5 and infiltrate, WBC <10,000
2	Temperature >38.5 and infiltrate and/ or WBC >10,000
3	Lobar consolidation on radiograph
4	Pneumonia or elevated temperature requiring hospitalization
	Dyspnea
0	None
1	Dyspnea on moderate exertion
2	Dyspnea with normal activity, walking on level ground
3	Dyspnea at rest
4	Requires supplemental oxygen
	Cough
0	None
1	Intermittent, no medication necessary
2	Intermittent, non-narcotic medication
3	Constant or requiring narcotic medication
4	Constant, requiring narcotic medication but without relief

is flawed and under-reported in most series because only absolute numbers are provided without factoring in patients who were not "at risk."

A literature review of the reported rates of fatal hemoptysis in patients undergoing either HDR or LDR endobronchial radiotherapy is presented in Tables 10 and 11. Overall, the average fatal hemoptysis rate for LDR, intermediate-dose-rate (IDR), or HDR do not appear to be significantly different, and the mean values are 5% and 8%. However, the HDR group appears to contain some significant "outliers." The exact causes for this variance have not totally been defined, but could include inaccurate reporting, variable follow-up, different patient populations, different prior, concomitant, and sequential therapeutic measures, different rates of follow-up bronchoscopy, biopsy (which could induce trauma), the total length treated, and total dose, as well as fractionation. These issues can only be sorted out in a prospective trial.

When the switch was made from LDR to HDR at the University of Wisconsin, radiobiological modeling was carried out in an attempt to limit this particular complication.[51] In the LDR group, a dose of 20 Gy at 2 cm was routinely prescribed, which equates to approximately 50 Gy at 1 cm. Using the α/β formulation, a 60% increase in late effects was predicted if a single equivalent fraction was to be utilized for HDR. A schema was chosen using four fractions of 4 Gy each at 2 cm delivered over 2 days with the catheter left in place for the duration. No significant differences in fatal hemoptysis were found using this approach.

Bedwinek et al.[62] noted a surprisingly high 32% rate of fatal hemoptysis in their series of 38 patients. In an attempt to sort out treatment related hemoptysis from tumor related hemoptysis, they constructed a time curve of cumulative probability of hemoptysis that suggested a >90% risk beyond 25 weeks. However, because a substantial number of these events occurred at such a short point in time following brachytherapy, the role of tumor progression in causing hemoptysis must be seriously evaluated. In fact, three of five patients undergoing bronchoscopic evaluation prior to hemoptysis were found to have tumor. This may in fact suggest that hemoptysis might even represent failure of therapy rather than a consequence![73] In a further analysis to identify risk factors for hemoptysis, Bedwinek noted that prior laser therapy, prior external radiation, and size of extrabronchial disease did not influence the rate of hemoptysis. Hemoptysis as a presenting symptom also did not influence the ultimate rate of hemoptysis. Interestingly, two of four (50%) patients who had two courses of brachytherapy died from hemoptysis, compared to a 29% rate for the single-course group. The factor most closely associated with a high risk was location, with the left upper lobe demonstrating a 75% (6/8) risk. Autopsy data on patients dying

Table 9.
Endobronchial Brachytherapy Data Sheet

Sympton Resolution

Patient name: _____

History number: _____

Date of implant: _____

Date of follow-up: _____

Symptom	Present	Absent	Improved	Worsened
Cough*				
Dyspnea*				
Pneumonia⊗				
Hemoptysis°				
Chest Pain∅				

*	Grade 0	Grade 1	Grade 2	Grade 3	Grade 4
Cough	None	Mild, dry, no meds	Persistent, requiring anti-tussives	Severe, unresponsive to narcotic anti-tussive	Severe, respiratory
Dyspnea	None	Mild dyspnea on exertion	Dyspnea with minimal effort, but not at rest	Dyspnea at rest, intermittent oxygen	Continuous oxygen necessary

⊗ Pneumonia:
  (a) Clinically obvious findings: antibiotics required.
  (b) Positive sputum cultures with elevated white count (≥1.5 × normal).
  (c) Radiographically obvious pneumonia.
° Hemoptysis: Present or absent
∅ Chest pain: Patient's perception

Table 10.
Fatal Hemoptysis Rates (LDR/IDR) Reported in the Literature

Author	Year	Technique	Patients	Number	% Fatal Hemoptysis
Lo[53]	1992	LDR	87	3	3
Locken[54]	1990	LDR	27	0	0
Mehta[51]	1992	LDR	66	4	6
Paradelo[55]	1992	LDR	32	3	9
Roach[52]	1990	LDR	17	0	0
Schray[42]	1988	LDR	65	7	11
Speiser[59]	1993	LDR	47	2	4
Susnerwala[56]	1992	LDR	14	0	0
Total	1988–1993		355	19	5

IDR = intermediate-dose-rate; LDR = low-dose-rate.

Table 11.
Fatal Hemoptysis rates (HDR) Reported in the Literature

Author	Year	Technique	Patients	Number	% Fatal Hemoptysis
Aygun[69]	1992	HDR	62	9	15
Bedwinek[62]	1992	HDR	38	12	32
Burt[60]	1990	HDR	50	0	0
Fass[61]	1990	HDR	15	0	0
Gauwitz[58]	1992	HDR	24	1	4
Khanavkar[75]	1991	HDR	12	6	50
Kohek[64]	1990	HDR	81	3	4
Macha[35]	1987	HDR	56	4	7
Mehta[51]	1992	HDR	31	1	3
Miller[63]	1990	HDR	88	0	0
Nori[57]	1987	HDR	15	0	0
Seagren[37]	1985	HDR	20	5	25
Speiser[59]	1993	HDR	295	23	8
Stout[65]	1990	HDR	100	0	0
Sutedja[66]	1992	HDR	31	10	32
Total	1985–1993		918	74	8

HDR = high-dose-rate.

from lung cancer not treated by brachytherapy reveal that the left upper lobe is in fact a "high-risk" site. Miller and McGregor,[74] in an autopsy series of 877 cases, found an overall incidence of fatal hemoptysis of 29/877 (3.3%), but the risk in the left upper lobe was 15/120 (12.5%). An additional risk factor in this autopsy study was the histologic type with squamous cell carcinoma having a 7.4% (24/326) risk. The authors recreated this situation for dosimetric evaluation and demonstrated that the wall of the pulmonary artery could fall within a "hot-spot" of 20–30 Gy with a single 6 Gy fraction, implying that the total numeric dose to it, including a prior median external beam dose of 60 Gy, could well be in the order of 150 Gy. Obviously, these data must be taken into consideration when retreating left upper lobar lesions. Bedwinek's final hypothesis was that the tumor had already created a fistula between the bronchus and the pulmonary artery, and the brachytherapy may simply have "unplugged" the tumor. Autopsy verification of such a phenomenon is lacking.

Another report with an alarmingly high hemoptysis rate is the one by Khanavkar et al.,[75] reporting a 50% (6/12) occurrence. Interestingly, squamous histology and left upper lobe location predominated in their fatal hemoptysis group. They noted that, although total radiation dose did not influence the occurrence of this complication, the length of irradiated segment of bronchus had some correlation. Patients who developed fatal hemoptysis had an average length of 5.3 cm treated compared to 3.5 cm (a 51% difference) for those not experiencing hemoptysis.

Radiation Bronchitis

Speiser and Spartling[76] have recently described an entity known as radiation bronchitis and stenosis. This was identified during follow-up bronchoscopy and was graded by severity. Grade 1 is mild mucosal inflammation with swelling, characterized by a thin whitish circumferential membrane without endoscopic or clinical evidence of obstruction. Grade 2 is represented by greater exudation from this membrane causing symptoms that might require endoscopic debridement or medical management consisting of steroid therapy both oral and aerosol, inhalation of alkalinized (with $NaHCO_3$ to reduce the viscosity of mucous) bronchodilators, oral mucolytic agents, and antitussives. Grade 3 is defined as a severe inflammatory response with a marked membranous exudate. Mehta et al.[77] have previously described this as "chronic mucosal sloughing" and suggested that a combination of factors such as high-dose external radiation, multiple laser treatments, and a high dose to the mucosa from brachytherapy may play a causative role. Such a reaction may require multiple debridements. The most severe or grade 4 reaction is characterized by significant fibrosis resulting in circumferential narrowing, which requires management with balloon or bougie dilatation, photoresection, or stent placement.

The overall incidence by grade in the report by Speiser and Spartling[76] was 29%, 22%, 20%, and 29% for grades 1 through 4, respectively. They found that risk factors for this complication included large cell histology, concomitant high-dose external beam radiotherapy, the addition of laser therapy, male gender, and longer survival. The risk of fatal hemoptysis was slightly higher in this group at 12% compared to 7% in those who did not develop radiation bronchitis.

Other Fistulae

The occurrence of fistulae at other locations such as the mediastinum or esophagus is less common. In several studies, the incidence of this has been reported to be between 1%–3%.[77] Although not as acutely fatal as tracheo-vascular fistulae, these fistulae are also ultimately fatal. Patients with tracheo-mediastinal fistulae develop lethal mediastinitis over several days to weeks, and patients with tracheo-esophageal fistulae develop aspiration pneumonia.

Other Methods of Treating Endobronchial Disease

Other potential complimentary and competing techniques to treat endobronchial disease are presented below.

Biopsy Recanalization

Endobronchial recanalization, using forceps biopsy via a rigid bronchoscope under general anesthesia, was reported to produce short-term success by Huzly.[78] However, the many disadvantages of this method include the inability to access lesions beyond the primary bronchi, the necessity for general anesthesia, the inability to control peribronchial tumor, and an unacceptably high hemoptysis

rate. For the most part, this method is no longer frequently used, although some "debulking and resection" is still performed at the time of bronchoscopy for placement of brachytherapy catheters. Usually, this does not amount to much beyond a biopsy and gentle suction.

Electrocoagulation

Endoscopic electrosurgery has been extensively used for the removal of colonic polyps. Limited reports of its application in the airways exist. The cautery probe can readily be passed through the accessory channel of the fiberoptic bronchoscope. Polypoid lesions can be rather readily sectioned out. The alternative approach is to vaporize the lesion, but the risk of fire in the bronchus exists.

Cryosurgery

The use of extreme variations in heat and temperature represent further physical methods of endobronchial tumor ablation that have now been used for several years. In general, these techniques also require rigid bronchoscopy and hence, general anesthesia. This limits the level of tumor that can be accessed easily. Additionally, these modalities have no impact on peribronchial tumor.

A prospective study was carried out by Walsh et al.[79] to assess the value of bronchoscopic cryotherapy for palliation of malignant airway occlusion. Symptoms, lung function, radiographic and bronchoscopic findings were recorded serially before and after 81 cryotherapy sessions in 33 consecutive patients. Most patients improved in terms of overall symptoms, stridor, and hemoptysis, and they had an overall improvement in dyspnea. Objective improvement in lung function was seen in 58% of patients. Bronchoscopic evidence of relief of obstruction was seen in 77% of patients and 24% showed improvement in degree of collapse on the radiograph. There were no major complications. These results compared favorably with the results in published series of patients having laser therapy, and it was concluded that bronchoscopic cryotherapy is valuable for the palliation of inoperable bronchial carcinoma.

Laser Therapy

At present, there are three laser systems used for photoablation of endobronchial tumor: the argon laser, the carbon dioxide laser, and the neodymium:yttrium-aluminum-garnet (YAG) laser.

The argon laser light is rapidly and efficiently absorbed by hemoglobin, thus severely limiting the penetration into tissue. When considerable hemorrhage is encountered, this technique can become considerably flawed. The CO_2 laser cannot be conducted using quartz monofilament fibers and thus requires rigid bronchoscopy, with all its limitations. The YAG laser, which can be used both with the rigid as well as the flexible fiberoptic bronchoscope, has tissue penetration of several millimeters up to several centimeters if the dose is increased and has, therefore, become a "favorite" in endobronchial photoresection.[80–89] Although the YAG laser may be used with the flexible bronchoscope, it has been the experience at the University of Wisconsin, as well as the experience reported by others, that the best results may be achieved with the rigid bronchoscope because it permits better visualization, ensures safety by allowing for passage of the bronchoscope beyond the tumor and laser-resecting only while withdrawing, and allows better hemostasis, suction, ventilation, and removal of large pieces of tumor.[90,91] As a consequence, laser-resection is ideally used for tracheal or proximal bronchial lesions beyond which the rigid bronchoscope can be passed.[92,93] Benign tumors as well as low grade malignancies are often well managed by this technique.[94]

The two primary effects of the YAG laser on tissue are thermal necrosis and photocoagulation. The latter effect provides hemostasis, thereby making it easy to remove relatively large tumor pieces once they have undergone thermal necrosis. However, these effects are also responsible for the possible hazards of laser resection, i.e., severe hemorrhage from vascular perforation and the formation of fistulae. Additionally, laser therapy requires that the proportion of oxygen in inhaled air be <50%; and, in compromised patients, this requirement may lead to hypoxemia. Brutinell and colleagues,[95] in an editorial in the journal Chest, warn that "The Nd:Yag laser in the treatment of a tracheo-bronchial neoplasm . . . can also be a dangerous one. After a treatment modality becomes accepted in clinical practice, there is a tendency to become complacent about the risks involved in its use." They report a risk of death from hemorrhage of 2%, fire in the tracheo-bronchial tree, pneumothorax, esophageal fistula, bronchial perforation, and hypoxemia.

The major advantage of laser photoresection is almost immediate relief of airway occlusion, resulting in dramatic symptomatic relief in most patients. For example, in a series of 47 patients undergoing laser resection at the Cleveland Clinic, immediate relief was documented in all 47 patients.[96] In fact, in that particular study, a survival advantage was suggested when laser photoresection preceded radiation therapy as compared to radiation only. However, because of the inherent limitations of laser resection, i.e., the inability to resect submucosal and peribronchial disease, the dramatic responses are typically quite short lived, requiring either multiple resections or the addition of endobronchial radiation. A recent study suggested that when compared with external beam radiation, "faster palliation with fewer side effects is probably achieved with laser therapy," but no supporting data were presented.[97] Although this combination is frequently used, it is unclear whether endobronchial radiation might not eventually achieve the same result, and some reports have even suggested that there may be a higher fistualization risk when the combination approach is used.[98]

Photodynamic Therapy

Photodynamic therapy involves the excitation of a photosensitizer chemical by light that results in the production of chemical species capable of interacting with oxygen to produce radicals that cause cellular death and damage.[99–102] The primary targets are believed to be cellular and mitochondrial membranes, but damage to nucleic acids and proteins is also involved.[103–107] Although several chemicals such as methylene blue, eosin, tetracycline, and chlorophylls have been described as possessing these properties, most interest has focused on the hematoporphyrin derivatives that tend to accumulate in neoplastic tissue after intravenous administration.[108] The half-life in neoplastic tissue is on the order of several days, probably as a consequence of hypervascularity and poor lymphatic drainage.[109]

For endobronchial photodynamic therapy, the commonly used photosensitizers include hematoporphyrin derivative and Photofrin-II. An argon-pumped dye laser producing red light at 630 nm is focused by optical fibers through a fiberoptic bronchoscope to the tumor. More than 300 patients with lung cancer have now been treated with this system, with the largest experience coming from Tokyo Medical College where in a series of 176 patients, a complete response rate of 78% was observed. Tumor size <1 cm appears to be a positive prognostic factor with 100% complete response rate. At the Mayo Clinic, 65 patients have undergone photodynamic endobronchial therapy with a complete response rate of 55% in patients with radiographically occult disease.[67] For more significant endobronchial disease, the current level of sophistication of photodynamic therapy is unlikely to produce significant tumor resolution.

Endobronchial Prosthesis

A number of tracheo-bronchial prosthetic devices have been designed to relieve airway occlusion when other therapeutic options have been exhausted. These include expandable wire stents[110] as well as molded silicone stents,[111,112] several models of which can actually be inserted using flexible bronchoscopes. Metallic stents, however, can also provide a framework for the development of expanding granulation tissue as well as tumor growth and are only indicated in patients with very short life expectancy. Silicone stents can become plugged with dried secretions and require bronchoscopic monitoring.

External Beam Radiotherapy

External beam radiation alone achieves successful reversal of atelectasis and pneumonitis ranging from 21%–61%.[97,113] In the largest reported series, Slawson and Scott[114] reported only a 23% rate of improvement in atelectasis following conventional external beam radiation in 330 patients. In the study by Chetty et al.,[97] all of the patients who responded received >50 Gy; whereas, no patient receiving <50 Gy had a favorable response. Even if patients reaerate with external beam radiation, the time required to achieve this is generally longer than with endobronchial radiation. Since a fair number of patients present with metastatic disease, an immunocompromised state, or a short median survival, waiting several weeks to achieve a palliative result is not optimal and frequently not feasible.

Summary

Local control rates for the majority of lung cancer patients have been poor, leading to substantial morbidity and mortality. Despite the encouraging preliminary data and theoretical rationale for interstitial lung brachytherapy in a number of clinical situations, the widespread use of these techniques has not occurred. Reasons include lack of a randomized trial in advanced disease demonstrating superior local control rates over external radiation alone, the technical demands of the procedure, as well as interest in less invasive radiation techniques.

Endobronchial brachytherapy is an effective technique to control symptoms for a sustained duration in the majority of patients with symptomatic endobronchial disease. Recent technological advances have helped to make this procedure more appealing to the physician and patient alike, which has contributed to its widespread use. Clinical trials are needed to better define the role of this modality in the face of competing and complimentary treatment methods.

References

1. Boring CC, Savires TS, Tong T. Cancer statistics, 1991, Ca-A. Cancer J Clin 1991;41:19–36.
2. Perez CA, Stanley K, Grundy G, et al. Impact of irradiation technique and tumor extent in tumor control and survival of patients with unresectable non-oat cell carcinoma of the lung. Cancer 1982;50:1091–1099.
3. Moylan D. Overview of endobronchial brachytherapy and review of literature. AERALTS II. New Orleans LA, 1987.

4. Cox JD, Yesner R, Mietlowski W, et al. Influence of cell type on failure pattern after irradiation for locally advanced carcinoma of the lung. From the Veterans' Administration Group (VALG). Cancer 1979;44:94–98.

5. Perez CA, Stanley K, Rubin P, et al. A prospective randomized study of various irradiation doses and fractionation schedules in the treatment of inoperable non-oat-cell carcinoma of the lung: Preliminary report by the radiation therapy oncology group. Cancer 1980;45: 2744–2753.

6. Cox JD, Pajak TF, Herskovic A, et al. Five-year survival after hyperfractionated radiation therapy for non-small-cell carcinoma of the lung: Results of RTOG protocol 81–08. Am J Clin Oncol 1991;14:280–284.

7. Emami B, Lyman J, Brown A, et al. Tolerance of normal tissue to therapeutic irradiation. Int J Radiation Oncol Biol Phys 1991;21:109–122.

8. Hancock SL, Hoppe RT, Horning SJ, et al. Intercurrent death after Hodgkin disease therapy in radiotherapy and adjuvant MOPP trials. Ann Intern Med 1988;109:183–189.

9. Graham EA, Singer JJ. Successful removal of an entire lung for carcinoma of the bronchus. JAMA 1933;101:1371–1374.

10. Henschke UK. Interstitial implantation in the treatment of primary bronchogenic carcinoma. AJR 1958;79:981–989.

11. Henschke UK, Hilaris BS, Mohan GD. Afterloading in interstitial and intracavitary radiation therapy. AJR 1963;90:386–395.

12. Hilaris BS, Holt G. Cancer therapy by interstitial and intracavitary radiation. Final report for Public Health Service Grant EC 00113, Bureau of Radiological Health, Rockville, Maryland, 1968.

13. Nori D. Role of intraoperative brachytherapy in non-small cell lung cancer. In: Nori D (ed). Proceedings of International Conference on Thoracic Oncology. Booth Memorial Medical Center, New York, 1991, pp. 43–55.

14. Hilaris BS, Nori D, Anderson LL. Brachytherapy treatment planning. In: Vaeth JM, Meyer J (eds). Frontiers of Radiation Therapy and Oncology, Vol. 21: Treatment Planning in Radiation Therapy of Cancer. 1987, pp. 94–106.

15. Nori D. Intraoperative brachytherapy in non-small cell lung cancer. Sem Surg Onc 1993;9: 99–107.

16. Nori D, Hilaris BS. Brachytherapy in lung, prostate and soft tissue sarcomas. Proceedings of the Endocurietherapy Research Foundation Meeting, Los Angeles, CA, 1984, pp. 115–130.

17. Hilaris BS, Nori D, Anderson LL (eds). An Atlas of Brachytherapy. Clinical Applications in Cancer of the Lung. Macmillan, New York, 1988, pp. 184–202.

18. Marchese M, Nori D, Anderson LL, et al. A versatile permanent planar implant technique utilizing I-125 seed embedded in Gelfoam. Int J Radiat Oncol Biol Phys 1981;194:747–751.

19. Greenblatt D, Nori D, Tankenbaum A, et al. Brachytherapy techniques utilizing I-125 seeds. Endocurie Hypertherm Oncol 1987;3: 73–80.

20. Nori D, Bains M, Hilaris BS, et al. New intraoperative brachytherapy techniques for positive or close surgical margins. J Surg Oncol 1989;42:54–59.

21. Hilaris BS, Nori D, Anderson LL: New approaches to brachytherapy. In DeVita V, Hellman S, Rosenberg S (eds): Principles and Practice of Oncology. Lippincott, Philadelphia, 1986.

22. Hilaris BS, Nori D, Martini N. Results of radiation therapy in stage I and II unresectable non-small cell lung cancer. Endocurie Hypertherm Oncol 1986;2:15–21.

23. Hilaris BS, Nori D, Beattie EJ Jr, et al. Value of perioperative brachytherapy in the management of non-oat cell carcinoma of the lung. Int J Radiat Oncol Biol Phys 1983;9: 1161–1166.

24. Hilaris BS, Martini N. Interstitial brachytherapy in cancer of the lung: 20 year experience. Int J Radiat Oncol Biol Phys 1979;5: 1956–1976.

25. Burt ME, Pomerantz AH, Bains MS, et al. Results of surgical treatment of stage III lung cancer invading mediastinum. Surg Clin North Am 1987;67:997–1000.

26. Nori D, Sundaresan A, Bains M, et al. Bronchogenic carcinoma with invasion of the spine: Treatment with combined surgery and perioperative brachytherapy. JAMA 1982;248: 2491–2492.

27. Hilaris BS, Martini N, Wong GY, et al. Treatment of superior sulcus tumor (Pancoast tumor). Surg Clin North Am 1987;67:965–977.

28. Yankeuer S. Two cases of lung tumour treated bronchoscopically. New York Med J 1922;21:741–742.

29. Kernan JD. Carcinoma of the lung and bronchus. Treatment with radon implantation and diathermy. Arch Otolaryngol 1933;17: 457–475.

30. Pancoast HK. Superior pulmonary sulcus tumor. JAMA 1932;99:1391–1396.

31. Ormerod FC. Some notes on the treatment of carcinoma of the bronchus. J Larynx Otol 1941;56:1–10.

32. Schlungbaum W, Blum H, Brandt HJ. Ergebnisse der endobronchialen strahlentherapie

des bronchialkarzinoms. Radiologie Austria 1962;XIII/3:201.

33. Bublitt G, Labitzke R. Ergenbnisse endobronchialer kontaktbestrahlung des bronchuskarzinomas mit Co 60 Perlen. Strahlentherapie 1967;134:332.

34. Henschke UK, Hilaris BS, Mahan GD. Remote afterloading for intracavitary applicators. Radiology 1964;83:344–345.

35. Macha HN, Koch K, Stadler M, et al. New technique for treating occlusive and stenosing tumours of the trachea and main bronchii: Endobronchial irradiation by high dose iridium-192 combined with laser canalization. Thorax 1987;42:511–515.

36. Rooney SM, Goldnier PL, Bains MS, et al. Anesthesia for the application of endotracheal and endobronchial radiation therapy. J Thorac Cardiovasc Surg 1984;87:693–697.

37. Seagren SL, Havvel JH, Havv RA. High dose rate intraluminal irradiation in recurrent endobronchial carcinoma. Chest 1985;88(6):810–814.

38. George PJM, Hadly JM, Mantell BS, et al. Medium dose rate endobronchial radiotherapy with Cesium 137. Thorax 1992;47:474–477.

39. Mendiondo OA, Dillon M, Beach LJ. Endobronchial brachytherapy in the treatment of recurrent bronchogenic carcinoma. Int J Radiat Oncol Biol Phys 1983;9:579–582.

40. Hilaris BS, Martini N, Loumanen RK. Endobronchial interstitial implantation. Clin Bull 1979;9:17–20.

41. Shahabi S, Mehta MP, Wiley AL, et al. The role of computed tomography in dosimetric evaluation of endobronchial implants. Endocurie/Hypertherm Oncol 1988;4:187–191.

42. Schray MF, McDougall JC, Martinez A, et al. Management of malignant airway compromise with laser and low dose rate brachytherapy. Chest 1988;93:264–269.

43. Joyner LR, Hauskins L. Iridium afterloading and Neodymium-YAG laser treatment of segmental and lobar intrabronchial malignant obstructions. Tumor Diagnostik Therapie 1986;7:183–187.

44. Korba AL, Spear RK, Howard D, et al. High dose fraction intrabronchial radiation therapy for non-small cell carcinoma of the lung. Presented at: Current Endobronchial Therapy: State of the Art, Phoenix, AZ, 1987.

45. Loeffler EL, Van der Laarse R. Technique and individual afterloading treatment planning simulating classic Stockholm brachytherapy for cervix cancer. In: Vahrson H, Rauthe G (eds). High Dose Rate Afterloading in the Treatment of the Uterus, Breast and Rectum.

Urban and Schwarzenberg, Munich, 1988, Supplement 82,83,89.

46. Loeffler EL. In: Rotte K, Kiffer J (eds). Changes in Brachytherapy, Quality Control in Brachytherapy. D.E. Wacholz KG, Nurenberg, 1989.

47. Van der Laarse R. In: Mould RF (ed). The Selectron Treatment Planning System. Nucletron, Leersum, 1985, pp. 176–186.

48. Speiser BL. High dose-rate endobronchial brachytherapy: Whither goest thou? Int J Radiat Oncol Biol Phys 1992;23:250.

49. Mehta MP. Endobronchial brachytherapy: Whither prescription point? Int J Radiat Oncol Biol Phys 1992;23:251.

50. Allen MD, Baldwin JC, Fish VJ, et al. Combined laser therapy and endobronchial radiotherapy for unresectable lung carcinoma with bronchial obstruction. Am J Surg 1985;150:71–77.

51. Mehta MP, Petereit DG, Chosy L, et al. Sequential comparison of low dose rate and hyperfractionated high dose rate endobronchial radiation for malignant airway occlusion. Int J Radiat Oncol Biol Phys 1992;23:133–139.

52. Roach M III, Leidholdt EM Jr, Tatera BS, et al. Endobronchial radiation therapy (EBRT) in the management of lung cancer. Int J Radiat Oncol Biol Phys 1990;18:1449–1454.

53. Lo TCM, Beamis JF Jr, Weinstein RS, et al. Intraluminal low-dose rate brachytherapy for malignant endobronchial obstruction. Radiother Oncol 1992;23:16–20.

54. Locken P, Dillon M, Patel P, et al. Palliation of locally recurrent non-small cell lung cancer with low dose rate Iridium-192 endobronchial implant combined with localized external beam irradiation. Endocurie/Hypertherm Oncol 1990;6:217–222.

55. Paradelo JC, Waxman MJ, Throne BJ, et al. Endobronchial irradiation with ^{192}Ir in the treatment of malignant endobronchial obstruction. Chest 1992;102:1072–1074.

56. Susnerwala SS, Sharma S, Deshpande DD, et al. Endobronchial brachytherapy: A preliminary experience. J Surg Oncol 1992;50:115–117.

57. Nori D, Hilaris BS, Martini N. Intraluminal irradiation in bronchogenic carcinoma. Surg Clin North Am 1987;67:1093–1102.

58. Gauwitz M, Ellerbroek N, Komaki R, et al. High dose endobronchial irradiation in recurrent bronchogenic carcinoma. Int J Radiat Oncol Biol Phys 1992;23:397–400.

59. Speiser BL, Spratling L. Remote afterloading brachytherapy for the local control of endobronchial carcinoma. Int J Radiat Oncol Biol Phys 1993;25:579–587.

60. Burt PA, O'Driscoll BR, Nortley HM, et al. In-

traluminal irradiation for the palliation of lung cancer with the high dose rate micro-Selectron. Thorax 1990;45:765–768.

61. Fass DE, Armstrong J, Harrison LB. Fractionated high dose rate endobronchial treatment for recurrent lung cancer. Endocurie/Hypertherm Oncol 1990;6:211–215.

62. Bedwinek J, Petty A, Bruton C, et al. The use of high dose rate endobronchial brachytherapy to palliate symptomatic endobronchial recurrence of previously irradiated bronchogenic carcinoma. Int J Radiat Oncol Biol Phys 1991;22:23–30.

63. Miller JI Jr, Phillips TW. Neodymium-YAG laser and brachytherapy in the management of inoperable bronchogenic carcinoma. Ann Thorac Surg 1990;50:190–196.

64. Kohek P, Pakisch B, Rehak P, et al. Nd-YAG laser debulking combined with ^{192}Ir HDR brachytherapy for obstructing cancer of the central bronchial airways: Technique and results. Selectron Brachyther J 1990;S1:45–47.

65. Stout R, Burt PA, O'Driscoll BR, et al. HDR brachytherapy for palliation and cure in bronchial carcinoma: The Manchester experience using a single dose technique. Selectron Brachyther J 1990;S1:48–50.

66. Sutedja G, Baris G, Schaake-Koning C, et al. High dose rate brachytherapy in patients with local recurrences after radiotherapy of non-small cell lung cancer. Int J Radiat Oncol Biol Phys 1992;24:551–553.

67. Edell ES, Cortese DA, McDougall JC. Ancillary therapies in the management of lung cancer: Photodynamic therapy, laser therapy, and endobronchial prosthetic devices. Mayo Clin Proc 1993;68:685–690.

68. Reddi RP, Marbach JC. HDR remote afterloading brachytherapy of carcinoma of the lung. Selectron Brachyther J 1992;6(1):21–23.

69. Aygun C, Weiner S, Scariato A, et al. Treatment of non-small cell lung cancer with external beam radiotherapy and high dose rate brachytherapy. Int J Radiat Oncol Biol Phys 1992;23:127–132.

70. Bastin KT, Mehta MP, Kinsella TJ. Thoracic volume radiation sparing following endobronchial brachytherapy: A quantitative analysis. Int J Radiat Oncol Biol Phys 1993;25:703–707.

71. Sutedja T, Zoetmulder F, Zandwijk N. High dose rate brachytherapy improves resectability in squamous cell lung cancer. Chest 1992;102:308–309.

72. Macha HN, Wahlers B. Adjuvant endobronchial irradiation with curative intent: A report of 17 patients. Presented at the 8th International Brachytherapy Conference, New York, April 1993.

73. Speiser B, Spratling L. Fatal hemoptysis: Complication or failure of treatment. Int J Radiat Oncol Biol Phys 1993;25:925.

74. Miller R, McGregor D. Hemorrhage from carcinoma of the lung. Cancer 1975;36:904–913.

75. Khanavkar B, Stern P, Alberti W, et al. Complications associated with brachytherapy alone or with laser in lung cancer. Chest 1991;99:1062–1065.

76. Speiser BL, Spartling L. Radiation bronchitis and stenosis secondary to high dose rate endobronchial irradiation. Int J Radiat Oncol Biol Phys 1993;25:589–597.

77. Mehta MP, Shahabi S, Jarjour NN, et al. Endobronchial irradiation for malignant airway obstruction. Int J Radiat Oncol Biol Phys 1989;17:847–851.

78. Huzly A. Bronchoskopie in Lokalanasthesie. In: Giesbach R, Muller RW (eds). Bronchoskopische Eingriffe. Verlag, Berlin, 1974.

79. Walsh DA, Maiwand MO, Nath AR, et al. Bronchoscopic cryotherapy for advanced bronchial carcinoma. Thorax 1990;45:509–513.

80. Arabian A, Spagnolo SV. Laser therapy in patients with primary lung cancer. Chest 1984;86:519–523.

81. Brutinel WM, Cortese DA, McDougall JC, et al. A two year experience with the neodymium-YAG laser in endobronchial obstruction. Chest 1987;91:159–165.

82. Cavaliere S, Foccoli P, Farina PL. Nd:YAG laser bronchoscopy: A five year experience with 1,396 applications in 1,000 patients. Chest 1988;94:15–21.

83. Gelb AF, Epstein JD. Nd-YAG laser in lung cancer. West J Med 1984;140:393–397.

84. Hetzel MR, Millard FJC, Ayesh R, et al. Laser treatment for carcinoma of the bronchus. Br Med J 1983;286:12–16.

85. McDougall JC, Cortese DA. Neodymium-YAG laser therapy of malignant airway obstruction: A preliminary report. Mayo Clin Proc 1983;58:35–39.

86. McElvein RB. Laser endoscopy. Ann Thorac Surg 1981;32:463–466.

87. Personne C, Colchen A, Bonnette P, et al. Laser in bronchology: Methods of application. Lung 1990;168(S):1085–1088.

88. Shapshay SM, Dumon JF, Beamis JF Jr. Endoscopic treatment of tracheobronchial malignancy: Experience with Nd-YAG and CO_2 lasers in 506 operations. Otolaryngol Head Neck Surg 1985;93:205–210.

89. Wolfe WG, Cole PH, Sabiston DC Jr. Experimental and clinical use of the YAG laser in the

management of pulmonary neoplasms. Ann Surg 1984;199:526–531.

90. Dumon JF, Reboud E, Garbe L, et al. Treatment of tracheobronchial lesions by laser photoresection. Chest 1982;81:278–284.

91. Toty L, Personne C, Colchen A, et al. Bronchoscopic management of tracheal lesions using the neodymium yttrium aluminum garnet laser. Thorax 1981;36:175–178.

92. Kvale PA, Eichenhorn MS, Radke JR, et al. YAG laser photoresection of lesions obstructing the central airways. Chest 1985;87:283–288.

93. Parr GVS, Unger M, Trout RG, et al. One hundred neodymium-YAG laser ablations of obstructing tracheal neoplasms. Ann Thorac Surg 1984;38:374–379.

94. Diaz-Jimenez JP, Canela-Cardona M, Maestre-Alcacer J. Nd:YAG laser photoresection of low grade malignant tumors of the tracheobronchial tree. Chest 1990;97:920–922.

95. Brutinell WM, Cortese DA, Edell ES, et al. Complications of Nd:YAG laser therapy. Chest 1988;94:902–903.

96. Desai SJ, Mehta AC, Medendorp SV, et al. Survival experience following Nd:YAG laser photoresection for primary bronchogenic carcinoma. Chest 1988;94:939–944.

97. Chetty KG, Sassoon CSM, Viravathana T, et al. Effect of radiation therapy on bronchial obstruction due to bronchogenic carcinoma. Chest 1989;95:582–584.

98. Mehta MP, Shahabi S, Jarjour N, et al. Effect of endobronchial radiation therapy on malignant bronchial obstruction. Chest 1990;97:662–665.

99. Mitchell JB, McPherson S, DeGraff W, et al. Oxygen dependence of hematoporphyrin derivative-induced photoactivation of Chinese Hamster cells. Cancer Res 1985;45:2008–2011.

100. Lee See K, Borbes LJ, Betts WH. Oxygen dependency and photocytotoxicity with hematoporphyrin derivative. Photochem Photobiol 1984;39:631–634.

101. Moan J, Sommer S. Oxygen dependence of the photosensitizing effect of hematoporphyrin derivative in NHIK 3025 cells. Cancer Res 1985;45:1608–1610.

102. Gibson SL, Hilf R. Interdependence of fluence, drug dose and oxygen on hemato-porphyrin derivative induced photosensitization of tumor mitochrondria. Photochem Photobiol 1985;42:367–373.

103. Gibson SL, Hilf R. Photosensitization of mitochondrial cytochrome c oxidase by hematoporphyrin derivative and related porphyrins in vitro and in vivo. Cancer Res 1983;43:4191–4197.

104. Hilf R, Warne NW, Smail DB, et al. Photodynamic inactivation of selected intracellular enzymes by hematoporphyrin derivative and their relationship to tumor cell viability in vitro. Cancer Lett 1984;24:165–172.

105. Foote CS. Mechanisms of photooxygenation. In: Doiron DR, Gomer CJ (eds). Porphyrin Localization and Treatment of Tumors. Liss, New York, 1984, pp. 3–18.

106. Fiel RJ, Datta-Gupta N, Mark EH, et al. Induction of DNA damage by porphyrin photosensitizers. Cancer Res 1981;41:3543–3545.

107. Moan J, Waksvik H, Christensen T. DNA single-strand breaks and sister chromatid exchanges induced by treatment with hematoporphyrin and light or by x-rays in human NHIK 3025 cells. Cancer Res 1980;40:2915–2918.

108. Doiron DR, Gomer CJ. In: Doiron DR, Gomer CJ (eds). Porphyrin Localization and Treatment of Tumors. Liss, New York, 1984, p. xxiii.

109. Bugelski PJ, Porter CW, Dougherty TJ, et al. Autoradiographic distribution of hematoporphyrin derivative in normal and tumor tissue of the mouse. Cancer Res 1981;41:4606–4612.

110. Simonds AK, Irving JD, Clarke SW, et al. Use of expandable metal stents in the treatment of bronchial obstruction. Thorax 1989;44:680–681.

111. Dumon JF. A dedicated tracheobronchial stent. Chest 1990;97:328–332.

112. Insall RL, Morritt GN. Palliation of malignant tracheal strictures using silicone T tubes. Thorax 1991;46:168–171.

113. Majid DA, Lee S, Khushalani S, et al. The response of atelectasis from lung cancer to radiation therapy. Int J Radiat Oncol Biol Phys 1989;17:847–851.

114. Slawson RG, Scott RM. Radiation therapy in bronchogenic carcinoma. Ther Radiol 1990;132:175–176.

Breast

Frank A. Vicini, M.D., Daniel Clarke, M.D.,
Alvaro Martinez, M.D., FACR

Overview

The use of breast conserving therapy (BCT) in the management of early stage breast cancer is now well established. The goals of this treatment approach are to excise the bulk of the primary tumor in the breast using a cosmetically acceptable surgical technique and to use moderate doses of irradiation to eliminate any residual cancer. In several randomized clinical trials with large numbers of patients and long-term follow-up, equivalent survival after mastectomy and BCT has been observed.[1,2] Retrospective reviews of clinical outcome with BCT have also shown low rates of local recurrence, high rates of satisfactory cosmetic results, and a very low rate of complications.[3–7] The recognition that breast conserving techniques are as effective as amputation has resulted in a gradual shift away from mastectomy and a declaration by the National Cancer Institute Consensus Development Conference in 1990, that lumpectomy plus radiation therapy should now be considered as the preferred treatment in the management of this disease.[8]

Though there is general agreement that BCT is an acceptable method of primary treatment for most patients with early stage breast cancer, what constitutes the most appropriate technique of BCT has yet to be agreed upon. Most of the debate regarding the optimal technique of BCT centers on two questions: 1) What is the most appropriate extent of surgical resection; and 2) How much radiation should be delivered? While each of these questions may, at first, appear to be independent, recent data have convincingly revealed that they are both interrelated and complementary.

Surgical options used to treat breast cancer include biopsy, gross local excision, wide excision, and quadrantectomy. In general, more limited surgeries produce the least cosmetic distortion but at the risk of a higher rate of local recurrence. Conversely, larger resections appear to produce improved local control rates but at the price of less satisfactory cosmetic results. Recent data from the Joint Center for Radiation Therapy, Boston, MA, clearly illustrate each of these points. Olivetto et al.[9] showed that the cosmetic result after BCT was adversely affected if the lumpectomy specimen exceeded 70 cm.[3] Vicini et al.,[10] when analyzing the same cohort of patients, demonstrated that the risk of local recurrence decreased as the extent of surgical resection increased. What then represents the optimal extent of breast resection to provide both adequate local control and an acceptable cosmetic result? Ideally, a wide excision or re-excision should be performed to obtain pathologically negative surgical margins prior to radiotherapy. From a practical point of

From Nag S (ed): *Principles and Practice of Brachytherapy.* © Futura Publishing Co., Inc., Armonk, NY, 1997.

Table 1.
Five-Year Actuarial Rate of Local Breast Recurrence in Relation to the Extent of Breast Resection and the Presence of EIC

	Tumor Size	Extent of Breast Resection			Probability Value
		Smallest	Intermediate	Largest	
EIC+	T1	29%	22%	10%	0.07
	T2	36%	26%	9%	0.04
EIC−	T1	9%	2%	0%	0.02
	T2	6%	2%	3%	NS

EIC = extensive intraductal component; NS = not stated.

view, however, histologic assessment of the adequacy of all margins is difficult to perform. Moreover, achieving pathologically negative margins may be most important in tumors with an extensive intraductal component (EIC) but considerably less so when an EIC is absent. In the analysis above by Vicini et al.[10] (Table 1), the impact of surgical resection on decreasing the risk of local recurrence was most pronounced in patients with an EIC. In patients without an EIC, local control was easily achieved with standard doses of whole breast radiation therapy (supplemented by a carefully designed boost) even in the case of focally positive margins or a small breast resection. In the presence of an EIC, standard doses of radiation were not as effective in controlling local disease and only in those patients with larger surgeries was the local control rate acceptable. Thus, the need for wide surgical margins and for re-excision should be carefully assessed and tailored to the individual case.

With respect to the optimal dose of radiotherapy in BCT, the literature is also controversial. Several investigators have shown a "dose-response relationship" between the tumor-bed dose and the rate of local control. Nobler and Venet[11] reported a better control rate in the breast with doses >60 Gy. A dose response was also noted by van Limbergen et al.[12] Clarke et al.[13] also reported a dose-response relationship; when a nominal standard dose (NSD) of <1840 ret was given to the tumor bed, a higher recurrence rate was noted. Other investigators have not shown this clear cut dose-response relationship. This controversy may, in large part, be explained by the findings published by Holland et al.,[14]

who performed a pathological and radiographic study on mastectomy specimens to assess the location of residual tumor in the breast after a simulated tumor excision. The authors found that 43% of patients had residual tumor remaining in the breast after tumor excision with a 2-cm margin. Of greater significance, however, was the fact that patients with an EIC were more likely to have a prominent amount of residual ductal carcinoma in situ (DCIS) remaining in the breast after tumor excision than patients without an EIC (44% vs 3%, P<0.0001).

What the above data imply is that much of the risk of tumor recurrence in the breast after BCT may be related to the volume of disease remaining in the breast after surgery. In patients with an EIC, either an increased breast resection or a higher tumor bed dose (or both) may be needed to overcome the effect of this risk factor. Thus, with the knowledge of what constitutes a high risk subgroup, and with an understanding of the extent of surgical resection that has been undertaken, the aggressiveness of breast irradiation can be appropriately tailored to improve outcome.

On the basis of the above data, the following recommendations can be made regarding treatment to the breast in patients managed with BCT. After adequate tumor excision is performed, whole breast irradiation to doses in the range of 45–50 Gy should be delivered. Though controversial, this is generally followed with a boost to the tumor bed. As discussed above, it has been observed that a dose effect with breast cancer does exist. In all of the studies where this has been demonstrated, it is the tumor bed dose, not the whole breast dose, that is most important. In patients without adverse histopathologic findings (e.g., negative margins, no EIC) a tumor bed dose of 50 Gy may be adequate.[1,15–17] However, there are currently no consistent data identifying which subset of patients do not need a boost and as a result many centers continue to recommend its use in all patients.[3,18] Patients with significant risk factors for local recurrence (e.g., high grade, an EIC that is inadequately excised, or young age), should be boosted more aggressively to at least 60 Gy. For these patients, an interstitial implant is advised since higher doses can be delivered with a good or excellent cosmetic result.

Interstitial Brachytherapy as Boost Treatment

Introduction

Interstitial implants remain an important and effective method of boosting patients treated with BCT. Table 2 lists the major cen-

Table 2A.
Low-Dose-Rate Brachytherapy As Boost Treatment: Perioperative Series

Institution	Number of Patients	Isotope	Boost Dose (Gy)	Total Dose (Gy)	Local Recurrence (5 Year Act)	Cosmetic Result (% Good/Excellent)
University of Kansas[19,63]	245	Ir-192	15–20	>60	3%	87
Thomas Jefferson University[20,53]*	655	Ir-192	20	>60	7%	88
Memorial Sloan Kettering[54]**	52	Ir-192	15–22	>60	0	+
Tygerberg Hospital Parowvallei C.P.[55]	126	Ir-192	25	>70	<2%	—
Syed[56]	30	Ir-192	25–30	70–80	0%	>75

* Overlapping series with University of Kansas.
** Pilot trial.
+ Mean "overall cosmesis" score of 8.0/10.0.

Table 2B.
Low-Dose-Rate Brachytherapy as Boost Treatment: Post-External Beam Radiotherapy Series 5

Institute	Number of Patients	Isotope	Boost Dose (Gy)	Total Dose (Gy)	Local Recurrence (%)	Cosmetic Result (% Good/Excellent)
William Beaumont Hospital[18]	86	I-125	15	>60	3	>90
	197	Ir-192	15–20	>60	4	>90
Tufts University[41]	81	Ir-192	20	>70	NS*	>85
Tata Memorial Hospital, Bombay, India[57,58]	273	Ir-192	15–30	60–75	14	81
Harvard Group[39]	145	Ir-192	20	>60	6	95
Institut Gustave-Roussy[58,59]**	138	Ir-192	25	>60	T_1-8 T_2-12	T_1-87 T_2-59
Group Hospitalier Pitie' Salpetrie're Paris, France[61]	169	Ir-192	15	60	6.0	96

* Not stated.
** T_1 and T_2 tumors only.

ters that currently use implant boosts. In general, interstitial implants are best used in patients with significant risk factors for local recurrence (either clinical and/or histopathologic) or in patients with deep seated tumors in large breasts not technically suitable for electron beam teletherapy. When a boost dose is applied, especially if the dose is over 14 Gy, an implant may offer both radiobiological and cosmetic advantages (see below). In most patients, the implant is performed 7–10 days after whole breast irradiation under local or general anesthesia. However, these implants can also be performed perioperatively (i.e., at the time of re-excision or axillary dissection), thus avoiding an additional anesthetic and allowing the surgeon's input in identifying the tumor bed.[19,20]

Traditionally, interstitial implants have been performed using several different low-dose-rate (LDR) techniques using the isotopes iridium-192 (Ir-192) or iodine-125 (I-125). Each interstitial implant system was derived from empiric data that were used to develop a series of rules and/or guidelines to aid the radiotherapist in constructing an implant that would deliver a predetermined total dose or dose rate to a specified point or reference volume. In Europe, the Paris system is the most commonly used dosimetry system for LDR interstitial breast implants. This system is well documented in both classic and current textbooks and will not be reviewed here.[21,22] In the United States, the traditional interstitial dosimetry system has been the Manchester or the Patterson Parker system.[21,23,24] As concepts in interstitial brachytherapy changed and as different isotopes became available, different dosimetry systems were developed (e.g., the dimension averaging system used for I-125).[25] Over the past decade, most centers have used modifications of the Memorial

system for implant construction.[26] More recently, implant techniques have been further modified in order to incorporate the advantages of high-dose-rate (HDR) treatment (i.e., elimination of radiation exposure to personnel, no hospitalization).

When an implant is constructed, either a rigid template or a freehand system of needle placement is used.[27,28] After the area to be implanted is identified on the skin of the breast (using a combination of mammography, surgical clips, ultrasonography, computed tomography, palpation, etc.), hollow stainless steel needles are inserted into the breast. These trocars are then replaced with afterloading tubes that accommodate either an LDR or HDR source. Depending upon the implant technique or isotopes chosen, these catheters remain in position from as little as several hours up to 4 or 5 days. For LDR implants, a dose of 15–20 Gy is generally prescribed at a dose rate of 30–70 cGy/hr. Recent data suggest that there may be a significant effect of dose rate on local control and cosmetic results for carcinoma of the breast treated with Ir-192 implants.[29] Dose rates outside of this range are not recommended. With HDR boosts, the optimal fractionation scheme has not yet been clearly defined. However, two of the centers with the largest number of patients deliver 1000 cGy in one fraction (Table 3). As discussed below, institutions using LDR techniques report excellent long-term local control and cosmetic results. Centers using HDR techniques also report good results; however, longer follow-up will be needed to assess the effectiveness of this technique compared with LDR brachytherapy.

At William Beaumont Hospital (WBH), interstitial implants have been used to boost patients treated with BCT since 1980. In 1986, I-125 seeds replaced Ir-192 seeds due to the

Table 3.
High-Dose-Rate Brachytherapy As Boost Treatment

Institution	Number of Patients	Dose/Fraction (Gy)	Total Dose (Gy)	% Local Recurrence	Cosmetic Result (% Good/Excellent)
Saarbrucker Winterbergkliniken[52]	224	10–15	60	4	81
Austria[60,64]	210	10	60	4	91

isotopes reduced shielding requirements, less patient and personnel radiation exposure, and significant dosimetric advantages. The long-term impact of interstitial boosts on the rate of local control and cosmetic results in patients treated with BCT at WBH will be reviewed with special emphasis on the isotope I-125.

Materials and Methods

From 1/1/80 to 12/31/87, 403 women with stage I and II breast cancer were treated with BCT at WBH, Royal Oak, Michigan. Surgery consisted of at least an excisional biopsy in all patients. Two hundred forty-six patients (61%) underwent re-excision, and 384 patients (95%) were treated with axillary dissection. All patients received whole breast irradiation with tangents to 45–50 Gy followed by a boost to the tumor bed to at least 60 Gy using either photons (4%), electrons (26%), or an interstitial implant with I-125 (21%) or Ir-192 (49%). Prior to 1986, patients who required a boost were treated with an interstitial implant using Ir-192 seeds (ribbons). In 1986, electron beam therapy became available at WBH and I-125 seeds replaced Ir-192 for all interstitial implants. Patients selected for I-125 implants constituted a group of women considered to be at greater risk of local recurrence (e.g., an EIC, uncertain or positive margins, young age, high grade, diffusely infiltrating tumors, etc.) or had large breasts not technically suitable for electron beam therapy. The electron beam and I-125 subgroups represented a more "modern era" population whereby histopathology was used to tailor treatment.

Tumor Bed Localization

All implants were performed in the operative suite under general or local anesthesia. The tumor bed was localized with the aid of mammography, ultrasonography, computed tomography, palpation, or input from the surgeon (i.e., surgical clips or direct visualization if performed perioperatively). The volume to be implanted consisted of the biopsy cavity plus a 2- to 3-cm margin. Patients with an EIC or tumors in close proximity to the nipple areolar complex were implanted with larger volumes that included that structure.

Implant Technique

The implant technique used has been previously reported.[30] After the boost volume was outlined on the breast, stainless steel 17 gauge trocars were inserted through the breast (without a template guide) using the same guidelines for ribbon and plane separation as used with Ir-192 (interplane and needle separation were generally 1–1.5 cm apart). Afterloading tubes were then pulled through the breast as the trocars were removed. Barium buttons were then positioned on the tubes to secure the implant. Postoperatively, patients were transported to the Radiation Oncology Department for localization films. "Dummy" seeds were introduced into the afterloading catheters and a film normal to the implant planes was taken to define treatment parameters (i.e., active length). An orthogonal pair (generally AP and lateral) was used for computerized reconstruction. Isodose distributions were calculated using the Nucletron Planning System (Nucletron, B.V., Loersum, The Netherlands). The standard policy after August 1986 was to deliver a minimal tumor dose of 1500 cGy at 62.5 cGy/hr over 24 hours.

Dosimetry I-125

Since I-125 ribbons are prepared by loading loose seeds (separated by spacers) into hollow ribbons, seed spacing was adjusted (based on the available seed activity) to deliver the desired dose rate to the target isodose line. In addition, individualized ribbon construction allowed interseed separation to be adjusted to "optimize" the dose distribution within a given region of an implant in cases with deviated catheters. Most commonly, seed spacing was adjusted in a single catheter to ensure that the 100% isodose line encompassed the entire implant volume. A dose of 15 Gy was prescribed as the minimum dose anywhere within the prescription volume, subject to the provision that the area (judged by the physician) of the 150% isodose line be 50% or less than the area of the prescription isodose line in the central plane isodose distribution.

Dosimetry Ir-192

With Ir-192 implants, the volume of the implant was preplanned and ribbons of a specified active length were ordered prior to the implant procedure. After implant construction, ribbons were cut at 1-cm intervals to correspond to the implant geometry (as needed). Since seed spacing is fixed with Ir-192 ribbons, the dose distribution could not be adjusted to "optimize" implants, as with I-125. In addition, since the dose rate is a function of the seed activity and implant volume (both of which are fixed values after the implant is constructed), it could not be adjusted to deliver the desired dose rate to the target volume line (as with I-125). A dose rate was chosen that optimally encompassed the treatment volume within the central plane of the implant, subject to the same provision listed above for I-125. (Dose rates generally ranged from 30–50 cGy/hr). Isodose distributions were calculated using the Theraplan Planning system.

Ribbons were afterloaded in the patient's room and were secured with Henschke buttons. With I-125 implants, thin flexible lead rubber was taped over the implant for shielding. Generally, shielding consisted of 1–1.5 mm of lead rubber (0.08- to 0.125-mm lead equivalent). Comparable shielding requirements for Ir-192 implants consisted of 5.0 cm of lead mounted on a portable rolling bedside shield. After 24 hours, the ribbons were removed, a survey completed and the implant tubes removed from the breast. Implant removal was well tolerated and rarely required postprocedure analgesia. As a result, the implant time for I-125 was commonly 24 hours and hospital stay was usually <36 hours. (Implant times for Ir-192 were generally 36–48 hours). Patients were discharged home shortly thereafter.

Results

With a median follow-up of 86 months, 25 patients have recurred in the treated breast for a 5- and 10-year actuarial rate of local recurrence of 3.8% and 8.9%, respectively. Table 4 lists the 10-year actuarial rates of local recurrences in the breast based upon the boost technique used. There were no statistically significant differences in the rate of local recurrence using either photons (25%), electrons (8.7%), Ir-192 (8.6%), or I-125 (2.6%).

The impact of boost technique on cosmetic outcome is shown in Table 5. Again, no significant differences in the percentages of patients obtaining good/excellent cosmetic results were noted between I-125 (93%), Ir-192 (88%), electrons (90%), or photons (81%), P = NS.

Discussion

These results demonstrate that interstitial implant boosts used in patients treated with BCT provide excellent rates of local control and cosmetic results. The 10-year actuarial rates of local recurrence in the breast were not significantly different between patients boosted with either I-125 (2.6%), Ir-192 (8.6%), electrons (8.7%), or photons (25%). These results also suggest that the use of interstitial implants does not significantly alter cosmetic outcome when compared with either electrons or photons. With median cosmetic follow-up of 46 months, 90% of all patients treated with interstitial implants have good/excellent cosmetic results.

Prior to the development of linear accelerators capable of generating high energy electrons, interstitial implants were the primary method for boosting patients treated with

Table 4.
Local Tumor Recurrence vs Boost Technique

Boost Technique	Number of Patients	Median F/U (Months)	% Distant Failure (10 Year Act)	% Local Recurrence (10 Year Act)
I-125	86	77	11	3
Ir-192	197	102	18	9
Electrons	105	75	17	9
Photons	15	81	0	25

F/U = follow-up.

Table 5.
Cosmetic Outcome vs Boost Technique

Boost Technique	Number of Patients	Cosmetic F/U (Months)	Cosmetic Results (% Good/Excellent)
I-125	86	40	93
Ir-192	197	48	88
Electrons	105	29	90
Photons	15	35	81

F/U = follow-up.

BCT.[31] However, due to the unique physical characteristics of electron beams (i.e., dose localization) and their ease of use, the indications for treatment with interstitial implants diminished and, at many institutions, are currently limited to patients with large breasts not optimally treated with electrons. More recently, however, the use of interstitial implants has generated new interest due to radiobiological data that suggest that the continuous LDR irradiation delivered by interstitial implants may be more efficacious than standard, brief exposure fractionated regimens as used with electron beam teletherapy boosts.[32] Glicksman and Leith[32] point out that the normal processes of radiobiological repair, repopulation, and redistribution enhance the effects of continuous LDR radiation therapy. In addition, the oxygen enhancement ratio (OER) has been shown to be approximately 20% lower with brachytherapy than in standard, fractionated external beam radiation therapy.[33]

Due to the superior dose localization properties of implants and their potential enhanced radiobiological effectiveness, some authors believe implants may be the treatment of choice both for patients with deep seated lesions in large breasts and/or in patients with significant risk factors for local recurrence.[34] The above data provide indirect evidence that patients treated with interstitial implants may have a higher rate of local tumor control, since 71% of patients boosted with I-125 had significant risk factors for local recurrence. However, since all potential risk factors for local recurrence have not yet been evaluated for the entire patient population (incomplete pathological review), no definite conclusion can be reached regarding the potential superiority of a brachytherapy

boost. These excellent results do demonstrate, however, that implants can provide a highly satisfactory level of local control even in patients with poor prognostic factors (e.g., an EIC, young age, close or positive margins, etc.).

Krishnan et al.[19] reported similar findings in their group of high risk patients treated with perioperative interstitial boost irradiation. Two hundred fifty patients received 15–20 Gy from a perioperative interstitial Ir-192 boost followed by 45–50 Gy external beam radiotherapy to the whole breast. At a median follow-up of 58 months, there was no statistically significant difference in the 10-year actuarial rate of local recurrence in the breast between patients with or without an EIC in their tumor (9% vs 5.2%, P = NS). The authors also point out that perioperative interstitial implants may have additional radiobiological advantages.[35] The delivery of continuous LDR irradiation immediately after debulking (i.e., lumpectomy) may have the advantage of damaging tumor cells before regrowth leads to tumor volumes greater than microscopic disease.

HDR techniques have also been used to boost patients treated with BCT. The major advantages of this treatment approach include: 1) the elimination of radiation exposure to staff and personnel; 2) the ability to treat women on an out-patient basis; and 3) optimized dose distributions within the implanted volume. Table 3 lists the centers currently investigating HDR interstitial boosts. Though the optimal fractionation schedule has not been defined, both the cosmetic outcome and local control rates reported are encouraging and the technique appears promising. However, longer follow-up will be needed to establish the equivalence of this technique compared to LDR brachytherapy.

Other investigators have previously reported inferior cosmetic results using interstitial implant boosts as compared to electron beam therapy.[36] It has been suggested that the diminished cosmetic results observed (particularly in large volume implants) may be related to inhomogeneity of dose distribution resulting in the development of fat necrosis and fibrosis.[37,38] The data above do not demonstrate any impairment in cosmetic outcome with I-125 interstitial implants (or Ir-192). This in part, may be related to the ability to optimize the dose distribution within an I-125 implant and the standardized implant technique. All implants were constructed to ensure that the most superficial plane was an acceptable distance from the skin surface (0.75–1.0 cm) and that seeds at the proximal and distal ends of each ribbon were at least 0.5–0.75 cm from the skin. In addition, strict dose homogeneity criteria were used in all implants in order to avoid excessive hot spots within the implanted volume. Using these guidelines, more than 93% of implanted breasts treated with I-125 and 88% with Ir-192 obtained good or excellent cosmetic results. The previously reported findings of significant telangiectasia, retraction, skin thickening, or fat necrosis were not seen with these techniques.

Part of the improvement in cosmetic results with I-125 may also be due to the isotopes unique dosimetric characteristics when compared to Ir-192. The average energy emission by I-125 is 30 KeV; and therefore, dose deposition results primarily from photoelectric interactions rather than Compton effects. This results in a 30%–40% reduction in dose absorption by fat cells with I-125 as compared to Ir-192.[23] This may lower the incidence of fat necrosis and may reduce the risk of later breast fibrosis.

More recent updates of cosmetic outcome with interstitial boosts at other institutions also do not suggest that this method of boost treatment results in inferior results.[39,40] Wazer et al.[41] recently reported their results with interstitial Ir-192 boosts of up to 20 Gy on selected patients treated with BCT. Despite the higher doses of irradiation, they found that the use of an interstitial implant resulted in a cosmetic result that was at least as good as that achieved with electron beam teletherapy.

They believed their excellent results were secondary to careful attention to dose homogeneity throughout the implant volume and total skin dose.

Conclusions

Data from multiple institutions with long-term follow-up clearly indicate that interstitial implant boosts provide excellent local control rates and cosmetic results in selected patients treated with BCT. These implants appear best suited for patients with significant risk factors for local recurrence or in patients with deep seated lesions in large breasts not technically suitable for electron beam teletherapy. LDR techniques have been the traditional method for implanting these patients, and a large experience now exists for both Ir-192 and I-125. HDR techniques have recently become available and preliminary data are encouraging. Both the LDR and HDR techniques are highly reproducible and offer clinicians an alternative, efficacious means of boosting early stage breast cancer patients treated with BCT.

Interstitial Brachytherapy as the Sole Radiation Modality

Introduction

As discussed above, BCT has become an accepted option in the treatment of most patients with stage I and II breast cancer. The major advantage of BCT is related to the superior cosmetic result and reduced psychological and emotional trauma resulting from this procedure compared to mastectomy. However, BCT also has relative disadvantages. The technique is a more complex and prolonged treatment regimen that requires approximately 5–7 weeks to complete. As a result, for patients who are elderly or live at a distance from treatment centers, logistical problems can prove prohibitive. In addition, with the more frequent use of adjuvant chemotherapy in both node negative and positive patients, substantial delays can be incurred prior to the initiation of either local breast irradiation or systemic chemotherapy. Thus, despite the obvious cosmetic and potentially emotional advantages of BCT, only 10%–40% of patients who are candidates for breast conservation actually receive it.[42]

Most of the logistical problems with BCT relate to the protracted course of external beam irradiation to the whole breast. Standard therapy after tumor excision generally includes 5 weeks of external beam irradiation to the whole breast (45–50 Gy) followed by a boost to the tumor bed with either an additional eight to ten fractions (days) of external beam radiotherapy or a 2- to 3-day interstitial implant. The rationale for this approach is based upon two principles. First, higher doses of irradiation are given to the "tumor bed" in an attempt to control residual small foci of cancer that may be left behind after excision alone. Second, whole breast irradiation is used to eliminate possible areas of occult multicentric in situ or infiltrating cancer in remote areas of the breast. That such remote, multicentric areas of cancer exist has long been established. However, the biological significance of these areas of occult cancer is unknown, and the necessity to prophylactically treat the entire breast has recently been questioned. For instance, there are now at least five prospective randomized trials comparing the outcome of patients treated with excisional biopsy alone or followed by whole breast irradiation.[43,44] In all of these trials, the majority of recurrences in the breast in patients who did *not* receive irradiation occurred at or in the area of the tumor bed. Thus, it would appear that radiotherapy after tumor excision exerts its maximal effect upon reducing breast cancer recurrence at or near the tumor site.

The implications of these observations form the basis for the following hypothesis: Can an acceptable outcome be achieved with irradiation delivered only to the vicinity of the tumor bed and can interstitial brachytherapy be used as the sole radiation modality in these patients? If this were so, brachytherapy alone could be delivered in only 3–5 days after tumor excision, thus significantly shortening the overall treatment time and potentially reducing health care costs. In order to ensure optimal rates of success with this approach, it is necessary to identify the most ideal candidates (i.e., patients with truly localized, non-multicentric disease). There are clinical and histopathologic markers that can predict (with reasonable certainty) the likelihood that a carcinoma is localized and has been ade-quately excised prior to radiotherapy. Mammography has successfully been used both pre- and postoperatively to assess the full extent of a carcinoma in a breast. Stomper and Connolly[45] have shown that the majority of infiltrating ductal carcinomas (59%–90%) associated with calcifications on mammography (especially if extensive) are likely to be associated with extensive intraductal cancer in the breast; whereas, carcinomas without mammographic calcifications likely do not (17%–24%). In addition, Holland et al.,[14] evaluated 217 mastectomy specimens in patients who underwent a "simulated" tumor excision. They found that the majority of patients who had prominent residual cancer outside of the tumor bed after simulated gross excision had an EIC (44%) in the original tumor while only 3% of patients without an EIC did (P<0.00001). Only in patients with an EIC was this cancer at a significant distance from the tumor bed. Thus, the ideal candidates for such an approach would be required to have mammographically acceptable lesions that were adequately excised and lacking an EIC.

An additional potential advantage of this treatment approach is that brachytherapy also provides a higher central dose and possibly more effective delivery of irradiation to the area most at risk for recurrence. As discussed in the previous section, there are radiobiological data that suggest that LDR radiotherapy (as provided by an interstitial implant) may be more effacious than standard, fractionated external beam irradiation.[32,33] In addition, brachytherapy should provide an acceptable cosmetic result in this setting. This is suggested by multiple trials combining an interstitial implant boost of the breast with standard whole breast irradiation and early results from trials in Europe and the United States exploring the use of an implant as the sole radiation modality.[46]

If feasible, interstitial brachytherapy alone can offer an alternative treatment for selected patients with early stage breast cancer that is intermediate between observation alone (after excisional biopsy) and full breast irradiation. There are currently several trials attempting to identify subsets of patients that may do well without added irradiation following excisional biopsy alone.[43,44,47–49] At the present time, however, no consistent

Table 6.
Brachytherapy Alone in Breast Conserving Therapy

Institution	Number of Patients	Dose/fx (cGy)	Total Dose (cGy)	% Local Recurrence	Cosmetic Result (% Good/Excellent)
		HDR			
Ochsner Clinic[62]	26	400 × 8	3200	0	67
Royal Devon/Exeter Hospital Exeter, England[52]	45	1000 × 2 700 × 4 600 × 6	2000 2800 3600	8.8	95
London Regional Cancer Center London, Ontario[65]	21	372 × 10	3720	0	>95
		LDR			
William Beaumont Hospital	33	52 cGy/hour	5000	0	>95
Guys Hospital[49]	27	40 cGy/hour	5500	7	83
Oshsner Clinic[62]	26	—	4500	0	76

fx = fraction; HDR = high-dose-rate; LDR = low-dose-rate.

subgroup of patients has been identified that has achieved a high enough rate of local control to eliminate all radiotherapy. Interstitial brachytherapy alone if successful, may give an alternative to selected low risk patients obviating the need for 5–7 weeks of external beam irradiation.

Institutions investigating interstitial brachytherapy alone following wide excision for early stage breast cancer are listed in Table 6. Both LDR and HDR protocols are being conducted. Most of these trials have slightly different selection criteria, surgical techniques, and radiotherapy schedules. However, preliminary data indicate that the concept is practical and early results are promising. At WBH, LDR interstitial brachytherapy has been used in selected early stage breast cancer patients as the sole radiation modality since early 1993. The preliminary findings (i.e., local control and acute toxicity) will be presented.

Materials and Methods

From 2/28/93 through 7/1/94, 33 women with early stage breast cancer were entered onto a protocol of tumor bed irradiation only using an LDR interstitial implant with I-125. Patients with infiltrating ductal carcinoma were eligible only if the tumor was <3 cm, margins were clear (>2 mm), there was no

EIC, a postoperative mammogram was performed, and the breast was technically suitable for implant. Patients with pure DCIS, infiltrating lobular carcinoma, or mammograms with diffuse calcifications extending over an area >3 cm were excluded. All patients underwent axillary dissection.

Tumor Bed Localization

The treatment volume was limited to the tumor bed plus a 2-cm margin. The biopsy cavity was localized by a combination of palpation, mammography, or, with implants performed perioperatively, with the guidance of the surgeon. Since the surgical scar can often be a poor indicator of the location of the underlying tumor bed,[50,51] ultrasonography was also used to define the three-dimensional tumor bed margins on the skin of the breast, if the implant was placed after lumpectomy (Figure 1). The superior, inferior, medial, lateral, and posterior border of the tumor bed were identified and marked on the skin surface. The implant volume was preplanned (based upon the ultrasound measurements) and the entrance and exit points of the needles were projected on the breast surface. When possible, surgical clips were also placed at the time of lumpectomy to aid in implant construction. Prior to the implant, pa-

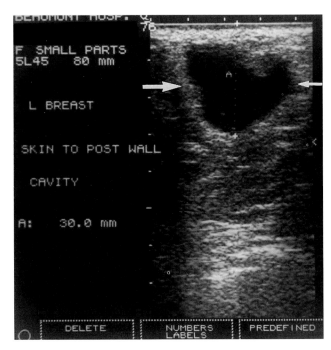

Figure 1. Ultrasound delineation of biopsy cavity: Arrows outline borders of biopsy cavity to be marked on skin surface. Cross indicates depth of biopsy cavity.

tients were taken to the simulator and the location of these clips was projected onto the skin surface to help define implant borders (clip location was also used to assess the adequacy of implant construction at simulation).

Implant Technique

Implants were placed in the operating suite under local or general anesthesia using a standardized template (Figure 2). Intercatheter separation on the template was fixed at 15 mm and the interplane separation was 14 mm. Templates of two or three planes were available depending upon the size of the breast and biopsy cavity. Since the entrance and exit points of the implant needles usually extend several centimeters beyond the implant volume outlined on the skin, the template length was adjustable and could be easily changed intraoperatively to accommodate separations from 10–18 cm. Ultrasonography was also used intraoperatively to ensure that the afterloading catheters encompassed the biopsy cavity (Figure 3).

Dosimetry

Patients received a total of 5000 cGy delivered at 52 cGy/hr over a period of 96 hours.

Since I-125 seeds were used, implants could be optimized (after construction) to improve homogeneity throughout the implant volume. A dose of 50 Gy was prescribed as the minimum dose anywhere within the prescription volume, subject to the provision that no contiguous area (i.e., confluent around multiple catheters) of 150% of the prescribed dose should exist in the central plane isodose distribution. Note that this provision is considerably more restrictive than the one used for the boost technique (see above). The more regular catheter spacing of a template technique allows more stringent dose specification criteria to be imposed. Perioperative complications, cosmetic outcome, and local control were assessed. Patient tolerance, reproducibility of the technique, and template stability during the treatment were also evaluated.

Results

The median follow-up is 12 months (range 2–16). Implants were well tolerated; two patients experienced mild pain that required nonnarcotic analgesics. No perioperative infections or significant skin reactions related to the implant were noted. Early cosmetic results

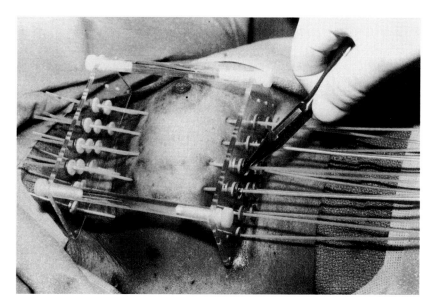

Figure 2. Breast template being secured with Henschke buttons. Interplane separation on template is 14 mm and intercatheter separation is 15 mm.

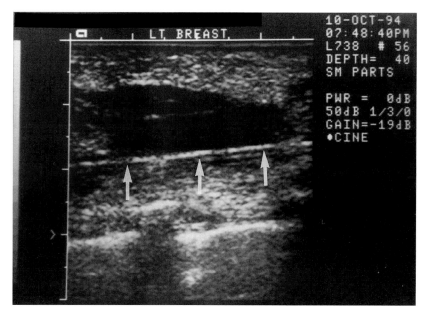

Figure 3. Intraoperative ultrasound-guided placement of afterloading catheters. Arrows indicate position of catheter at posterior border of biopsy cavity.

revealed minimal changes to the treated breast, consisting of transient hyperpigmentation at the puncture sites and temporary induration in the tumor bed. All ten patients with a minimum follow-up of 6 months had good-to-excellent cosmetic results. Seventeen patients had negative follow-up mammograms, and all patients are clinically free of disease.

Discussion

Brachytherapy alone in the management of early stage breast cancer appears to be a well tolerated, reproducible, and convenient method of treating selected patients with this disease. Early results suggest that this treatment approach may provide an acceptable alternative therapy intermediate between conventional, fractionated radiotherapy (to 50–60 Gy), and observation alone after lumpectomy. Though results are preliminary, sufficient data are available to suggest that this technique may prove efficacious.

Several centers have used both LDR and HDR techniques when treating patients alone with brachytherapy (Table 6). One of the trials using LDR brachytherapy with the longest follow-up is from Guys Hospital in London.[46] Twenty-seven patients received an LDR interstitial implant using a rigid template. The tumor bed plus a 2-cm margin was implanted with iridium wire delivering 55 Gy over 5.5 days to 85% of the basal dose rate as defined by the Paris system. With a median follow-up of 27 months, two patients developed an isolated recurrence in the breast, and two failed in the breast and systemically, concurrently. Eighty-three percent of patients obtained a good or excellent cosmetic result.

Other centers have used HDR techniques with varying fractionation schemes. At the present time, the optimal radiation schedule for HDR brachytherapy remains undefined. At the Royal Devon and Exter Hospital, Exter, England, three different fractionation schedules were used to treat patients with T1 and T2 tumors with clear or close margins after lumpectomy (without axillary dissection).[52] Using a rigid template and needle system to compress the breast into a well defined and reproducible volume, patients received either: 1) 20 Gy in two fractions (22 patients);

2) 28 Gy in four fractions (17 patients); or 3) 32 Gy in six fractions (8 patients).

With a median follow-up time of 18 months (range 6–36 months), four patients developed a local recurrence (two had synchronous axillary failures) and three patients developed new primaries in separate quadrants of the breast. Cosmetic outcome was rated as excellent in 95% of patients (regardless of fractionation schedule).

The data above indicate that treatment of a limited breast volume alone with either LDR or HDR interstitial brachytherapy provides an excellent cosmetic outcome and may be appropriate for certain patients. However, strict clinical and histopathologic eligibility criteria need to be followed (i.e., negative margins, no EIC, axillary dissection) in order to ensure optimal success with this approach. In addition, meticulous tumor bed localization must be performed (using either surgical clips, ultrasonography, or computed tomography), since a limited breast volume is irradiated.

Conclusion

Interstitial brachytherapy as the sole radiation modality for selected patients with early stage breast cancer is currently being investigated due to the potential reduction in overall treatment time, improvements in patient convenience, and possible reductions in medical costs this technique offers. Several pilot trials with both LDR and HDR techniques have been completed and early results are encouraging. However, criteria for patient eligibility and optimal dose/fractionation schemes have yet to be defined; longer follow-up will be required to establish the equivalence of this approach to standard BCT.

References

1. Fisher B, Anderson S. Conservative surgery for the management of invasive and non-invasive carcinoma of the breast: NSABP Trials. World J Surg 1994;18:63–69.
2. Veronesi U, Banfi A, Salvadori B, et al. Breast conservation is the treatment of choice in small breast cancer: Long-term results of a randomized trial. Eur J Cancer 1990;26:668–670.
3. Vicini F, Recht A, Abner A, et al. Recurrence in the breast following treatment of patients with early stage breast cancer with conserva-

tive surgery and radiation therapy. J Natl Cancer Inst Monogr 1992;11:33–39.

4. Stotter A, McNeese, Ames FC, et al. Predicting the rate and extent of locoregional failure after breast conservation therapy for early breast cancer. Cancer 1989;64:2217–2225.

5. Clark R, Wilkinson R, Miceli P, et al. Breast cancer. Experiences with conservative therapy. Am J Clin Oncol 1987;10:461–468.

6. Spitalier J, Gambarelli J, Brandone H, et al. Breast-conserving surgery with radiation therapy for operable mammary carcinoma: A 25-year experience. World J Surg 1986;10:1014–1020.

7. Fourquet A, Campana F, Zafrani B, et al. Prognostic factors of breast recurrence in the conservative management of early breast cancer: A 25-year follow-up. Int J Radiat Oncol Biol Phys 1989;17:719–725.

8. National Institutes for Health Consensus Conference: Treatment of early-stage breast cancer. JAMA 1991;265:391–395.

9. Olivetto LA, Rose MA, Osteen RT, et al. Late cosmetic outcome after conservative surgery and radiotherapy: Analysis of causes of cosmetic failure. Int J Radiat Oncol Biol Phys 1989;17:747–753.

10. Vicini FA, Eberlein TJ, Connolly JL, et al. The optimal extent of resection for patients with stages I and II breast cancer treated with conservative surgery and radiotherapy. Ann Surg 1991;214:200–208.

11. Nobler MP, Venet L. Prognostic factors in patients undergoing curative irradiation for breast cancer. Int J Radiat Oncol Biol Phys 1985;11:1323–1331.

12. van Limbergen E, van den Bogaert W, van der Schueren E, et al. Tumor excision and radiotherapy as primary treatment of breast cancer: Analysis of patient and treatment parameters and local control. Radiother Oncol 1987;8:1–9.

13. Clarke DH, Le MG, Sarrazin D, et al. Analysis of local-regional relapses in patients with early stage breast cancers treated with excision and radiotherapy: Experience of the Institut Gustave-Roussy. Int J Radiat Oncol Biol Phys 1985;11:137–145.

14. Holland R, Connolly J, Gelman R, et al. Nature and extent of residual cancer in the breast related to the intraductal component in the primary tumor. Int J Radiat Oncol Biol Phys 1988;15:182–183.

15. Hartsell W, Galinsky D, Griem K, et al. Lumpectomy with negative margins: Is a boost dose to the tumor bed necessary? (Abstract) Int J Radiat Oncol Biol Phys 1994;30(Suppl):246.

16. Bedwinek JM, Perez CA, Kramer S, et al. Irradiation as the primary management of Stage I and II adenocarcinoma of the breast. Analysis of the RTOG breast registry. Cancer Clin Trials 1980;3:11–18.

17. Pezner RD, Lipsett JA, Desai K, et al. To boost or not to boost: Decreasing radiation therapy in conservative breast cancer treatment when "inked" tumor resection margins are pathologically free of cancer. Int J Radiat Oncol Biol Phys 1988;14:873–877.

18. Vicini FA, White J, Gustafson G, et al. The use of iodine-125 seeds as a substitute for iridium-192 seeds in temporary interstitial breast implants. Int J Radiat Oncol Biol Phys 1993;27(3):561–566.

19. Krishnan L, Jewell WR, Krishnan EC, et al. Breast cancer with extensive intraductal component: Treatment with immediate interstitial breast irradiation. Radiology 1992;183:273–276.

20. Mansfield CM, Kamarnicky LT, Schwartz GF, et al. Perioperative implantation of Ir-192 as the boost technique for Stage I and II breast cancer: 10 year results in 655 patients. Radiology 1994;192:33–36.

21. Pierquin B, Dutreix CH, Paine D, et al. The Paris System in interstitial radiation therapy. Acta Radiol Oncol 1978;17(Fasc. 1):33–48.

22. Shalek RJ, Stovall M. Dosimetry in implant therapy. In: Radiation Dosimetry. Attix, Roesch, Tochilin, New York Academic Press, 1969.

23. Johns HE, Cunningham JR. Appendices A. Basic data. Table 3c and 3e. In: The Physics of Radiology. Fourth Edition, 1983, pp. 714–725.

24. Meredith WS (ed). Radium Dosage, The Manchester System. E and Livingston S, Edinburgh, 1947.

25. Hilaris BS (ed). Handbook of Interstitial Brachytherapy. Publishing Sciences Group, Inc., Action, Massachusettes, 1975.

26. Anderson LL, Hilaris BS, Wagner LK. A nomograph for planar implant planning. Endocurie/Hypertherm Oncol 1985;1:9–15.

27. Johnson DW. An adjustable breast bridge for use in multi-plane breast implants. Br J Radiol 1984;57:159–162.

28. Martinez A, Goffinet D. Irradiation with external beam and interstitial radioactive implants as primary treatment for early carcinoma of the breast. Surg Gynecol Obstet 1981;152:285–290.

29. Mazeron JJ, Simon JM, Crook J, et al. Influence of dose rate on local control of breast carcinoma treated by external beam irradiation plus iridium-192 implant. Int J Radiat Oncol Biol Phys 1991;21(5):1173–1177.

30. Clarke DH, Edmundson CK, Martinez A, et al. The utilization of I-125 seeds as a substitute for Ir-192 seeds in temporary interstitial im-

plants. An overview and a description of the William Beaumont Hospital technique. Int J Radiat Oncol Biol Phys 1988;15:1027–1033.

31. Leung S, Otmezquine Y, Calitchi E, et al. Locoregional recurrences following radical external beam irradiation and interstitial implantation for operable breast cancer: A 23-year experience. Radiother Oncol 1986;5:1–10.

32. Glicksman AS, Leith JT. Radiobiological considerations of brachytherapy. Oncology 1988; 2(1):25.

33. Hall EF, Lam YM. The renaissance in low dose rate interstitial implants. Radiobiological considerations. In: Vaeth J (ed). Frontiers of Radiation Therapy and Oncology. Karger Ag, Basil, Switzerland, 1978, pp. 21–234.

34. Clarke DH, Martinez A. Identification of patients who are at high risk for locoregional breast cancer recurrence after conservative surgery and radiotherapy: A review article for surgeons, pathologists, and radiation and medical oncologists. J Clin Oncol 1992;10:474–483.

35. Krishnan EC, Krishnan L, Cytaki E, et al. Radiobiological advantages of an immediate interstitial boost dose in conservative treatment of breast cancer. Int J Radiat Oncol Biol Phys 1990;18(2):419–424.

36. Rose M, Olivetto J, Cady B, et al. Conservative surgery and radiation therapy for early stage breast cancer. Long-term cosmetic results. Arch Surg 1989;124:153–157.

37. Stefanik D, Brereton HD, Lee TC. Fat necrosis following breast irradiation for carcinoma; Clinical presentation and diagnosis. Breast 1982;8(4):4–6.

38. Clarke D, Martinez A, Cox RS. Analysis of cosmetic results and complications in patients with stage I and II breast cancer treated by biopsy and irradiation. Int J Radiat Oncol Biol Phys 1983;9:1807–1813.

39. de la Rochefordiere A, Abner AL, Silver B, et al. Are cosmetic results following conservative surgery and radiation therapy for early breast cancer dependent upon technique? Int J Radiat Oncol Biol Phys 1992;23(5):925–931.

40. Denham JW, Hamilton CS, Cross P. Breast conservation, the problem of treating the excision site effectively: Physical criteria for the choice of technique used. Clin Oncol 1991;3:250–256.

41. Wazer DE, DiPetrillo T, Schmidt-Ullrich R, et al. Factors influencing cosmetic outcome and complication risk after conservative surgery and radiotherapy for early-stage breast carcinoma. J Clin Oncol 1992;10:356–363.

42. Farrow DC, Hunt WC, Samet JM. Geographic variation in the treatment of localized breast cancer. N Engl J Med 1992;326:1097–1101.

43. Fisher B, Redmond C. Lumpectomy for breast cancer: An update of the NSABP experience. National Surgical Adjuvant Breast and Bowel Project. Monogr Natl Cancer Inst 1992;11:7–13.

44. Liljegren G, Holmberg L, Adami H-O, et al. Sector resection with or without postoperative radiotherapy for stage I breast cancer: Five-year results of a randomized trial. J Natl Cancer Inst 1994;86:717–722.

45. Stomper PC, Connolly JL. Mammographic features predicting an extensive intraductal component in early stage infiltrating ductal carcinoma. Am J Roentgenol 1992;158:269–272.

46. Fentiman IS, Poole C, Tong D, et al. Iridium implant treatment without external radiotherapy for operable breast cancer: A pilot study. Eur J Cancer 1991;27:447–450.

47. Clark RM, McCulloch PB, Levine MN, et al. Randomized clinical trial to assess the effectiveness of breast irradiation following lumpectomy and axillary dissection for node-negative breast cancer. J Natl Cancer Inst 1992;84: 683–689.

48. Stewart HJ, Prescott RJ, Forrest PA. Conservative therapy of breast cancer. (Letter) Lancet 1989;2:168–169.

49. Veronesi U, Luini A, Del Vecchio M, et al. Radiotherapy after breast preserving surgery in women with localized cancer of the breast. N Engl J Med 1993;328:1587–1591.

50. Machtay M, Lanciano R, Hoffman J, et al. Inaccuracies in using the lumpectomy scar for planning electron boosts in primary breast carcinoma. Int J Radiat Oncol Biol Phys 1994;30(1): 43–48.

51. Denham JW, Sillar RW, Clarke D. Boost dosage to the excision site following conservative surgery for breast cancers: It's easy to miss. Clin Oncol 1991;3:257–261.

52. Clarke DH, Vicini FA, Jacobs H, et al. High dose rate brachytherapy for breast cancer. In: Nag S (ed). High Dose Rate Brachytherapy: A Textbook. Futura Publishing Company, Inc., Armonk, NY, 1994, pp. 321–329.

53. Mansfield CM. Intraoperative Ir-192 implantation for early breast cancer—techniques and results. Cancer 1990;66:1–5.

54. McCormick B, Waesson MF, Cox L, et al. Iridium-192 implants for primary breast cancer: Experience with placement at the time of wide local excision. Int J Radiat Oncol Biol Phys 1988;15:745–748.

55. Van Zyl JA, Muller AGS. Breast-conserving treatment for stage I and II cancer. S Afr Med J 1989;75:519–523.

56. Syed AMN, Puthawala A, Fleming P, et al. Combination of external and interstitial irradiation in the primary management of breast carcinoma. Cancer 1980;46:1360–1365.

57. Sarin R, Dinshaw KA, Shrivastava SK, et al. Therapeutic factors influencing the cosmetic outcome and late complications in the conservative management of early stage breast cancer. Int J Radiat Oncol Biol Phys 1993;27(2): 285–292.

58. Deore SM, Dip RP, Sarin R, et al. Influence of dose-rate and dose per fraction on clinical outcome of breast cancer treated by external beam irradiation plus iridium-192 implants: Analysis of 289 cases. Int J Radiat Oncol Biol Phys 1993;26(4):601–606.

59. Pierquin B, Huart J, Raynal M, et al. Conservative treatment for breast cancer: Long-term techniques and results (15 years). Radiother Oncol 1991;20:16–23.

60. Hammer J, Track C, Pakisch B, et al. The impact of boost type (E-, Ir-192 HDR) on the cosmetic result in conservative breast cancer treatment. Radiother Oncol 1994;31(Suppl):7.

61. Touboul E, Beklacemi Y, Ozsahin M, et al. Conservative surgery and radiation therapy in the treatment of stage I and II breast cancer: Influence of type of boost (electrons vs iridium 192 implant) on local control. (Abstract) Int J Radiat Oncol Biol Phys 1994;30(Suppl 1): 245–246.

62. Kuske R, Bolton J, Wilenzick R, et al. Brachytherapy as the sole method of breast irradiation in Tis, T_1, T_2, N_{0-1} breast cancer. (Abstract) Int J Radiat Oncol Biol Phys 1994;30(Suppl 1):245.

63. Krishnan L, Jewell W, Mansfield CM, et al. Early stage breast cancer: Local control after conservative surgery and radiation therapy with immediate interstitial boost. Radiology 1993; 187:95–98.

64. Hammer J, Seewald DH, Track C, et al. Breast cancer: Primary treatment with external-beam radiation therapy and high-dose-rate iridium implantation. Radiology 1994;193:573–577.

65. Perera F, Chisela F, Engel J, et al. Method of localization and implantation of the lumpectomy site for high dose rate brachytherapy after conservative surgery for T1 and T2 breast cancer. Int J Radiat Oncol Biol Phys 1995;31(4).

Chapter 18

Extrahepatic Bile Duct and Liver Cancer

Beth Erickson, M.D., Subir Nag, M.D.

Introduction

For the purpose of this chapter, extrahepatic bile duct carcinomas will include those located in the main hepatic duct junction, the common hepatic duct, the supraduodenal common bile duct, and diffusely throughout the bile ducts and exclude those in the intrapancreatic bile duct, ampulla, and gallbladder. These tumors pose a challenge because they spread by direct extension either within the ducts or by extraductal involvement of surrounding organs, and they are often multicentric, placing the entire biliary tree at risk. The rich lymphatic network and the thin walls of the extrahepatic bile ducts allow early extension through the walls into the submucosal lymphatics and to lymph nodes in the portahepatis and celiac axis, which are involved in 40%–50% of patients.[1–3]

Surgical extirpation is the treatment of choice. However, as a result of the pattern of spread of these tumors, 70%–80% are unresectable upon presentation, due to invasion of the portal vein, hepatic artery, or involvement of the secondary and tertiary bile duct tributaries in both hepatic lobes.[2–4] Even after successful gross tumor removal, margins are often tenuous or positive due to intraductal spread, indicating the need for adjunctive treatment to decrease the risk of recurrence

after resection alone.[1,2,5] When margins are positive, resection must be considered palliative. As a rule, survival is poor but depends in part on the location of the tumor, resectability, margin status, and the ability to sustain biliary drainage. A median survival of 12–24 months and a 5-year survival of 0%–15% is achieved in some resected patients; whereas, a median survival of 6 months and a survival of <5% is achieved in unresectable patients.[1,3,5–9] It is locoregional, rather than distant disease that is most often the cause of death, usually as a result of liver failure secondary to progressive obstruction, complicated by cholangitis and sepsis.[1,2,5,7,8,10] Therefore, increasing survival by securing local control should be the objective of treatment. These treatment goals must, however, be balanced against the knowledge that, despite aggressive locoregional treatment, many patients will succumb to their disease and that, in realistic terms, treatment will be essentially palliative. Therefore, duration and morbidity of treatment must be compared with its benefit.

Methods

Although supporting data are lacking, extrahepatic biliary tumors have been thought to be radioresistant. More recently, proof to the contrary has been emerging and a role

From Nag S (ed): *Principles and Practice of Brachytherapy.* © Futura Publishing Co., Inc., Armonk, NY, 1997.

Table 1.
Extrahepatic Bile Duct

Author	Number of Patients	Def Post-Op	Ext Xrt	Pre Post I.C.	I.C. Dose Prescription	Margin/Source Length
Bethune, et al, 1981 (23)	1	Def-1	3000 cGy/10 FX EXT + 1330 cGy intra-op e-'s	Post	1230 cGy/45 hours at 1 cm from tube at 27 cGy/hour	
Buskirk, et al, 1984 (22)	5	Def-5	4500 cGy (large) 500 cGy (boost)	Post	2000–2500 cGy at 0.5–1.0 cm from source	1.5 cm beyond lesion
Chitwood, et al, 1982 (3)	10	Def-8 Post-op-2	None or 4600 cGy/23 FX-7 pts EXT & I.C.-7 I.C. only-3	Pre	5000 cGy/21–100 hours at inner surface of bile duct (Effective dia = 1.0 cm) Mean of 5489 cGy ± 636 cGy	
Ede, et al, 1989 (31)	14	Def	0	I.C.: 2 weeks after catheter insertion	6000 cGy/85 hours at 0.5 cm from source at 71 cGy/hour	1 cm margin
Fields & Emami, 1987 (15)	8	Def-7 Post-op-1	2160–5040 cGy EXT & I.C.-8	Post: Break of 3–4 weeks after external	949–2567 cGy at 1.0 cm from source	
Fletcher, et al, 1983 (27)	18	Def	0	I.C.: 10–14 days after tube placement	Mean = 4470 cGy/55.3 hours at 0.5 cm from source at 80 cGy/hour	
Fletcher, et al, 1981 (25)	8	Def	0	I.C.: 10–14 days after tube placement	4000–4800 cGy/48 hours at 0.5 cm from source at 83–100 cGy/hour	
Flickenger, et al, 1991 (8)	12	Def Post-op	None or 2600–6000 cGy EXT & I.C.-9 I.C. only-3	Post	I.C. only: 2800, 2960, 5500 cGy at 0.5 cm from source; boost: 1400–4500 cGy at 0.5 cm from source	
Fogel & Weissberg, 1984 (24)	3	Def	4400–5400 cGy	Post: 3–4 weeks	1800–3800 cGy at 1.5 cm from source at 40 cGy/hour	3–4 cm source length

Low Dose Rate Series

Activity Ir	Number Sources	Number Insertions	Stents	Local Control	Survival	Complications
		1	T-tube	1/1 (100%)	2 years	
	1–2	1	Perc	4/5 (80%)	2/5 NED 7–20 months 1 DSD at 18 months	2 UGI bleeds 2° to gastric and duodenal ulcers
5.7–25.5 mCi (mean of 9.5 mCi ± 1.5 mCi)	1–2	1–2 if disease persists	Perc	6/10 (60%) at 3–13 months	5/10 alive 1–12 months after XRT; Resected and radiated (2): (6 & 13 months). Def EXT & I.C. XRT (3): (19, 22, 26 months)	0
	1	1	Nasobiliary		10.5 months after implant	Cholangitis-2
	1–2	1	Perc		Median of 15 months after XRT (1.5–34.5 months) 2/8 NED at 24 and 34.5 months	Fatal sepsis-2 Bile duct stenosis & sepsis-1 Gastric ulcer with SBO-1 Liver abscess-1
	1	1 or 2 if disease recurs	Perc-2 U&T-tubes-6		11 months median; 9 pts surv ≥ 12 months (4–38 months)	
	1	1 or 2 if disease recurs	Perc-2 U&T-tubes-6	2/8 (25%)	11 months median 2 pts NED at 2 years 6/8 alive 2, 4, 5, 16, 22, & 23 months	
		1				
26.6 mCi– 28.8 mCi	1	1	Perc-2 Transhepatic-1	18–19 months Biliary drainage d/c after 1.5 years	19 months 21 months	

(continued)

Table 1.
(*continued*)

Author	Number of Patients	Def Post-Op	Ext Xrt	Pre Post I.C.	I.C. Dose Prescription	Margin/Source Length
Gonzalez, et al, 1990 (7)	27	Def-12 Post-op-15	I.C. & EXT-23 I.C. only-4		1.0 cm from source	
Hayes, Sapozink,& Miller, 1988 (30)	10	Def	None or 4100–6020 cGy I.C. & EXT-8 I.C. only-2	Post: Break of 2 weeks after external	1310–5800 cGy at 0.5 cm from outside of catheter	8–12 seeds/ ribbon with 1.0 cm spacing
Herskovic, Engler, & Noell, 1985 (13)	16	Def Post-op	None or 3600–5000 cGy (12 pts) EXT & I.C.-12 I.C. only-4	Pre: Several days or weeks after catheter placed	1060–10,000 cGy at 0.5 cm from source (0.15–0.6 cm) at 37–240 cGy/hour	>5 cm margin
Herskovic, et al, 1981 (11)	10	Def-8 Post-op-2	None or 4600 cGy/23 FX-7 pts EXT & I.C.-7 I.C. only-3	Pre	5000 cGy/21–100 hours at inner surfacer of bile duct (Effective dia = 1.0 cm)	42 mm-1 pt
Johnson, Safai, & Goffinet, 1985 (29)	7	Def	4000–5500 cGy EXT & I.C.-7	Post: Break of 2–3 weeks after external	3100–10,647 cGy at 0.5 cm from source at 101 cGy/hour	4–15 cm source length
Jones, et al, 1983 (12)	10	Def-8 Post-op-2	None or 3600–5000 (mean of 4554 cGy) EXT & I.C.-7 I.C. only-3	Pre	4750–10,000 cGy/ 21–162 hours (mean of 60.1 hours ± 11.2) calc radius of 1.5–5.8 mm (mean = 3.8 ± 0.4 mm)	

Activity Ir	Number Sources	Number Insertions	Stents	Local Control	Survival	Complications
	1–2		Perc U&Y tube-16 Nasobiliary-1 Other-10		Median surivival 18.7 months with EXT & I.C. XRT after resection (15 pts) and 12.3 months after biliary drainage, (9 pts)	Duodenal ulcers-5 Pyloric stenosis-3
44–52 mBQ/ seed; 8–12 seeds/ ribbon	1–2	1	Perc		I.C. only: 11.9 & 13.8 months EXT & I.C.: Median = 13.2 months (7.4–30.3)	Sepsis-75%; Cholangitis-62%; Abscess-30%; GI bleed-50%; Hemobilia-38%; Duodenal ulcer-38%; Gastric outlet obstr.-25%
1.1 mCi/seed 8–21 seeds	1–3	1–2 if disease persists	Perc-14 T-tube-2	13/15 (81%) 3 marginal recurrences	1 pt NED at 30 months 15/16 dead (10/16 DC̃D)	Cholangitis-5 Duodenal & gastric ulcers-2
5.7–25.5 mCi (mean of 9.5 mCi ± 1.5 mCi)	1–2	1–2 if disease persists	Perc	6/10 (60%) at 3–13 months	5/10 alive 1–12 months after XRT; Resected and radiated (2): (6 & 13 months); Def EXT & I.C. XRT (3): (19, 22, 26 months)	0
	1	1–2	Perc U&T-tubes	4/7 (57%)	Mean = 8.3 months after XRT; 3 alive at 5, 5.5, 13 months (2 NED)	Duodenal ulcer-1
5.7–25.5 mCi (mean of 9.5 mCi ± 1.5 mCi)	1–2	1–2 if disease persists	Perc	6/10 (60%) at 3–13 months	Resected & radiated-2: (6 & 13 months) Definitive EXT & I.C.-3: (19, 22, 26 months)	0

(continued)

Table 1.
(*continued*)

Author	Number of Patients	Def Post-Op	Ext Xrt	Pre Post I.C.	I.C. Dose Prescription	Margin/Source Length
Karani, et al, 1985 (28)	30	Def	0	I.C.: 10–14 days after tube placement	4000–5000 cGy/48 hours (Mean = 4470 cGy/55.3 hours) at 0.5 cm from source at 83–104 cGy/ hour (Mean = 90 cGy/hour)	
Kumar, Good, & McCaul, 1986 (38)	5	Def	None or 4000 cGy (4/5)	Pre	6000 cGy to a volume over 120 hours at 50 cGy/ hour (4.0–7.0 cm)	10 cm & 5 cm (10 & 5 seeds spaced 1 cm apart)
Levitt, et al, 1988 (33)	7	Def	3000 cGy/10 FX	Pre: EXT XRT 1–4 weeks after	6000 cGy/90 hours at 0.5 cm from source (70–109 hours) at 66.6 cGy/hour	1.5 × length of stricture
Mahe, et al, 1991 (10) Gerard, et al, 1991 (18)	25	Def-13 Post-op-12	None or 4250 cGy (17 pts) (Curative) 2000 cGy/5 FX- (Palliative); EXT & I.C.-17 I.C. only-8	Pre: External beam follows after 3 weeks	3000–6000 cGy at 0.5–1.0 cm from source-(I.C. only); 1000—1500 cGy at 1 cm from source, (curative boost) or 2000–3000 cGy at 1 cm from source, (palliative boost)	4–8 cm 1.5–2.0 cm margin beyond lesion
Meyers & Jones, 1988 (14)	27	Def-24 Post-op-3	None or 3000–4500 cGy EXT & I.C.-22 I.C. only-5	Pre	3000–5000 cGy at 0.5 cm from source	5 cm margin
Minsky, et al, 1991 (36)	5	Def	5000 cGy/25 FX with 1500 cGy boost	Post	1000–2000 cGy/ 33.3–53.8 hours at 1 cm from source	

Activity Ir	Number Sources	Number Insertions	Stents	Local Control	Survival	Complications
	1	1 or 2 if disease recurs	Perc U&T-tubes		Median = 16.8 months (1–66) 21 pts alive > 1 year 5 pts alive > 2 years 2 pts alive > 4 years 1 pt alive > 6 years	
4–10 mCi per seed (10 in 1 catheter, 5 in other)	2	1–2	Perc	4/5 (80%)	3/5 alive at 6, 10, 25 months	Fatal hepatic venous bleed-1
	1–2	1–2 if disease persists	Nasobiliary		Median = 10 months after XRT	Cholangitis-30%
4–12 mCi/cm	1–2	1	Perc or via lap		Gross resection 2 pts EXT & I.C. DCD 7 & 14 months 2 pts I.C. only DCD 58 & 60 months	Cholangitis-3
	1–3	1–2 if disease persists	Perc-23 T-tube-4		Median survival 11.5 months after XRT (1–58 months) (I.C. only = 3.6 months; I.C. & EXT = 14.3 months) resected: (8, 15, & 53 months); unresected ave survival of 5.8 months vs 14.1 months with resection	Cholangitis-21/27 Hemobilia-4 Periductal absecess-9 Abscess + Choledochoduo- denal fistula-1
	1	1	Perc		Median: 17 months; 4 year actuarial = 36%	Gastric ulcer-1 Hepatic abscess-1

Table 1.
(*continued*)

Author	Number of Patients	Def Post-Op	Ext Xrt	Pre Post I.C.	I.C. Dose Prescription	Margin/Source Length
Minsky, et al, 1990 (35)	4	Def	5000 cGy/25 FX with 1500 cGy boost	Post: 4 weeks after external	1000–2000 cGy/ 33.3–53.8 hours at 1 cm from source	
Molt, et al, 1986 (34)	7	Def	None or 3000–3300 cGy/10–11 FX EXT & I.C.-6 I.C.-1	Post	1320–6000 cGy/ 48–177 hours at 0.5 cm from source	12 Ir-192 seeds spaced at 1 cm intervals
Montemaggi, et al, 1992 (54)	5		0	Def	5000 cGy at 1 cm from source	
Mornex, et al, 1984 (17)	7	Def-5 Post-2	None or 2000 cGy/5 FX-5000 cGy/25 FX	Pre: External beam follows 4–8 weeks	1000–6000 cGy at 0.5 cm from source	4–6 cm source length 1 cm margin either end
Trodella, et al, 1991 (37)	8	Def	None or 2600–2850 cGy EXT & I.C.-2 I.C. only-6	Pre	Mean: 4800 cGy at 1 cm from source (2000–5000 cGy) at 42.8 cGy/hour (30–61)	6.1 cm source length (1–15 cm)
Veeze-Kuijpers, et al, 1990 (16)	30	Def-31 Post-op-11	None or 3000–4000 cGy/15–16 FX I.C. only-4	Pre & Post: 2 weeks before & after external	1500 cGy × 2/75 hours at 1 cm from source or 2500 cGy × 1 at 1 cm from source at 20 cGy/hour	Positioned 2 cm proximal to tumor in duodenum
Wheeler, et al, 1981 (26)	5	Def	EXT & I.C.-1 I.C. only-4	I.C.: 10–14 days after tube placement	4000–4800 cGy/48 hours at 0.5 cm from source at 83–100 cGy/ hour	

* AĈD = alive with disease; BID = twice per day; DĈD = dead with disease; Def = definitive irradiation; Dia = diameter; DŜD = dead without disease; EXT = external beam; FX = fraction; IC = intracavitary; IR = Iridium 192; NED = no evidence of disease; Perc = percutaneous; Post-op = post-operative irradiation; TID = three times per day.

for radiation therapy for both resectable and unresectable tumors has been established.

Postoperative External Beam Radiation Therapy and Brachytherapy

Whenever possible, resection should be attempted. After this, every attempt must be made to enhance the durability of locoregional control. To this purpose, both external beam radiation therapy (EBRT) and brachytherapy may be combined to minimize late complications and to target areas where margins may be close or positive. EBRT doses in the range of 45–50 Gy with brachytherapy dose of about 15–25 Gy (at 1 cm) are commonly used.[3,7,8,10–21]

Definitive External Beam Radiation Therapy and Brachytherapy

More typically, the disease is unresectable and definitive radiation is required.[5] The goals of treatment in unresectable disease are, at a minimum, to alleviate pain, to relieve obstruction, to provide tumor regression, and

Activity Ir	Number Sources	Number Insertions	Stents	Local Control	Survival	Complications
	1	1	Perc	3/4 (75%)	3 pts NED at 16, 48, 52 months; 1 pt DCD at 16 months	Gastric ulcer-1 Hepatic abscess-1
	1–2	1–3	Perc U&T-tube straight		Median: 3.75 months (2–13 months) after I.C. & EXT XRT	UGI bleeds (1 hemobilia & 1 duodenal ulcer)-2
		1	Perc Nasobiliary	4/5 (80%) Jaundice controlled	11.5 months after XRT	
4–8 mCi/cm	1	1	Perc T-tube		4/7 NED at 4, 5, 8, & 12 months	Cholangitis-1
2.04–4.79 mCi/cm with total of 30.6–47.8 mCi	1	1	Perc-3 Nasobiliary-5	Jaundice ↓ pain ↓ 7/8	Overall = 13.1 months (2–43 months) 2 pts survived >12 months; 1 pt NED at 43 months	Gastroduodenal bleed-3
	1	1–2	Perc		Median = 10 months 3 pts >30 months 16% at 3 years	Cholangitis-6/38 Gastritis and duodenal ulcers-3
= to 15 mg RA eq	1	1 or 2 if disease recurs	Perc-2 U&T-tubes-6	2/8 (25%)	11 months median 2 pts NED at 2 years 6/8 alive 2, 4, 5, 16, 22, & 23 months	

possibly to improve survival. With unresectable disease, the challenge of definitive irradiation is to deliver adequate doses to eradicate gross tumor while respecting the tolerance of the surrounding normal tissues (liver, kidneys, GI tract, and spinal cord). If treatment is with "curative intent," doses in excess of 60 Gy are needed, but this often exceeds the tolerance of the adjacent normal organs. The high rate of locoregional recurrence after definitive EBRT points to the need for techniques to deliver higher doses of radiation. Intraluminal brachytherapy may provide this option, providing access and additional dose delivery to the tumor while sparing the surrounding normal tissues.[3,7,8,] [10–19,21–44] EBRT usually precedes brachytherapy[8,15,16,19,20,22–24,29,30,32,34–36,39–41,43] to decrease tumor bulk before implantation so that residual disease is encompassed by the limited range of the intraluminal radiation. At some institutions, implantation has preceded EBRT, decreasing the likelihood of catheter loss through dislodgment and expediting internal drainage conversion.[3,10–14,16–19,33,37,38]

EBRT doses ranging from 20–60 Gy have been reported in the literature, but typical doses range from 45–50 Gy (Tables 1 and 2).[2,5,45–49] The fields must encompass the tumor or tumor bed, abdominal wall and drain sites, and regional lymph nodes (including those along the biliary tree, portahepatis,

Table 2.
Extrahepatic Bile Duct

Author	Number of Patients	Def Post-Op	Ext Xrt	Pre Post I.C.	I.C. Dose Prescription	Margin/Source Length
Haffty, et al, 1987 Gamma Med (39)	1	Def	5400 cGy/32 FX	Post	480 cGy at 0.5 cm from lumen surface	6 cm length
Yoshimura, et al, 1989; RALS (40)	1	Def	3200 cGy/16 FX	Post	3750 cGy/5 FX at 1 cm from source	
Yoshimura, et al, 1992; RALS (41)	15	Def	3000–3200 cGy	Post	3000–6000 cGy/ 4–6 FX/2 per week at 1 cm from source	
Urban, et al, 1990 Nucletron (42)	2	Def	0	Def	300–1000 cGy/FX up to 2000 cGy over 2 days at 1 cm from source	
Pavlou, et al, 1990 Nucletron (19)	8	Def Post-op ((-)margins)	None or 4500 cGy	Pre-post	No EXT: 3000 cGy/ 6 FX/BID at 1 cm from source/ 3 days EXT: 2000 cGy/4 FX/BID at 1 cm from source/ 2 days or 3000 cGy/5 FX/ 1 week or 1000 cGy/3 FX/ TID at 1 cm from source	
Kurisu, et al, 1991; RALS (20)	5	Post-op	None or 2000–4200 cGy/10–21 FX	Post	1000 cGy/1FX-1 1150 cGy/1FX-1 2000 cGy/1FX-1 2100 cGy/1FX-1 4000 cGy/4FX at 1 cm from source-1	
Nori, et al, 1993 (43)	15	Def	None or 4500–5000 cGy/25–28 FX	Post	EXT: 1500–2000 cGy/3–4 FX/1 week apart at 1 cm from source; No EXT: 3000 cGy/6 FX/BID/3 days at 1 cm from source	5–7 cm (2–3 cm margin either side)
Pakisch, et al, 1992 Nucletron (44)	9	Def	None or 5040 cGy/25 FX EXT & IC-6 IC only-3		1000 cGy at 0.75 cm from source	
Ryu, et al, 1988; RALS (21)	6	Def-5 Post-op-1	None or 5000 cGy EXT & IC-4 IC only-2		500 cGy × 5 at 1.5 cm from source	
Classen & Hagenmuller, 1987 (62)	17				3000 cGy at 1 cm from source	

Def = definitive irradiation; Post-op = post-operative irradiation; Perc = percutaneous; EXT = external beam; IC = intracavitary; Dia = diameter; NED = no evidence of disease; ACD = alive with disease; DSD = dead without disease; DCD = dead with disease; BID = twice per day; TID = three times per day; FX = fraction.

High Dose Rate Series

Activity	Number Sources	Number Insertions	Stents	Local Control	Survival	Complications
10 Ci Ir 192	1	2, 10 days apart	Perc	Lesion ↓		
4 Ci Co60	1	5, 2 per week	Perc			
4 Ci Co60		4–6, 2 per week	Perc	Tube Free-7 months; 12/13 able to d/c perc tube	Ave = 9.0 months 2/15 alive at 26.8 & 32.2 months after XRT	Hemobilia-1
10 Ci Ir 192	1–2		Nasobiliary			0
10 Ci Ir 192	1–2	1–6 given 1–3 per day over 1–5 days	Nasobiliary-6 Perc-2			0
4 Ci Co60		1–4	Perc T-tube		2/5-Alive 36–41 months after XRT	Fatal Sepsis-1 Cholangitis-5
10 Ci Ir 192	1–2	1 FX per week x 3–4; 6 FX/BID/3 days; 4 FX/BID/2 days	Perc Nasobiliary		8 NED at 6–24 months	Sepsis-1
10 Ci Ir 192			Nasobiliary	9/9 maintance of bile flow ↓ puritis 7/9 palliated for 7l5 month	7.5 months	
4 Ci Co60			5, 1–2 per week	Perc	5/6 resolution of stricture	
10 Ci Ir 192			Perc Nasobiliary (LDR)		3 months (1–10) 4 NED at 3–16 months (Def XRT) 1 DSD at 7 months 1 NED at 9 months (Post-op XRT)	

celiac axis, and pancreaticoduodenal area) with generous margins to allow for undetected spread throughout the biliary tree remote from the tumor. The target volume is often difficult to define due to the intrahepatic spread of these tumors, and radiological imaging studies including the percutaneous transhepatic cholangiograms (PTC), CAT, MRI, ultrasound, and endoscopic retrograde cholangiopancreatography (ERCP) should be used whenever possible to define suitable radiation portals. In addition, the information documented at laparotomy should also be available to help define the irradiated volume. Surgeons should be made aware that placement of surgical clips at tumor margins is invaluable for treatment planning.

Brachytherapy Alone

A third treatment option for stented patients is intraluminal irradiation alone. Because this approach has certain limitations (i.e., bulky tumor will not be encompassed by the limited penetration of the intraluminal sources), brachytherapy alone is reserved for palliation.[3,7,8,10–14,16–21,25–28,30–32,34,37,38,42–44,50–54]

Brachytherapy Techniques

Intraluminal brachytherapy is particularly suited to this disease site as one can take advantage of the anatomical lumens where these tumors originate to place radioactive materials. Plastic catheters can be placed at the time of radiological studies, laparotomy, or endoscopy for external or internal biliary drainage and are used to provide access to the biliary tract. The percutaneous transhepatic technique is the technique most commonly used at our institutions and is recommended.

Transhepatic Catheter Placement

Transhepatic or percutaneous catheter insertion (ring, pigtail) is performed by an interventional radiologist and entails guiding a catheter into the dilated intrahepatic bile ducts, through the obstructing tumor, and into the duodenum, over a guide wire positioned during percutaneous cholangiography. This procedure provides both internal biliary drainage across the tumor and external drainage via the proximal end of the catheter.[32,51,55–58] Occasionally, if the obstructive tumor initially prevents entry into the duodenum, a few days of external percutaneous drainage alone will relieve the edema; and, typically, a second attempt at duodenal entry will be successful. It is possible that intraluminal irradiation to the proximal obstructed site may help to open up the obstruction.[32,55,59]

Intraoperative Catheter Placement

Biliary catheters (T-tubes, U-tubes, Y-tubes, silastic transhepatic biliary stents) can also be placed by a surgeon intraoperatively, after biopsy, bypass, or resection.[4,6,51] It is important to discuss with the surgeon the location of the catheters in relationship to the tumor or tumor margins and segments of the GI tract so that sources can be placed strategically. When remote afterloading techniques are used, the surgeon should also be aware of the difficulties in loading acutely angled afterloading catheters. In the series of Fletcher et al.,[25] four patients underwent T-tube placement with the long horizontal limb placed through the tumor from below, high into the proximal hepatic duct. Later, it proved difficult to manipulate the iridium wire into position because of the acute angle between the vertical and horizontal limbs of the T-tube.

Endoscopic Catheter Placement

Catheter insertion through stents or prosthesis is accomplished endoscopically by a gastroenterologist at the time of the ERCP.[7,19,31,33,37,42–44,53,54,60–62] The preceding endoscopic sphincterotomy and placement of the prosthesis through the stricture allows internal drainage of bile. This technique, therefore, avoids percutaneous puncture through the liver or a laparotomy for catheter placement and may decrease complications and patient discomfort. The in-dwelling prosthesis is thought to decrease the risk of papillitis and ampullary stricture when traversed by iridium.[61] It is important for the gastroenterologist to avoid forming a redundant loop in the duodenum, which is difficult to negotiate with a cable-driven high-dose-rate (HDR) source.[19,42,43] Anchoring of the catheter in the biliary tree may also be problematic.

Biliary Drainage Catheter

Regardless of drainage technique, it is important to place a biliary drainage catheter of adequate diameter (usually an 8–10Fr for low-dose-rate [LDR] and a 10–14Fr for HDR) to allow placement of the brachytherapy catheter. The exact diameter of biliary drainage catheter depends upon whether an LDR, 5Fr, or 6Fr HDR afterloading catheter is used. Further, the higher internal friction of soft drainage catheters, which are more comfortable for the patients, requires use of a larger diameter catheter compared to stiff catheters. We generally insert the afterloading catheter to be used into the drainage catheter to confirm its easy passage before the procedure. It is also important to understand the relationship of the catheters to the duodenum or other adjacent portions of the GI tract to avoid unnecessary irradiation of these vulnerable structures.

Radioactive Sources: Low-Dose-Rate/High-Dose-Rate

The first sources used for intraluminal irradiation were radium needles, housed in plastic tubes and inserted through drainage catheters. Walters and Olson[63] reported successful palliation of jaundice by using of two 5-mg radium needles placed in the hepatic ducts after incomplete resection. Kaplan[64] treated an incisional recurrence with a combination of external radiotherapy and a 3000 mg/hr radium implant. Conroy et al.,[50] placed radium needles enclosed in a catheter in an 8Fr percutaneous ring catheter positioned with the aid of fluoroscopy and with the number of needles inserted determined by the length of the obstructed segment imaged on the cholangiogram. The 72-hour implant delivered 140 Gy to the wall of the bile duct. Radium was subsequently replaced by "low activity" iridium-192 in most series (Table 1)[6,32,37,51–53, 55–58,60,62,65] and, more recently, by "high activity" iridium-192 (10 Ci) and cobalt-60 (4 Ci) (Table 2).

Afterloading Techniques

Two brachytherapy techniques have been implemented for the treatment of extrahepatic biliary tumors: 1) manual afterloading LDR (Table 1); and 2) remote afterloading HDR (Table 2). The techniques are similar with regards to the dose prescription points, the effective source length, and margins chosen, but differ in total dose, dose rate, number of fractions, and duration of treatment. In addition, a larger diameter catheter (10–14Fr) than the 8–10Fr catheter used for LDR techniques is required for HDR techniques. The advantages of LDR irradiation are that typically only one insertion and a smaller diameter catheter are required. In-patient care and radiation exposure to caregivers are inherent disadvantages, as is the potential for interference with bile drainage while the sources occupy the drainage catheter. HDR techniques can be delivered on an out-patient basis with complete radiation protection for individuals involved, with the added advantage of the ability to optimize the dose distribution. Also, the likelihood of catheter-related sepsis and catheter dislodgment is minimized; however, multiple insertions are required. In cases in which the HDR source cannot negotiate sharp curves within the catheterized biliary system, an LDR technique is required.[19,42,43]

Transhepatic (Percutaneous) Technique. The following steps are required for intraluminal insertion of radioactive sources into catheters with external access that are placed percutaneously or at the time of surgery. Before intraluminal irradiation, the diagnostic radiologist, gastroenterologist, or surgeon reviews the pretreatment cholangiogram and ERCP and identifies the site and length of obstruction (Figures 1 and 2). For LDR techniques, this step will initiate ordering of the appropriate length and activity of iridium. For HDR techniques, it is important to verify that a biliary drainage catheter of adequate diameter (usually No. 10–14Fr) is in place to accommodate the HDR catheter identified for biliary procedures. For either mode of delivery, planning and insertion of the afterloading catheter and dummy sources can be performed in the radiation oncology, diagnostic radiology, or endoscopy suite. Fluoroscopy and orthogonal radiography must be available. Using sterile precautions, the biliary drain is opened, the orifice cleaned, and the catheter is flushed with sterile normal saline. A sterilized blind-ended catheter (with a stainless steel guide

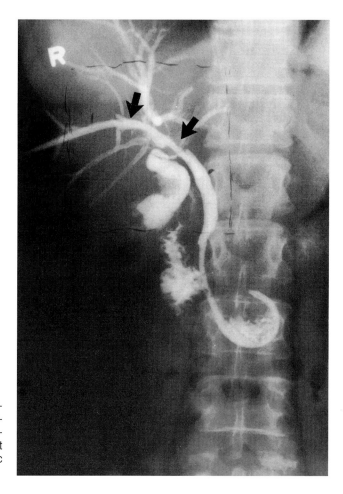

Figure 1. Transhepatic cholangiogram of a patient with cholangiocarcinoma. Arrows indicate level of obstruction at the junction of the right hepatic duct and common hepatic duct.

wire/obturator that prevents kinking) is inserted into the drainage catheter and advanced to the desired position in the biliary tree under fluoroscopy, often using biliary contrast to define the stricture. The guide wire is then replaced by a dummy source train. Orthogonal radiographs for computerized dosimetry are taken (Figure 3). For LDR applications, the iridium source train length is determined, factoring in a sufficient margin (usually 2–3 cm) on either side of the stricture. The unsterilized iridium ribbon or wire is then inserted into the location in the biliary tree determined initially with the dummy sources. The iridium source train is secured in place for the duration of the implant. Certain types of biliary drainage tube adapters (e.g., Tuohy-Borst) will allow external and internal bile drainage during the implant duration, and

the necessary drainage bags must be placed if external drainage is required.[10,13,17,18,34,43,55] The source train and catheter are subsequently removed at the bedside after the typical 24- to 72-hour implant. For HDR techniques, the treatment length is determined from the x-rays using the radiopaque markers on the dummy source train to identify the number and location of dwell positions, including an adequate margin on either side of the stricture (Figure 3). Total dose and fraction size are determined. Computerized dosimetry follows and may be optimized to shape the dose distribution, if required. The HDR brachytherapy catheter is connected to the remote afterloading device with a special metal adapter previously placed on the external end of the biliary HDR catheter, and treatment is delivered. After treatment deliv-

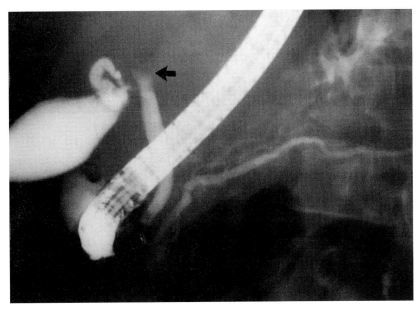

Figure 2. Endoscopic retrograde cholangiopancreatography (ERCP) of the same patient. Arrow indicates the distal level of obstruction in the common hepatic duct, just proximal to the junction with the cystic duct.

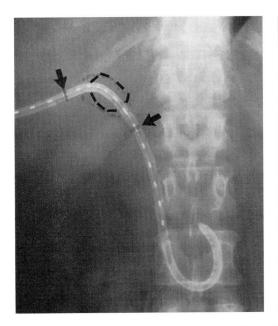 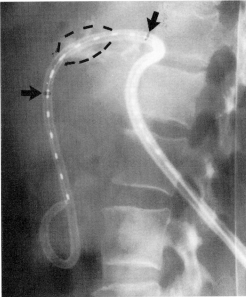

Figure 3. Localization radiographs of the patient with dummy source train in the afterloading catheter. Tumor volume is marked, and the area to be irradiated is indicated by arrows. 3A) Anterio-posterior radiograph; 3B) lateral radiograph.

ery, for both HDR and LDR techniques, the catheter is removed, and the biliary drainage catheter is flushed and capped. The patient is discharged home on antibiotics with recommendations for temperature monitoring.

Endoscopic Techniques. Endoscopic techniques are usually initiated in the endoscopy suite. Typically the biliary system has already been evaluated by ERCP and a sphincterotomy performed to provide access for a large caliber prosthesis.[31,33,53,61] Though the stent is often removed, some suggest leaving it in place during intraluminal irradiation to decrease the risk of cholangitis.[33] A guide wire is loaded into an appropriately sized (6–10Fr) catheter, passed transorally through the duodenum into the bile duct via the sphincterotomy and is advanced through the malignant stricture. Biliary contrast is often injected during this process. Under fluoroscopy, this catheter is removed, and the guide wire is left in place. A 10–14Fr straight nasobiliary tube is threaded over the guide wire through the scope channel, and the nasobiliary tube is advanced beyond the stricture and into the biliary tree. The endoscope is then slowly withdrawn during fluoroscopy; the proximal end of the tube is rerouted from the mouth to the nose, and the nasobiliary drainage tube secured. After removal of the guide wire, an extra long (130–150 cm) No. 5–6Fr afterloading catheter with an inner radio-opaque dummy source train is passed through the 10Fr nasobiliary tube and advanced through the lesion under fluoroscopy. The patient may then be transferred to the radiation oncology department or remain in the endoscopy suite where orthogonal films are taken for computerized dosimetry. Determination of the fraction size and corresponding number of dwell positions and dwell times ensues.

When determining the length of biliary tree to irradiate with either LDR or HDR sources, it is important to avoid irradiation of the duodenal mucosa. Veeze-Kuijpers et al.,[16] recommended positioning the iridium about 2 cm proximal to the duodenum. The dummy source train is removed, and the nasobiliary catheter is connected to the HDR remote afterloader using the special metal adapter. After the treatment is completed, the nasobiliary tube is removed and the patient is re-

turned to the endoscopy suite where an ERCP is again performed, and a large caliber endoprosthesis is reinserted for biliary drainage, if this was previously removed. The patient is then admitted to the hospital for intravenous antibiotics and monitoring and typically is discharged the next day. Alternatively, more than one fraction may be given per day over several days before the catheter is removed.[42–44] One disadvantage of the endoscopic approach is that a preexisting stent must be removed, necessitating another ERCP to replace the stent after irradiation and posing further risk associated with additional sedation and failure to subsequently replace the stent. Furthermore, it is sometimes difficult for the HDR source to negotiate the duodenalampullary curve. For these reasons, the transhepatic approach is often preferred for both LDR and HDR insertions. Techniques allowing retention of the stent during irradiation need to be developed. Though most frequently implemented with HDR techniques,[18,19,42,43,62] the endoscopic approach is also possible for LDR techniques,[7,31,33,37,53,54,60–62] although the tolerance of the nasobiliary catheter may be limited and the in-dwelling source may obstruct bile flow. A variation of the endoscopic technique for LDR applications described by Siegel et al.,[53] uses a double lumen catheter, preloaded with iridium, inserted after sphincterotomy and guide wire placement, and placed endoscopically, rather than through a nasobiliary catheter, thus avoiding the discomfort of the nasal catheter and allowing internal rather than external drainage (duodenal biliary drainage). Double-lumen catheters are also available with one lumen carrying the iridium wire and the other maintaining bile drainage.[62]

Systemic antibiotics are typically recommended before, during, and after manipulation of the LDR and HDR catheters to avoid cholangitis.[13,16,19,30–31,33,42,43,59] Oral ciprofloxacin is an effective choice due to its high concentration in bile, broad spectrum of activity, and out-patient availability. Sterile techniques should always be used when the in-dwelling catheter is entered. Daily catheter irrigation with 50 cc of normal saline, without aspiration is recommended before and after, but not during, the LDR insertions[13,30,59] and at the completion of HDR procedures.[19,42,43]

Patients should be advised to monitor their temperatures for at least 24 hours after the insertion and to report temperatures higher than 101.5°F.

Dose Specification

Bile duct diameters range from 3–25 mm.[13] An approximation of their size can be made from the initial cholangiogram. Minsky et al.,[66] recently reported the use of endoluminal ultrasound to help define both intraluminal and extraluminal tumor volume. A major limitation of traditional imaging of the biliary tree is the difficulty in accurately defining the proximal, distal, and lateral extent of tumor, which can lead to the great disparity in prescription points and the active lengths treated. Due to this uncertainty, various prescription points have been chosen for these insertions, and this has led to great differences in the reported delivered dose and dose rates (Tables 1 and 2). With a single line source, prescription points at 0.5 cm from the radioactive source train[51,56,60] or 1.0 cm from the radioactive source train[32,52] are typically cited in the literature. Other prescription points have included: 0.75 cm and 1.5 cm from the radioactive source; 0.5 cm, 1 cm, and 1.5 cm from the exterior catheter wall; the inner surface of the bile duct (determined from cholangiogram with an effective diameter of 1 cm, and range of radii of 1.5–5.8 mm); or unspecified.[6,38,53,57] This wide variation in dose prescription points makes comparisons difficult and it is recommended that doses be prescribed at 1 cm from the source.[55]

The use of two radioactive source trains rather than just one has also been described, typically for lesions involving the paired hepatic ducts or bifurcation lesions.[3,7,10–15,18,19,22,30,32–34,38,42,43,55] In these cases, after taking care to ensure that the second source train does not overlap the first source train, the source trains are arranged in a Y-shaped fashion to irradiate the left, right, and common hepatic ducts. This Y-shaped configuration can cover lesions at the bifurcation more adequately than is possible with a single line source. The use of three sources has also been described.[13,14] The choice of a dose prescription point and subsequent dosimetric analysis

when using more than one line source are not well described in the literature.

Source Length

The length of the source trains or number of dwell positions will depend on the length of the stenosis, which is determined at the time of the initial cholangiogram and also at the time of fluoroscopy during catheter insertion (Tables 1 and 2). Margins of at least 1 cm and as large as 5 cm on either side of the stricture have been reported.[10,13,14,17,18,22,31,32,43,61] Because of several initial marginal recurrences, Herskovic, Engler, and Noell[13] recommended irradiating a margin even larger than 5 cm and extending the source length to include the bile duct and the ampulla to at least 5 cm proximal to the hepatic bifurcation.[14] Levitt et al.,[33] recommend a source length 1.5 times that of the length of the stricture. In general, we have found a margin of 2–3 cm on either side of the stricture to be adequate.

Dose/Fractionation Schemes

Reports of the timing of LDR insertions with respect to external irradiation vary (Table 1). In general, intervals of 2–4 weeks between initial external and intracavitary irradiation are reported in the literature,[15,16,24,29,30,35,36] although there is no data to mandate any break between the two. Likewise, intervals of 1–8 weeks between initial intraluminal irradiation and ensuing EBRT,[10,16–18,33] and time spans of several days to several weeks after establishment of biliary drainage (percutaneous or endoscopic) before intraluminal irradiation are also reported.[13,25–28,31,51] A second LDR insertion for persistent disease at varying intervals[3,11–14,25–28,33,51] and planned multiple LDR insertions, typically 1 or 2 weeks apart, are reported in some series.[34,52] For HDR, the fractionation scheme may vary because of the type of existent stenting. Patients with internal stenting may receive their fractions once or twice a day over 2–3 days to expedite removal of the nasobiliary tube; however, patients with percutaneous stenting will typically receive 1–2 fractions per week. Reports of HDR schedules also vary, but generally 2–6 fractions are delivered over several days to weeks (Table 2).

Fraction size and total intraluminal dose vary by series, depending in part on the use of EBRT and upon whether LDR or HDR techniques are implemented (Tables 1 and 2). Definitive intraluminal doses of 40–60 Gy with LDR techniques and 10–30 Gy with HDR techniques versus boost doses of 7–100 Gy with LDR techniques and 5–60 Gy with HDR techniques are cited in the literature. The High Dose Rate Brachytherapy Working Group (HIBWOG) has proposed a dose of definitive EBRT of 45 Gy with an HDR brachytherapy boost of 20 Gy (5 Gyx4) specified at 1 cm from the source. For palliative intraluminal irradiation, 30 Gy (5 Gyx6) (HDR) was proposed.[32] For LDR, we use 25–30 Gy brachytherapy (at 1 cm) to boost 45 Gy EBRT for definitive treatments and 40 Gy LDR brachytherapy alone for palliation. The seed activity and total activity chosen vary greatly from series to series (Tables 1 and 2). The doses are difficult to compare because the prescription points and dose rates vary.

Other Techniques

Although liver tumors are most commonly implanted using the intraluminal techniques described above, unresectable liver tumors (usually metastatic from a colorectal primary) can also be implanted using intraoperative iodine-125 (I-125) seeds,[35,36,67–70] or intraoperative interstitial HDR brachytherapy.[71,72]

Iodine-125 seeds are implanted under direct vision into unresectable liver tumors using a Mick Applicator (Mick Radio-Nuclear Instruments, Bronx, NY, USA) at laparotomy. If the tumor is resected with close margins, I-125 seeds in Vicryl sutures or in Surgicel are used in a planar implant. Doses of about 160 Gray are generally delivered. Armstrong et al.[70] reported a median survival of 18 months, with 42% of patients surviving 3 years or more. However, extrahepatic metastasis occurred in 83% of patients.

Another technique described by Thomas et al.[71,72] involved using ultrasound to guide the intraoperative insertion of hollow needles into unresected liver tumors. HDR brachytherapy doses of 20–30 Gy were then delivered to the periphery of the tumor. The needles were removed after treatment (about 1 hour). Although single lesions are commonly treated, multiple lesions (up to 11) were also treated, the largest median diameter being 5 cm. They reported a 25% local control at 26 months (median time of progression = 8 months). In 87% of patients, new sites of disease developed in the remainder of the liver.[71]

The liver is a vascular organ and is not generally implanted interstitially. However, as shown above, it is possible to implant these tumors interstitially with minimal morbidity.

Results

Local Control

Long-term local control is an important end-point in this disease and is achievable in some patients.[3,11–13,22,23,25,26,29,35,38,54] Relief of biliary obstruction, evidenced by a decline in liver enzymes and jaundice and improved quality of life, is one cited palliative end-point.[3,11,25,37] However, it is difficult to distinguish the contribution of the drainage catheter from that of the brachytherapy. Whether the biliary drainage catheter can be discontinued after irradiation is unclear. Pakisch et al.[44] noted unrestrained bile flow in nine of nine patients treated with definitive intraluminal HDR with or without EBRT, with palliation lasting as long as the survival time (7.5 months) in seven of the nine patients. Hayes et al.[30] noted no cases of recurrent biliary obstruction after intracavitary HDR with or without EBRT with removal of the drainage catheter in one patient. In five patients with unresectable carcinoma, Ryu et al.[21] reported that the bile duct stricture resolved, allowing removal of the external drainage catheter after HDR intraluminal irradiation with or without EBRT; whereas, Molt et al.[34] reported that all patients retained their catheters after irradiation and that no change was seen on post-treatment cholangiograms. Yoshimura et al.[41] reported an average tube-free period of 7 months after definitive intraluminal HDR with or without EBRT, with 12 of 13 patients who were treated able to discontinue percutaneous drainage. Fogel and Weissberg[24] were able to discontinue percutaneous drainage in one patient for 1.5 years after definitive external and intracavitary irradiation.

Survival

There is some suggestion that the patency of drainage secured by radiation may enhance survival. Wheeler et al.,[26] using definitive external and intracavitary versus intracavitary irradiation alone suggested that radiation enhanced the effect of tube drainage, thereby reducing the number of early mortalities and giving a significantly increased chance of surviving 9 months than with surgical drainage alone (P<0.01). Radiation was concluded to improve survival over bile drainage alone, with a median survival of 11 months and with two patients NED at 2 years.[25,26] In a follow-up of the Wheeler series, a mean survival of 16.8 months (1–66 months) was achieved with the addition of intraluminal irradiation, and survival time compared to that associated with bypass surgery or percutaneous biliary drainage alone was doubled.[27,28,51] Jones et al.[12] noted a mean survival of 10.6 months in patients stented and irradiated (postoperatove and definitive) versus 3.5 months for those with stenting alone. One of the ten patients treated had removal of the stent "for a time."[3,11]

As shown in Tables 1 and 2, survival seems to be increased, though not in all series, in patients who have undergone resection and have subsequently received postoperative irradiation. Langer et al.[9] recommend resection whenever possible even when margins are positive and report an increase in mean survival to 32 months versus 8–10 months for those with bypass or intubation alone. Gonzalez et al.,[7] noted a median survival for surgery alone versus surgery and postoperative irradiation of 8.25 and 19 months, respectively, and 1-, 2-, and 3-year survival rates of 36%, 18%, and 10% for surgery alone versus 85%, 42%, and 31% for surgery and postoperative irradiation (P = 0.0005). Survival was also superior to that of patients who were treated with biliary drainage and irradiation, with a median survival of 12.3 months with 1-, 2-, and 3-year survivals of 46%, 15%, and 12%.[7]

Data supporting the ability of the combination of external and intraluminal brachytherapy to enhance local control and survival through delivery of higher doses are inconclusive.[7] There is a suggestion that the combination may be superior to EBRT alone, perhaps because of the higher cumulative doses delivered.[14,15,22,30] Long-term survival of patients treated with a combination of EBRT and brachytherapy boost has been reported.[17,20,35–37,41,43]

Complications

The frequency of complications after irradiation is recorded in Tables 1 and 2. Transient cholangitis is the most frequent complication after intraluminal irradiation. Fatal sepsis is reported in several series. Perihepatic abscesses have been observed in several series (some autopsy), typically near the drainage catheter.[59] Perhaps one of the most worrisome outcomes is GI tract injury after irradiation, which is most often observed when both external and intracavitary irradiation are combined.[7,13,15,16,22,29,30,34,35,37] Excessive bleeding or hemobilia through the drainage catheter is a particularly worrisome complication and can be fatal. It is unclear if intraluminal radiation increases this risk or if the presence of drainage catheters alone is enough to create fistulous tracts between the blood vessels and bile ducts. Most cases cited in the literature followed the combination of external and intracavitary irradiation.[14,30,34,38,41,73] Herskovic, Engler, and Noell[13] recommended 50 Gy at 0.5 cm from the source, often with supplemental external irradiation of 50 Gy, and reported no instances of fistulization, ductal perforation, or bile peritonitis.

That delivery of such large doses to the biliary ducts will result in a high incidence of biliary strictures is to be expected. It would not seem efficacious to replace malignant strictures with radiation-induced strictures. Hence, most authors leave an in-dwelling stent for a few months after radiation to minimize the risk of biliary strictures. Bile duct strictures or fibrosis were reported in one patient treated with external and intracavitary irradiation in the series of Fields and Emami.[15] Bile duct fibrosis was specifically denied in the series of Veeze-Kuijpers et al.,[16] which was treated with external and intracavitary irradiation, and in the series of Kumar et al.[38]

Discussion

Considering the known spread pattern of these lesions throughout the biliary tree and to the regional lymphatics, it would seem that using a combination of EBRT to treat the primary tumor and adjacent tissues at risk and intraluminal radiation to "boost" the bulky luminal and periluminal disease or areas of close or positive margins to higher doses would be a reasonable approach.[2] This will allow a decrease in the external dose, thereby minimizing side effects, and it will shorten the course of treatment for these patients who have a limited survival. The major problem with exclusive intraluminal irradiation is that the diameter of irradiated volume measures only 1–2 cm in diameter, but the tumor volume often exceeds this range.[38] Hence, EBRT is used to treat the entire target volume, and the brachytherapy is used as a boost.

Several authors have hypothesized a dose-response relationship for tumors of the extrahepatic biliary tree. Mittal, Deutsch, and Iwatsuki[74] observed a median survival of 11 months in patients receiving an EBRT dose >70 TDF (>45 Gy/4.5 weeks) as compared to 4.4 months in patients receiving <70 TDF. Nine of 13 patients (69%) who completed a radiation dose >70 TDF survived >9 months, whereas all of those receiving <70 TDF died within 9 months. However, a follow-up of the University of Pittsburgh experience, including the use of brachytherapy and increasing doses of EBRT, failed to confirm the effect of dose on survival. Only extrahepatic duct primaries, increasing calendar year of treatment, and liver transplantation with postoperative radiation were significantly associated with an increase in survival.[8] Other dose-response data is available from Hishikawa et al.,[75] who reported an improvement in prognosis with doses above 40 Gy EBRT (10.3 months vs 3 months survival), as did Smoron,[47] reporting an average survival of 15 months versus 2.5 months with EBRT doses >40 Gy versus <40 Gy. Pilepich and Lambert[46] noted improved local control of disease in two patients with unresectable common bile duct carcinomas treated with 60 Gy/30 fractions of EBRT compared to local control in those treated with 40–43 Gy. Gonzalez et al.,[7] noted a dose response effect above 40 Gy, but not 50 Gy.

Survival appears to be closely related to surgical intervention that is dictated by tumor extent at presentation: laparotomy alone,

mean survival of 5.6 months; stenting with a Y- or T-tube, mean survival of 9.9 months; transhepatic stenting, mean survival of 18.6 months; and tumor resection, mean survival of 22.2 months.[3,6,7,9,18,48] Biliary decompression alone appears to improve the mean survival of patients with extrahepatic biliary tumors from 3 months with no treatment to approximately 9 months.[8,28] The impact of radiation on survival is debated. Selection factors may affect the choice of therapy and lead to differences in survival. Differences in survival between patients surgically resected with or without postoperative irradiation and those who present with unresectable disease requiring definitive irradiation are debatable, as is the impact of radiation dose and technique, i.e., use of exclusive EBRT or intracavitary irradiation or a combination of the two. In the largest series of patients reviewed, Gonzalez et al.,[7] reported the results of various treatment regimens for 112 patients with proximal bile duct cancer treated at seven EORTC institutions (mean or median survival after resection with positive margins = 7–23 months and a 3-year survival rate ranging from 10%–18%). Adding their series to other series in the literature, the mean survival was 13.9 ± 5 months with a mean survival at 3 years of 13% in 179 patients. In 79 patients, who subsequently received adjunctive postoperative irradiation, the median or mean survival varied from 15.7–28 months with a 3-year survival rate between 25%–31% and a mean survival of 21.5 ± 5 months. Patients with tumor resection and postoperative irradiation had a significantly better survival rate than those treated with surgery alone or with biliary drainage and irradiation. No conclusion could be reached about the addition of intraluminal irradiation. In a review of the literature of 300 patients treated with biliary drainage and irradiation without resection, the median or mean survival varied from 7–27 months with survival rates at 1 and 3 years varying between 10%–63% and 0%–30% and a mean survival of 12.5 ± 4 to 8 months versus 10 months without the addition of radiation.

The effect of radiation on normal tissue and tumor observed at autopsy include: considerable fibrosis with a few nests of necrotic-appearing tumor cells,[50] fibrocollagenous tissue with scattered hemorrhagic foci of tumor cells,[29] cancer cells in the liver but not in the area irradiated,[41] and marked fibrosis around the common hepatic duct with biopsies revealing only fibrosis and some tumor cells with pyknotic nuclei.[52] Sindelar, Tepper, and Travis[76] delivered 20, 30, and 45 Gy to a 5-cm circle in a canine model with intraoperative electrons and observed fibrosis and thickening of the common duct as early as 6 weeks after irradiation, which was dose-related.

There is little information in the literature concerning complications associated with long-term percutaneous biliary drainage, regardless of intraluminal brachytherapy. Hemobilia, cholangitis, and intrahepatic abscesses have been reported apart from radiation, and the impact of radiation on their development is unknown. Langer et al.[9] reported a 56% incidence of cholangitis in catheterized patients without irradiation. The risk of cholangitis with endoscopic techniques appears to diminish if radiation is delayed at least 2 weeks after biliary endoprosthesis insertion.[65] Fletcher et al.[25,27] recommended frequent irrigation of exteriorized drainage tubes to decrease the risk of cholangitis, but speculated that the risk of cholangitis was directly related to the placement and maintenance of the drainage tubes, rather than to the insertion of the iridium. The use of antibiotics 12–24 hours before and 48–72 hours after catheter manipulation or replacement is recommended. Patients with subsequent signs of cholangitis should be treated with antibiotics for 10–14 days. Frequent tube irrigation without aspiration (organisms drawn from GI tract) with clean techniques are recommended. Fever developing in this setting usually means that the tube has become occluded with sludge or dislodged and needs cleaning or replacement. Oral antibiotics are then prescribed, and fevers should subside within 24 hours. Prolonged fever should raise the suspicion of liver abscess, the frequency of which is increased after 8 months of external drainage, and the patients should be admitted for work-up and potential drainage to avoid fatal sepsis.[30,59]

Significant complications are primarily related to incidental irradiation of the GI tract. Buskirk et el.[22] preferred to give an EBRT boost rather than an intraluminal boost to patients with formation of a choledocho- or hepaticoenterostomy because of the proximity of the small intestine to tumor and the risk of necrosis and ulceration. They also recommend not exceeding 55 Gy to the distal stomach and duodenum, unless the volumes to be treated were small. Planning with contrast material in the stomach, esophagus, and duodenum was recommended. Gerard et al.[18] recommend brachytherapy dose specification at 0.5 cm rather than 1.0 cm from the source, particularly if near a surgical anastomosis, because of the very high dose that is produced in the first few millimeters. Higher doses may be possible when the catheter is in the middle of an unresected tumor. With the nasobiliary approach, there has been speculation that the in-dwelling prosthesis decreases the risk of papillitis and ampullary stricture distancing the mucosa from the in-dwelling iridium, although irradiation of the duodenum is typically avoided by appropriate source length if tumor is not close to the duodenum.[61] Veeze-Kuijpers et al.[16] recommended positioning the iridium 2 cm proximal to the duodenum. The University of Pittsburgh experience could not correlate ulcer-free survival with the treatment variables of total dose or the use of brachytherapy or EBRT. They suggested that other factors such as biliary drainage catheters or surgical biliary diversion may contribute.[8]

Radiological studies often demonstrate biliary stenosis after radiation. Radiation-induced stricture formation is of concern particularly when intraluminal techniques are used, and the question of whether, after radiation, a malignant stricture is not simply replaced by a fibrotic stricture is important since all such strictures may be life-threatening. Nag speculates that intraluminal brachytherapy may lead to ductal fibrosis and strictures and recommends leaving the catheters in place several months after intraluminal therapy to avoid this.[32] Veeze-Kuijpers et al.[16] reported no bile duct fibrosis with postoperative definitive external and intracavitary irradiation, but kept the stents in to prevent problems. Molt et al.,[34] who also kept the stents in after irradiation, was reluctant to remove them because one patient had recurrence of jaundice in 6 weeks. If the patient is anxious to have external drainage catheters removed, it is possible to convert from external to internal drainage. Strictures may develop and may require dilation or reintubation of the ducts.[13]

The efficacy of chemotherapy, particularly 5-FU remains controversial, as documented in multiple retrospective series.[1,2,4,5,7,8,10,14,15,17,22,24,29,34–36,43,45,47–49,54,74,77–79] Further research is needed to confirm the role of systemic agents.

Additional areas of investigation include the use of hyperthermia in association with intraluminal iridium, extensive liver resection, liver transplantation, and whole liver irradiation.[80–82]

A cooperative prospective randomized trial at John Hopkins and two other centers is underway to evaluate the role of EBRT and intracavitary irradiation after curative or palliative resection.[4] Only large prospective trials can lead to resolution of some of the questions yet unsolved in treatment of these challenging malignancies.

Conclusions

Intraluminal brachytherapy may be a useful and ingenious technique to deliver higher doses of radiation to tumors of the extrahepatic bile ducts. Techniques should be implemented with care to make them not only effective but safe. The long-term efficacy of this mode of radiation should be studied further.

References

1. Kopelson G, Harisiadis L, Tretter P, et al. The role of radiation therapy in cancer of the extrahepatic biliary system: An analysis of thirteen patients and a review of the literature of the effectiveness of surgery, chemotherapy and radiotherapy. Int J Radiat Oncol Biol Phys 1977; 2:883–894.

2. Kopelson G, Gunderson LL. Primary and adjuvant radiation therapy in gallbladder and extrahepatic biliary tract carcinoma. J Clin Gastroenterol 1983;5:43–50.

3. Chitwood WR, Meyers WC, Heaston DK, et al. Diagnosis and treatment of primary extrahepatic bile duct tumors. Am J Surg 1982;143: 99–106.

4. Cameron JL. Proximal cholangiocarcinomas. Br J Surg 1988;75:115–1156.

5. Kopelson G, Galdabini J, Warshaw AL, et al. Patterns of failure after curative surgery for extra-hepatic biliary tract carcinoma: Implications for adjuvant therapy. Int J Radiat Oncol Biol Phys 1981;7:413–417.

6. Cameron JL, Broe P, Zuidema GD. Proximal bile duct tumors surgical management with silastic transhepatic biliary stents. Ann Surg 1982;196:412–419.

7. Gonzalez D, Gerard JP, Maners AW, et al. Results of radiation therapy in carcinoma of the proximal bile duct (Klatskin tumor). Semin Liver Dis 1990;10:131–141.

8. Flickinger JC, Iwatsuki S, Starzl TE. Radiation therapy for primary carcinoma of the extrahepatic biliary system. Cancer 1991;68:289–294.

9. Langer JC, Langer B, Taylor BR, et al. Carcinoma of the extrahepatic bile ducts: Results of an aggressive surgical approach. Surgery 1985; 98:752–759.

10. Mahe M, Romestaing P, Talon B, et al. Radiation therapy in extrahepatic bile duct carcinoma. Radiother Oncol 1991;21:121–127.

11. Herskovic A, Heaston D, Engle MJ, et al. Irradiation of biliary carcinoma. Radiology 1981; 139:219–222.

12. Jones RS, Chitwood WR, Heaston DK, et al. The combined use of percutaneous transhepatic drainage and irradiation for carcinoma of the extrahepatic bile ducts. Contemp Surg 1983;22:59–64.

13. Herskovic AM, Engler MJ, Noell KT. Radical radiotherapy for bile duct carcinoma. Endocurie Hypertherm Oncol 1985;I:119–124.

14. Meyers WC, Jones RS. Internal radiation for bile duct cancer. World J Surg 1988;12:99–104.

15. Fields JN, Emami B. Carcinoma of the extrahepatic biliary system—results of primary and adjuvant radiotherapy. Int J Radiat Oncol Biol Phys 1987;13:331–338.

16. Veeze-Kuijpers B, Meerwaldt JH, Lameris JS, et al. The role of radiotherapy in the treatment of bile duct carcinoma. Int J Radiat Oncol Biol Phys 1990;18:63–67.

17. Mornex F, Ardiet JM, Bret P, et al. Radiotherapy of high bile duct carcinoma using intracatheter iridium-192 wire. Cancer 1984;54:2069–2073.

18. Gerard JP, Ardiet JM, Mahe M, et al. Intraluminal iridium-192 LDR brachytherapy in extrahepatic bile duct carcinoma. Brachytherapy J 1991;5:69–74.

19. Pavlou WJ, Vikram B, Urban MS, et al. The use of high dose rate remote brachytherapy in the treatment of malignant biliary obstruction. Brachytherapy J 1991;5:13–16.

20. Kurisu K, Hishikawa Y, Taniguchi M, et al. High-dose-rate intraluminal brachytherapy for bile duct carcinoma after surgery. Radiother Oncol 1991;21:65–66.

21. Ryu M, Sato S, Watanabe K, et al. Intraluminal irradiation using remote after loading system

for advanced biliary tract cancer. J JPN Biliary Assoc 1988;2:127–137.

22. Buskirk SJ, Gunderson LL, Adson MA, et al. Analysis of failure following curative irradiation of gallbladder and extrahepatic bile duct carcinoma. Int J Radiat Oncol Biol Phys 1984; 10:2013–2023.

23. Bethune W, Roux V, Anderson J, et al. Extrahepatic bile duct carcinoma: A case report. J Natl Med Assoc 1981;73:547–549.

24. Fogel TD, Weissberg JB. The role of radiation therapy in carcinoma of the extrahepatic bile ducts. Int J Radiat Oncol Biol Phys 1984;10: 2251–2258.

25. Fletcher MS, Brinkley D, Dawson JL, et al. Treatment of high bileduct carcinoma by internal radiotherapy with iridium-192 wire. Lancet 1981;2:172–174.

26. Wheeler PG, Dawson JL, Nunnerley H, et al. Newer techniques in the diagnosis and treatment of proximal bile duct carcinoma—an analysis of 41 consecutive patients. Q J Med 1981;199:247–258.

27. Fletcher MS, Brinkley D, Dawson JL, et al. Treatment of hilar carcinoma by bile drainage combined with internal radiotherapy using ^{192}iridium wire. Br J Surg 1983;70:733–735.

28. Karani J, Fletcher M, Brinkley D, et al. Internal biliary drainage and local radiotherapy with iridium-192 wire in treatment of hilar cholangiocarcinoma. Clin Radiol 1985;36:603–606.

29. Johnson DW, Safai C, Goffinet DR. Malignant obstructive jaundice: Treatment with external beam and intracavitary radiotherapy. Int J Radiat Oncol Biol Phys 1985;11:411–416.

30. Hayes JK, Sapozink MD, Miller FJ. Definitive radiation therapy in bile duct carcinoma. Int J Radiat Oncol Biol Phys 1988;15:735–744.

31. Ede RJ, Williams SJ, Hatfield ARW, et al. Endoscopic management of inoperable cholangiocarcinoma using iridium-192. Br J Surg 1989; 76:867–869.

32. Nag S. Intraluminal brachytherapy of the biliary tract and esophagus. In: Dinshaw KA, Chaudhury AJ (eds). Technology Transfer Program in Brachytherapy. Professional Education Division, Bombay, 1987, pp. 163–169.

33. Levitt MD, Laurence BH, Cameron F, et al. Transpapillary iridium-192 wire in the treatment of malignant bile duct obstruction. Gut 1988;29:149–152.

34. Molt P, Hopfan S, Watson RC, et al. Intraluminal radiation therapy in the management of malignant biliary obstruction. Cancer 1986;57: 536–544.

35. Minsky BD, Wesson MF, Armstrong JG, et al. Combined modality therapy of extrahepatic biliary system cancer. Int J Radiat Oncol Biol Phys 1990;18:1157–1163.

36. Minsky BD, Kemeny N, Armstrong JG, et al. Extrahepatic biliary system cancer: An update of a combined modality approach. Am J Clin Oncol 1991;14:433–437.

37. Trodella L, Mantini G, Barina M, et al. External and intracavitary radiotherapy in the management of carcinoma of extrahepatic biliary tract. RAYS 1991;16:71–75.

38. Kumar PP, Good RR, McCaul GF. Intraluminal endocurietherapy of inoperable Klatskin's tumor with high-activity ^{192}iridium. Radiat Med 1986;4:21–26.

39. Haffty BG, Mate TP, Greenwood LH, et al. Malignant biliary obstruction: Intracavitary treatment with a high-dose-rate remote afterloading device. Radiology 1987;164:574–576.

40. Yoshimura H, Sakaguchi H, Yoshioka T, et al. Afterloading intracavitary irradiation and expanding stent for malignant biliary obstruction. Radiat Med 1989;7:36–41.

41. Yoshimura H, Ohishi H, Tamada T, et al. Cobalt-60 HDR intralumenal brachytherapy for advanced biliary tract cancer. In: Mould RF (ed). International Brachytherapy, Programme & Abstracts 7th International Brachytherapy Working Conference. Nucletron International B.V., The Netherlands, 1992, pp. 495–498.

42. Urban MS, Siegel JH, Pavlou W, et al. Treatment of malignant biliary obstruction with a high-dose rate remote afterloading device using a 10 F nasobiliary tube. Gastrointest Endosc 1990;36:292–296.

43. Nori D, Nag S, Rogers D, et al. Remote afterloading high dose rate brachytherapy for carcinoma of the bile duct. In: Nag S (ed). High Dose Rate Brachytherapy: A Textbook. Futura Publishing Co., Inc., Armonk, NY, 1994, pp. 331–338.

44. Pakisch VB, Klein GE, Stucklschweiger G, et al. Metallgeflecht-endoprothese und intraluminare high-dose-rate-^{192}iridium-brachytherapie zur palliativen behandlung maligner gallengangsobstruktionen. Fortschr Rontgenstr 1992; 156:592–595.

45. Green N, Mikkelsen WP, Kernen JA. Cancer of the common hepatic bile ducts—palliative radiotherapy. Radiology 1973;109:687–689.

46. Pilepich MV, Lambert PM. Radiotherapy of carcinomas of the extrahepatic biliary system. Radiology 1978;127:767–770.

47. Smoron GL. Radiation therapy of carcinoma of gallbladder and biliary tract. Cancer 1977;40: 1422–1424.

48. Black K, Hanna SS, Langer B, et al. Manage-

ment of carcinoma of the extrahepatic bile ducts. Can J Surg 1978;21:542–545.

49. Hanna SS, Rider WD. Carcinoma of the gallbladder or extrahepatic bile ducts: The role of radiotherapy. CMA J 1978;118:59–61.

50. Conroy RM, Shahbazian AA, Edwards KC, et al. A new method for treating carcinomatous biliary obstruction with intracatheter radium. Cancer 1982;49:1321–1327.

51. Nunnerley HB, Karani JB. Intraductal radiation. Radiol Clin North Am 1990;28:1237–1240.

52. Prempree T, Cox EF, Sewchand W, et al. Cholangiocarcinoma a place for brachytherapy. Acta Radiol Oncol 1983;22:353–359.

53. Siegel JH, Lichtenstein JL, Pullano WE, et al. Treatment of malignant biliary obstruction by endoscopic implantation of iridium 192 using a new double lumen endoprosthesis. Gastrointest Endosc 1988;34:301–306.

54. Montemaggi P, Luzi S, Caspiani O, et al. Intralumenal brachytherapy in the treatment of neoplastic jaundice. In: Mould RF (ed). International Brachytherapy. Nucletron International B.V., The Netherlands, 1992, pp. 492–494.

55. Nag S, Tai DL, Gold RE. Biliary tract neoplasms: A simple management technique. South Med J 1984;77:593–595.

56. Son YH, Nori D, Leibel SA, et al. Biliary tree. In: Interstitial Collaborative Working Group. Interstitial Brachytherapy, Programme & Abstracts 7th International Brachytherapy Working Conference. Raven Press, New York, 1990, pp. 153–156.

57. Ikeda H, Kuroda C, Uchida H, et al. Intraluminal irradiation with iridium-192 wires for extrahepatic bile duct carcinoma. Nippon Igaku Hoshasen Gakkai Zasshi 1979;39:1356–1358.

58. Koster R, Schmidt H, Greuel H. Bestrahlung von malignen gallengangsverschlussen in afterloading-technik. Strahlentherapie 1982;158:678–680.

59. Pennington L, Kaufman S, Cameron JL. Intrahepatic abscess as a complication of long-term percutaneous internal biliary drainage. Surgery 1982;91:642–645.

60. Phillip J, Hagenmuller F, Manegold K, et al. Endoskopische, intraduktale strahlentherapie hochsitzender gallengangskarzinome. Dtsch Med Wschr 1984;109:422–426.

61. Venu RP, Geenen JE, Hogan WJ, et al. Intraluminal radiation therapy for biliary tract malignancy—an endoscopic approach. Gastrointest Endosc 1987;33:236–238.

62. Classen M, Hagenmuller F. Endoprosthesis and local irradiation in the treatment of biliary malignancies. Endoscopy 1987;19:25–30.

63. Walters W, Olson PF. Papillary colloid adeno-

carcinoma of the extrahepatic bile ducts. Minn Med 1935;18:460–462.

64. Kaplan II. Clinical Radiation Therapy. Second Edition. Paul B. Hoeber Inc., New York, 1949, p. 495.

65. Novell JR, Hilson A, Hobbs KEF. Therapeutic aspects of radio-isotopes in hepatobiliary malignancy. Br J Surg 1991;78:901–906.

66. Minsky B, Botet J, Gerdes H, et al. Ultrasound directed extrahepatic bile duct intraluminal brachytherapy. Int J Radiat Oncol Biol Phys 1992;23:165–167.

67. Dobelbower RR, Merrick HW, Ahuja RK, et al. ^{125}I interstitial implant, precision high-dose external beam therapy, and 5-FU for unresectable adenocarcinoma of pancreas and extrahepatic biliary tree. Cancer 1986;58:2185–2195.

68. Nag S. Radiotherapy and brachytherapy for recurrent colorectal cancer. Sem Surg Oncol 1991;7:177–180.

69. Donath D, Nori D, Turnbull A, et al. Brachytherapy in the treatment of solitary colorectal metastases to liver. J Surg Oncol 1990;44:55–61.

70. Armstrong JG, Anderson LL, Harrison LB. Treatment of liver metastases from colorectal cancer with radioactive implants. Cancer 1994;73:1800–1804.

71. Thomas DS, Dritschilo A. Interstitial high dose rate irradiation for hepatic tumors. In: Nag S (ed). High Dose Rate Brachytherapy: A Textbook. Futura Publishing Co, Inc., Armonk, NY, 1994, pp. 339–346.

72. Thomas DS, Nauta RJ, Rodgers JE. Intraoperative high dose rate interstitial irradiation of hepatic metastases from colorectal carcinomas: Results of a phase I-II trial. Cancer 1993;71:1977–1981.

73. McLean GK, Ring EJ, Freiman DB. Therapeutic alternatives in the treatment of intrahepatic biliary obstruction. Radiology 1982;145:289–295.

74. Mittal B, Deutsch M, Iwatsuki S. Primary cancers of extrahepatic biliary passages. Int J Radiat Oncol Biol Phys 1985;11:849–854.

75. Hishikawa Y, Shimada T, Miura T. Radiation therapy of carcinoma of the extrahepatic bile ducts. Radiology 1983;146:787–789.

76. Sindelar WF, Tepper J, Travis EL. Tolerance of bile duct to intraoperative irradiation. Surgery 1982;92:533–540.

77. Lees CD, Zapolanski A, Cooperman AM, et al. Carcinoma of the bile ducts. Surg Gynecol Obstet 1980;151:193–198.

78. Hudgins PT, Meoz RT. Radiation therapy for obstructive jaundice secondary to tumor malignancy. Int J Radiat Oncol Biol Phys 1976;1:1195–1198.

79. Hashmonai M, Lev L, Schramek A, et al. Long survival following combined treatment of inoperable cholangiocarcinoma: Surgery, radiotherapy, and chemotherapy. J Surg Oncol 1980;13:231–235.

80. Wong JYC, Vora NL, Chou CK, et al. Intracatheter hyperthermia and iridium-192 radiotherapy in the treatment of bile duct carcinoma. Int J Radiat Oncol Biol Phys 1988;14:353–359.

81. Nobler MP. Treatment of cholangiocarcinoma with brachytherapy teletherapy, hyperthermia, and chemotherapy. Endocurie Hypertherm Oncol 1991;7:63–66.

82. Coughlin CT, Wong TZ, Ryan TP. Interstitial microwave-induced hyperthermia and iridium brachytherapy for the treatment of obstructing biliary carcinomas. Int J Hypertherm 1992;8: 157–171.

Chapter 19

Cancer of the Pancreas

Chitti R. Moorthy, M.D., Basil S. Hilaris, M.D.,
FACR

Introduction

Carcinoma of the pancreas has climbed from relative obscurity to the fifth leading cause of cancer mortality in the United States, exceeded only by cancer of the lung, colon, breast, and prostate. The incidence and the age specific death rates from this cancer are on the rise. The American Cancer Society estimates that 27,000 new cases (13,000 males and 14,000 females) will be diagnosed and 25,900 (12,400 males and 13,500 females) will die of this disease in the year 1994.[1] Despite the sophistication of surgical techniques and advances in the radiation therapy and chemotherapy modalities, the results are distressingly poor with a <2% 5-year survival.[2,3] This poor prognosis is related to the fact that at the time of diagnosis in over 85% of the patients, the cancer has already spread outside the gland, and in two-thirds of the patients, metastasis is already evident.[4-6] Both locoregional control and distant metastases represent a challenging management problem.

Management with Surgery

Curative surgical procedures such as pancreatoduodenectomy (Whipple's procedure) and total pancreatectomy, which at one time were considered as the only hope for cure, have consistently failed to demonstrate 5-year survival rates of >5%. The associated high morbidity and mortality rates (50% and 20%, respectively) did not improve with the increased sophistication of surgical techniques.[2] Furthermore, the resectability rate is very low at <20% even in patients with stage I disease; and, of those undergoing resection 85% fail locoregionally.[7-9]

Management with Chemotherapy

The use of chemotherapy in pancreatic cancer is at a very early stage of development. The reported response rates with 5-Fluorouracil (5-FU), the most extensively studied single drug, vary in the literature from 0%–67% (average 28%). The results of combination chemotherapy are somewhat more encouraging with response rates in the range of 12%–48%.[10]

Management with External Beam Radiation Therapy

Attempts at radical radiation therapy have been in general unsuccessful. Radiosensitive structures adjacent to the pancreas (liver, kidney, spinal cord, intestine) have limited the amount of radiation to only palliative doses.[11]

Dobelbower,[12] at Thomas Jefferson University Hospital (TJUH), has described a precision high-dose technique, using 45 MV photon and 15–40 MeV electron beam to a dose of

From Nag S (ed): *Principles and Practice of Brachytherapy*. © Futura Publishing Co., Inc., Armonk, NY, 1997.

6000–7000 rads in 7–9 weeks. Forty patients with pancreatic cancer were treated in this fashion. The median survival from diagnosis was 12 months, while 12 patients who received adjuvant chemotherapy had a median survival of 15 months. However, it is discouraging to note that even at each high dose of radiation, the locoregional control rate is <50%.[12] High linear energy transfer (LET) and charged particle radiation trials have failed to demonstrate increased survivals.[13–17] Intraoperative radiation therapy (IORT) studies have not validated the initial optimism.[17–23]

Two general conclusions are possible regarding surgery, external beam radiation, or IORT: 1) none of these techniques is adequate; and 2) improved local tumor control with more aggressive therapy will not necessarily translate into significantly better long-term survival because of the high probability that pancreatic cancer will metastasize independently of local tumor control.

Combined Modality Management

The high proclivity of systemic disease from pancreatic cancer demands systemic therapy in addition to locoregional therapies. The Gastrointestinal Tumor Study Group (GITSG) documented a survival advantage for postoperative chemoradiotherapy (5-FU + 4000 cGy) in resectable cases, with over 40% of patients alive at 2 years compared to 18% for surgury alone.[24] The superior survival was also evident for unresectable cases treated with moderate dose (4000 cGy) or high dose (6000 cGy) when 5-FU was added.[25] However, the final outcome in terms of survival and locoregional control remains far from being satisfactory.

Thus, the inherent clinical limitations of surgery and/or external beam radiation modalities with or without systemic therapy, in achieving uncomplicated cures or local controls have prompted the search for viable alternatives. Intraoperative interstitial brachytherapy (BRT) into localized unresectable pancreatic tumors has been suggested as a means of achieving palliation of pain and local control without significant complications or operative mortality.

History of Brachytherapy for Pancreatic Cancer

The first attempt at radiation treatment for cancer of the pancreas was reported by Upcott in 1911.[26] He introduced a capsule of 5 mg of radium through the cholecystostomy opening and left it in place for 6 hours; the next day he repeated the application for 4 hours. A month later, the sinus was healed and the patient appeared well. Abel,[27] in 1924, reported a similar application of radium at the time of a third exploration in a patient with adenocarcinoma of the pancreas; 6 months later the patient was well and had gained weight. In 1925, Handley[28] treated seven patients using radium-226 tubes, which were inserted into the tumor and anchored with sutures. These remained in place for 5 days, delivering a dose of 700–1000 mg hrs.

The first permanent implant of pancreatic cancer with radon seeds was performed by George Pack[29] in 1926 at Memorial Hospital. In 1933, Leven[30] implanted radon seeds in the head of the pancreas of dogs and observed marked atrophy of parenchyma and fibrosis in the area around the seeds.

In 1956, Ulrich Henschke[31] reported the use of gold-198 for permanent interstitial implantation of pancreatic tumors. One of these patients, a 60-year-old male had an unresectable papillary adenocarcinoma of the ampulla of Vater. He was implanted in 1954 with 59 seeds of 4 mCi each and received about 10,000 rads to a volume of 65 cm. This patient was alive and well 20 years after implantation. Subsequently, several authors reported their experience with gold grain implants for pancreatic cancer.[42] The list of the authors, the year of the first report, and the isotopes used are given in Table 1.

Table 1.
History[25–27]

Author	Year	Isotope	Form
Upcott	1911	Ra-226	capsules
Abel	1924	Ra-226	capsules
Handley	1925	Ra-226	capsules
Pack	1926	Rn-222	seeds
Henschke	1954	Au-198	seeds
Henschke	1957	Ir-192	seeds
Hilaris	1969	I-125	seeds

Table 2.
TNM Staging of Carcinoma of the Pancreas

Primary Tumor (T)

TX	Primary tumor cannot be assessed
T0	No evidence of primary tumor
T1	Tumor limited to the pancreas
	T1a Tumor 2 cm or less in greatest dimension
	T2b Tumor >2 cm in greatest dimension
T2	Tumor extends directly to the duodenum, bile duct, or peripancreatic tissues
T3	Tumor extends directly to the stomach, spleen, colon, or adjacent large vessels

Regional Lymph Nodes (N)

NX	Regional lymph nodes cannot be assessed
N0	No regional lymph node metastases
N1	Regional lymph node metastases

Distant Metastasis (M)

MX	Presence of distant metastasis cannot be assessed
M0	No distant metastasis
M1	Distant metastasis

Stage Grouping

Stage I	T1	N0	M0
	T2	N0	M0
Stage II	T3	N0	M0
Stage III	ANY T	N1	M0
Stage IV	ANY T	ANY N	M1

Table 3.
Indications and Criteria for Selection

1. Biopsy proven adenocarcinoma
2. Tumor size: 5 cm or less
3. Unresectable locally advanced lesions
4. Resectable lesions in patients who do not tolerate radical surgery
5. No evidence of disseminated peritoneal disease
6. No evidence of distant metastases

Methods

Indications and Criteria of Selection

Accurate evaluation of the extent of the disease and determination of the stage (AJC staging classification) (Table 2) are vital in the proper selection of the patients for BRT procedure. The pretreatment work-up should include angiography to assess the involvement of the blood vessels, CT scan and/or MRI scan, a chest x-ray, bone scan, endoscopic retrograde pancreatography (ERCP), and biopsy confirmation of the diagnosis.

Patients with biopsy proven, unresectable, locally advanced lesions with or without lymph node metastases can be considered for brachytherapy. Patients with diffuse omental, peritoneal, or distant metastases, with an expected median survival of <3 months are not suitable candidates. Large primary tumors (over 5 cm) require significantly high radioactivity to be implanted and, therefore an acceptable therapeutic ratio may not be possible (Table 3). Distant spread occurs mainly to the liver, lungs, and with a lesser frequency to bones, the brain, and other anatomical sites.

Brachytherapy is recommended for tumors localized to the pancreas or having minimal direct peripancreatic extension (Figure 1). If regional nodal metastases (mainly celiac) are present and the implant of the primary site is feasible, a palliative interstitial implant may be done only in order to relieve pain. Supplementary external beam radiation may be considered in the latter case to increase the chance of local control.

Brachytherapy Techniques

Intraoperative permanent interstitial implantation is the standard technique that is widely practiced in several centers. Routine use of temporary implantation in this location involves technical difficulties with proper catheter placement and subsequent removal and, therefore, is not a recommended procedure.[32–35]

Permanent Interstitial Implantation Procedure

Under general anesthesia, an exploratory laparotomy is performed. The laparotomy allows real-time determination of the extent of disease within the pancreas and into adjacent peripancreatic tissues or to other areas in the abdomen beyond the line of potential resection, making possible a decision as to the resectability of the tumor or the alternative option of permanent interstitial implantation

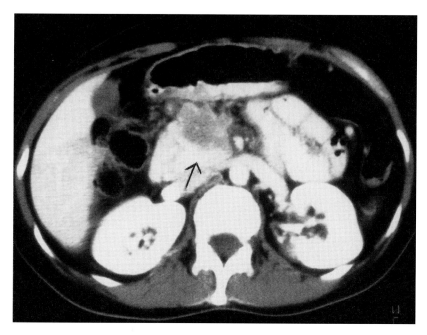

Figure 1. CT scan showing a mass in the head of the pancreas (pretreatment planning is based on the tumor volume derived from the CT scan).

with radioactive iodine-125 (I-125) sources. Furthermore, it allows as physiologically normal as possible restoration of the continuity of the biliary, pancreatic, and gastrointestinal passages.

Mobilization of the duodenum in lesions of the head of the pancreas (Kocher's maneuver) will facilitate the determination of the posterior extent of the tumor.

Once the tumor extent is determined, the three mutually perpendicular dimensions of the tumor are measured. The length and width of the tumor are usually measured using a caliper provided in the permanent implant kit. The anteroposterior dimension (depth) is measured by carefully placing a 15 cm long, 17 gauge implantation needle (supplied with Mick permanent implant applicator kit [Mick Radio-Nuclear, Bronx, NY, USA]) into the tumor. The length of the needle extending above the pancreas is measured with a stainless steel ruler, and this value is subtracted from the total length of the needle with the difference obtained indicating the depth of the tumor.

Prior to implantation, mobilization of the stomach and upward retraction will expose the anterior surface of the pancreas and facilitate the subsequent insertion of the implantation needles. The portal vein above the pancreas and the superior mesenteric vessels below the pancreas must be identified to avoid their injury.

The total activity to be implanted, the number of sources, and the spacing of the sources along each needle are determined using the permanent I-125 implantation nomograph. The predetermined number of needles (obtained by dividing the total number of sources by the number of sources per needle) is inserted into the pancreatic tumor until the tips can be felt by a finger placed behind the pancreas (Figure 2). Generally, the preferred distance between the needles is about 1–1.5 cm. If bleeding secondary to puncture of small pancreatic vessels occurs during the insertion of the needles, the needle is retracted and pressure is applied using a sponge stick for a minute or longer if necessary. The needles should be placed as parallel to each other as possible. After the insertion, the operator should make sure that none of the needle tips have gone through the pancreas, which will result in loss of sources into the peritoneal

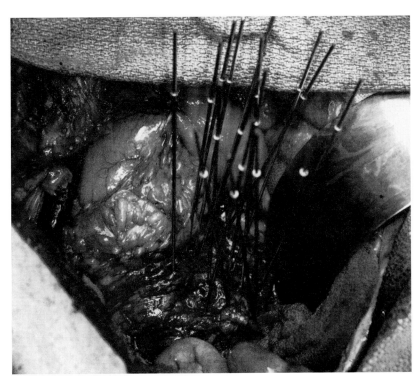

Figure 2. Insertion of the needles: the stainless steel needles are inserted into the pancreatic tumor until their tips can be sensed by the examining finger placed behind the pancreas. Needles are placed parallel to each other as much as possible.

cavity. After all the needles are in place, the Mick applicator is attached to one needle at a time with the aid of an Adson clamp (Figure 3). Then, the I-125 sources are inserted into the pancreatic tumor through each needle at the predetermined spacing and the needle is carefully withdrawn. During this procedure, a careful record is kept of the number of I-125 sources implanted, the activity in mci per source, and the spacing between sources.

To avoid radiation damage to the adjacent stomach and duodenum, it is advisable to place the radioactive sources at a distance of about 0.5–1.0 cm from the surface of the pancreas. Whenever feasible, at the end of the procedure, a segment of the omentum is mobilized and positioned over the anterior surface of the implanted tumor in the pancreas to increase the distance between the implanted sources and the bowel, as well as to prevent leakage of pancreatic fluid and resultant peritonitis.

A choleystojejunostomy and/or gastrojejunostomy should be performed at the completion of brachytherapy in the presence of biliary or gastrointestinal obstruction. Small surgical hemoclips should be placed on the anterior surface of the pancreatic tumor to define and outline the region on future localization films for dosimetry evaluation. The surgeon then closes the incision in the usual manner.

In addition, for patients presenting with pain, we recently implemented a new technique of neurolytic celiac plexus block in an attempt to provide quick and sustained pain relief. After the completion of BRT procedure, epidural needles are used to advance fine catheters through the crura of the diaphragm alongside of the aorta. The catheters are sutured in position on either side, and their free ends are brought out percutaneously to be sutured to the skin. The position of the catheters to the splanchnic nerves is confirmed by injection of radio-opaque dye. Then, initially

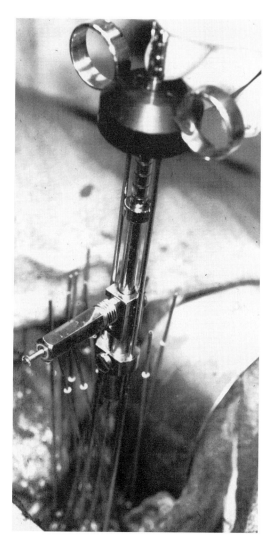

Figure 3. Loading the needles with radioactive sources using Mick applicator: the applicator is attached to one needle at a time while steadying the needle with an Adson clamp. Then, I-125 seeds are deposited into the pancreatic tissue at precalculated spacing along the needle, which is then retracted and detached from the applicator.

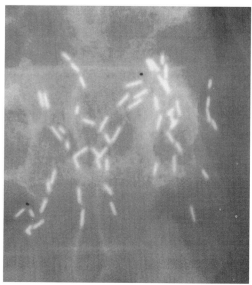

Figure 4. Anteroposterior film showing radioactive sources.

lidocaine and later permanent chemical neurolytic agents (Bupivicaine) are injected postoperatively for pain relief.[36]

Source Localization and Computerized Dosimetry

Localization orthogonal radiographs are taken as soon as the patient becomes ambulatory, usually the third to fourth postoperative day (Figure 4). Isodose contours can be computer generated, and a minimum and maximum tumor dose can be calculated. The dose is determined from the volume-dose information supplied by the computer. The usual recommended tumor dose with I-125 BRT is 16,000 cGy over the period of total decay. Palladium-103 has been used as a substitute for I-125 because of its shorter half-life and higher initial dose rate. The recommended tumor dose with Pd-103 is 11500 cGy. Computerized dose calculations are displayed on orthogonal films as well as the appropriate CT transverse sections (Figure 5). Three-dimensional dosimetry capability, when available, would provide opportunity for pretreatment planning and more accurate evaluation of the dosimetry in relation to the target volume and adjacent anatomy (Figure 6).

Postimplant Evaluation and Follow-Up Care

Patients are seen at 2- to 3-month intervals for the first year. Local tumor control is assessed by repeat localization radiographs to evaluate the tumor regression by determining

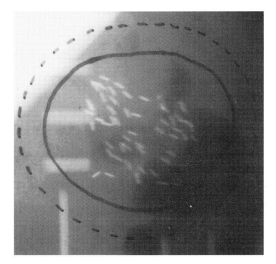

Figure 5. Lateral radiograph with dosimetry superimposed. The inner continuous contour represents 16,000 cGy and the outer contour the 50% isodose line.

the approximation of the sources or by utilizing CT and/or MRI scans.

Postimplant Adjuvant Therapy

Postoperative external beam irradiation to the primary and regional lymphatics may be given with or without chemotherapy. Complete wound healing must be achieved before initiating radiation therapy (usually 3–6 weeks). The radiation is delivered through 3-field or 4-field technique, delivering tumor dose in the range of 4000–4500 cGy at 180–200 cGy per fraction.[33] The most common chemotherapy agent used is 5-FU with or without mitomycin-C and CCNU.

Results

Intraoperative brachytherapy has received limited emphasis. Since the introduction of iodine-125, permanent implantation for pancreatic cancer by us (Basil S. Hilaris, et al.) at Memorial Sloan-Kettering Cancer Center in

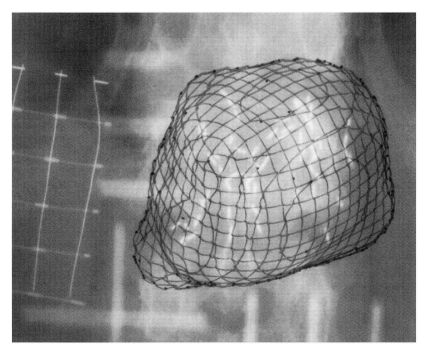

Figure 6. Three-dimensional isodose distribution (100% isodose) superimposed on lateral radiograph.

Table 4.
Comparative Results

Author	Year	Treatment	% of Patients	Local Control	Median Survival (months)	Complications
		Surgical Combinations				
Shapiro[7]	1975	S	—	—	13.9	21% mort
Moertel, et al.[24]	1987	S	—	—	10.5	
		S + XRT + 5FU	—	—	21.0	
		XRT Combinations				
Abel, et al.[19]	1981	IORT (20–40 GY)	108	40%	6.0	
Moertel[25]	1981	60 Gy	25	—	5.5	
		60 Gy + 5FU	83	—	10.0	
		40 Gy + 5FU	83	—	10.0	
		Intraoperative Combinations				
Barone, et al.[38]	1975	Radon seeds + FUDR	8	—	8.2	13%
Shipley, et al.[36]	1980	45 GY + I125	12	—	11.0	42%
Syed, et al.[39]	1983	40 Gy + I125	18	—	14.0	22%
Mohiuddin, et al.[40]	1988	60 Gy + I125	13	77%	5.5	31% mort
		55 Gy + I125 + Chemo	19	85%	11.3	
		5 Gy + I125 + 50 Gy + Chemo	54	87%	12.5	7% mort
Peretz, Hilaris, et al.[45]	1989	T1N0M0 I125	30	—	11.6	
		T1N0M0 I125 + Chemo		—	18.9	
		T1N1M0 I125 + Chemo ± XRT	14	—	8.0	
		T2–T3N0M0 I125 ± Chemo ± XRT	47	—	5.9	28%
		T2–T3N1M0 I125 ± Chemo ± XRT	7	—	5.25	
Hilaris, Moorthy, et al.[47,48]	1991	T3N0M0 I125 + 5FU	10	—	10.0	6%
		T2–T3N1M1 I125 + 5FU	6	—	5.5	

FU = follow-up; S = surgery; XRT = external beam irradiation; IORT = intraoperative radiotherapy; mort = mortality.

1969, several authors have reported their experience with this procedure with or without the addition of postoperative external beam radiation or chemotherapy (Table 4).[32,37–41]

At the Massachusetts General Hospital (MGH), Shipley and his coworkers treated 12 patients with locally advanced pancreatic carcinoma with a combination of I-125 implantation (calculated dose of 16,000 cGy) and external beam radiation (4500 cGy in 5 weeks) delivered to the primary tumor and regional lymph nodes. The median survival in this se-

ries was 11 months, with one patient surviving for 30 months. Pancreatic fistula developed in two patients.[37]

From 1974–1987, 98 patients at Memorial Sloan-Kettering Cancer Center with biopsy proven unresectable adenocarcinoma of the pancreas were treated with I-125 implantation at laparotomy. The majority of patients had primary tumor located in the head of the pancreas (64 patients), and 30 patients had T1N0 disease. The median survival for the whole group was 7 months. The median survival of patients with stage T1N0 was significantly longer than that of patients with T2–3N0 (11.6 vs 6.1 months).[43–45]

Patients with T1N0 disease who received postoperative chemotherapy had the longest median survival of 18.9 months after the implant. Patients with T1 disease who had >30% regression of the implanted volume had also the longest median survival of 15.5 months. A multivariate analysis of factors affecting survival, including sex, age, location of the primary, nature of operating procedure, presenting symptoms, tumor dose, volume of implant, postoperative radiotherapy, postoperative chemotherapy, stage of disease, and reduction of the volume of the implant, was performed with Cox proportional regression hazard model. Four prognostic factors were found to significantly contribute to long-term survival. These included T stage (P = 0.002), N stage (P = 0.017), the degree of tumor response as determined by the reduction in implant size (P = 0.03), and administration of postoperative chemotherapy (P = 0.002).

Pain relief was the most significant subjective response affected by the implant. Significant pain relief was observed in 37 of 57 patients presenting with pain (65%) that lasted for 5–47 months. Nineteen patients experienced postoperative complications. These included bilary fistula (4), gastrointestinal bleeding (3), gastrointestinal obstruction (6), sepsis (5), and deep vein thrombophlebitis (4). One patient (1%) died on postoperative day 32 with pancreatic fistula and sepsis.

The survival advantage of postoperative chemotherapy as an adjuvant to brachytherapy was also evident in a series of sequential trials conducted by Mohiuddin et al.[41] from (TJUH). Between 1978–1986, 86 patients with unresectable adenocarcinoma of the pancreas were treated with I-125 brachytherapy and postoperative external beam radiation with or without chemotherapy (5-FU, mitomycin-C, and CCNU). Group 1 was comprised of 13 patients treated with postoperative external beam radiation (6000 cGy in 6 weeks). Group 2 (19 patients) received chemotherapy in addition to external beam radiation 5500 cGy, and Group 3 (54 patients) received preoperative external beam radiation 500 cGy, perioperative chemotherapy, and postoperative external beam radiation 5000 cGy followed by further chemotherapy. Clinical local tumor control was excellent in all three groups (84%). In spite of adjuvant chemotherapy, 64% of the patients had distant metastases, especially to the liver. The median survival in the three groups of patients was 5.5, 11.3, and 12.5 months, and the corresponding 2-year actuarial survival was 0%, 15%, and 22%. The perioperative mortality was reduced from 31% (10/32) in groups 1 and 2 to 7% (4/54) in group 3 by improvements in the technique, nutritional support, and early ambulation.

While the superior results obtained with adjuvant chemotherapy are promising, the true contribution of external beam irradiation to the primary and regional lymph nodes (after brachytherapy) has not been clearly evaluated. In an attempt to address this question, a pilot study was conducted at our institution (New York Medical College/Westchester Medical Center). From 1988–1990, 16 patients with unresectable pancreatic carcinoma were treated with intraoperative brachytherapy followed by postoperative chemotherapy (5-FU) but without external beam irradiation. Of these, ten patients with stage II disease (T3N0M0) had a median survival of 10 months and 2-year actuarial survival of 15%. This compares favorably with results obtained for similar groups of patients in other series (TJUH, MSKCC) that included postoperative external beam irradiation. Our preliminary experience with a limited number of patients suggests no survival advantage to adding postoperative external beam irradiation to brachytherapy and chemotherapy.

Mortality and Morbidity

The major long-term complications of the treatment include GI bleeding, ulceration of the bowel, pancreatic fistula, enterocutaneous fistula, and abscess formation.[46–48] The high morbidity (6%–42%) and perioperative mortality (3%–31%) can be minimized by careful pretreatment planning, proper intraoperative technique, and follow-up care (Tables 4 and 5).[39–41]

Conclusions

The management of unresectable carcinoma of the pancreas continues to pose a sig-

Table 5.
Steps to Minimize Complications

1. Plan the implant preoperatively using CT or MRI scans
2. Minimize the number of needles to be implanted
3. Avoid trauma to the blood vessels (SMA, SMV, PV, etc)
4. Monitor the tip of the needle (not to go through the pancreas)
5. Establish hemostasis at each step
6. Use omental flap over the implanted region
7. Maintain appropriate antibiotic coverage

SMA = superior mesenteric artery; SMV = superior mesenteric vein; PV = portal vein.

nificant challenge in spite of innovations in surgery, radiation therapy, and chemotherapy. Used alone, none of these modalities is adequate, and improved local tumor control alone with more aggressive therapy will not necessarily translate into significantly better long-term survival because of higher probability that pancreatic cancer will metastasize independent of local tumor control. Although surgery remains the treatment of choice for early lesions, brachytherapy followed by chemotherapy appears to be an acceptable modality for locoregionally advanced tumors. The gain in survival from this procedure in unresectable cases is modest; however, the palliation of pain is significant. The addition of conventional external beam radiation after an adequate implant may be of limited value, although it is associated with increased morbidity and interferes with subsequent administration of chemotherapy. Therefore, this requires further investigation.

Novel treatment strategies, such as preoperative split course chemoradiotherapy similar to the GITSG regimen, may debulk the tumor before brachytherapy and needs to be investigated. Three-dimensional treatment planning will allow improvement of therapeutic ratio and may have beneficial impact on local control and survival.

References

1. Cancer Facts and Figures, American Cancer Society, 1994, pp. 5–6.
2. Gudjonsson B. Cancer of the pancreas: 50 years of surgery. Cancer 1987;60:2284–2303.
3. Connolly MM, Dawson PJ, Michelassi F. Survival in 1001 patients with pancreatic carcinoma. Ann Surg 1987;206:366–373.
4. Biometry Branch National Cancer Institute, Axtel LM, Cutler SJ, Myers MH (eds). End Results in Cancer, Report No. 4. DHEW Pub No. 73–272 End Results Section, 1972, pp. 81–84.
5. Branch National Cancer Institute, Axtel LM, Myers MH (eds). Recent Trends in Survival of Cancer Patients, 1960–1971. DHEW Pub No. 75–767. End Results Section, 1974, p. 30.
6. Cubilla AL, Fitzgerald PJ. Pancreas cancer. 1. Duct cell adenocarcinoma. In: Pathology Annual, Part 1. Appleton-Century-Crofts, New York, 1978, pp. 241–287.
7. Shapiro T. Adenocarcinoma of the pancreas: A statistical analysis of biliary bypass vs. whipple resection in good risk patients. Ann Surg 1975; 82:715–721.
8. Tepper J, Nardi G, Suit H. Carcinoma of the pancreas: Review of MGH experience from 1963–1987, analysis of surgical failure and implications for radiation therapy. Cancer 1976; 37:1519–1524.
9. Morrow N, Hilaris B, Brennan MF. Comparison of conventional surgical resection, radioactive implantation and bypass procedure for exocrine carcinoma of the pancreas, 1975–1980. Ann Surg 1984;199:1–5.
10. Harter W, Dritschillo A. Cancer of the pancreas: Are chemotherapy and radiation appropriate? Clin Oncol 1989;3:27–37.
11. Haslam JB, Cavanaugh PJ, Stroup SL. Radiation therapy in the treatment of unresectable adenocarcinoma of the pancreas. Cancer 1973;32: 1341–1345.
12. Dobelbower RR Jr. The radiotherapy of pancreatic cancer. Semin Oncol 1979;6:378–389.
13. Kaul R, Cohen L, Hendrickson F, et al. Pancreatic carcinoma: Results with fast neutron therapy. Int J Radiat Oncol Biol Phys 1981;7: 173–178.
14. Smith FP, Schein PS, Macdonald JS, et al. Fast neutron irradiation for locally advanced pancreatic cancer. Int J Radiat Oncol Biol Phys 1981;7:1527–1531.
15. Al-Abdulla ASM, Hussey DH, Olson MH, et al. Experience with fast neutron therapy for unresectable carcinoma of the pancreas. Int J Radiat Oncol Biol Phys 1981;7:165–172.
16. Castro JR, Quivey JM, Lyman JT, et al. Current status of clinical particle radiotherapy at Lawrence Berkeley Laboratory. Cancer 1980;46: 633–641.
17. Kligerman MM, Sala JM, Smith AR, et al. Tissue reaction and tumor response with negative pi mesons. J Can Assoc Radiol 1980;31:13.
18. Goldson AL, Ashaveri E, Espinoza MC, et al.

Single high-dose intraoperative electrons for advanced stage pancreatic cancer: Phase I pilot study. Int J Radiat Oncol Biol Phys 1981;7:869.

19. Abe M, Takahashi M. Intraoperative radiotherapy: The Japanese experience. Int J Radiat Oncol Biol Phys 1981;7:863.

20. Nishamura A, Nakano M, Otsu H, et al. Intraoperative radiotherapy for advanced carcinoma of the pancreas. Cancer 1984;54:2375.

21. Shipley WU, Wood WC, Tepper JE, et al. Intraoperative electron beam irradiation for patients with unresectable pancreatic carcinoma. Ann Surg 1984;200:289.

22. Tepper JE, Shipley WU, Warshaw AL, et al. The role of Misonidazole combined with intraoperative radiation therapy in the treatment of pancreatic carcinoma. J Clin Oncol 1987;5:579.

23. Gunderson LL, Martin JK, Kvols LT, et al. Intraoperative external beam irradiation ± 5-FU for locally advanced pancreatic cancer. Int J Radiat Oncol Biol Phys 1987;13:319.

24. Gastrointestinal Tumor Study Group. Further evidence of effective adjuvant combined radiation and chemotherapy following resection of pancreatic cancer. Cancer 1987;59:2006–2010.

25. Moertel CG, Frytak S, Hahn RG, et al. Gastrointestinal Tumor Study Group. Therapy of locally unresectable pancreatic carcinoma: A randomized comparison of high dose (6000 rads) radiation alone, moderate dose radiation (4000 rads + 5-Fluorouracil), and high dose radiation + 5-Fluorouracil. Cancer 1981;48:1705–1710.

26. Upcott H. Tumors of the ampulla of vater. Ann Surg 1912;56:710–725.

27. Abel L. Carcinoma of papilla of Vater. South Med J 1924;17:24–27.

28. Handley WS. Pancreatic cancer and its treatment by implanted radium. Ann Surg 1934;100:215–223.

29. Pack GT, McNeer G. Radiation treatment of pancreatic cancer. Am J Roentgenol 1938;40:708–714.

30. Leven NL. Primary carcinoma of the pancreas. Am J Cancer 1933;18:852–874.

31. Henschke UK. Interstitial implantation with radioisotopes. In: Hahn PF (ed). Therapeutic Use of Artificial Radioisotopes. John Wiley and Sons, New York, 1956.

32. Hilaris BS, Roussis K. Cancer of the pancreas. In: Hilaris BS (ed). Handbook of Interstitial Brachytherapy. Acton Publishing Science Group, Inc., Acton, 1975, pp. 251–262.

33. Hilaris BS, Anderson LL, Tokita N. Interstitial implantation of pancreatic cancer. In: Voeth JM (ed). Frontiers of Radiation Therapy Oncology. S. Karger. Besel, 1978, pp. 62–71.

34. Hilaris BS, Nori D, Anderson L. Brachytherapy for cancer of the pancreas. In: Hilaris BS (ed). An Atlas of Brachytherapy. Macmillan Publishing Company, New York, 1988, pp. 204–244.

35. Hilaris B, Moorthy C, Kim J. Radiotherapeutic management of pancreatic cancer at Memorial Sloan-Kettering Cancer Center. In: Conn I (ed). Pancreatic Cancer: New Directions in Therapeutic Management. Masson, New York, 1980, pp. 251–262.

36. DelGuercio LRM, Hilaris BS, Moorthy CR, et al. Brachytherapy and splanchnisectomy for pain control in unresectable pancreatic carcinoma. Updating course on pancreatic diseases. Proceedings of "Updating Course on Pancreatic Disease, Genoa, Italy, 1992, p. 114.

37. Shipley WU, Nardi GL, Cohen AM, et al. Iodine-125 implant and external beam irradiation in patients with localized pancreatic cancer. A comparative study to surgical resection. Cancer 1980;45:709–714.

38. Barone RM. Treatment of carcinoma of the pancreas with radon seed implantation and intra-arterial infusion of 5-FUDR. Surg Clin North Am 1975;55:117–128.

39. Dobelbower RR, Merrick HW, Ahuja RK, et al. I-125 interstitial implant precision high dose external beam therapy and 5-FU for unresectable adenocarcioma of pancreas and extrahepatic biliary tree. Cancer 1986;58:2185–2195.

40. Syed AMN, Puthawala AA, Neblett DL. Interstitial iodine-125 implant in the management of unresectable pancreatic carcinoma. Cancer 1983;52:808–813.

41. Mohiuddin M, Cantor RJ, Biermann W, et al. Combined modality treatment of localized unresectable adenocarcinoma of the pancreas. Int J Radiat Oncol Biol Phys 1988;14:79–84.

42. Borgelt B. Radiation therapy with either gold grain implant or neutron beam for unresectable adenocarcinoma of the pancreas. In: Cohn I (ed). Pancreatic Cancer: New Directions in Therapeutic Management. Masson, New York, 1980, pp. 55–63.

43. Brennan M, Manolatos S, Genest P, et al. Brachytherapy in the management of pancreatic cancer. In: Hilaris BS, Nori D (eds). Brachytherapy Oncology Update, 1984. Memorial Sloan-Kettering Cancer Center, New York, 1984, pp. 29–41.

44. Manolatos S, Hilaris, BS, Nori D, et al. Intraoperative brachytherapy in the management of locally advanced pancreatic cancer, identification of prognostic factors. In: The Proceedings of the American Endocurietherapy Society Annual Meeting, vol 2, no 4, 1986, pp. 217.

45. Peretz T, Nori D, Hilaris BS, et al. Treatment of primary unresectable carcinoma of the pan-

creas with I-125 implantation. Int J Radiat Oncol Biol Phys 1989;17:931–935.

46. Whittington R, Dobelbower R, Borgelt B, et al. Combined iodine-125 implantation and precision high-dose radiotherapy in the treatment of unresectable pancreatic carcinoma. In: Cohn I (ed). Pancreatic Cancer: New Directions in Therapeutic Management. Masson, New York, 1980.

47. Hilaris BS, Moorthy C, DelGuercio L, et al. Per-manent I-125 brachytherapy and 5-Fluorouracil in unresectable adenocarcinoma of the pancreas: Treatment results. Endocurie/Hypertherm Oncol 1991;7:85.

48. Lebovics E, Mittelman A, Delguercio LR, et al. Pancreaticobiliary fistula and obstructive jaundice complicating I-125 implants for pancreatic cancer: Endoscopic diagnosis and management. Gastrointest Endosc 1990;36:610–611.

Chapter 20

Endocavitary and Brachytherapy Techniques in the Conservative Management of Anorectal Cancers

Subir Nag, M.D., Jean-Pierre Gerard, M.D.

Introduction

Abdominal perineal resection (APR) was the mainstay for therapy of lower colorectal cancers since 1908 when Miles[1] performed the first resection. Various modifications of the procedure have been tried with only minor improvement of results.[2] Since there is major morbidity of APR and since radiation therapy has become available, the value of APR has been questioned.[3]

Endocavitary iridium has been used for the radiotherapeutic management of colorectal cancers since 1914.[4] However, because of the limitations of the early radiotherapy equipment, colorectal cancers were considered to be relatively radioresistant. The advent of high megavoltage radiation showed that patients with colorectal cancers could be cured by radiation therapy alone.[5] The last decade has seen a major trend toward organ preservation in the treatment of various cancers, including breast, larynx, and prostate. Conservative management of the anorectal area has been popularized, especially in France, by Papillon et al.[6–12] Various techniques of radiotherapy, including external beam radiotherapy (EBRT), endocavitary contact therapy, brachytherapy, and intraoperative radiation therapy, have been attempted. Although adenocarcinoma of the rectum is primarily treated by surgery, selected cases can be curatively treated with irradiation alone. Squamous cell carcinomas of the anal canal are now primarily treated by irradiation (often along with concurrent chemotherapy).

Endocavitary Contact Radiation Therapy Alone

Early stage rectal adenocarcinoma has a low incidence of lymphatic involvement and, therefore, can be treated with local excision, electrocoagulation, or primary radiotherapy while preserving the rectal function. Endocavitary radiation for early rectal cancers was used as early as the 1940s by Lamarque and Gros.[13] Using a 50-KV Phillips contact x-ray machine, they obtained a 5-year survival rate of 42% in a series of 26 patients.

Techniques

The method was made popular by Papillon of the Centre Leon Berard, Lyon, France. A 50 KV Phillips contact machine producing 10–20

From Nag S (ed): *Principles and Practice of Brachytherapy.* © Futura Publishing Co., Inc., Armonk, NY, 1997.

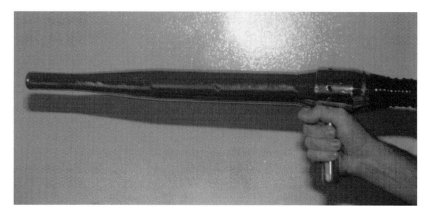

Figure 1A. A 50-kV Phillips contact machine.

Gy per minute output is used. This machine has a short (4 cm) source-to-skin distance (SSD), with a depth dose of about 25% at 1 cm. A 0.5-mm aluminum filter is used, and the effective treatment diameter is 3 cm. After an enema, the patient is treated in the knee-chest position. The radiation oncologist holds the contact x-ray machine (wearing a leaded rubber glove and leaded apron for radiation protection) directly over the rectal tumor (Figures 1A and 1B). These applications deliver 30 Gy at the surface and take about 2 minutes. The procedure is performed on an out-patient basis, and usually four treatments are given (total of about 120 Gy in 6–8 weeks with about 2 weeks between treatments). This high superficial dose produces rapid shrinkage of an exophytic tumor and the tumor is destroyed layer by layer. This prolonged duration of treatment allows the tumor to regress (Figures 2A-C and 3A-C).

Patient Selection Criteria

1. Well to moderately differentiated adenocarcinoma. Poorly differentiated

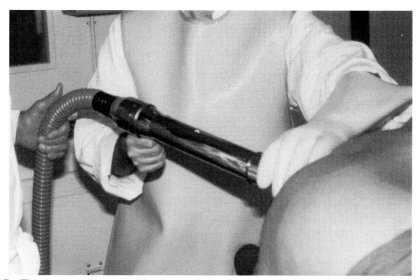

Figure 1B. The contact x-ray machine is applied to the rectal tumor with the patient in the knee-chest position.

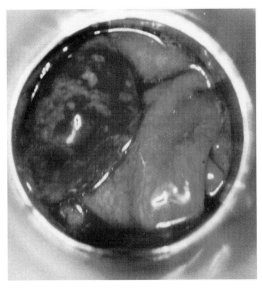

Figure 2A. Well differentiated adenocarcinoma of rectum, T1 N0, 2.5 cm in diameter, before treatment by contact x-ray.

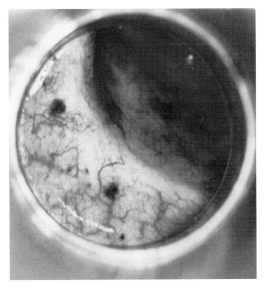

Figure 2C. The same patient 2 years after the end of contact x-ray treatment, which delivered 85 Gy/4 fractions/48 days.

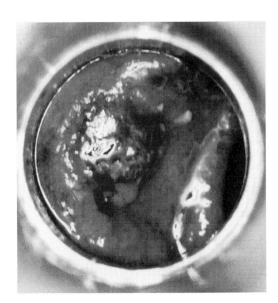

Figure 2B. The same tumor 7 days after the first dose of 35 Gy by contact x-ray (50 kV).

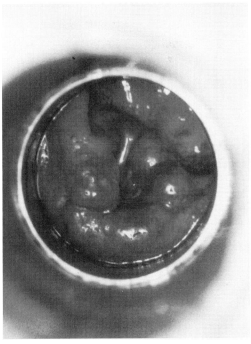

Figure 3A. Moderately well differentiated adenocarcinoma of rectum, T2 N0, 2.5 cm in diameter, before treatment by contact x-ray.

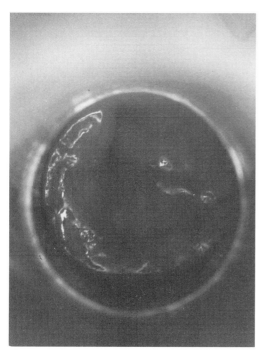

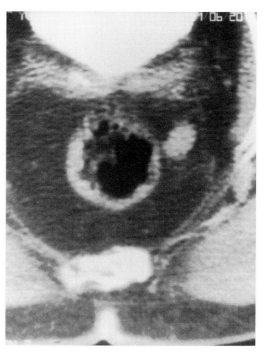

Figure 3B. The same patient 1 year later, after the end of treatment with a dose of 110 Gy of contact x-ray, 50 kV, in five fractions and 69 days. Complete remission.

Figure 3C. Two and one-half years after treatment, a hard nodule was felt in the pararectal wall. CT scan very clearly showed a 1-cm nodule. Abdominoperineal resection was performed, and the operative specimen was histologically confirmed to be a metastatic lymph node (adenocarcinoma). The patient died of intercurrent disease 3 years after surgery.

tumors and melanomas are not suitable candidates.

2. Size of lesion. Small tumors (<3 cm) are preferred, although tumors up to 5 cm in diameter can be treated.

3. Tumors should be preferably exophytic with minimal rectal wall penetration. Transrectal ultrasound (TRUS) should be used to assess the depth of penetration. If muscularis propria is involved, contact x-ray alone is not suitable. The tumors should not be fixed.

4. The tumors should be accessible to the contact therapy machine and hence should be <10–12 cm from the anal verge.

5. Absence of pathologically involved lymph nodes. TRUS is better than digital examination to detect small, metastatic, pararectal lymph nodes. Pathologically involved (N1) lymph nodes

are a contraindication for contact therapy alone.

6. Nonulcerative lesions are preferred.

7. Can be used as prophylactic treatment after removal of a malignant polyp.

8. The patient must be reliable and agree to close follow-up.

Morson[14] showed that well differentiated and moderately well differentiated adenocarcinomas have a low incidence of lymph node metastases. Hermanek et al.[15] showed that incidence of lymphatic spread is also dependent on the depth of invasion, being 0%, 3%, 24%, and 38% when the tumor is limited to the submucosa, inner part of the muscular layer, outer muscular layer, or perirectal spread, respectively. Although deep digital palpation can be used, transrectal ultrasound is the most reliable technique for measuring the depth of invasion and for assessing the presence of small (<1 cm), metastatic, pararectal lymph nodes.

Pretreatment Evaluation

1. Careful digital rectal examination and proctoscopy of an empty ampulla in the knee-chest position.
2. Transrectal ultrasound to assess depth of penetration and pararectal lymph nodes.
3. CT scan of the abdomen and pelvis.
4. CEA level.
5. Colonoscopy to rule out synchronous chronic lesions.

Results

Papillon's and Berard[16] series at the Centre Leon Berard is by far the largest, with 312 patients treated and followed for more than 5 years, with no patients lost to follow-up. All patients had invasive, mobile, well differentiated, or moderately differentiated adenocarcinoma; 209 cases were polypoid and 103 cases were ulcerative. The mean age was 65, range 25–91 years. The treatments were well tolerated, with slight proctitis in 10% of patients. Superficial radionecrosis was rare (5%), and most healed spontaneously. Occasional bleeding occurred. Stricture or rectal narrowing was not a problem.

The 5-year disease-free survival was 74%, with 7.7% dying of cancer, 17% dying of intercurrent disease, and 1.3% dying postoperatively. Of the 231 patients who were alive and disease-free, 96% had normal anal function. Four percent (8 patients) had a permanent colostomy after APR.

Experience in the United States has been more limited. Sischy[17] reported on 129 patients of rectal carcinoma treated with endocavitary radiation using a technique similar to Papillon's. He observed limited local morbidity and no systemic side effects. Anal sphincter and sexual function were preserved. Recurrences were observed in six out of the 129 patients within 18 months of treatment. The local control rate was 95%. Palliation was effectively obtained in 83% of 87 patients.

Myerson et al.,[18] at Washington University, St. Louis, reported 52 patients treated either by endocavitary radiation only or 45 Gy EBRT followed by endocavitary radiation. Ideal tumors (defined as being <3 cm in diameter, freely mobile, and having no nodes), were well controlled either with endocavitary radiation alone or endocavitary radiation plus EBRT (18 out of 22 local control with irradiation, 100% local control with salvage surgery). The more extensive tumors showed improved local control with the addition of EBRT (2/10 locally controlled without EBRT vs 14/18 locally controlled with EBRT). There was no major symptomatic complications of treatment. Nine patients experienced minor proctitis or bleeding referable to the endocavitary radiation. Hence, Myerson et al.[18] advocate the addition of EBRT to the endocavitary irradiation if the tumors are marginal, that is, mobile and 3–4 cm in diameter, or tethered.

Lavery et al.,[19] reported on 62 patients treated by contact therapy at The Cleveland Clinic, Cleveland, Ohio. Sixteen of these patients also had excisional biopsies. The median tumor dose was 120 Gy delivered in four fractions at monthly intervals. At a mean follow-up of 31 months, 90% of the patients were disease-free at the time of review or death. Eighteen percent developed local recurrence. The local recurrence rate was higher in the ulcerated tumors (29%) versus polypoid tumors (14%). Only minor morbidity was observed, consisting mainly of rectal bleeding and urgency. No fistulae or stricture injuries were noted. Two patients required temporary colostomies for radiation proctitis.

Kovalic[20] used endocavitary radiation to treat 52 patients in Milwaukee, Wisconsin. The dose used was somewhat lower (80 Gy in four treatments over 6 weeks). The patients treated included 32 patients with adenocarcinoma and 19 patients with villus adenoma. Of the 32 patients with adenocarcinoma, the overall local recurrence rate was 24%. The 1-, 2-, and 3-year determinant disease-free survival rates were 90%, 79%, and 74%, respectively. There was minimal morbidity associated with the treatment. The patients with villous adenoma did not fare as well as those with adenocarcinoma; and, therefore, Kovalic[20] hypothesized that adenomas were more radioresistant and would require higher doses.

Roth et al.[21] reported the Dijon experience

with 91 patients with limited rectal tumors treated with intracavitary radiotherapy alone or associated with interstitial brachytherapy using techniques similar to Papillon. Of these, 72 had adenocarcinoma and 19 had villous adenomas. Seventy-six percent (69 out of 91) had local tumor control. After salvage surgery, the local tumor control was 91%, with sphincter function preserved in 85%. The local relapse-free survival at 5 years was 97% for T_{1A}, 77% for T_{1B}, 65% for T_{2A}, and 60% for T_{2B}. The tumors of the anterior rectal wall had a better local control rate compared to that of tumors in a lateral or posterior location (100% vs 63% vs 67%, respectively). They advocated use of contact therapy alone for stage T_{1A}, with the addition of interstitial brachytherapy for T_{1B}, T_{2A}, and T_{2B}.

Combined Endocavitary Radiation and External Beam Radiation Therapy

Endocavitary radiation is only applicable to T_1 or small T_2 tumors, which represent only <10% of cancers of the lower rectum. More advanced tumors have a higher risk of lymph node involvement and have deeper lesions, which do not receive sufficient radiation from the endocavitary technique. These patients receive EBRT to the pelvis, with the endocavitary radiation being used as a boost.

Technique

The posterior pelvic arc technique of EBRT used by Papillon consists of a posterior 120° arc rotation to a limited field using cobalt-60, with the patient in the prone position. A similar dose distribution as the arc technique can be obtained with a linear accelerator using a 3-field technique and a concomitant boost.[12]

1. A dose of 30 Gy is delivered in ten fractions within 12 days. The advantage of this technique is the limited target volume, which includes the regional spread of rectal cancer.
2. The satisfactory protection of the small bowel is achieved by bladder distention.
3. There is good tolerance, with proctitis relieved by steroid enema.

4. The hot spot of 35 Gy is given to the tumor area.
5. Endocavitary radiation is given 2 months later, consisting of contact therapy of 25 Gy and/or an iridium-192 implant of 20–30 Gy.[22] Contact therapy can be given before EBRT on the exophytic portion of the tumor. After EBRT the rectal mucosa is often edematous and contact therapy is more difficult on a retracted, infiltrating residual tumor. Iridium implant is always given as the last treatment on the tumor bed after maximal shrinkage by EBRT and contact x-ray therapy.

Results

Seventy-six patients with T_2-T_3 tumors of the distal rectum were treated. Among the 67 patients followed for more than 5 years, the disease-free survival was 60%, with 12% dying of cancer and 27% dying of intercurrent disease. Of the 40% alive and well after more than 5 years, 39 had normal anal function and one patient had a permanent colostomy after APR for local recurrence.

Low-Dose-Rate Iridium Brachytherapy for Primary Rectal Cancers

Endocavitary contact therapy delivers a high dose of radiation to the surface of the tumor. Since there is a small source-to-skin distance (4 cm), there is only limited penetration. Therefore, it is effective for exophytic tumors, treating the tumor layer by layer. Endocavitary radiation is, therefore, not effective in treating deeply penetrating tumors or tumors >4 cm in diameter. These patients are better treated with a combination of interstitial implants after EBRT or a combination of EBRT and endocavitary radiation. This procedure combines the advantages of EBRT (homogenous dose to a large volume), of endocavitary radiation (a large dose to the surface of the tumor), and of interstitial brachytherapy (delivery of a large dose inside the tumor with sparing of normal tissues) while localiz-

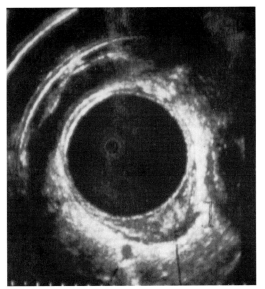

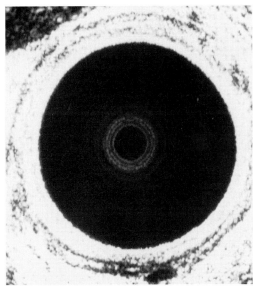

Figure 4A. Patient with a T3 N1, low rectal adenocarcinoma stage by transrectal ultrasound, which was inoperable because of cardiorespiratory insufficiency. Treatment by irradiation alone: 1) 80 Gy contact x-ray; 2) EBRT (39 Gy/13 F/17 days) and 1 Gy × 4 with concomitant boost (field within the field); 3) iridium-192 perineal implant (20 Gy/24 hours). Treatment was performed in 1989.

Figure 4B. The same patient, alive and well in 1994 with normal anorectal function.

ing the highest radiation dose within the tumor (Figures 4A and 4B).

Techniques

The anus and rectum do not tolerate high doses of radiation. Hence, the following precautions must be followed:

1. The brachytherapy should be used as a boost rather than as the sole treatment.
2. The implant should always be performed in a single plane rather than multiple planes to minimize the volume irradiated.
3. To prevent strictures, only a part of the circumference of the rectum (not the entire circumference) should be implanted.
4. Preferably, the dose should be limited to 15–20 Gy, up to a maximum of 30 Gy.

Papillon et al.[11] have developed a crescentic plastic template with holes 1 cm apart (Arplay, Inc., Izeure, France). The template is sutured to the perineal skin. Steel hollow needles are implanted through the holes in the template through the perineal skin into the site of the tumor (parallelism is confirmed fluoroscopically) and are loaded with iridium-192 wires of 1.5–2.5 mCi per cm (Figures 5A-C). Doses of 15–20 Gy are used 2 months after completion of EBRT.[11] A steel fork technique can also be used. The hollow prongs are 4 cm long and 1.6 cm apart (Arplay, Inc.).[11] The implant is performed under local anesthesia with the patient in the knee-chest position. The fork is inserted 1 cm below the tumor area, pushed superiorly parallel to the axis of the rectal ampulla, and kept in place by a rubber drain sutured to the skin of the anal margins. A 20–30 Gy dose is delivered using the Paris system. Iridium-192 wires (4–7 mCi per cm) are used, and treatment time does not exceed 36 hours.

In the United States, the technique used by Syed et al.[23] (using a Syed template to place two implants that each deliver a minimum tumor dose of 15–20 Gy in 25–40 hours) is usually implemented after delivery of 40–50 Gy of EBRT to the primary and regional nodes

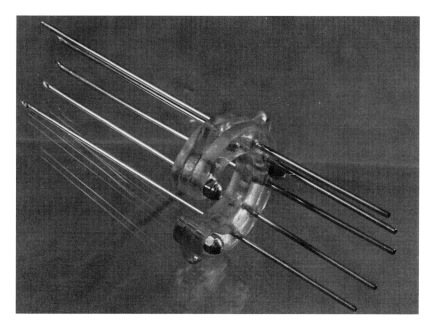

Figure 5A. Template and stainless needle for anorectal perineal implant.

over 5–6 weeks. The interval between the completion of external radiation and first implant, as well as that between the first and second implant, is 2–3 weeks. The total dose to the primary site, with the combination of the EBRT and two interstitial implants, ranges from 70–90 Gy. We prefer a single implant with the dose restricted to 25–30 Gy with a single plane implant not encompassing greater than two thirds of the circumference of the rectum.

Delclos uses a rectal plug in the anus to keep it distended and a large Foley catheter through the rectal plug to keep the normal rectum and anus away from the implanted site.[24] A dose of 60–65 Gy is given in 5–7 days when treating low risk tumors with interstitial brachytherapy alone. Borderline and larger tumors are treated with 40 Gy in 3–4 days with 40 Gy EBRT in 20 fractions over 4 weeks.

Results

In 90 patients with T_1-T_2 invasive adenocarcinoma of the rectum, Papillon et al.[11] reported on the use of iridium-192 brachytherapy after four applications of contact x-ray therapy. The rate of control was 84%. In 62 elderly poor risk patients with T_2-T_3 tumors

treated with combined EBRT at the dose of 30–35 Gy in ten fractions, followed by iridium-192 implants, the rate of death due to treatment failures was 14.5%, and among the patients controlled, 97% had normal anal function.[11] Careful patient selection and techniques must obviously be followed.

Puthawala et al.[23] reported their experience with 40 patients treated with a combination of external beam and two interstitial implantations. They obtained complete local tumor control of 70%. After salvage surgery, the local control was 75%. Disease-free survival was 60% with an average follow-up period of 3 years. The overall complication rate was 20%.

Vider et al.[25] reported on a flexible implant technique using tygone tubes that allows the patient to move freely in the room. They reported encouraging preliminary results on four patients, but the maximum follow-up was only 6 months. Jackson[26] reported on 36 patients treated with EBRT and iridium-192 implants. Four patients with recurrent rectal cancer received additional permanent I-125 seeds at the time of laparotomy. The most severe complication was uncontrolled diarrhea with incontinence and stenosis. Two patients developed severe necrosis. The complica-

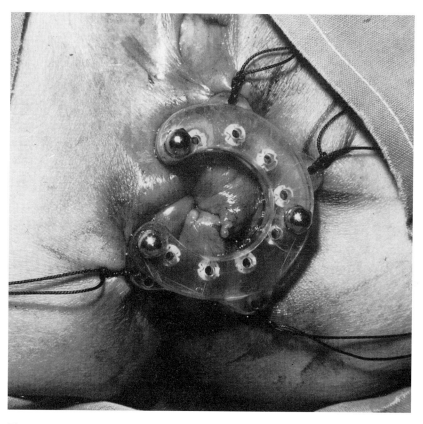

Figure 5B. Template fixed to the perineum.

tions were more severe in those treated with excision followed by immediate implant, and with those lesions that were treated with a single high-dose (40–50 Gy) implant.

Interstitial Implant for Recurrent Disease

Patients with recurrent colorectal carcinoma have a poor prognosis and high morbidity because they have had previous abdominal surgeries and EBRT. Brachytherapy techniques can be used in the treatment of these recurrent colorectal cancers.

Technique

Permanent Iodine-125

Depending on the accessibility and site of the recurrence, the implantation can either be performed transperineally or under direct vi-

sion at laparotomy. If possible, the tumor is debulked and the tumor bed implanted. Since these patients have frequently previously received EBRT, brachytherapy is most commonly used alone. Iodine-125 seeds can be implanted into the tumor using a Mick applicator (Mick Radio-Nuclear Instruments, Bronx, NY, USA) (Figures 6A and 6B). Doses of about 160 Gy to total decay are delivered. Whenever possible, omentum is placed over the tumor area to reduce the radiation dose to the bowel.

Radioimmunoguided Brachytherapy

Nag et al.[27] described a radioimmunoguided brachytherapy technique (RIGBY) to implant the microscopic tumor bed. In this technique, patients were injected with I-125 labeled antibody. A hand-held gamma-detecting probe was used to detect and resect areas of high radioactivity representing tumor.

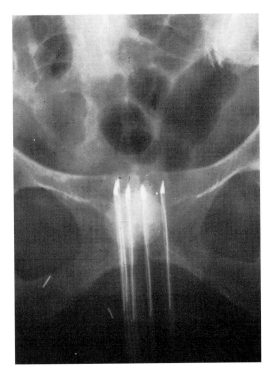

Figure 5C. Control x-ray of an implant for an anal canal carcinoma with five iridium-192 wires 5 cm long.

Areas with persistent high probe counts after resection represented the areas of occult residual disease and were then implanted with a median dose of 160 Gy I-125 using the Mick applicator. The gamma-detecting probe was used to demarcate the occult tumor volume (Figures 7A-C). Clinical assessment showed that local control was achieved in 73%. The median survival was 17.5 months, with a 1-year survival of 73%. The RIGBY procedure did not significantly increase the morbidity seen in recurrent colorectal patients undergoing major surgery.[27] If there is insufficient underlying tissue to hold the I-125 seeds, or if the underlying vessels will not allow interstitial placement of I-125 seeds, the seeds are embedded in gelfoam, surgicel, or vicryl sutures and sutured on the tumor bed.[28] It is important to place an omental, peritoneal flap to prevent normal bowel from coming in contact with areas receiving high-dose radiation. We attempt to deliver a minimum peripheral dose of 160 Gy to the tumor or tumor bed and have

used this technique to implant I-125 seeds in recurrent disease in the pelvic side wall, presacrum, periaortic areas, and the liver.[29]

Removable Iridium-192 Brachytherapy

Hollow, blind-ended, afterloading catheters are placed parallel to each other about 1 cm apart in a single plane and sutured to the tumor bed by absorbable sutures (Figure 8). The catheters are brought out of the body cavity through the abdominal wall or perineum and sutured to the skin with buttons. Normally radiosensitive organs, such as the small bowel, are displaced from the radiation field by using omental or peritoneal flaps. The catheters are loaded with iridium-192 ribbons 3–5 days after surgery to allow adequate healing. Doses of 45–60 Gy are delivered over 2–6 days if brachytherapy is used alone, or 20–30 Gy if brachytherapy is used to boost the EBRT dose. The catheters are removed after the brachytherapy dose has been delivered.

Results

Fourquet et al.[30] reported the Memorial Sloan-Kettering experience with 51 patients. The patients were treated with either I-125 or iridium-192 implants. The median survival of the patients was 14 months, with a 1-year actuarial survival rate of 57%. The local control rate at 6 months was 81%, and at 12 months was 64%. In general, the therapy was well tolerated, with 6% of patients developing severe complications when interstitial implant was combined with extensive surgery.

Endocavitary High-Dose-Rate Brachytherapy

High-dose-rate (HDR) brachytherapy has been used to deliver brachytherapy on an outpatient basis with elimination of radiation exposure hazards. Kaufman et al.[31] described an intraluminal HDR brachytherapy technique in which rectal cylinders (2-cm diameter) were used with a central radioactive source. Doses were prescribed at 0.5 cm from the applicator. Treatment length varied from 3–10 cm. Dose per fraction ranged from 4.4–8.4 Gy. One to four fractions were given at weekly intervals. The patients were treated on an out-patient

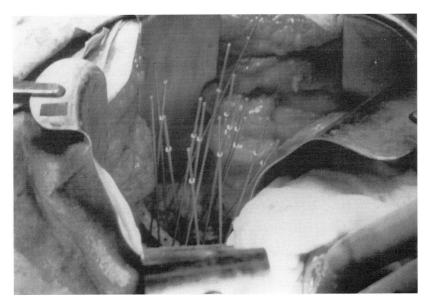

Figure 6A. Hollow needles (17 gauge) are implanted into the tumor bed in the presacral area after resection of recurrent rectal tumor.

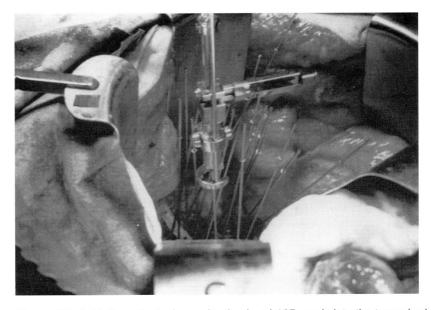

Figure 6B. A Mick applicator is used to implant I-125 seeds into the tumor bed.

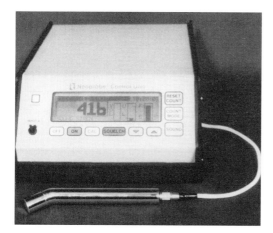

Figure 7A. A hand-held gamma-detecting probe: the Neoprobe 1000.

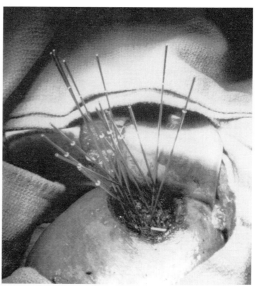

Figure 7C. Under guidance of the probe, 17 gauge, hollow needles are used to implant I-125 seeds into the tumor bed after resection of the liver metastasis.

basis using topical anesthesia and an HDR remote afterloading source with iridium-192 to give the treatments in a few minutes. Twenty-eight patients were treated, with three patients being boosted with EBRT. Of 27 available patients, the overall actual 5-year survival was 50%, and the overall local disease-free survival was 36% at 5 years. Kaufman et al.[31] reported that 71% of the 15 patients receiving elective brachytherapy achieved local control, whereas only five (39%) of the 13 patients with recurrent disease achieved local control. Eleven percent developed grade three complications requiring surgical intervention. The complication risk increased with increased

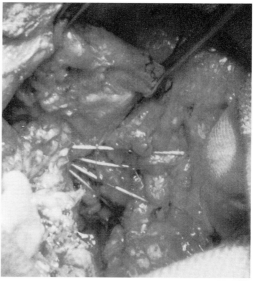

Figure 8. Afterloading catheters for iridium-192 brachytherapy are implanted on the tumor bed after resection of recurrent rectal tumor in pelvis.

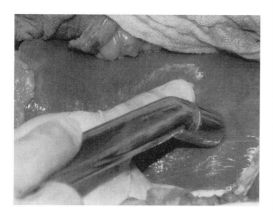

Figure 7B. The Neoprobe is used to localized the tumor.

treatment length, high brachytherapy dose per fraction, and high total cumulative dose.

Doss et al.[32] reported on eight patients treated with HDR brachytherapy; 180° internal tungsten shielding was used to shield half of the rectal mucosa circumference. In their preliminary analysis, tumor regression was noted in all patients with a complete response seen in two patients. There was palliation of bleeding and pain in all patients.

Kamikonya et al.[33] reported treating 52 patients with rectal cancer with preoperative HDR intraluminal brachytherapy. The cylinders were 1 or 2 cm in diameter, and the irradiation source could be placed centrally or eccentrically. The cylinder was held to the perineum by means of a plastic hip shell prepared individually for each patient. The dose was prescribed at 0.5 cm depth within tissue.

Fifteen patients were given a preoperative dose of 50–80 Gy, 35 patients received 30–40 Gy, and two patients received 16–20 Gy. Forty-six out of 52 patients were alive and well at the median follow-up of 3.3 years. These patients underwent surgery. Major complications of fistula, pelvic abscess, and anastomotic leakage were significantly more frequent in the high-dose group (5/15 patients vs 1/35 patients in the medium-dose group, and 0/2 for the low-dose group), leading to the conclusion that optimum results were obtained with 30–40 Gy intraluminal brachytherapy.[33]

Intraoperative High-Dose-Rate Remote Brachytherapy

Intraoperative electron beam radiotherapy (IORT) has been used to deliver a localized

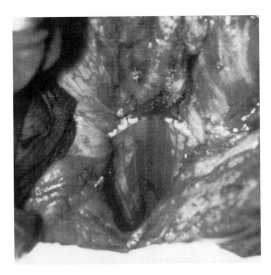

Figure 9B. The flab is applied over the tumor bed in the sacral hollow after resection of recurrent tumor. Note that the bowel is retracted away from the implant site.

boost radiation in locally advanced colorectal cancers.[34] There are many locations, such as the prepubic area, pelvic side walls, and deep in the sacral hollow, where electron beam IORT is not feasible. We have used intraoperative HDR remote brachytherapy to deliver a single intraoperative radiation dose in these circumstances[35] (Figures 9A and 9B). This technique affords the additional advantage of being able to retract or shield radiosensitive sources from the high-dose radiation area. Furthermore, the radiation is applied directly to the tumor bed, minimizing risk of geographical miss. To minimize the risk of infection, catheters are not left in the patient. Treatments are usually given through HDR catheters, parallel and 1 cm apart, incorporated in templates or gelatinous flabs. Doses of 10–20 Gy are delivered at 0.5 cm depth within the tissue. A disadvantage of this technique is that a shielded operating room is required. Out of a group of 61 patients with colorectal carcinomas treated, 30 patients with >6-month follow-up were evaluated. Recurrences were observed in one of 16 primary rectal tumors (6%) and in three of 14 recurrent tumors (21%). Of the 16 patients with primary rectal cancers, the 3-year actuarial survival rate was 85% if the lymph nodes

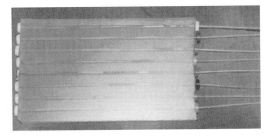

Figure 9A. The intraoperative HDR brachytherapy applicator is made of 1-cm thick supermold flab with afterloading catheters inserted 1 cm apart.

were negative, and 50% if the lymph nodes were positive. The postoperative complication rate (both minor and major) was 47%, similar to the 48% complication rate for the patients treated with surgery alone.[35]

Combined Modality Therapy for Anal Canal Cancers

Combination chemotherapy and radiotherapy is considered the standard treatment for anal canal cancers.[11,36–42] The techniques of EBRT and brachytherapy have been described previously in this chapter. Chemotherapy, usually with 5-Fluorouracil (5-FU) and mitomycin-C is usually used; 5-FU and Cis-platinum can also be used. A local excision biopsy is usually performed for T_1 lesions. A limited inguinal dissection is performed for palpable inguinal lymph nodes.

Results

Papillon et al.[11] reported that of the 221 patients with epidermoid carcinoma of the anal canal treated with iridium, the rate of death related to treatment failures was 20%; and, among the patients cured, >90% retained normal sphincter function.

Kin et al.[43] reported on 32 patients with anal canal cancers treated with EBRT and iridium-192. The survival rates at 3 and 5 years were 78% and 61%. The local control rate was 75%. Severe radionecrosis occurred in 6%.

A complete response was seen in 104 of the 108 patients (96%) treated by Wagner et al.[44] The overall 5-year survival was $64\% \pm 6\%$, and specific survival was $72\% \pm 8\%$. Patients treated with chemotherapy showed a tendency for a better survival rate. Anal preservation was possible in 65% of the patients. Nine APRs were performed for recurrence, and seven for severe necrosis.

Conclusion

Radiotherapy plays an important role in the conservative management of low rectal and anal canal cancers. Radiotherapy can be given by external beam, endocavitary radiation, interstitial implantation, or intraoperative radiation therapy. Patients suitable for conservative procedure include those with:

1. Low grade, well to moderately differentiated tumors;
2. Limited rectal wall penetration (confirmed by palpation and transrectal ultrasound);
3. Tumors <4 cm in diameter;
4. Absence of metastasis to lymph nodes.

Small, superficial exophytic rectal adenocarcinomas can be treated by endocavitary contact radiation therapy alone. When treating T2-T3 adenocarcinomas in inoperable patients, the addition of external beam and/or brachytherapy is required. Primary irradiation (possibly along with concurrent chemotherapy) is the treatment of choice for squamous cell carcinoma of the anal canal. Salvage surgery should be reserved for local failures. Conservative management can give the patient the optimal chance of a cure with good quality of life. Close cooperation between the radiation oncologist and surgeon is required for optimal results.

References

1. Miles EW. A method of performing abdominoperineal excision for carcinoma of the rectum and of the terminal portion of the pelvic colon. Lancet 1908;2:1812.
2. Nichols RJ. Surgery. In: Duncan W (ed). Recent Results in Cancer Research. Springer-Verlag, Berlin, 1982, pp. 101–112.
3. Rider MB. The 1975 Gordon Richards Memorial Lecture: Is the Miles operation really necessary for the treatment of rectal cancer? J Can Assoc Radiol 1975;26:167–175.
4. Symonds CJ. Cancer of the rectum: Excision after application of radium. Proc Roy Soc Med 1914;7:152.
5. Wang CC, Schuylz MD. The role of radiation therapy in management of carcinoma of the sigmoid, rectosigmoid, and rectum. Radiology 1962;79:1–5.
6. Papillon J. The future of external beam irradiation as initial treatment of rectal cancer. Br J Surg 1987;74:449–454.
7. Papillon J. Role do la radiotherapie dans la preservation anale pour le cancer du bas rectum. Lyon Chir 1991;87:21–14.
8. Papillon J. Intracavitary irradiation of early rectal cancers for cure: A series of 186 cases. Cancer 1975;36:696–701.
9. Papillon J. Rectal and Anal Cancers. Conservative Treatment by Irradiation—An Alternative

to Radical Surgery. Springer-Verlag, Berlin, 1982.

10. Papillon J. New prospects in the conservative treatment of rectal cancer. Dis Colon Rectum 1984;27:695–700.

11. Papillon J, Montbarbon JF, Gerard JP, et al. Interstitial curietherapy in the conservative treatment of anal and rectal cancers. Int J Radiat Oncol Biol Phys 1989;17:1161–1169.

12. Gerard JP. The use of radiotherapy for patients with low rectal cancer: An overview of the Lyon experience. Aust J NZ J Surg 1994;64:457–463.

13. Lamarque PL, Gros CG. La radiotherapie di contact des cancers du rectum. J Radiol Electrol 1946;27:343.

14. Morson BC. Factors influencing the prognosis of early cancer of the rectum. Proc Roy Soc Med 1966;59:607.

15. Hermanek P, Altendorf A, Gneselmann W. Pathomorphologische Aspekte zu kontinenzerhaltenden Therapieverfahren bei Mastdarmkrebs. In: Riefferscheid H, Langer S (eds). Der Mastdarmkrebs. Thieme, Stuttgart, 1980, pp. 1–12.

16. Papillon J, Berard Ph. Endocavitary irradiation in the conservative treatment of adenocarcinoma of the low rectum. World J Surg 1992;16:451–457.

17. Sischy B. The use of endocavitary irradiation for selected carcinomas of the rectum: Ten years experience. Radiother Oncol 1985;4:97–101.

18. Myerson RJ, Walz BJ, Kodner IJ, et al. Endocavitary radiation therapy for rectal carcinoma: Results with and without external beam. Endocurie Hypertherm Oncol 1989;5:195–200.

19. Lavery IC, Jones IT, Weakley FL, et al. Definitive management of rectal cancer by contact (endocavitary) irradiation. Dis Colon Rectum 1987;30:835–838.

20. Kovalic JJ. Endocavitary irradiation for rectal cancer and villous adenomas. Int J Radiol Oncol Biol Phys 1988;14:261–264.

21. Roth SL, Horiot JC, Calais G, et al. Prognostic factors in limited rectal cancer treated with intracavitary irradiation. Int J Radiol Oncol Biol Phys 1989;16:1445–1451.

22. Papillon J. Present status of radiation therapy in the conservative management of rectal cancer. Radiother Oncol 1990;17:275–283.

23. Puthawala AA, Syed AMN, Gates TC, et al. Definitive treatment of extensive anorectal carcinoma by external and interstitial irradiation. Cancer 1982;50:1746–1750.

24. Delclos L. The place of brachytherapy in conservative treatment of small tumors of the anal canal and low rectum. Proceedings of The 3rd International Brachytherapy and Remote Afterloading Symposium and Workshop, May 19–21, 1993, U. of Texas, Anderson Hospital and Tumor Institute, pp. 95–102.

25. Vider M, Lim N, Ditlow R, et al. The flexible implant in treatment of rectal carcinomas. J Surg Oncol 1982;20:157–160.

26. Jackson BR. Iridium implants in treatment of anorectal carcinoma. Dis Colon Rectum 1980;23:145–150.

27. Nag S, Ellis RJ, Martin EW, et al. A feasibility study of radio-immunoguided iodine-125 brachytherapy for metastatic colorectal cancer. Radiat Oncol Invest 1995;2:230–236.

28. Nori D, Bains M, Hilaris BS, et al. New intraoperative brachytherapy techniques for positive or close surgical margins. J Surg Oncol 1989;42:54–59.

29. Nag S. Radiotherapy and brachytherapy for recurrent colorectal cancer. Sem Surg Oncol 1991;7:177–180.

30. Fourquet A, Enker WE, Shank B, et al. The value of interstitial radiation in advanced and recurrent colorectal cancer. Endocurie Hypertherm Oncol 1985;1:113–117.

31. Kaufman N, Nori D, Shank B, et al. Remote afterloading intraluminal brachytherapy in the treatment of rectal, rectosigmoid, and anal cancer: A feasibility study. Int J Radiat Oncol Biol Phys 1989;17:663–668.

32. Doss LL, Schaffner SJ, Lange BJ, et al. Remote afterloading brachytherapy in rectal and anorectal carcinoma. Selectron Brachyther J 1992;6:58–62.

33. Kamikonya N, Hishikawa Y, Izumi M, et al. Preoperative radiotherapy for rectal cancer using intralumenal HDR brachytherapy. In: Mould RF, Batterman JJ, Martinez AA, et al. (eds): Brachytherapy from Radium to Optimization. Nucletron International BV, Veenendaal, The Netherlands, 1994, pp. 216–219.

34. Abuchaibe O, Calvo FA, Azinovic I, et al. Intraoperative radiotherapy in locally advanced recurrent colorectal cancer. Int J Radiol Oncol Biol Phys 1993;26:859–867.

35. Nag S, Lukas P, Thomas DS, et al. Intraoperative high dose rate remote brachytherapy. In: Nag S (ed). High Dose Rate Brachytherapy. Futura Publishing Co., Inc., Armonk, NY, 1994, pp. 427–445.

36. Cummings BJ, Keane TJ, O'Sullivan B, et al. Epidermoid anal cancer: Treatment by radiation alone or by radiation and 5 Fluorouracil with and without Mitomycin C. Int J Radiat Oncol Biol Phys 1991;21:1115–1125.

37. Doggett SW, Green JP, Cantril ST. Efficacy of radiation therapy alone for limited squamous

cell carcinoma of the anal canal. Int J Radiat Oncol Biol Phys 1988;15:1069–1072.

38. Eschwege P, Lasser P, Chavy A, et al. Squamous cell carcinoma of the anal canal: Treatment by external beam irradiation. Radiother Oncol 1987;3:145–150.

39. Glimelius B, Pahlmann L. Radiation therapy of anal epidermoid carcinoma. Int J Radiat Oncol Biol Phys 1987;13:305–312.

40. Hughes LL, Rich TA, Delclos L, et al. Radiotherapy for anal cancer: Experience from 1979–1987. Int J Radiat Oncol Biol Phys 1989; 17:1153–1160.

41. John MJ, Flam M, Lovalvo L, et al. Feasibility of nonsurgical definitive management of anal canal carcinoma. Int J Radiat Oncol Biol Phys 1987;13:299–303.

42. Nigro ND, Vaitkevicius VK, Considine B. Combined therapy for cancer of the anal canal. Dis Colon Rectum 1974;27:763–766.

43. Ng Ying Kin NYK, Pigneux J, Auvray H, et al. Our experience of conservative treatment of anal canal carcinoma combining external irradiation and interstitial implant: 32 cases treated between 1973 and 1982. Int J Radiat Oncol Biol Phys 1988;14:253–259.

44. Wagner J-P, Mahe MA, Romestaing P, et al. Radiation therapy in the conservative treatment of carcinoma of the anal canal. Int J Radiat Oncol Biol Phys 1994;29:17–23.

Chapter 21

Brachytherapy for Prostate Cancer

Subir Nag, M.D., Vladimir Pak, M.D.,
John Blasko, M.D.,
Peter D. Grimm, D.O.

Introduction

Carcinoma of the prostate is the most common male malignancy in the United States constituting 36% of all nonskin cancers in the male.[1] Approximately 317,100 new prostate cancers are expected in 1996. There are various treatment options for localized early prostate cancer including radical prostatectomy, modified radical prostatectomy, external beam radiation therapy (EBRT), brachytherapy, cryotherapy, hormonal therapy, and careful observation. A consensus development panel for the management of clinically localized prostate cancer sponsored by the National Institute of Health resulted in disagreement over several aspects of management for early prostate cancer.[2] This chapter will not attempt to discuss the details of the controversy about optimal treatment of early prostate cancer.

Radical prostatectomy provides excellent local control. However, it has significant morbidity, especially with impotence (90%–100%), urinary incontinence (15%–33%), and urethral strictures (10%). Many men avoid radical prostatectomy fearing this morbidity. A nerve-sparing operation, as devised by Walsh[3] results in a much lower rate of impotence. EBRT given daily over 7–8 weeks has been used with success for stages A-C prostate carcinoma. It can be delivered by standard techniques or by three-dimensional conformal therapy, which allows delivery of higher doses.[4] High doses of radiation concentrated within a small volume, sparing surrounding normal tissues, can be achieved by brachytherapy. Historical developments in brachytherapy will be reviewed, and details of the transperineal, ultrasound-guided, permanent brachytherapy techniques will be discussed in more depth since this is the most widely used brachytherapy now. Other techniques such as removable iridium implants and high-dose-rate (HDR) brachytherapy will be outlined.

Historical Review

The use of brachytherapy for treatment of prostate cancer is not new. Pasteau and Degrais[5] reported on the use of radium in prostate cancer treatment as early as 1913. The earliest brachytherapy for prostate cancer involved the introduction of a silver tube into the urethra through which radium was inserted with a long wire. Later, with the use of a cystoscope, it became possible to introduce radium into the bladder as well. Radium-containing needles were subsequently developed for both curative attempts and palliation of symptoms. Other techniques included using the rectum as a channel for insertion of radium tubes and placement of sources surgically through the perineum or the bladder. These approaches with radium use resulted in severe bowel and bladder irritation and ulcerations, which prompted a search for more locally acting radiation sources.[6] Flocks et al.[7] described the use of radioactive gold (Au-198) in the form of colloidal solution injections. It was felt to be promising due to its short half-life (2.7 days) and emission of short-distance beta radiation (3 mm) in addition to gamma radiation. Its distribution in the tissue and migration of small quantities (10%) into the lymphatics could potentially treat microscopic metastases. Au-198 also allowed for rapid delivery of radiation at a relatively high-dose rate. Due to the technical difficulties involved with using colloidal solutions, Au-198 seeds were developed to be used either alone or in combination with EBRT. Since Au-198 had high energy emission, only a small number of seeds (about 6–30), depending on the implant volume, seed activity, and EBRT dose, were required to deliver 20–35 Gy brachytherapy dose. The results achieved using permanent Au-198 implantation were comparable to EBRT alone.[7–9] However, the radiation exposure hazard associated with the high energy of Au-198 prevented it from ever becoming very popular. The advent of megavoltage radiation and the high morbidity of early brachytherapy techniques further reduced the interest in brachytherapy in the 1960s.

The introduction of a low energy radionuclide, iodine-125 (I-125), renewed the interest in brachytherapy for prostate carcinoma. Hilaris and Whitmore[10] at Memorial Sloan-Kettering Cancer Center popularized the implantation of iodine-125 seeds. I-125 has a half-life of 60 days and emits both photons and electrons (with the electrons being absorbed by the titanium wall of the seeds). The energy of the photons is low (28 KeV), and this virtually eliminates exposure problems for staff. The implant was performed using a retropubic approach combined with a modified bilateral pelvic lymph node dissection. The pelvic node dissection was mainly a staging procedure rather than a therapeutic one, because the prognosis is closely related to the status of the pelvic lymph nodes. The endopelvic fascia was incised and the prostate mobilized and exposed for implantation under direct vision by a suprapubic approach. The patient had to be hospitalized for a few days.

The largest series using I-125 implantation was reported from the Memorial Sloan-Kettering Cancer Center, New York. From 1970–1980, 606 patients were treated. Overall 5-year survival was 79%. When analyzed by stage, the 5-year survival was 96%, 76%, 69%, and 13% for T1, T2, T3, and T4, respectively. Local recurrence was present in 10%, and distant metastases occurred in 30% of cases. Recurrence rate was higher in patients with positive nodes (66%) than in patients with negative nodes (26%). Recurrence rate was also strongly associated with tumor grade: 21% for GI, 40% for GII, and 92% for GIII.[11]

Morton and Peschel[12] compared 141 patients treated with retropubic I-125 implant to 166 patients treated with EBRT for stages A2, B, and C tumors at the same institution (Yale University, New Haven, CT, USA). The 9-year disease-free survival rates were 88%, 62%, and 30% for implant and 74%, 63%, and 37% for EBRT for stages A2, B, and C, respectively.

In another series, Schellhammer and associates[13] used I-125 retropubic implants as definitive treatment in 115 patients. The actuarial 5-year disease-free survival was 100%, 81%, 49%, and 41% for A2, B, C, and D1 disease. By grade, the actuarial 5-year disease-free survival was 95%, 65%, and 34% for well, moderate, and poorly differentiated lesions, respectively. Results of these reviews indicated that retropubic I-125 implantation was comparable to EBRT for selected, low to moderately differentiated tumors limited to the prostate.

Complications of retropubic iodine-125 implantation include dysuria, incontinence, proctitis, impotence, and intraoperative complications. Fowler et al.,[14] in 1979, published a review of operative, postoperative, and late complications in 300 patients treated with pelvic lymphadenectomy and retropubic I-125 implant. Intraoperative complications were most commonly nerve injury (4%) and excessive bleeding (2%). Postoperative complications occurred in 23% of the cases, most commonly in the pelvis (10%). These included lymphoceles, hematomas, abscesses, cellulitis, and wound complications. Cardiovascular complications (primarily pulmonary embolism) accounted for another 7%. Eight patients (3%) required transurethral resection of prostate (TURP) 2–7 months postoperatively because of obstructive symptoms or retention. One hundred seventy-seven patients were followed for 6 months or more. Late morbidity (>6 months) was noted in 28% of these patients. This included voiding symptoms (12%), lower extremity lymphedema (5%), rectal symptoms (3%), and transient gross hematuria (2%). Late wound complications occurred in 4% of cases. Incidence of treatment related impotence was 7%.

A major problem with the retropubic technique was difficulty in achieving homogenous implantation of the gland, especially the apex, due to its location deep in the pelvis, with access impaired by the pubic symphysis. Poor distribution of seeds achieved by the retropubic approach has been reported as an important factor in lack of local control; whereas, significant correlation has been documented between good implant quality and negative rebiopsy rates as well as reduction in follow-up prostate specific antigen (PSA) levels.[15,16] Poor long-term clinical control achieved by the retropubic I-125 technique and the development of the nerve-sparing technique of radical prostatectomy caused a loss of interest in prostate brachytherapy in the early 1980s. However, in the late 1980s, introduction of new technologies, such as transrectal ultrasound (TRUS) for guidance and new isotopes with a short half-life such as palladium-103 (Pd-103), allowed implantation via a transperineal (rather than retropubic) approach and interest in prostate brachytherapy was revived.

Transperineal Permanent Brachytherapy

As early as 1980, Charyulu[17] described a transperineal interstitial implant technique that did not require a surgical exploration. All patients were initially given EBRT (5720 cGy in 31 treatments). The patients were then given a boost dose of 3200 cGy with radon (Rn-222) seeds. This technique was used to treat 23 relatively advanced stage C carcinoma

of the prostate that produced 96% local disease control, and 15 patients were alive and disease free, with a minimum of 2-year follow-up. The position of the needles was guided by a template (with holes 1 cm apart), and the tip of the needle was positioned at the level of the Foley bulb as seen on the radiograph.

In 1981, Kumar et al.[18] improved the technique by guiding the needles with C-arm fluoroscopy. A major impetus to prostate brachytherapy came with the introduction of TRUS guidance by Holm et al.[19] in 1983. They used a TRUS probe attached to a perspex template to permanently implant I-125 seeds. This allowed a more uniform implantation of the prostate gland since the needles could be inserted parallel to each other, unobstructed by the pubic arch. Nag[20] combined the advantages of the TRUS and fluoroscopy to implant the prostate transperineally in 1985. Over the last decade, this technique has been refined and popularized, especially by the Seattle, Washington group.[21–26] Another major impetus to prostate brachytherapy has been the publicity in the lay press that has prompted many men to explore their treatment options.

The transperineal brachytherapy technique is becoming a popular alternative for the patient since it offers the following advantages:

1. It avoids morbidity of laparotomy;
2. It is an out-patient procedure and avoids hospitalization;
3. It allows early recovery and early return to normal activity for the patient;
4. It allows for precise placement of the seeds and results in a more uniform seed distribution throughout the prostate, including the apex;
5. There is minimal bleeding from the procedure;
6. It has a relatively low long-term morbidity;
7. It is a one time procedure;
8. It is well tolerated by older patients in poor medical condition.
9. It results in maintenance of sexual potency in a high percentage of patients.

Technique of Transperineal I-125/Pd-103 Brachytherapy

This is an outline of the general procedure. The details of technique used varies at different centers, depending on whether it is based on the use of TRUS, CT scan, fluoroscopy, or a combination of the above.[20,24]

Preoperative Work-Up

1. PSA.
2. Digital rectal examination (DRE).
3. TRUS of the prostate.
4. Chest x-ray.
5. Bone scan, if indicated.
6. CT scan of the abdomen and pelvis.

Patient Selection

1. The patient should have a biopsy proven carcinoma of the prostate.
2. Patients with clinical stages A and B are candidates. Selected stage C patients may be implanted with this technique, especially if they are boosted with EBRT or downstaged with hormonal therapy.
3. There should be no evidence of distant metastases on bone scan, radiograph, or CT scan. Patients with known pelvic nodal metastasis in CT scan have poor prognosis and are not suitable candidates for brachytherapy.
4. Previous TURP is a relative contraindication, because a large TURP defect will allow loss of the radioactive seeds. In addition, the patient is at a higher risk for urethral necrosis, stricture, and incontinence. Hence, we generally avoid implanting a patient after TURP. In those cases who are implanted after a TURP, it is prudent to wait at least 2–3 months to allow some tissue regeneration in the defect.
5. Advanced age is **NOT** a contraindication.
6. Patients with large volume glands are not good candidates for an implant, because the pubic arch can interfere with the needle insertion and because of the large number of seeds required for the implant. Selected patients who still prefer a seed implantation may be evaluated for implantation if the prostate size can be reduced by a few months of hormonal therapy or if the brachytherapy is used as a boost to EBRT.
7. Extensive prostate calcification is a relative contraindication since it results in a poor ultrasound image, thereby hindering accurate needle placement.

Therapeutic options, including radical prostatectomy, external beam radiation, brachytherapy, and careful observation, should have been explained to the patient.

Choice of Radioisotopes

Permanent prostate brachytherapy is generally performed using I-125 or Pd-103. The recommended dose is 115–120 Gy for Pd-103 and 150–160 Gy for I-125 for brachytherapy as a sole modality. The brachytherapy doses are reduced by 25–50% if 40–50 Gy external beam is added for larger sized (>60 gm) or high grade (>6 Gleason score) tumors. The low-dose rate of I-125 may be a possible disadvantage in faster growing tumors and has been suggested as a contributing factor in failure of local control.[27] Pd-103 has a shorter half-life of 17 days, and delivers a higher dose rate (22 cGy/hr); therefore it may be more suitable for faster growing tumors. This advantage of Pd-103 over I-125 has been demonstrated in a rapidly proliferating rat prostate tumor model[28] but has not been seen with slower growing animal tumor models.[29] Therefore, some authors use Pd-103 to implant the poorly differentiated, faster growing tumors and I-125 to implant the well differentiated, slower growing tumors; however, to date, there is no clinical confirmation of this radiobiological hypothesis and animal data. Gold (Au-198) and radon (Rn-222) have higher energy emission and the interseed spacing is less critical. However, they are rarely used now since their higher energy pose greater radiation exposure hazards to medical care givers.

Preplanning

The preplan can be based on a CT scan or an ultrasound. In the ultrasound technique, an initial ultrasound is performed using a "stepping unit," which allows movement of the probe at 0.5-cm increments. Cross-section images are obtained 0.5 cm apart from the base to the apex of the prostate. Once the dimensions of the prostate are outlined, the computer program automatically calculates the volume. The patient should be scanned in the lithotomy position, mimicking the position during the operation, and the ultrasound probe should be securely stabilized. The target volume includes the entire prostate with a small periprostatic area. The number of seeds required to achieve the desired peripheral dose can then be obtained from either a nomogram or, more commonly, from a commercially available brachytherapy planning computer program that can optimize dose distributions to conform to the size and shape of the prostate. Although some centers prefer to implant the entire prostate gland homogeneously, others prefer to weight the distribution peripherally. This avoids implantation of seeds close to the urethra, thereby reducing the urethral dose and minimizing potential urinary morbidity.

The preplanning can also be done using a CT scan. This is especially suitable for departments that have a dedicated CT scanner. A flat table top insert is used for the CT scan, and the patient is in a semilithotomy position mimicking the position in the operating room. A Foley catheter is inserted into the bladder, and the Foley bulb is inflated with contrast material. About 30 cc of very dilute contrast is inserted into the bladder to better visualize the bladder. The Foley catheter is pulled inferiorly such that the bulb is at the bladder neck. A rectal tube is inserted in the rectum to better identify the rectum. A CT scan (a coned-down view of the prostate and periprostatic area) is obtained throughout the entire prostate gland at 0.5-cm intervals. CT scan images are then used to obtain the dimensions of the prostate and the number of seeds needed is determined using a nomogram, as above. We prefer to order 5%–10% extra seeds to be on the safe side in the event of any seed loss during the implantation procedure or to accommodate differences in prostate dimensions seen between the preplan and the implantation procedure.

Preoperative Preparation

Preadmission testing, including complete blood counts, blood chemistries, chest x-ray,

and electrocardiogram are done if they have not been previously done. The patients are on a clear liquid diet for 48 hours, and are fasting (NPO) after midnight. An enema is given on the morning of the procedure. Antibiotics are given prophylactically.

Implantation Procedure

These procedures are performed on an outpatient basis under general or spinal anesthesia with the patient in a lithotomy (or semilithotomy) position. TRUS and C-arm fluoroscopy are available (Figure 1). Stability and security of the guidance apparatus and ultrasound probe are very important. As a result, many institutions have devised custom mounting apparatus that securely attaches the probe/template/stepper unit complex to the

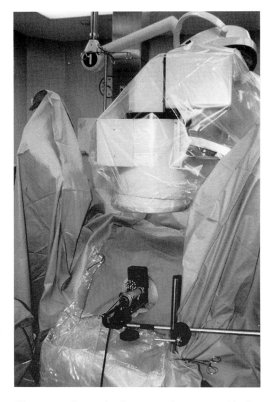

Figure 1. Setup in the operating room with the patient draped in the lithotomy position, with C-arm fluoroscope (above patient) and the transrectal ultrasound probe (in the rectum) attached to the stepping unit and stabilization plate.

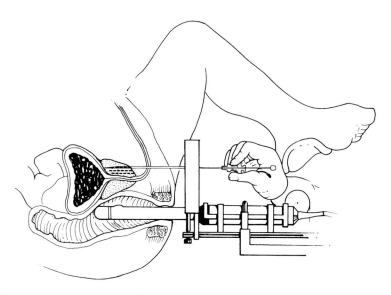

Figure 2. Diagram illustrating the TRUS transducer in the rectum at the apex of the prostate. It is attached to the stepping unit. A needle is inserted through the template (which in turn is attached to the stepping unit) into the prostate gland.

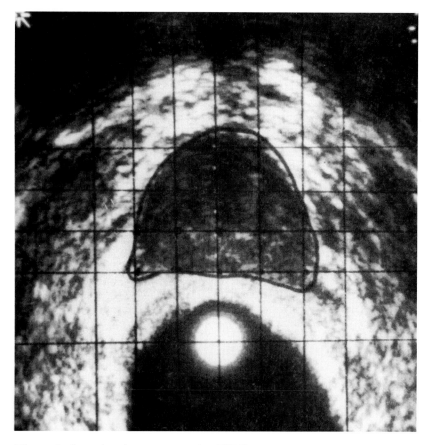

Figure 3. Scanning the prostate using TRUS.

operating room table so that inadvertent movement does not occur during the implant (Figure 2). The perineum is prepared and draped. The scrotum is retracted anteriorly out of the field and sutured suprapubically. In some approaches, a Foley catheter is inserted into the bladder, and the Foley bulb inflated with dilute hypaque. A flexible metal guide-wire placed through the Foley catheter helps with the identification of the urethra during TRUS and fluoroscopy. The "stepping unit" of the ultrasound probe is then attached to the stabilization device. The ultrasound probe is attached to the stepping unit and the prostate is scanned (Figure 3). The probe is then set at the most superior plane of the implant.

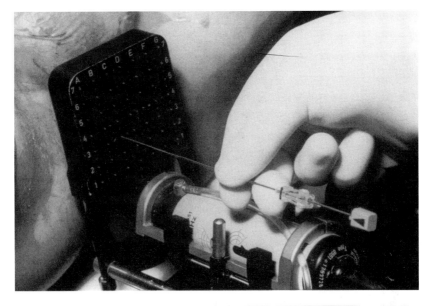

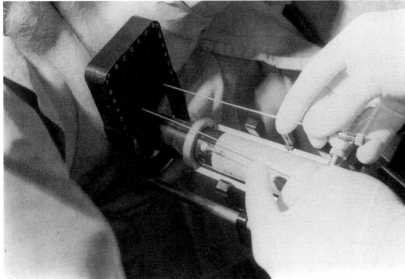

Figure 4. The first needle is inserted through the template into the prostate. This needle (and the subsequent one on the contralateral side) serve to anchor the prostate and prevent prostate rotation.

The template is then secured to the ultrasound probe 2–3 cm from the perineum. The dots seen on the electronically produced grid of the ultrasound image correspond to the template holes, thereby guiding the needle placement. The ultrasound probe is aligned such that the first horizontal row on the grid is parallel to the posterior margin of the prostate through all transverse images and such that every 5-mm image is identical to the preimplant volume study, if one was performed. If a nomogram approach is used, the prostate volume is confirmed and the required number of I-125 or Pd-103 seeds is determined. If a preplanned approach is used, the alignment is now correct to carry out the plan.

A needle is inserted into the template hole corresponding to the position chosen from the matrix pattern of the area of the prostate to be implanted (Figure 4). The probe is advanced to a transverse scan plane between the base and apex of the prostate in the mid-prostate area. The needle tip is inserted until its image, the "acroflash," is seen on the image (Figure 5). The prostate is then scanned in the longitudinal position, and the needle is advanced to the final position at the base of the prostate. Fluoroscopy can be used to verify the precise location of the base of the prostate, its relationship to the hypaque-filled Foley bulb, and the relationship of the apex of the prostate to the inferior pubic arch. Using a similar technique, the entire prostate is implanted with needles 1.0 or 0.5 cm apart (Figure 6). Care is taken to avoid placement of seeds within or immediately adjacent to the urethra. Seeds adjacent to the urethra contribute to high urethral dose that leads to excessive urinary morbidity, and loss of a substantial number of seeds through the urethra can lead to underdosing. The position of the needles are then reconfirmed using fluoroscopy at some centers (Figure 7).

A Mick applicator model No. TP-200 (Mick

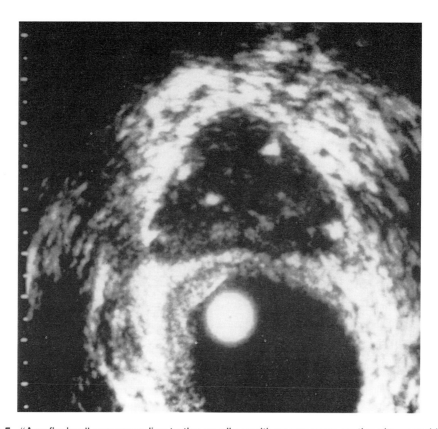

Figure 5. "Acroflashes" corresponding to the needle positions are seen on the ultrasound image.

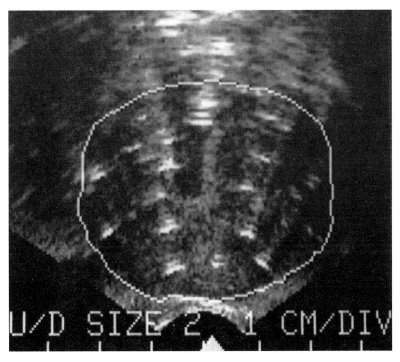

Figure 6. TRUS at the completion of needle insertion, showing the position of the needles within the prostate gland.

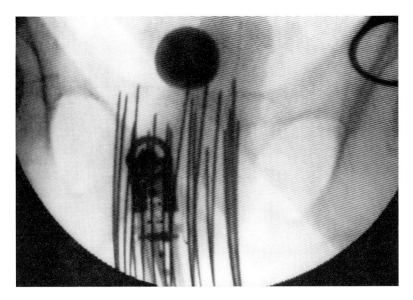

Figure 7. Fluoroscopy on completion of needle insertion confirms the relationship of the needle tips to the Foley bulb. The prostate is scanned from the base to the apex while fluoroscopy is used to identify the relationship of the prostate base to the Foley catheter and that of the prostate apex to the pubic arch. This technique delineates the superior and inferior extent to be implanted.

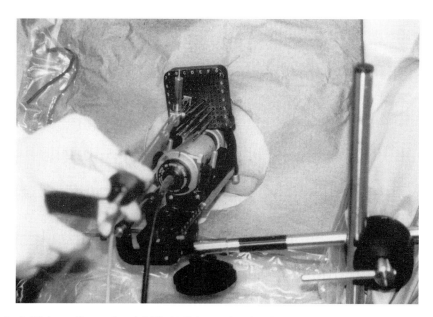

Figure 8. A Mick applicator (model TP-200) is used to implant the I-125 or Pd-103 seeds into the prostate. Alternatively, needles preloaded with I-125 or Pd-103 seeds can be used.

Radio-Nuclear Instruments, Bronx, NY, USA) is then attached sequentially to each needle, and the I-125 or Pd-103 seeds are inserted 1 cm apart (Figure 8). The position of the seeds implanted can be verified with fluoroscopy. Alternatively, some centers prefer to use pre-loaded needles. Prior to the procedure, 21 cm long, 18-gauge needles, are preloaded with I-125 or Pd-103 seeds and spacers such that the seeds are placed 1 cm apart. The spacers are made of #3 chromic catgut. Each needle tip is sealed with a plug of bone wax to prevent dislodging the seeds. A stylet is used to push the seeds and spacers into the prostate gland.

Another alternative is to use rapid strands (Medi-Physics, Arlington Heights, IL, USA) in which ten I-125 seeds spaced 1 cm apart are incorporated in an absorbable rigid suture material. The advantage of the rapid strand is that the seeds will remain 1 cm apart. The advantages of using the Mick applicator are its flexibility and the ability to place the seeds and make changes as required on the operating room table. The disadvantage is that the procedure requires more time (especially in inexperienced hands). The stylet must be withdrawn slowly to avoid displacing or suctioning back the seeds.

Fluoroscopy, which is used to confirm the needle and implanted seed positions, is particularly useful when a poor image is obtained on the ultrasound due to prostatic calcifications or reflections from the other needles. It is important to bear in mind that the prostate is not a perfect cylinder, but more walnut-shaped. The posterior portion extends more superiorly at the base of the prostate and the prostate narrows inferiorly at the apex.

During the procedure, an assistant (brachytherapy technologist or nurse) keeps a record of each seed and each template position being implanted. Occasionally, the needle position may have to be adjusted manually to reach the exact coordinate. This is especially important when trying to implant the anterior and superior lateral portions of the prostate in a patient with a narrow pubic arch by angling the needle anterio-laterally. Alternatively, some centers use an orthopedic drill to penetrate the pubic bone and implant the peripheral, anterio-lateral needles obstructed by a narrow pubic arch. As an added precaution, a digital rectal examination is performed before inserting the seeds to ensure that none of the needles are in or close to the rectum. This is especially important if there were some technical difficulties with the ultrasound imaging. The fluoroscopy and manual needle insertion can help fill any "cold" spot if required. All the needles are then surveyed for any residual activity, and any retrieved seeds can be reimplanted into the prostate. A cystoscopy may be performed to check for any seed dislodgment in the urethra or bladder.

Postimplantation Procedures

The patient is left with an in-dwelling Foley catheter until recovery from anesthesia. The catheter is then removed and surveyed for dislodged seeds. Orthogonal localization anterio-posterior and lateral radiographs and a CT scan of the prostate (at 5-mm intervals from the base to the apex) are obtained (Figures 9 and 10). Computerized dosimetry calculations (at multiple planes) are then performed by the physicists and compared with the post-implant CT scans. If the dosimetry suggests significant underdosage in some portion of the prostate, the patient is evaluated for addi-

tional EBRT or a second implant. This, however, is rarely required. A chest radiograph is also obtained to scan the lungs for embolized seeds (Figure 11). Oral antibiotics (e.g., ciprofloxacin, 500 mg, BID for 1 week; pyridium, 200 mg TID) are prescribed, and the patients are routinely discharged home on the same day. Some patients may require hytrin or ditropan for relief of urinary spasms.

Radiation precautions are explained to the patients. They are advised to avoid prolonged close contact with children (under 18 years) and pregnant women for 2 months (for Pd-103) or 6 months (for I-125). After the procedure, the patient may sleep in the same bed with the spouse and sex may be resumed in a few weeks after the implant, although it may be uncomfortable initially. The patients are advised to wear condoms initially to prevent the unlikely dislodgment of seeds into the vagina. A written copy of the guidelines is given to the patient, as well as a "medical alert" wrist bracelet to be worn for the duration of the radiation precaution. Details of radiation pre-

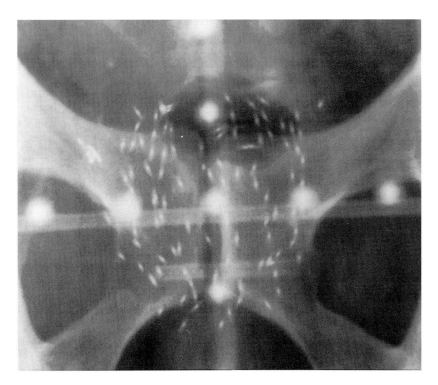

Figure 9. An anterio-posterior localization radiograph demonstrates homogeneous distribution of the seeds within the prostate gland.

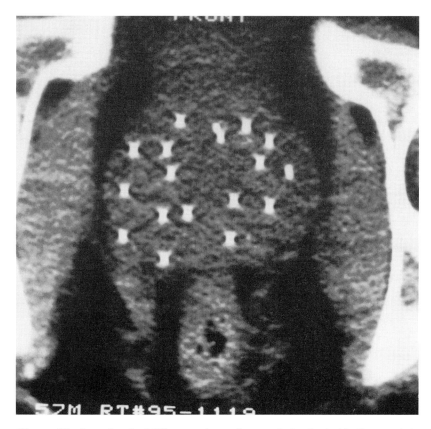

Figure 10. A postimplant CT scan shows the seeds implanted in the prostate.

cautions are given in the chapter on radiation safety.

Close postoperative follow-up is essential. The patient is jointly followed by the urologist and the radiation oncologist, with digital rectal examinations and PSA at regular intervals (usually at 1, 3, 6, 12, 18, and 24 months). Ultrasound-guided biopsies may be done routinely at some centers, or, more commonly, are performed if a recurrence is suspected (elevated PSA, palpable nodule on DRE).

Results

The largest experience with transperineal permanent brachytherapy of the prostate was reported by Blasko et al.[25] and has been summarized in Table 1. In the brachytherapy alone series, 320 patients with clinical stage T1 (23%) or T2 (77%) carcinoma of the pros-

tate were treated with either I-125 or Pd-103 between January 1988 and June 1993. These patients were followed for a minimum of 24 months (median follow-up = 45 months; range = 24 to 88 months). Gleason score at initial biopsy revealed 40% well differentiated, 50% moderately differentiated, 7% poorly differentiated, and 3% ungraded. Mean PSA at presentation was 7.9 ng/mL, range 0.2–74.6. Twenty-seven percent of the PSAs were normal (<4.0 ng/mL) at presentation. Average patient age was 70 years. All patients were followed prospectively for PSA response, histologic sterilization as indicated by posttreatment biopsy, complications, and clinical disease progression.

Local failure (i.e., either a positive digital examination or a positive biopsy with a PSA>1.0 ng/mL) occurred in five of 320 patients (6-year actuarial control rate of 97%); distant failure (i.e., a positive bone scan) oc-

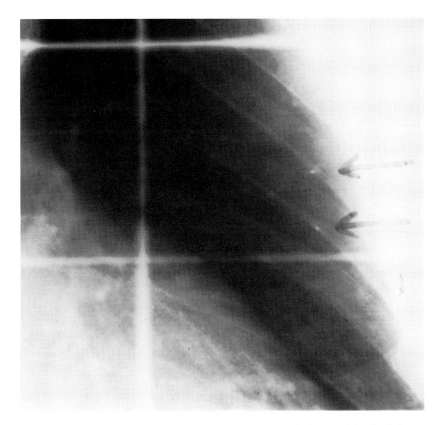

Figure 11. Anterio-posterior chest radiograph shows two seeds (arrows) in the left upper lobe of the lung.

curred in ten patients (6-year actuarial control rate of 93%). A 6-year actuarial PSA progression-free (nonrising PSA) rate of 83% was observed. A PSA nadir ≤1.5 ng/mL was achieved by 97% of the study population. Postimplant biopsies were obtained in 190/320 (59%) of patients between 12–60 months after treatment. Negative biopsies were obtained in 154 (81%) and positive biopsies in six (3%). The remaining 30 (16%) biopsies were indeterminate. Experience suggests that the majority of indeterminate biopsies convert to negative on subsequent biopsy, with PSA profiles resembling those of negative biopsy patients.

In the combined EBRT with brachytherapy series, 188 patients with clinical stage T1 (11%), T2 (83%), or T3 (6%) carcinoma of the prostate were treated between January 1987 and June 1993 with 45 Gy EBRT to the prostate and a limited pelvic field and a brachytherapy boost with either I-125 (120 Gy MPD) or Pd-103 (90 Gy MPD).[25] These patients were followed for a minimum of 24 months (median = 50 months; range = 24 to 94 months). Gleason score histology revealed 11% well differentiated, 53% moderately differetiated, 36% poorly differetiated tumors. Mean PSA at presentation was 15.7 ng/mL (Hybritech), range = 0.4 to 138. Eighteen percent of the PSAs were followed prospectively for PSA response, histologic sterilization as indicated by post-treatment biopsy, complications, and clinical disease progression.

Local failure (i.e., either a positive digital examination or a positive biopsy with a PSA >1.0 ng/mL) after this combined therapy occurred in 11 of 188 patients (6-year actuarial control rate of 92%); distant failure (i.e., a positive bone scan) occurred in 19 patients (6-year actuarial control rate of 86%). A 6-year actuarial PSA progression-free (nonrising PSA) rate of 72% was observed. A PSA nadir

Table 1.
I-125/Pd-103 Brachytherapy of the Prostate at the Northwest Tumor Institute[25]

	I-125/Pd-103 Brachytherapy Alone	I-125/Pd-103 Brachytherapy + EBRT
Number of patients	320	188
External beam dose (Gy)	0	45
Target I-125 dose (Gy)	160	120
Target Pd-103 dose (Gy)	115	90
Minimum follow-up (months)	24	24
Median follow-up (months)	45	50
Mean PSA at presentation (ng/mL)	7.9	15.7
Average age (years)	70	69
Results:		
Local failure	5/320 (2%)	11/188 (6%)
6 year actuarial local control	97%	92%
Distant failure	10/320 (3%)	19/188 (10%)
6 year actuarial distant disease-free rate	93%	86%
6 year actuarial PSA progression-free rate	83%	72%
6 year PSA <1.0 ng/mL	76%	67%
PSA Nadir ≤1.5 ng/mL	97%	92%
6 year Median PSA (ng/mL)	0.1	0.1
5 year PSA progression-free survival rate:		
Initial PSA <10.0 ng/mL	95%	82%
Initial PSA 10.1–20.0 ng/mL	84%	76%
Initial PSA >20.0 ng/mL	68%	65%
Negative biopsy	81%	77%
Positive biopsy	3%	9%
Intermediate biopsy	16%	15%
Morbidity:		
Grade 3 urinary complications	8%	7%
Grade 4 urinary complications	1.5%	1%
6 Year actuarial incontinence rate:		
In patients with prior TURP	48%	29%
In patients with no prior TURP	0%	0%
Proctitis	2%	6%
Loss of potency at 3 years	25%	30%
Diminished potency	30%	30%
Loss of potency in those <65 years of age	15%	20%

EBRT = external beam radiotherapy; PSA = prostate specific antigen; TURP = transurethral resection of prostate.

≤1.5 ng/mL was achieved by 92% of the study population. Postimplant biopsies were obtained in 128/188 (68%) of patients between 12 and 60 months after treatment. Negative biopsies were obtained in 98 (77%) and positive biopsies in 11 (9%). The remaining 19 (15%) biopsies were indeterminate. Experience suggests that the majority of indeterminate biopsies convert to negative on subsequent biopsy, with PSA profiles resembling those of negative biopsy patients.

At the recent American Urologic Association meeting, Blasko et al.[26] also reported on

treating 97 patients with Pd-103. With a median follow-up of 37 months, there were no clinical failures; the 4-year actuarial freedom-from-relapse rate was 95%.

Beyer[30] reported on 250 patients implanted for stages A and B prostate carcinoma: 227 with I-125 and 23 with Pd-103 (for higher grade lesions). PSA levels progressively decreased from a median of 7.1 at presentation to a median of 1.5 at 6 months and 0.8 at 12 months (86% and 93% normal, respectively). In another series, Brosman and Tokita[31] reported on 80 patients implanted with Pd-103 transperineally. With a mean follow-up of 11.8 months, PSA level became normal or decreased by >50% in all patients.

Morbidity

The patients generally experience some degree of perineal soreness immediately after the implantation. This pain generally resolves after several days. Most patients complain of some degree of urinary irritation (frequency, urgency, diminished stream) due to prostate inflammation, beginning at 1–2 weeks after implant and lasting for a few weeks. Generally, these symptoms resolve without treatment; however, in a few cases, they may become very severe, requiring medication (e.g., hytrin) or temporary bladder catheterization. Transurethral incision of the prostatic urethra or hospitalization for relief of obstructive symptoms are rarely required.

Blasko et al.[25] in reporting on patients treated by transperineal I-125/Pd-103 implantation alone noted that grade 3 complications (mostly mild to moderate) occurred in 8%. This included incontinence, irritative uropathy, and proctitis. Grade 4 complications occurred in 1.5% (two patients who required urinary diversion). Urinary morbidity was strongly associated with TURP: the 6-year actuarial incontinence rate for patients with a prior TURP was 48%, for those without a prior TURP it was 0%. The details of these morbidity results are given in Table 1.

In patients treated by EBRT with transperineal I-125/Pd-103 implantation as a boost, Blasko et al.[25] report that grade 3 complications (mostly mild to moderate) occurred in 7%. This included incontinence, irritative uropathy, and proctitis. Grade 4 complications occurred in 1% (one patient who developed a vesicorectal fistula requiring urinary diversion and temporary colostomy). Again, urinary morbidity was associated with TURP: the 6-year actuarial incontinence rate for patients with a prior TURP was 29%, for those without a prior TURP was 0%. The details of these morbidity results are given in Table 1.[25]

Nag et al.[32] implanted 32 patients transperineally with Pd-103. With a median follow-up of 20 months, 88% experienced some urinary symptoms and 18% had grade 3 or 4 toxicity

(severe dysuria, frequency 7–10 times per night, gross hematuria, or obstruction requiring hospitalization). Most symptoms, however, were grade 1 or 2 and transient. Of 3213 seeds implanted, only seven migrated to the lungs, and none caused symptoms.

Arteberry et al.[33] reported on 21 patients treated with CT-based transperineal I-125 and found that nearly all patients developed symptoms including substantial dysuria, increased nocturia, and frequency, 2–24 weeks following implantation with symptoms usually resolving within 4–6 months of implantation. At 6–7 months, only three patients had persistent mild dysuria. Only one out of 18 patients developed new onset of impotence.

Low-Dose-Rate Iridium-192

Iridium 192 (Ir-192) emits gamma radiation with an average energy of 380 KeV and a half-life of 74 days. The removable Ir-192 technique as popularized by Syed and associates[35] uses a template to implant needles transperineally into the prostate at the time of laparotomy, along with a modified pelvic lymph node dissection. The radioactive iridium is kept in place for 2–3 days and then removed. Doses of EBRT vary from 40–50 Gy with a brachytherapy boost of 30–35 Gy at a dose rate of 0.5–0.9 Gy/hr, which is delivered either before or after EBRT.

The use of temporary low-dose-rate (LDR) Ir-192 implants has resulted in good local control rates. In a study of 321 patients with localized carcinoma of the prostate treated by modified pelvic lymphadenectomy, Ir-192 implant and external beam radiation, Khan et al.[34] reported an overall 5-year disease-free survival of 69%. When broken down by stage, the 5-year disease-free survival was 90%, 90%, 65%, and 45% and local control rates were 95%, 93%, 84%, and 73% for stages A2, B1, B2, and C, respectively. Reported rate of GI and GU complications was 13% for RTOG grades 2 and 3 and none for grades 4 and 5. Histologic grade and nodal status were strongly associated with 5-year disease-free survival. Rates of 81%, 66%, and 45% for grades 1, 2, and 3, were noted. Disease-free survival was 77% for negative nodes versus 33% for positive nodes.

In another large review, Syed et al.[35] looked

at 200 patients with stages A2-C adenocarcinoma of the prostate treated in this manner. The actuarial 5-year survival was 85% with a 91% rate of clinical control and a positive rebiopsy rate of 16% among the 74 patients who underwent biopsies. Sixteen patients (8%) died with distant metastases, while 14 (7%) died of causes unrelated to prostate cancer. In the first 100 patients, the incidence of moderate to severe complications was 11%; however, modifying the dose distribution to reduce the rectal dose and reducing the total dose in patients who previously underwent TURP reduced the complication rate to 4% in the second group of 100 patients. Results of LDR Ir-192 treatment appear superior to treatment with EBRT alone or permanent I-125 seeds, particularly for stage B and C disease and high grade tumors.

High-Dose-Rate Iridium-192

Technique

Development of brachytherapy using HDR Ir-192 delivered with remote afterloaders has eliminated the exposure risks to staff. It offers the advantages of reduced treatment time and expense, and allows for treatment to be delivered in the out-patient setting. Finally, it has an increased potential for optimizing dosage because the dose distribution for HDR can be adjusted better than for LDR by varying the dwell times of the Ir-192 source. Experience with gynecological tumors and estimation of fractionation and dosage based on the linear quadratic equation have facilitated the substitution of HDR Ir-192 for LDR Ir-192 in treatment of prostate carcinoma.

HDR Ir-192 brachytherapy used at Kiel University involved a scheme that added conventional EBRT to areas of subclinical disease. Two HDR Ir-192 boosts were given interspersed during the course of EBRT to reduce overall treatment time.[36] The dose of EBRT was 50 Gy and the two implants were 15 Gy each. Special dose-modifying blocks were used during EBRT to limit the total prostate dose to 70 Gy. This scheme required two separate implantation procedures. Each HDR Ir-192 boost was preplanned using TRUS imaging with the outer capsule of the prostate marked as the target volume. Six to 12 needles

were inserted via a grid template and the patient was then afterloaded using a GammaMed II HDR afterloader (Isotopen-Technik Dr. Sauerwein GMBH, Haan, Germany). The total time elapsed for implantation and treatment ranged from 50–80 minutes.

Mate and associates[37] in Seattle modified the above technique by using a single implantation procedure and delivering fractionated HDR after a course of EBRT. Their treatment design was meant to parallel other commonly designed treatments for gynecological and head and neck tumors (i.e., using EBRT followed by an interstitial boost). External beam radiation was used to deliver 50–54 Gy via 120° lateral arcs using small 8x8 cm fields, or a 4-field pelvic technique using 10x10 cm fields. Two or 3 weeks following completion of EBRT, four consecutive HDR treatments were delivered over 3 days via afterloaded Ir-192. Following insertion of the needles, the template was sutured to the perineum to hold the needles in position. The needle position was verified by postoperative CT scanning. CT was used to outline prostate capsule as the target volume. HDR dosing was initially 3 Gy per fraction to a total of 12 Gy and later increased to 4 Gy per fraction to a total of 16 Gy. Needle placement was preferentially designed to increase the implant dose at the periphery, particularly at postero-lateral portions of the prostate, which are the major sites of tumor.

At the Royal Oak Hospital in Michigan, stages B2 and C prostate adenocarcinoma were given 4560 cGy whole pelvic EBRT with HDR Ir-192 implant boosts done during weeks 1, 2, and 3 of EBRT.[38] Implant doses were 550 cGy in 29 patients and 600 cGy in nine patients. Transperineal needle implants were done on an out-patient basis using real-time ultrasound guidance with on-line isodose distributions. The target volume included the entire prostate gland and the medial aspects of seminal vesicles.

Results

The Kiel group looked at 99 patients with a mean follow-up of 38 months. Thirty-six had surgical or hormonal debulking prior to radiation therapy. Out of 68 patients with available pretreatment PSA levels, 53 were above normal (4 ng/mL). At 12-months follow-up, 62 patients had normal PSA levels. Fourteen patients had high risk T2G3 tumors and 20 patients had T3G3 tumors. Follow-up TRUS-guided biopsies demonstrated tumor regression in 60% of the high risk lesions, another 22% were indeterminate, and 18% had evidence of tumor. Systemic progression was found in ten patients.[36] In Seattle, 75 patients with prostate carcinoma stages A-C were entered in the study. Out of 55 patients with a minimum follow-up of 1 year, 48 had PSA return to normal levels. In seven cases, serum PSA level reached a trough and then rose again.[37] At the William Beaumont Hospital in Michigan, 38 patients were treated for stages B2 and C prostatic adenocarcinoma. The mean follow-up was 6 months and the serum PSA levels obtained at 3 months were reduced by 50% or more in 83% of patients.[38]

Side Effects

In the Kiel study, 30% of the patients developed dysuria, but only 5% had severe dysuria. Urethral stricture developed in eight patients of whom seven had previous TURP or adenectomy. Advanced cystitis occurred in seven cases and six of them required electrocoagulation or TURP. Proctitis of >1-year duration occurred in 25% and 10% had severe symptoms related to proctitis. Three out of 99 developed rectal ulceration and all healed following conservative management. Thirty of 73 patients developed new erectile dysfunction; however, 11 of these also received hormonal therapy.[36] In the Seattle group of 75 patients, no significant intraoperative complications were observed. Acute (occurring within 90 days) RTOG grade 3–4 urologic or rectal toxicity was not observed. In the 55 patients with a minimum follow-up of 1 year (mean 22 months), no clinically significant cystitis, urethritis, proctitis, or incontinence developed. Urethral stricture developed in three cases. Two patients developed urinary retention without established etiology and one patient developed mild rectal bleeding with proctitis.[37] At the Royal Oak Hospital in Michigan, where 38 patients were implanted with a mean follow-up of 6 months, no significant intraoperative or perioperative complications occurred. Two patients developed grade

3 dysuria and one grade 3 diarrhea. Reported side effects included urinary retention (41%), perineal pain (27%), hemorrhagic cystitis (18%), hematospermia (18%), and bladder spasms (5%).[38]

Management of Local Recurrences

After brachytherapy, the PSA levels are closely monitored. A consistent rise in PSA level indicates that the patient may have failed locally, distally, or both locally and distally. A biopsy of the prostate and metastatic work-up is obtained. There is a small subset of patients who will have a histologically proven local prostatic recurrence without evidence of distal metastasis. These patients may be candidates for a radical or nerve-sparing, modified radical prostatectomy or cystoprostatectomy.[39–41] Only small numbers of patients with recurrent tumors have been thus treated. Thompson et al.[39] reported that salvage surgery was a viable option in five patients who had failed radiation therapy (two of whom had I-125 brachytherapy). Neerhut et al.[40] performed salvage radical prostatectomy in 16 patients failing radiation therapy. Although there was no operative mortality, major complications included rectal injury, ureteral transection, anastomotic stricture, and urinary incontinence. There were positive surgical margins (usually at the apex) in six of the 16 patients. Mador et al.[41] reported on their experience with cystoprostatectomy or radical prostatectomy in seven patients. Significant morbidity included two patients with rectal lacerations, two with temporary urinary incontinence, and one with idiopathic thrombocytopenia. Hence, although salvage surgery is possible, it is difficult and is associated with substantial morbidity.

Brachytherapy can be used as salvage after failure of EBRT or for isolated recurrence after prior brachytherapy.[42,43] Cumes et al.[42] reported the Stanford University experience with 14 patients who were treated with I-125 brachytherapy after failing EBRT treatment. Major morbidity occurred in nine of these 14 patients including bladder incontinence, enuresis, diarrhea, rectourethral fistula, rectal stenosis, and rectal ulcer. Wallner et al.[43] reported the Memorial Sloan-Kettering experience with a repeat I-125 implant in 13 patients failing brachytherapy. Six of the patients had complete regression of palpable disease; however, there was a 100% actuarial rate of distant metastasis at 6 years.

Since poor results and high morbidity are obtained with salvage surgery or brachytherapy, we generally advise hormonal therapy to patients who fail brachytherapy.

Discussion and Conclusion

The rationale of brachytherapy is to deliver a high dose of radiation to a confined volume with relative sparing of surrounding normal tissue. Although this concept is appealing, poor results with primitive implant techniques in the past has resulted in skepticism regarding brachytherapy for prostate carcinoma. However, intermediate-term PSA-based results with transperineal, ultrasound-guided template techniques suggest that modern brachytherapy is capable of achieving outcomes equivalent to those of radical prostatectomy or external beam irradiation.

Modern transperineal brachytherapy techniques using ultrasound guidance with either iodine-125, palladium-103, LDR iridium, or HDR iridium brachytherapy offer good alternatives for management of localized prostate cancer in appropriately selected patients. This modality allows delivery of a higher localized radiation dose than that achievable by conventional EBRT; and it is an effective alternative to surgery for those patients who, for reasons of advanced age or poor medical condition, may be unable to undergo surgery. The nonsurgical, out-patient basis of permanent, ultrasound-guided transperineal prostate brachytherapy has high patient appeal and offers minimal morbidity in appropriately selected patients. Brachytherapy is convenient and cost effective, and it generally results in minimal impairment of the patient's lifestyle.

The role of brachytherapy in the treatment of carcinoma of the prostate appears to be either as monotherapy for early stage lesions or as a boost after modest doses of external beam irradiation for patients with more advanced stages. Select advanced cases may be downsized with hormonal therapy and then be evaluated for brachytherapy. Recurrent cases after EBRT or prostatectomy are not good candidates for brachytherapy, due to poor local control and higher morbidity.

The accurate performance of today's implants has been aided by technological improvements, but quality implants still require skill, adequate training, and extreme attention to detail. Whether acceptable prostate brachytherapy can be performed in the community or whether it will be limited to centers of excellence remains to be demonstrated. Since prostate cancer is a relatively slow growing malignancy, a longer (10–15 years) follow-up is needed to determine the eventual efficacy of this treatment. Although the final place of prostate brachytherapy in the armamentarium of prostate cancer treatment will await the maturation of long-term, controlled clinical trials, the future appears bright.

References

1. Parker SL, Tong T, Bolden S, et al. Cancer statistics, 1996. Ca Cancer J Clin 1996;46:5–28.
2. Consensus Conference. The management of clinically localized prostate cancer. JAMA 1987; 258:2727–2730.
3. Walsh PC. Radical retropubic prostatectomy with reduced morbidity: An anatomic approach. NCI Monogr 1983;7:133–137.
4. Hanks GE, Corn BW, Lee R, et al. External beam irradiation of prostate cancer. Cancer 1995;75:1972–1977.
5. Pasteau O, Degrais Dr. The radium treatment of cancer of the prostate. Arch Roentg Ray 1914;28:396–410.
6. Young H. Technique of radium treatment of cancer of the prostate and seminal vesicles. Surg Gynecol Obstet 1922;34:93–98.
7. Flocks RH, Kerr HD, Elkins HB, et al. Treatment of carcinoma of the prostate by interstitial radiation with radioactive gold (Au-198): A preliminary report. J Urol 1952;68:510–522.
8. Lannon SG, el-Araby AA, Joseph PK, et al. Long-term results of combined interstitial gold seed implantation plus external beam irradiation in localised carcinoma of the prostate. Br J Urol 1993;72:782–791.
9. Crusinberry RA, Kramolowsky EV, Loening SA. Percutaneous transperineal placement of gold-198 seeds for treatment of carcinoma of the prostate. The Prostate 1987;11:59–67.
10. Whitmore WF Jr, Hilaris B, Grabstald H. Retropubic implantation of iodine-125 in the treatment of prostatic cancer. J Urol 1972;108: 918–920.

11. Batata MA, Hilaris BS, Whitmore WF Jr. Factors affecting tumor control. In: Hilaris BS, Batata MA (eds). Brachytherapy Oncology—1993. Memorial Sloan-Kettering Cancer Center, New York, 1983, pp. 65–72.

12. Morton JD, Peschel RE. A detailed analysis of the chronic complications from iodine-125 implant vs external beam irradiation for prostate cancer. Endocurie/Hypertherm Oncol 1988;4: 113–118.

13. Schellhammer PF, El-Mahdi AE, Ladaga LE, et al. [125]Iodine implantation for carcinoma of the prostate: 5-year survival free of disease and incidence of local failure. J Urol 1985;134: 1140–1145.

14. Fowler JE Jr, Barzell W, Hilaris BS, et al. Complications of [125]iodine implantation and pelvic lymphadenectomy in the treatment of prostatic cancer. J Urol 1979;121:447–451.

15. Sogani P, et al. Carcinoma of the prostate: Treatment with pelvic lymphadenectomy and iodine-125 implants. Clin Bull 1979;9:24–31.

16. Kandzari S, Belis J, Kim J-C, et al. Clinical results of early stage prostatic cancer treated by pelvic lymphadenectomy and [125]iodine implants. J Urol 1982;127:923–927.

17. Charyulu KKN. Transperineal interstitial implantation of prostate cancer: A new method. Int J Radiat Oncol Biol Phys 1980;6:1261–1266.

18. Kumar PP, Bartone FF. Transperineal percutaneous I-125 implant of prostate. Urology 1961; 17:238–240.

19. Holm HH, Juul N, Pedersen JF, et al. Transperineal [125]iodine seed implantation in prostatic cancer guided by transrectal ultrasonography. J Urol 1983;130:283–286.

20. Nag S. Transperineal iodine-125 implantation of the prostate under transrectal ultrasound and fluoroscopic control. Endocurie/Hypertherm Oncol 1985;1:207–211.

21. Blasko JC, Radge H, Schumacher D. Transperineal percutaneous iodine-125 implantation for prostatic carcinoma using transrectal ultrasound and template guidance. Endocurie/Hypertherm Oncol 1987;3:131–139.

22. Blasko JC, Grimm PD, Radge H. Brachytherapy and organ preservation in the management of carcinoma of the prostate. Sem Radiat Oncol 1993;3:240–249.

23. Blasko JC, Radge H, Grimm PD. Transperineal ultrasound-guided implantation of the prostate: Morbidity and complications. Scand J Urol Nephrol Suppl 1991;137:113–118.

24. Grimm PD, Blasko JC, Radge H. Ultrasound-guided transperineal implantation of iodine-125 and palladium-103 for the treatment of early-stage prostate cancer—technical concepts in planning, operative technique, and evaluation. Atlas Urol Clin North Am 1994;2: 113–125.

25. Blasko JC, Radge H, Grimm PD, et al. Transperineal ultrasound-guided brachytherapy with I-125 or Pd-103 for prostate cancer: The Seattle experience in 508 patients. 37th Annual Meeting of the American Society for Therapeutic Radiology and Oncology, Miami Beach, FL, October 8–11, 1995.

26. Blasko JC, Radge H, Grimm PD, et al. Transperineal ultrasound-guided brachytherapy for prostate carcinoma. Presented at the 90th Annual Meeting of the American Urological Association, Las Vegas, NV, Abstract No. 626, April 23–28, 1995.

27. Schellhammer PF, el-Mahdi AM, Higgins EM, et al. Prostate biopsy after definitive treatment by interstitial ^{125}I implant of external beam radiation therapy. J Urol 1987;137:897–901.

28. Nag S, Sweeney PJ, Wientjes MG. Dose-response study of iodine-125 and palladium-103 brachytherapy in a rat prostate tumor (Nb AI-1). Endocurie/Hypertherm Oncol 1993;9: 97–104.

29. Nag S, Ribovich M, Cai JZ, et al. Palladium-103 vs. iodine-125 brachytherapy in a slow-growing rat prostate tumor. Radiother Oncol 1995;35(Suppl 1):58.

30. Beyer DC. Early prostate-specific antigen response to radioisotope implantation. Endocurie/Hypertherm Oncol 1992;8:181–186.

31. Brosman SA, Tokita K. Transrectal ultrasound-guided interstitial radiation therapy for localized prostate cancer. Urology 1991;38: 372–376.

32. Nag S, Scaperoth DD, Badalament R, et al. Transperineal palladium-103 prostate brachytherapy: Analysis of morbidity and seed migration. Urology 1995;45:87–92.

33. Arterbery VA, Wallner K, Roy J, et al. Short-term morbidity form CT-planned transperineal I-125 prostate implants. Int J Radiat Oncol Biol Phys 1993;25:661–667.

34. Khan K, Thompson W, Bush S, et al. Transperineal percutaneous iridium-192 interstitial template implant of the prostate: Results and complications in 321 patients. Int J Radiat Oncol Biol Phys 1992;22:935–939.

35. Syed AMN, Puthawala A, Austin P, et al. Temporary iridium-192 implant in the management of carcinoma of the prostate. Cancer 1992;69: 2515–2524.

36. Mate TP, Kovács G, Martinez A. High dose rate brachytherapy of the prostate. In: Nag S (ed). High Dose Rate Brachytherapy. Futura Publishing Co., Inc., Armonk, NY, 1994, pp. 355–371.

37. Mate TP, Gottesman J, Anderson K, et al. Frac-

tionated HDR iridium-192 conformal prostatic brachytherapy: The Seattle method. In: Mould RF (ed). International Brachytherapy—Proceedings of the 7th International Brachytherapy Working Conference, Baltimore, September 6–8, 1992. Nucletron International, Veenendaal, The Netherlands, 1992, pp. 359–362.

38. Martinez AA, Edmundson GK, Gonzalez J, et al. Combined external beam radiation & conformal HDR real time iridium-192 brachytherapy dosimetry for locally advanced adenocarcinoma of the prostate. In: Mould RF, Batterman JJ, Martinez AA, et al. (eds). Brachytherapy from Radium to Optimization. Nucletron International, Veenendaal, The Netherlands, 1994, pp. 220–229.

39. Thompson IM, Rounder JB, Spence R, et al. Salvage radical prostatectomy for adenocarcinoma of the prostate. Cancer 1988;61: 1464–1466.

40. Neerhut GJ, Wheeler T, Cantini M, et al. Salvage radical prostatectomy for radiorecurrent adenocarcinoma of the prostate. J Urol 1988; 140:544–549.

41. Mador DR, Huben RP, Wajsman Z, et al. Salvage radical prostatectomy following radical radiotherapy for adenocarcinoma of the prostate. J Urol 1985;133:58–60.

42. Cumes DM, Goffinet DR, Martinez A, et al. Complications of ^{125}iodine implantation and pelvic lymphadenectomy for prostatic cancer with special reference to patients who had failed external beam therapy as their initial mode of therapy. J Urol 1981;126:620–622.

43. Wallner KE, Nori D, Morse MJ, et al. ^{125}Iodine reimplantation for locally progressive prostatic carcinoma. J Urol 1990;144:704–706.

Bladder

A.J. Wijnmaalen, M.D., P.C.M. Koper, M.D.,
A.G. Visser, Ph.D., J.J. Battermann, M.D., Ph.D.

Introduction

The estimated number of new cases of bladder cancer in the United States in 1994 was 51,200 (4.2% of all cancer cases).[1] In The Netherlands the number of patients with newly diagnosed invasive bladder cancer in 1990 was 1963 (3.5% of all cancers).[2] Various risk factors for the development of bladder cancer have been identified.[3,4]

Transitional cell carcinoma comprises about 90% of all malignant bladder tumors.[5] In a small number of cases, a squamous cell carcinoma or adenocarcinoma is found, whereas the occurrence of other histologies is very rare.

The first clinical classification of bladder cancer was developed in 1946 by Jewett and Strong.[6] They showed a relationship between the depth of tumor infiltration in the bladder wall and the risk of developing regional and distant metastases. This classification was adjusted by Marshall into an 0, A, B, C, and D system, based upon bimanual examination of the bladder under anesthesia and the infiltration depth at microscopic evaluation of biopsy specimens.[7] The Tumor-Node-Metastases (TNM) system of the International Union against Cancer and the American Joint Committee appears to be the most widely accepted accurate clinical staging system at the moment.[8]

Generally, the work-up of patients with a bladder tumor consists of urine cytology, cystoscopy, biopsy or a transurethral resection (TUR) of visible tumor, multiple random biopsies if considered necessary, bimanual palpation prior to and directly following resection of (all) visible tumor, intravenous pyelography, echography, and, dependent on T-category, chest x-ray, CT-scan of abdomen and pelvis, and bone scintigraphy.

Besides T-category of tumors without nodes or distant metastases, various other factors appear to be of prognostic value: grade of differentiation, multiplicity, concomitant urothelial dysplasia and carcinoma in situ, tumor morphology, tumor size, completeness of resection, tumor recurrence, vascular invasion, ureteric obstruction, performance status, and hemoglobin level.[9,10]

The definitive treatment is chosen mainly based on tumor stage and general condition of the patient: TUR only, TUR followed by intravesical chemo- or immunotherapy, partial or radical cystectomy with or without preoperative external beam radiotherapy (EBRT), interstitial radiotherapy (IRT) only or in combination with EBRT, EBRT only, radiation in combination with chemotherapy, neoadjuvant chemotherapy followed by surgery or radiation, and, in case of distant metastases, systemic chemotherapy or palliative measures only.

Early in this century, it was recognized that IRT could deliver a higher dose to malignant

From Nag S (ed): *Principles and Practice of Brachytherapy.* © Futura Publishing Co., Inc., Armonk, NY, 1997.

tumors without unacceptable damage to surrounding normal tissues, as compared to the external beams available at that time. Since then, several reports have emerged from centers throughout Europe and the United States concerning different techniques of IRT in bladder cancer. Permanent implantation of radon seeds[11–17] and gold grains[16,18,19] through a cystoscope, under cystoscopic control by suprapubic or vaginal puncture, or directly after performing a cystotomy has been reported. For temporary implants, techniques were developed using radium needles,[14,20–23] cobalt needles,[24] or tantalum[19,24–26] or iridium wires.[27] Generally, these sources were placed after cystotomy; but, in some cases, needles were placed transvaginally.[14] An afterloading technique using iridium wires was first described in 1969.[28]

The interpretation of the early series is difficult because of the low number of cases reported in some instances, a poor description of selection criteria, lack of tumor classification, lack of uniform pathology criteria, and poor dosimetry and statistics. Nevertheless, through the years it has become clear that interstitial radiation in bladder cancer can cure a certain number of patients. Tumors should be solitary and <4–5 cm in diameter and a single plane implant should be used.

Later on, the number of centers where IRT in bladder cancer was applied decreased, apparently due to the development of super- and megavoltage EBRT that provided better dose distribution and less toxicity, and better surgical procedures and pre- and postoperative care.

Centers in The Netherlands and in France, however, continued the use of low-dose-rate (LDR) IRT in selected patients with bladder cancer. In France, the afterloading iridium wire technique has been used since 1969; whereas, in The Netherlands radium or cesium needles were gradually replaced by a similar afterloading technique later on. The radium/cesium needle technique and the iridium wire afterloading technique and their results will be dealt with in detail separately.

Methods

Radium and Cesium Needle Technique

The use of radium needles in the treatment of bladder cancer patients was introduced by

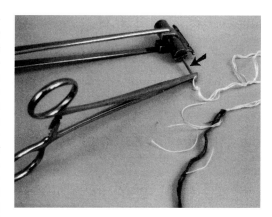

Figure 1. Cesium needle (arrow) taken in a needle holder and partly extracted from a small safe.

Breur and De Waard[23] in 1951 in the Rotterdam RadioTherapy Institute (RRTI, presently Dr. Daniel den Hoed Cancer Center, DDHCC) and later on in the Antoni van Leeuwenhoek Ziekenhuis/Nederlands Kanker Instituut (AvL/NKI) in Amsterdam. Some smaller centers in The Netherlands adopted this technique as well. In 1983, cesium needles replaced the radium needles.

Needles were available with an active length of 2, 3, and 4 cm (Figure 1). The real length of the needles was 1 cm more because the solid point and the eyelet, necessary for the introduction in the bladder wall and for the attachment of threads, respectively, did not contain radioactive material.

The source strength of the radium needles was previously expressed in terms of "mg Ra equivalent" (mgRaeq) and the needles for the bladder implants ranged from 2–4 mgRaeq. In present day terms, the source strength would be specified in terms of the reference air-kerma rate (RAKR), i.e., the air-kerma rate at a reference distance of 1 m, ranging from 14.5–29 μGy/hr.

Both the radium and cesium needles were encapsulated in platinum with a wall thickness of 0.5 mm. Advantage of platinum over stainless steel as encapsulating material is the better visibility on the x-ray radiographs made for reconstruction of the implant. The active length and the source strength of the cesium needles (1.5–3 mgRaeq, i.e., an RAKR ranging from 10.8–21.7 μGy/hr) were close to those of the radium needles.

The implantation of the needles required a certain degree of force, which could result in bending of a needle. Bent needles were taken out of clinical use because of the presumed increased risk of leaking of active material. For instance, in 1979 the entire stock of radium needles in the DDHCC consisted of 117 needles, of which 17 were taken out of use because of bending.

The surgical part of the whole procedure was the responsibility of the (referring) urologist; whereas, the radiation oncologist performed the actual implantation. After opening the abdominal wall by a lower median abdominal incision or a Pfannenstiel incision, the bladder, usually filled with a few hundred cc of NaCl 0.9% solution in advance, was opened through a median incision in the anterior wall. Care was taken to keep the peritoneal cavity closed. A paramedian area of the bladder was chosen for the incision in case the tumor was localized in the anterior wall itself, the dome of the bladder, or at the junction from the side wall to the anterior wall.

For the implantation, the needles were placed in a holder at 45°, 90°, 135°, or 180°, dependent upon the site of the tumor. Needles were implanted so that the solid point and eyelet were in the lumen of the organ, the rest of the needle being in the bladder wall parallel to the mucosa. Needles spaced ±1 cm apart, were inserted parallel to each other covering the whole target area sufficiently, the outer two placed just outside the target area. Finally, needles crossing the points and eyelets at each side were placed in order to avoid underdosage in those areas. For geometry, the rules of the Manchester or Paterson & Parker system were followed, although no correction was made for the size of the implantation area or for noncrossing needles, and all needles had the same radiation intensity.[29]

Generally, during the implantation procedure considerable edema of the mucosa developed, which made it necessary to insert the needles within the shortest possible time in order to avoid misinterpretation of the geometry. Of course, for radiation protection, it was also important to perform the implantation as quickly as possible. During the implantation procedure, the bladder wall was relatively stretched, making it necessary for the radiation oncologist to anticipate changes in the position of the needles after closing the bladder, in order to avoid unacceptable violations of the rules of geometry. After completion of the implantation, the bladder and abdominal wall were closed, while the threads attached to the needles were passed through a drain in the wounds (Figure 2). Due to the rather large diameter this drain was a potential porte d'entrée for bacteria. A suprapubic or transurethral bladder catheter and wound drains were left behind.

Implantation is very difficult if the tumor is located in the anterior wall or dome of the bladder, or in a diverticulum. Therefore, in those cases usually a partial bladder resection or diverticulectomy is performed first, generally followed by implantation from outside after closing the bladder.

As soon as possible after the operation, the patient was transported to one of the simulators for two orthogonal radiographs of the bladder area, which were used to create a three-dimensional reconstruction of the position of the needles (Figures 3 and 4). The dose specification procedure as used in Rotterdam was described by Vaeth and Meurk[30] in 1963. Points of expected minimum and maximum dose rates at 0.5 cm from the implanted surface were selected. Subsequently, these points were indicated in the model of the implant by placing thin tubes of different color with the tips at the required positions. Next, the dose rate in each point was calculated by measuring the distances of a point to the ends of the active lengths of all needles. To calculate the dose rate, it was assumed that the isodoses around a line source are approximated by ellipses. By taking the sum of the distances of a point to both ends of a needle, the dose-rate contribution from that needle could be read from a table. Summing the dose-rate contributions from all needles gave the actual dose rate in that point.

The accuracy of this dose calculation using the spatial reconstruction of the implant has been investigated by Van Kleffens and Star[31] by comparing the results with dose calculations made using stereo x-ray photogrammetry and with direct dose measurement with thermoluminescence dosimetry (TLD) probes

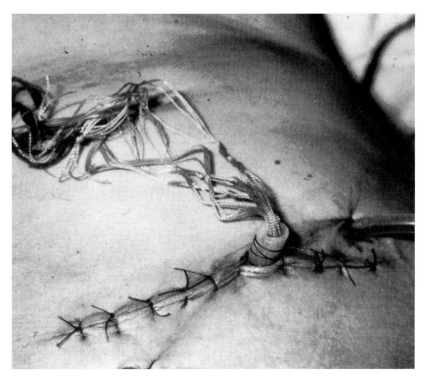

Figure 2. Situation after cesium needle implantation of the bladder. Threads attached to the needles are passed through a drain around which the bladder and abdominal wall are closed.

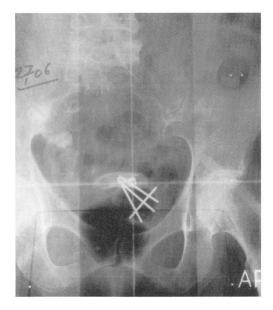

Figure 3. Anterior-posterior radiograph showing the position of cesium needles in the bladder.

in a gelatin phantom containing eight radium needles. The accuracy of the dose calculations made with the reconstruction technique was found to be satisfactory, the maximum difference with the TLD dose being 7%, the dose averaging over ten TLD probe positions being in close agreement.

After calculation of the dose rates in the chosen reference points, the minimum dose rate found was used to determine the application time.

In Rotterdam, a dose-rate correction similar to the one in the TDF model[32] was applied using the following iso-effect function:

$$D = c \, T^{0.3}$$

where D is the physical dose, T is the application time, and c is the proportionality constant. The intention of this dose-rate correction was to give a dose equivalent to 65 Gy in 7 days (168 hrs), i.e., a standard dose rate of 38.7 cGy/hr. If the dose rate of the actual implant is d (cGy/hr), the application time to

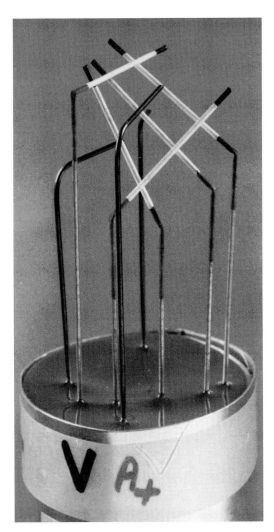

Figure 4. Reconstruction of the position of cesium needles, used for dose-rate calculations.

give a dose equivalent to 65 Gy in 168 hours is then given by:

$$T = 168 \left[\frac{d}{38.7} \right]^{-1.43}$$

This dose-rate correction factor results in rather large corrections: for instance, at a dose rate of 50 cGy/hr, a physical dose of 58.2 Gy is given (i.e., 10% lower compared to the reference dose of 65 Gy), for higher dose rates the correction is even higher. Because needles of uniform source strength were

used, larger implants generally resulted in higher dose rates and, as a consequence of the dose-rate correction applied, in lower physical doses.

In Amsterdam, the radiographs were used to determine the spatial coordinates of the needles in order to compute isodose distributions; the dose was given at an isodose curve covering a margin of about 0.5 cm around the tumor. A dose of 60 Gy was delivered without correction for dose rate.[33]

During treatment the patient had to remain in bed in a specially shielded room and no visitors were allowed. When the application time was over, the needles were removed one by one through the drain by pulling the threads, after which the drain itself was taken out. Secondary healing of the drain opening could be slow, regularly causing temporary urine leakage or even a vesicocutaneous fistula.

One of the main disadvantages of using radioactive needles is the radiation hazard to the personnel. Table 1 gives the mean value of radiation exposure (μSv) on several sites of the body of the urologist, the radiation oncologist, the radiotherapy technician, the theater nurse, and the anesthesiologist, measured during three bladder implantations. As could be expected, the urologist, the radiation oncologist, and the theater nurse received the highest doses. The radiation oncologist was only present during a short period, explaining the lower level of radiation in his/her case. The dose to the eyes and thyroid of the radiotherapy technician was extremely high during one operation, because of prolonged exposure caused by difficulties in source preparation. Based upon these data and the maximum allowed exposure limits at that time (1990), a urologist can perform up to 680 implantations per annum.

Afterloading Iridium Wire Technique

The first paper on an afterloading technique with iridium in bladder cancer was published in 1969 by Gros et al.[28] from Bordeaux. Subsequently, different centers in France adopted this technique to deliver radiation in the bladder interstitially.[34–36] In The Netherlands, the afterloading technique was introduced in Deventer in 1984,[37] in Amsterdam

Table 1.
Mean Radiation Exposure (μSv) Measured During Three Bladder Implantations
with Cesium Needles on Several Sites of the Body of Personnel Involved

	Eyes	Thyroid	Chest	Groin	Left Wrist	Right Wrist
Urologist	180	195	374	297	694	540
Radiation oncologist	96	109	152	68	308	307
Radiotherapy technician	247	246	103	103	87	156
Theater nurse	120	145	197	227	384	194
Anesthesiologist	28	24	19	17	15	26

in 1987,[38] and later on in Utrecht[39] and in Rotterdam.[40] In this technique, hollow plastic tubes, which are loaded with iridium afterwards, are placed in the target area in the bladder.

Generally, a lower median abdominal incision is performed and the bladder is opened in the midline of the anterior wall, unless the tumor site requires a paramedian incision. For insertion of the hollow plastic tubes, different methods are used. In French centers, hollow needles are inserted in the bladder wall in the desired position under constant monitoring by a palpating finger, bringing the point of the needle through the bladder mucosa at the opposite side of the target volume. A nylon thread, firmly attached to a tube, is then inserted into the needle, and subsequently the needle and the tube are pulled through the bladder wall. Battermann and Boon[39] attached the leading thin ends of their tubes to ordinary surgical needles; however, in Rotterdam open ended plastic tubes are fixed to needles that have a screwthreading to ensure anchorage of the tubes (Figure 5). In all centers, needles of various lengths and curvatures are available for optimal implantation in all anatomical conditions possible.

The number of tubes necessary to cover the target area are inserted parallel to each other, 1–1.5 cm apart, the outer two lying just outside the area to be irradiated. In case of a partial cystectomy usually two tubes are inserted, one on each side and parallel to the incision, either before or after closing of the wound; preferably, the wound is closed transversally. The tubes have in-dwelling plastic or metal guide wires in order to prevent kinking. Metal markers can be introduced in the bladder wall at both ends of the incision or around the tar-

get area in other cases in order to check the length and position of the dummy wires on localization radiographs. The length of the iridium wire in each tube is defined after insertion of all tubes needed to cover the target area. Since only parallel sources are used, about 15% of the length of the iridium wires (about 1–1.5 cm) should be outside the target area to avoid underdosage at both ends. After the tubes have been inserted, they are fixed in the bladder wall with catgut stitches and the bladder wall and abdominal wall are closed around them. Another possibility is to thread the ends of the tubes separately at both sides through the bladder wall and abdominal wall laterally to the incision. In those cases, the tubes are fixed to the skin with buttons (Figure 6).

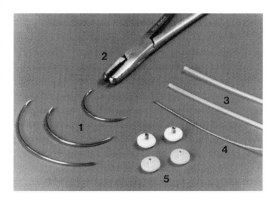

Figure 5. Material used for the iridium wire afterloading technique. 1) curved needles of various sizes with a threading at their ends; 2) needle holder; 3) hollow plastic tubes; 4) metal guidewire; and 5) buttons, used for fixation of the tubes to the skin.

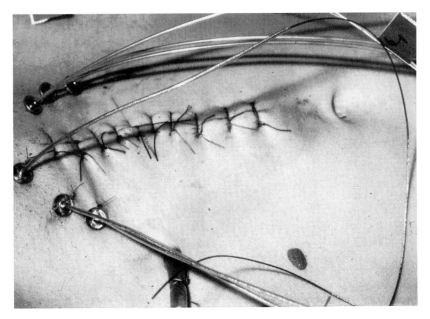

Figure 6. Situation after implantation of three tubes. The tubes are threaded through the abdominal wall separately at both sides, laterally of the incision.

After completion of the operation orthogonal or stereoshift radiographs of the implanted area are made with dummy sources in the tubes (Figure 7). After digitizing the radiographs, dose distributions are calculated, usually in three planes, i.e., the central plane (defined as the plane through the geometric center of the implant and perpendicular to the main direction of the implanted catheters) and two planes parallel to the central plane through the distal ends of the implant (Figure 8).

The radiation oncologist chooses a reference isodose (i.e., a reference dose rate) from the dose distributions calculated. This reference isodose should encompass the whole target area in all isodose planes without causing overdosage in the center of the implant. This choice of the reference isodose still contains a somewhat subjective element. Therefore, a dose specification similar to that of the Paris system is recommended[41]: the local dose minima between the intersections of the line sources with the central plane are calculated and the reference dose is then chosen to a percentage of the average value of these dose minima. In the Paris system the reference dose is chosen to be 85% of the "basal dose" (i.e., the average over the local dose minima in the central plane). Even if a different percentage was to be used, this method of dose specification has the distinct advantage that the specification is based on a dose calculated in a region with minimal dose gradient (instead of choosing an isodose in a strong gradient region at the tumor periphery). Furthermore, the choice of the percentage of the "basal dose" gives some indication of the level of overdosage of the central part of the implant relative to the periphery.

Iridium wires with a uniform source strength are cut to the required length, which is determined during surgery and the localization procedure. After being cut they are sealed inside nylon catheters and loaded in a storage container from which they can be loaded in the afterloading device or directly in the tubes. A remote afterloading device is preferable, but manual loading is also possible.

In France, the iridium is inserted in the tubes after 4–7 days; in Holland, the interstitial radiation starts on the day of surgery or on the following day. During treatment, the patient remains in a shielded room. Visitors

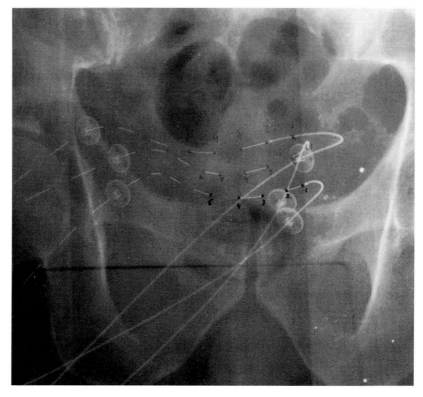

Figure 7. Anterior-posterior radiograph after implantation of tubes. Metal guidewires have been introduced at one end, whereas dummy sources with alternating pieces of lead and nylon of 1 cm length have been inserted from the other side.

are only allowed when a remote afterloading system is used so that the sources can be retracted into a safe temporarily. When the application time has expired, the iridium wires are first removed from the tubes. The tubes are removed separately by gently pulling, if applicable after removing external fixation material. Removing the material is well tolerated and does not require sedation or anesthesia.

The afterloading technique has several advantages over the radium/cesium needle technique. First, there is considerably less radiation exposure to the personnel involved. Second, the whole implantation procedure can be performed in a more relaxed way. Finally, there is the possibility of some dose optimization in case of disappointing geometry of the tubes; the length of the iridium wires can be adjusted, iridium wires of different ac-

tivity can be used, and even the application time per wire can be chosen differently.

Results

Radium/Cesium Technique

Because interstitial radiation by radium and cesium needles seems to be restricted to The Netherlands, the evolution of the technique and the results from Dutch centers only will be discussed.

Generally, selection of patients was based upon joint cystoscopies by the urologist and radiation oncologist. Patients with a solitary T1, T2, or T3 tumor with a diameter not exceeding 5 cm, were considered eligible for IRT. Tumors in the bladder neck were generally excluded because of poor accessibility. Another criterion was that the part of the bladder to be irradiated could be satisfactorily cov-

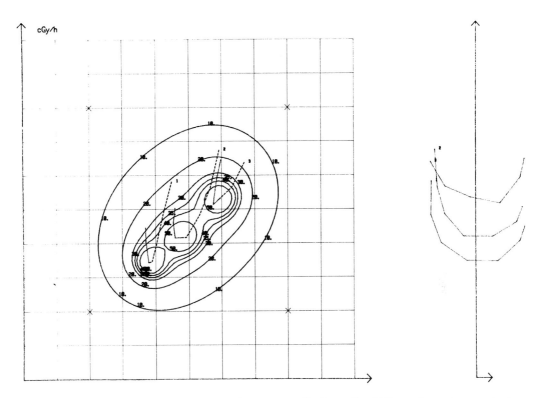

Figure 8. Isodose pattern in the central plane perpendicular to the iridium wires; plane and wires are shown on the right side of the diagram.

ered by a one plane implant. Of course, the patient should be fit enough to undergo surgery. No random biopsies, nor standard lymphadenectomy were performed. Follow-up was done at joint clinics every 3 months during the first 2 years; follow-up intervals were extended thereafter.

In Rotterdam, Van der Werf-Messing[42] noticed scar metastases after IRT; and in order to prevent these, postoperative irradiation to the scar area (200-250 kV, 1050–1500 r skin dose in three to four fractions) was introduced in 1956. To prevent other iatrogenic metastases, in 1962 this postoperative radiation was replaced by preoperative radiotherapy to the true pelvis through two opposed fields with a dose of 10.5 Gy in three fractions calculated in the midplane.[43] Comparison with previous series showed that adding postoperative scar irradiation reduced the risk of scar metastases in T2 and T3 tumors, whereas after introduction of preoperative radiation the incidence was reduced to zero; in T1 tumors scar metas-

tases were never observed. Furthermore, it appeared that the prognosis in T3 tumors and to some extent in T2 tumors was improved by the addition of preoperative radiation, mainly due to a reduced incidence of distant metastases.[44] Since the results in T3 tumors were considered unsatisfactory, a new approach was introduced in 1977, to sterilize possible lymph node metastases in the pelvis. After 3x3.5 Gy EBRT the application time for IRT, necessary to deliver the biological equivalent of 65 Gy in 168 hours was reduced to 55%. Three weeks later an additional 30 Gy EBRT in 15 fractions was delivered to the true pelvis.[45] The results of this approach were encouraging, though generally there was a large time interval between IRT and the additional 30 Gy EBRT. Therefore, the treatment schedule was changed to 40 Gy (20x2 Gy) EBRT, followed by IRT after 1–2 weeks at a reduced dose of 50%.[46]

Meanwhile, a nonrandomized comparative study showed that the addition of IRT to a

Table 2.
Results of Radium/Cesium Needle Interstitial Radiation in T_1 Bladder Cancer

Author	Ref. No.	Treatment	n	FU (m)	Bladder Relapse (%)	Distant Metastasis (%)	Overall 5-Year Survival (%)	Corrected 5-Year Survival (%)
Werf-Messing	42	IRT equiv. 65 Gy (full dose)*	23	19	5†	n.s.	64	n.s.
Werf-Messing	47	10.5 Gy EBRT + IRT full dose	195	79	18	13	n.s.	80
		IRT full dose						
Battermann	33	10.5 Gy EBRT + 60 Gy IRT	34	60	19	6	72	n.s.
		30 Gy EBRT + 40 Gy IRT						
Wijnmaalen	51	51 Gy IRT	127	72	30	10	80	89
		10.5 Gy EBRT + 51 Gy IRT						
		40 Gy EBRT + 27 Gy IRT						
De Neve	52	12 Gy EBRT + 53 Gy IRT	13	69	15	23	74*	74*
Veen	37	10.5 Gy EBRT + 60 Gy IRT	15	60	13	7	n.s.	n.s.

n = number of patients; m = months; corrected survival = for intercurrent death corrected survival; IRT = interstitial radiotherapy; * equiv. 65 Gy = dose equivalent to 65 Gy in 168 hours = full dose; EBRT = external beam radiotherapy; † = pure local recurrence; n.s. = not stated; * = DeNeve, personal communication.

TUR in T1 tumors could reduce the bladder relapse rate from 75% to 18%; moreover, the risk of metastases was reduced and survival increased.[47]

In an analysis of 328 T2 and 63 T3 tumors factors negatively influencing the prognosis in T2 tumors were identified: >1 TUR, poorly differentiated tumor, vascular invasion, and ureter obstruction.[48] Therefore, the policy for T2 tumors with these poor prognostic factors was changed to 40 Gy EBRT and 50% IRT, as in all T3 tumors. Indeed, analysis of this approach showed an improved survival.[49]

Thus, since 1983 the policy for T1 tumors in Rotterdam is full-dose IRT; for T2 tumors without poor prognostic factors 3x3.5 Gy EBRT plus full-dose IRT; and for T2 tumors with poor prognostic factors and all T3 tumors 20x2.0 Gy EBRT plus reduced IRT (50%).

In Amsterdam, treatment policy was changed in 1978 from 3x3.5 Gy EBRT plus 60 Gy IRT to 15x2 Gy EBRT plus 40 Gy IRT.[33,50] It appeared that by this change the risk of distant metastases was reduced from 32% to 13%. From 1982 until 1984 a lymph node dissection was performed in 34 consecutive patients. In four patients node metastases were observed. Since the value of this additional information was considered limited, node dissection was discontinued. Because it is difficult to exactly define the difference between T2 and T3A tumors, they are both evaluated as T2 in the Amsterdam series. Results of the different series from Rotterdam and Amsterdam, as well as three reports from other centers are summarized by T-category in Tables 2, 3, and 4.[33,37,42,46–53]

The mean number of needles per patient as published in two series was six.[33,51] Mean dose rates of 43, 60, and 70 cGy/hr have been reported in three series resulting in mean application times of 114, 90, and 86 hours, respectively.[37,51,52]

Fifty to 80% of the bladder relapses occurred at the original tumor site, whereas 20%–50% developed outside the treated area.[33,42,47,50]

In the postoperative phase, urinary infection, urine leakage, and delayed wound healing frequently occurred; lethal complications were seen in 0%– 2%.[33,42,43,48–53]

During follow-up, necrosis in the implanted area was seen in up to 50% of the patients, leading to symptoms in only a minority.[42,48,49,52,53] Stone formation in the scar area in the bladder, and the development of telangiectasia was also frequently seen, although causing symptoms in only a few patients.[33,42,48,49,51,52]

The mean hospitalization period in six reports varied from 18–38 days.[33,37,40,42,50,53]

Afterloading Iridium Wire Technique

Since the afterloading iridium wire technique was first described in 1969,[28] reports on

Table 3.
Results of Radium/Cesium Needle Interstitial Radiation in T_2 Bladder Cancer

Author	Ref. No.	Treatment	n	FU (m)	Bladder Relapse (%)	Distant Metastasis (%)	Overall 5-Year Survival (%)	Corrected 5-Year Survival (%)
Werf-Messing	42	IRT equiv. 65 Gy (full dose)*	81	19	27†	n.s.	34	n.s.
Werf-Messing	48	10.5 Gy EBRT + IRT full dose	328	24	16	17ˣ	58	75
Battermann	50	10.5 Gy EBRT + 60 Gy IRT 30 Gy EBRT + 40 Gy IRT	120	84	18	15	60	n.s.
Werf-Messing	49	40 Gy EBRT + IRT reduced dose (50%)	48@	27	13	13	72	78
Wijnmaalen	51	10.5 Gy EBRT + 51 Gy IRT 40 Gy EBRT + 27 Gy IRT	139	72	29	19	50	68
De Neve	52	12 Gy EBRT + 53 Gy IRT	19	69	32	0	78˙	86˙
Roesink	53	Low-dose EBRT + 60 Gy IRT	75	68	n.s.	n.s.	67	71
Veen	37	10.5 Gy EBRT + 60 Gy IRT	31	60	26	32	n.s.	n.s.

n = number of patients; m = months; corrected survival = for intercurrent death corrected survival; IRT = interstitial radiotherapy; * equiv. 65 Gy = dose equivalent to 65 Gy in 168 hours = full dose; EBRT = external beam radiotherapy; † = pure local recurrence; n.s. = not stated; ˣ = metastasis without local recurrence only; @ = T_2 tumors with poor prognostic factors; ˙ = DeNeve, personal communication.

this technique of applying interstitial radiation emerged from several French centers.[34–36,54–58] Generally, standard treatment in these series consisted of low-dose preoperative EBRT (3x3.5 Gy, 2x6.0 Gy, 2x6.5 Gy, or 1x8.5 Gy), followed by a unilateral or bilateral external iliac lymph node dissection, partial cystectomy or tumorectomy, and 45–60 Gy IRT, starting on day 4–7 after surgery.

In one center, the IRT dose is increased from 40–60 Gy in case of positive margins of the partial cystectomy specimen.[55] Reduction of the IRT dose and additional postoperative EBRT is reported in case of lymph node metastases or pT3 tumors.[35,36,54]

In 1992, Rozan et al.[59] published the results from eight centers in France; all patients received low-dose EBRT, followed by node dissection in 59% and partial cystectomy plus IRT in 58%, or tumorectomy plus IRT (42%). Small series have been reported by two American centers.[60,61] Results from Utrecht[62] and Amsterdam[38] have been published recently. Finally, preliminary data are available from Rotterdam (Wijnmaalen, personal communication).

The selection criteria are not essentially different from those in the radium/cesium needle technique: solitary T1, T2, and T3 tumors with a diameter not exceeding 4–5 cm.

Table 4.
Results of Radium/Cesium Needle Interstitial Radiation in T_3 Bladder Cancer

Author	Ref. No.	Treatment	n	FU (m)	Bladder Relapse (%)	Distant Metastasis (%)	Overall 5-Year Survival (%)	Corrected 5-Year Survival (%)
Werf-Messing	42	IRT equiv. 65 Gy (full dose)*	42	19	61†	n.s.	10	n.s.
Werf-Messing	46	10.5 Gy EBRT + IRT reduced dose (50%) + 30 Gy EBRT	41	12	n.s.	n.s.	57@	74@
Werf-Messing	48	10.5 Gy EBRT + IRT full dose	63	24	28	21ˣ	38	62
Werf-Messing	49	40 Gy EBRT + IRT reduced dose (50%)	42	27	14	12	54	84
Wijnmaalen	51	10.5 Gy EBRT + 51 Gy IRT 40 Gy EBRT + 27 Gy IRT	44	72	37	20	61	71

n = number of patients; m = months; corrected survival = for intercurrent death corrected survival; IRT = interstitial radiotherapy; * equiv. 65 Gy = dose equivalent to 65 Gy in 168 hours = full dose; EBRT = external beam radiotherapy; † = pure local recurrence; n.s. = not stated; @ = 3-year data; ˣ = metastasis without local recurrence only.

Table 5.
Results of Afterloading Iridium Wire Interstitial Radiotherapy in T_1 Tumors

Author	Ref. No.	Treatment	n	FU (m)	Bladder Relapse (%)	Distant Metastasis (%)	Overall 5-Year Survival (%)	Corrected 5-Year Survival (%)
Rozan	59	11 Gy EBRT + 50 Gy IRT	98*	51	15	10@	77	93
Moonen	38	30 Gy EBRT + 40 Gy IRT	12	40	0	8	86#	n.s.
Battermann	62	30 Gy EBRT + 40 Gy IRT	4	30	0	0	75	100
Wijnmaalen	pers.comm.	60 Gy IRT	26	26	23	15	86˙	n.s.

n = number of patients; m = months; corrected survival = for intercurrent death corrected survival; EBRT = external beam radiotherapy; IRT = interstitial radiotherapy; * = pathological T classification (pT); @ = all pT categories together; # = T_1, T_2; and T_{3A}; n.s. = not stated; ˙ = 2-year survival.

In France, apparently mainly tumors in the mobile part of the bladder are selected for IRT since in the majority of patients a partial cystectomy or tumorectomy is performed. In the Dutch centers, the indications for partial cystectomy remained unchanged after changing the IRT technique. Lymph node dissection is not routinely performed in The Netherlands. Results of IRT by the afterloading iridium wire technique by T-category are presented in Tables 5, 6, and 7.[38,59-62]

In case of partial cystectomy, generally two tubes are implanted,[59] the number in other cases varying from three to five.[38,60-62] The dose rate is reported in three series, varying from 30–65 cGy/hr.[60-62] The mean application time for 40 Gy IRT was 110 hours in one series.[38]

Twenty-six to 60% of the reported bladder relapses occurred at the original tumor site; in 40%–62% a relapse elsewhere in the bladder developed.[38,54-56,58,59] Postoperative lethal complications have been reported in 0%–2.6%.[38,58,59,62] Other acute complications reported were mainly urinary infection, delayed wound healing, and vesicocutaneous fistula. Rozan et al.[59] reported complications in the postoperative phase in 58 patients (28%): 4.4% thrombosis, 16.6% locoregional problems, 10.7% complications outside the treated area, and 1.5% postoperative death. Group II complications (more serious or persistent complications requiring hospitalization) were seen in 29 patients (8 hematuria, 17 chronic cystitis, 2 impaired capacity, and 11 fistula), whereas in one additional patient surgery was necessary for correction of a fistula; six patients developed a ureteral stenosis; in one of them surgery was necessary.

In the Utrecht series[62] postoperative complications consisted of psychological decompensation (8%), ileus (5%), and cardiovascular problems (5%). One patient died postoperatively. During follow-up, a ureter obstruction developed in two patients (5%); in one patient, a reimplantation had to be per-

Table 6.
Results of Afterloading Iridium Wire Interstitial Radiotherapy in T_2 Tumors

Author	Ref. No.	Treatment	n	FU (m)	Bladder Relapse (%)	Distant Metastasis (%)	Overall 5-Year Survival (%)	Corrected 5-Year Survival (%)
Rozan	59	11 Gy EBRT + 50 Gy IRT	66*	51	18§	10@	63	81
Strauss	60	Various schemes	9	22	22	33	n.s.	n.s.
Moonen	38	30 Gy EBRT + 40 Gy IRT	28†	40	21	18	86#	n.s.
Battermann	62	30 Gy EBRT + 40 Gy IRT	28	30	14	21	65	76
Wijnmaalen	pers.comm.	40 Gy EBRT + 30 Gy IRT	37	26	14	27	55˙	n.s.

n = number of patients; m = months; corrected survival = for intercurrent death corrected survival; EBRT = external beam radiotherapy; IRT = interstitial radiotherapy; * = pathological T classification (pT); § = pT_2 and pT_{3A} together; @ = all pT categories together; n.s. = not stated; † = T_2 and T_{3A} together; # = T_1, T_2 and T_{3A} together; ˙ = 2-year survival.

Table 7.
Results of Afterloading Iridium Wire Interstitial Radiotherapy in T_3 Tumors

Author	Ref. No.	Treatment	n	FU (m)	Bladder Relapse (%)	Distant Metastasis (%)	Overall 5-Year Survival (%)	Corrected 5-Year Survival (%)
Rozan	59	11 Gy EBRT + 50 Gy IRT	35*	51	18§	10@	47	62
Grossman	61	45 Gy EBRT + 19 Gy IRT	7	40	29	14	n.s.	n.s.
Battermann	62	30 Gy EBRT + 40 Gy IRT	6	30	17	17	67	67
Wijnmaalen	pers.comm.	40 Gy EBRT + 30 Gy IRT	9	26	22	33	63˙	n.s.

n = number of patients; m = months; corrected survival = for intercurrent death corrected survival; EBRT = external beam radiotherapy; IRT = interstitial radiotherapy; * = pathological T classification (pT); § = pT_2 and pT_{3A} together; @ = all pT categories together; n.s. = not stated; ˙ = 2-year survival.

formed. No other severe late complications have been recorded.

Moonen et al.[38] reported wound infection in 8%, urine leakage in 8%, psychological problems in another 8%, accidental perforation of the sigmoid in one patient, and osteomyelitis of the pubic bone in another patient. Late severe complications were not recorded, but during follow-up ulceration in the irradiated area was common (53%), leading to symptoms in only 10% of the patients. The mean hospitalization period varied from 13–26 days.[38,59,62]

Conclusions and Recommendations

LDR IRT in patients with T1, T2, and T3 bladder cancer with a diameter not exceeding 5 cm yields good to excellent results in terms of local control and survival (Tables 2–7).

It is difficult to define the exact place of this treatment modality within the arsenal of approaches in bladder cancer patients. IRT is applied in a highly selected group of patients, and there are no comparative (randomized) studies. Finally, the experience with brachytherapy in bladder cancer is limited to those few centers in which modern brachytherapy facilities are available and in which an excellent cooperation exists between urologists and radiation oncologists.

For IRT, the afterloading iridium wire technique is presently the standard treatment because of radiation protection, the possibility of dose optimization to some extent and of postoperative intensive care, if necessary.

Preferably, patients should be selected by

the urologist and the radiation oncologist together. Under anesthesia, a cystoscopy has to be performed, as well as a bimanual examination of the bladder area; a TUR of all visible tumor should be performed, followed by a repeated digital rectal examination. For accurate determination of the T category, the resected material must contain muscular tissue. If a tumor mass that cannot be sufficiently irradiated by a one plane implant remains palpable, or when the tumor is located at or extends into the bladder neck, the patient should be considered unsuitable for brachytherapy. Of 2146 patients referred for radiotherapy in Rotterdam, 29% could be accepted for IRT.[44] In two other Dutch series, this was only 10% and 12%.[38,52]

It remains a matter of debate whether random biopsies from normal looking mucosa should be taken in order to exclude patients with dysplasia or carcinoma in situ elsewhere in the bladder. In the large Dutch centers, random biopsies are not routinely taken; but in France, random biopsy appears to be part of the work-up.[58,59] Considering that about 50% of the bladder relapses occur outside the original tumor site, dysplasia or carcinoma in situ may play a role in the development of recurrences. Van der Werf-Messing et al.[44] demonstrated the presence of carcinoma in situ or invasive carcinoma at 2 cm from the visible tumor in 17%, 13%, and 34% in T1, T2, and T3 tumors, respectively. Yet, there appeared to be no correlation between these findings and the incidence of local recurrences. In a series of 85 patients in whom random biopsies were taken before definitive treatment, 62% of the recurrences developed outside the original tumor area.[58] This fact neither supports the hypothesis that by exclusion of patients with carcinoma in situ or dysplasia outside the tumor area the risk of a bladder relapse outside the treated volume will decrease.

Although in principle only solitary tumors are accepted, IRT may be considered when multiple tumors are confined to an area of <5 cm in diameter in an easily accessible part of the bladder.

In T1 carcinoma the prognosis does not appear to be improved by the addition of preoperative EBRT.[44] Low-dose preoperative EBRT is given in all T categories in French centers to prevent iatrogenic metastases, whereas the Dutch centers apply a dose of 30 or 40 Gy in T2 and T3 tumors, in order to sterilize subclinical disease outside the tumor area as well. We believe that EBRT should be delivered to a small field covering the true pelvis only.

In our experience, tubes can be inserted under epidural anesthesia without any problem. Accessibility is best through a midline lower abdominal incision.

The role of lymphadenectomy has not been established. The chance of lymph node metastases appears to be low in this selective group of patients; in five series the incidence was <10%,[50,54-56,59] whereas in one series 18% of the patients appeared to have developed lymph node metastases before definitive treatment.[36] We consider lymphadenectomy a diagnostic procedure not indicated in this selective group of patients, since the chance of finding metastases is low and the operation is extended, theoretically increasing the risk of complications. If, however, at lymphadenectomy positive nodes are found, we support the concept of reducing the dose of IRT and adding postoperative EBRT if no or low-dose EBRT has been applied.[35,36,54,56] In cases where 30 Gy or 40 Gy EBRT has been applied preoperatively, the treatment should be completed as planned beforehand.

A partial cystectomy, with a very limited margin, should only be performed for practical reasons and should not be a selection criterion in itself.

Proximity of a ureter ostium is not a contraindication for IRT. Reimplantation of the ureter in the dome or insertion of a ureter catheter can be considered if the tubes for IRT must be placed through the area of a ureter ostium. Whether this prevents acute and late complications is unclear. In our experience, the development of a ureter stenosis is rare; on the contrary, a rigid ostium remaining open is seen regularly.

Although the number of patients with adenocarcinoma or squamous cell carcinoma is low, we have the impression that these histologies do not influence prognosis negatively; they should not be excluded from IRT protocols.

Unless the location of the tumor requires another incision, the bladder is opened in the midline. Subsequently, the bladder mucosa is carefully inspected, and the bladder wall is palpated to confirm the solitary character of the tumor.

Plastic tubes are introduced in the bladder wall as parallel as possible, with proper spacing and coverage of the target area (see iridium wire afterloading technique above). Preferably, the tubes are inserted under constant monitoring of a palpating finger. Generally, three to four tubes will be sufficient. When a partial cystectomy has been performed, two tubes are placed at both sides of the suture. Insertion of an extra tube should be considered when doubt exists regarding the parallelism. Subsequently, the decision of which tubes to load to obtain optimal dose distribution can be made; even partial loading of the tubes may be considered.

In our opinion, the number of perforations in the bladder wall should be kept as restricted as possible in order to prevent urine leakage. This means inserting the tubes in the bladder wall from outside, not perforating the mucosa. Often this will not be possible; and, at least at one side, the tubes will have to be introduced from outside into the bladder before insertion in the target area is possible. We advise threading the tubes through the abdominal wall separately at both sides of the lower abdominal incision and not through the cystotomy and abdominal wound, in order to reduce the risk of infections, urine leakage, and delayed wound healing.

Metal markers can be placed in the bladder wall at the margins of the target area to define the position and length of the iridium wires. Metal guide wires may also be used for this purpose; each wire should be retracted into the margin at one side and fixed in the tube by clamping a button used for fixation of the tube to the abdominal wall; subsequently, the unfixed end of the wire is introduced into the other end of the same tube until it touches the fixed end; by retracting the wire up to the margin at the other side of the target area, the exact length of the iridium needed is defined. After surgery there is no need to delay IRT, unless the histology report in case of a partial cystectomy influences the dose to be given.

The risk of death because of postoperative complications (mainly cardiovascular and pulmonary) will not exceed 3%.[38,40,49–51,53,59,62] According to Battermann[62] and Moonen, et al.[38] both the incidence of nonserious acute complications and the hospitalization period are reduced by the afterloading iridium wire technique in comparison to IRT with radium or cesium needles. Wijnmaalen et al.,[40] however, could not show a significant difference between both techniques. Serious late complications are rare.

The development of necrosis or ulceration at the interstitially irradiated side is quite common during follow-up. In the majority of the patients these complications do not cause any complaints.[38,42,48,49,52,53] This phenomenon may well resemble tumor recurrence, but if urine cytology remains negative, additional biopsies or TURs should generally be avoided, since healing might be delayed. Also, telangiectasia and stone formation in the scar area may develop, but these cause complaints in only a minority of patients.

Follow-up consists of cystoscopies and cytologic urine examination every 3 months during the first 2 years and less frequently thereafter.

Future Developments

Pulsed-Dose-Rate Brachytherapy

Pulsed-dose-rate (PDR) brachytherapy is a new type of afterloading IRT in which a continuous LDR treatment is simulated by a series of "pulses," i.e., fractions of short duration (10–20 minutes) with time intervals between fractions of 1 to a few hours. The concept of simulating LDR brachytherapy with a series of small fractions has been proposed by Brenner and Hall.[63]

The incentive in initiating PDR brachytherapy and testing its feasibility in relation to "classical" LDR brachytherapy is to combine the mainly radiobiological advantages of LDR brachytherapy with the mainly physical, logistic, and practical advantages of modern high-dose-rate (HDR) afterloaders using a single iridium source "stepping" through a range of dwell positions in an implant to produce a dose distribution. Specifically, the advantages of PDR brachytherapy would be:

1. Maintaining the radiobiological advantages of LDR brachytherapy (i.e., a high level of local control in combination with optimum sparing of normal tissues), but offering the patient the possibility to receive visitors and proper nursing care during the intervals.
2. The possibility to freely choose the effective dose rate of the treatment, independent of the implant volume and the strength of available sources.
3. The possibility of optimizing the dose distribution through dwell time variations,[64] especially in cases where the position of the tubes deviates.
4. No more need of preparing individual iridium source lines (wires or ribbons) for each implant.

In view of the extensive experience with LDR interstitial radiation of bladder cancer obtained, it seems appropriate to consider PDR as a possible replacement of the present LDR treatments. The schedules applied for PDR brachytherapy in Rotterdam in head and neck implants involve a fraction dose of 1.0 or 1.5 Gy (depending on whether a boost is given or a full treatment), an interval of 3 hours, i.e., eight fractions per day. Testing similar schedules for PDR brachytherapy of bladder cancer is being considered.

Integrated Brachytherapy Unit

The terminology "Integrated Brachytherapy Unit" (IBU) was recently introduced for a setup including a shielded operating room, equipped with a dedicated simulator suitable for use during surgical procedures, coupled to a computer planning system for direct use of fluoroscopy images for on-line planning, if needed for intraoperative applications.

Three categories of applications are foreseen in an IBU:

1. placement of tubes during surgery, on-line planning, and one single irradiation in the IBU, while displacing normal tissues (intraoperative brachytherapy);
2. idem, but the tubes stay in place and the patient is treated with either fractionated HDR, PDR, or LDR brachytherapy afterwards (i.e., intraoperative and perioperative brachytherapy);
3. the IBU-system is only used for reconstruction, no intraoperative irradiation is applied.

The application of intraoperative irradiation (i.e., categories 1 or 2) of implanted bladder cancers is not foreseen in Rotterdam, since the use of a single high irradiation dose during surgery could presumably result in an increased probability of normal tissue damage. The present results with LDR brachytherapy do not appear to warrant the application of intraoperative irradiation.

X-ray imaging may be used during surgical procedures in selected patients in whom the geometry of the implant is expected to be less than optimal or in whom the implant geometry might change after closing of the bladder. In these cases, this imaging capability will allow evaluation of the resulting geometry during the surgical procedure so that corrective measures may be taken when needed.

References

1. Boring CC, Squires TS, Tong T, et al. Cancer statistics, 1994. CA Cancer J Clin 1994;44:7–26.
2. Visser O, Coebergh JWW, Schouten LJ. Incidence of cancer in The Netherlands 1990. Second report of the Netherlands Cancer Registry. SIG Health Care Information, Utrecht, 1990.
3. Morrison AS, Cole P. Urinary tract. In: Schottenfeld D, Fraumeni JF Jr. (eds). Cancer Epidemiology and Prevention. W.B. Saunders Company, Philadelphia, PA, 1982, pp. 925–937.
4. Wall RL, Clausen KP. Carcinoma of the urinary bladder in patients receiving cyclophosphamide. N Engl J Med 1975;293:271–273.
5. Rosai J. Bladder and urethra. In: Rosai J (ed). Ackerman's Surgical Pathology. The C.V. Mosby Company, St. Louis, MO, 1989, pp. 898–922.
6. Jewett HJ, Strong GH. Infiltrating carcinoma of the bladder: Relation of depth of penetration of the bladder wall to incidence of local extension and metastases. J Urol 1946;55:366–372.
7. Marshall VF. The relation of the preoperative estimate to the pathologic demonstration of the extent of vesicle neoplasms. J Urol 1952; 68:714–723.
8. Hermanek P, Sobin LH. TNM Classification of Malignant Tumours. Fourth Edition. Springer-Verlag, Berlin, 1987.
9. Aso Y, Bouffioux C, Flanigan R, et al. Prognostic factors in Ta, T1 (superficial) bladder cancer. In: Niijima T, Aso Y, Koontz W, et al. (eds). Consensus Development in Clinical Bladder Cancer Research. Proceedings of the Second and Third International Consensus Development Symposia. SCI, Paris, 1993, pp. 176–186.
10. Fosså SD, Koontz W, Matsumoto K, et al. Prognostic factors in muscle-invasive bladder cancer. In: Niijima T, Aso Y, Koontz W, et al. (eds). Consensus Development in Clinical Bladder Cancer Research. Proceedings of the Second and Third International Consensus Development Symposia. SCI, Paris, 1993, pp. 187–198.
11. Watson EM. The management of bladder tumors, particularly the inoperable type. J Urol 1925;14:509–517.
12. Barringer BS. Twenty five years of radon treatment of cancer of the bladder. JAMA 1947;135: 616–618.
13. Hutchison RG. Measured dosage in the radium treatment of the urinary bladder. Br J Surg 1935;22:663–670.
14. Herger CC, Sauer HR. Radium treatment of cancer of the bladder. Report of 267 cases. Am J Roentgenol 1942;47:909–915.
15. Millen JLE. Carcinoma of the bladder. III. Treatment by radon seed implantation and deep X-ray therapy. Br J Radiol 1949;22:402–405.
16. Carver JH. Interstitial radiation in the treatment of selected cases of cancer of the bladder. Br J Urol 1959;31:313–316.
17. Dix VW, Shanks W, Tresidder GC, et al. Carcinoma of the bladder; treatment by diathermy snare excision and interstitial irradiation. Br J Urol 1970;42:213–228.
18. Munro AI. The results of using radioactive gold grains in the treatment of bladder growths. Br J Urol 1964;36:541–548.
19. Williams GB, Trott PA, Bloom HJG. Carcinoma of the bladder treated by interstitial irradiation. Br J Urol 1981;53:221–224.
20. Lenz M, Cahill GF, Melicow MM, et al. The treatment of cancer of the bladder by radium needles. Am J Roentgenol 1947;58:486–492.
21. Jacobs A. Symposium: Carcinoma of the blad-

der. I. The treatment of cancer of the bladder by radium. Br J Radiol 1949;22:393–398.

22. Darget R. Tumeurs malignes de la vessie. Traitement par la radium thérapie à vessie ouverte. Masson, Paris, 1951.

23. Breur K, De Waard T. De radio-chirurgische behandeling van blaascarcinoom. Ned Tijdschr Geneeskd 1956;100:1052–1062.

24. Sahatchiev A, Kirov S, Tcheretchanski P, et al. Résultats de la curiethérapie interstitielle du cancer de la vessie. Ann Radiol 1971;14: 643–648.

25. Wallace DM, Stapleton JE, Turner RC. Radioactive tantalum wire implantation as a method of treatment for early carcinoma of the bladder. Br J Radiol 1952;25:421–424.

26. Bloom HJG. Treatment of carcinoma of the bladder. A symposium. I. Treatment by interstitial irradiation using tantalum 182 wire. Br J Radiol 1960;33:471–479.

27. Pizzi GB, Calzavara F, Cauzzo C, et al. Endocuriethérapie du cancer de la vessie. Proposition d'une nouvelle technique par fils d'[192]Iridium en tubes de Cyponil. J Radiol 1979;60:715–718.

28. Gros Ch, Bollack C, Keiling R. Curiethérapie par Iridium 192. Préparation inactive des petits cancers de la vessie. J Radiol Electrol 1969;50: 437–439.

29. Meredith WJ. Radium dosage. The Manchester System. Compiled from articles by Paterson R, Spiers FW, Stephenson SK, et al. E & S Livingstone LTD, Edinburgh, 1949.

30. Vaeth JM, Meurk ML. Use of the Rotterdam radium reconstruction device. Am J Roentgenol 1963;89:87–90.

31. Van Kleffens HJ, Star WM. Application of stereo X-ray photogrammetry (SRM) in the determination of absorbed dose values during intracavitary radiation therapy. Int J Radiat Oncol Biol Phys 1979;5:557–563.

32. Orton CG. Time-dose factors (TDF) in brachytherapy. Br J Radiol 1974;47:603–607.

33. Battermann JJ, Tierie AH. Results of implantation for T_1 and T_2 bladder tumours. Radiother Oncol 1986;5:85–90.

34. Pierquin B, Chassagne DJ, Chahbazian CM, et al. Chapter X-Genitourinary system. In: Brachytherapy. Warren H Green, Inc, St. Louis, MO, 1978, pp. 198–201.

35. Chassagne DJ, Court B, Gerbaulet A, et al. Technique d'endocuriethérapie par fils d'Iridium[192] avec ou sans cystectomie partielle associee. In: Kuss R, Rozan R, Giraud B (eds). Le Traitement Conservateur dans le Cancer de Vessie (Symposium Proceedings). Laboratoires Sandoz, Paris, 1982, pp. 92–99.

36. Gérard JP, De Laroche G, Ardiet JM, et al. La curiethérapie à l'iridium dans le traitement conservateur des cancers infiltrants de vessie. J d'Urol 1985;91:139–144.

37. Veen RE. Applicators for interstitial radiotherapy, "the Deventer system" (thesis). 1994.

38. Moonen LMF, Horenblas S, Van der Voet JCM, et al. Bladder conservation in selected T1G3 and muscle invasive T_2-T_{3a} bladder carcinoma using combination therapy of surgery and iridium-192 implantation. Br J Urol 1994;74: 322–327.

39. Battermann JJ, Boon TA. Remote-controlled afterloading technique for the treatment of bladder cancer. Endocurie Hypertherm Oncol 1991;7:151–154.

40. Wijnmaalen AJ, Boeken Kruger CGG, Helle PA, et al. Interstitial irradiation in bladder cancer: Feasibility and complications of two different techniques. (Abstract). Int J Radiat Oncol Biol Phys 1991;21;(Suppl 1):218.

41. Dutreix A, Marinello G, Wambersie A. Dosimetrie et Curietherapie. Masson, Paris, 1982.

42. Van der Werf-Messing BHP. Treatment of carcinoma of the bladder with radium. Clin Radiol 1965;16:16–26.

43. Van der Werf-Messing BHP. Carcinoma of the bladder treated by suprapubic radium implants. The value of additional external irradiation. Eur J Cancer 1969;5:277–285.

44. Van der Werf-Messing BHP. Cancer of the urinary bladder treated by interstitial radium implant. Int J Radiat Oncol Biol Phys 1978;4: 373–378.

45. Van der Werf-Messing BHP, Star WM, Menon RS. $T_3N_xM_0$ carcinoma of the urinary bladder treated by the combination of radium implant and external irradiation. A preliminary report. Int J Radiat Oncol Biol Phys 1980;6:1723–1725.

46. Van der Werf-Messing BHP, Menon RS, Hop WCJ. Carcinoma of the urinary bladder category $T_3N_xM_0$ treated by the combination of radium implant and external irradiation: Second report. Int J Radiat Oncol Biol Phys 1983; 9:177–180.

47. Van der Werf-Messing BHP, Hop WCJ. Carcinoma of the urinary bladder (category $T_1N_xM_0$) treated either by radium implant or by transurethral resection only. Int J Radiat Oncol Biol Phys 1981;7:299–303.

48. Van der Werf-Messing BHP, Menon RS, Hop WCJ. Cancer of the urinary bladder category T_2, T_3, (N_xM_0) treated by interstitial radium implant: Second report. Int J Radiat Oncol Biol Phys 1983;9:481–485.

49. Van der Werf-Messing BHP, Van Putten WLJ. Carcinoma of the urinary bladder category $T_{2,3}N_xM_0$ treated by 40 Gy external irradiation followed by cesium[137] implant at reduced dose

(50%). Int J Radiat Oncol Biol Phys 1989;16: 369–371.

50. Battermann JJ, Boon TA. Interstitial therapy in the management of T2 bladder tumors. Endocurie Hypertherm Oncol 1988;4:1–6.

51. Wijnmaalen AJ, Van Putten WLJ, Hofman F, et al. LDR brachytherapy with radium or caesium-137 needles for bladder cancer: Results for 312 patients. In: Mould RF (ed). International Brachytherapy, Proceedings 7th International Brachytherapy Working Conference, Baltimore/Washington, USA, 6–8 September 1992. Veenendaal: Nucletron International BV, 1992, pp. 397–400.

52. De Neve W, Lybeert MLM, Goor C, et al. T1 and T2 carcinoma of the urinary bladder: Long term results with external, preoperative, or interstitial radiotherapy. Int J Radiat Oncol Biol Phys 1992;23:299–304.

53. Roesink JM, De Ru VJ, Hofman P, et al. Interstitiële radiotherapie bij het blaascarcinoom: voor en na mei 1988. Tijdschr Kanker 1993;17: 28–31.

54. Botto H, Perrin JL, Auvert J, et al. Treatment of malignant bladder tumors by iridium-192 wiring. Urology 1980;16:467–469.

55. Mazeron JJ, Housset M, Calitchi E, et al. Bilan de l'endocurietherapie des épithéliomas de la vessie a l'Iridium 192: expérience des hopitaux Henri Mondor et Necker. In: Kuss R, Rozan R, Giraud B (eds). Le Traitement Conservateur dans le Cancer de Vessie (Symposium Proceedings). Laboratoires Sandoz, Paris, 1982, pp. 100–106.

56. Mazeron JJ, Marinello G, Leung S, et al. Treatment of bladder tumors by iridium 192 implantation. The Créteil technique. Radiother Oncol 1985;4:111–119.

57. Mazeron JJ, Abbou CC, Chopin D, et al. Traitement conservateur des épithéliomas vésicaux par cystectomie partielle et endocuriethérapie par Iridium 192. Ann Urol 1987;21:175–178.

58. Mazeron JJ, Crook J, Chopin D, et al. Conservative treatment of bladder carcinoma by partial cystectomy and interstitial Iridium 192. Int J Radiat Oncol Biol Phys 1988;15:1323–1330.

59. Rozan R, Albuisson E, Donnarieix D, et al. Interstitial iridium-192 for bladder cancer (A multicentric survey: 205 patients). Int J Radiat Oncol Biol Phys 1992;24:469–477.

60. Straus KL, Littman P, Wein AJ, et al. Treatment of bladder cancer with interstitial iridium-192 implantation and external beam irradiation. Int J Radiat Oncol Biol Phys 1988;14:265–271.

61. Grossman HB, Sandler HM, Perez-Tamayo C. Treatment of T3a bladder cancer with iridium implantation. Urology 1993;41:217–220.

62. Battermann JJ: Bladder implantation: Fact or fiction? In: Mould RF, Battermann JJ, Martinez AA, et al. (eds). Brachytherapy from Radium to Optimization. Nucletron International B.V., Veenendaal, The Netherlands, 1994, pp. 230–238.

63. Brenner DJ, Hall EJ. Conditions for the equivalence of continuous to pulsed low dose rate brachytherapy. Int J Radiat Oncol Biol Phys 1990;20:181–190.

64. Kolkman-Deurloo IKK, Visser AG, Niël CGJH, et al. Optimization of interstitial volume implants. Radiat Oncol 1994;31:229–239.

Cancer of the Female Urethra

Subir Nag, M.D., Rodney E. Ellis, M.D.

Introduction

Cancers of the female urethra, while rare, can be traced as far back in the medical literature as 1833.[1] Carcinoma of the female urethra accounts for only 0.02% of all cancers in females, and 0.1% of all gynecological malignancies. The average age at diagnosis of carcinoma of the female urethra ranges between 50–80 years of age (average 60–61 years). There is a 3:1 ratio of whites to blacks.[2,3] Although the traditional treatment approach has been surgical, in the past several decades, techniques have been developed for application of brachytherapy to treat these lesions. These techniques have often been combined with either external beam radiotherapy (EBRT) or a limited surgical excision.

Methods

Treatment modalities for carcinoma of the female urethra vary depending on the extent of disease. Small, well differentiated lesions with minimal infiltration may often be removed surgically; however, as the size of the lesion or depth of the infiltration increases, the risk of stress incontinence or total incontinence increases. Limited lesions of the distal urethra are best treated with brachytherapy alone. For lesions involving the entire length of the urethra, a total urethrocystectomy or primary EBRT have been attempted; however, both treatment modalities yield poor results. The combination of EBRT followed by a brachytherapy boost or a urethrocystectomy 5–6 weeks after completion of EBRT may possibly result in improved control.[2]

Selection Criteria for Brachytherapy

Patients with cancer of the urethra suitable for treatment with brachytherapy include the following:

1. Those with small lesions of the distal urethra, which can be treated by brachytherapy alone; or
2. Those with larger lesions involving the proximal urethra or entire urethra, which are best treated by a combination of EBRT and brachytherapy.

Patients with tumors >4 cm or those with inguinal lymph node involvement are not good candidates for brachytherapy.

External Beam Radiation Therapy

EBRT is generally given to the entire pelvis for advanced lesions or lesions involving the proximal urethra. Doses of 45–50 Gy are generally used over 5 weeks if given as a preoperative dose or if used in combination with brachytherapy. If the patient is treated by EBRT alone, a cone down boost is given to deliver a total dose of 60–70 Gy in 6–7 weeks.[1–6]

From Nag S (ed): *Principles and Practice of Brachytherapy.* © Futura Publishing Co., Inc., Armonk, NY, 1997.

Brachytherapy Techniques

A template technique is generally used. Memorial Sloan Kettering Cancer Center in New York has described a urethral plexiglas template.[7] We generally use a Syed template (Figure 1). The patient is implanted in the lithotomy position under spinal or general anesthesia. A Foley catheter is inserted into the bladder, and the Foley bulb inflated with dilute hypaque. Seventeen gauge needles are implanted through the template to adequately cover the target volume in a single or double plane, usually in a circular fashion. Lesions of the distal urethra are performed without a

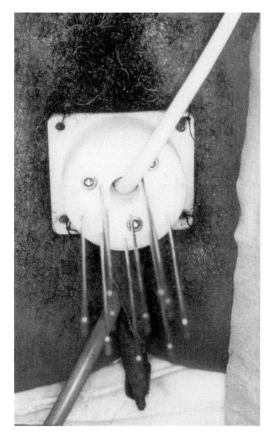

Figure 1. Patient with carcinoma of the posterior urethra being treated with a two plane Ir-192 implant with ten needles in a Syed template. A Foley catheter is placed through the center of the template into the bladder and gauze distends the vagina. A rectal catheter is placed for identification on the localization radiograph.

suprapubic cystotomy. However, for lesions of the proximal urethra, or the entire length of the urethra, it is preferable to add a suprapubic cystotomy to rule out bladder invasion and guide needle placement. For lesions of the anterior urethra, the needles are loaded so that the sources extend 1–2 cm beyond the urethra.

Although a variety of sources (radium-226, cesium-137, iridium-192) have been used, we generally use iridium-192 seeds in plastic ribbons. Iridium-192 forks in single or double gutter can also be used, especially for the distal lesions. To reduce morbidity, it is important that the vagina be distended using an empty vaginal cylinder or gauze packing to displace the posterior and lateral vaginal walls from the high-dose area.

Dose

Limited lesions of the distal urethra can be treated by a brachytherapy dose of about 60 Gy in 5–7 days. In more advanced lesions, when EBRT of 45–50 Gy has been delivered to the pelvis, the brachytherapy dose is limited to 30–40 Gy in 3–4 days. The brachytherapy is generally given after the EBRT has been used to shrink the larger tumors. Smaller tumors can be treated with an initial brachytherapy boost followed by EBRT.

Results

Treatment Summary (Table 1)

Komaki reported on a nonrandomized series of 13 patients treated for carcinoma of the female urethra. For cases with risk of lymph node involvement, EBRT was given to the pelvis to deliver 42–50 Gy in combination with an additional brachytherapy boost using iridium hairpins. Clinically localized disease was treated with primary implantation without external beam nodal radiotherapy. The brachytherapy doses ranged from 30–73 Gy depending on whether the brachytherapy was being given as a boost or as primary treatment. Local control was 82%. Survival data showed a 45% disease-free survival at 5–10 years. No complications were noted.[1]

Delclos et al.[9] reported on a nonrandomized series of 38 patients treated between

Table 1.
Carcinoma of the Female Urethra: Results of Brachytherapy

Author	Number of Patients	EBRT Dose (Gy)	Brachy Dose (Gy)	Local Control	Actuarial Survival	Complications
Komaki[1]	13	42–50 in 4–5 weeks	30–73 Ir 192 implants	9/11, 82%	5/11, 45% NED 5–10 years	—
Delclos[9] (1948–1972)	38	60–70 / 40–50 in 4–5 weeks +	30–40 / 50–70 in 4–7 days	29/38, 78% for all three groups combined	14/37, 37% at 5 years	—
Garden, Delclos[4]	86	EBRT + Brachy (35 patients) / 40–70 EBRT alone (21 patients)	20–70 (med 30) 30 patients brachy alone / 45–75 (med 60)	72% at 1 year / 65% at 2 years / 64% at 5 years (overall)	41% at 5 years / 31% at 10 years / 22% at 15 years (overall)	Urethral stenosis (11/86) 13% / Cystitis/hemorrhage (6/86) 7% / Fistula/necrosis (10/86) 12%
Klein, Kersh[10]	3	40–50	27–30	3/3, 100% @ 27–37 months	2/3, 67%	None
Nori, et al.[7]	12	20–40 in 2–5 weeks	40–60 in 4–7 days	67% 5 years	67% 5 years (88–100% 5 years for anterior lesion <4 cm with low hist. grade)	Urethral stricture, 1 patient (8%) / Urinary incontinence, 1 patient (8%)
Prempree[11]	14	40–45	15–20	78%	77% 5 years	Urethral stenosis, 2 patients (4%) / Leg edema, 1 patient (stage IVa) (14%)

EBRT = external beam radiation therapy; NED = no evidence of disease.

1949 and 1972 for carcinoma of the female urethra. Patients received either 60–70 Gy of EBRT or 40–50 Gy of EBRT combined with a 30–40 Gy brachytherapy boost, or primary interstitial brachytherapy to deliver 50–70 Gy in 4–7 days. Overall, local control was obtained in 76% of the cases. Survival at 5 years was 37%. Tumor extension to the bladder, paraurethral tissue, or vulva was felt to worsen prognosis.[10]

A second nonrandomized, retrospective study from M.D. Anderson Medical Center, by Garden et al.,[4] looked at a total of 86 patients treated between 1955–1989. Twenty-one patients received 40–71 Gy of EBRT; 35 patients received 20–70 Gy (median dose = 46 Gy) external beam combined with a brachytherapy boost of 20–70 Gy (median dose = 30 Gy). Thirty patients were treated with primary interstitial radiation to 45–75 Gy (median dose = 60 Gy). Local control rates in the combined treatment group were 72% at 1 year, 65% at 2 years, and 64% at 5 years. Actuarial survival rates were 41% at 5 years, 31% at 10 years, and 22% at 15 years. Extension of tumor to adjacent structures, fixation of the primary lesion, or involvement of the entire urethra all resulted in worse survival (P<0.05); involvement of the entire urethra also resulted in worse local control. Complications resulted from therapy in 49% of the patients who had obtained local control, and their data show that increasing the dose results in increased complications but does not improve the local control rate.

Klein et al.[10] reported on three patients with urethral carcinoma treated with EBRT and interstitial iridium-192 with a template technique. Three patients received 40–50 Gy of EBRT combined with a 27–30 Gy brachytherapy boost. Local control was 100% at 27–37 months; the survival rate was 67%. No complications were reported.

Nori et al.[7] and Hilaris et al.,[8] at Sloan Kettering Memorial Hospital, reported on 12 patients with urethral carcinoma treated with interstitial iridium-192 to deliver a dose of 40–60 Gy to the primary tumor in 4–7 days. In some patients, the pelvic lymph nodes received 20–40 Gy of EBRT as well, if they were believed to be at high risk of developing metastatic disease. The local control and actuarial survival rates at 5 years were both 67%. However, for anterior lesions <4 cm in size and of low histologic grade, the survival rates at 5 years were as high as 88%–100%. Complications were seen in only two patients, including one urethral stricture and one patient with urinary incontinence.

Prempree et al.[11] reported on 14 nonrandomized patients with carcinoma of the urethra treated with radiotherapy. Three stage I patients received 50–65 Gy of brachytherapy alone; ten patients with stage II-III disease received 40–45 Gy of EBRT combined with a 15–20 Gy brachytherapy boost. One patient with stage IVb cancer received 50 Gy of EBRT over 5.5 weeks. Local control was obtained in 78%, and the 5-year survival rate was 77%. Complications were noted as "rare" (two urethral strictures and one case of leg edema in a patient who had been treated with EBRT and surgery). Poor prognostic factors were bladder neck involvement, parametrial extension, and inguinal node involvement.

Discussion

Local control achieved by brachytherapy ranges between 64%–100%, with actuarial survival ranging from 37%–100% at 5 years (Table 1). Narayan and Konety[12] reported a 5-year survival rate of 47% (32%–100%) after surgical treatment of tumors limited to the anterior female urethra, in comparison to a survival rate of 11% (0%–21%) for treatment of lesions of the entire urethra, with local control. They also report a recurrence rate of 66%–100%.

Sequelae of Treatment

Complications related to treatment of carcinoma of the female urethra can be difficult to manage and care must be taken to minimize them. Reported complication rates vary from 0%–42%, including urethral stenosis, incontinence, cystitis, bowel obstruction, fistulization, and postoperative mortality.[3] Immediate reactions, such as mucositis, can be expected to peak at 10 days to 2 weeks after removal of the implant and may last from 4–8 weeks; the severity may be decreased by using an empty vaginal cylinder and rolled sponges or pads to displace the adjacent normal tissues. Acutely, urethral irritation including dysuria and urinary frequency may be expected as well. Long-term complications, such as vaginal synechia, urethral stenosis, fistulization, and necrosis, may also occur. Vaginal synechia may be minimized by appropriate hygiene combined with the use of a vaginal dilator. Urethral stenosis can often be treated with dilatations as needed. Fistulization, which may occur as a result of tumor regression or due to irradiation-induced tissue necrosis, may be decreased with careful treatment planning and implantation technique and is best managed conservatively with sitz baths and frequent hydrogen peroxide irrigation.[2]

Summary

Brachytherapy administered as primary treatment or adjuvently with external radiation or surgery has been found to be an effective method to treat cancers of the female urethra. The techniques afford results comparable to those achieved with surgical management, while maintaining organ function.

References

1. Komaki R. Female urethra. In: Pierquin B, Wilson JF, Chassagne D (eds). Modern Brachytherapy. Masson Publishing, New York, 1987, pp. 215–219.
2. Delclos L. Carcinoma of the female urethra: Interstitial irradiation. In: Johnson DE, Boileau MA (eds). Genitourinary Tumors: Fundamental Principles and Surgical Techniques. Grune & Stratton, New York, 1982, pp. 275–286.
3. Perez CA, Pilepich MV. Female urethra. In: Perez CA, Brady LW (eds). Principles and Practice of Radiation Oncology. J.B. Lippincott, Co, New York, 1992, pp. 1059–1066.
4. Garden AS, Zagars GK, Delclos L. Primary carcinoma of the female urethra: Results of radiation therapy. Cancer 1993;71:3102–3108.
5. Forman JD, Lichter AS. The role of radiation therapy in the management of the male and female urethra. Urol Clin North Am 1992;19: 383–389.
6. Delclos L, Wharton JT, Flether GH, et al. The role of brachytherapy in the treatment of primary carcinoma of the vagina and female urethra. In: Frederick WG III (ed). Modern Interstitial and Intracavitary Radiation Managment. Masson Publishing, New York, 1981, pp. 78–82.
7. Nori D, Leibel SA, Son YH. Urethral cancer. In: Anderson LL, Nori D, Nath R, et al. (eds). Interstitial Brachytherapy: Physical, Biological, and Clinical Considerations. Raven Press, New York, 1990, pp. 213–216.
8. Hilaris BS, Nori D, Anderson LL. Brachytherapy in cancer of the female urethra. In: Hilaris BS (ed). An Atlas of Brachytherapy. Macmillan Publishing, New York, 1988, pp. 286–292.
9. Delclos L, Wharton JT, Rutledge FN. Tumors of the vagina and female urethra. In: Fletcher GH (ed). Textbook of Radiotherapy. Lea & Febiger, Philadelphia, 1980, pp. 826–828.
10. Klein FA, Ali MM, Kersh R. Carcinoma of the female urethra: Combined iridium Ir-192 interstitial and external beam radiotherapy. South Med J 1987;80:1129–1132.
11. Prempree T, Amornmarn R, Patanaphan V. Radiation therapy in primary carcinoma of the female urethra. Cancer 1984;54:729–733.
12. Narayan P, Konety B. Surgical treatment of female urethral carcinoma. Urol Clin North Am 1992;19:373–382.

Chapter 24

Brachytherapy for Cancer of the Penis

Subir Nag, M.D., Rodney J. Ellis, M.D.

Introduction

Carcinoma of the penis is rare in the United States, occurring mainly in uncircumcised males after the age of 50. Primary surgical treatment of carcinoma of the distal penis requires partial or total amputation of the penis, resulting in psychological trauma of emasculation and sexual dysfunction. Hence, radiation therapy is the treatment of choice if a comparable control rate can be achieved. The radiation can be given by external beam, brachytherapy, or a combination.

Methods

An initial circumcision is performed to accurately evaluate the tumor extension and reduce the mobility of swelling and secondary infection.

External Beam Radiation Therapy

External beam radiation therapy (EBRT) can be given by orthovoltage radiation for fairly superficial lesions. More invasive tumors are treated using megavoltage irradiation (cobalt-60 or 4–6 MeV x-rays). Specialized techniques, including tissue equivalent bolus, have to be used to ensure homogeneity. Doses of 60–70 Gy are generally given in 30–35 fractions. These doses are restricted to 50–55 Gy if a smaller number of fractions are used. Another option is to use a moderate dose of EBRT (40–45 Gy) followed by a 20–25 Gy boost with brachytherapy.

Interstitial Brachytherapy

Interstitial brachytherapy was commonly performed using radium needles. This had the disadvantage of radiation exposure and, therefore, an afterloading iridium-192 technique is now commonly used. Unless the lesion is very superficial, a two plane implant is commonly used. The procedure is performed under spinal or general anesthesia. A Foley catheter is inserted into the bladder. Hollow needles are then introduced, parallel and 1 cm apart (Figure 1). Templates may be used to maintain the parallel spacing of the implant. We prefer to use button-ended catheters instead. Gauze is used to hold the penis in a perpendicular position. This also serves to displace the testes, thereby minimizing the radiation dose to the testes. Care has to be taken to ensure the entire tumor is implanted with sufficient margins. Smaller lesions, <0.5-cm thick, may be implanted by a single plane, taking care to extend the implant beyond the lesion.

Doses of 60–70 Gy are delivered over 4–8 days. The Foley catheter is kept in for the entire duration of the implant and removed 1–2

From Nag S (ed): *Principles and Practice of Brachytherapy.* © Futura Publishing Co., Inc., Armonk, NY, 1997.

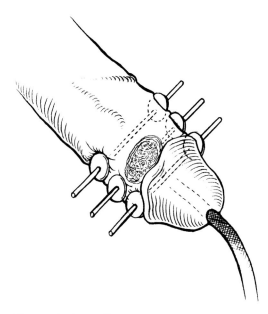

Figure 1. A small superficial carcinoma of the penis, implanted with Ir-192 by three catheters inserted in a single plane. A Foley catheter is inserted into the bladder.

days after completion of the brachytherapy. Antibiotic coverage (for example 1-gm Ancef) is advised during the procedure and maintained for a few days after removal of the implant. Proper skin care is maintained.

Mold Technique

An alternative technique that can be used for superficial tumors is the use of a cylindrical mold placed over the penis. The mold is worn by the patient for about 10–12 hours daily and is removed to allow the patient to urinate and sleep. The mold is placed in a lead lined box when not used. The patient keeps track of the total time worn. This technique, therefore, requires a very cooperative patient who is able to maintain radiation safety and is able to keep track of the total duration of use. Since it is difficult to maintain quality assurance and due to stringent radiation safety requirement in the United States, we prefer not to use this technique.

Indications for Brachytherapy

1. Brachytherapy is usually used for well circumscribed small tumors <3 cm in diameter with tumors limited to the glans penis and/or prepuce. The tumor may extend into the shaft, but there should be no nodal metastases.
2. If there are palpable inguinal lymph nodes, an inguinal lymphadenectomy is performed with postoperative EBRT (45–50 Gy) added if the lymph nodes are pathologically involved.
3. Patients with larger tumors are not good candidates for brachytherapy and are preferably treated by an amputation. However, if they refuse an amputation, EBRT and brachytherapy is an alternative.

Results

A number of centers, mainly in Europe, have retrospectively reported their results treating cancer of the penis with brachytherapy and have shown good local control ranging from 67%–93%, with actuarial survival rates from 58%–89% (Table 1). Organ function was retained in 67%–80% of the cases. These results compare favorably with other series that have reported comparable results for surgery or radiotherapy for T1 and T2 lesions.[1]

Neave et al.[2] reported a nonrandomized retrospective analysis of 44 patients with penile carcinomas who were treated with radiotherapy at the Royal London Hospital. Twenty patients received 50–55 Gy with EBRT while 24 patients received brachytherapy with an iridium-192 mold. The brachytherapy dose was prescribed to deliver 55.6 Gy to the surface and 46.3 Gy to the central axis of the penis. Local control was 67% overall, with a 53% control rate for the external beam group verses 79% for the brachytherapy group. The higher rate of control for the group treated with iridium was attributed to a treatment bias favoring brachytherapy for more favorably staged lesions. Actuarial survival rates for the combined groups were 87.9% at 2 years, 85.1% at 5 years, and 72.3% at 10 years. Both the response rate and the actuarial disease-free survival were equal for both groups for stage I patients. Complete response rates were related to the Jackson stage, with 80% response for stage I, 56% for stage II, and 0% for stages III and IV. Complications of therapy were limited to urethral strictures, 10% for ex-

Table 1.
Carcinoma of the Penis: Results of Radiotherapy

Author[ref]. (Institution)	Number of Patients	EBRT Dose (Gy)	Brachy Dose (Gy)	Local Control	Actuarial Survival	Complications	% Retaining Organ Function
Neave, et al.[2] (Royal London)	44	50–55 20–22 fx (20 patients)	Ir mold: 55.6 surface 46.3 central axis (24 patients)	Complete response 67% overall (79% Brachy 53% EBRT)	87.9% 2 years 85.1% 5 years 72.3% 10 years	Stricture 10% EBRT 13% mold	Not stated
Danczak-Ginalska[5] (Warsaw)	48	N.A.	Ra mold: 60–80 (30 patients) Ir: 70–90 (18 patients)	Ra 93% 3 years Ir 89% 3 years	Ra 93% 3 years Ir 89% 3 years	Ra 50% necrosis 7% stricture Ir 16% necrosis 0% stricture	72% overall, both groups combined
Delannes[4] (Centre Claudius Regaud)	51	N.A.	50–65 (mean 60)	91% T1–T2	71.8% 5 years 62.4% 10 years	23% necrosis 45% stenosis	67% overall 75% for T1–T2 tumors
Raynal, et al.[6] (Gustave Roussy/Henri Mondor)	45	55–60 for (+) pelvic L.N.	65–70	<30 mm 4 years = 86% >30 mm–40 mm 4 years = 83% >40 mm 4 years = 0%	58% 4 years	Delayed cicatrization Sclerosis	Not stated
Mazeron, et al.[7] (Henri Mondor)	50	50–60 for (+) L.N. Mixed beam	60–70 (mean 65)	89% T1, 78% T2, 71% T3 Post salvage 100% T1, 96% T2, 79% T3	59% 5 years	15% necrosis 5% sclerosis 20% stenosis	74%
Haile, Delclos, et al.[3] (M.D. Anderson)	20	45–50 to L.N. if at high risk	60Co mold: 60 Ra implant: 70–71	90%	—	20% necrosis 15% stenosis	80%
Rozan, et al.[8] Grp. A (Brachy) Grp. B (Brachy + EBRT)	259 184 75	40.5 (26 patients)	192Ir wire Group A: 63 Group B: 50	Local control = 85% overall	66% 5 years 52% 10 years	61% overall 30% stricture	78% Group A 64% Group B

EBRT = external beam radiation therapy; LN = lymph node; pts = patients.

ternal beam and 13% for brachytherapy; there was no reported necrosis.

Haile and Delclos[3] reported the M.D. Anderson experience with 20 patients who were treated with a variety of methods including superficial radiotherapy, external beam, radium implants, and a mold technique using cobalt-60. They obtained a 90% local control rate and reported that organ function was preserved in 80% of the patients; they did not report survival rates. Complications included urethral stenosis (15%) and necrosis (20%). Furthermore, they concluded that elective lymph node dissections were not warranted and that elective nodal radiation was recommended only for high risk patients in whom the groin was not clinically involved.

Delannes et al.[4] reported the Centre Claudius Regaud experience with a nonrandomized series of 51 patients with penile carcinoma treated with brachytherapy implants using iridium-192. Doses ranged between 50–65 Gy. Local control was 91% for T1 and T2 lesions, and survival rates were 71.8% and 64.2% at 5 and 10 years, respectively. The penis was conserved in 67% of the cases, with 75% conservation for T1 and T2 lesions. Complications included a 45% urethral stenosis rate and a 23% necrosis rate.

Danczak-Gilanlska[5] reported the Warsaw data on a nonrandomized series of 48 patients. Thirty patients treated with a radium mold received 60–80 Gy while the other 18 patients received iridium-192 implants delivering 70–90 Gy. Survival and local control were equal for both groups at 3 years; for those treated with radium molds, the local control rate was 93% and the survival rate was 83%, compared to 89% for both local control and survival at 3 years for the implanted group. Overall, 72% retained organ function; however, the iridium group had higher retained organ function. Complication rates were also lower in the implanted group, with 23% necrosis and 0% stenosis in the iridium group compared to 50% necrosis and 7% stricture in the radium group.

Raynal et al. reported on 45 nonrandomized patients with penile carcinoma treated with radiotherapy at the Institute Gustave Roussy and the Henri Mondor Hospital. Patients received 65–70 Gy to the primary lesion with afterloaded iridium-192; if the pelvic lymph nodes were involved, they also were treated with 55–60 Gy of EBRT. Data regarding local control at 4 years revealed that patients with lesions <30 mm in size (T1 or T2) had 86% local control at 4 years; that those with lesions >30 mm but <40 mm (T3a) showed an 83% control rate; and that those with lesions >40 mm in size (T3b and T4) had 0% local control at 4 years. Overall survival at 4 years was 58%, and complications included delayed cicatrization and sclerosis.[6]

In another nonrandomized series at Henri Mondor, Mazeron et al.[7] reported the radiotherapy results of 50 patients treated for penile carcinoma. These patients received between 60–70 Gy (mean 65 Gy) to the tumor via iridium-192 implants. If the lymph nodes were involved, they also were treated using a mixed beam of photons and electrons to deliver 50–60 Gy of EBRT. Local control was 89% for T1 lesions, 78% for T2 lesions, and 71% for T3 lesions. Post-treatment failures were salvaged with surgery to obtain 100% local control for T1 tumors, 96% for T2, and 79% for T3. Survival at 5 years was 58%. Organ function was retained in 74% of the cases.

Recently, Rozan et al.[8] reported results from a multicenter survey of 259 patients who received brachytherapy for penile carcinoma. Group A consisted of 184 patients treated with brachytherapy alone (63 Gy mean dose) using an afterloading Ir-192 wire technique. Group B consisted of 75 patients treated with surgery and brachytherapy (50 Gy mean dose); 26 patients in this group also received EBRT (40.5 Gy). Overall survival was 66% and 52% at 5 and 10 years, respectively. Local control was 85% overall. Organ function was retained in 78% of group A patients and in 64% of group B patients.. Tumor volume influenced complications, and the presence of lymph node involvement was found to affect survival; however, systematic lymph node dissection was not recommended. A second analysis of surgery and EBRT is pending, which should help to further define the role of radiotherapy in treating carcinoma of the penis.

Discussion

Complications due to radiotherapy of penile carcinomas are both acute and long term.

The immediate reaction, consisting of erythema, dry to moist desquamation, and subcutaneous swelling, is often mild and may last from 4–8 weeks. A 4- to 5-day course of antibiotics should be given after removal of the implant, and careful hygiene of the area should be maintained, including cleansing with mild soap and water and hydrogen peroxide and application of cortisone ointment.[9] Telangiectasia occurs as a late effect in most patients but is usually asymptomatic. Urethral stenosis has been reported (0%–40% frequency).[10] Most often, the urethral stenosis can be relieved through dilatation. Necrosis should first be managed conservatively but may, as a last resort, require amputation. Fistulization or recurrences are best managed surgically.[9]

Summary

Brachytherapy as primary treatment or in combination with EBRT or surgery has been found to be an effective method to treat cancers of the penis. The techniques afford efficacy comparable to that achieved by surgical management, and the improved cosmetic, psychological, and functional results brachytherapy provides make it an attractive alternative to other modalities.

References

1. Gerbaulet A, Lambin P. Radiation therapy of cancer of the penis: Indications, advantages, and pitfalls. Urol Clin North Am 1992;14:325–332.

2. Neave F, Neal AJ, Hoskin PJ, et al. Carcinoma of the penis: A retrospective review of treatment with iridium mould and external beam irradiation. Clin Oncol 1993;5:207–210.

3. Haile K, Delclos L. The place of radiation therapy in the treatment of carcinoma of the distal end of the penis. Cancer 1980;45:1980–1984.

4. Delannes M, Malavaud B, Douchez J, et al. Iridium-192 interstitial therapy for squamous cell carcinoma of the penis. Int J Radiat Oncol Biol Phys 1992;24:479–483.

5. Danczak-Ginalska Z. Treatment of penis carcinoma with interstitially administered iridium: Comparison with radium therapy. In: Grundman E, Vahlensieck W (eds). Tumors of the Male Genital System: Recent Results in Cancer Research. Springer-Verlag, New York, 1977, pp. 127–133.

6. Raynal M, Chassagne D, Baillet F, et al. Endocurietherapy of penis cancer. In: Grundman E, Vahlensieck W (eds). Tumor of the Male Genital System: Recent Results in Cancer Research. Springer-Verlag, New York, 1977, pp. 135–139.

7. Mazeron JJ, Langlois D, Lobo PA, et al. Interstitial radiation therapy for carcinoma of the penis using iridium-192 wires: The Henri Mondor experience (1970–1979). Int J Radiat Oncol Biol Phys 1984;10:1891–1895.

8. Rozan R, Albuisson E, Giraud B, et al. Interstitial brachytherapy for penile carcinoma: A multicentric survey (259 patients). Radiother Oncol 1995;36:83–93.

9. Delclos L. Interstitial irradiation of the penis. In: Johnson, Barlean (eds). Genitourinary Tumors. Grune & Stratton, New York, 1982, pp. 219–225.

10. Perez CA, Pilepich MV. Penis and male urethra. In: Perez CA, Brady LW (eds). Principles and Practice of Radiation Oncology. J.B. Lippincott Co, New York, 1992, pp. 1131–1142.

Chapter 25

Low-Dose-Rate Intracavitary Brachytherapy for Carcinoma of the Uterine Cervix

Kathryn E. Dusenbery, M.D., Bruce J. Gerbi, Ph.D.

Introduction

Megavoltage external beam pelvic radiation therapy (EBRT) combined with intracavitary brachytherapy is the standard radiotherapeutic management for patients with carcinoma of the cervix. Low-dose-rate (LDR) brachytherapy has been used since the early 1900s, but starting in the late 1950s with the cathetron cobalt-60, high-dose-rate (HDR) brachytherapy has become an acceptable treatment modality.[1-3] Although there are few randomized trials comparing the advantages and disadvantages of each approach, one major advantage to LDR is the extensive clinical experience and accumulated data that exists that demonstrates its efficacy and safety. Additionally, radiobiological data suggests that LDR may enhance the therapeutic ratio, possibly sparing the late effects in the bowel or bladder. This is particularly important for patients with gynecological malignancies since most of these patients will be cured of their cancer and will survive long enough to be at risk for developing late complications. This chapter focuses on the medical and technical considerations of LDR brachytherapy in cervical cancer. The relative advantages of LDR and HDR therapy are not discussed, but are outlined in Table 1.

Overview of the Treatment Plan

Design of the radiation treatment program depends on the extent and volume of the tumor. Staging (clinical or surgical) consists of a complete history and physical examination, a number of laboratory studies (complete blood count, blood chemistry, and urinalysis), a chest x-ray, and either an intravenous pyelogram or CT scan of the abdomen and pelvis along with an examination under anesthesia (EUA). The EUA allows the radiation oncologist to physically determine the size and consistency of the cervix, as well as with any extension beyond the cervix to the parametrium, pelvic side wall, or vagina. Disease extent should be carefully documented with detailed notes or diagrams. These diagrams can be referred to at the time of the first brachytherapy application, when significant tumor shrinkage may have occurred and the full extent of disease is not so obvious. During the EUA, a cystoscopy and proctoscopy may be done to determine if there is extension to the bladder or rectum. Additionally, some in-

From Nag S (ed): *Principles and Practice of Brachytherapy.* © Futura Publishing Co., Inc., Armonk, NY, 1997.

Table 1.
Advantages of Low- and High-Dose-Rate Brachytherapy

Low-Dose-Rate Advantages	
Patient	Long history of use
	Ability to predict rate of late complications
Clinical	Improves chances of catching tumors in sensitive phase of cell cycle
Physical	Longer treatment times allows for leisurely review of and potential modifications to the treatment plan prior to the delivery of a significant portion of treatment
	Favorable dose-rate effect on repair of normal tissues
	Infrequent replacement and calibration of sources because of long isotope half-life
High-Dose-Rate Advantages	
Patient	No short- or long-term confinement to bed
	No indwelling bladder catheters
	Not labeled "radiation risk zone" to relatives, visitors, and staff
	Avoid several anesthesias (possibly)
Clinical	Maintain position of the sources during the brief treatment
	Patient preparation
	No specialized nursing
	Ability to treat greater patient loads (high output of patients on each machine)
Physical	Short treatment times and minimal radiation protection problems
	Possibility of optimizing dose distribution by altering the dwell times of the source at different locations

Modified from Joslin, C.A.[67]

stitutions add an extraperitoneal pelvic and periaortic lymph node sampling,[4,5] which provides prognostic information and may help in designing the limits of the EBRT fields.

Most patients receive a combination of external beam treatments and brachytherapy, although very early lesions may be treated with brachytherapy alone. The ratio of external beam dose relative to brachytherapy dose can be determined by general guidelines, although experience provides optimal treatment determinations. In general, advanced tumors require more EBRT because the rapid decrease in dose occurring at a distance from the brachytherapy implant may result in inadequate treatment of the peripheries of large tumors. For advanced tumors, most or all of the EBRT is given prior to brachytherapy to shrink the tumor. This leads to a technically superior brachytherapy application and may result in radiobiological advantages,[6] such as better oxygenated and, therefore, more radio-sensitive tumor cells.

The first brachytherapy application is performed 3–4 weeks after the start of EBRT. The second application is usually performed 2 weeks later. Two implants are generally considered to be superior to a single implant.[7] During the intervening 2 weeks between

brachytherapy applications, the remainder of the whole pelvis (with or without periaortic nodal chain) and split pelvis irradiation may be given. The entire course of treatment, including both brachytherapy applications, usually takes 6–7 weeks. Protracted treatment times are associated with decreased local control and survival rates.[7a-7c]

Design of the external beam fields takes into account the predictable manner in which cancer of the uterine cervix usually spreads, first laterally into the paracervical nodes, then to the internal iliac, common iliac, and finally into the periaortic nodes. In patients with early disease, the nodes are often not involved. For larger tumors, the risk of nodal spread beyond the pelvis increases. Knowledge of nodal involvement is important when designing EBRT fields. In institutions where lymph nodes are surgically sampled, the number and distribution of involved nodes are known with some certainty. If surgical staging is not performed, the CT scan, lymphangiogram, or pelvis MRI scan may help identify suspicious nodes, which often can be biopsied under CT guidance.

In general, the EBRT includes the pelvis for patients with small tumors and with no evidence of spread to the pelvic lymph nodes.

We usually extend the field to include the low periaortic nodes (to the level of the second lumbar vertebrae) for patients with pathologically confirmed spread to the pelvic (but not periaortic) nodes. For patients with periaortic nodal spread, we include the entire periaortic chain (to the level of the tenth thoracic vertebra).[8–11] In patients who are not surgically staged and have no clinical evidence of pelvic or periaortic nodal spread, the limits of the EBRT are individualized, but for patients with large cervical tumors or extension into the parametrium, we generally extended the EBRT field to at least the low perioaortic nodal area. The prophylactic use of extended fields remains controversial.[12–14]

In addition to the initial whole pelvic or whole pelvic and periaortic EBRT, it is often desirable to continue to treat the nodal areas while blocking the central area where the high dose from the brachytherapy application is concentrated. Fields that have the central area blocked are called split pelvis fields. Some institutions design partial transmission blocks that correspond to the isodose lines of the brachytherapy application. At the University of Minnesota, our split pelvis block is generally 4.5 cm wide. The height of the block is determined by the height of the tandem and roughly corresponds to the height of the 30 cGy/hr isodose line.

Low-Dose-Rate Brachytherapy

Patients undergo a preoperative history and physical examination prior to the application of brachytherapy since medical conditions may have changed since initiating the EBRT and may influence the brachytherapy application. A complete blood count, electrolyte profile, and creatinine are obtained. For patients older than 40 years, a recent ECG is recommended. Patients should have had a chest x-ray at the time of diagnosis, so this is not repeated unless an abnormality was seen. If the patient is on coumadin, the anticoagulation is usually not reversed, but the level of anticoagulation is ascertained and adjusted as necessary.

For patients with an intact uterus, three intracavitary application types can be considered: 1) an intrauterine tandem with vaginal ovoids; 2) an intrauterine tandem (only) with a protruding vaginal source; or 3) an intrauterine tandem with a vaginal cylinder. The majority of patients will be candidates for an intrauterine tandem and vaginal colpostats. However, if more than 2–3 cm of the vagina is involved, the colpostats will not be adequate to cover the extent of vaginal disease. In such cases, a vaginal cylinder in conjunction with the intrauterine tandem should be considered. In patients with bulky (>2- to 3-cm long and >0.5 cm thick) vaginal involvement that does not respond to the initial 3–4 weeks of EBRT, an interstitial application should be considered.

For patients who have undergone a hysterectomy, brachytherapy alone or in conjunction with EBRT is often recommended.[15–21] Brachytherapy is recommended for patients at high risk for vaginal recurrence. The indications for a vaginal brachytherapy application after hysterectomy include patients who have undergone less than a modified radical hysterectomy (often because the cervical cancer was not suspected preoperatively) and patients who have a close or involved margin either at the parametrium or vagina at the time of the hysterectomy. Adjuvant EBRT either alone or in addition to brachytherapy is recommended for patients at high risk of pelvic failure after hysterectomy and include:

1. patients with lymph nodes involvement;
2. patients with large tumors (>4 cm);
3. patients with high grade tumors or tumors with lymph vascular space involvement.

Obviously, an intrauterine tandem cannot be used after a hysterectomy has been performed. Posthysterectomy patients without palpable residual central disease receive either a vaginal colpostat application or a vaginal cylinder. In the rare situation where a subtotal hysterectomy has been performed and a radical parametrectomy is contraindicated (i.e., tumor adheres to the bladder or rectum and nodes are positive), an interstitial application should be performed (as covered in another chapter).

Equipment

Manual afterloading Fletcher-Suit-Delcos tandem and vaginal colpostats are used for

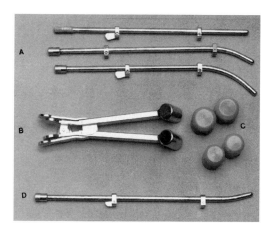

Figure 1. Fletcher-Suit-Delclos tandems, ovoids, and caps for ovoids. A) Tandems available curved or without curvature. B) Rectangular handled ovoids. Each ovoid has a 2.0-cm diameter. C) Caps available in two sizes resulting in ovoid diameters of 2.5 and 3 cm, respectively. D) Most frequently used tandem (#1 curvature), embossed at 2-cm intervals corresponding to eventual location of the cesium. Isodose distribution at 1.5 cm above and of effect of shielding around the colpostats.

the majority of cervical cancer patients at the University of Minnesota (Figure 1). Over 100 other applicators are available worldwide. LDR remote afterloading systems, which minimize the exposure to medical personnel, are available from manufacturers in several countries. For both manual and remote afterloading, the clinical, radiobiological, and physics principles of LDR are the same. Only the size of the applicators, radiation protection features, and possibly the ability to limit applicator movement during treatment differs. Integral to the applicator itself is an implantation system that has evolved around the use of those applicators. Paramount to performing LDR brachytherapy is a familiarity and comfort with the brachytherapy implantation system as well as the specifics of the applicators chosen by the radiation oncologist.

Fletcher-Suit-Delclos Colpostats

The original Fletcher colpostats were introduced in the early 1950s to replace the then standard Manchester radium tubes and ovoid applicators. Rectal and bladder shielding were provided but the colpostats needed to be preloaded. A subsequent modification by Suit in the later 1950s (Fletcher-Suit rectangular handled afterloading colpostat) allowed for afterloading, but modifications to the shielding were needed because of mechanical difficulties. These mechanical difficulties were corrected and the original shielding design is available for afterloading use (Fletcher-Suit round handled afterloading colpostat). Figure 2 illustrates the position of the tungsten shields and the resultant isodose distribution at 1 cm above and 1.5 cm below the ovoids.[22] The clinical significance of these shielding differences has not been determined.

Fletcher Intrauterine Tandems

The stainless steel intrauterine tandems are available without curvature (#0) or with three curvatures (#1, #2, and #3) that fit the majority of uterine cavities. The #1 curvature is most often used, but the more curved #2 or #3 tandems are appropriate for a significantly anteverted uterus or for a long intrauterine canal. Embossed lines are present at 2-cm intervals along the tandem, corresponding to the eventual location of the cesium sources that will be loaded into the tandem. The stainless steel collar (flange) is placed at the line corresponding to the length of the intrauterine canal. When sutured to the external os, it prevents the tandem from sliding further into the uterus (and therefore preventing fundal perforation). When sutured to the cervix, it serves as a radiographic marker of the position of the cervix.

Vaginal Cylinders

Vaginal cylinders that are afterloaded are used in conjunction with an intrauterine tandem to irradiate the vagina when the disease extends from the uterine cervix along the vaginal walls (Figure 3). A cylinder alone may be used after a radical hysterectomy if there is a close or positive vaginal margin. A vaginal cylinder is also useful for a patient with a very narrow vagina in whom it is technically difficult to secure the collar on the intrauterine tandem to the cervix. A small vaginal cylinder may be used for these patients, since the ring that fits over the cylinder can be sutured to

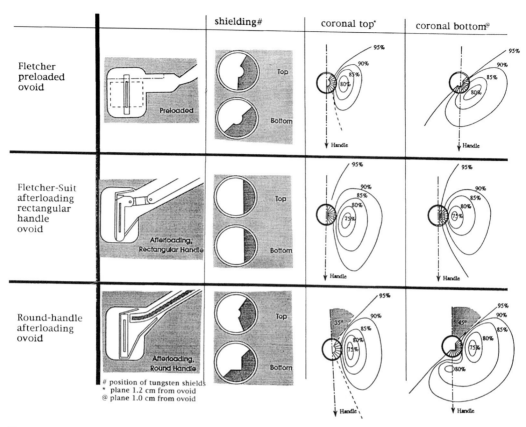

Figure 2. Three generations of Fletcher ovoids demonstrating the tungsten shielding design and resultant isodose distributions at 1.2 cm above and 1.0 cm below the ovoids. (Modified from Haas et al.[22] and Radium Accessories Services, Inc, Marathon, FL, USA; both with permission.)

the vulva to secure the intrauterine tandem. Cylinders are available in various diameters (1–5 cm) and lengths to fit any vaginal width and length. Some cylinders have hollow channels within them that allows for the option of inserting tungsten shields into one or more of the hollow channels to partially shield one or more of the vaginal walls.

Radioisotope

Most LDR intracavitary brachytherapy systems use cesium as the implanted radioisotope. One advantage of cesium-137 over radium-226 is the elimination of radon gas leakage. Another advantage is less required shielding for radiation protection because of the lower energy emitted from the photons, 0.662 MeV versus 0.8 MeV average (2.2 MeV maximum). Cesium may be purchased encapsulated asymmetrically in either platinum or stainless steel. The potential dosimetric consequences of this asymmetry is usually ignored.[23] The physical characteristics of one brand may differ somewhat from another. A commonly used cesium source has a physical length of 2 cm, physical width of 0.31 cm, and an active length of 1.4 cm (Figure 4).

General Procedure

At the University of Minnesota the insertion of these applicators is usually performed jointly with the gynecological oncologist. Although insertion of these appliances is often considered a "minor" surgical procedure, it is advantageous to have an experienced gynecological oncologist present. Often the tumor

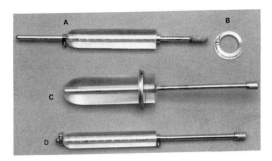

Figure 3. Vaginal cylinders are available in a variety of lengths and sizes. A) Arrangement for use on an intrauterine tandem and vaginal cylinder with collar sutured to the cervical os. B) Ring is placed around the cylinder, tightened at the appropriate position, and is sutured to the vulva at four sites. C. Custom vaginal cylinder designed to obviate the need for the collar at the vaginal apex[68] as seen in D.

has obliterated normal anatomy and finding the uterine canal without creating a false passage or perforating the uterus is difficult.

For insertion of the Fletcher-Suit-Delclos tandem and ovoids, the patient can choose either spinal or general anesthesia. Spinal anesthesia has the advantage that it wears off slowly, usually not until after completion of the simulation and after the patient has been transported to her room. By then other analgesics are available allowing for a smooth transition to either oral or parenteral pain control. Since the patient will be on bed rest for up to 3 days, preventing the development of a deep venous thrombosis is important. At the University of Minnesota, we use sequential pneumatic devices (pneumoboots) and low-dose (5000 units twice daily) subcutaneous heparin. Routine antibiotics are not prescribed unless the cervix is extremely necrotic or we suspect that the uterine wall was inadvertently perforated or a false passage created during the insertion.

Insertion of the Fletcher-Suit Tandem and Ovoids

In addition to the brachytherapy equipment, additional surgical equipment (usually found in a standard dilatation and curettage tray) is necessary for insertion of the tandem and ovoids (Figure 5). The patient is placed

in the dorsal lithotomy position and given an EUA. The extent of disease is delineated and compared to the preradiation therapy examination. It is particularly important to feel the position of the uterus. In most, but not all patients, the uterus is slightly anteflexed. Knowing the uterine position will help guide the

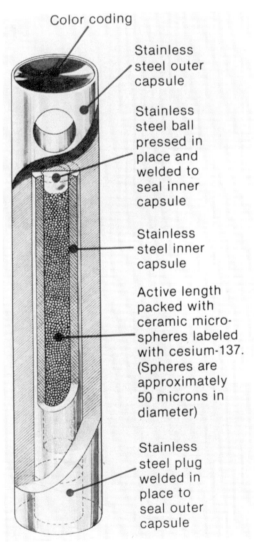

Figure 4. Cesium-137 tubes consist of asymmetrically placed cesium-labeled ceramic microspheres packed within a stainless steel or platinum casing. The eyelet is usually color coded to correspond to the nominal strength of the cesium. (From Medical Products Division/3M, St. Paul, MN, USA. Used with permission.)

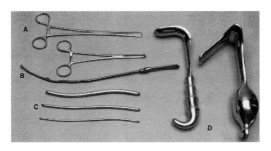

Figure 5. A dilatation and curettage tray usually has the major surgical equipment necessary for a tandem and ovoid application including an Allis clamp or single tooth tenaculum to grasp the cervical lip (A), a uterine sound (B), Hegar dilators to dilate the uterine canal (C), and a retractor and weighted speculum to help visualize the cervix (D).

sounding of the uterine canal. The perineum and vagina are then prepped with an antiseptic solution. The field is draped with sterile towels. A Foley catheter is placed into the bladder and the balloon filled with 7 cc of radiopaque contrast material (diatrizoate meglumine Hypaque[R]). A weighted speculum is placed in the vagina. The anterior cervical lip is grasped with a single tooth tenaculum or Allis clamp. The uterine canal is

sounded with a uterine sound and its length noted. Care is taken not to perforate through the uterine wall. If the uterine canal is difficult to find, ultrasound guidance can provide assistance (Figure 6). Serial dilatation of the cervical os is performed. A size of #7 Hegar (or #16 Hanks) is usually adequate to insert the tandem.

The collar on the tandem is placed at the mark on the tandem corresponding to the length of the uterine canal. Cesium sources are generally 2 cm in length, and since the aim is to have the lowest cesium source in the tandem at the level of the cervix, it is convenient if the uterus sounds to an even length (i.e., 6 or 8 cm). The collar then can be set at the 6- or 8-cm mark (Figure 7). If the uterus sounds to an odd length (i.e., 5 or 7 cm) the mark closest (but shorter) than the sounded length should be used. If the uterine canal sounds to a length of >8 cm, we generally set the cervical collar at the 8-cm mark.

At the University of Minnesota, we routinely suture the collar to the cervix using nonabsorbable suture material to ensure that the tandem will not dislodge. The suture is either run through the small tunnel at the collar and tied at the cervix, or a second collar is placed more distally (Figure 8) and the suture is run

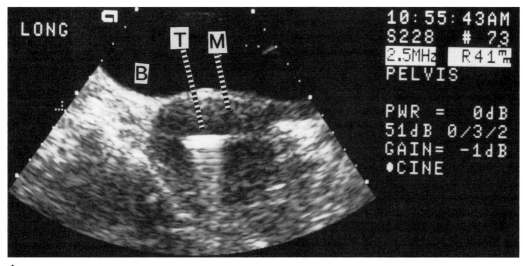

A

Figure 6. A) Longitudinal ultrasound image through the uterus demonstrating bladder (B), myometrium (M), and correct position of tandem within the uterine cavity (T).

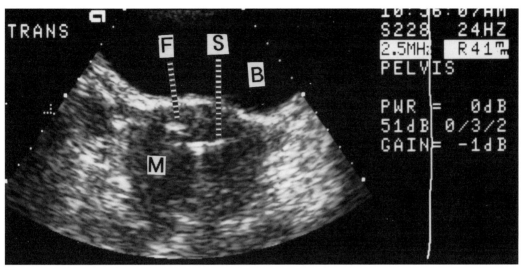

B

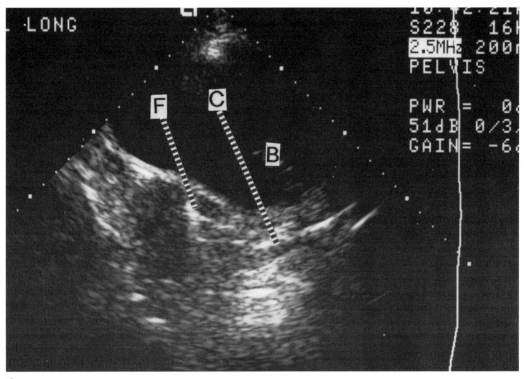

C

Figure 6. *(continued)* B) Longitudinal ultrasound image showing two echogenic stripes consisting of the tandem in a false passage (F) and endometrial stripe (S) where tandem should be. C) Transverse ultrasound image through the uterus demonstrating a false passage (F) that was inadvertently created and the true uterine canal (C).

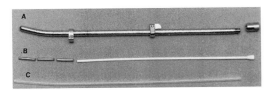

Figure 7. A) The proximal collar on the tandem is secured at the appropriate embossed line that will correspond to the eventual position of the cesium within the tandem. B) "Dummies" are oriented eyelet distally. A plunger that keeps the cesium sources at the apex of the tandem. C) The cesium sources are placed in a hollow nylon tube, followed by the plunger.

through both collars and tied at the distal collar. The knot is cut long to facilitate removal.

One of the advantages of the Fletcher-Suit tandem and ovoid applicators is that the tandem is inserted separately from the ovoids. By using various size caps and angles on the ovoids and curvatures on the tandem, the application can be customized to the patient's tumor and anatomy. The aim is to achieve a high-dose rate within the tumor and a low-dose rate in the critical normal tissues (bladder and rectum). This is usually accomplished by trying to orient the tandem relative to the ovoids so that the resultant isodose distribu-

tion around the application bears the typical pear-shaped distribution with the bottom of the pear encompassing the tumor. Achieving this distribution is referred to as optimizing the geometry of the application. This idealized geometry does not always correspond to the distribution of the tumor, and what appears to be a less than ideal geometry may actually yield a dose distribution around the tumor that is ideal.

After the tandem is secured, the colpostats are inserted. The size of the vaginal vault dictates what size caps (if any) can be placed on the colpostats. The colpostats should fit snugly against the vaginal fornices. In general, the largest caps that fit and still result in good geometry should be used. This optimizes the depth dose ratio. If the colpostats are too large, they do not fit into the vaginal fornices and are displaced into the distal vagina (caudally). It is sometimes difficult (especially for the novice) to tell if the colpostats are displaced caudally after the tandem and ovoids are in the patient. Therefore, prior to insertion of the tandem into the patient, a useful "trick" is to put the tandem next to the ovoids and to visualize where the proximal collar should be relative to the ovoids (Figure 9) and then set the second collar exactly at the point the ovoid handles come together. This distal collar will then serve as a marker for whether the ovoids are too cranial or too caudal relative to the tandem.

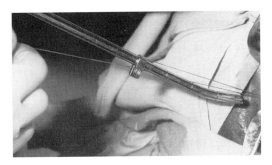

Figure 8. To prevent the tandem from dislodging, the proximal collar is sutured to the cervix by placing a suture through the cervix and running the suture through the hollow channel on the collar. Instead of securing the knot at the proximal collar, the suture can be threaded through a second collar placed more distally along the tandem and the knot tied at the distal collar. This facilitates removal of the tandem at the completion of the implant.

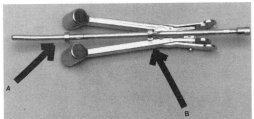

Figure 9. Since it is difficult to ascertain whether the ovoids are too proximal or distal relative to the cervix, the tandem and ovoids are placed in their desired orientation and the second collar is conveniently placed at the position where the ovoid handles come together prior to inserting them into the patient. Thus when the tandem and ovoids are in the patient, the distal marker helps determine if the geometry is good.

For a narrow vault in which the standard size colpostats will not fit, minicolpostats can be considered. However, at the University of Minnesota we prefer to use a protruding vaginal source (also called a hanging tandem) because of a higher incidence of bladder and rectal complications reported with the use of minicolpostats.[24] When the colpostats are in place, the tandem needs to be secured to the ovoids. We use a sterilized rubber band, but umbilical tape also can be used to tie the colpostats to the tandem. Alternatively, some systems have a yoke that secures the tandem to the colpostats and helps align the tandem relative to the colpostats to potentially improve the geometry.

Packing is used to optimize the geometry of the application and to displace the rectum posteriorly and bladder anteriorly away from the colpostats. Rolled gauze soaked in an antibacterial solution (Acroflavin, Spectrum Quality Products, Inc., Gardena, CA, USA) is used at the University of Minnesota. A metallic ribbon in the gauze helps outline the relative position of the vagina to the bladder and rectum. Because of the weight of the colpostats, there is a tendency for them to displace posteriorly. For that reason, the packing usually begins posteriorly, pushing the colpostats anteriorly. Packing anteriorly may be used at the midline to push the bladder anteriorly.

Representations of the desired geometric relationship between the tandem and ovoids are shown in Figure 10. An orthogonal pair of radiographs of a Fletcher-Suit tandem and ovoid application with good geometry is shown in Figure 11. In general, the aim is to have the tandem bisect the two ovoids. On anterior view, approximately one-third of the ovoid should be superior to the cervical collar and two-thirds should be inferior to the cervical collar. On lateral view, the colpostats should bisect the tandem, although most of the time the ovoids are slightly posterior to the tandem.

After the packing is completed, a Foley catheter is placed in the rectum and the balloon filled with contrast material (Hypaque). To confirm that a good geometry has been obtained, anterior and lateral x-rays are taken. This is usually accomplished with a portable x-ray unit. A C-Arm can also be used, but this is not possible with all operating room tables.

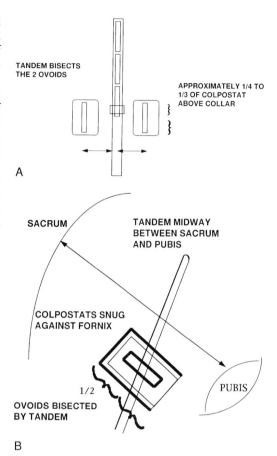

Figure 10. A) Diagram illustrating the desired orientation of the tandem relative to the ovoids as seen on an anterior view. B) Diagram illustrating the desired orientation of the tandem relative to the ovoids as seen on a lateral view.

If the applicator geometry is not "good," the packing is removed and the patient is repacked. The process is repeated as necessary. Examples of poor geometry implants are shown in Figure 12. Every attempt should be made to optimize the relationship between the tandem and ovoids. Further repacking is not necessary if after one or two attempts of repacking there is no improvement in geometry either because of the patient's anatomy or tumor extent; at this point, a decision must be made about how to load the tandem and ovoids. In general, if the distorted geometry leads to a higher tumor dose with an acceptable rectal and bladder dose, it is usually loaded with cesium as usual. If this is not the case, alternate loadings, or waiting an additional 1–2 weeks for more tumor shrinkage, is advisable.

Occasionally the vault is narrow and although the colpostats (without caps) can be inserted into the vagina, the x-ray reveals that they are inferior to the cervical collar. Repacking will not be of benefit in this situation since the problem is not with the alignment of colpostats relative to the tandem, but with the patient's anatomy (narrow vagina). Some authors have advocated minicolpostats in this situation. Minicolpostats have a diameter of 16 mm (regular colpostats 20 mm) and a flat inner surface. Early models had no shielding, although newer models are commercially available with tungsten shields. When loaded

with 10-mg cesium, minicolpostats deliver roughly the same vaginal surface dose as the small colpostats. When combined with the tandem, however, the bladder and rectal dose rates may be prohibitive. High bladder and rectal complication rates have been reported with minicolpostats.[24,25] An alternative to minicolpostats for patients with narrow vaginas is to load the tandem with a source that protrudes below the cervical collar into the upper vagina. This protruding vaginal source increases the dose rate within the cervical tumor without leading to prohibitively high bladder or rectal dose rates. The disadvantages to using the protruding vaginal source are that the distribution of dose near the cervix is not expanded inferiorly as is obtained with the addition of ovoids, that a longer im-

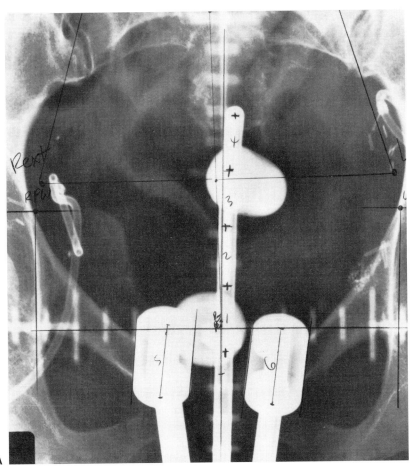

Figure 11. Radiographs of desired orientation of the tandem and ovoids. A) Anterio-posterior.

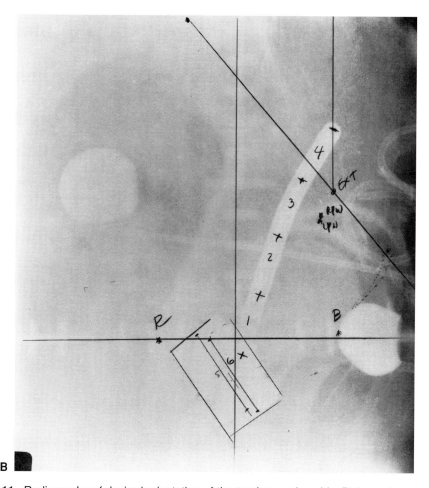

Figure 11. Radiographs of desired orientation of the tandem and ovoids. B) Lateral.

plant duration is required to achieve a certain total point A dose, and that the mg-hr prescription system cannot be used to determine implant duration. Additionally, bowel and bladder complications may be higher than with standard sized ovoids.[26] Alternatively, some institutions use intersititial brachytherapy in these cases (see Chapter 27).

Insertion of the Intrauterine Tandem and Vaginal Cylinder

The intrauterine tandem is inserted as previously described. The appropriate diameter vaginal cylinder is introduced over the intrauterine tandem and secured with a second collar. A metal ring slides over the cylinder and is tightened just distal to the introitus. The ring has four holes in it to suture the cylinder to the vulva at the corresponding four positions.

Insertion of the Vaginal Colpostats

Colpostats alone are used in patients at risk for a vaginal cuff recurrence. The length of vagina effectively treated with colpostats is relatively short (1–3 cm). Therefore, colpostats are usually not adequate for patients with vaginal cancer or a vaginal recurrence (e.g., from endometrial cancer). The same procedure in positioning, examining, prepping, and draping is carried out as above. The blad-

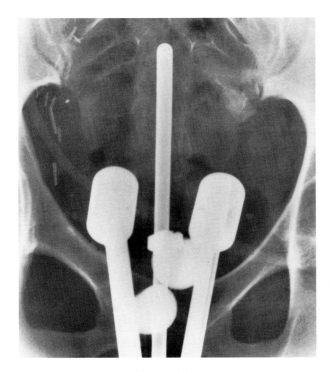

Figure 12A

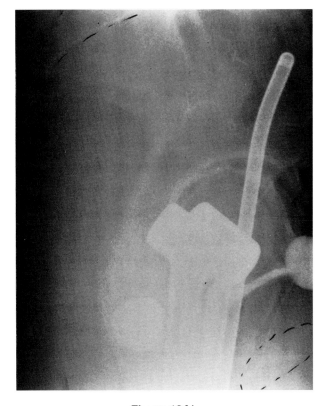

Figure 12A′

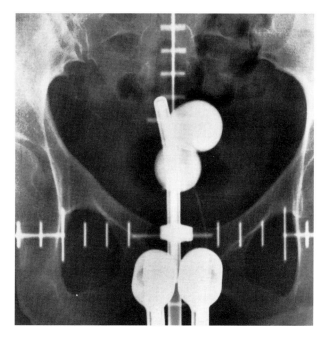

Figure 12B

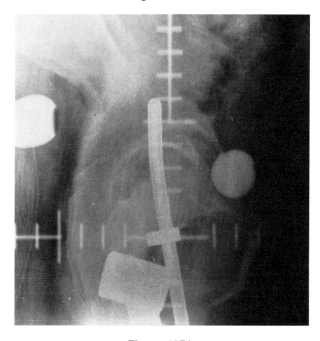

Figure 12B′

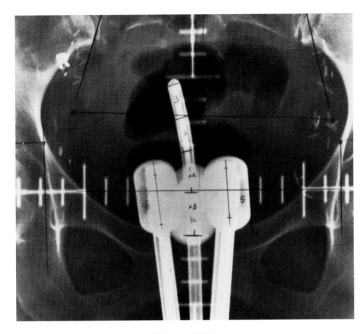

Figure 12C

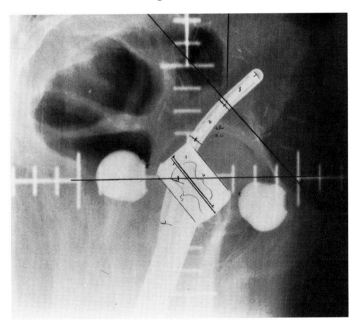

Figure 12C′

Figure 12. Radiographic examples of poor geometry. A and A′) Portable x-ray taken in the operating room demonstrating ovoids that are placed too inferior and posterior relative to the tandem. Repacking is indicated. Note that the ovoids are widely spaced and placing caps on the ovoids may help. B and B′) Radiograph demonstrating ovoids that are too inferior and posterior relative to the tandem. If caps are on the ovoids, removing them might improve the geometry. C and C′) The ovoids are anterior relative to the tandem resulting in a very high bladder dose rate.

der Foley catheter is inserted and the balloon filled with Hypaque. The size of the vaginal vault is estimated and the colpostats with the largest, most snugly fit caps are inserted. The goal is to secure the colpostats against the vaginal wall. Packing is used to hold the applicator in place and to push the rectum and bladder posteriorly and anteriorly away from the colpostats without increasing the distance between the area at risk for recurrence and the ovoid. To prevent the colpostats from dislodging in patients with short vaginas, the colpostat handles may be sutured to the vulva.

Insertion of the Vaginal Cylinders

When treating a longer segment of vaginal involvement, a vaginal cylinder is used instead of the colpostats. The same procedure is followed, but instead of colpostats, a vaginal cylinder is placed in the vagina. The cylinder with the greatest diameter, that produces a snug, but not tight fit, is used. This serves to optimize the dose at depth relative to the surface dose. A ring placed over the distal end of the cylinder is secured to the cylinder by means of a screw. The ring is then sutured to the vulva in four locations corresponding to holes in the ring at the 2, 4, 8, and 10 o'clock positions using nonabsorbable suture material.

Simulation

After insertion of the applicator, "dummy" cesium sources are loaded into the afterloading appliances and an orthogonal pair of radiographs are taken. The isocenter is set at the center of the collar for Fletcher-Suit tandem with ovoid applications or at the center of the application for other types of implants. The isocenter is set at the center of the two ovoids for the ovoids and, for the vaginal cylinder, at the center of the cylinder midway between the most proximal and most distal cesium "dummy" source. An anterior and lateral pair of orthogonal simulation films are taken. The "dummy" sources and rectal balloon are removed and the patient is transported back to her hospital room.

Applicator Loading Determination

After reviewing the orthogonal films, the "preliminary written directive" for loading the

cesium sources is decided upon. It is unusual for the final plan to differ from this preliminary plan, but occasionally this will occur. The Nuclear Regulatory Commission requires that the radiation oncologist provide a "preliminary written directive" that includes the patient's name, identifying information, radioisotope, number of sources, source strength, and date. This must be signed by the authorized user physician before the cesium can be loaded into the patient (Figure 13).

The standard loading for a 6-cm (3 sources) intrauterine tandem is 15 mg, 10 mg, 10 mg and for an 8-cm (4 sources) tandem is 15 mg, 10 mg, 10 mg, 10 mg. The standard loading for the vaginal ovoids are 15 mg for 2-cm diameter ovoids (with no caps); 20 mg for 2.5-cm diameter ovoids (with small caps); and 25 mg for 3.0-cm diameter ovoids (with large caps). Exceptions to these guidelines are for patients who have a "barrel-shaped" cervix. These patients have considerable tumor bulk in the expanded lower uterine segment. It is reasonable to put a more active source lower in the tandem for example, 15 mg, 15 mg, 10 mg (or 10 mg, 15 mg, 10 mg) in a 6-cm tandem loading and 15 mg, 15 mg, 10 mg, 10 mg (or 10 mg, 15 mg, 15 mg, 10 mg) in an 8-cm tandem loading, respectively.

A 15 mg source is never placed just above the cervical collar because the contribution of the ovoids to the dose in that area is considerable and the bladder and rectum are close. If ovoids cannot be used because of a narrow vagina, a single protruding vaginal source of 10 mg is added below the collar. Although minicolpostats are available, a high rate of rectal and bladder complications have been reported with their use.[24,25] We prefer the protruding vaginal source (e.g., 15 mg, 10 mg, 10 mg, 10 mg in a 6-cm tandem loaded), even though a higher risk of bladder and rectal complications may be seen in this instance as well.[26]

If a vaginal cylinder is used, the activity of the cesium put into the cylinder depends on the cylinder diameter. A computer plan can provide vaginal surface dose rate. However, since the computer plan often takes several hours to complete, and the patients are anxious to complete the implant, it is useful to know the approximate vaginal surface dose rate with a certain diameter cylinder loaded

UNIVERSITY OF MINNESOTA HOSPITAL AND CLINIC
DEPARTMENT OF THERAPEUTIC RADIOLOGY
BRACHYTHERAPY TREATMENT

WRITTEN DIRECTIVE

PATIENT IDENTIFICATION PLATE

I. PRIOR TO IMPLANTATION

PATIENT'S NAME		U of M HOSPITAL #
DIAGNOSIS	TREATMENT SITE	
STATION	REFERRING PHYSICIAN	

ISOTOPE USED
Cs-137 ☐   Ir-192 ☐   I-125 ☐   Other ☐   BATCH #

APPLICATOR(S) USED

# Ribbons	#Seeds/Ribbon	Total # seeds
mg. Ra. Equiv. per seed	Total mg. Ra. Equiv.	

DIAGRAM OF APPLICATION	TANDEM? YES ___ NO	NUMBER OF SOURCES
	COLPOSTATS? YES ___ NO	DIAMETER OF COLPOSTATS cm
	VAGINAL CYLINDER? YES ___ NO	DIAMETER OF CYLINDER cm

STAFF SIGNATURE:

II. PRIOR TO COMPLETION OF IMPLANT

TOTAL HOURS	DOSE [mg. hrs] (1.07 FILTRATION FACTOR INCLUDED)		
DOSE **(cGy)**	Point A	Point B	BLADDER	RECTUM
	VAGINAL SURFACE		

STAFF SIGNATURE:	PHYSICS SIGNATURE:

INSERTED	DATE	TIME	BY
REMOVED	DATE	TIME	BY

MR 307. DEC 93   WHITE-MEDICAL RECORD   YELLOW AND PINK-THERAPEUTIC RADIOLOGY DEPT.

Figure 13. Prior to placing the cesium in the patient a preliminary written directive must be completed and signed by the radiation oncologist. Prior to the completion of the implant, the final written directive must be completed.

a certain way so that the "preliminary written directive" can be completed and the cesium loaded into the applicator without delay. "Up and away" tables are useful in this regard (Table 2).

Another useful rule of thumb is that a 2-cm diameter cylinder with four sources loaded with 10 mg, 10 mg, 10 mg, 10 mg sources will yield a vaginal surface dose rate (at midimplant) of approximately 100 cGy/hr, and a dose rate at 0.5-cm deep to the surface of 60 cGy/hr. Larger diameter cylinders will give correspondingly lower dose rates. For example, a 3-cm diameter cylinder loaded identi-

Table 2.
Surface Dose Rates as a Function of Cylinder Diameter and Number of Sources

Diameter of Cylinder (mm)	Cesium (mg)	Number of Sources	Effective Length of Vagina Treated (mm)	Lateral Vaginal Surface Dose Rate (cGy/Hour)
20	10	1	16	71
"	10	2	34	87
"	10	3	51	108
"	10	4	65	102
26	15	1	19	64
"	15	2	32	91
"	15	3	52	110
"	15	4	62	118
32	20	1	18	57
"	20	2	32	88
"	20	3	48	107
"	20	4	57	116
36	25	1	22	60
"	25	2	33	92
"	25	3	47	115
"	25	4	62	123

Modified from Johnson and Potish with permission.[68]

cally will yield a 60 cGy/hr vaginal surface dose rate. Since the dose fall off is almost linear with distance at very close distances to the brachytherapy applicators, an approximation is possible of the corresponding vaginal surface dose rate. The preliminary written directive can be filled out accordingly, then modified depending on the computer plan.

After the "preliminary written directive" is completed, the cesium can be prepared for transportation to the patient's hospital room. A plastic straw, with a smaller diameter than the tandem, holds the cesium sources in tandem. A plunger keeps the sources at the apex of the straw. Since the cesium is positioned asymmetrically in the stainless steel capsule, the correct orientation for the cesium in the straw (in the tandem) and in the ovoids is illustrated in Figure 14.

We use a series of double checks to make sure the correct strength cesium sources are prepared for the patient. The lead pigs that are used to transport the cesium to the patients room are labeled with the patient's name. A "cesium transport card" accompanies the cesium (Figure 15). Before administering the brachytherapy dose, the identity of the patient must be verified by two independent means by checking the name of the pa-

tient against the name printed on the written directive. Moveable shields are placed on both sides of the patient's bed. After the cesium is placed in the applicator, the date and time of the loading are indicated on the cesium transport card and on the patient's hospital chart, which should also include a diagram of the loading and total source strength.

A survey of the room and surrounding area measure the exposure in mR/hr to assure that exposure rates are within acceptable limits to

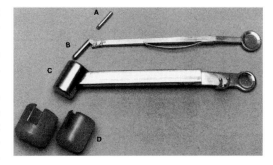

Figure 14. The cesium (A) is placed with the eyelet down in the holder (B), which is then slid into the ovoid (C). The two cap sizes are shown (D), which increase the ovoid diameter from 2.0 cm to 2.5 cm and 3.0 cm, respectively.

hospital personnel and patients who might be in adjoining rooms. The exposure rate at the patient's door and at the wall closest to the patient in adjoining rooms must be below 2 mR/hr. If not, additional shielding is placed until these limits are met. Signs on the patient's door alert others to the presence of radioactivity.

Computer Planning: Dose Calculations

For all brachytherapy implants, computerized dosage calculations are performed using the orthogonal film pair to provide the positional data of the sources and the applicators. To accomplish this, a variety of software packages are available. The general procedure includes digitizing the following points on the orthogonal x-rays into the computer planning system:

1. Tips and ends of the cesium sources.
2. Bladder reference point. Foley balloon is filled with 7 cc of radio-opaque fluid (Hypaque) and pulled down towards the bladder neck. On the lateral radiograph the reference point is obtained by drawing a line through the center of the balloon and the posterior surface of the balloon is used as the reference point. On the anterior radiograph the reference point is taken at the center of the balloon (Figure 16).
3. Rectal reference point. The International Commission Radiological Units and Measurements (ICRU) rectal reference point is obtained by drawing an anterior-posterior line on the lateral radiograph from the lower end of the intrauterine source (or from the middle of the intravaginal sources). The rectal point is taken at a depth of 0.5 cm, posterior to the point where this line traverses the posterior vaginal wall (the vaginal wall is identified by intravaginal radio-opaque gauze). The anterior coordinates of the rectal

UNIVERSITY OF MINNESOTA HOSPITAL AND CLINIC
DEPARTMENT OF THERAPEUTIC RADIOLOGY–RADIATION ONCOLOGY

ISOTOPE TRANSPORT CARD CESIUM ☐ IRIDIUM ☐ OTHER ☐

PATIENT NAME:	HOSPITAL NO.

APPLICATION NO. ☐ 1 ☐ 2 ☐ 3 ☐ 4 ☐ 5

DIAGRAM OF IMPLANT

APPLICATOR: mg. RA. EQ. IF IR-192:

☐ TANDEM ________ Batch #: ____________
☐ COLPOSTATS ________ NO. of SEEDS________
☐ CYLINDER ________ mg.Ra.Eq./SEED on________=________ (date)
☐ SIMON'S CAPSULES ________
☐ NEEDLES ________ Batch #: ____________
☐ OTHER: ____________ ________ NO. of SEEDS________
mg.Ra.Eq./SEED on________=________ (date)

TOTAL ACTIVITY ________

INSERTED	DATE	HOUR	No. of Sources	BY
REMOVED	DATE	HOUR	No. of Sources	BY

TOTAL HOURS	EQ.MG. HRS.
RADIOISOTOPE CURATOR	STAFF

23424, NOV 93

A

Figure 15. A) Cesium transport card accompanies movement of the cesium outside the radioisotope safe.

APPENDIX A-IV
PATIENT ROOM SURVEY FORM
University of Minnesota

Patient Identified by two independent means (Yes/No): _____

Diagram of implant, isotope, number of sources, and total activity in hospital chart (Y/N): _____

INITIAL ROOM SURVEY   Room Number: _____
(following insertion of sources)

Instrument used for the survey:

      Ionization Survey Meter_____ ; GM Survey Meter_____

EXPOSURE RATE: mR/hr

			Less than 2 mR/hr	
(A)	1 m from patient (unshielded):	_____		
(B)	At bedside (behind shield):	_____	Yes	No
(C)	Door to room:	_____	____	____
(D)	Wall closest to patient, in adjoining room:	_____	• ____	____
(E)	Wall farthest from patient, in adjoining room:	_____	• ____	____
(F)	Chair at foot of bed (if applicable):	_____	____	____

Patient in adjoining room(s); Room No(s). _____, _____

- If exposure rate for (C) through (E) is greater than 2 mR/hr, reposition the bed and/or shields to reduce the exposure rate to ≤2 mR/hr. If the exposure rate cannot be reduced to ≤2 mR/hr, notify the Therapeutic Radiology physicist on call or a member of the Radiation Protection Staff (see cesium or iridium emergency procedures for contact numbers).

*This need not be done if radioisotopes are present in the adjoining room.

Signature _____ Date/Time _____

FINAL ROOM SURVEY (following removal of the sources)

Instrument used for the survey:

      Ionization Survey Meter_____ ; GM Survey Meter_____

EXPOSURE RATE:

Patient _____mR/hr; Room _____mR/hr; Walls _____mR/hr

If exposure rate is greater than 2 mR/hr, indicate the reason: _____
_____

- If reason is a dislodged or missing source, immediately contact the physician/resident and Radiation Protection staff member on call (see cesium or iridium emergency procedures for contact numbers).

- If the exposure rate is greater than 2 mR/hr due to a radiation patient in an adjacent room, reposition the bed and/or shields in the adjacent patient's room to reduce the exposure rate to ≤2 mR/hr. If the exposure rate cannot be reduced to ≤2 mR/hr, notify the Therapeutic Radiology physicist on call or a member of the Radiation Protection Staff (see cesium or iridium emergency procedures for contact numbers).

B Signature _____ Date/Time _____

Figure 15. *(continued)* B) A convenient place to document some of the quality management program items is on the back of the cesium transport card, including the initial room survey (which is done after the cesium is loaded into the patient to assure low exposure rates for nurses and patients in adjoining rooms) and the final room survey (done as a double check to make sure the radioisotope has been removed).

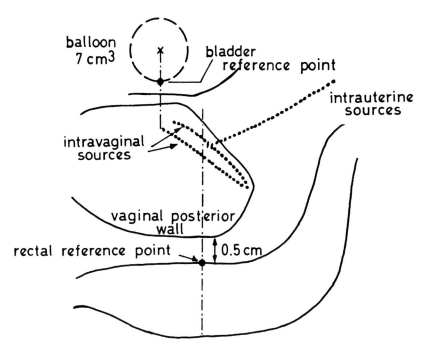

Figure 16. Location of bladder and rectum points as specified by the ICRU.[33] (From ICRU Report No. 38. Bethesda, MD: International Commission on Radiation Units and Measurements, 1985. Used with permission.)

point is at the lower end of the intra-uterine source or at the middle of the intravaginal sources at midline (Figure 16).

4. The Fletcher Lymphatic Trapezoid Points. A line is drawn from the junction of S1-S2 to the top of the symphysis. Then a line is drawn from the middle of that line to the middle of the anterior aspect of L4. A trapezoid is constructed in a plane passing through the transverse line in the pelvic brim plane and the midpoint of the anterior aspect of the body of L4. A point 6-cm lateral to the midline at the inferior end of this figure is used to give an estimate of the dose rate to the midexternal iliac nodes. At the top of the trapezoid, points 2-cm lateral to the midline at the level of L4 are used to estimate the dose to the low para-aortic nodes. The midpoint of a line connecting these two points is used to estimate the dose to the low common iliac nodes (Figure 17).

5. The Pelvic Wall Points. Pelvic wall reference points can be visualized on an AP and lateral radiograph and related to fixed bony structures. This point is intended to be representative of the absorbed dose at the distal part of the parametrium and at the obturator lymph nodes. On an AP radiograph, the pelvic-wall reference point is intersected by a horizontal line tangential to the highest point of the acetabulum and a vertical line tangential to the inner aspect of the acetabulum. On a lateral radiograph, the highest points of the right and left acetabulum, in the craniocaudal direction, are joined and the lateral projection of the pelvic-wall reference point is located at the middistance of these points (Figure 18).

Implant Duration

Milligram-Hours

When only radium sources were available in the precomputer era, gynecological

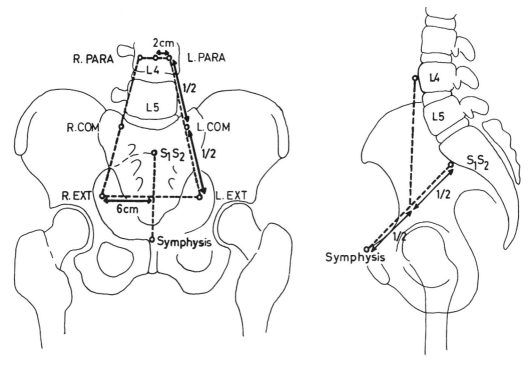

Figure 17. Determination of reference points corresponding to the lymphatic trapezoid of Fletcher.[33] (From ICRU Report No. 38. Bethesda, MD: International Commission on Radiation Units and Measurements, 1985. Used with permission.)

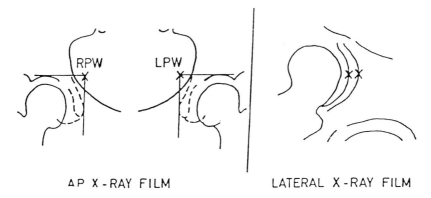

Figure 18. Definition of pelvic wall points.[33] Position of right pelvic wall (RPW) and left pelvic wall (LPW) are diagrammed. (From ICRU Report No. 38. Bethesda, MD: International Commission on Radiation Units and Measurements, 1985. Used with permission.)

brachytherapy applications were specified by the simple mathematical product of the number of milligrams of radium times the duration (in hours) of the implant. Thus an implant with five 10-mg radium sources left in place for 48 hours would yield a dose of 2400 mg-hrs (10 × 5 × 48). Since its initial use in the early 1900s in Europe, a dose prescription system evolved and was refined at M.D. Anderson hospital by Dr. Gilbert Fletcher.[27] Results obtained at M.D. Anderson are among the best in the world. At the University of Minnesota we depend heavily on the Fletcher mg-hr system to specify dose. A 7% correction factor (8.25/7.71) is used to convert the Fletcher mg-hrs to ICRU mg-hrs, since the mg-hrs recommended by Dr. Fletcher are for implants with radium encapsulated in 1-mm platinum (exposure rate constant 7.71 R/cm $2h^{-1 \, mg-1}$) and the ICRU specifies that radium sources with 0.5-mm platinum filtration be used as the standard (exposure rate constant 8.25 R/cm^2 h^{-1}mg^{-1}).

Although the mg-hr system is easy to use, this method does not provide information about the dose distribution around that application. The system works because it specifies a particular geometry between the tandem and ovoids and the sources are loaded in a rigidly prescribed manner. It is only applicable when both the tandem and ovoids are implanted. For a tandem loaded with a protruding vaginal source (no ovoids), the mg-hr dose specification is not applicable.

Point A

The second dose prescription system that evolved specifies the dose to four specific points in space around the applicator, points A, B, bladder, and rectum. Originally developed in Manchester England, this system is often referred to as the Manchester system. Point A was initially defined as the point 2 cm superior to the vaginal fornix and 2 cm lateral to the cervical canal. Point B was 3 cm lateral to point A. Points A and B were said to represent critical anatomical structures, point A representing the site where the uterine vessels crossed the ureter and point B representing the location of the more lateral pelvic nodes.

Although point A is usually described as 2 cm superior and 2 cm lateral to a specified origin, the definition of the point of origin is not standardized. Since the initial description of point A, many different origins have been defined without a clear consensus as to which origin is standard (Figure 19).[28] Depending on which origin is chosen, the point A dose can vary widely, especially if the ovoids are displaced either superiorly or inferiorly. A relatively small displacement of the ovoids superiorly results in a large increase in the dose rate to point A. Since dose rates fall off very rapidly with distance from the brachytherapy sources, any point surrounding the applicator will be expected to be in a rapid dose fall-off area, another disadvantage of using point A. For small tumors, point A may even lie outside the tumor volume, whereas for larger tumors, the tumor may extend significantly more lateral than point A. Since some definitions of point A are radiographic, point A may end up outside of the cervix all together.

At the University of Minnesota, we specify either point A_v or A_o to attempt to better specify the radiographic location of point A. The subscripts o and v refer to the os and vaginal fornix, respectively. In most situations, point A_v is used with the vertical origin determined on lateral radiograph at the point where the colpostat cap crosses the tandem and is 2 cm superior to this point along the axis of the cervical source, then 2 cm lateral. When colpostats are unable to be used (most often due to narrow vaginal vault), A_v cannot be specified (since with the absence of the ovoids, the vaginal fornix is not radiographically outlined), and instead A_o is specified as the vertical origin determined on anterior radiograph at top of the cervical collar 2 cm superior to this point along the axis of the cervical source, then 2 cm lateral.

Association Between Point A, Point B, and Milligram-Hours

In a perfect Fletcher-Suit implant loaded as described above, point A almost always lies between 50–60 cGy/hr. Point B usually lies between 10–20 cGy/hr and is largely dependent on the source strength in the ovoids. Because these dose rates for point A and B are usually confined to a narrow range, as are implant durations, it is not surprising that there is an association between these total point

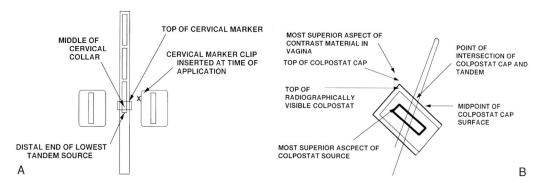

Figure 19. A) Possible origins of point A on anterior view. B) Possible origins of point A on lateral view.

doses and mg-hrs.[28-32] In an evaluation of almost 100 brachytherapy applications performed at the University of Minnesota, we found a fairly high correlation between mg-hrs of radium and doses at point A and point B (correlation coefficients of 0.73 and 0.89, respectively).[30] However, point A dose was markedly affected by the position of the colpostats relative to the tandem, and considerable interpatient variability made the routine translation between Fletcher and Manchester systems too unpredictable for clinical use. Despite these limitations, it is useful to roughly translate mg-hrs into point A or point B doses. Bhatnager[32a] has suggested a formula that roughly calculates the point A dose based on the milligrams of radium loaded.

$$\text{Point A(cGy/hr)} = 1.1\{(\#\text{mg in tandem}) + (\#\text{mg in ovoids}/2)\} \text{ cGy/hr}^{32a}$$

Likewise, the following formula roughly converts mg-hrs into the total point B dose.

$$\text{Point B (total dose in cGy)} = (\text{total mg-hrs in 2 implants}) \div 4$$

International Commission on Radiological Units and Measurements

In 1985, the ICRU recommended a system of LDR brachytherapy dose and volume specifications aimed at redefining and standardizing brachytherapy reporting terminology.[33] Three reporting approaches were proposed

to specify intracavitary applications (Table 3). Since specification of dose in brachytherapy involves complex three-dimensional gradients that do not lend themselves to simple reporting, it was suggested that all three methods be used to complement each other. These methods of dose specification were to report: 1) reference air-kerma rate; 2) absorbed dose at certain reference points; and 3) isodose reference volume.

The reference air-kerma rate was proposed

Table 3.
ICRU Reporting Data

Description of Technique
Source used (radionuclide, reference air kerma rate, shape and size of source, and filtration)
Simulation of linear source for point or moving sources
Applicator geometry (rigidity, tandem curvature, vaginal uterine connection, source geometry, shielding material)
Total Reference Air Kerma
Time Dose Pattern (Application Duration)
Description of Reference Volume
Reference isodose level
Isodose width, height, and thickness
Dose at Reference Points
Bladder
Rectum
Lymphatic trapezoid (lower periaortic, common iliac, external iliac)
Pelvic wall

ICRU = International Commission on Radiological Units and Measurements.

to introduce international units into the brachytherapy reporting. The reference air-kerma rate is expressed in mGy/hr at 1 m. The total reference air-kerma is therefore the sum of the products of the reference air-kerma rate and the duration of the application. The Fletcher mg-hrs can be easily converted into reference air-kerma by the following formula[34]:

1 mg hr = 6.5 mGy total reference air kerma (for filtration 1 mm PT)

Total reference air-kerma therefore has the same limitations as mg-hr dose specification.

The ICRU also recommended calculating absorbed dose at certain reference points (rectal, bladder, pelvic wall, trapezoid node points), but fell short of trying to standardize definitions for point A or B.

The most radical change proposed by the ICRU report was to specify reporting parameters for the pear shaped reference volume. The report states that "an absorbed dose level of 60 Gy is widely accepted as the appropriate reference level for classical low-dose-rate brachytherapy" and therefore the 60 Gy isodose reference volume was suggested. This reference volume is determined by measuring the width, height, and thickness tissue encompassed by the 60 Gy isodose curves. The method to measure these dimensions are as follows: The height (dh) is the maximum dimension along the intrauterine source and is measured in the frontal plane. The width (dw) is the maximum dimension perpendicular to the intrauterine source measured on the same frontal plane. The thickness (dt) is the maximum dimension perpendicular to the intrauterine source measured in the plane 90° lateral to the frontal plane (sagital plane).

The height (dh), thickness (dt), and width (dw) of a 60 Gy isodose reference volume, the product of which is the reference volume, are illustrated in Figure 20. The ICRU chose to subtract any EBRT from this 60 Gy reference volume. To choose the relevant isodose surface, the EBRT is subtracted from the 60 Gy volume and the remainder is divided by the implant duration to obtain the isodose surface by which to calculate the reference volume. For instance if a patient has received 40 Gy EBRT and 80 hours of brachytherapy, the 25

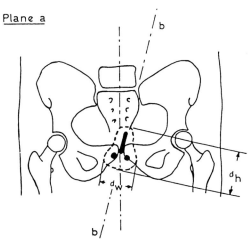

Figure 20. ICRU reference volume is determined by finding the reference isodose surface dimensions, dw (width), dh (height), and dt (thickness). (From ICRU dose and volume specification for reporting intracavitary therapy in gynecology.[33] ICRU Report No. 38. Bethesda, MD: International Commission on Radiation Units and Measurements, 1985. Used with permission.)

cGy/hr isodose surface is chosen to calculate the reference volume:

60 Gy-40 Gy = 20 Gy

20 Gy ÷ 80 hours = 0.25 Gy/hr

The 25 cGy/hour isodose surface is chosen.

The ICRU recommendation was an attempt to use the reference volume to further describe the brachytherapy application and shed light on the volume of tissue receiving a particular level of dose. Unfortunately, instead of being a helpful concept, it has only caused confusion and criticism and has been helpful neither for specification nor for reporting.[31]

The ICRU report 38 specifies a variety of points and volumes that can be reported but it does not address the question of dose prescription (implant duration). It simply gives recommendations for reporting doses, not prescribing them. The prescription of dose needs to be considered in the framework of the particular implant system being used.

The University of Minnesota Dose Specification Guidelines

At the University of Minnesota, we rely heavily on the Fletcher mg-hr dose specification system.[27] When mg-hrs are inappropriate (protruding vaginal source, vaginal cylinder) point calculations (A_v, or vaginal surface dose) are used (Table 4). The ICRU points are calculated for all patients, but are not routinely used to specify dose. We find them useful as a double check to assure ourselves that both an adequate tumor dose has been achieved (remembering that point A may

have little relationship to the tumor) and that bladder or rectal tolerances have not been exceeded (remembering that a point dose to the rectum or bladder provides no information about the dose to the rest of the rectum or bladder received).

Microinvasive (FIGO IA) tumors are unlikely to have spread to the pelvic lymph nodes. These patients may be treated with intracavitary therapy alone. Doses of up to 10,000 mg-hrs in two applications are used. For small (1–2 cm) IB tumors, up to 2,000 cGy pelvis EBRT is given depending on the extent of disease. The extent of intracavitary therapy depends on the amount of external beam whole pelvis therapy. If 2000 cGy EBRT is used, up to 8000 mg-hrs of cesium may be added in two implants. If 3000 cGy EBRT is used, up to 6500 mg-hrs of cesium may be used in two implants. The parametrial areas may be boosted with an additional 1000–2000 cGy EBRT using a split pelvis field, either with a straight split pelvis block (usually 4.5 cm in diameter) or with a step wedge block. For tumors 2–5 cm in size, 2500–3500 cGy EBRT

Table 4.
General Guidelines for Treatment of Carcinoma of the Cervix in Surgically Staged Patients

FIGO Stage	Parametrial Extension*	Tumor Size (cm)	Whole Pelvis EBRT Dose (cGy)**	Point A◆ (cGy)	Maximum mg-hour‡	Maximum Hours§	Point B† (cGy)
IB, IIA	no	<2	1000–2000	7000–7500	8000	72-2 week-48	5000–5500
		2–5	2500–3500	7500–8000	6500–7500	48-2 week-48	5500–6000
		5+	3500–4500	8000–9000	5000–6000✚	48-2 week-48	6000
IIB	yes	<2	3000	8000–9000	6000–6500	48-2 week-48	6000
		2–5	3000–3500	8000–9000	6000–6500	48-2 week-48	6000
		5+	3500–4500	8000–9000	5000–6000	48-2 week-48	6000
III	yes		4000–5000	8500–9500	5500–6000	48-2 week-48	6000
IVA	yes		individualize				

* If there is also vaginal extension, the length of vagina involved and bulk of cervical and vaginal tumor are used to determine whole pelvis EBRT dose. Since an intrauterine tandem and vaginal cylinder or iridium application are often used for patients with vaginal involvement, the mg-hour and maximum hour guidelines do no apply and dose must be individualized.

** Dose to the whole pelvis (± periaortic nodes) given with EBRT given depends on bulk of tumor, FIGO stage, and amount of regression at the time of the first brachytherapy application. If the periaortic nodes are included, periaortic nodal EBRT doses range from 4000–5000 cGy.

† Point "B" is boosted to 6000 cGy for all patients with pathologically proved involvement of pelvic nodes or tumors >2 cm in size. A split pelvis block is 4.5 cm wide with height determined by height of the tandem is used.

‡ Given in two applications, with tandem and ovoids 2 weeks apart. Does not take into account 1.07 filtration factor correction for cesium in 0.5 mm platinum.

§ This maximum is when nominal strengths of cesium of 10, 15, 20, and 25 mgs are used. If cesium of lower activity are used, the hours may be increased accordingly.

✚ Alternatively treat with a single intracavitary insertion of approximately 3000 mg-hour followed by an extrafascial hysterectomy.

◆ Point A_v is used unless ovoids cannot be used; then A_o is used.

EBRT = external beam therapy given at 175 cGy/day.

is given, and the two brachytherapy applications deliver 6500–7500 mg-hrs. For larger tumors, more whole pelvis (±periaortic nodal) EBRT is given (3000–4500 cGy), and the two brachytherapy applications are shorter (5000–6000 mg-hrs). When 4000–5000 cGy of whole pelvis EBRT has been given, between 4000–6000 mg-hrs of brachytherapy in two applications may be given. Once whole pelvis EBRT doses of over 4000 EBRT are exceeded, however, it is difficult to add significant amounts of brachytherapy. Therefore, an EUA is performed at the 4000 cGy dose level. If there has been good tumor shrinkage, the first implant is performed at that time. If the tumor is still large after an initial 4000 cGy whole pelvis EBRT and there is concern that the implant will not have good geometry, additional EBRT (with doses up to 1000 cGy) may be given.

For tumors with significant vaginal involvement, the implantation volume should include the extent of disease in the vagina. Usually the EBRT leads to shrinkage of the vaginal involvement so that at the time of the first brachytherapy application there is little palpable tumor left. Often the previous tumor is replaced with vague induration. We usually use a vaginal cylinder if this induration is minimal (<0.5 cm thick). If there is more tumor than 0.5 cm of induration remaining, implanting the vaginal component of the tumor with iridium should be considered. Tolerance of the vaginal wall to high doses of radiation probably depends on the length of vagina treated as well as on the total dose and dose rate. In general, the vaginal apex tolerates more than the distal vagina, with the apex tolerating doses of 10,000 cGy or more. More distal portions of the vagina should probably not receive more than 7000–8000 cGy.

Many institutions prefer to specify dose to "point A," as shown in Table 4. Although we usually prescribe by mg-hrs, we also carry the "point A_v" dose. We use the point A_v dose column primarily to reassure ourselves that neither an excessive nor an inadequate dose to point A_v has been delivered, keeping in mind that the point A_v dose may have little relationship to the cervical tumor dose. In the setting of a protruding vaginal source (no colpostats), the rules for mg-hrs do not apply. We therefore prescribe to point A_o in this situation.

For patients who have undergone a hysterectomy, the dose of external beam and brachytherapy need to be individualized for each patient, type of hysterectomy performed, and the surgical pathological findings (Table 5). If gross disease remains, interstitial therapy is usually given. For microscopic residual disease, intracavitary therapy is considered. The risk of bowel and bladder complications is high in this setting,[35–38] and care must be taken to minimize the risk of a late radiation complication as much as possible.

Dose to Bladder and Rectum

The ICRU suggests a method to choose which point to calculate the rectal and bladder dose. These point doses may have little relationship to the dose received by other parts of the bladder or rectum and may not

Table 5.
Post-Hysterectomy Dose Guidelines

	Dose (cGy)	
Situation	External Beam Therapy*	Brachytherapy
At risk for pelvic recurrence	4500–5000	none
At risk for vaginal recurrence	none	8–10,000 VSD (6500–7500 to 0.5 cm depth)
At risk for both pelvic and vaginal recurrence	4500–5000	4–5,000 VSD (2500–3500 to 0.5 cm depth)

* 175–200 cGy/day, volume treated individualized to the clinical and histopathological findings at the time of hysterectomy.
VSD = vaginal surface dose.

be the highest dose area. The localization of the bladder and rectum can be achieved by either placing Hypaque in a Foley catheter balloon that has been placed in the bladder or rectum, or by the use of rectally inserted ionization chambers. This method, however, is probably no more reliable than the point calculation method.

Generally, the bladder can tolerate more radiation than the rectum. No absolute point dose limit can be set, but it is preferable to keep the bladder point dose below 8000 cGy and the rectal point dose below 7000 cGy. Therefore, it is optimal if the rectal dose rate is lower than the bladder dose rate for the brachytherapy application. Additionally, it is also desirable for the dose rate to the bladder point to be 0.8 or less than that of the dose rate to point A.

Patient Care During the Implant

At the University of Minnesota, following insertion of the applicator, patients are monitored in the recovery room, then transported to the radiation therapy department where an orthogonal pair of simulator films is taken. The patient is then transported to her hospital room. The sources are subsequently loaded either manually or by remote afterloading techniques.

Adequate analgesia while the applicator is in place is crucial. We usually order oral narcotics for patients with colpostats or cylinders and parenteral narcotics for patients with intrauterine tandems. Since the prolonged bed rest is stressful, benzodiazepines are given as needed to help sedate patients. The anesthesia sometimes causes nausea postoperatively and antiemetics are routinely prescribed. For the duration of the implant, the subcutaneous heparin is continued and the sequential pneumatic stockings used. Daily inspection of the brachytherapy appliance should be performed to assure that it has not dislodged.

It is important that good nursing care continue despite the presence of the radioactivity. To accomplish this, nurses need to be educated about the level of radiation they are exposed to in the patient's room and how to keep that exposure to within acceptable limits. Patients containing radioactive sources should receive the same medical monitoring as any other hospitalized patients.

Despite careful attention to the care of these patients in the operating room and afterwards while the sources are in place, up to 7% of patients will have life-threatening complications.[39] In the event of a medical emergency during the implant, emergency care can be administered with the sources in the patient until the sources can be safely removed by trained personnel. The emergency care team should follow the proper precautions and maximize their distance from and minimize their time near the patient. At the University of Minnesota, film badges are distributed in a medical emergency to document the exposure to emergency personnel. If CPR is necessary, the person giving chest compressions is alternated at 10-minute intervals. The radiation oncologist should be immediately called and informed of the nature of the emergency and will decide if it is necessary to remove the radioactive sources. The radiation protection officer for the hospital should also be called.

Implant Removal

Prior to implant removal, patients are premedicated with either oral or parenteral narcotics. We also make use of intravenous short acting benodiazepines (for example midazolam [Versed[R]]), which are anxiolytic and often cause a retrograde amnesia for the removal.

At the scheduled removal time, the cesium sources are removed, returned to their lead pigs that are put into a lead lined cart, and transported back to the radiation oncology department for storage in the radioisotope safe. After the cesium has been removed, the afterloading appliance may be removed from the patient. For a cylinder, this merely involves cutting the sutures holding the cylinder ring to the perineum and gently pulling the cylinder free. For colpostats, the packing is removed, then the screw holding the colpostats together is removed and each colpostat individually withdrawn from the vagina. For patients with a tandem and ovoid application, the packing and ovoids are removed first, then the suture holding the tandem to the cervix is cut. The tandem then can be slipped out of the intrauterine canal.

Sequelae

Acute sequelae including diarrhea, cystitis, fatigue, and lowered peripheral blood counts are common, but usually resolve within weeks after treatment. Ovarian failure occurs in nearly all patients, unless ovarian transposition outside the pelvis has been performed.[40,41] Shrinkage of the vagina can be minimized by daily use of a dilator during and after a course of radiation therapy.

The risk of developing a major complication depends on multiple factors. Patient related factors include the stage and extent of the disease, weight, age,[42] smoking history,[43] and number of previous abdominal surgical procedures.[44,45] Treatment related factors include the volume of EBRT field treated, fraction size, the dose of EBRT, the brachytherapy used, and the technique of implantation used.[26,46-51]

The Patterns of Care study reported that from 8%–15% of patients treated for cervical cancer with definitive irradiation required hospitalization for a complication, half of which required a surgical intervention. Others have reported similar percentages. In a recent review of 1784 patients treated at M.D. Anderson Hospital with FIGO stage IB cervix cancer, the risk of a major complication was 9.3% at 5 years and 14.4% at 20 years.[52] The most common gastrointestinal complications include proctitis, rectal ulceration, sigmoid stricture, or small bowel obstruction. Urinary complications include cystitis, or ureteral stricture. Rectovaginal or vesicovaginal fistulae are uncommon.

Results

The Patterns of Care Study reported 4-year disease-free survivals of 87%, 66%, and 28% for FIGO stages I, II, and III, respectively.[44] Results from other individual institutions are shown in Table 6. Although results are often reported by FIGO stage, other prognostic factors such as tumor volume or extent of nodal spread may be more important prognosticators of outcome, not currently reflected in the clinical staging system of FIGO. Patients with FIGO stage IA or small IB disease have an excellent prognosis with 5-year disease-free survival estimates from 80%–100%.[50,53-56] For larger IB lesions, 5-year disease-free survival estimates range from 75%– 90%. Stage IIB disease-free survival results range from 60%–75%[57-59] and with IIIB, the 5-year disease-free survival rates drop to 30%–50%.[59,60]

The in-field failure rate increases with increasing initial FIGO stage (Table 7). For stage I patients an in-field recurrence rate of 5%–9% has been reported.[45,59,61-64] For stage II pa-

Table 6.
Five-Year Disease-Free Survival Rates Reported For Carcinoma of the Cervix

Author [Reference]	Total Number of Patients	Stage				
		IB	IIA	IIB	III	IVA
Perez [69]	970	85	70	68	45	—
Petterson [70]	32,428	78	—		57	8
Coia [44]	565	74	—	56	33	—
Horiot [58]	1,383	9	85	75	50	20
Montana [56, 57, 71]	533	83	76	62	33	—
Potish [72]	153	67	71	70	—	—
Leibel [60]	119	—	—	—	—	—
Gerbaulet [53]	441	89	78	—	—	—
Kramer [73]	48	—	—	—	—	18
Mendenhall [55]	264	70*	71	70*	—	—
		68**		43**		
Kim [59]	569	82	78	65	48	27
Thoms† [74]	371	56**	49**	53**	—	—
Willin [54]	168	88	77	68	—	—

* = <6 cm; ** = >6 cm; † = 5-year survival.

Table 7.
Percentage of In-Field Failure Rates

Author [Reference]	FIGO Stage			
	I	II	III	IV
Coia [44]	12	27	51	—
Kim [59]	11.2	8.2 (IIA)	52	69
		30 (IIB)		
Horiot [58]	8	12 (IIA)	37 (IIIA)	82
		20 (IIB)	43 (IIIB)	
Montana [57, 71, 75]	11	16 (IIA)	61 (IIIA)	—
		34 (IIB)	47 (IIIB)	

UNIVERSITY OF MINNESOTA HEALTH SYSTEM   Hospital No.:
Department of Therapeutic Radiology – Radiation Oncology   Patient Name:

BRACHYTHERAPY QMP CHECKLIST   Dates of Implantation:

I.   BEFORE INSERTION OF RADIOACTIVE SOURCES INTO THE PATIENT

1. Preliminary written directive signed and on file (radioisotope, number of sources, and source strengths).

_____
attending physician   (initial and date)

2. Patient positively identified by two independent methods.

_____
attending physician   (initial and date)

3. Verification that source preparation is in agreement with signed preliminary written directive.

_____
curator/resident physician   (initial and date)

4. Position of sources within patient verified radiographically.

_____
attending physician   (initial and date)

II.   AFTER INSERTION BUT PRIOR TO COMPLETION OF TREATMENT

5. Recording of actual source loading sequence in patient's chart.

_____
resident physician   (initial and date)

6. Final written directive signed and on file (radioisotope, treatments site, total source strength, and exposure time).

_____
attending physician   (initial and date)

7. Check of dose calculations, computerized treatment plan, computations in the Daily Dose Record, and the planned implant duration.

_____
physicist   (initial and date)

8. Daily physical inspection of implant position.

_____
physician   (initial and date)

_____
physician   (initial and date)

_____
physician   (initial and date)

III. AFTER SOURCE REMOVAL

9. Sources removed at the planned time (temporary implants).

_____
resident physician   (initial and date)

10. Check that administered dose agrees with final written directive dose to within ± 10%*.

_____
attending physician   (initial and date)

* If delivered dose differs from final written directive by more than ± 10% but less than or equal to ± 20%, this is a recordable event. Notify the physician and physics staff for the required action.

If delivered dose differs from final written directive by more than ± 20%, this is a misadministration. The physician and physics staff need to be notified immediately.

_____   _____
ATTENDING PHYSICIAN ADMINISTERING THERAPY (signature)   DATE

05272, JAN 95   B1b

Figure 21. A checklist of tasks that need be completed for every patient undergoing a brachytherapy application is a helpful tool to document that these tasks were performed and as a double check to ensure that nothing is overlooked.

tients the in-field recurrences range is between 10%–23%, and for stage III patients up to a 61% in-field recurrence rate has been reported.

Quality Management Program

A quality management program (QMP) is crucial to the safe functioning of a brachytherapy program.[65] This cannot be accomplished without a dedicated physics support. The various components of a QMP are covered in another chapter and may be found in the AAPM Task Group 40 Report.[66] However, several issues relative to intracavitary cesium applications deserve emphasis. To assure accurate preparation of the sources that are to be loaded into the patient, a series of double checks should be in place. We use color-coded cesium sources, and check each source in a well-ionization chamber; also, two people must prepare the sources to double check each other. Sources must be logged in and out of the department (along with a visual count of the remaining sources left in the cesium safe) and all sources leaving the isotope room are always accompanied by a cesium transport card (Figure 15). Regulations mandated by the Nuclear Regulatory Commission are followed. We have found it helpful to have a checklist to ensure compliance with these regulations with every brachytherapy application (Figure 21).

Quality assurance (QA) tests for the brachy-therapy applicators need to be performed intermittently. A rattling noise when the ovoids are gently shaken suggests that the rectal or bladder shields have dislodged and the applicator should be radiographed immediately to verify this. Reports of tandem tips coming off while implanted and remaining within the uterine cavity make it prudent to check the integrity of the tandem tip with each insertion. The American Association of Physicists in Medicine Task Group 40 recommended QA procedures for brachytherapy applicators[66] as outlined in Table 8. In addition to these tests, we radiograph the applicators yearly to confirm correct position of the shields.

Conclusions

In early stages, cancer of the uterine cervix is highly curable with either surgery or radiation therapy. As the tumor advances, however, the best chance of cure is with aggressive, definitive radiation therapy consisting of a combination of external beam treatments and brachytherapy applications. Both of the components are important, however it is probably the skilled use of intracavitary brachytherapy that is the most crucial to a successful outcome. This skill is achieved through experience as well as meticulous attention to the details of the treatment outlined here.

References

1. Nag, S, Abitbol AA, Anderson LL, et al. Consensus guidelines for high dose rate remote brachytherapy in cervical, endometrial, and endobronchial tumors. Clinical Research Committee, American Endocurietherapy Society. Int J Radiat Oncol Biol Phys 1993;27:1241.
2. Sarkaria JN, Petereit DG, Stitt JA, et al. A comparison of the efficacy and complication rates of low dose-rate versus high dose-rate brachytherapy in the treatment of uterine cervical carcinoma. Int J Radiat Oncol Biol Phys 1994;30:75.
3. Brenner DJ, Hall EJ. Fractionated high dose rate versus low dose rate regimens for intracavitary brachytherapy of the cervix. I. General considerations based on radiobiology [see comments]. Br J Radiol 1991;64:133.
4. LaPolla, JP, Schlaerth JB, Gaddis O, et al. The influence of surgical staging on the evaluation

Table 8.
Quality Assurance Tests for Intracavitary Brachytherapy Applicators: Frequency of Performance and Acceptable Tolerance Limits

Test	Frequency	Tolerance
Source location	I, Y	D
Coincidence of dummy and active sources	I	1 mm
Location of shields	I, Y*	D

I = initial use or following malfunction and repairs; Y = yearly; D = documented and correction applied or noted in report of measurement when appropriate.

* Before each use, the applicator may be shaken to listen for loose parts [66].

and treatment of patients with cervical carcinoma. Gynecol Oncol 1986;24:194.

5. Heaps JM, Berek JS. Surgical staging of cervical cancer. (Review). Clin Obstet Gynecol 1990; 33:852.

6. Paterson R, Russell MH. Clinical trials in malignant disease. VI. Cancer of the cervix uteri: Is x-ray therapy more effective given before or after radium? Clin Radil 1962;13.

7. Maracial LV, Marcial JM, Krall JM, et al. Comparison of 1 vs 2 or more intracavitary brachytherapy applications in the management of carcinoma of the cervix with irradiaton alone. Int J Radiat Oncol Biol Phys 1991;20:81.

7a. Lanciano RM, Pajak TF, Martz K. The influence of treatment time on outcome for squamous cell cancer of the uterine cervix treated with radiation: A patterns of care study. Int J Radiat Oncol Biol Phys 1993;25:391–397.

7b. Perez CA, Grigsby PW, Catro-Vita H, et al. Carcinoma of the uterine cervix. I. Implact of prolongation of overall treatment time and timing of brachytherapy on outcome of radiation therapy. Int J Radiat Oncol Biol Phys 1995;25:391–397.

7c. Petereit DG, Karkaria JM, Chappell R, et al. The adverse effect of treatment prolongation in cervical carcinoma. Int J Radiat Oncol Biol Phys 1995;32:1301–1307.

8. Podczaski E, Stryker JA, Kaminski P, et al. Extended-field radiation therapy for carcinoma of the cervix. Cancer 1990;66:251.

9. Potish RA, Twiggs LB, Adcock LL, et al. The utility and limitations of decision theory in the utilization of surgical staging and extended field radiotherapy in cervical cancer. Obstet Gynecol Surv 1984;39:555.

10. Rubin SC, Brookland R, Mikuta JJ, et al. Paraaortic nodal metastases in early cervical carcinoma: Long-term survival following extended-field radiotherapy. Gynecol Oncol 1984;18:213.

11. Nori D, Valentine E, Hilaris BS. The role of paraaortic node irradiation in the treatment of cancer of the cervix. Int J Radiat Oncol Biol Phys 1985;11:1469.

12. Rotman M, Pajak TF, Choi K, et al. Prophylactic extented field irradiation of para-aortic lymph nodes in stages IIB and bulky IB and IIIa cervical carcinomas: Ten year treatment results of RTOG 79–20. JAMA 1995;274:387.

13. Rotman M, Choi K, Guse C, et al. Prophylactic irradiation of the para-aortic lymph node chain in stage IIB and bulky stage IB carcinoma of the cervix, initial treatment results of RTOG 7920 [see comments]. Int J Radiat Oncol Biol Phys 1990;19:513.

14. Haie C, Pejovic MJ, Gerbaulet A. Is prophylactic para-aortic irradiation worthwhile in the treatment of advanced cervical carcinoma? Radiother Oncol 1988;11:101–102.

15. Alvarez RD, Soong SJ, Kinney WK, et al. Identification of prognostic factors and risk groups in patients found to have nodal metastasis at the time of radical hysterectomy for early-stage squamous carcinoma of the cervix. Gynecol Oncol 1989;35:130.

16. Barter JF, Soong SJ, Shingleton HM, et al. Complications of combined radical hysterectomy—postoperative radiation therapy in women with early stage cervical cancer. Gynecol Oncol 1989;32:292.

17. Gonzalez GD, Ketting BW, van BB, et al. Carcinoma of the uterine cervix stage IB and IIA: Results of postoperative irradiation in patients with microscopic infiltration in the parametrium and/or lymph node metastasis. Int J Radiat Oncol Biol Phys 1989;16:389.

18. Photopulos GJ, Vander ZR, Miller B, et al. Vaginal radiation brachytherapy to reduce central recurrence after radical hysterectomy for cervical carcinoma. Gynecol Oncol 1990;38:187.

19. Rettenmaier MA, Casanova DM, Micha JP, et al. Radical hysterectomy and tailored postoperative radiation therapy in the management of bulky stage 1B cervical cancer. Cancer 1989;63:2220.

20. Russell AH, Tong DY, Figge DC, et al. Adjuvant postoperative pelvic radiation for carcinoma of the uterine cervix: Pattern of cancer recurrence in patients undergoing elective radiation following radical hysterectomy and pelvic lymphadenectomy. Int J Radiat Oncol Biol Phys 1984;10:211.

21. Soisson AP, Soper JT, Clarke PD, et al. Adjuvant radiotherapy following radical hysterectomy for patients with stage IB and IIA cervical cancer. Gynecol Oncol 1990;37:390.

22. Haas JS, Dean RD, Mansfield CM. Dosimetric comparison of the Fletcher family of gynecologic colpostats 1950–1980. Int J Radiat Oncol Biol Phys 1985;11:1317.

23. Sharma SC, Williamson JF, Khan FM, et al. Dosimetric consequences of asymmetric positioning of active source in Cs 137 and Ra 226 intracavitary tubes. Int J Radiat Oncol Biol Phys 1981;7:555.

24. Kuske RR, Perez CA, Jacobs AJ, et al. Minicolpostats in the treatment of carcinoma of the uterine cervix. Int J Radiat Oncol Biol Phys 1988;14:899.

25. Paris KJ, Spanos WJ, Day TG, et al. Incidence of complications with mini-vaginal colpostats in carcinoma of the uterine cervix. Int J Radiat Oncol Biol Phys 1991;21:911.

26. Crook JM, Esche BA, Chaplain G, et al. Dose-volume analysis and the prevention of radia-

tion sequelae in cervical cancer. Radiother Oncol 1987;8:321.

27. Fletcher GH. Female pelvis: Squamous cell carcinoma of the uterine cervix. In: Textbook of Radiotherapy. Saunders, London, 1973, p. 620.

28. Potish RA, Gerbi BJ. Cervical cancer: Intracavitary dose specification and prescription. Radiology 1987;165:555.

29. Esche BA, Crook JM, Isturiz J, et al. Reference volume, milligram-hours and external irradiation for the Fletcher applicator. Radiother Oncol 1987;9:255.

30. Potish RA, Diebel RC, Khan FM. The relationship between milligram-hours and dose to point A in carcinoma of the cervix. Radiology 1982;145:479.

31. Potish RA, Gerbi B. Role of point A in the era of computerized dosimetry. Radiology 1986;158.

32. Potish RA. The effect of applicator geometry on dose specification in cervical cancer. Int J Radiat Oncol Biol Phys 1990;18:1513.

32a. Bhatnager JP, Kaplan C, Specht R. A rule of thumb for dose rate at point A for the Fletcher-Suit applicator (correspondence). Br J Radiol 1980;53:511–512.

33. ICRU, ICoR. Dose and volume specification for reporting intracavitary therapy in gynecology. ICRU Report 38, 1, 1985.

34. Wilkinson JM, Ramachandran TP. The ICRU recommendations for reporting intracavitary therapy in gynaecology and the Manchester method of treating cancer of the cervix uteri. Br J Radiol 1989;62:362.

35. Jacobs AJ, Perez CA, Camel HM, et al. Complications in patients receiving both irradiation and radical hysterectomy for carcinoma of the uterine cervix. Gynecol Oncol 1985;22:273.

36. Perez CA, Kao MS. Radiation therapy alone or combined with surgery in the treatment of barrel-shaped carcinoma of the uterine cervix (stages IB, IIA, IIB). Int J Radiat Oncol Biol Phys 1985;11:1903.

37. Kim RY, Salter MM, Shingleton HM. Adjuvant postoperative radiation therapy following radical hysterectomy in stage IB CA of the cervix—analysis of treatment failure. Int J Radiat Oncol Biol Phys 1988;14:445.

38. Farquharson DI, Shingleton HM, Soong SJ, et al. The adverse effects of cervical cancer treatment on bladder function. Gynecol Oncol 1987;27:15.

39. Dusenbery KD, Carson LF, Potish RA. Perioperative morbidity and mortality of gynecologic brachytherapy. Cancer 1991;67:2786.

40. Husseinzadeh N, Nahhas WA, Velkley DE, et al. The preservation of ovarian function in young women undergoing pelvic radiation therapy. Gynecol Oncol 1984;18:373.

41. Belinson JL, Doherty M, McDay JB. A new technique for ovarian transposition. Surg Gynecol Obstet 1984;159:157.

42. Kucera H, Genger H, Wagner G, et al. Prognosis of primary radiotherapy of cervix cancer in younger females. Geburtshilfe und Frauenheilkunde 1986;46:800.

43. Kucera H, Enzelsberger H, Eppel W, et al. The influence of nicotine abuse and diabetes mellitus on the results of primary irradiation in the treatment of carcinoma of the cervix. Cancer 1987;60:1.

44. Coia L, Won M, Lanciano R, et al. The patterns of care outcome study for cancer of the uterine cervix. Results of the Second National Practice Survey. Cancer 1990;66:2451.

45. Potish RA, Twiggs LB. An analysis of adjuvant treatment strategies for carcinoma of the cervix. Am J Clin Oncol 1989;12:430.

46. Unal A, Hamberger A, Seski J, et al. An analysis of the severe complications of irradiation of carcinoma of the uterine cervix: Treatment with intracavitary radium and parametrial irradiation. Int J Radiat Oncol Biol Phys 1981;7: 999.

47. Deore SM, Shrivastava KV PS, Dinshaw KA. The severity of late rectal and recto-sigmoid complications related to fraction size in irradiation treatment of carcinoma cervix stage IIIB. Strahlenther Onkol 1991;167:638.

48. Hanks GE, Herring DF, Kramer S. Patterns of care outcome studies. Cancer 1983;51:959.

49. Montana GS, Fowler WC. Carcinoma of the cervix: Analysis of bladder and rectal radiation dose and complications. Int J Radiat Oncol Biol Phys 1989;16:95.

50. Perez CA, Breaux S, Bedwinek JM, et al. Radiation therapy alone in the treatment of carcinoma of the uterine cervix. II. Analysis of complications. Cancer 1984;54:235.

51. Pourquier H, Delard R, Achille E, et al. A quantified approach to the analysis and prevention of urinary complications in radiotherapeutic treatment of cancer of the cervix. Int J Radiat Oncol Biol Phys 1987;13:1025.

52. Eifel PJ, Levenback C, Wharton T, et al. Time course and incidence of late complications in patients treated with radiation therapy for FIGO Stage IB carcinoma of the uterine cervix. Int J Radiat Oncol Biol Phys 1995;32:1289.

53. Gerbaulet AL, Kunkler IH, Kerr GR, et al. Combined radiotherapy and surgery: Local control and complications in early carcinoma of the uterine cervix—the Villejuif experience, 1975–1984. (Review). Radiother Oncol 1992; 23:66.

54. Willen H, Eklund G, Johnsson JE, et al. Invasive squamous cell carcinoma of the uterine cervix.

VIII. Survival and malignancy grading in patients treated by irradiation in Lund 1969–1970. Acta Radiol Oncol 1985;24:41.

55. Mendenhall WM, Thar TL, Bova FJ, et al. Prognostic and treatment factors affecting pelvic control of Stage IB and IIA-B carcinoma of the intact uterine cervix treated with radiation therapy alone. Cancer 1984;53:2649.

56. Montana GS, Fowler WC, Varia MA, et al. Analysis of results of radiation therapy for stage IB carcinoma of the cervix. Cancer 1987;60:2195.

57. Montana GS, Fowler WC, Varia MA, et al. Analysis of results of radiation therapy for Stage II carcinoma of the cervix. Cancer 1985;55:956.

58. Horiot JC, Pigneux J, Pourquier H, et al. Radiotherapy alone in carcinoma of the intact uterine cervix according to G.H. Fletcher guidelines: A French cooperative study of 1383 cases. (Review). Int J Radiat Oncol Biol Phys 1988;14:605.

59. Kim RY, Trotti A, Wu CJ, et al. Radiation alone in the treatment of cancer of the uterine cervix: Analysis of pelvic failure and dose response relationship. Int J Radiat Oncol Biol Phys 1989; 17:973.

60. Leibel S, Bauer M, Wasserman T, et al. Radiotherapy with or without misonidazole for patients with stage IIIB or stage IVA squamous cell carcinoma of the uterine cervix: Preliminary report of a Radiation Therapy Oncology Group randomized trial. Int J Radiat Oncol Biol Phys 1987;13:541.

61. Adcock LL, Potish RA, Julian TM, et al. Carcinoma of the cervix, FIGO stage IB: Treatment failures. Gynecol Oncol 1984;18:218.

62. Eifel PJ, Morris M, Oswald MJ, et al. Adenocarcinoma of the uterine cervix. Prognosis and patterns of failure in 367 cases. Cancer 1990; 65:2507.

63. Montana GS, Martz K, Hanks G. Patterns and sites of failure in cervix cancer treated in the USA in 1978. Int J Radiat Oncol Biol Phys 1991; 20:87.

64. Sommers GM, Grigsby PW, Perez CA, et al. Outcome of recurrent cervical carcinoma following definitive irradiation. Gynecol Oncol 1989;35:150.

65. Dawson J, Roy T, Abrath F, et al. Comprehensive quality management program for radiation oncology. Radiother Oncol 1994;31:187.

66. Kutcher GJ, Coia L, Gillin M, et al. Comprehensive QA for radiation oncology: Report of AAPM radiaton therapy committee task group 40. Med Phys 1994;21:581.

67. Joslin CA. A place for high dose rate brachytherapy in gynaecological oncology: Fact or fiction. Act Select Brachyther J 1991;(Suppl)2: 3.

68. Johnson JM, Johnson RAP. The provision of a uniform vaginal surface dose rate by a novel afterloading vaginal cylinder. Med Dos 1991; 16:193.

69. Perez CA, Camel HM, Kuske RR, et al. Radiation therapy alone in the treatment of carcinoma of the uterine cervix: A 20-year experience. Gynecol Oncol 1986;23:127.

70. Pettersson F. The 19th FIGO Annual Report on the results of treatment in Gynecological Cancer. Radiumhemmet, 1985.

71. Montana GS, Fowler WC, Varia MA, et al. Carcinoma of the cervix stage III: Results of radiation therapy. Cancer 1986;1:148.

72. Potish RA, Downey GO, Adcock LL, et al. The role of surgical debulking in cancer of the uterine cervix. Int J Radiat Oncol Biol Phys 1989; 17:979.

73. Kramer C, Peschel RE, Goldberg N, et al. Radiation treatment of FIGO stage IVA carcinoma of the cervix. Gynecol Oncol 1989;32:323.

74. Thoms W, Eifel P, Smith L, et al. Bulky endocervical carcinomas: A 23 year experience. Int J Radiat Oncol Biol Phys 1992;23:491.

75. Montana GS, Fowler WC Jr, Varia MA, et al. Carcinoma of the cervix stage IB: Results of treatment with radiation therapy. Int J Radiat Oncol Biol Phys 1983;9:45.

— Chapter 26 —

High-Dose-Rate Brachytherapy for Cervical Carcinoma

Judith Anne Stitt, M.D.

Introduction

The development of radioactive isotopes to treat cervical cancer began during the early days of radiation oncology history. The effectiveness of plaque therapy and intracavitary radium for treating cancer demonstrated its usefulness long before external radiation therapy became part of radiation oncology practice. In 1939, A. James Larkin[1] stated, "The complete destruction of cervical carcinoma in many cases of all types and stages has brought radium to the point where it is the agent of choice in the treatment of all but the early operable cases."

Radium-226 loaded in the applicator and then placed into the patient while in the operating suite was the earliest form of source handling. Radium-226 in sealed sources consists of the isotope and daughter products, including radon gas, sealed in a platinum tube. Shortcomings of preloaded brachytherapy include exposure not only to the physician who inserts and positions the applicator and isotope, but also nursing and other personnel in the procedure suite. A major radiation safety issue results from the relatively soft platinum encased tubes that can be broken, releasing radon gas. With a half-life of 1620 years, a radium accident is a major safety problem.

Several European centers devised systems for treatment of cervical cancer that specified the applicator, source strength, source distribution in the uterus and cervix, dose rate, and total treatment time. These systems have come to be known by the city where each was developed and used extensively.[2–4] The Stockholm, Paris, and Manchester systems of gynecological brachytherapy described in Table 1 serves as the basis for our current style of practice in modern brachytherapy.

Afterloading applicators were developed during the 1950s to allow the applicator to be placed in the patient and positioned as needed prior to loading active sources for treatment.[5,6] Cesium-137 became a common substitute for radium primarily because of radiation safety issues of leaky or broken radium sources. Applicators developed for preloaded radium use were commonly modified for afterloading cesium. A variety of instruments, including the Fletcher-Suit, Henschke, and Ter-Pogossian applicators, were developed by their namesakes and have been used extensively.[7,8]

Remote afterloading, initially developed at the Radiumhemmet to further decrease radiation exposure by performing source handling through mechanical means,[9] eliminated personnel exposure for all portions of the procedure and source loading process. Customization of therapy by remotely controlling the

From Nag S (ed): *Principles and Practice of Brachytherapy.* © Futura Publishing Co., Inc., Armonk, NY, 1997.

Table 1.
Gynecological Brachytherapy Systems

Stockholm, 1918:	60–80 mg radium in uterine rod & cervical box. 2–3 applications of 30 hours over 3 weeks.
Paris, 1920:	Semi-fixed applicator, low total radium activity. Uterine:vaginal sources at 1:1 over 6–8 days.
Manchester, 1929:	Semifixed applicator, higher radium activity. Uterine:vaginal sources at 1:1.5 over 140 hours.
Madison, 1989:	Fixed applicator, high-dose-rate iridium. Redefined dose specification points. Altered time/dose/fractionation course.

source position became feasible. Remote afterloading can be performed with low-dose-rate (LDR), medium-dose-rate (MDR), or high-dose-rate (HDR) sources. Remote afterloading with high intensity sources was introduced by Ulrich Henschke and Basil Hilaris.[10,11] The Japanese have treated large numbers of patients with the cobalt-60 Ralstron.[12] Other units include the cesium-137 Curietron and the iridium-192 Buchler.[13] The microSelectron uses 4-mm long iridium sources with infinitely variable source dwell positions, allowing a high level of dose optimization unattainable with radium, cesium, or cobalt pellets.[14] The elaborate computer hardware and sophisticated software that are used provide a degree of accuracy unavailable in the past with other gynecological systems.

LDR brachytherapy with radium, cesium, cobalt, or iridium sources has traditionally been given at dose rates of 0.4–0.8 Gy/hr. The pioneers of radiation therapy used these isotopes to develop highly successful treatment schedules for cervical cancer. HDR intracavitary radiation (HDR-ICR) refers to dose rate of 0.5–5.0 Gy/min, a rate commonly administered with linear accelerators during external beam radiation therapy (EBRT). Isotopes that can be produced in a nuclear reactor in this dose-rate range for medical application include cobalt, cesium, and iridium.

This change in dose rates introduces additional radiobiological factors into fractionation schedules necessitating careful evaluation of fraction size, length of treatment courses, and total dose of external plus intracavitary brachytherapy for cervical cancer. Selective loading of dwell positions can be used to improve the dose distribution for both LDR and HDR remote afterloading units to achieve optimum tumor dose distribution while limiting normal tissue exposure. However, LDR remote afterloading applicators are still subject to the same degree of mobility in the pelvis during a course of therapy. During HDR therapy, instruments are positioned and stabilized in place with packing or retraction. Treatment is given to a specified tumor volume over several minutes of treatment time with essentially no change in the position of the applicator or surrounding vulnerable normal tissues.

Clinical Experience in High-Dose-Rate Brachytherapy for Cervical Carcinoma

HDR-ICR for treatment of cervical cancer, which has developed clinically over the past 15–20 years in Europe and Asia, has only recently become an important treatment modality in North America. Brachytherapy given at dose rates of 0.5–5.0 Gy/min means that an intracavitary procedure that previously required hospitalization and bed rest for several days can be administered over a short time on an out-patient basis. This treatment modality has brought about changes in both the technical and the clinical aspects of brachytherapy. Computer-controlled treatment planning and treatment delivery units have been developed and brachytherapy applicators have been modified. Techniques for management of out-patient therapy have been devised; new dose schedules that combine external beam and intracavitary treatments have been implemented and dose specification definitions have been revised.[9,10,15–20]

Table 2.
Advantages of High-Dose-Rate Brachytherapy for Cervical Carcinoma

Multiple fractions can be given on an outpatient basis.
Complete radiation protection for staff.
No general anesthetic or bed rest needed.
Accuracy of source and applicator position.
Individualized treatment with source optimization.
Ability to treat large clinical patient volume.

Practical as well as medical factors are involved in making a decision to change a brachytherapy program to HDR therapy. Table 2 summarizes the major factors to be considered when contemplating the move to HDR brachytherapy technology. From the medical perspective, out-patient therapy for gynecological malignancies lessens the incidence of general anesthesia complications during or after LDR procedures. Perioperative and postoperative complications resulting from prolonged bed rest can be eliminated. Life-threatening perioperative complications from LDR intracavitary brachytherapy occurred in 6.4% of 327 patients at the University of Minnesota undergoing LDR brachytherapy procedures. Fatal complications occurred in three women. These events included thromboembolic, cardiac, and pulmonary morbidities resulting from general anesthesia and/or bed rest.[21]

The radiation safety benefits of HDR or LDR remote afterloading programs are considerable for institutions with a large volume brachytherapy practice. Cost containment issues of out-patient versus in-patient therapy are valid arguments in favor of developing HDR treatment programs. There is a cost-shift toward the radiation oncology department and away from the hospital that results from HDR out-patient programs.[22]

The biological factors involved in HDR brachytherapy may result in adverse effects to the normal tissues. A high dose per fraction directed at the cancer, if given to rectal or bladder mucosa, may result is late sequelae of fibrosis or fistula. Early clinical trials moving from LDR to HDR demonstrated higher bladder and bowel complications if time-dose

effects on normal tissues were not meticulously observed.[23] Geometry of applicator insertion and stabilization can be used to overcome this relative radiobiological disadvantage. Another concern in beginning HDR therapy for cervical carcinoma is the issue of local tumor control. The world experience in treating cervical carcinoma has been with LDR brachytherapy combined with EBRT. HDR brachytherapy must uphold the same tumor control results as LDR treatment before this technique can be said to be an acceptable alternative. Institutions that treat a relatively low number of patients with cervical cancer must be wary of making a switch in technique, particularly to one that requires a high level of staffing and experience. The risks of using HDR brachytherapy lie not only in irretrievable treatment error because such high doses of irradiation are delivered in seconds, but also in failing to control tumor or increasing late normal tissue effects.

Clinical experience with HDR-ICR has been developed and reported by numerous institutions. Although there are threads of common practice, institutions have unique practice patterns and characteristics that identify their HDR programs.[11,24–31] Insertion techniques including applicator selection, positioning, and stabilization, use of sedation, specifics of dosimetry films, and calculations for selected institutions are described in *High Dose Rate Brachytherapy: A Textbook.*[32]

Cardiff, England

Joslin et al.[11] initiated an HDR brachytherapy program for cervical cancer in the late 1960s using high activity cobalt-60 in a Cathetron unit. EBRT is initiated prior to adding brachytherapy. Prescribed doses are the same for all stages of cervical disease. A central wedge that does not protect the lower vagina is used during external therapy. Treatment philosophy is that early stage disease should be treated with a radical dose limited only by normal tissue tolerance.

Applicator insertion is performed with sufficient anesthesia to allow cervical dilation. The procedure is carried out in the operating theater and the patient is transported on the same cart to the treatment room for HDR therapy. A posterior retractor is used with Man-

Table 3.
Cardiff Technique of High-Dose-Rate
Brachytherapy for Cervical Carcinoma

External Beam Technique	Intracavitary Technique
24 Gy in 12 fractions	Four fractions of 10 Gy to point A
Telecobalt AP-PA	Tandem and small ovoids
Central wedge	Retractor to keep rectal dose at 60% of point A

Table 4.
McGill University Technique
of High-Dose-Rate Brachytherapy
for Cervical Carcinoma

External Beam Technique	Intracavitary Technique
46 Gy in 23 fractions	Three weekly fractions of 8–10 Gy to point A
4-field, 4–10 MV photons	Tandem and Manchester ovoids
No central block	In vivo bladder and rectal dosimetry

chester ovoids to decrease the dose to the anterior rectal wall. Rectal dose is recorded at the treatment sessions and can be kept at 60% of the point A dose.[23] Table 3 summarizes the technical aspect of therapy.

McGill University

Patients with cervical carcinoma are treated with a combination of EBRT and HDR intracavitary brachytherapy. The dose from EBRT and intracavitary treatment does not vary by stage. Central blocking of the tissues receiving HDR therapy is not done. HDR treatment is given with a Selectron cobalt-60 unit. The HDR fractionation schedule was developed empirically from time-dose fractionation calculations of prior LDR brachytherapy experience and in keeping with the Joslin dose fractionation system.[24]

Brachytherapy is given as out-patient treatment with spinal anesthesia. Vaginal packing is used to maximize the distance between the sources and the anterior bladder and posterior rectal walls. In vivo measurement of maximum bladder and rectal dose rates are obtained prior to the HDR treatment by using low activity cobalt-60 sources in a configuration identical to that used with high activity sources. A probe containing a diode detector is introduced into the bladder and rectum and maximum dose rates are recorded as the probe is withdrawn.[25] Table 4 shows the integration of EBRT and intracavitary HDR treatment at McGill University.

Wayne State University

The Wayne State University gynecological HDR treatment program has been under way

since 1987. The institution uses a highly fractionated HDR treatment course with up to 8–12 HDR fractions (Table 5). Brachytherapy is started 2–4 weeks after initiation of EBRT. A customized central step wedge is used during the HDR treatment period to shield central pelvic tissue while treating peripheral pelvic lymph nodes. The patient population tends toward higher stages of cancer with 30% of patients presenting with stages IIB-IVA disease.[26]

The highly fractionated schedule was chosen for several reasons. It was decided to reduce the rectal dose for each HDR fraction to 200–250 cGy to be close to doses considered tolerable for fractionated teletherapy. The linear-quadratic (L-Q) model was used to determine how many HDR fractions would be equivalent to an LDR regimen of 60 Gy at point A.[27] The intracavitary technique utilizes an intrauterine stent so that applicators can

Table 5.
Wayne State University Technique
of High-Dose-Rate Brachytherapy
for Cervical Carcinoma

External Beam Technique	Intracavitary Technique
1.8–2.0 Gy/fraction initial whole pelvis to 19.8 Gy	3.86 Gy/fx to point A; 3 fractions/ week for 8–12 fractions
Then, central step wedge used during high-dose-rate to 39.6 Gy	Ring applicator with cervical stent; no sedation or anesthesia use

be placed quickly without cervical dilatation with little or no sedation. A tandem and ring applicator or tandem and cylinder facilitates this process because of ease of reproducibility from one insertion to another. Treatment planning is performed on the initial insertion and is duplicated for all fractions by verifying the applicator position with C-arm fluoroscopy or radiographs.

University of Wisconsin

HDR brachytherapy is integrated into the EBRT schedule early in the course of therapy for stage I and II cervical carcinoma patients. External beam dose, intracavitary dose, and use of a central block vary according to the stage and volume of disease. The central dose at point M and the pelvic side wall dose at point E, are in the higher range of doses used for cervical cancer. For patients with larger volume of central disease, HDR brachytherapy is started after several weeks of whole pelvis irradiation to allow shrinkage of the cervical disease. Intracavitary therapy may be performed twice weekly after EBRT is completed.[28]

The dose fractionation schedules developed for HDR therapy were designed to produce equivalent tumor control and, with special attention to treatment geometry, late complication rates as the previous LDR therapy schedules, based on the L-Q model.[16] Brachytherapy is accomplished with conscious sedation as an out-patient. Nursing staff manages the IV sedation and vital signs during the procedure. Applicator insertion, radiographs for dosimetry, treatment planning, and HDR treatments are performed in the same room without moving the patient. Optimized treatment planning is performed for each insertion. Treatment techniques at the University of Wisconsin are summarized in Table 6.

Results

Joslin's group in England has treated 371 patients over 6 years. The 5-year survival is stage I: 94.4%, stage II: 62%, and stage III: 37.2%. There are very few long-term survival rates—for patients treated by the Cardiff group the 15-year survival rate is stage I: 93%, stage II: 54.3%, and stage III: 33.6%. Central disease recurrence developed in three of 95 (3%) stage I patients, in 23 of 170 (14%) stage II patients, and 30 of 106 (28%) patients with stage III disease over 8 years. Recurrent disease developed over a 6- to 10-year period.[23]

At McGill University 187 patients have been followed for a minimum of 35 months. Patterns of recurrence show that 26 patients developed pelvic recurrence. Of all patients with distant and local failure, 88% were manifest within 24 months of completing treatment. Five-year actuarial survival for stage IB is 72%, for stage IIA is 65%, for stage IIB is 66%, for stage IIIA is 66%, and for stage IIIB is 45%.[25]

The results at Wayne State University with 88 patients treated from August 1988 to December 1992 show 5-year survival rates for

Table 6.
University of Wisconsin Technique of High-Dose-Rate Brachytherapy for Cervical Carcinoma

External Beam Technique	Intracavitary Technique
1.7 Gy/fraction, 4 fractions/week	4.3 to 9.1 Gy/fraction to point A, one fraction/week for 5 fractions
4-field, 10 MV photons	
Total dose varies by volume/volume	Tandem and Manchester ovoids
Central block varies by stage/volume	Rectal dose at 80% of point A dose

Stage		Total Dose (Gy)	
		Point M	Point E
IB 60 Gy to parametrium	9.1 Gy pt A/5 fractions	45.5	60
IIB 51 Gy to whole pelvis	4.9 Gy pt A/5 fractions	75.5	60
IIIB 60 Gy to whole pelvis	4.3 Gy pt A/5 fractions	81.5	60

stage IB/IIA: 83%, stage IIB-IIIA: 69%, and stage IIB-IVA: 56%. There were 56 African-American and 32 Caucasian patients. No difference in mortality between the ethnic groups was demonstrated. Local control was achieved in 71/88 (80%) patients. Central and pelvic failure occurred in 12 patients, with distant relapse only in 17, and combination of local and distant disease recurrence in five patients. In patients with recurrent and/or distant disease recurrence, 82% died within 2 years.[27]

Patients treated with HDR brachytherapy and EBRT for cervical cancer were compared with those treated with LDR therapy at the University of Wisconsin. One hundred ninety-eight stage IB-IIIB patients treated with LDR from 1977–1989 were compared with 40 patients treated with the HDR regime from 1989–1991. Both patient groups were comparable with regard to age, weight, stage distribution, bulk of disease, and histology. No significant difference in survival was found between the LDR and HDR groups. Actuarial overall 3-year survival for LDR and HDR groups was 66% and 77%, respectively. Disease control in the pelvis was similar for the LDR and HDR patient groups. Three-year actuarial pelvic control was 80% and 77% for LDR and HDR patients, respectively. Overall, 74 of 198 (37%) LDR patients and 11 of 40 (28%) HDR patients failed either locally or distantly.[30]

Side Effects and Complications

The large patient population from the Cardiff series and the long duration of follow-up provides important data regarding late effects of HDR brachytherapy combined with EBRT for cervical carcinoma. No case of rectovaginal fistula has been seen at up to 15 years. This is a result of limiting the dose to the rectum to a maximum total dose of <45 Gy. Ten patients (2.7%) had one or more episodes of rectal bleeding developing at a median of 17.5 months. Two patients required surgery for sigmoid stricture. Bladder symptoms of hematuria in the absence of recurrent disease was seen in 15 patients (4%) in periods ranging up to 107 months. Cystoscopic findings were usually telangiectasia of the bladder base. No

surgical intervention was required. Vaginal stenosis or shortening was noted in 93 cases (25%) and was usually an asymptomatic finding.[23]

Acute complications at McGill University consisted mainly of grade 1 and 2 gastrointestinal and urinary toxicities. No increase in frequency or the nature of acute toxicities was observed when compared to their LDR experience. Late complications were seen in 14.7% of HDR patients, with 7.6% of patients experiencing grade 3 or 4 complications. Late radiation proctitis developed at a median of 15 months. Four patients developed rectal ulceration with three requiring colostomy.[25]

Complications attributable to pelvic radiotherapy and HDR brachytherapy in the Wayne State University series occurred in 11 of 88 patients. Those effects included six patients with recurring grade 2 diarrhea and two patients with grade 2 rectal symptoms. Grade 3 and 4 sequelae occurred in three patients (3.4%). These complications included vaginal-vesical fistula following surgery for recurrent tumor, small bowel obstruction, and severe vaginal stenosis.[27]

Late complications in patients treated with LDR brachytherapy were comparable to patients receiving HDR brachytherapy at the University of Wisconsin. No grade 4 small bowel, large bowel, or urinary sequelae developed in the HDR treatment group. One patient developed grade 4 radiation proctitis requiring resection and colostomy.[30]

Development of a High-Dose-Rate Program for Cervical Carcinoma

Instituting an HDR brachytherapy program requires considerable organization, discussion, and commitment by clinicians, physicists, and management of the radiation oncology department. Use of dose equivalency equations to devise new treatment schedules creates a myriad of clinical time-dose fraction schedules that may be confusing to the practitioner interested in establishing a program. The American Brachytherapy Society has published a consensus report of its Clinical Research Committee that can provide a focus point for departmental discussions of a new program.[33] Some issues to be considered should include patient load, cancer sites, and stages seen in practice. For example, in the United Sates, the number of patients treated for endometrial cancer exceeds the number treated for cervical cancer. A department may decide to use HDR vaginal cuff irradiation to treat women with endometrial cancer postoperatively, but to continue to use LDR brachytherapy for patients with cervical cancer. The disease control and late sequelae with LDR therapy of cervical cancer have been well described. For departments treating only a few cervical cases per year, a change to HDR brachytherapy might be ill advised due to the initial learning curve. Discussions of demographics, disease stages, and technical expertise of the staff are important considerations in the decision to initiate an HDR program.

Factors affecting the fiscal aspects of starting an HDR program include:

1. The types of procedures to be performed;
2. Staffing issues, i.e., the number of physicians, physicists, and department staff required;
3. Equipment costs including: the initial cost of an HDR unit; applicators; dummy sources; source calibration devices; quality assurance equipment; and the quarterly cost for source replacement for iridium HDR units.

Additionally, the cost of room renovation, shielding, and electrical, audio-visual, and radiographic equipment must be considered. The logistics of scheduling treatment, staffing for nursing and radiation therapy technologist (RTT) personnel, and coordination of treatment with other departments must be addressed.

In changing from LDR to HDR treatment for cervical carcinoma, the following factors must be considered.

External Beam Dose/ Brachytherapy Dose

Traditionally, carcinoma of the cervix has been treated with a combination of EBRT and intracavitary brachytherapy. The ratio of the EBRT dose to the brachytherapy dose depends on the volume and stage of the disease.

As the stage of the disease increases, the EBRT dose given increases, compared to that with brachytherapy, whether LDR or HDR techniques are used. If HDR brachytherapy is to be added to the department's armamentarium, the clinicians and physicists must decide on the treatment protocol to be used (a decision in which review of the literature can be helpful). The stages to be treated, when and how EBRT will be combined with HDR brachytherapy, and the time-dose fractionation schedules of the proposed treatment protocols must be discussed. HDR brachytherapy is easily integrated into the EBRT schedule through substitution for an EBRT session. This allows for shortening of the overall treatment course and may possibly lead to increased tumor control.

Fractionation

The optimal fractionation scheme for HDR brachytherapy is unknown. The L-Q equation is a common model used by experienced centers as a guideline to formulate treatment regimens for HDR cervical cancer brachytherapy programs. Since the radiological effect of HDR differ from those of LDR treatment, a greater number of HDR fractions is required to achieve an equivalent therapeutic ratio. Each institution is encouraged to adopt its own treatment policies and to apply them in a consistent fashion to document treatment outcome and sequelae. It must be emphasized that the L-Q model is to be used only as a guideline and that caution must be exercised.

Procedure

One advantage of HDR brachytherapy is that treatment can be given on an out-patient basis. Conscious sedation for the procedure requires close monitoring of the patient and intensive nursing care. The medical, nursing, and physics staffs must work efficiently and with great intensity to complete the insertion, filming, and treatment planning for HDR brachytherapy procedures.

Dose Specification

Description of the dose delivered to the treatment area and to normal tissues in the brachytherapy volume must be specified. Localization films and dose calculations are necessary for each application. A well defined method of specifying the doses and dose points should be part of the treatment protocol. Ideally, localization films should be taken, the applicator should be inserted, and the treatment should be performed without moving the patient.

Optimization

With HDR brachytherapy, the opportunity exists for computerized dose optimization. The position and dwell time of each dwell site for the source can be manipulated to achieve modest alterations in the isodose curves. However, optimization requires increased treatment planning time and experienced physics and dosimetry staffs to perform the optimization procedure. Optimization of a treatment plan is not an acceptable means of accounting for poor applicator position.

Discussion and Conclusions

HDR brachytherapy for carcinoma of the cervix developed over 10–20 years is now moving into a phase of greater sophistication, particularly regarding dose specification and integration of brachytherapy with EBRT. Evaluation of initial studies of HDR brachytherapy for cervical cancer show that investigators who moved from LDR to HDR brachytherapy have increased the number of HDR fractions during a treatment course while decreasing the dose per fraction. This approach should achieve decreased long-term bladder and bowel complications while maintaining or improving local tumor control. As institutions proceed with HDR gynecological programs, they are reporting their past LDR experience of survival and complications compared to their current HDR program results. It is difficult to compare HDR brachytherapy results from one institution to those of another because of variations in dose specification, treatment schedules, and toxicity grading. Within the same institution, sequential LDR and HDR studies and a few prospective, randomized trials suggest that the move to HDR brachytherapy can be accomplished safely while maintaining excellent disease control and the

expected incidence of normal tissue toxicity sequelae. It is unlikely that multi-institutional, randomized, controlled trials will be performed to evaluate the effectiveness of HDR compared with LDR brachytherapy for cervical cancer. Institutions proficient at HDR brachytherapy have developed their own novel approaches for combining external beam irradiation with intracavitary HDR therapy that may enhance the therapeutic ratio and lead to increased tumor control rates without altering late sequelae. Innovations in treatment unit design and refinement of hardware and software for treatment planning facilitate treatment techniques that advance research in HDR brachytherapy.

References

1. Larkin AJ. Radium in General Practice. Paul B. Hoeber, New York, 1939, p. 72.
2. Kottmeier HL. Surgical and radiation treatment of carcinoma of the uterine cervix. Acta Obst Gynecol Scand 1964;43:2.
3. Lamarque P, Coliez R. Electroradiotherapie. L. Delherm, Paris, 1951, p. 2549.
4. Paterson R. The Treatment of Malignant Disease by Radium and X-Rays. Edward Arnold, London, 1948.
5. Fletcher G. Cervical radium applicators with screening in the direction of the bladder and rectum. Radiology 1953;60:77–84.
6. Suit H. Modification of the Fletcher ovoid system for afterloading using standard sized radium tubes. Radiology 1963;81:126–131.
7. Henschke U. Afterloading application for radiation therapy of carcinoma of the uterus. Radiology 1960;87:834.
8. Simon N, Silverstone S. Intracavitary radiotherapy of endometrial cancer by afterloading. Gynecol Oncol 1972;1:13.
9. Sievert RM. Two arrangements for reducing irradiation dangers in teleradium treatment. Acta Radiol 1937;18:157–162.
10. Henschke UK, Hilaris BS, Mahon GD. Intracavitary radiation therapy of cancer of uterine cervix by remote afterloading with cycling sources. Am J Roentgenol 1966;96:45–51.
11. Joslin CAF, O'Connell D, Howard N. The treatment of uterine carcinoma using the Cathetron: III. Clinical considerations and preliminary reports on treatment results. Br J Radiol 1967;40:895–904.
12. Inoue T, Hori S, Miyata Y, et al. High versus low dose rate intracavitary irradiation of carcinoma of the uterine cervix. Acta Radiol Oncol 1978;17:277–282.

13. Taina E. A comparison of clinical results following high dose rate intracavitary afterloading irradiation with Co-60 and conventional radium therapy for stage I-II endometrial cancer. Acta Gynecol Scand 1981;103(Suppl): 1–71.

14. Van't Hooft E. Recent Advances in Brachytherapy Physics. American Institute of Physics, New York, 1981, pp. 167–177.

15. Fu KK, Phillips TL. High dose rate versus low dose rate intracavitary brachytherapy for carcinoma of the cervix. Int J Radiat Oncol Biol Phys 1989;19:791–796.

16. Stitt JA. High-dose-rate intracavitary brachytherapy for gynecologic malignancies. Oncology 1992;6:59–79.

17. Koga K, Wantanabe K, Kawano M, et al. Radiotherapy for carcinoma of the uterine cervix by remotely controlled afterloading intracavitary system with high dose rate. Int J Radiat Oncol Biol Phys 1983;9:351–356.

18. Shigematsu Y, Nishiyama K, Masake N, et al. Treatment of carcinoma of the uterine cervix by remotely controlled afterloading intracavitary radiotherapy with high dose rate: A comparative study with a low dose rate system. Int J Radiat Oncol Biol Phys 1983;9:351–356.

19. Himmelman A, Holmberg E, Oden A, et al. Intracavitary irradiation of carcinoma of the cervix stage IB and IIA: A clinical comparison between a remote high dose rate afterloading system and a low dose rate manual system. Acta Radiol Oncol 1985;24:139–144.

20. Teshima T, Chatani M, Hata K, et al. High dose rate intracavitary therapy for carcinoma of the uterine cervix: I. General figures of survival and complication. Int J Radiat Oncol Biol Phys 1987;13:1035–1041.

21. Dusenbery KE, Carson LF, Potish RA. Perioperative morbidity and mortality of gynecologic brachytherapy. Cancer 1991;67:2786–2790.

22. Bastin K, Buchler D, Shanahan T, et al. Cost efficiency of HDR brachytherapy for gynaecological cancer. Activity 1992;6(2):67.

23. Utley JF, von Essen CF, Horn RA, et al. High dose rate afterloading intracavitary therapy in carcinoma of the cervix. Int J Radiat Oncol Biol Phys 1984;10:2259–2263.

24. Joslin CAF. High activity source afterloading in gynecologic cancer and its future prospects, Ulrich Henschke Memorial Lecture. Endo Hyper Oncol 1989;5:69–81.

25. Roman TN, Souhami L, Freeman CR, et al. High dose rate afterloading intracavitary therapy in carcinoma of the cervix. Int J Radiat Oncol Biol Phys 1991;20:921–926.

26. Selke P, Roman TN, Souhami L, et al. Treatment results of high dose rate brachytherapy in patients with carcinoma of the cervix. 1993; 27:803–809.

27. Ahmad K, Kim YH, Ezzell G, et al. Reproducibility of multifractionated outpatient high dose rate brachytherapy in carcinoma of the cervix using the Ahmad-Kim positioner. Endo Hyper Oncol 1992;8:171–173.

28. Han I, Malviaya V, Orton C, et al. Multifractionated high dose rate brachytherapy with concurrent daily teletherapy for cervical cancer. Gynecol Oncol, In Press.

29. Stitt JS, Fowler JF, Thomadsen BR, et al. High dose rate brachytherapy in carcinoma of the cervix-clinical and biological considerations. Int J Radiat Oncol Biol Phys 1992;24:335–348.

30. Thomadsen BR, Shahabi S, Stitt JA. High dose rate brachytherapy in carcinoma of the cervix—physics and dosimetry considerations. Int J Radiat Oncol Biol Phys 1992;24:349–357.

31. Sarkaria JN, Petereit DG, Stitt JA, et al. A comparison of the efficacy and complication rates of low-dose-rate versus high-dose-rate brachytherapy in the treatment of cervical carcinoma. Int J Radiat Oncol Biol Phys 1994;30:75–82.

32. Abitbol AA, Stitt JA, Schwade JG, et al. High dose rate brachytherapy for carcinoma of the cervix. In: Nag S (ed). High Dose Rate Brachytherapy: A Textbook. Futura Publishing Co., Inc, Armonk, NY, 1994, pp. 373–383.

33. Nag S, Abitbol AA, Anderson LL, et al. Consensus guidelines for high dose rate remote brachytherapy in cervical, endometrial, and endobronchial tumors. Int J Radiat Oncol Biol Phys 1993;27:1241–1244.

Chapter 27

Interstitial Implantation of Gynecological Malignancies

Beth Erickson, M.D., Michael T. Gillin, Ph.D.

Introduction

Transperineal interstitial implantation of gynecological tumors offers an alternative to intracavitary techniques in the setting of bulky disease or anatomical distortion. The theoretical benefits of interstitial implantation contrast the limitations of intracavitary techniques and include treating the disease precisely in its anatomical location, independent of volume and anatomical distortion, and providing a wider, more uniform distribution of radiation in the pelvis.[1]

Over the last 80 years, interstitial implantation techniques have evolved concomitantly with intracavitary techniques in the treatment of gynecological malignancies. Beginning as early as 1914,[2] interstitial sources were implanted in concert with intracavitary, and through the years, were used extensively in the definitive treatment of vaginal and cervical carcinomas or as a preoperative or postoperative adjuvant or occasionally for vulvar carcinomas or recurrent gynecological malignancies. External beam irradiation was used increasingly over time. Initially, freehand transvaginal or laparotomy-guided radon and radium needle implantation was used to improve the distribution of radiation within the parametria. Intraoperative permanent seed implantation was also used for disease not en-

compassable by needles. With both needle and seed implantation, source positioning was somewhat unpredictable even in the best of hands.

Templates (Perspex stabilizers) for radium needles were described in 1942 by Green and Jennings[3] for use in accessible sites such as the vagina.[4] Template-guided techniques for the insertion of cobalt-60 needles were subsequently introduced by Barnes, Morton, and colleaugues[5–9] at Ohio State in the years 1948–1951 for use in multiple pelvic malignancies. The template concept allowed for a more predictable distribution of the needles than possible with freehand radium needle implantation. Rather than inserting all of the needles through the vagina, the needles could be inserted across the entire perineum. Disadvantages included the inaccessibility of the vagina through which to palpate tumor and guide needle placement and the inability to displace the bladder and rectum with packing. The plastic template was designed to fulfill the "ideal" needle arrangement recommended by Corscaden et al.[10] for transvaginal implantation of cervical carcinoma, with concentric cylinders accommodating up to 36 cervical, paracervical, and parametrial needles in addition to a tandem or plastic guide to hold the sources in the endocervical canal. The cobalt-60 needles used were available in a much

From Nag S (ed): *Principles and Practice of Brachytherapy*. © Futura Publishing Co., Inc., Armonk, NY, 1997.

greater array of lengths and activities than radium needles. Interstitial implantation techniques were previously limited by the stock of lengths and strengths of radium needles available. The longest active length of a radium needle available was 6 cm (range 1–6) because longer needles were too brittle for insertion. This sometimes led to inadequate coverage of tumor. Complications were more frequent with the high intensity (10–13 mg) rather than the preferred low intensity radium needles (1–5 mg). Unlike radium needles, different strength cylinders of cobalt could be loaded into the same needle so as to individualize treatment. The diameter of the needles was also much smaller than that of radium needles making them easier to insert but also causing some divergence despite the template. Animal studies as well as laparotomy-guided implantation confirmed the safety of these template-guided insertions. No vascular or visceral injuries were observed in animals or humans even if the bladder was penetrated. Septic events were not documented in the presence of antibiotics given prior to and during the implant. The adoption of cobalt needle implantation, however, at other institutions was limited because of the disadvantage of the short half-life of the source.[11]

The concept of afterloading of template-guided needles was proposed by Mowatt and Stevens.[12] Hollow stainless steel needles were inserted through a Perspex stabilizer and later afterloaded with varying units of radium, radon seeds in gold capillary tubing, or cobalt seeds. A dumbbell loading of the needles was possible if indicated.

A further development in interstitial implantation that had a significant impact on present day techniques was the emergence of Ir-192 sources made available by Henschke et al.[13] at Memorial. Liegner[14,15] reported transperineal insertion of Ir-192 in 1958 for extensive and recurrent centrally located pelvic malignancies. Needles were inserted through the perineum until the tips touched the bony sacral hollow, and were subsequently replaced by 17-gauge tubing and afterloaded with Ir-192 and Co-60. The needles were as long as 20 cm and spaced approximately 1.0 cm apart without the use of a template. Bladder, artery, or vein penetration

with the needles was not thought to represent an imminent risk to the patient. The use of Ir-192 in addition to Co-60 at M.D Anderson was also reported by Suit et al.[16] in 1961 and Fletcher et al.[17] in 1962 for treatment of cervical stump carcinomas and residual disease in the parametria or lateral pelvic wall after external and intracavitary irradiation for cervical carcinoma.[18] Both the use of Ir-192 and the afterloading marked the progression into present day implantation techniques.

Several tenants of interstitial implantation from these early series would guide future interstitial implantation. Low activity sources widely distributed are essential with a needle spacing of 1–2 cm in a specified relationship to the tandem. Differential needle strength and length is required across the implanted volume to achieve a homogeneous dose distribution. Interstitial and intracavitary techniques are usually combined and must be dealt with in dose specification. External beam must be used conservatively and integrated carefully with the implant. Despite some initial trepidation, laparotomy established the safety of the process. There was a trend toward improved control of disease with a potential for an increase in complications with interstitial techniques.

Due to advances in external beam techniques during the 1960s-1970s, interstitial implantation fell into relative disuse. A resurgence of interest in interstitial implantation emerged through the work of Goffinet, Martinez, and colleagues[19] in 1974 at Stanford University. Use of a prefabricated perineal template, the MUPIT (Martinez Universal Perineal Interstitial Template), through which steel needles were inserted and subsequently loaded with Ir-192 or I-125 for implantation of multiple gynecological malignance was subsequently reported.[20] Concurrent to Martinez, Feder, Syed, and Neblett reported revival of Waterman's approach[21] of interstitial implantation of extensive cervical carcinomas and vaginal carcinomas utilizing the Syed-Neblett transperineal template and needle system.[22–24] A "butterfly" configuration, as described by Corscaden et al.,[10] that encompassed the parametria with relative sparing of the bladder and rectum was achieved. It was the evolution of these two systems utilizing templates and Ir-192 that had a significant impact on the development of the current transperineal interstitial implantation techniques to be detailed.

Methods

Indications for Interstitial Implantation

1. Cervical carcinoma—A) Bulky disease (including IVA); B) Narrow vagina; C) Loss of endocervical canal; D) Distal vaginal involvement or extensive proximal vaginal involvement (>0.5 cm thick); E. Cervical stump; F) Persistent disease after external beam and intracavitary implantation.
2. Advanced vaginal carcinoma (vaginal disease thicker than 0.5 cm).
3. Advanced endometrial carcinoma.
4. Recurrent gynecological carcinoma after surgery or prior radiation.

Applicators

The two well known template systems that were first implemented in 1974 for interstitial implantation of perineal tumors include the MUPIT and the Syed-Neblett system. A formal description of the MUPIT for treatment of prostatic, anorectal, and gynecological (cervical, endometrial, vaginal, and vulvar lesions) malignancies was published in 1983 and subsequent years.[20,25–29] One template accommodates multiple pelvic-perineal malignancies rather than designing separate templates for each site. The MUPIT consists of a flat acrylic template and a flat acrylic cover plate, two sets of acrylic cylinders of different diameters to accommodate differences in anatomy, obturators, screws, and 17-gauge stainless steel blind-ended needles of different lengths (may use varying lengths in same patient). Three large holes are located along the vertical centerline of the template to accommodate a bladder catheter, vaginal cylinder, and rectal cylinder. The template is bolted to these cylinders to fix the system. The template is also fixed to the patient's perineum through use of two suture holes. Around the three large holes in the template are a bilaterally symmetric array of small holes that served as trocar guides such that the inserted needles lie in parallel horizontal planes perpendicular

to the plane of the template. These planes are spaced vertically at 1-cm intervals. The horizontal rows of holes are of two types: type I—holes are perpendicular to the template; and type II—holes are oblique to the template angled approximately 13° laterally outward. The use of type II holes allows a wider volume of parametrial tissues to be covered without interference from the ischium (use of the angled holes has been discontinued due to the complex dosimetry that results). The holes in each row are spaced 1.25 cm apart. A volume of 4 cm to either side of midplane can be covered by the use of only type I holes and 7 cm with type II. The vaginal and rectal cylinders comprise the intracavitary component of the system and are available in two sizes. The vaginal and rectal cylinder can accommodate either an intrauterine tandem or drainage tube. Each of the cylinders also has an inner flange that carries an array of eight continuous guide holes for the placement of needles located on a circle with a slightly smaller diameter than the diameter of the cylinder facilitating placement of needles near but not immediately next to the mucosa of the vaginal or rectal walls. Use of the MUPIT is reported at several institutions[30,31] with modification for high-dose-rate (HDR) techniques for vaginal and cervical carcinomas reported by Donath et al.[32] Commercialized applicators are available through Nucletron Corporation (Columbia, MD, USA) for HDR insertions.

The original Syed-Neblett fenestrated template used for treatment of cervical, vaginal, vulvar, and other pelvic malignancies consists of five concentric rings or arcs (the larger circles are missing portions of their superior and inferior arcs) in 1-cm radial increments, including a central grooved needle-holding vaginal obturator (2-cm diameter, 15 cm long), through which a maximum of 44 needles (17 gauge, 20 cm in length) can be inserted, accompanied by a central uterine tandem of medium curvature. The holes of each arc are separated by 1 cm and each arc is separated from an adjacent arc by 1 cm. The template consists of two lucite plates each 1.2-cm thick held together by Allen-head screws, drilled identically to accept the needles. A large central opening accepts the grooved plastic obturator, which can be threaded over a tandem. O-rings are placed in the walls surrounding the guide needles and are flattened when the template is screwed together fixing all of the needles in place.[22,23] Currently there are three Syed-Neblett templates of varying size and shape for use in implantation of gynecological malignancies (GYN 1-36 needles; GYN 2-44 needles; GYN 3-54 needles), as well as templates for implantation of the rectum, prostate, and urethra (Figure 1) (Best Industries, Springfield, VA, USA;

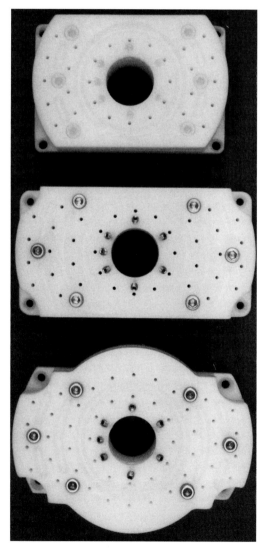

Figure 1. Syed-Neblett templates (top to bottom): GYN 1, GYN 2, GYN 3.

Alpha-Omega Services, Inc., Bellflower, CA, USA). Use of the Syed-Neblett system is reported at multiple institutions.[1,22–24,29,33–69]

Several modifications of these standard templates have also evolved. Shahabi et al.[66] has added lead shielding posteriorly to the Syed-Neblett vaginal obturator to decrease the rectal dose. Branson et al.[55] utilizes a modified and laterally enlarged Syed-Neblett applicator for the treatment of cervical, vaginal, and other gynecological malignancies called the Hammersmith Hedgehog. John et al.[70] have modified the Syed-Neblett template for treatment of cervical carcinoma because of several limitations: 1) the inability to insert the needles through the peripheral rows of the template because of the pelvic bones; 2) the convergence of the cephalad ends of the needles; 3) the 1-cm spacing that led to a large number of needles. To address these limitations, angled holes have been added to the standard Syed-Neblett template and the number of needles required has decreased by 40% (36 to 24) due to an increase in interneedle spacing (1.5 cm). Iridium seed strengths >60% used for a typical Syed implant are used to maintain the same activity as that used for the Syed but the amount of Cs-137 in the tandem has been increased to 35 mg Ra eq to yield a 2:1 ratio of dose to points A and B. A modified Syed-Neblett type of perineal template, with needle spacing of 2.0 cm, has been designed by Hockel and Muller[71] for HDR interstitial brachytherapy of cervical, vaginal, and vulvar carcinomas that can be disassembled after the insertion of the central needles to allow for cystoscopic and rectoscopic control of the needle positions. HDR techniques for cervical carcinoma using a disposable Syed-Neblett template have also been reported by Herskovic et al.[72]

Other innovative templates have also been designed that have been used at single institutions. At Memorial, the Nori-Hilaris-Anderson template is used for advanced or recurrent carcinoma of the cervix. It consists of a perineal template with removable parts, corresponding to the superior (urethral) and inferior (rectal) portions of the template with a vaginal obturator, uterine tandem, and stainless steel needles with stylets.[73] Bentel et al.[74] have fabricated customized templates for multiple gynecological sites following CT scanning with the obturator in the vagina. The obturator is used as a reference structure for aligning the target contour from each image to form a composite two-dimensional contour of maximum tumor extent in a plane perpendicular to the obturator. Dose distributions are calculated to determine the optimum placement of Ir-192 needles in the template. Osian et al.[75] have also created customized templates based on CT for recurrent cervical and other pelvic tumors as have LaVigne, Schoeppel, and McShan.[76] Angled needles were often necessary to avoid perforation of the rectum, bladder, or pubic bone. Leung and Sexton[77,78] have created "Paris system" templates in horseshoe and hexagonal configurations accommodating 6-, 8-, and 10-cm long Ir-192 sources for patients with vaginal carcinomas or positive vaginal margins following hysterectomy for cervical carcinoma. No central tandem is used. Perforations in the template are spaced 18 mm apart in a triangular cross-sectional array with a separation of 15 mm between each row of perforations. Most templates require 13 or fewer sources unlike the 20–32 required with the Syed and Martinez systems. A simple circular vaginal template has been designed by Choy et al.[79] for use in patients with vaginal stenosis and for patients with inadvertent hysterectomy as a substitute for intracavitary techniques for cervical carcinoma. The plastic applicators of diameter 2–3.5 cm hold 6–8 Cs-137 needles on the periphery or eight peripheral needles and one central needle. Many institutions fabricate their own templates. Use of such templates for vulvar, vaginal, and cervical carcinomas have been reported in several series.[59,80–92]

Insertion Techniques

Preoperative Preparation

A complete preop evaluation is undertaken prior to implantation including an ECG, chest x-ray, complete blood count, PT, PTT, and serum chemistries. Patients must have a bowel-clearing schedule the day before the procedure. At our institution patients are instructed to eat a low residue diet the day prior to the implant and are NPO after midnight. One to two L of Go-lytely are taken until the bowels are clear. Other bowel regimens may

include magnesium citrate, stool softeners, fleets or soap suds enemas, sometimes in combination with antibiotics (neomycin) to rid the GI tract of bacteria.[25,29] Some of these bowel cleansing routines require admission the night before implantation whereas with the Go-lytely prep patients can be admitted the day of the procedure. A betadine vaginal and perineal prep are given once the patient is in the operating room. A three-way bladder catheter with a 30-cc balloon attached to a TURY (Baxter, Mcgaw Park, IL, USA) set for infusion of saline into the bladder is used at our institution. The large 30-cc bulb and three-way catheter system are needed for bladder filling (150–200 cc of saline) to enable transabdominal ultrasound imaging during insertion of the anterior needles. The bulb is filled with a solution of dilute Hypaque® for future visibility on orthogonal x-rays. Following needle insertion, the catheter bulb is deflated to 7 cc so that the contrast does not create artifact on the CT images that follow implantation. Patients are also given 3 g of Unasyn IV during implantation. Thigh high Ted hose are usually worn during the implant with or without sequential compression devices on the legs to prevent thrombus formation.

Anesthesia

When possible, our patients undergo epidural catheter placement prior to needle implantation.[30,35,36,57,72,75,93,94] Relative contraindications to epidural anesthesia include anatomical deformity such as a meningomyelocele or bony deformities impeding catheter insertion; anticoagulation (excluding aspirin and short-term subcutaneous heparin) unless reversal is possible; conditions such as liver disease resulting in an uncorrectable PT, PTT; or elevated intracranial pressure. The epidural not only contributes to pain control during needle insertion, but is also used for postoperative pain management in preference to IV, IM, or oral pain medications. It is important to explain and discuss the procedure with the anesthesiologists prior to the implant so that they realize that pain management will be needed 24 hours per day postinsertion as well as during the insertion. Our patients meet with the anesthesiologists the week before the procedure so that an effective pain strategy can be planned well ahead of time. It is imperative to have good catheter placement at the onset, taped securely in place, as it is exceedingly difficult to replace the catheter once the patient has been implanted and loaded. On the morning of implantation, induction of an adequate level block (T10-S5) using a lidocaine or bupivacaine infusion with or without fentanyl is established prior to implantation so that it is effective when the patient becomes aroused after the procedure is complete. Monitored anesthesia (propofol) usually accompanies the epidural to relax the patient during needle insertion. General endotracheal anesthesia is only necessary if laparoscopy or laparotomy are used to guide needle placement. At some institutions, the use of spinal anesthesia has also been described.[38,39,44,45] General anesthesia is still used at many institutions.[23–25,30,35,38–41,44,45,55,68,74]

Insertion

Insertion of the Syed-Neblett system is performed in the operating room at our institution. Allen stirrups are used to place the patient in the dorsal lithotomy position with the pelvis in a more neutral position than achieved with candy cane stirrups. A pelvic examination under anesthesia is performed to assess tumor dimensions and extensions, the proximity of other pelvic organs, and the position of the uterus. Sounding of the uterus and dilatation of the endocervical canal follow, and a pair of stainless steel balls are sewn on the anterior and posterior lips of the cervix and/or the upper and lower boundaries of the vaginal lesion of interest for reference on future orthogonal radiographs. For patients with a patent endocervical canal, a Fletcher-Suit stainless steel tandem without a sail is inserted. If a tandem cannot negotiate the endocervical canal, a 25-cm guide needle is inserted instead[54] and held in place with a custom-built obturator insert with a set screw fabricated at our institution. The Syed-Neblett obturator is then threaded over the tandem. A "sleeve" also fabricated at our institution, is placed over the obturator when needles are to be inserted into the obturator surface grooves, to prevent their direct contact with the vaginal mucosa.[95] The Syed-Neblett template is then threaded over the obturator, and positioned flush with the perineal surface. It is important to ascertain that the template is appropriately centered on the perineum and that the perineum is relatively flat through careful patient positioning. Rotation of the template from its typical horizontal position is sometimes needed to encompass vaginal or vulvar disease. Insertion of the 17-gauge needles that measure 20–25 cm in length follows. The 25-cm needles are often needed on the obturator surface (15 cm long) in patients with deep vaginas or for patients with deep-seated intrapelvic disease. The needles used at our institution are closed tipped to reduce the risk of infection and have a funneled proximal end to make source loading easier. The closed-tipped needles do not, however, alert the physician if an artery has been entered. Plastic flexi-guides have been used in several patients at our institution though bending of the needles and broken needle tips have discouraged their use. The use of plastic flexi-guides with templates has been previously reported.[30,52,74,96,97]

Choice of Template Holes

It is not necessary to use all of the template holes but rather, the choice should be based on the location of the tumor volume. It is important to realize that needles must be inserted beyond the tumor both laterally and in a cephalocaudal direction to adequately cover the tumor volume.[98] Template holes nearest the bladder and rectum (11, 12, 1, 5, 6, and 7 o'clock positions of paracervical ring) are often avoided unless there is tumor extension so mandating such as vesicovaginal or rectovaginal septal involvement or urethral involvement (Figure 2). Interference from the pubic bones may preclude use of some needle holes anteriorly and laterally.

Both symmetric and asymmetric loading of the template have been described by Martinez et al.[25–28] for patients with circumferential or unilateral extension of paracervical disease. Erickson et al.[37] also recommend selective use of key template holes. Symmetric loading of the template is practiced by Syed.[35,36] Aristizabal et al.[38–41] recommend filling the entire template whenever possible.

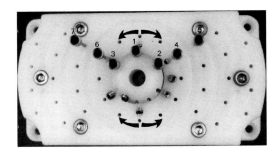

Figure 2. Template holes typically left unloaded near rectum and bladder (curved arrows) and needles inserted with ultrasound guidance (1–7).

Depth of Needle Insertion

Before placing the first needle, the preradiation MRIs are reviewed and the distance from the perineum to the uterine fundus is measured so as to estimate the appropriate depth of needle insertion. Problematic anatomical situations are also identified including an anteverted uterus overlying the bladder dome, suprauterine sigmoid, pelvic small bowel, a deviated or "horned" bladder, or massive disease. An estimate of needle depth insertion can also be made by referencing the needle depth insertion to the intrauterine tandem once the uterine sounding depth is known. It may not be necessary to insert all of the needles to the same depth as the tandem but this will subsequently require dealing with different rather than uniform source lengths, which can be problematic both during loading and dosimetrically.[55] We typically insert at least the obturator needles to the same depth as the tandem. Once the bladder is filled with 150–200 cc of saline, intraoperative transabdominal ultrasound is also performed to guide needles close to the bladder, and to further confirm the appropriate depth of needle insertion by visualizing the endocervical canal, cervico-uterine junction, and uterine fundus, and their relationship to the advancing needles.[99] Ultrasound is most helpful during placement of the most anterior needles on the obturator surface and the anterior lateral holes of the template (7–10 needles) (Figure 2). If the initial needles are advanced too far cephalad, they will touch the sacrum and are necessarily retracted. After several needles are in place, an intraoperative

x-ray is obtained, confirming the desired relationship of the needles to the tandem and marker balls. Adjustments as needed are then made and films repeated if necessary. After the depth of insertion has been determined and documented by measuring the needle protrusion from the template, similar placement of the remaining needles is accomplished once the bladder is drained. Those needles nearest the rectum are inserted with a guiding rectal finger to avoid penetration. Cystoscopy and proctosigmoidoscopy are used at some institutions to rule out rectal and bladder penetration at the end of the procedure.[60,71] If ultrasound or cystoscopy are not used for guiding needle insertion near the bladder, methylene blue or indigo carmine dye instillation into the bladder can be used to rule out bladder penetration by the needles.[60] Konski et al.[45] routinely fill the bladder with saline during the implant to displace bowel from the pelvis and decrease the risk of perforation. Needle depth can also be determined with the aid of laparoscopy or laparotomy. This is strongly recommended in the posthysterectomy setting when bowel may be adherent to and freed from the vaginal cuff. Use of laparoscopy is reported in several series,[24,51,60,74] though we have found this sometimes discourages optimum needle placement because of the fear of penetrating intervening bowel loops. Additionally, it is not always possible to visualize all of the needles that may be buried in the pelvic tissues or bladder. Use of laparotomy is particularly helpful as the needles can be manually guided by two teams from the perineum to the lower abdominal cavity.[24,27,30,34,37–39,48,55,57,60–62,74,77] This may be especially helpful for patients with problematic anatomies as previously described or for patients with adherent pelvic bowel or prior hysterectomy. Disaia, Syed, and Puthawala[57] reported use of an open implant technique for patients with vaginal disease following prior hysterectomy. Guidance of the needles following laparotomy as well as the placement of an omental carpet to displace bowel from the needle tips were the advantages of the technique. There is generally, however, reluctance on the part of surgeons to perform laparotomies for needle placement due to the concern over submitting the patient to a major abdominal procedure in addition to the interstitial implant.[60]

Perhaps the best method of confirming optimum needle depth insertion is through the use of CT following needle insertion, as practiced at our institution and described under "Dosimetry."[67]

The depth of needle insertion varies greatly by institution. Through use of laparotomy, digital examination including rectal exam and orthogonal films, the depth of needles insertion in Martinez's series ranged from 6.5–13.5 cm. The superior extension of tumor determined the depth to which the needles were placed and the inferior extent determined the number of sources per ribbon. No intention was made to implant disease above the lower uterine segment unless mandated by tumor extension.[25–28] Fu et al.[29] describe a preplanning process in which the patient undergoes CT or MRI with the vaginal obturator in place, such that from the dimensions of tumor shown on the CT or MRI one can determine how far the needles should extend beyond the tip of the vaginal obturator to encompass the tumor volume with margin. A similar system using CT is described by Bentel et al.,[74] Osian et al.,[75] and LaVigne et al.[76] Corn et al.[60] also reported preplanning of vaginal implants by obtaining MRIs with the vaginal obturator in place. An endorectal coil was used to improve image quality. Fluoroscopic guidance during needle insertion has been reported in several series to ensure parallelism and the optimum depth of insertion (S. Nag personal communication).[48,54]

As the dose decreases near the tips of the needles, the needles must be inserted several centimeters beyond the target volume when possible to ensure adequate coverage.[55,100] Neblett et al.[98] suggest that the sources extend 1–2 cm beyond the target volume. Branson et al.[55] recommended that the needles be inserted 1 cm beyond the tumor volume. Leung[77] suggested needle insertion 1–1.5 cm beyond the tumor volume, and Kumar et al.[53,54] suggested 1 cm distal to tumor in the cervix. In Syed's series, the needles were inserted approximately 2–4 cm into the cervix and parametrial tissues.[22,23,29] Aristizabal et al.[38–41] recommended needle insertion 3–4 cm beyond the cervix. In the series of Choy et al.,[79] the depth of insertion was typically 2–3 cm into the cervix or 2 cm into the vaginal cuff. We have not been convinced that insertion 2–3 cm into the cervix is adequate as there is rapid fall-off of dose near the needle tips, which are essentially inactive. This results in an inadequate distribution near the level of "point A," which is 2 cm up from the cervical marker balls. We use the Paris system guidelines such that the sources are inserted 15%–20% longer on each end than the target length.[77] This may be somewhat problematic at the superior aspect of the implant in the presence of intervening bowel and must be balanced against morbidity.

Use of the Vaginal Obturator Surface

When first introduced in 1974, the Syed-Neblett vaginal obturator surface was routinely loaded, usually in association with a central intrauterine tandem.[22–24,34,56] Long-term follow-up, however, revealed a substantial incidence of rectovaginal and vesicovaginal fistulae, and vaginal necrosis.[34,56] Mucosal injury related to the direct proximity of the obturator needles to the vaginal mucosa and compression of the vaginal mucosa between the obturator sources and the sources occupying the first ring of the template was speculated.[38–40] Tandem sources in close proximaty to the obturator sources created a central "hot spot" that added to mucosal injury leading eventually to vaginal necrosis and fistulae.[1] Ensuing recommendations concluded that the obturator needles should not be loaded in the presence of protruding vaginal sources in the tandem,[35–37] or even in the absence of a tandem,[38–40] and that concomitant tandem sources be omitted if the obturator surface needles were to be loaded.[1,37]

Such recommendations pose a dilemma, both for irradiation of uterine and vaginal disease. The Syed-Neblett system is particularly suited for treatment of vaginal disease due to the presence of a vaginal obturator that can carry needles in close approximation to disease. These central obturator needles can be strategically loaded to encompass disease from the fornices to the introitus as needed. Additionally, the obturator needles can be advanced directly into the cervix and may be essential in delivering tumoricidal doses of radiation to the cervix by preventing a central "cold spot," especially in the absence of an intrauterine tandem.[101]

Though controversial, use of the vaginal obturator surface is routine at our institution due to a modification of the Syed-Neblett obturator. A vaginal obturator "sleeve" is placed over the obturator and needles in the obturator grooves.[95] The sleeve distances the mucosa of the vagina from the surface of the needles thereby preventing "hot spots" in the vaginal mucosa.

This same concept of distancing of the needles from the surface of the vagina is achieved with the MUPIT vaginal obturator where the needles are arranged in a circle inside the vaginal obturator.[25]

Use of a Tandem

Use of a central tandem is also controversial because of the potential for a central hot spot and resultant inhomogeneity within the implanted volume. A tandem is used at our institution whenever the endocervical canal is negotiable for patients with cervical carcinoma. A tandem is not always necessary when treating vaginal carcinomas if there is not cervical involvement. A departure of our technique from others previously reported is the use of Ir-192 in the tandem rather than Cs-137, which is available in a much greater variety of lengths and activities. The Ir-192 source is typically twice the activity of the other central sources. After careful scrutiny of the dosimetry, this does not result in a central hot spot but rather avoids a central cold spot. It must be remembered that in standard intracavitary insertions, the cervical dose is typically $2 \times$ the point A dose.[101,102] A certain amount of "inhomogeneity" within the implanted volume may be needed to adequately address disease within the cervix. A similar concern over underdosing of the central tumor volume in the absence of a tandem and particularly with differential loading was published recently by Deore et al.[101] speculating that this may be responsible for the significant rate of local failure in some series. Prempree[103] also reported improved local control when a tandem was used in association with radium needles in comparison to the absence of a tandem.

In the series by Martinez and Schray,[27] a central tandem loaded with Cs-137 was recommended only when there was involvement of the lower uterine segment when uterine sources needed to be inserted beyond the needles. The use of an intrauterine tandem was otherwise discouraged as it disrupted the homogeneity of dose distribution and produced a much higher central dose with a resultant increase in rectal and bladder doses. Needles alone were necessarily used when the endocervical canal could not be located (50% of IIIB cases). Tandems were used in 55% of Syed et al's cases.[22–24,35,36,56] Syed et al. recommended decreasing the activity of the cesium sources in the tandem (20–35 mg Ra eq) and discontinuation of loading of the surface of the vaginal obturator when a tandem was used.[34–36] A significant decrease in complications was observed with these and other modifications.[35,36] Use of a central tandem loaded with Cs-137 was not statistically correlated with complications in the series of Ampuero et al.[1] although the percentage area "hot spot" within the implanted volume did correlate significantly with the presence of serious complications. To minimize this inhomogeneity, Ampuero et al.[1] recommended that a tandem not be used routinely. In a follow-up series by Erickson et al.,[37] it was stressed that if a tandem (20 mg Ra eq, Cs-137) was necessary, the central obturator surface should not be loaded. Aristizabal et al.[38–41] also recommended use of the central tandem (35 mg Ra eq) without loading of the vaginal obturator sources. Branson et al.[55] used a tandem if the inner most ring of the template was not loaded. Fontanesi et al.[42] used tandems loaded with Cs-137 when the endocervical canal was patent. The absence of a tandem did not correlate with an increased risk of recurrence. The use of tandems is also reported in other series.[74]

Fixation

Once the needles have been inserted to satisfaction, the needles are fixed in place by tightening the large template screws. It is important to tighten the obturator set screws prior to inserting needles through the template as it is difficult to gain access to these screws once the template needles are in place. The uterine tandem set screw is tightened last once it is confirmed that the tandem is inserted to its initial depth. A measurement of needle protrusion from the template confirms the intended depth of needle insertion and uniformity of depth of insertion of the needles. Both the MUPIT and Syed-Neblett template are sutured to the perineum through small holes placed at the four corners of the template. It is not always necessary to use all of the suture holes and usually the anterior holes are more easily accessed at the time of removal of the system. We use prolene sutures and attempt to suture through an adequate amount of cutaneous and subcutaneous tissue so that there is not excessive tension on a small area of skin that can cause necrosis. Xerofoam gauze, which is embedded with an antibiotic emulsion, is packed between the perineal skin and the template both anteriorly and posteriorly to discourage bacterial growth. Gauze 4 × 4s are placed between the thighs and the template to avoid pressure necrosis. Two ABD pads are taped together to "envelope" the system. A 16Fr red rubber catheter is placed in the rectum for future rectal contrast. The patient is taken down from the dorsal lithotomy position and placed in a frog legged position on pillows to avoid tension on the system. In obese patients it is important to prevent the thighs from displacing the system as the patients legs are lowered from the dorsal lithotomy position. The patient is transferred to the recovery room and epidural anesthesia optimized. Sources are not typically loaded until the day after needle insertion to allow time for patient care and source arrival.

Use of Rectal and Bladder Distention

At some institutions, a large rectal tube with or without a balloon is used to displace the posterior wall of the rectum and drain secretions.[29,81] With the MUPIT, a rectal cylinder is placed to assure a fixed distance between the vagina and rectum and to displace the posterior rectal wall. A rectal tube is used to evacuate flatus and secretions. Bladder distension as reported by Martinez et al.[25–28] is also used during implantation to decrease the bladder dose and displace small bowel. We do not use bladder distention as we fear it may push parts of the bladder closer to the needles.

Pain Control and Postoperative Care of the Patient

Epidural anesthesia is used at our institution for postoperative pain management. The lidocaine or bupivacaine infusion initiated in the operating room is continued, with or without morphine or fentanyl supplementation, throughout the duration of the implant. Once on the hospital ward, the patient's vitals and oxygen saturation must be monitored regularly while the epidural is in place. The nurses caring for these patients must have formal instruction in care of patients with epidurals. The pharmacy must also be accustomed to mixing the appropriate concentration of medications for the infusion. Additionally, at our institution the anesthesiologists write all of the orders for pain management while the epidural is in place and the addition of oral, IV, or IM pain medications by other physicians is discouraged. Such efforts require the availability of well trained anesthesiologists 24 hours per day. Supplemental epidural boluses may be needed PRN. In preference to an epidural, oral, IM, or IV (including patient controlled analgesia) pain medications are used at some institutions.[45,72] No matter what the choice, it is important to assure that the patient is comfortable as uncontrolled pain can quickly become a crisis for these patients. An air bed is also used to provide further comfort, with the head of the bed kept at 30° or less. Elastic Ted hose and sequential compression devices are maintained on the legs to reduce the risk of thromboembolic events. At some institutions, subcutaneous heparin is also used. Patients are log-rolled once per shift to change their underlying chucks and to check for signs of fecal material or pressure decubiti. A clean chuck is placed every shift so that the patient's skin is not exposed to irritating secretions. A low residue diet and scheduled lomotil 3–4 times/day are given to prevent bowel movements. If the patient does stool, it must be quickly cleansed from the skin and template. A spray bottle may be helpful in removing stool from the template. The gauze 4 × 4s and ABD pads are changed at least once per day. The patient is kept frog-legged but is allowed to move her legs and bend her knees. Three grams of IV unasyn are given every 6 hours. If the patient becomes febrile on this regimen, other appropriate antibiotics to cover additional anaerobes, gram negatives, staphylococcus, and streptococcus are added. Nausea sometimes accompanies the epidural and antiemetics are made available if needed. Occasionally the patient will develop an ileus from the narcotics and lomotil and this must be recognized should abdominal distention and nausea develop. Incentive spirometry is used to reduce the risk of fever due to atelectasis. Routine radiation precautions are put into effect once the patient is loaded. Depending on the number and activity of sources, the implant activity may be quite high making surveying of adjacent rooms and hallways even more important.

Applicator Removal and Postimplant Care

When an epidural is in place, a bolus can be given 15–30 minutes prior to needle removal. If other forms of pain control have been used, IV or IM pain medication can be given 20–30 minutes prior to removal.[25,35,36] The applicator is removed at the bedside with the patient in a frog-legged position. The sutures are clipped to free the template from the perineal skin. At some institutions the template, needles, and tandem are removed as a unit over several minutes.[24,25,35,36] If a curved tandem has been inserted, the system must be removed with care to avoid trauma to the cervix. Our preference is to remove some of the more peripheral needles individually so that there is not so much resistance and tension on the cervix during removal. Bleeding may be more of a problem if the removal is traumatic. Should bleeding occur, pressure applied to the perineum with ABD pads is usually effective in controlling it. Following removal, the perineum is washed with a mild soap followed by Neosporin applications. A perineal pad is placed in the event of bleeding. Activity is increased gradually, from supine, to sitting, to leg dangling, to walking with assistance, after the epidural effects have dissipated. Once ambulating, the sequential compression devices and bladder catheter are removed and a dilute betadine or hydrogen peroxide douche are given. The IV unasyn is changed to oral augmentin or another appropriate antibiotic that the patient will take for a week as an out-patient. The scheduled lo-motil is changed to PRN to promote stooling prior to discharge. The patient is usually monitored at least one shift prior to discharge. The patient is instructed to sitz bathe 2 times/day, followed by perineal Neosporin applications. Once discharged, the patient is instructed to call with temperatures above 101.50, resurgence of vaginal bleeding, or difficulty with voiding. Pain medication is usually not required. The patient is usually seen the week after the implant at the time of initiation of external pelvic side-wall boosting for assessment of acute reactions. A small amount of vaginal discharge and some discomfort with voiding are expected. Inflammation around the suture sites is typical but quickly resolves with proper care. Perineal cellulitis is a rare occurrence if proper perineal care and antibiotics have been used.

Dosimetry

Traditionally, interstitial implantation has been guided by published systems, referring to a set of rules taking into account the source strengths, geometry, and method of application in order to obtain suitable dose distributions over the volumes to be treated. Prior to computerized dosimetry, early interstitial techniques relied on Paterson-Parker and Quimby tables, as well as, film dosimetry for analysis of the dose distribution. Though guidelines for volume implants were laid down in the Quimby and Paterson-Parker systems, these rules were designed for radium sources, and certainly do not apply to the rigid source distribution defined by template applications. The Paris system, though often applied to planar, template defined implants, does not address volume implants greater than two planes.[104] The large volume implants of the pelvis here described defy all traditional rules, with needle and source placement rigidly determined by the template holes, without the ability to cross sources, and with few guidelines for selection of source activity.

Both the MUPIT and the Syed-Neblett applicators were introduced in 1974 in concert with computerized dosimetry.[20,22,23,25–28] Originally, preplanned computerized dosimetry plots that relied on the fixed and ideal relationship of the template and needles were published by Neblett et al. and available for users of the Syed-Neblett perineal template system.[105] These were used for preplanning as well as following implantation without generation of dosimetry for each individual patient. These dose-rate distribution plots have subsequently been taken out of circulation due to the high central dose rates produced with the activity and uniformity of sources suggested (DL. Neblett, written communication, 1994).

The concept of preplanning was introduced with the development of template techniques due to the predictability of dose distribution as a result of the fixed positions of the sources in the template. This preplanning process, which enabled the generation of dose-rate distributions prior to implantation to guide the selection of source length, position, and activity and allow modifications prior to needle insertion, has been suggested in many series.[25,27,29,45,48,54,60,74,75,106] Once in the operating room, the needles ideally pass through the template into tissue and result in a specific intended geometrical arrangement inside the patient. If this is in fact accomplished, these preplanned dose-rate plots can be used for the final dosimetry. If the anticipated positioning is not realized, postimplant dosimetry should be altered as needed allowing optimization of the dosimetry for each patient.[25,27,106]

A further step in the dosimetric analysis of these complex implants, used in most current series, has been computer-generated orthogonal film-based dosimetry.[1,24,25,29,30,34–36, 38–42,44–46,55,56,60,68,74,77,100,107] This model predicts individual source locations from the orthogonal films following implantation, assuming that the source guides are straight, perpendicular to the template, and placed at equal depths in tissue. The X-Y-Z coordinates are determined after orthogonal films are taken with the cervical os as the geometric origin. The computer is given the number of source guides in the template and their location; the number of iridium seeds per guide and their activity and separation; and the tandem source number, activity, and spacing. The computer then calculates a dose rate at any desired geometric point within the tumor mass by summating the dose contributions from all of the sources and incorporating the inverse square law and a correction factor for attenuation.[34,107]

While computer-assisted dosimetry following implantation better represents individualized treatment parameters than precalculated dosimetry, both assume ideal positioning of sources internally. Ideal positioning is seldom achieved and frequently, significant deviation of the needles from their anticipated course is found on the radiographs.[107] Additionally, a true understanding of the dose distribution as it relates to tumor volume and critical normal structures has remained elusive utilizing orthogonal film-based dosimetry. The relationship of the needles and dose distribution to the implanted cervical marker, bladder catheter bulb, rectal contrast, and pelvic sidewall structures can be established, but soft tissue structures such as the uterus as well as the entire bladder and rectosigmoid cannot be imaged. One must rely on point doses to make treatment decisions along with superimposition of the isodose curves on the implant film. Such two-dimensional orthogonal film-based dosimetry appears inadequate in the setting of large volume interstitial implants.

Despite years of clinical use, a system for dosimetric analysis has not been formalized for use with the transperineal implants. Few rules have been established to guide the insertion and interpret the dosimetry. When using the Syed-Neblett applicator, the choice of source strength, number, and location as well as interpretation of the resultant dosimetry has been left to the discretion of the brachytherapist, with little guidance as to selection of the appropriate dose rates, prescription isodose, and uncertainty as to the significance of the volume of tissue treated to selected doses. Often times, the isodose that encompasses the needles, unrelated to anatomy, is chosen as the reference isodose, with a resultant dose-rate gradient across the volume and central hot spots. As a result, these large volume implants have been criticized for dose distribution inhomogeneity and dose rates higher than those recommended in traditional low-dose-rate (LDR) systems, with a resultant increase in complications. No published guidelines exist for dose limitations for the bladder, rectum, or medial parametria, nor is there a recorded maximum or average homogeneous tumor dose per unit volume beyond which an intolerable complication rate exists.[34] It has also been a challenge to evaluate and describe the completed implant that is characterized by multiple source lengths and activities, as well as to understand the dose distribution to structures of interest.

At our institution, to address these limitations and criticisms, we have pursued the use of CT-guided dosimetry in the planning and analysis of interstitial implants of gynecological malignancies.[67] Despite reports of CT scanning following needle placement in several series,[32,50,54,74,75,108,109] a comprehensive approach to its use has not been previously published nor has any dosimetric system for the planning and analysis of these large volume implants been adequately addressed. We have used CT imaging following needle implantation to identify tumor volume and critical normal structures, to confirm the adequacy of needle placement in relation to these structures and the need for adjustment, to analyze and manipulate the dose distribution as it relates to these structures, and to assist with dose specification and the integration of external beam irradiation. The phases of this process will be described.

Sources

Both Cs-137 microspheres and Ir-192 ribbons or wires can be accommodated by the needles in the MUPIT and the Syed-Neblett templates.[38–41,110] Low activity Ir-192 is most frequently used although recently use of high activity Ir-192 has also been reported.[32,71,72] The use of radium and cesium needle sources has also been described for the uncommon situations when Ir-192 is not available.[97]

Source Length, Activity, and Differential Loading

At our institution, Ir-192 source ordering is accomplished the day of the implant with loading the following day. The user must first determine the number of source trains needed, an estimate of the active length of the trains, and the desired activity and spacing of the Ir-192 seeds. The number of sources required is determined by viewing the intraoperative x-ray and CT, and confirming this

with the needle count taken in the operating room. The number of 20- and 25-cm needles must be distinguished. A source train must also be ordered for the tandem or central needle. Dosimetric preplanning is performed prior to implantation once the desired reference dose rate is specified. By entering different source activities and lengths into various template and obturator positions using the line source computer program (Theratronics computerized systems, Kanata, Ontario, Canada), the optimum dose-rate and dose distributions can be selected by manipulating source activity, length, and location. This will guide needle placement in the operating room and facilitate source ordering. A general rule is that linear activities of <1 mCi/cm are desired. Differential source activity is the rule, with the core sources typically 1/2 to 1/3 the activity of the peripheral sources (0.13 mCi/seed vs 0.37 mCi/seed). Equal source strengths will result in a large section of the interior portion of the implant receiving a high dose when compared to the reference isodose, perhaps accounting for the high rate of late complications in series recommending uniform loading patterns. In reality, the ordered activity may vary from that which is received due to availability. Seed spacing center to center is typically 0.5 cm rather than 1.0 cm to allow small incremental adjustments in length.

The exact length of the source trains is determined the day following needle insertion when the patient is brought to the simulator for needle identification films. The length of the sources is determined by the relationship of needle tips to the location of the stainless steel cervical marker balls. Potential overlap of the tandem and needle source trains must be evaluated, as must the amount of vagina included within the implant. A minimum extension of the active length of the sources of 2 cm beyond the cervical marker balls or vaginal disease is established (Figure 3). Typical source train lengths are 7.3 cm (range 4–12 cm).

Source loading is accomplished within the department and a confirmatory radiograph taken with all sources in place. Modifications of the planned source placement, based upon the location of specific needles and critical structures, can be made prior to loading the

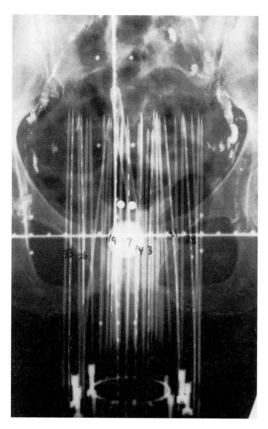

Figure 3. AP radiograph Syed-Neblett template, needles, and tandem. Note: Cervical marker balls above bladder catheter bulb. "Dummy" sources are in several central and peripheral needles.

patient or during the implant. A physicist and physician load the template together and follow a diagram that is color-coded by source activity. It also indicates which needles are to be left unloaded. Plastic caps are placed over the ends of the needles to avoid source dislodgment and the system is subsequently enveloped with an ABD pad.

Selection of source activity for the MUPIT was intended to produce narrowing of the treatment volume near the longitudinal midplane of the patient to avoid overdosage of the bladder and rectum. For asymmetric tumors, the distribution could be narrowed on the uninvolved side by selectively avoiding insertion of needles in these locations. To achieve this, the use of full (0.6 mg Ra eq) and half-strength (0.3 mg Ra eq) sources was

recommended such that the activity of the central sources was 1/2 to 1/3 that of the activity of the peripheral sources. Approximately eight Ir-192 seeds/needles and 100 mg Ra eq per implant were used for the straight needles and two or three seeds for the oblique needles.[20,25–29] In the original Syed-Neblett system, each needle held five or six seeds, spaced 1 cm apart over a 4 or 5 cm length. The seed strengths chosen were in the range of 0.30–0.45 mg Ra eq. No attempt was made to implant the entire parametria homogeneously, which differs from the Martinez approach. Instead, each group of parametrial needles (on opposite sides of the template) was looked upon as a laterally displaced "colpostat" carrying 15–25 mg Ra eq of Ir-192. Instead of being oriented like traditional colpostats in X-Z or AP planes, they were oriented in X-Y or a cephalad-caudad plane. Each needle group was located relatively away from the bladder and rectum and nearer to the lateral pelvic wall. They were much more likely to irradiate the nodal volume of interest while minimizing the dose to the bladder and rectum than the traditionally located colpostats.[23] The average implant consisted of 20–30 ribbons of Ir-192 or 40–70 mg Ra eq in the "colpostat" sources and 35 mg Ra eq Cs-137 in the tandem for cervical carcinomas and six to nine seeds/ribbon for vaginal carcinomas.[22–24,56] Later, lower Ir-192 activities of 0.25–0.40 mg Ra eq/seed were recommended with differential loading of the peripheral versus central sources. Seven seeds were inserted per needle and only 20–35 mg Ra eq of Cs-137 was inserted in the tandem.[35,36] Other authors have also encouraged the use of differential source loading.[1,37,42,45,48,65,74,111] Erickson et al.[37] chose seed strengths of 0.25–0.40 mg Ra eq using six to eight seeds/ribbon except if there was vaginal involvement with a total activity of 20 mg Ra eq of Cs-137 in the tandem. Bentel et al.[74] used seed activities of 0.5 mCi and 0.25 mCi, and Konski et al.[45] used seed activities of 0.45–0.47 mCi and 0.2–0.25 mCi/seed for the peripheral and central sources, respectively. In the series by Aristizabal et al.,[38–41] the typical number of needles used was 30 with active lengths of Ir-192 sources of 6.0 cm with an activity of 2.2 mg Ra eq/source. The tandem held 35 mg Ra eq of Cs-137.

Computerized Dosimetry

Following needle insertion, either the day of or following, the patient undergoes a pelvic CT scan with intravenous and rectal contrast with the unloaded needles in place. Thirty to 40 axial images spaced 5 mm apart are obtained. The axial images are then formatted and reviewed by the diagnostic radiologist, radiation oncologist, and physicist. This will readily identify problems such as a pelvic hematoma, perforated tandem, or the need for adjustment of the depth of needle insertion early in the time course of events. Reconstructed sagittal and coronal views are available that give further insight into the appropriateness of needle depth insertion.

Orthogonal films are next taken to identify the implanted needles following the CT scan. Dummy sources are placed in four to six needles at a time and orthogonal films are successively repeated (Figure 3). These films can then be used to identify the needles on the CT images or to directly digitize the sources into the planning computer.

The CT study is read into the computer (Theraplan V.5B [Theratronics]) and source locations are entered onto the CT images. There are several methods of source entering, all of which make use of the orthogonal films. One method is to digitize the source locations from the films. This is time consuming for large implants containing hundreds of seeds. Additionally, if the patient moves during the simulation between films, then the relative position of the patient moves and the relative positions of the sources will be changed. A second method lessens the digitalization time by approximating the seed strands as continuous line sources and digitizing the two endpoints only.[68] A third method uses the preplan jig program. The preplan jig requires the position coordinates (x,y) of each source strand in a single axial CT plane. The user enters the number of seeds in the strand and the program positions the seeds on that slice and on other CT slices. This method assumes the same x and y coordinates throughout the strand. It does not account for needle curvature. To adjust for this, the x and y coordinates must be found for several CT levels and a single strand broken into several jigs. The simulator films are necessary to identify the

needles on the CT images and which needles are deviated from the horizontal plane to predict where they would lie on the CT images at different levels. Often at the cephalic end of the implant, needles converge in groups and must be individually identified in order to assign their correct activity.

The software is limited to 500 seeds or 30 line sources per plan and if this number is exceeded, two plans must be calculated and summed.

The spatial relationship between the needles and normal anatomy can be clearly defined on the CTs despite the presence of some artifact from the metal needles and marker ball. CT confirms the adequacy of needle and tandem placement through its display of the needles in the patient's anatomy. Because of the epidural, the needles and tandem can be manipulated after the patient leaves the operating room if necessary. It is possible to delineate both the cervix and uterus to some degree though difficult to distinguish tumor from normal uterus. If perforation of the uterus has occurred, the tandem can be retracted to an intrauterine position (Figure 4A). Likewise, if the needles have advanced into small bowel, the needles can be retracted appropriately (Figure 4B). It is easy to see the proximity of the needles to the bladder and rectum and if there is inadvertent penetration of the rectosigmoid or bladder, these needles may be removed or left unloaded (Figures 4C and 4D). Contrast in the rectosigmoid along it circuitous course makes it distinguishable on each slice (Figure 5A). It is important to use a dilute contrast in the rectum so that the needles near or potentially in the rectal wall are not obscured by the contrast. Air is also a suitable contrast agent. Though contrast is routinely placed in the Foley catheter bulb, it is also possible to see the entire bladder and the outline of the posterior wall due to the excreted IV contrast (Figure 5B). It is quite apparent that the dose calculation points based on orthogonal films may underestimate the actual doses to the rectum and bladder. The bladder and rectum are often "draped" across the nearby needles exposing a larger surface area to nearby sources than revealed on plain films (Figure 5B). Modification of the planned source placement based upon the location of specific needles

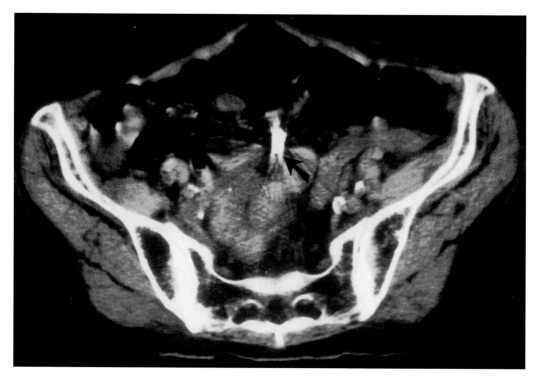

Figure 4A

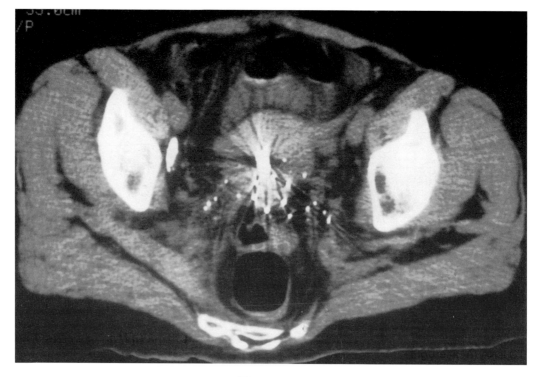

Figure 4B

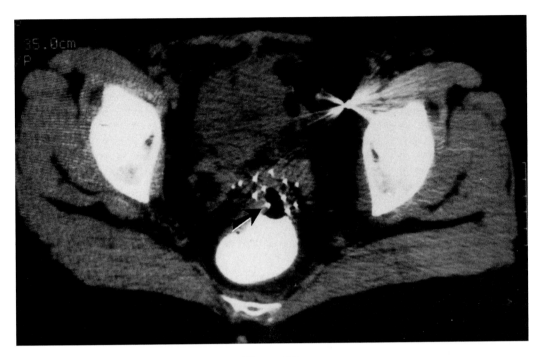

Figure 4C

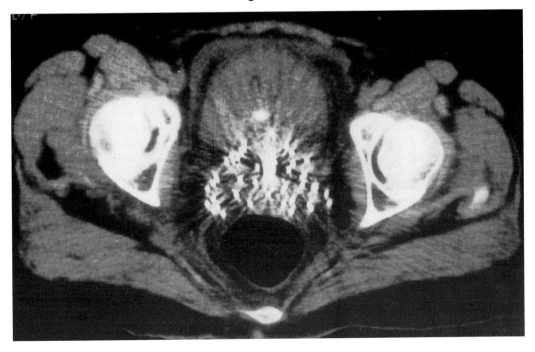

Figure 4D

Figure 4. A) Axial CT demonstrating perforated uterine tandem (arrow). B) Axial CT demonstrating needles in small bowel near the cephalad end of the implant. C) Axial CT demonstrating needle in wall of contrast-filled rectum (arrow). D) Axial CT demonstrating intended insertion of needles into posterior bladder wall in a patient with bladder invasion by tumor.

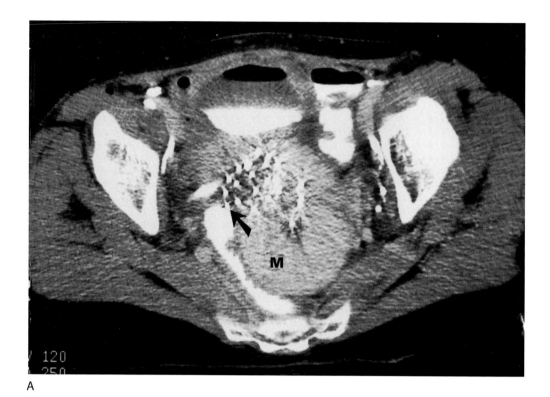

A

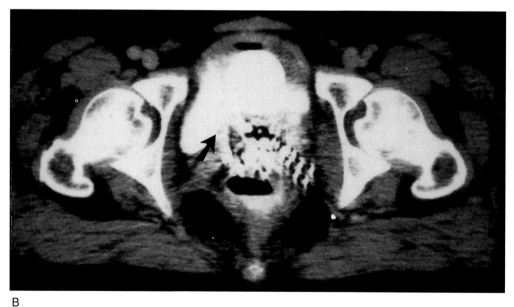

B

Figure 5. A) Axial CT demonstrating circuitous rectosigmoid distinguished with contrast. Note: needle (arrow) in close proximity to rectum that was not loaded. Note: Large uterine myoma that is not traversed by needles (M). B) Axial CT demonstrating the contrast filled bladder that is draped laterally near the peripheral needles (arrow). These needles were loaded with sources of lower activity because of this proximity. Contrast is also present in the rectosigmoid.

and critical structures can therefore be made before or after source loading (Figures 5A and 5B).

Contours of the rectosigmoid, bladder, and tumor volume are delineated and entered on each appropriate axial image through use of a track ball both for ease of identification of these structures on isodose distributions and for dose volume histogram analysis. A contour is also drawn around the needles. The tumor volume is assumed to be within the contour though this may not always be true. Comparison of the location of the needles and the preimplant MRI is sometimes helpful in making a more accurate determination of tumor volume. Subsequently, dose rate and total dose distributions are displayed with the anatomy on the axial CT images.

Dose Rate

Dose rate and total dose distributions are displayed with the appropriate anatomy on axial CT images and on reconstructed sagittal and coronal images, enabling direct visualization of the dose distribution throughout the tumor volume, as well as the rectum and bladder (Figures 6A-C and 7A-C). There is a much clearer understanding of the dose distribution as it relates to both the tumor volumes and critical normal organs with this CT-guided approach. Multiple points of dose specification for the rectum and bladder are easily defined on the CT. The isodose curve that intersects with a significant amount of the rectum and bladder is chosen as the normal tissue dose rate. The dose and dose rates to the tumor volume (reference isodose), point A (Figures 6A-C), the vaginal mucosa (obturator surface) (Figures 7A-C) and pelvic sidewall (Figure 6C) are also assessed from the dosimetry display. The point A slice is defined as 2 cm up and over from the stainless steel cervical marker balls, and is used to relate intracavitary dose prescription to interstitial. Printed isodose distributions are also produced for the "central plane," "point A slice," cervical marker ball, and inferior and superior limits of the implant.

The homogeneity of the dose-rate distribution can be assessed, as well as the location and dimensions of "hot spots" within the distribution. Selection of the "reference isodose" is possible when viewing the distribution and displaying various dose-rate surfaces. The concept of a reference isodose and hyperdose sleeve are borrowed from the Paris system though not defined as strictly as in the Paris system. The reference isodose is defined as the isodose surface, which, in the central plane, surrounds all of the needles with some restrictions. Various criteria have been developed to select an appropriate reference isodose. A dose-rate gradient across the implant >20% to significant volumes is avoided. In the central plane of the implant, the isodose surface whose value is <125% of the reference isodose should not be contiguous and should have dimensions <2 × 2 cm. A maximum of two times the reference isodose (hyperdose sleeve) is acceptable in direct proximity to the needles, but its diameter should be <1 cm. Such criteria can be applied by viewing the dose distribution superimposed upon the anatomy on multiple axial CT slices, as well as the two-dimensional isodose distributions (Figures 6B and 7B).

At our institution, traditional low-dose rates are the goal, achieved through differential loading of low activity sources as described, including reference dose rates of 60–80 cGy/hr, point A dose rates of 50–80 cGy/hr, obturator surface dose rates of 80–100 cGy/hr, and bladder and rectal dose rates <80% of the reference dose rate. The dose distribution can be manipulated, altering the dose rates, homogeneity, and shape of the distribution by selectively changing the activity associated with a particular needle or needles by selectively unloading, either immediately or during the implant, strategic needles, or by changing the number of seeds in each needle. In addition to the multiplanar dose distributions, a simple independent hand calculation is also performed to confirm the dose at a specific point.

Martinez et al.[25–28] recommended dose rates encompassing the tumor volume of 75 cGy/hr (maximum hot spot of 100–110 cGy/hr or 125% isodose around needles only), with bladder and rectal dose rates of 40 cGy/hr. In the original Syed-Neblett system, a minimum dose rate to the lateral parametria (point B) of 40–80 cGy/hr with a maximum dose rate of 80–120 cGy/hr to the medial parametria (point A) was considered ideal with the bladder and rectum receiving 30–50 cGy/

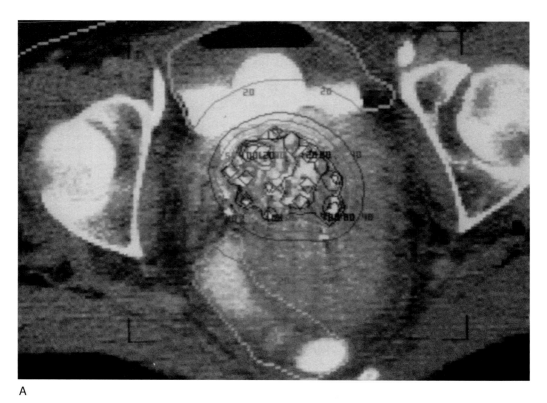

A

Figure 6. A) Axial CT at level of point A with superimposed dose-rate distribution. Note: Contrast-defined bladder and rectum intersected by the isodose distribution. B) Two-dimensional isodose distribution corresponding to this same axial CT slice. Note: Contour of rectum and bladder (R, B). C) Axial CT at level of point A with total dose superimposed. Note: pelvic side-wall distribution, as well as, distribution through the rectum and bladder.

hr.[22–24,56] Later, modified dose rates of a maximum of 80 cGy/hr to point A, 50 cGy/hr to point B, and 25 cGy/hr to the rectum and bladder were recommended.[35,36] Ampuero et al.[1] recommended traditional low-dose rates to the treatment volume of 30–60 cGy/hr as complications were observed at 100 cGy/hr. Erickson et al.[37] suggested a maximum dose rate of 100 cGy/hr with a mean value of 80 cGy/hr. The dose rate to the implanted volume in the series of Choy et al.[79] ranged from 13–16 Gy/day over 4 days and Branson et al.[55] recommended that the dose rate to the treated volume should not exceed 10 Gy/24 hours. Fontanesi et al.[42] chose source activities and loadings so as not to exceed 60 cGy/hr to the tumor volume. Bentel et al.[74] used customized templates and differential source loading to achieve 50 cGy/hr to the target volume. Dose rates in the series by Konski et al.[45] were approximately 52–60 cGy/hr. Potish and Williamson[68] recommend traditional low-dose rates of 35–55 cGy/hr with the dose rate varying by only 5–10 cGy/hr throughout the treatment volume.

Dose and Dose Specification Points

Typically at our institution, total doses to the tumor volume or reference isodose from the implant range from 25–40 Gy over 2–4 days. Total doses to the isodose line 20% higher than the reference isodose are also recorded as are total doses to point A, the rectosigmoid, bladder, obturator surface, and pelvic side wall. Use of a point A dose is not strictly compatible with interstitial volume implants but is used as a guide to relate intracavi-

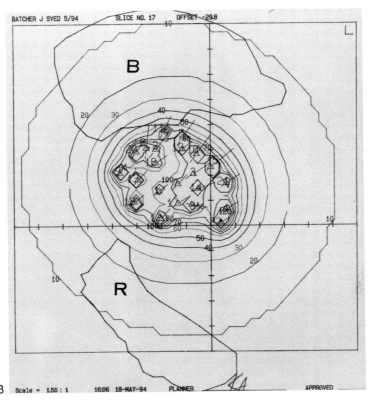

B

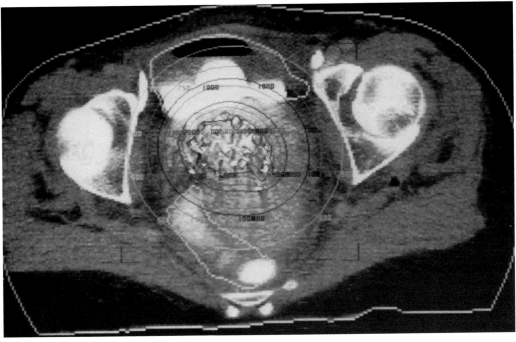

C

Figure 6. *(continued)*

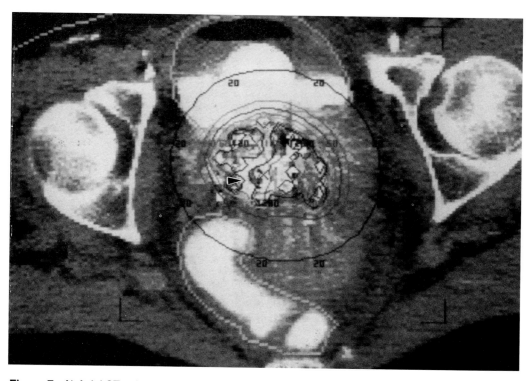

Figure 7. A) Axial CT at level of posterior cervical marker ball with superimposed dose-rate distribution. Note: Contrast-defined bladder and rectum intersected by the isodose distribution and vaginal obturator (arrowhead). B) Two-dimensional isodose distribution corresponding to the axial CT slice. Note: Contour of bladder, rectum, and vaginal obturator (R, B, arrowhead). C) Axial CT at same level with total dose superimposed. Note: Vaginal obturator (arrowhead) distribution, as well as, distribution through the rectum and bladder.

tary doses to interstitial and has been used in several series.

The total implant dose to the lateral parametria (point B) in Syed et al's first report was 30 Gy.[22,23] In their follow-up series, Syed et al. reported 40–60 Gy to point A with two implants, with total cumulative external and implant doses of 80–100 Gy to point A and 55–75 Gy to point B for cervical carcinoma.[35,36] For vaginal carcinomas, 45–50 Gy was delivered over 24–36 hours with a total minimum dose of 80–100 Gy (external + implant) suggested.[24,56] Dose specification in Aristizabal et al.'s[38–41] series was 48 Gy to point A, 24 Gy to point B, and 17 Gy to the rectum and bladder over the 48-hour implant. Fontanesi et al.[42] recommended doses to point A and point B from external beam and implantation not to exceed 100 Gy and 65 Gy, respectively, with maximum rectal doses of

75 Gy and bladder doses of 80 Gy. Kumar et al.[53,54] delivered 90 Gy to point A through a combination of external beam (40 Gy) and interstitial implantation (50 Gy). Use of point A and B was also used in the series of Vermund et al.[44] and John et al.[70] Potish and Williamson[68] recommended that cumulative external beam and implant doses of 85 Gy to point A and 60 Gy to point B should not be exceeded with interstitial implantation. Gaddis et al.[34] considered use of points A and B to be of insignificant value when calculating dose rates for the templates. Instead, Gaddis recommends consideration be given to the homogeneous maximum, minimum, and average tumor dose within a given tumor volume. However, for large volume interstitial implants, no published guidelines exist for dose limitations for the bladder, rectum, or medial parametria, nor is there a recorded

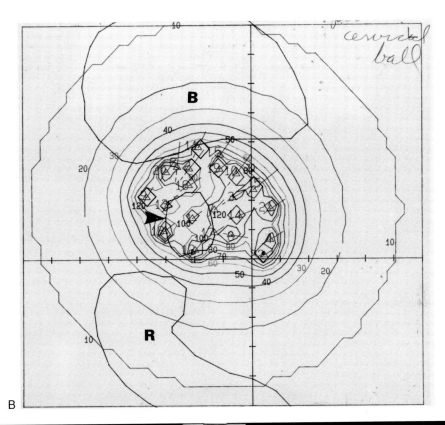

B

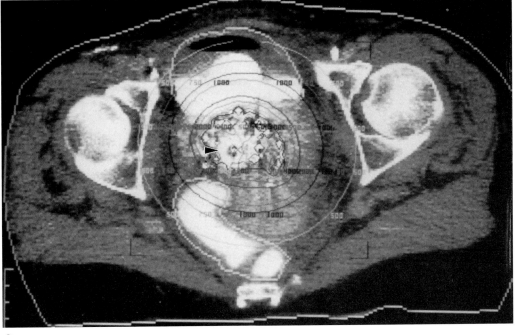

C

Figure 7. *(continued)*

maximum or average homogeneous tumor dose per unit volume beyond which an intolerable complication rate exists.[34] With the MUPIT, the implant dose defined at the cross-sectional plane at the center of the implant was 35–37 Gy.[25–28] Hughes-Davies, Silver, and Kapp[30] prescribed the dose to dose rate contours that included the estimated tumor volume (40–100 cGy/hr) with a median prescribed dose of 30 Gy (6–60 Gy). Ampuero et al.[1] delivered an additional 15–35 Gy/implant (maximum of 40 Gy for two implants). In the series by Erickson et al.,[37] one or two implants were performed (cesium implant 25–40 Gy) interstitial (20–30 Gy). Rush et al.[48] prescribed 30–45 Gy with one implant with total cumulative external and implant doses of 60–90 Gy. Leung[77] recommended 20–30 Gy to the reference isodose. Konski et al.[45] recorded mean implant doses of approximately 31–32 Gy.

Integration with External Beam

The CT-based dosimetry system at our institution also enables entry of the external beam fields and doses, so that cumulative implant and external dose distributions can be produced. This can be very helpful in the design of the midline blocks or for the reduced pelvic side-wall boosts. Multiple implants can also be summated in this way.

At our institution, external whole pelvic irradiation (39.6–45 Gy) precedes implantation, which follows a 1-week break. Following the implant, external irradiation resumes the following week with placement of a midline block corresponding to the lateral boundaries of the needles (not traditional 4–5 cm) delivering 45–50.4 Gy through AP-PA split pelvic fields alone. Reduced AP-PA pelvic side-wall boosts are sometimes given to total doses of 59.6 Gy. The tumor volume receives combined implant and external beam doses of 70–85 Gy over 8 weeks.

Most series recommend limiting whole pelvis doses to 35–45 Gy (20–60 Gy) with subsequent midline blocking and parametrial-lateral pelvic side-wall boosts of 10–20 Gy.[1, 20, 22–28, 30, 34, 35, 37–42, 44, 45, 48, 53, 54, 56, 77, 79] Though midline blocks of 4 cm are described in some series[38–41] wider and more customized blocks are usually needed, corresponding to the needle volume.[20,25–28] Increasing

complications have been associated with higher external beam doses.[20,25–28,45] Hyperfractionated radiation has been reported in one series.[42]

Implant Number/Sequencing

At our institution, only one interstitial implant is planned unless there is persistent disease at least 6–8 weeks following the first implant or poor placement of the first implant. It has been our experience that it is difficult to get patients to agree to two implants. Some have had preceding intracavitary implants. In the series by Martinez et al.,[20,25–28] one or two interstitial implants followed whole pelvis irradiation by 2 weeks with subsequent pelvic side-wall boosts 2 weeks after the implant. In the series by Syed et al.,[22–24,34–36,56] one or two Ir-192 interstitial implants (spaced 2 weeks apart and 2 weeks after external treatment) or one intracavitary followed by one interstitial implant followed external beam. External beam preceded one or two implants in Ampuero et al.'s[1] series (both interstitial or one interstitial and intracavitary). Implantation followed external beam by 10 days in Aristizabal et al.'s[38–41] series using either one intracavitary tandem and ovoid implant and one interstitial, or two interstitial implants at 2-week intervals. Fontanesi et al.[42] reported use of one intracavitary and one interstitial implant or one to two interstitial implants 2 weeks after external beam. Kumar et al.[54] used two interstitial implants of 25 Gy/implant at a minimum interval of 2 weeks. Vermund et al.[44] performed one interstitial implant 2 weeks after external beam, and Rush et al.[48] performed one implant 2–3 weeks after external beam. Gaddis et al.[34] correlated the use of two interstitial implants with increased complications. Erickson et al.[37] recommended one implant for this reason unless preceding intracavitary irradiation was used.

Results

Results using the Syed-Neblett or MUPIT systems for multiple gynecological sites are listed in Table 1 detailing local control, survival, and complications in larger published series.

Table 1.
Results of Transperineal Interstitial Implantation

Series	Site	Number Patients	Local Control	Survival	Complications
Feder, Syed, Neblett (23) 1974–1976 Pre-Modification Syed-Neblett	Cervix / III / IVA	38 / 35 / 3	60% at 24 mo. (ave F/U) / 0% at 24 mo. (ave F/U) (16–40 mo.)	60% NED at 24 mo.	8% *Necrosis of cervix—2* Paravaginal abscess—1
Gaddis et al (34) 1975–1979	Cervix	75	70.7% at med F/U 17 mo. (3–60 mo.)		Adverse 21.3%—(16/75)
	IB	14	64.3%		*Fistulae—(10/75)—13.3%*
	IIA	8	100%	Stage II—68% at 24 mo.	Median time = 11 mo. (5–19 mo.)
	IIB	25	80%		*Grade III non-fistulous—* (6/75)—8%
Pre-Modification	III	26	53.8%	Stage III—38.5% at 12 mo.	(Proctosigmoiditis; cystitis, vault necrosis)
Syed-Neblett	IVA	2	100% Median time to recurrence 6 mo. (1–28 mo.)		Grade II (13/75)—17%
Syed et al (35) 1977–1982	Cervix	60	78% at median F/U 48 mo.	58% overall actuarial disease free	Serious—3%
	IB	6	100% (Minimum F/U = 36 mo.)	83%	*Fistulae (2/60)—3%*
	IIA	2	100%	100%	Cystitis (3/60)—5%
Post-Modification	IIB	21	72%	67%	Proctitis (3/60)—5%
Syed-Neblett	IIIB	26	77%	50%	
	IVA	5	80%	20%	
Aristizabel et al (38)	Cervix	21	85% at 26 mo. (15–48) mean F/U		*Grade II & III (7/21)—33%*
1978–1981	IB	2	100%		*Fistulae—(3)—1.5%*
	IIB	3	100%		*Vag. Necrosis—(1)*
Pre-Modification	IIIB	15	86%		Proctitis & Cystitis—(3)
Syed-Neblett	IVA	1	0%		
Aristizabel et al (40)	Cervix	118			*Grade III—(14/118)—12%*
	IIB	41	76%		*Fistulae—8%*
1978–1982	IIIB	77	74%		*Grade II—(11/118)—9%*
Post-Modification			at mean F/U 29 mo. (24–64 mo.)		*Grade I—33%*
Syed-Neblett Vermund et al (44)	Cervix	27		41% (11/27) (NED)	*Major 33%—(9/27)*
	IB	4		1/4	*RV fistula—(3)—1.1%*
1985–1991	IIA	1		0/1	*Vag Fistula—(1)*
	IIB	8		4/8	*Colostomy—(3)—1.1%*
	IIIA	3		1/3	(proctitis & abscess)
Syed-Neblett	IIIB	11		5/11	Sigmoid stricture—(1) Ureteral stenosis—(2) (With urinary incontinence—1)
Fleming et al (24)	Vagina	13	77% at 3–20 mo.	10/13 NED at 3–20 mo.	23%—(3/13)
	I	3			Vag. Ulcer—(1) at 1 mo.
1976–1978	II	9			*Vag necrosis—(2) at 4—12 mo.*
Pre-Modification Syed-Neblett	III	1			
Puthawala et al (56)	Vagina	27	85% at median 50 mo (40–84)	56% NED at median of 50 mo.	*Major—15%—(4/27)*
1976–1979	I	1	100%		*RV fistula—(2)—7%*
	IIA	7	100%	37% distant metastases	*Necrosis—(4)—15% at 8–14 mo*
	IIB	9	78%		Superficial vag necrosis—(7) at 4–8
Pre-Modification	III	9	78%		wks after XRT
Syed-Neblett	IV	1	100% Local failure at 8–40 mo.		Vag stenosis—(3)

(continued)

Table 1.
(continued)

Series	Site	Number Patients	Local Control	Survival	Complications
Ampuero et al (1) 1978–1980	*Cervix*	24	54% at 25–41 mo.	25% (6/24) NED at 25–41 mo.	37.5%—(9/24)
	IB	1	0%		*RV fistula*—(1)
	II	6	30%		Rectal stricture—(4)
	III	11	63.6%		Hemorrhagic proctitis—(4)
	IV	3	66.7%		*Colostomy*—(1)
Pre-Modification	*Recur*	3	33%		(7–24 mo. after XRT—Median 12 mo.)
Syed-Neblett	*Vagina*	4	100% at 49–51 mo.	75% (3/4) NED at 49–51 mo.	
				1/4 DSD at 5 mo.	75%—(3/4)
	I	1			*Rectal stricture with colostomy —* (1)
	II	1			
	III	1			Hemorrhagic proctitis—(1)
	IV	1			*Vag. necrosis*—(1)
Erickson et al (37) 1978–1987	*Cervix*	32	74% at 17 mo med F/U (2–58 mo)		8%—(4/51)
	IB	4	100%		Radiation colitis—(1)
	IIA	1	100%		(Colostomy at 10 mo. (2%))
	IIB	10	86%		
	IIIA	5	40%		Proctitis and bleeding—(2) at 9–10
Post-Modification	IIIB	12	73%		mo.
Syed-Neblett	*Vagina*	9	72% at 16 mo med F/U (2–62 mo)		
	I	3			
	II	6			
	Sarcoma	3	67% at 14 mo med F/U (11–32 mo)		
	IIA	1			
	IIIA	2			
	Myometrium	1			
	Recurrent	6	1/6		
		51	70% at med 18 mo. (2–62)		
Konski et al (45)			87% (all pts.)	Mean survival time = 16 mo.	*Major*—17%—(4/23)
1990–1993	*Cervix*	17	88%	(1.2–31.0)	VV Fistula—(1)
	Vagina	5	80%		RV Fistula—(1)
	Endometrium	1	100%		Rectal ulcer with bleeding—(2)
			mean time to failure = 8.5 mo. (0.8—30.1 mo.)	Mean survival time = 20 mo. (5.7–34)	*Minor* 26%—(6/23)
Syed-Neblett	*Recurrent*	7	100%		Rectal bleeding—(6) Mean 8.4 mo. (2.5–16.5 mo.)
	Vulva			17% distant failure	Hematuria—(1)
	Endometrium				Ureteral stricture—(1)
Fontanesi et al (42)			83% (26/30) (all pts.)	60% (18/30) NED at 36 mo.	*RV fistula and/or colostomy* (6/ 30)—20% at 6–16 mo.
1984–1991	Cervix	24	87% at median F/U 36 mo. (4–84)	(4–84 mo.)	
	II	5			*Vag. necrosis*—(2) at 8–12 mo.
	III	16			Hematuria—(1) at 40 mo.
Syed-Neblett	IV	3			Radiation proctitis (9/30)—30%
	Vagina	6	100% at median F/U 36 mo. (4–84)		
	III	1	interval to recur = 5–9 mo.		
	IV	5			
Kumar et al (53–54)	*Cervix*	3	33% (1/3) at 12 mo.)		SBO with ileal resection—1
1979–1985	(stump)		2 failures at 5 and 7 mo.		
Syed-Neblett	*Recurrent* Cervix	4			

(continued)

Table 1.
(*continued*)

Series	Site	Number Patients	Local Control	Survival	Complications
Rush et al (48)			69% (11/16) (all pts.)		25%—(4/16)
1988–1990	*Cervix*	5	80% at 10–23 mo.		*Enteric fistula*—(1)
	Vagina	2	50% at 28–44 mo.		*Other fistula*—(2)
	Endometrium	1	0% at 6 mo.		*Necrosis*—(1)
	Recurrent	8			
	Cervix	2	100% at 24–49 mo.		
	Vulva	3	66% at 12–30 mo.		
Syed-Neblett	Endometrium	*3*	66% at 12–30 mo.		
		16			
Puthawala et al (61)	*Recurrent*	26	62% (16/26)	NED	15%
1975–1978	Cervix	14	50%	29% (4/14)	
	Endometrium	5	100%	40% (2/5)	
	Vagina	5	60%	20% (1/5)	
Pre-Modification	Ovary	2	50%	50% (1/2)	
Syed-Neblett			MInimum F/U = 24 mo.		
Monk et al (62)	*Recurrent*	28	71% at median F/U 44 mo.	36% (10/28) NED at med. 44 mo	11%—(3/28)
1984–1989	Cervix	18		33%—(4/10)	*VV + RV fistula* — (1)
	Endometrium	10		40%—(6/18)	*SBO + Ureteral stricture*—(1)
Syed-Neblett					*Ureterointestinal fistula*—(1)
Martinez et al (26, 28)	*Cervix*	37	83.8% at 1–7.5 yr		5.4%
1976–1983	IIB				*Urinary diversion*—(1)
	IIIB				*Rectal ulcer*—1 at 14 mo.
Stanford/Mayo Clinic	*Vaginal-Urethral*	26	80.8% at 1–7.0 yr		8%
MUPIT					*Colostomy*—(1)
			All local failures within 15 mo.		*Urinary Diversion*—1
Hughes-Davies, Silver,	*Cervix*	70	25% (all pts.)	DFS at 5 years—22%	*Fistula*—(18)—13%
Kapp (30)	IB/IIA	10			*Bladder*—(17)—12%
1977–1992	IIB/Barrel	28	22%	36% 3 years	*Bowel (Colostomy)*—(28)—20%
	IIIA	5			*Late Mortality*—(3)—2%
Stanford/Harvard	IIIB	21	44%	18% 3 years	
	IVA	6			
MUPIT	*Vagina/vulva*	20			
	Recurrent	37			
	Cervix	23	36% 3 years	26% 3 years	
	Endometrium	14			

Pts = patients; Mo = month; Wks = weeks; F/U = follow-up; Ave = average; Med = median; NED = no evidence of disease; DSD = dead without disease; DFS = disease free survival; Recur = recurrence; Vag = vaginal; RV = rectovaginal; VV = vesicovaginal; SBO = small bowel obstruction.

Cervix

Local Control

Prognostic indicators of local control were addressed in the series of Aristizabal et al.[40] Pelvic control rates were similar irrespective of tumor size and degree of parametrial or vaginal involvement, but higher rates of recurrence were seen in patients with a barrel cervix, hydronephrosis, and frozen pelvis. Unilateral versus bilateral parametrial involvement did not impact on local control. In the series of Fontanesi et al.,[42] statistical evaluation of various patient and treatment related issues including use of an intracavitary implant prior to interstitial, conventional versus hyperfractionated external beam, and use of a tandem loaded with Cs-137, all failed to correlate with local control. In the series of Hughes-Davies, Silver, and Kapp,[30] there was no relationship of dose to local control or complications.

Complications

In the series of Gaddis et al.[34] (premodification), the overall treatment related fistula rate was 13.3% and the overall adverse complication rate was 21.3% (16/75 patients), most commonly affecting the rectosigmoid (66%)

followed by the bladder (16.7%) and vagina (necrosis) (16.7%). To better explain the high incidence of complications, a review of dosimetry disclosed that some patients had received point A doses in excess of 120 Gy; bladder and rectal doses in excess of 86 Gy; and dose rates to point A of up to 200 cGy/ hr with loading of both the obturator needles and tandem. Additionally, a high and uniform activity of Ir-192 was used (0.84 mg Ra eq) delivering 150–200 mg/hr to point A. Most patients with morbidity had received 110 and 130 Gy to point A. The use of a tandem and central guides increased the dose to the rectum and bladder. The tandem sometimes slipped into the vagina with higher rectal doses. When the tandem could not be used the central guides were loaded with a greater number of seeds, with higher rectal and bladder doses. Additionally, computerized dosimetry was not available making dose determination more uncertain, typically based on mg/ hr with resultant increased doses to the rectum. An increase in complications was observed with one versus two template insertions. The injury to the rectosigmoid was speculated to have also been due to the linear arrangement of sources near the rectum and the posterior slant of the needles.[34–36] In the subsequent series of 60 patients with cervical carcinoma treated from 1977–1982 (postmodification) reported by Syed et al.[35,36] in 1986, several modifications were recommended to reduce complications: 1) if the intrauterine tandem is utilized, then none of the central six source guides along the vaginal obturator surface should be used; 2) in the absence of bulky disease, the anterior three and posterior three guides in the second diameter of the perineal template should not be used to reduce the dose to the bladder and rectum; 3) if the central six guides are implanted in place of the tandem, then only four or five seeds should be loaded in these guides; 4) the activity of the Ir-192 seeds should be in the range of 0.25–0.35 mg Ra eq so that the dose rate to point A does not exceed 80 cGy/hr; 5) differential unloading of the tandem and the central guides should be used when necessary to achieve higher point B doses, or higher activity seeds (0.40 mg Ra eq) should be used in the lateral guides; 6) to prevent slipping of the tandem into the va-

gina, the tandem should be fixed at the conclusion of the procedure rather than the beginning; and 7) the tandem source activity should be decreased to 20–35 mg Ra eq and seven (nine to ten if vaginal involvement) seeds loaded in the needles, spaced 1 cm apart from center to center. With these modifications, serious complications were decreased from 8% in their first reported series to 3% (two rectovaginal fistulae).

In the series of Ampuero et al.[1] (premodification), 24 patients with advanced cervical carcinoma (including cervical stump) and four with vaginal carcinomas were treated from 1978–1980 using the techniques described by Feder prior to the Syed modifications (equal source activities; obturator loaded). Complications developed in nine of the 24 (37.5%) patients with cervical carcinoma. Eleven variables were studied for prediction of complications: 1) dose from implant; 2) dose rate in prescribed volume of template; 3) number of seeds in implant; 4) radium equivalent of Ir-192 and Cs-137; 5) individual Ir-192 seed strength; 6) template volume; 7) percentage area of "hot spot" in template; 8) external treatment dose; 9) Ir-192 in obturator ring trocars; 10) tandem loaded with Cs-137; and 11) number of seeds per ribbon. The only variable that appeared to significantly (P = 0.06) impact on the probability of complications was the percentage area of "hot spot" in the template (1.5 times reference isodose). The percentage hot spot represented the degree of nonuniformity of dose rate across the implant volume. Dose-rate uniformity could be maximized by manipulating the seed strengths, and seed and ribbon number. To minimize inhomogeneity, Ampuero et al.[1] recommends that a tandem not routinely be used. Additionally, if the percentage area hot spot is significant, on the order of 20% or above, the dose rate should be altered by adjusting seed activities (differential loading) and ribbons. A follow-up series by Erickson et al.[37] (postmodification) stressed that: 1) the maximum dose rate for the prescribed tumor volume should be 100 cGy/hr with a mean dose rate of 80 cGy/hr in the 51 patients studied; 2) additionally, hot spots exceeding 25% of the implant volume with >10% dose gradient should be avoided; 3) the central obturator should not be loaded if a tandem is used;

4) load only as many needles as needed; 5) seed strengths of 0.25–0.40 mg Ra eq were suggested; 6) six to eight seeds/ribbon were suggested except if vaginal involvement exists; 7) <3 Cs-137 sources (total activity of 20 mg Ra eq) should be used in the tandem; and 8) one implant rather than two should be performed. In the follow-up series spanning from 1978–1982, an overall rate of complications of 8% (4/51) was reported, representing a significant decrease from the 42% in the first series by Ampuero et al.[1] with the modifications specified.

Aristizabal et al.[40] (postmodification) reported grade 2 and 3 complications in 9% and 12% of patients, respectively, which was a significant decrease from prior studies due to several important modifications. Previously, a high incidence of grade 2 and 3 complications were observed in patients in whom needles were loaded on the surface of the obturator (80%).[38,39] The use of obturator needles has subsequently been discontinued and the fistulae formation rate decreased to 8%. They have also discontinued use of the three most anterior and posterior needles on the first ring of the template as these added significantly to bladder and rectal doses. The incidence of complications also increased from 6% to 20.5% as mg-hrs increased from <4500 to >4500. With the modifications described, the serious complication rate has dropped from 33% to 16% without a decrease in local control.[40]

In the series of Fontanesi et al.,[42] ten patients developed complications. The only statistically significant variable that correlated with these complications was rectal dose rates >60 cGy/hr that were present in five out of six patients with fistulae and/or small bowel obstruction. Five out of 13 patients with rectal hourly doses in excess of 60 cGy/hr developed rectovaginal fistulae and/or small bowel obstruction compared with one of 17 with hourly doses between 35–60 cGy/hr (P = 0.05). Konski et al.[45] reported a serious complication rate of 17% (4/23). A statistical difference in the combined external beam and implant dose to the rectum was noted between those patients who had rectal complications compared with those who did not (66.82 Gy vs 53.65 Gy [P = 0.02]) and current

recommendations are to limit the external beam rectal dose to 40 Gy.

Kumar, Good, and Jones[54] attributed the high complications rates with transperineal interstitial implantation to the inability to pack the rectum and bladder away from the needles, the convergence of needles close to the rectum, and the use of Cs-137 in the tandem. Rectal dose rates were often identical to those at point A. Bellotti et al.[64] also speculated that the increase in rectal complications was due to convergence of the needles near the rectum and the posterior angulation of the system. Vermund et al.[43,44] noted a significant increase in major complications with external beam and interstitial implantation (33%) versus external beam and intracavitary irradiation (13%) for cervical carcinoma. Complications of the bowel were the most frequent although many patients had multiple complications. This increase in complications was attributable to the higher doses to point B with interstitial versus intracavitary techniques. Despite this increase in dose, interstitial brachytherapy did not improve tumor control in advanced cases (41%) when compared with intracavitary brachytherapy (65%).

A follow-up of the Bentel[112] series including 12 patients with a primary cancer of the cervix or vagina and 12 with recurrent disease of the cervix or rectum reported actuarial local control and survival at 3 years of 46% and 31%, but 40% had severe late normal tissue morbidity (10/24 patients) requiring hospitalization or surgery (RV, VV fistulae-4, SBO-1, necrosis-5). Chemotherapy was implicated as perhaps contributing to moribity as five patients who received concurrent chemotherapy developed a significant complication (P = 0.02).

In the series of Hughes-Davies, Silver, and Kapp,[30] there were three treatment related deaths and two patients developed pathological fracture of the pubic ramus. Acute complications occurred in 14 patients, four of which were infectious. Antibiotics were not routinely given during the implant.

Vagina

Nori et al.,[81] using single and double plane plastic tube or needle implants, recommend that interstitial implantation of vaginal lesions should be restricted to those involving no more than half the circumference of the vagina to avoid possible extensive necrosis and that the uninvolved tissue should be kept away from the implanted region either by packing or by use of an obturator. Such limitations have not been specified using the Syed-Neblett and MUPIT systems. Additionally, for lesions of the posterior wall, Nori et al.[81] recommend that the rectal ampulla should be kept distended either with a 30-mL Foley catheter bulb or a rectal obturator. The target dose is calculated at a depth of 0.5 cm or the maximum tumor depth.

Leung and Sexton[78] reviewed the experience at their institution from 1970–1989 using the Paris system template for positive vaginal margins following hysterectomy for cervical carcinoma as well as for primary vaginal carcinomas. The use of interstitial implantation of Ir-192 in 15 stage I and II patients correlated with an increase in local control over use of intracavitary techniques with 13/15 locally controlled. Two out of 15 developed serious complications of proctitis, rectovaginal fistula, and colostomy at 14 months and perineal necrosis at 7 months.

Vulva

There are no large series currently reporting use of Ir-192 interstitial implantation for vulvar malignancies listed in Table 1, but only small series with others reported in the literature. Goffinet et al.[19] reported the Stanford University experience with transperineal interstitial implantation of Ir-192 through steel needles or plastic tubes with or without I-125 permanent seed implantation and with or without a template for vulvar carcinomas from 1974–1977. A follow-up series from 1974–1978 by Martinez, Herstein, and Portnuff[20] again reported the use of I-125 (120–140 Gy) or Ir-192 in suture or within template-guided needles (30–60 Gy) following resection or external beam irradiation (45–50 Gy). Seven of the nine were locally controlled at 6–62 months with one local failure at 6 months. A subsequent series by Hughes-Davies, Silver, and Kapp[30] from Stanford and Harvard also reported vulvar implantation. Carlino et al.[69] reported use of the Syed-Neblett approach combined with exter-

nal beam irradiation with or without surgery in the treatment of 17 patients with advanced vulvar carcinomas with lesions near the urethra or clitoris. The best results were achieved when surgery and interstitial irradiation were combined (67%–72% NED at 5 years) versus interstitial and external beam alone (25% NED at 5 years). At Memorial Sloan Kettering, radiation therapy rather than surgical extirpation is reserved for select small lesions in medically inoperable patients, for technically unresectable lesions, and for recurrent lesions. External beam doses of 40–50 Gy are followed by single or two plane implants using plastic catheters or the customized template technique afterloaded with Ir-192 or I-125 with dose rates in the central plane of 40–80 cGy/hr delivering 30–40 Gy.[59,80,82,113,114] Use of Ir-192 for patients with locally advanced or recurrent vulvar lesions are reported in several additional series, using the Syed-Neblett system or other template systems or freehand plastic tube techniques.[45,48,59,87,115–118] Hockel and Muller[71] also treated vulvar lesions with a Syed-Neblett template modified for HDR Ir-192 and Jacobs[119] with freehand HDR Ir-192 implants.

Recurrent Disease

Several small series of patients treated for recurrent gynecological malignancies following surgery or irradiation are listed in Table 1. The concept of reirradiation of recurrent gynecological malignancies following prior radiation with or without surgery was introduced by Syed[33] in 1975. Subsequently, Puthawala et al.[61] reported use of salvage interstitial implantation of temporary Ir-192 and permanent I-125 in the setting of recurrent cervical, vaginal, endometrial, and ovarian malignancies following prior to irradiation (Table 1). Laparotomy was performed in the majority of these patients treated from 1975–1978. The advantages of laparotomy included: 1) direct observation of tumor recurrence with biopsy; 2) separation of bowel adhesions; 3) tumor reductive surgery; 4) placement of afterloading needles under direct vision and palpation; 5) ability to perform permanent I-125 seed implants for disease not encompassed by needles; and 6) ability to separate small bowel from the needles with an omental pedicle graft. Doses of 40–50 Gy given in two separate transperineal Ir-192 implants or 120–160 Gy over 1 year with I-125 were delivered. Puthawala et al.[56] also described implantation of vaginal carcinomas following hysterectomy or definitive irradiation for cervical carcinoma. For patients with disease involving the upper vagina following hysterectomy (recurrent cervical carcinoma after hysterectomy or vaginal recurrence of endometrial carcinoma), Disaia, Syed, and Puthawala[57] subsequently described an open implant technique at the time of laparotomy to achieve optimum placement of the needles. The advantages of this technique included: 1) evaluation of the size and extent of the recurrent disease; 2) separation of bowel and bladder adhesions; 3) precise placement of the implant guides utilizing direct vision and palpation; and 4) interposition of an omental pedicle graft to separate the bladder and rectum from the tumor and overlying bowel from the needle tips. Implant doses of 20–25 Gy per implant on one or two occasions with external beam doses of 34–50 Gy were recommended. Subsequent results reported by Monk et al.,[62] from that same institution, for patients with locally recurrent uterine corpus or uterine cervix cancers after primary surgery using open interstitial implantation are recorded in Table 1. Ten patients (29%) suffered acute postoperative complications. Patients with one rather than two interstitial implants, with side-wall involvement, with tumors >6 cm, with a history of previous pelvic irradiation or with persistent disease after open interstitial implant were not salvaged. All eight patients with persistent disease at the completion of salvage therapy died of disease after a median of 7 months (2–19 months). Nine patients developed a second recurrence and died at a median of 19 months (7–42 months). Two implants were performed in most patients unless they had a previous history of radiation, distant metastases, or problem with the first implant. Twenty-two patients received whole pelvis treatment with 21 receiving a second closed interstitial application. Dose intensity was predictive of survival with all long-term disease-free survivors receiving a total dose of 80–90 Gy to their recurrent tumor after external beam, open implant, and a second

closed implant. Corn et al.[60] performed laparotomy or laparoscopy as well as MRI to guide needle placement in patients with apical vaginal tumors recurring after hysterectomy. The median dose to the isodose covering the tumor volume was 40 Gy (31–50 Gy), which was encompassed by the 60 cGy/hr isodose line. External beam doses of 45–50.4 Gy were used. Kumar et al.[53,54] reported the use of the Syed-Neblett system for the treatment of central recurrences of cervical carcinoma following prior irradiation or surgery and Randall et al.[46,47] and Sears et al.[120] reported retreatment of recurrent cervical, endometrial, and vaginal carcinomas after prior definitive irradiation with or without hysterectomy. More lateral disease inaccessible to the needles was treated with transperineal insertion of I-125 seeds. Angel et al.[63] also reported use of the Syed-Neblett system for treatment of recurrent endometrial carcinomas as did Bellotti et al.[64] in combination with external irradiation for recurrent endometrial and cervical carcinomas. Branson et al.[55] used the modified Syed-Neblett template to treat recurrent vulvar carcinomas and recurrent cervical carcinomas after hysterectomy. Martinez et al.[20,26] reported the use of the MUPIT system for treatment of recurrent endometrial presenting in the vagina and other recurrent gynecological malignancies. A follow-up series from both Harvard and Stanford reported use of the MUPIT for recurrent cervical and endometrial carcinomas.[30] Bentel et al.[74] described fabrication of customized templates based on pelvic examination and CT to optimally address bulky recurrences of cervical carcinoma presenting after hysterectomy and persistent cervical carcinoma after external beam as did Osian et al.[75] for recurrent cervical carcinoma. Choy et al.[79] reported use of their circular template afterloaded with Cs-137 for the treatment of recurrent cervical carcinoma after irradiation in the presence of a narrow vagina. Hockel and Muller[71] suggested the use of HDR Ir-192 interstitial techniques using a modified Syed-Neblett template as did Donath et al.[32] for the treatment of recurrent cervical carcinoma following initial definitive irradiation. Hockel, Knapstein, and Kutzner[108] reported treatment of recurrent cervical, endometrial, and vulvar malignancies following radiation with or without prior surgery that had infiltrated the pelvic wall with resection followed by implantation of plastic catheters afterloaded with high activity Ir-192 using remote afterloading HDR techniques. Treatment of recurrent disease is reported in other series with plastic tube techniques.[113,114,116,121–125]

Discussion

Though the focus of this review has been the use of template-guided interstitial implantation of gynecological malignancies, freehand insertion of plastic tubes or needles in single or double planes, afterloaded with Ir-192 or I-125, is preferred at many institutions.[11,13–20,48,59,80–82,91,113–119,121–136] Skill is required to insert the needles in a parallel and uniform direction. Absence of the template does allow direct palpation of disease through the vagina to guide implantation and placement of packing to displace the uninvolved vagina, bladder, and rectum. Limitations of such techniques include convergence or divergence of the needles or tubes and a nonfixed relationship between the interstitial and intracavitary components of the system. It may be dosimetrically more difficult to deal with the dose distribution at the interface between the vaginal ovoids or cylinder and the parametrial and paravaginal needles and there is the potential for greater inhomogeneity within the treatment volume due to this nonfixed relationship. It is also difficult to implant large volumes of disease with single and double planes. Such techniques may however be invaluable in patients with small residuum after external beam, periurethral disease, or perineal disease.

Permanent seed implantation also suffers from some of the same unpredictability of dose distribution but may be helpful in disease sites such as the pelvic wall, which is inaccessible to needle implantation, particularly when laparotomy is used.[11,14,15,17,19,20,46,53,54,61,88–90,113,114,120–124,137–141]

Conclusions

Interstitial implantation of gynecological malignancies is an invaluable tool in the setting of extensive or large volume disease, anatomical distortion, and recurrent disease. Implementation of such techniques is a necessary component of the brachytherapy services available to patients as results with external beam alone or inadequate intracavitary applications compromise both local control and survival. It is, however, extremely important to understand the potential for morbidity with interstitial techniques. Control and manipulation of dose rate and total dose through selection of needle site insertion, source activity, dose specification, and duration of implantation are essential in producing a favorable end result, as is careful integration with external beam.

The dose rate, volume of tissue irradiated, and total dose delivered through the interstitial implant as well as the external beam volume and dose may have a significant impact on both local control and complications. Separation of the significance of these factors predictive of local control and morbidity remains to be further analyzed. The integration and efficacy of chemotherapy are also under consideration.[48,112] Future work should be focused on these issues as well as techniques that will limit the number and depth of needles inserted. In the future, better tumor volume delineation may be made possible through the use of MRI rather than CT.[29,60,142] Given the dosimetric complexity of transperineal interstitial implants various tools including dose volume histograms should be developed and tested in attempt to further evaluate and summarize this procedure.

References

1. Ampuero F, Doss LL, Khan M, et al. The Syed-Neblett interstitial template in locally advanced gynecological malignancies. Int J Radiat Oncol Biol Phys 1983;9:1897–1903.
2. Stevenson WC. Preliminary clinical report on a new and economical method of radium therapy by means of emanation needles. Br Med J 1914;9–10.
3. Green A, Jennings WA. New techniques in radium and radon therapy. J Facul Radiol 1951;2:206–233.
4. Mead KW. Methods of increasing accuracy in radon and radium implants. Med J Aust 1955;2:232–235.
5. Holzaepfel JH. Results of treatment of squamous cell carcinoma of the cervix. Cancer 1951;4:251–254.

6. Barnes AC, Morton JL, Callendine GW. The use of radioactive cobalt in the treatment of carcinoma of the cervix. Am J Obstet Gynec 1950;60:1112–1120.

7. Morton JL, Callendine GW, Myers WG. Radioactive cobalt[60] in plastic tubing for interstitial radiation therapy. Radiology 1951;56:553–559.

8. Morton JL, Barnes AC, Callendine GW, et al. Individualized interstitial irradiation of cancer of the uterine cervix using cobalt 60 in needles, inserted through a lucite template. Am J Roentgenol Rad Ther 1951;65:737–747.

9. Morton JL, Barnes AC, Hendricks CH, et al. Irradiation of cancer of the uterine cervix with radioactive cobalt 60 in guided aluminum needles and in plastic threads. Am J Roentgenol Rad Ther 1953;69:813–825.

10. Corscaden JA, Gusberg SB, Donlan CP. Precision dosage in interstitial irradiation of cancer of the cervix uteri. Am J Roentgenol Rad Ther 1948;60:522–534.

11. Delclos L. Are interstitial radium applications passe? Front Radiat Ther Onc 1978;12:42–56.

12. Mowatt KS, Stevens KA. Afterloading—a contribution to the protection problem. J Facul Radiol 1956;8:28–31.

13. Henschke UK, Hilaris BS, Mahan GD. Afterloading in interstitial and intracavitary radiation therapy. 1963;90:386–395.

14. Liegner LM. "Blind end" technique for iridium[192] removable nylon ribbon interstitial implants: Applicable to carcinoma of rectum and vagina. J Nucl Med 1962;3:255–267.

15. Liegner LM. Radon and radioactive seed volume implants for extensive recurrent vaginal-pelvic cancer. Radiology 1964;82:786–793.

16. Suit HD, Shalek RJ, Moore EB, et al. Afterloading technic with rigid needles in interstitial radiation therapy. Radiology 1961;76:431–437.

17. Fletcher GH, Stovall M, Sampiere V. Radiotherapy of cancers of the cervix uteri. In: Carcinoma of the Uterine Cervix, Endometrium, and Ovary. Year Book Medical Publisher, Chicago, 1962, pp. 69–148.

18. Chau P. Radiotherapeutic management of malignant tumors of the vagina. AJR 1963;89(3):502–523.

19. Goffinet DR, Martinez A, Pooler D, et al. Perineal brachytherapy. Front Radiat Ther Onc 1978;12:72–81.

20. Martinez A, Herstein P, Portnuff J. Interstitial therapy of perineal and gynecological malignancies. Int J Radiat Oncol Biol Phys 1983;9:409–416.

21. Pitts HC, Waterman GW. The treatment of

cancer of the cervix uteri at the Rhode Island Hospital. Surg Gynec Obstet 1937;64:30–38.

22. Syed AMN, Feder BH. Technique of afterloading interstitial implants. Radiol Clin 1977;46:458–475.

23. Feder BH, Syed AMN, Neblett D. Treatment of extensive carcinoma of the cervix with the "transperineal parametrial butterfly." Int J Radiat Oncol Biol Phys 1978;4:735–742.

24. Fleming P, Syed AMN, Neblett D, et al. Description of an afterloading ^{192}Ir interstitial-intracavitary technique in the treatment of carcinoma of the vagina. Obstet Gynecol 1980;55:525–530.

25. Martinez A, Cox RS, Edmundson GK. A multiple-site perineal applicator (MUPIT) for treatment of prostatic, anorectal, and gynecologic malignancies. Int J Radiat Oncol Biol Phys 1984;10:297–305.

26. Martinez A, Edmundson GK, Cox RS, et al. Combination of external beam irradiation and multiple-site perineal applicator (MUPIT) for treatment of locally advanced or recurrent prostatic, anorectal, and gynecologic malignancies. Int J Radiat Oncol Biol Phys 1985;11:391–398.

27. Martinez A, Schray MF. Template and other extended techniques for pelvic and perineal implants. ASTRO Refresher Course, October 2, 1985.

28. Martinez A, Edmundson GK, Clarke D. The role of transperineal template implants in gynecological malignancies. Brachytherapy J 1991;5:107–113.

29. Fu KK, Sneed PK, Leibel SA, et al. Carcinoma of the cervix. In: Interstitial Collaborative Working Group (eds). Interstitial Brachytherapy. Raven Press, Ltd, New York, 1990, pp. 179–188.

30. Hughes-Davies L, Silver B, Kapp DS. Parametrial interstitial brachytherapy for advanced or recurrent pelvic malignancy: The Harvard/Standford Experience. Gynecol Oncol 1995;58:24–27.

31. Spirtos NM, Doshi BP, Kapp DS, et al. Radiation therapy for primary squamous cell carcinoma of the vagina: Stanford University experience. Gynecol Oncol 1989;35:20–26.

32. Donath D, Clark B, Kaufmann C, et al. HDR interstitial brachytherapy of lower gynecological tract cancer. In: Mould RF (ed). International Brachytherapy Programme & Abstracts 7th International Brachytherapy Working Conference. Nucletron International BV, The Netherlands, 1992, pp. 219–225.

33. Syed ANM, Feder BH, George FW, et al. Management of extensive residual cancer with interstitial iridium implant: A preliminary re-

port. In: Hilaris BS (ed). Afterloading 20 Years of Experience 1955–1975. New York, NY, 1975, pp. 119–124.

34. Gaddis O, Morrow CP, Klement V, et al. Treatment of cervical carcinoma employing a template for transperineal interstitial Ir^{192} brachytherapy. Int J Radiat Oncol Biol Phys 1983;9: 819–827.

35. Syed AMN, Puthawala AA, Neblett D, et al. Transperineal interstitial-intracavitary "syed-neblett" applicator in the treatment of carcinoma of the uterine cervix. Endocurie/Hypertherm Oncol 1986;2:1–13.

36. Syed AMN, Puthawala AA. Interstitial-intracavitary "syed-neblett" applicator in the treatment of carcinoma of the cervix. In: Nori D, Hilaris BS (eds). Radiation Therapy of Gynecological Cancer. Alan R. Liss, Inc, New York, 1987, pp. 297–307.

37. Erickson KR, Truitt JS, Bush SE, et al. Interstitial implantation of gynecologic malignancies using Syed-Neblett template: Update of results, technique, and complications. Endocurie/Hypertherm Oncol 1989;5:99–105.

38. Aristizabal SA, Surwit EA, Hevezi JM, et al. Treatment of advanced cancer of the cervix with transperineal interstitial irradiation. Int J Radiat Oncol Biol Phys 1983;9:1013–1017.

39. Aristizabal SA, Surwit E, Valencia A, et al. Treatment of locally advanced cancer of the cervix with transperineal interstitial irradiation. Am J Clin Oncol 1983;6:645–650.

40. Aristizabal SA, Valencia A, Ocampo G, et al. Interstitial parametrial irradiation in cancer of the cervix stage IIB-IIIB. Endocurie/Hypertherm Oncol 1985;1:41–48.

41. Aristizabal SA, Woolfitt B, Valencia A, et al. Interstitial parametrial implants in carcinoma of the cervix stage II-B. Int J Radiat Oncol Biol Phys 1987;13:445–450.

42. Fontanesi J, Dylewski G, Photopulos G, et al. Impact of dose on local control and development of complications in patients with advanced gynecological malignancies treated by interstitial template boost technique. Endocurie/Hypertherm Oncol 1993;9:115–119.

43. Vermund H. Evolution of brachytherapy in the treatment of uterine cervical carcinoma: A review. Endocurie/Hypertherm Oncol 1995; 11:1–8.

44. Vermund H, Alqaisi ME, Chenier T, et al. Interstitial and intracavitary brachytherapy in carcinoma of the uterine cervix. Endocurie/Hypertherm Oncol 1995;11:43–55.

45. Konski A, Mueller W, Marsa G, et al. Interstitial volume implantation of gynecologic tumors: Indications and efficacy. Endocurie/Hypertherm Oncol 1995;11:25–30.

46. Randall ME, Evans L, Greven KM, et al. Interstitial reirradiation for recurrent gynecologic malignancies: Results and analysis of prognostic factors. Gynecol Oncol 1993;48:23–31.

47. Randall ME, Barrett RJ. Interstitial irradiation in the management of recurrent carcinoma of the cervix. NCMJ 1988;49:306–308.

48. Rush S, Lovecchio J, Gal D, et al. Comprehensive management including interstitial brachytherapy for locally advanced or recurrent gynecologic malignancies. Gynecol Oncol 1992;46:322–325.

49. Meerwaldt JH, Koper PCM, Visser AG, et al. Interstitial radiotherapy for advanced stage cervical cancer. In: Mould RF (ed). Brachytherapy 2. Nucletron International BV, The Netherlands, 1989, pp. 317–323.

50. Montemaggi P, Smaniotto D, Valentini V, et al. Decreased side effects for locally advanced cervical carcinoma using CT & optimization. In: Mould RF (ed). International Brachytherapy Programme & Abstracts 7th International Brachytherapy Working Conference. Nucletron International BV, The Netherlands, 1992, pp. 173–175.

51. Childers JM, Brainard P, Rogoff EE, et al. Laparoscopically assisted transperineal interstitial irradiation and surgical staging for advanced cervical carcinoma. Endocurie/Hypertherm Oncol 1994;10:83–86.

52. Bourland JD, Reynolds KL, Chaney EL, et al. An integrated system for interstitial ^{192}Ir implants. Int J Radiat Oncol Biol Phys 1987;13: 455–463.

53. Kumar PP, Taylor J, Scott JC, et al. Indication for interstitial brachytherapy in carcinoma of the uterine cervix. J Natl Med Assoc 1984;76: 721–725.

54. Kumar PP, Good RR, Jones EO. Dosimetry comparison between interstitial and intracavitary irradiation in the treatment of uterine cervix cancer. Radiation Med 1986;4:89–96.

55. Branson AN, Dunn P, Kam KC, et al. A device for interstitial therapy of low pelvic tumours—the Hammersmith perineal hedgehog. Br J Radiol 1985;58:537–542.

56. Puthawala A, Syed AMN, Nalick R, et al. Integrated external and interstitial radiation therapy for primary carcinoma of the vagina. Obstet Gynecol 1983;62:367–372.

57. Disaia PJ, Syed AMN, Puthawala AA. Malignant neoplasia of the upper vagina. Endocurie/Hypertherm Oncol 1990;6:251–256.

58. Manetta A, Gutrecht EL, Berman ML, et al.

Primary invasive carcinoma of the vagina. Obstet Gynecol 1990;76:639–642.

59. Phillips TL, Nori D, Peschel RE. Carcinoma of the vagina and vulva. In: Interstitial Collaborative Working Group (eds). Interstitial Brachytherapy. Raven Press, Ltd, New York, 1990, pp. 189–197.

60. Corn BW, Lanciano RM, Rosenblum N, et al. Improved treatment planning for the Syed-Neblett template using endorectal-coil magnetic resonance and intraoperative (laparotomy/laparoscopy) guidance: A new integrated technique for hysterectomized women with vaginal tumors. Gynecol Oncol 1995;56: 255–261.

61. Puthawala AA, Syed AMN, Fleming PA, et al. Re-irradiation with interstitial implant for recurrent pelvic malignancies. Cancer 1982;50: 2810–2814.

62. Monk BJ, Walker JL, Tewari K, et al. Open interstitial brachytherapy for the treatment of local-regional recurrences of uterine corpus and cervix cancer after primary surgery. Gynecol Oncol 1994;52:222–228.

63. Angel C, DuBeshter B, Dawson AE, et al. Recurrent stage I endometrial adenocarcinoma in the nonirradiated patient: Preliminary results of surgical "staging." Gynecol Oncol 1993;48:221–226.

64. Bellotti JE, Kagan AR, Wollin M, et al. Application of the ICRU report 38 reference volume concept to the radiotherapeutic management of recurrent endometrial and cervical carcinoma. Radiother Oncol 1993;26:254–259.

65. Thomadsen B, Shahabi S, Mehta M, et al. Differential loadings of brachytherapy templates. Endocurie/Hypertherm Oncol 1990;6: 197–202.

66. Shahabi S, Mehta M, Kubsad S, et al. Technical modification of perineal templates to reduce rectal mucosal dose from pelvic interstitial brachytherapy. Endocurie/Hypertherm Oncol 1991;7:57–61.

67. Erickson B, Albano K, Gillin M. CT-guided interstitial implantation of gynecologic malignancies. Submitted to Int J Rad Onc Biol Phys 1996;36(3):699–709.

68. Potish RA, Williamson JF. Clinical and physical aspects of interstitial template therapy in gynecologic malignancy. In: Levitt, Khan, Potish (eds). Technological Basis of Radiation Therapy. 1992, pp. 155–170.

69. Carlino G, Parisi S, Montemaggi P, et al. Interstitial radiotherapy with Ir-192 in vulvar cancer. Eur J Gynaec Oncol 1984;3:183–185.

70. John B, Scarbrough EC, Nguyen PD, et al. A diverging gynecological template for radioactive interstitial/intracavitary implants of the cervix. Int J Radiat Oncol Biol Phys 1988;15: 461–465.

71. Hockel M, Muller T. A new perineal template assembly for high-dose-rate interstitial brachytherapy of gynecologic malignancies. Radiother Oncol 1994;31:262–264.

72. Herskovic TM, Pineda A, Pereira M, et al. Hyperfractionated template treatment of cancer of cervix using the microselecton high dose rate remote afterloader. Endocurie/Hypertherm Oncol 1995;11:97–99.

73. Hilaris BS, Nori D, Anderson LL. Brachytherapy in cancer of the cervix. In: Hilaris BS, Nori D, Anderson LL (eds). Atlas of Brachytherapy. Macmillan Publishing Co, New York, 1988, pp. 244–256.

74. Bentel GC, Oleson JR, Clarke-Pearson D, et al. Transperineal templates for brachytherapy treatment of pelvic malignancies—a comparison of standard and customized templates. Int J Radiat Oncol Biol Phys 1990;19:751–758.

75. Osian AD, Anderson LL, Linares LA, et al. Treatment planning for permanent and temporary percutaneous implants with custom made templates. Int J Radiat Oncol Biol Phys 1989;16:219–223.

76. LaVigne ML, Schoeppel SL, McShan DL. The use of CT-based 3-D anatomical modeling in the design of customized perineal templates for interstitial gynecologic implants. Med Dosim 1991;16:187–192.

77. Leung S. Perineal template techniques for interstitial implantation of gynecological cancers using the paris system of dosimetry. Int J Radiat Oncol Biol Phys 1990;19:769–774.

78. Leung S, Sexton M. Radical radiation therapy for carcinoma of the vagina-impact of treatment modalities on outcome: Peter MacCallum cancer institute experience 1970–1990. Int J Radiat Oncol Biol Phys 1993;25:413–418.

79. Choy D, Wong RLC, Sham J, et al. Vaginal template implant for cervical carcinoma with vaginal stenosis or inadvertent diagnosis after hysterectomy. Int J Radiat Oncol Biol Phys 1993;28:457–462.

80. Hilaris BS, Nori D, Anderson LL. Brachytherapy in cancer of the vulva. In: Hilaris BS, Nori D, Anderson LL (eds). Atlas of Brachytherapy. Macmillan Publishing Co, New York, 1988, pp. 276–284.

81. Hilaris BS, Nori D, Anderson LL. Brachytherapy in cancer of the vagina. In: Hilaris BS, Nori D, Anderson LL (eds). Atlas of Brachytherapy. Macmillan Publishing Co, New York, 1988, pp. 266–274.

82. Nori D. Principles of radiotherapy in the treatment of cancer of the vulva. In: Nori D, Hilaris BS (eds). Radiation Therapy of Gynecological Cancer. Alan R. Liss, Inc, New York, 1987, pp. 191–198.

83. Perez CA, Kuske R, Glasgow GP. Review of brachytherapy techniques for gynecologic tumors. Endocurie/Hypertherm Oncol 1985;1: 153–175.

84. Perez CA, Camel HM, Galakatos AE, et al. Definitive irradiation in carcinoma of the vagina: Long-term evaluation of results. Int J Radiat Oncol Biol Phys 1988;15:1283–1290.

85. Perez CA. Uterine cervix. In: Perez CA, Brady LW (eds). Principles and Practice of Radiation Oncology. Lippincott Co, Philadelphia, 1992, p. 1171.

86. Perez CA. Vagina. In: Perez CA, Brady LW (eds). Principles and Practice of Radiation Oncology. Lippincott Co, Philadelphia, 1992, pp. 1264–1265.

87. Perez CA, Grigsby PW. Vulva. In: Perez CA, Brady LW (eds). Principles and Practice of Radiation Oncology. Lippincott Co, Philadelphia, 1992, p. 1278.

88. Nori D, Hilaris BS, Stanimir G, et al. Radiation therapy of primary vaginal carcinoma. Int J Rad Oncol Biol Phys 1983;9(10):1471–1475.

89. Nori D. Principles of radiation therapy in the treatment of vaginal tumors. In: Nori D, Hilaris BS (eds). Radiation Therapy of Gynecological Cancer. Alan R. Liss, Inc, New York, 1987, pp. 173–190.

90. Stock RG, Mychalczak B, Armstrong JG, et al. The importance of brachytherapy technique in the management of primary carcinoma of the vagina. Int J Radiat Oncol Biol Phys 1992; 24:747–753.

91. Stock RG, Chen ASJ, Seski J. A 30-year experience in the management of primary carcinoma of the vagina: Analysis of prognostic factors and treatment modalities. Gynecol Oncol 1995;56:45–52.

92. Lee WR, Marcus RB, Sombeck MD, et al. Radiotherapy alone for carcinoma of the vagina: The importance of overall treatment time. Int J Radiat Oncol Biol Phys 1994;29:983–988.

93. Shaves M, Barnhill D, Bosscher J, et al. Indwelling epidural catheters for pain control in gynecologic cancer patients. Obstet Gynecol 1991;77:642–644.

94. Blythe JG, Hodel KA, Wahl TM, et al. Continuous postoperative epidural analgesia for gynecologic oncology patients. Gynecol Oncol 1990;37:307–310.

95. Erickson B, Albano K, Withnell J, et al. Modification of the Syed-Neblett template system to enable loading of the vaginal obturator. Endocurie/Hypertherm Oncol 1996;12(1): 7–15.

96. Boyer AL, Wang CC, Gitterman M. A luer lock afterloading device for iridium-192 brachytherapy. Int J Radiat Oncol Biol Phys 1980;6: 511–512.

97. Aristizabal SA, Williamson JF. Interstitial brachytherapy using standard radium-226 or cesium-137 needles and modern brachytherapy techniques. Endocurie/Hypertherm Oncol 1987;3:193–199.

98. Neblett DL, Syed AMN, Puthawala AA, et al. An interstitial implant technique evaluated by contiguous volume analysis. Endocurie/Hypertherm Oncol 1985;1:213–222.

99. Erickson B, Foley WD, Gillin M, et al. Ultrasound-guided transperineal interstitial implantation of pelvic malignancies: Description of the technique. Presented at the American Endocurietherapy Society, December 8, 1993. Endocurie/Hypertherm Oncol 1995;11:107–113.

100. Chu J, Fong K. Endocurietherapy dosimetry for a cylindrical template applicator. Endocurie/Hypertherm Oncol 1985;1:83–89.

101. Deore SM, Ahmad M, Yaparpalvi R, et al. Five dosimetric considerations in perineal templates: Regarding Kavanagh et al. Int J Radiat Oncol Biol Phys 1995;32:555.

102. Maruyama Y, Van Nagell JR, Wrede DE, et al. Approaches to optimization of dose in radiation therapy of cervix carcinoma. Radiology 1976;120:389–398.

103. Prempree T. Parametrial implant in stage IIIB cancer of the cervix. Cancer 1983;52:748–750.

104. Deore SM. Different perspectives in dosimetry of iridium-192 implants. Endocurie/Hypertherm Oncol 1988;4:49–50.

105. Neblett DL, Harrop R, Haymond HR, et al. Interstitial-intracavitary (Syed-Neblett applicator) dose-rate distribution plots. Lac/USC Med. Ctr USC School of Med Publ 1978;1: 1–24.

106. Sandor J, Palos B, Goffinet D, et al. Dose calculations for planar arrays of ^{192}Ir and ^{125}I seeds for brachytherapy. Appl Radiol 1979;8: 41–47.

107. Forell BW. Ideal versus actual dosimetry for iridium-192 template procedures. Phys Med Biol 1983;28:417–420.

108. Hockel M, Knapstein PG, Kutzner J. A novel combined operative and radiotherapeutic treatment approach for recurrent gynecologic malignant lesions infiltrating the pelvic wall. Surg Gynecol Obstet 1991;173:297–302.

109. Shahabi S, Mehta M, Wiley AL, et al. Computed tomographic dosimetric planning for optimization of pelvic interstitial implants. Endocurie/Hypertherm Oncol 1990;6:47–52.

110. Williamson JF, Seminoff T. Template-guided interstitial implants: Cs-137 reusable sources as a substitute for Ir-192. Radiology 1987;165: 265–269.

111. Richards MJS, Lewis HL, Bruckman JE, et al. The use of differential loading with iridium-192 interstitial brachytherapy. Endocurie/Hypertherm Oncol 1988;4:245–252.

112. Kavanagh BD, Bentel GC, Montana GS. Soft tissue complication rates after low dose rate brachytherapy using customized perineal templates. Int J Radiat Oncol Biol Phys 1994; 30:508.

113. Nori D, Hilaris BS, Kim HS, et al. Interstitial irradiation in recurrent gynecological cancer. Int J Radiat Oncol Biol Phys 1981;7: 1513–1517.

114. Nori D, Hilaris BS. Role of interstitial implantation in gynecological cancer. In: Nori D, Hilaris BS (eds). Radiation Therapy of Gynecological Cancer. Alan R. Liss, Inc, New York, 1987, pp. 283–296.

115. Battermann JJ. Is there a role for brachytherapy in the management of vulva cancer? In: Mould RF (ed). International Brachytherapy Programme & Abstracts 7th International Brachytherapy Working Conference. Nucletron International BV, The Netherlands, 1992, pp. 226–228.

116. Prempree T, Amornmarn R. Radiation treatment of recurrent carcinoma of the vulva. Cancer 1984;54:1943–1949.

117. Cuccia CA. Radiation therapy in the treatment of carcinoma of the vulva. In: Lewis GC, Wentz WB, Jaffe RM (eds). New Concepts in Gynecological Oncology. Davis, Philadelphia, 1966, pp. 405–416.

118. Pirtoli L, Rottoli ML. Results of radiation therapy for vulvar carcinoma. Acta Radiol Oncol 1982;21:45–48.

119. Jacobs H. Interstitial brachytherapy for advanced cancer of the vulva: A case report. Brachytherapy J 1992;6:37.

120. Sears JD, Greven KM, Hoen HM, et al. Prognostic factors and treatment outcome for patients with locally recurrent endometrial cancer. Cancer 1994;74:1303–1308.

121. Russell AH, Koh WJ, Markette K, et al. Radical reirradiation for recurrent or second primary carcinoma of the female reproductive tract. Gynecol Oncol 1987;27:226–232.

122. Kuten A, Grigsby PW, Perez CA, et al. Results of radiotherapy in recurrent endometrial carcinoma: A retrospective analysis of 51 patients. Int J Radiat Oncol Biol Phys 1989;17: 29–34.

123. Evans SR, Hilaris BS, Barber HRK. External vs. interstitial irradiation in unresectable recurrent cancer of the cervix. Cancer 1971;28: 1284–1288.

124. Mandell LR, Nori D, Hilaris B. Recurrent stage I endometrial carcinoma: Results of treatment and prognostic factors. Int J Radiat Oncol Biol Phys 1985;11:1103–1109.

125. Potter ME, Alvarez RD, Gay FL, et al. Optimal therapy for pelvic recurrence after radical hysterectomy for early-stage cervical cancer. Gynecol Oncol 1990;37:74–77.

126. Dancuart F, Delclos L, Wharton JT, et al. Primary squamous cell carcinoma of the vagina treated by radiotherapy: A failures analysis—The MD Anderson Hospital experience 1955–1982. Int J Radiat Oncol Biol Phys 1988; 14:745–749.

127. Perticucci S. Diagnostic, prognostic, and therapeutic considerations in invasive carcinoma of the vagina. Obstet Gynecol 1972;40: 843–850.

128. Prempree T, Viravathana T, Slawson RG, et al. Radiation management of primary carcinoma of the vagina. Cancer 1977;40:109–118.

129. Prempree T, Amornmarn R. Radiation treatment of primary carcinoma of the vagina. Acta Radiol Oncol 1985;24:51–56.

130. Kavadi VS, Eifel PJ. Figo stage IIIA carcinoma of the uterine cervix. Int J Radiat Oncol Biol Phys 1992;24:211–215.

131. Chu AM, Beechinor R. Survival and recurrence patterns in the radiation treatment of carcinoma of the vagina. Gynecol Oncol 1984;19:298–307.

132. Pierquin B, Wilson JF, Chassagne D. Vagina. In: Pierquin B, Wilson JF, Chassagne D (eds). Modern Brachytherapy. Masson Publishing USA, Inc, Paris, France, 1987, pp. 211–214.

133. Rubin SC, Young J, Mikuta JJ. Squamous carcinoma of the vagina: Treatment, complications, and long-term follow-up. Gynecol Oncol 1985;20:346–353.

134. Reddy S, Lee MS, Graham JE, et al. Radiation therapy in primary carcinoma of the vagina. Gynecol Oncol 1987;26:19–24.

135. Reddy S, Saxena VS, Reddy S, et al. Results of radiotherapeutic management of primary carcinoma of the vagina. Int J Radiat Oncol Biol Phys 1991;21:1041–1044.

136. Kirkbride P, Fyles A, Rawlings GA, et al. Carcinoma of the vagina—experience at the Prin-

cess Margaret Hospital (1974–1989). Gynecol Oncol 1995;56:435–443.

137. Bloedorn FG, Munzenrider JE, Tak WK, et al. The role of interstitial therapy in present day radiotherapy. Am J Roentgenol Rad Ther 1977;128:291–297.

138. Tak WK. Interstitial therapy in gynecological cancer. Gynecol Oncol 1978;6:429–437.

139. Greenblatt DR, Nori D, Tankenbaum A, et al. New brachytherapy techniques using iodine-125 seeds for tumor bed implants. Endocurie/Hypertherm Oncol 1987;3:73–80.

140. Nori D, Son YH, Fu KK. Bladder and pelvic recurrences. In: Interstitial Collaborative Working Group (eds). Interstitial Brachytherapy. Raven Press, Ltd, New York, 1990, pp. 171–178.

141. Sharma SK, Forgione H, Isaacs JH. Iodine-125 interstitial implants as salvage therapy for recurrent gynecologic malignancies. Cancer 1991;67:2467–2471.

142. Erickson BA, Erickson SJ, Prost RW, et al. Magnetic resonance imaging following interstitial implantation of pelvic malignancies. Radiat Oncol Invest 1995;2:295–300.

Chapter 28

Brachytherapy for Endometrial Carcinoma

Judith Anne Stitt, M.D., Andre A. Abitbol, M.D.

Endometrial carcinoma is the most common gynecological malignancy, exceeding the number of new cases of both cervical and ovarian carcinomas diagnosed in the United States each year. However, endometrial cancer has the lowest mortality rate of the gynecological cancers, primarily because it commonly presents as early stage disease and is curable with surgery and/or radiation therapy. American Cancer Society statistics estimate that more than 32,000 new cases of endometrial cancer will be diagnosed in 1995. Since 80% of endometrial cancer presents as stage I disease confined to the lining of the uterus, approximately 26,000 women will be diagnosed with early stage disease annually.[1]

Surgical management with total abdominal hysterectomy with bilateral salpingo-oophorectomy (TAH-BSO) for endometrial cancer provides primary therapy for this disease, as well as supplying information necessary for staging and determining the need for adjuvant irradiation. Although survival from endometrial cancer is 85%–95% with appropriate therapy, it is important to identify groups of patients who have risk factors for local recurrence or distant disease and formulate an appropriate treatment plan. The decision to recommend adjuvant irradiation depends on the histologic grade, level of invasion into the myometrium, volume of myometrial disease, and microscopic involvement of the cervix. The decision to use pelvic irradiation for high risk of pelvic nodal disease, and/or vaginal cuff irradiation to decrease the incidence of cuff recurrence is also based on the knowledge of surgical findings, extent of disease, and the likelihood of micrometastatic disease. Identification of the prognostic variables that affect outcome allow an institution to develop policies for treatment of endometrial cancer by stage of disease.[2]

In 1929, Larkin[3] wrote that "Malignant disease of the body of the uterus is commonly treated by hysterectomy with the possibility that radium before or after the operation tends to decrease the number of recurrences, or at least, to defer them for a longer time." Specific combinations of surgery, external beam therapy, or brachytherapy can be used in a rational fashion to tailor treatment of a patient's disease. TAH-BSO, peritoneal washings, and lymph node sampling is indicated as primary surgical therapy for women with stage I and occult stage II endometrial cancer. Patients with deep myometrial invasion or high grade tumors are given postoperative external beam irradiation with or without an intracavitary boost to the vaginal apex using low-dose-rate (LDR) or high-dose-rate (HDR) isotopes. Vaginal cuff brachytherapy alone is indicated for patients with more superficial myometrial dis-

From Nag S (ed): *Principles and Practice of Brachytherapy.* © Futura Publishing Co., Inc., Armonk, NY, 1997.

ease. For patients with gross involvement of the cervix, combination therapy with preoperative irradiation using external beam treatment alone or in combination with brachytherapy is indicated.

Adjuvant Brachytherapy for Operable Endometrial Cancer

The Mallinckrodt Experience

Treatment policies at the Mallinckrodt Institute of Radiology (MIR) advocate preoperative brachytherapy for stage I, grade 2 and 3 tumors based on data showing that these patients have a poor prognosis.[4] LDR insertions are performed preoperatively for these patients using a combination of intrauterine tandem and vaginal ovoids with preload radium Heyman capsules or afterloading cesium Simon-Heyman capsules. The lower uterine segment and the endocervical canal are irradiated via the capsules and tandem. The vaginal vault is always irradiated with vaginal colpostats. If risk factors that portend a higher rate of recurrence are identified in the hysterectomy specimen, postoperative irradiation is added to the treatment program. These prognostic factors include deep myometrial invasion, cervical extension, and pelvic lymph node metastasis. For women with stage II disease, both microscopic endocervical glandular involvement or cervical stromal involvement, preoperative irradiation with external beam and brachytherapy is always given using MIR guidelines.

Materials and Methods

Preoperative brachytherapy given for stage I, grade 2 and 3 endometrial cancers utilizes Simon-Heyman capsules in the uterine cavity with a central tandem combined with vaginal colpostats.[5] One intracavitary insertion is used to deliver 3500–4000 mgh (milligram-hour) to the body of the uterus and 1800 mgh (60 Gy) to the vaginal mucosa. Surgery with TAH-BSO is performed 1–2 weeks following preoperative intracavitary brachytherapy.

For patients treated with TAH-BSO, postoperative irradiation is added for stage I, grade 2 and 3 adenocarcinoma and those with deep myometrial invasion. Whole pelvis irradiation

to 20 Gy plus parametrial irradiation for an additional 30 Gy using a midline block is given.[6]

External beam therapy is combined with LDR brachytherapy using vaginal ovoids. Postoperative intracavitary vaginal cuff irradiation is performed with paired colpostats of 2.0-, 2.5-, or 3.0-cm diameter. Treating the length of the vagina with cylinders is not necessary. Cesium-137 with activity of 20-, 25-, or 30-mg radium equivalents is loaded depending on the colpostat diameter used for the insertion. A dose of 60–70 Gy is delivered to the vaginal mucosa surface.[7]

Results

A series of 858 patients with clinical stage I carcinoma of the endometrium were treated with definitive irradiation and TAH-BSO. Most women received preoperative intracavitary brachytherapy using Heyman capsules and tandem followed by surgery within 3 days up to 6 weeks. The 5-year overall survival rate for all patients was 84%. Patients receiving <2500 mgh to the uterine cavity had a 49% 5-year progression-free survival rate compared with 63% for 2500–3500 mgh, and 87% for those who received >3500 mgh.[6]

Seventy-eight patients with stage II disease received preoperative or postoperative brachytherapy combined with external beam irradiation. Pelvic recurrence developed in 10% of these patients with involvement of the endometrium and cervix. Actuarial disease-free 5-year survival was 75%.[7]

Side Effects and Complications

For 334 stage I patients treated with preoperative brachytherapy, immediate TAH-BSO, and no postoperative external beam therapy, the severe complication rate was zero. In contrast, the overall severe complication rate (grades 2, 3, and 4) was 10% in 75 stage I patients receiving postoperative external beam irradiation. Vaginal stenosis was reported in only two of the 858 patients.[6]

The University of Wisconsin Experience

A percentage of women with surgically staged and treated adenocarcinoma of the en-

Table 1.
Adjuvant Therapy for Surgically Staged Endometrial Cancer

Stage Ia, Grade 1,2	Stage Ia, Grade 3 Stage Ib, Grade 1,2*	Stage Ib, Grade 3 Stage Ic, Grade 1,2,3 Stage Ia,b, Grade 1,2,3
No further therapy	Vaginal cuff irradiation	Whole pelvis irradiation + cuff XRT

* Treat stage Ib, grade 2 tumor volume greater or equal to 2 cm with whole pelvis XRT.

dometrium are candidates for adjuvant pelvic or vaginal cuff irradiation to prevent local or local/regional recurrence. At the University of Wisconsin no further therapy is given to patients with stage IA, grade 1 or 2 cancers if their tumors are smaller than 2 cm. For early stage disease with tumors larger than 2 cm and those with stage IB, grade 1 or 2 disease, vaginal cuff irradiation is recommended (Table 1). Whole pelvis irradiation is performed for stage IB, grade 3, stage IC, grades 1, 2, 3, and stages IIA and IIB. Vaginal cuff irradiation may be added to the whole pelvis depending on the tumor volume, location in the uterus, and degree of cervical involvement.[8]

Materials and Methods: Adjuvant Vaginal Cuff Irradiation

The Madison system of HDR gynecological brachytherapy for adjuvant cuff irradiation prescribes just two HDR fractions of 16.2 Gy per fraction to the vaginal apex using vaginal colpostats (Table 2). This HDR fractionation is equivalent to 60 Gy total dose as a single treatment session using LDR brachytherapy. The decision to use so few fractions was based upon patient convenience in accordance with reasonable radiobiological princi-

Table 2.
Adjuvant Brachytherapy for
Operable Endometrial Cancer:
Vaginal Cuff Irradiation

Dose to Vaginal Surface (Gy)		
Total Dose	Dose/Fraction	Number of Fractions
32.4 Gy	16.2 Gy	2

ples. Patients begin treatment approximately 4 weeks after surgery. Vaginal colpostats rather than cylinders are used for adjuvant therapy to avoid treating too long a segment of the vagina. Additionally, because of the anisotropy of iridium-192 when used in cylinders, the dose at the vaginal apex is less than at the cylinder sides, and could, theoretically, be the cause of under dosing this region. Anisotropy in colpostats serves to lower the dose to the bladder trigone and to the anterior rectal wall.

Techniques of applicator insertion, fluoroscopy, and radiography for treatment planning films have been developed and modified from LDR to accommodate the characteristics of HDR therapy. Ovoid insertions are performed in the department in a shielded procedure suite. Nursing personnel monitor the patient's vital signs and oximetry during the procedure. Pelvic examination, insertion of the applicator, and HDR treatments are performed using conscious sedation with intermittent intravenous doses of fentanyl and midazolam (Table 3). Modifications in the procedure table and in radiographic equipment allow for applicator insertion, evaluation of applicator position via fluoroscopy, dosimetry filming, and HDR treatment to be accomplished without moving the patient from the dorsal lithotomy position or out of the procedure room. Treatment is specified to the vaginal surface. Because 16.2 Gy is being given per fraction it is mandatory to achieve technically meticulous insertions and perform dosimetry for each of the two treatments. Several methods of decreasing the dose to critical normal structures are used to protect the bladder and rectum. A posterior retractor is always used underneath the colpostats to displace the anterior rectal wall further from the

Table 3.
Intravenous Sedation for
Out-Patient Gynecological Procedures

1. Radiation oncology nurse makes assessment for allergies, current medication, baseline vital signs, level of alertness and records information on IV sedation flow sheet. Nurse inserts heparin well for IV access.
2. The nurse under the supervision of the attending physician administers fentanyl and midazolam and continuously monitors the patient's condition.
3. During IV sedation the patient's blood pressure, pulse, and oxygen saturation are monitored every 3–10 minutes throughout the sedation procedure.
4. Initial doses of fentanyl, 50 mcg, and midazolam, 2 mg are used. (Dose reductions for elderly or frail patients are 25 mcg fentanyl and 1 mg midazolam). Additional doses are titrated to achieve patient comfort. All doses are recorded on the flow sheet.
5. If the oxygen saturation falls below 90%, oxygen will be administered by mask. Further drug administration is withheld until the oxygen saturation returns to >90%.
6. Naloxone and flumazenil are available in the room in case over-sedation occurs.
7. The patient is discharged only after vital signs and oxygen saturation are stable and preprocedure level of alertness has returned.

ovoids. Saline soaked packing is placed anterior to the applicator to raise the bladder base away from the applicator. The bladder and rectal dose calculation points can be kept to approximately 80% of the prescription dose via these means (Figure 1).

Treatment planning for vaginal ovoids has been streamlined as a result of a recent study performed at the University of Wisconsin evaluating a variety of treatment planning factors that relate to ovoid dosimetry. For the first insertion, dosimetry films are evaluated for ovoid size, position, and relationship to the bladder and rectum. After assuring that the medial aspects of the ovoids are touching as assessed by radiograph, the treatment uses standard treatment parameters for each dwell position by activating dwell position numbers 2, 4, 6, and 8 of the treatment unit using a 2.5-mm step size. A pretreatment physics check sheet confirms the appropriate ovoid size, po-

sition on dosimetry films, offset of sources, and step size. This short form of dosimetry is confirmed by standard treatment planning methods prior to the second of the two ovoid fractions. Doses to the bladder and rectum are calculated and recorded.

Materials and Methods: Whole Pelvis and Vaginal Cuff Irradiation

Following TAH-BSO, peritoneal washings, and lymph node sampling, if the hysterectomy specimen reveals a stage I, grade 3 lesion, deep myometrial invasion, or stage II disease with cervical involvement, then postoperative external irradiation of 50 Gy to the whole pelvis is administered over 6 weeks. Vaginal cuff therapy may be combined with whole pelvis irradiation depending on the tumor volume, location in the uterus, and degree of cervical involvement. When the cervix or lower uterine segment is involved, a boost to the vaginal apex is added after completion of external beam treatment. The equivalent of 10- or 20-Gy LDR is given using 4.5 or 7.8 Gy to the vaginal surface for each of two HDR fractions. Vaginal colpostats are used with the technique described previously (Table 4).

Results

An evaluation of the first 63 patients with early stage endometrial carcinoma treated with vaginal cuff HDR brachytherapy at the University of Wisconsin showed no vaginal cuff recurrences at median follow-up of 1.6 years (range 0.75–4.3 years). One regional recurrence at the pelvic side wall occurred at 1.2 years. This patient is alive without evidence of disease 1.5 years after completion of salvage pelvic irradiation.[9]

Side Effects and Complications. Acute effects of the applicator insertion and intravenous sedation are minimal. Patients are conscious at the end of the procedure and usually do not require medication for comfort once the applicator insertion has been completed and planning is under way. Following the procedure patients are discharged from clinic ambulatory with normal vital signs and are able to continue their daily routine.

Late effects of therapy were evaluated for

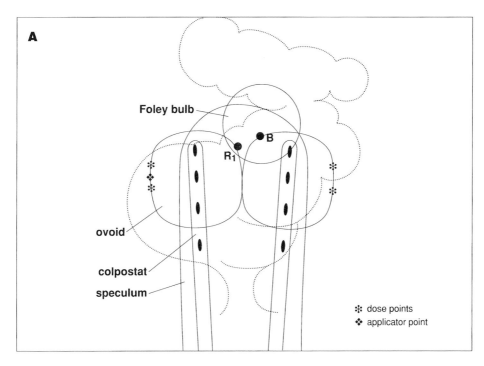

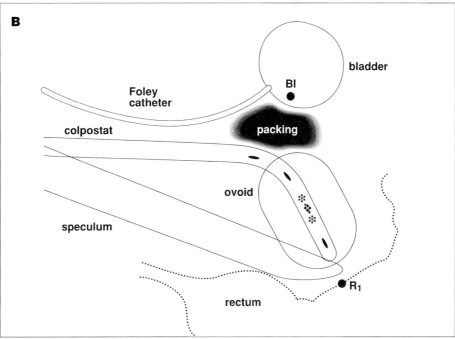

Figure 1A and 1B. Location of bladder, rectum, and vaginal surface dose points for the Madison System.

Table 4.
Adjuvant Brachytherapy for
Operable Endometrial Cancer:
Whole Pelvis + Vaginal Cuff Irradiation

Dose to Vaginal Surface (Gy)		
Total Dose	Dose/Fraction	Number of Fractions
9.0 Gy	4.5 Gy	2
15.6 Gy	7.8 Gy	2

Postoperative external beam irradiation to 50 Gy whole pelvis over 6 weeks plus high-dose-rate brachytherapy as described above.

patients in this phase II trial. Fourteen of the 63 patients (22%) experienced vaginal apex fibrosis documented by physical exam, which was clinically asymptomatic in four patients. Two women reported stress incontinence, however, these symptoms were noted prior to their HDR therapy. One patient died 2.4 years after HDR therapy from cardiovascular disease without evidence of cancer at autopsy.[9]

Materials and Methods: Preoperative Irradiation

At the University of Wisconsin, women who have operable stage II disease with cervical stromal invasion are managed by giving 40-Gy whole pelvis external beam therapy over 5 weeks using 4-field technique and custom blocking. Five HDR brachytherapy fractions using an intrauterine tandem and vaginal colpostats are interdigitated into the external beam treatment schedule giving one HDR treatment per week. The LDR equivalent of 25 Gy to the paracervical region (point M in the Madison System of dose specification) is given using 4.3 Gy per fraction HDR brachy-

therapy for each of the five fractions. The dose to the vaginal surface is the LDR equivalent of 30 Gy specifying 4.9 Gy to the vaginal surface for each of the five fractions (Table 5).

TAH-BSO, peritoneal washings, and periaortic lymph node sampling is performed 4–6 weeks after completion of preoperative irradiation.

The University of Miami Experience

Materials and Methods: Adjuvant Irradiation

Adjuvant treatment for endometrial carcinoma at the University of Miami is given using external beam pelvic irradiation to 39.6 Gy in 22 fractions with 4-field box technique. After the placement of a midline vaginal block, an additional 5.4 Gy in three fractions is given using AP/PA technique. HDR brachytherapy is started after 39.6 Gy of external beam therapy. Brachytherapy is performed using a single line source placed centrally in a vaginal cylinder. The largest diameter of cylinder that comfortably fits the vagina is used. The length of vagina irradiated is usually limited to the superior portion of the vagina. Three insertions using 5 Gy per fraction prescribed at 0.5-cm depth are performed 1 week apart. If the initial vaginal length treated is 5–6 cm, it is advisable to reduce the length of the treated volume for the subsequent applications. A useful therapeutic strategy is to use a pair of ovoids or a ring applicator to accomplish the volume reduction and to decrease dose inhomogeneity at the apex of the vagina.[10]

The University of Miami has developed an HDR vaginal applicator with a variable diameter (3, 3.5, and 4 cm). The applicator is designed with a minimal 3-cm diameter cylinder and optional additional sleeves of 0.25- or 0.5-cm thickness that allow placement of six pe-

Table 5.
Preoperative Irradiation for Operable Endometrial Cancer:
Whole Pelvis + Vaginal Cuff Irradiation

	Total Dose	Dose/Fraction	Number of Fractions
Dose to paracervical point M-Gy	21.5 Gy	4.3 Gy	5
Dose to vaginal surface-Gy	24.5 Gy	4.9 Gy	5

Preoperative external beam irradiation to 40 Gy whole pelvis over 5 weeks plus high-dose-rate brachytherapy as described above.

ripheral catheters and a central tandem. The Houdek (University of Miami) applicator has the advantage of enhanced dose distribution optimization achieved by positioning the peripheral catheters more closely to the vaginal surface. It is possible to deliver a relatively lower vaginal surface dose for an equivalent depth dose by using optional additional sleeves (Figure 2). Moreover, the problem of anisotropy is considerably reduced because of the dose contribution of the peripheral catheters to the apex of the vagina. When using the Houdek applicator for the treatment of primary vaginal carcinoma or recurrent endometrial carcinoma of the vaginal cuff, the dose distribution can be shaped according to the tumor involvement by selective use of the peripheral catheters alone or combined with the central catheters. This application is particularly useful for boosting the dose to a localized region of the vaginal wall.[10]

Materials and Methods: Preoperative Irradiation

Patients treated preoperatively for endometrial carcinoma at the Univeristy of Miami receive 30.6 Gy at 1.8 Gy per fraction to the pelvis. At this point a midline block is placed and the first of three HDR brachytherapy insertions is performed. A dose of 6 Gy to a point on the myometrial surface using a uterine tandem and ring applicator is prescribed. External irradiation 4 days per week is continued to a total of 45 Gy. After 3 weeks rest, a conservative hysterectomy is performed.

The Memorial Sloan-Kettering Experience

Women with high grade endometrial cancer (grades 2 and 3), and/or greater than one-third invasion of the myometrium in the surgi-

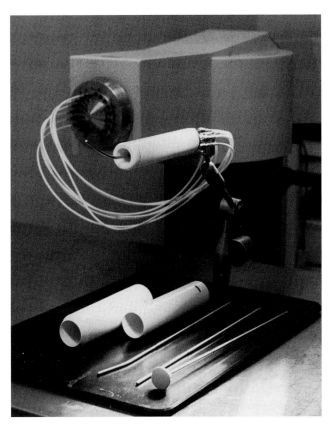

Figure 2. Houdeck (University of Miami) uterovaginal applicator with central tandem and six peripheral catheters in vaginal cylinder.

cal specimen, and all FIGO stage II patients receive preoperative or postoperative irradiation. A combination of external beam therapy and HDR intracavitary brachytherapy is used.

Materials and Methods

External beam irradiation of the whole pelvis is prescribed to 40 Gy over 4 weeks using 4-field technique. Treatment is given using high energy photons via two nonopposing fields a day, with the dose calculated at the midplane. Postoperative treatment to the vaginal vault is given using HDR brachytherapy with 2.0-, 2.5-, or 3.0-cm vaginal cylinders. Patients are treated supine in the dorsal lithotomy position. No sedation is required for the treatment. A total dose of 21 Gy is given at 0.5 cm from the vaginal mucosal surface treating 5 cm of vaginal length. Three applications of 7 Gy per fraction at 2 week intervals are given over 4 weeks. Increasing the number of fractions to deliver the total dose minimizes vaginal mucosal toxicity and the late effect of vaginal stenosis when the 2-cm diameter cylinder is used.[11]

An evaluation of two dose schedules of HDR brachytherapy comparing a total dose of 21 Gy in 7-Gy fractions given every 2 weeks over 4 weeks with a total dose of 15 Gy in 5 Gy fractions was done to determine if local control could be maintained with a further reduction in overall complications. All doses were prescribed at 0.5 cm from the vaginal surface. Following 40-Gy external beam pelvic irradiation, 200 patients were treated with one of these two dose levels.[12]

Results

Three hundred patients with stage IA, IB, and II endometrial cancer have been treated with a combined approach of preoperative or postoperative external beam irradiation plus HDR vaginal vault irradiation using the 21-Gy fractionation schedule. The 5- and 10-year disease-free survival for stage IA patients is 96% and 91%, respectively; for stage IB patients is 83% and 75%, respectively; and for stage II patients is 77% and 71%, respectively. No difference in survival was seen between the patients treated with preoperative therapy versus postoperative irradiation.[12]

Six patients developed local recurrence. Greater than 90% of patients who developed local disease did so within 36 months of adjuvant therapy.

Evaluation of the different vaginal brachytherapy dose schedules showed the 5-year survival for stage I patients treated with 21 and 15 Gy to be 88.7% and 88.5%, respectively. Survival for stage II patients was 82% for the 21- and 15-Gy treatment groups. The local failure rate was 6% for both groups. The complication rate was 6% in the 21-Gy group and 2% in the 15-Gy group. Thus a lower total dose of vaginal brachytherapy can be used to achieve the same local control while decreasing the sequelae of cystitis and vaginal stenosis.[12]

Complications

Complications were mild to moderate in nature. Nine percent of the 300 patients experienced symptoms that included cystitis in 4.5%, vaginal stenosis in 2.5%, and proctitis 1.5%. All complications were managed with conservative treatment and did not require surgical intervention.[12]

Brachytherapy for Inoperable Endometrial Carcinoma

A small number of women with carcinoma of the endometrium are medically inoperable because of significant cardiac or pulmonary disease, or are unresectable because of locally advanced cancer. Patients who are not candidates for general anesthesia and extrafascial hysterectomy commonly have cardio-respiratory illness complicated by diabetes, hypertension, and/or obesity. These same risk factors increase the possibility of bowel complications from external beam radiation making some of these patients poor candidates for pelvic irradiation. Aggressive radiotherapy alone with external beam and intracavitary brachytherapy can provide curative treatment for these patients, however, there is a 10%–15% decrease in survival compared to results with primary surgical management. Factors that account for the lower survival probably relate to the general health of these patients and decreased ability to adequately stage their disease.[13] Many of the conditions that are associated with endometrial cancer patients that preclude surgery also place these patients at added risk for anesthesia and prolonged bed rest used with LDR brachytherapy. The incidence of thromboembolic events and cardiac decompensation during LDR brachytherapy can be significant.[14]

Primary irradiation is indicated for patients with locally advanced unresectable disease, or those with distant metastatic disease at diagnosis. External beam treatment and intracavitary brachytherapy can be used alone or in combination to manage these patients.

The Mallinckrodt Experience

Women who are deemed medically inoperable because of significant medical illness that precludes surgery are treated with a combination of intracavitary irradiation using Simon-Heyman afterloading capsules and Fletcher-Suit tandem and ovoids in combination with external beam irradiation. Patients selected for intracavitary radiation alone are generally older and have well to moderately well differentiated tumors. Those who are treated with intracavitary radiation plus external beam therapy tend to be younger and may have poorly differentiated disease.

Materials and Methods

Patients treated with radiation alone for medically inoperable endometrial cancer receive uterine packing with Simon-Heyman afterloading capsules with an intrauterine tandem in the lower uterine cavity and vaginal colpostats at the vaginal apex.[15] The dose is specified in mgh with the uterus receiving an average dose of 4837 mgh and the vaginal mucosa 2050 mgh.

Another technique combines intracavitary brachytherapy with pelvic irradiation using the LDR brachytherapy technique of uterine packing and vaginal colpostats with the doses described above, plus whole pelvis irradiation with or without a parametrial boost. Patients are treated with AP/PA technique using 18- to 25-MV photons at 1.8–2.0 Gy per fraction, 5 days a week. The total dose of pelvic irradiation is 20 Gy to the whole pelvis with an additional 25 Gy to the parametria using a midline shield.

The University of Wisconsin Experience

Treatment protocols for women with inoperable stage I or II endometrial cancer have been developed at the University of Wisconsin using HDR remote afterloading brachytherapy exclusively. No external beam irradiation is combined with brachytherapy for this select group of patients.[16] The morbidity of pelvic irradiation in patients who are grossly obese and have coexisting vascular medical conditions is felt to be greater than the potential for positive lymph node disease.

Materials and Methods

Tandem and ovoid insertions for inoperable endometrial cancer are performed in the department in a shielded procedure suite. Nursing personnel monitor the patient's vital signs and oximetry during the procedure with intravenous sedation using intermittent doses of fentanyl and midazolam. Modifications in radiographic equipment and the procedure table allow us to perform insertions, evaluate their position with fluoroscopy and ultrasound, take dosimetry films, and give HDR treatment without moving the patient from the dorsal lithotomy position or out of the procedure room.

Pelvic ultrasound utilized during the placement procedure will verify the uterine location and extent of disease as well as the actual location of the tandem. Large uterine size contributes to difficulty in locating the superior extent of the corpus.[17] The tandem may feel as though it is in place, when actually lodging against the anterior wall, even though the instrument is many centimeters into the uterus. The ultrasound hard copy can be used in conjunction with dosimetry radiographs to identify dose and make adjustments in the specification points for treatment planning (Figure 3).

Several methods of decreasing the dose to critical normal structures are used to protect the bladder and rectum. A posterior retractor is always used underneath the colpostats to move the anterior rectal wall further from the ovoids. Saline soaked packing is placed anterior to the applicator to raise the bladder base away from the applicator. Seven cubic centimeters of contrast is used in the bladder cathe-

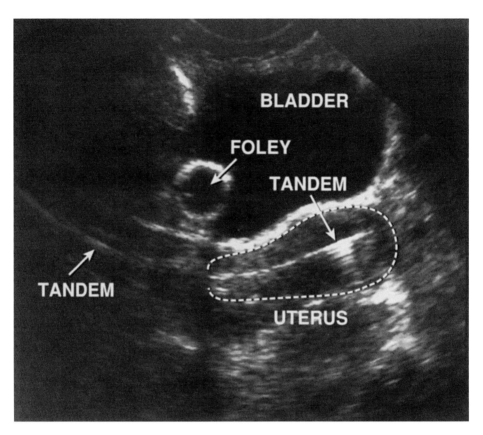

Figure 3. Ultrasound for inoperable endometrial carcinoma.

ter balloon and very dilute barium is placed in the rectum to identify critical dose regions of these normal structures. A biplane fluoroscopic and radiographic system allows us to obtain AP and lateral images without moving the patient or x-ray equipment. Evaluation of the applicator position by fluoroscopy determines if adjustments should be made before taking dosimetry films. If the patient is moved to take dosimetry films and returned to the room for treatment, the applicator position and location of normal tissues may be altered enough to invalidate the accuracy of treatment.

The Madison system of dose specification for inoperable endometrial carcinoma prescribes five HDR intracavitary fractions of 9.5 Gy each to the paracervical region-point M, at weekly intervals. Dose to the vaginal surface is 8.2 Gy per fraction for each of the five fractions. No external beam therapy is used

(Table 6). This fractionation scheme was developed based on LDR Heyman capsule packing that delivered 7000 mg in two fractions 1 week apart. The HDR dose specification system defines critical dose points to reflect the structures of interest for inoperable endometrial cancer (Figure 4). Dose specification for the paracervical region is designated as point M and lies 2 cm lateral to the center of the uterine canal and 2 cm cephalad from the center dwell position of the vaginal colpostat. The myometrium is represented by point W laterally and point S superiorly. Point W lies 2 cm caudad from the midline of the uterine cavity apex and 3 cm lateral to the uterine tandem in uteri sounding <10 cm and 4 cm lateral to the tandem for uteri >10 cm. With this protocol of dose specification, it is recommended that a single tandem be used for uteri sounding >10 cm, two 15° tandems for 10- to 12-cm uteri, and a triple tandem (two 30° and

Table 6.
Primary Brachytherapy for Inoperable Endometrial Cancer Stage I & II

Dose Point	Total Dose	Dose per Fraction	Number of Fractions
Point M	46 Gy	9.2 Gy	5
Point W	35 Gy	7 Gy	5
Point S	28.5 Gy	5.7 Gy	5
Vag Surface	41 Gy	8.2 Gy	5

See Figure 4 for location of Points M, W, S, Vaginal Surface.

a central 15°) for uteri >12 cm. Optimization of treatment planning using these dose specification points ensures adequate coverage of the myometrium and allows doses to the bladder and rectum to be minimized.

The University of Miami Experience

Materials and Methods

For patients treated with brachytherapy alone, the University of Miami uses 5 weekly

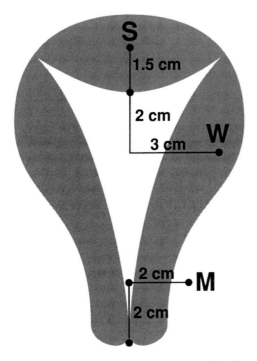

Figure 4. Madison System of inoperable dose specification. ● demonstrates point M, W, S.

fractions each delivering 7 Gy at the deep uterine myometrium. For patients treated with combined external beam therapy and HDR brachytherapy, external beam treatment is initiated using a 4-field box technique delivering 19.8 Gy with 1.8-Gy fractions to the whole pelvis. At this point, HDR brachytherapy is interdigitated with the external beam treatment. Four weekly applications are performed, each delivering 6–7 Gy to the deep myometrium. External beam therapy continues 4 days per week using an AP/PA technique with a progressively enlarging midline bar to a total external dose of 45–50.4 Gy.

Although a variety of applicators may be used for HDR applications, the simplest is a uterine tandem and vaginal colpostats, but this has the limitation of not irradiating the uterine surface homogeneously. A "Y" shaped applicator, comprised of two abutting tandems, is easy to use and irradiates the fundus more evenly by allowing the tip of each tandem to lodge in each cornu (Figure 5). The dose is specified at 2.0 cm inferiorly from the fundus in the midline and 2 cm laterally. To ensure a more homogeneous dose to the entire myometrium and dose optimization, a preplanning MRI of the uterus and intraoperative ultrasound are used.

Results

The 5-year survival rates for endometrial carcinoma treated with radiotherapy alone vary from a low rate of 28.3% in Gusberg's series to a high rate of 78% in the Landgren series.[13,18] This wide range in results is probably related to the heterogeneity of patients. Some reports include women who are inoperable because of locally advanced stage III and IV disease as well as those with early stage disease who are inoperable because of medical contraindications. Without surgical staging as part of patient evaluation, a clear definition of the extent and grade of disease and stratification for analysis is difficult.

Primary irradiation as treatment of endometrial cancer seems to be a less effective treatment when compared to surgical series. Clinical staging of endometrial cancer does not separate out the different prognostic factors that correlate well with outcome. It is likely that many patients who do not have surgical

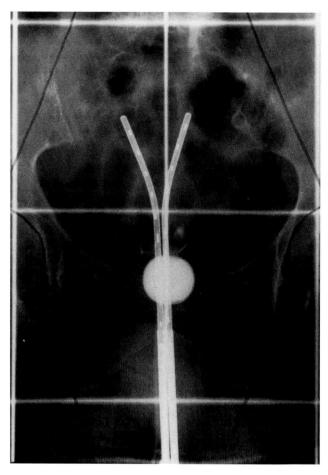

Figure 5. "Y" shaped uterine applicator. The tip of each detachable tandem lodges in the cornu of the uterine fundus.

staging are actually understaged. Joelsson et al.[19] reported a 5-year survival rate of 90% for more than 500 patients treated with surgery and radiation therapy compared to survival of 71% for 197 women treated with primary radiation.

However, with adequate doses of irradiation and geometrically appropriate brachytherapy, radiation therapy as primary treatment for inoperable endometrial cancer can produce local control and survival similar to surgical series. The Mallinckrodt data demonstrates that treatment of stage I inoperable endometrial cancer with aggressive radiation therapy alone approaches that of patients treated with surgery and irradiation.[15] For patients receiving a combination of external beam irradiation and brachytherapy the overall survival at 5 years is 85.7%. Patients with more severe medical illness are treated with brachytherapy only and have an overall survival of 62.5% at 5 years.

Wang et al.[20] described improved local control with higher brachytherapy doses. Local control of 95% was achieved with doses >7000 mgh using Heyman capsules and external beam therapy versus 63% local control when doses were <7000 mgh.

Side Effects and Complications

Sequelae of therapy in the Mallinckrodt patients were genitourinary and intestinal in nature. All serious complications occurred in patients receiving combined high dose external beam irradiation and brachytherapy.[15] Five of 49 patients experienced major treatment related effects with repeated occurrences requiring hospitalization for diagnosis and management of proctitis and urinary incontinence. Three of 49 women required major surgery for correction of fistulae or rectal stricture.

Rotte et al.[21] have compared their results using LDR and HDR brachytherapy regimen using historic controls and found no difference in survival stage for stage. Interestingly, they noted a decreased rate of thromboembolic events from 7.5% to 0% when switching from an LDR to an HDR regimen. This effect is presumed to be a result of ambulatory HDR brachytherapy that avoids prolonged bed rest.

Management of Vaginal Recurrence in Endometrial Carcinoma

Nearly 50% of patients that develop recurrence after surgery alone for endometrial carcinoma will fail in the pelvis. Half of these local recurrences are in the vagina. The view that a vaginal recurrence is often a solitary metastasis is supported by improved 5-year survival rates, with estimates quoted in the literature ranging from 33%–50%.[22] Factors that influence prognosis of vaginal recurrence from endometrial carcinoma include site of disease recurrence and the interval to relapse following primary treatment. Upper vaginal lesions have been associated with improved survival compared with lesions of the anterior, suburethral, and lower vaginal walls. Recurrences that occur in the vaginal vault can be treated successfully with surgery, radiation therapy, or a combination of the two. External beam therapy is commonly combined with brachytherapy to achieve tumor control.

The Memorial Sloan-Kettering Experience

Interstitial irradiation is used at Memorial Sloan-Kettering Hospital as a method of treatment for patients with unresectable recurrent gynecological malignancies.[23] Iridium-192 is used for removable implants to deliver a total dose of 40–50 Gy over 4–5 days prescribed at 0.5 cm from the plane of the implant. Iodine-125 seeds are used for permanent brachytherapy to deliver a minimal peripheral dose of 130–160 Gy. Brachytherapy may be supplemented with external beam treatment depending on prior therapy as well as tumor and patient characteristics.

The University of Wisconsin Experience

Treatment of vaginal recurrence depends on the site of the recurrence, the volume of tumor, normal tissues that are involved, and prior therapy that may have been given. For patients with local disease of the vagina who received no prior irradiation we recommend 50 Gy to the whole pelvis over 5–6 weeks followed by vaginal irradiation with HDR ovoids, cylinders, or interstitial techniques. A total dose of 70–80 Gy from the combined external beam and isotope therapy is recommended. When using HDR brachytherapy with external beam with HDR therapy the vaginal boost is 4.9 Gy for each of five fractions for a total brachytherapy dose of 24.5 Gy (Table 7). For patients who have received prior external beam therapy to the pelvis, interstitial or intracavitary brachytherapy may be used alone.

The University of Miami Experience

Treatment for pelvic recurrence of endometrial carcinoma is initiated with external beam irradiation to 45 Gy at 1.8 Gy per fraction using the 4-field box technique to the whole pelvis. HDR brachytherapy begins after 30 Gy. A Houdak cylinder applicator is used for 4 weekly applications prescribing 6

Table 7.
Brachytherapy for
Recurrent Endometrial Cancer

Dose to Vaginal Surface (Gy)		
Total Dose	Dose per Fraction	Number of Fractions
24.5 Gy	4.9 Gy	5

External beam irradiation to 50 Gy whole pelvis over 6 weeks plus high-dose-rate brachytherapy as described above.

Gy per fraction at 0.5 cm from the applicator surface. This applicator is particularly suited for conforming the dose to vaginal apex and vaginal wall involvement.

Results, Side Effects, and Complications

Locally recurrent gynecological malignancies present complex management problems for the surgical and radiation oncology teams. Unlike other sites of recurrent disease, treatment of recurrence in the female pelvis may be successful because of the potential to deliver high doses to disease via brachytherapy. Results from different institutions vary depending on method of prior treatment, whether the recurrence is multifocal, central, or peripheral, and retreatment techniques and doses used.

At Memorial Sloan-Kettering, 45% of patients treated for recurrence of cervical, endometrial, vaginal, and urethral carcinomas survived without disease for 5 years or longer following interstitial implantation as treatment for recurrent disease.[23] They identified a more favorable group of patients who benefited from interstitial salvage therapy. These patients include women with disease detected during routine follow-up examination, central vaginal recurrences, and unilateral localized pelvic side-wall disease. Patients with pelvic pain, leg edema, multiple sites of pelvic recurrence, and positive para-aortic nodes were less likely to benefit from retreatment.

At the MIR, 28 of 34 patients with loco-regional recurrence of endometrial cancer treated with a combination of surgery, external beam irradiation, and/or LDR brachytherapy showed complete tumor regression of the vagina.[24] Eighteen patients achieved loco-regional control. The 5- and 10-year actuarial survival rates for 51 patients, including those with concurrent local disease and distant metastasis, were 18% and 12.5%, respectively. There were no survivors beyond 1.5 years among patients with pelvic recurrence.

Complications of treatment for local recurrence are related to the nature of the therapy, site of recurrence, volume of tumor, and normal tissues. In 69 patients at Memorial Sloan-Kettering treated for recurrence, acute effects included two patients with thromboembolic events, one death from pulmonary embolism postoperatively, two patients with perineal cellulitis, and two patients with bladder symptoms.[23] Late complications observed in five patients included partial bowel obstruction, rectovaginal fistula, and radiation proctitis, all requiring management with surgical intervention.

References

1. Wingo PA, Tong T, Bolden S. Cancer Statistics. CA-A Cancer J Clin 1995;45:8–31.
2. Creasman WT, et al. Surgical pathologic spread patterns of endometrial cancer: A Gynecologic Oncology Group Study. Cancer 1987;60: 2035–2041.
3. Larkin AJ. Radium in general practice. In: Gynecological Diseases. Paul B. Hoeber, New York, 1929, p. 74.
4. Bedwinek J, Galakatos A, Camel M, et al. Stage I, grade III adenocarcinoma of the endometrium treated with surgery and irradiation: Sites of failure and correlation of failure rate with irradiation technique. Cancer 1984;54:40–47.
5. Silverstone SM, Simon N. Afterloading with miniaturized cesium-137 sources in the treatment of cancer of the uterus. Int J Radiat Oncol Biol Phys 1976;1:1017–1021.
6. Grigsby PW, Perez CA, Kuten A, et al. Clinical stage I endometrial cancer: Results of adjuvant irradiation and patterns of failure. Int J Radiat Oncol Biol Phys 1991;21:379–385.
7. Grigsby PW, Perez CA, Kuten A, et al. Clinical stage I endometrial cancer: Prognostic factors for local control and distant metastasis and implications for the new FIGO surgical staging system. Int J Radiat Oncol Biol Phys 1992;22: 905–911.
8. Stitt JA. High-dose-rate intracavitary brachytherapy for gynecologic malignancies. Oncology 1992;59:79.
9. Noyes WR, Bastin KT, Edwards SA, et al. Postoperative vaginal cuff irradiation using high-dose-rate remote afterloading: A phase II clinical protocol. Int J Radiat Oncol Biol Phys, accepted for publication, 1995.
10. Houdek PV, Schwade JG, Abitbol AA, et al. HDR transvaginal brachytherapy: Applicator design and dosimetry. Activity 1991;2(Suppl): 28–31.
11. Mandell L, Nori D, Anderson L, et al. Postoperative vaginal radiation in endometrial cancer using a remote afterloading technique. Int J Radiat Oncol Biol Phys 1985;11:473–478.
12. Nori D, Hilaris BS, Tome M, et al. Combined surgery and radiation in endometrial carci-

noma: An analysis of prognostic factors. Int J Radiat Oncol Biol Phys 1987;13:489–497.

13. Gusberg SB, Jones HC, Tovell HM. Selection of treatment for corpus cancer. Am J Obstet Gynecol 1960;80:374–380.

14. Dusenberry K, Carson L, Potish R. Perioperative morbidity and mortality of gynecologic brachytherapy. Cancer 1991;67:2786–2790.

15. Grigsby PW, Kuske RR, Perez CA, et al. Medically inoperable stage I adenocarcinoma of the endometrium treated with radiotherapy alone. Int J Radiat Oncol Biol Phys 1987;13:483–488.

16. Stitt JA. Dose specification for inoperable endometrial carcinoma: The Madison system. Activity/Int Selec Brachytherapy J 1991;2(Suppl): 32–34.

17. McGinn CJ, Stitt JA, Buchler DA, et al. Intraoperative ultrasound guidance during high dose rate intracavitary brachytherapy of the uterine cervix and corpus. Endocurietherapy/Hyperthermia Onc 1992;8:101–104.

18. Landgren RC, Flecher GH, Delclos L, et al. Irradiation of endometrial cancer in patients with medical contraindication to surgery or with unresectable lesions. Am J Roentgenol 1976;126: 148–154.

19. Joelsson I, Sandri A, Kottmeier HL. Carcinoma of the uterine corpus: A retrospective survey of individualized therapy. Acta Radiol 1973; 334(Suppl):3–63.

20. Wang M, Hussey D, Vigliotti A, et al. Inoperable adenocarcinoma of the endometrium: Radiation therapy. Radiology 1987;165:561–565.

21. Rotte K. Technique and results of HDR afterloading in cancer of the endometrium. In: Martinez A, Orton CG, Mould RF (eds). Brachytherapy HDR and LDR. Nucletron, columbia, MD, 1990, pp. 68–79.

22. Rubin P, Gerle RD, Quick RS, et al. Significance of vaginal recurrence in endometrial carcinoma. Am J Roentgenol Radium Ther Nucl Med 1963;89:91–100.

23. Nori G, Hilaris BS, Kim HS, et al. Interstitial irradiation in recurrent gynecological cancer. Int J Radiat Oncol Biol Phys 1981;7:1513–1517.

24. Kuten A, Grigsby PW, Perez CA, et al. Results of radiotherapy in recurrent endometrial carcinoma: A retrospective analysis of 51 patients. Int J Radiat Oncol Biol Phys 1989;17:29–34.

Chapter 29

Cancer of the Vagina

David Donath, M.D., FRCP(C)

Introduction

Primary carcinoma of the vagina represents only 1%–3% of all gynecological malignancies.[1-3] The vagina is surrounded by several organs, such as the cervix, rectum, and bladder. A primary malignancy involving any one of these adjacent organs is substantially more common than a primary malignancy of the vagina. As a result, inflexible diagnostic criteria ruling out a concomitant primary malignancy of the same histology and originating from the neighboring organs, particularly the cervix, must be fulfilled prior to the diagnosis of a primary vaginal malignancy. These include colposcopy and multiple biopsies of the cervix. An additional example pertains to the positive exclusion of endometrial carcinoma prior to the diagnosis of primary adenocarcinoma of the vagina.

If one of these separate organs was previously involved by a malignancy of the same histology, there must be at least a 5-year tumor-free period prior to the diagnosis of a primary vaginal cancer. Perez et al.[4] have reported that when a vaginal tumor is detected more than 5 years after treatment of a cervical cancer without evidence of local recurrence in the cervix, the results after therapy are comparable to those of de novo primary vaginal carcinoma, and these patients should be treated with curative aim.

More than 90% of primary vaginal tumors are squamous cell carcinoma.[4] Other pathological types in decreasing frequency include adenocarcinomas arising from the Bartholin's submucosal glandular epithelium, clear cell adenocarcinoma in young patients, sarcomas, and melanoma.

Natural History and Patterns of Spread

Early detection and a routine gynecological follow-up are critical. A prior hysterectomy should not rule out the diagnosis of vaginal cancer as in some series about 50% of patients with vaginal cancer had undergone a prior hysterectomy for benign disease or cervical intraepithelial neoplasia.[2] Vaginal cytological screening is still deemed essential in women who have had a hysterectomy.

Fifty-one percent of all cases occur in the upper third of the vagina while 57% of all cases occur on the posterior wall.[5] In over 50% of cases, more than two thirds of the full length of the vagina is involved.[6] When less than two thirds of the vagina is involved, the lower part of the vagina is more frequently involved when the tumor is located anteriorly, and the upper part of the vagina in posteriorly located tumors.[6]

Not only is the vagina closely encircled by several other organs, but there also lacks an anatomical barrier between the vagina and these entities. As such, primary vaginal tumors can easily spread into surrounding tis-

From Nag S (ed): *Principles and Practice of Brachytherapy.* © Futura Publishing Co., Inc., Armonk, NY, 1997.

sue. Anterior lesions can penetrate the vesico-vaginal septum. Posterior lesions can easily extend into the rectovaginal septum. Laterally, these tumors can expand into paravaginal tissue and parametrium before reaching the pelvic side walls.

The examination should include careful manipulation of the vaginal speculum to ensure that the entire vaginal mucosa is visualized.[7] The diagnostic evaluation should also include bimanual pelvic and rectal examinations, cystoscopy, and proctosigmoidoscopy. The bimanual examinations should be done under anesthesia and should be clearly recorded as this will form the basis for staging and selection of treatment modalities.

About 5%–20% of patients with primary vaginal cancer will have clinically positive nodes.[5,8] Lesions of the upper third drain to the same lymph node groups as carcinoma of the cervix while those lesions involving the lower two thirds tend to disperse to inguinal and femoral lymph nodes before reaching the pelvic nodes.[9] Due to the multifocal nature of this disease within the vagina and the tendency for submucosal spread, any of the nodal groups may be involved regardless of where the lesion is located. CT and/or MRI should be done to complete the diagnostic evaluation to determine the extent of loco-regional spread and lymph node involvement. MRI accuracy for primary or metastatic cancer of the vagina is over 90% with similar impressive figures for sensitivity and specificity.[10]

The clinical stage of the vaginal carcinoma, as determined by the depth of penetration into the vaginal wall or surrounding tissues, is

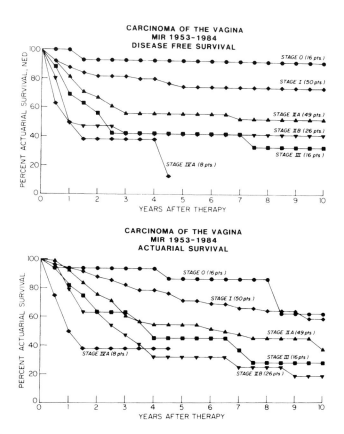

Figure 1. A) Tumor-free survival for all patients with primary carcinoma of the vagina (stages 0 through IVA). B) Overall survival of all patients by stage. (From: Perez CA, Camel HM, Galakatos AE, et al. Definitive irradiation in carcinoma of the vagina: Long-term evaluation of results. Int J Radiat Oncol Biol Phys 1988;15:1285.)

the most important determinant of prognosis. This is well shown in Figure 1.[6,8,11] In one series, no correlation was found between treatment results and the following factors: age of patient, amount of mucosal involvement, and location.[4,11] In other series, vaginal wall location and increasing length of vaginal involvement had a significant bearing on disease-free survival irrespective of the clinical stage.[6,12,13] Less than one-third length involvement was associated with 75% disease-free survival.[6] Poor outcome was seen when multiple walls were involved.[6] As for tumor location, tumors localized to the upper third had a better survival as compared to tumors in the lower third.[6,14] The presence of inguinal lymphadenopathy was generally found to be an important prognostic factor.[6,14] Some found tumor grade to be a prognostic factor,[13,14] while others have not.[6,15] Finally, in one series the presence of symptoms was also found to be of prognostic significance. Patients with presenting symptoms had a cure rate of 37%, whereas 61% of asymptomatic patients survived.[14]

In the International Federation of Gynecology and Obstetrics (FIGO) staging system, those tumors that are confined to the vaginal mucosa, are stage I. Those tumors that have extended beyond the mucosa into the paravaginal and parametrial tissues but not the pelvic side wall are considered stage II. Once the tumor reaches the side wall, it is classified as stage III. Tumors extending beyond the true pelvis or involving the bladder or rectum are considered stage IV. About 80% of patients presenting without symptoms to their physicians will have stage I disease, while 75% with symptoms will have advanced disease.[6,14]

General Management

Radiation therapy is often considered the treatment of choice due to the favorable tumor control achieved with radiation and the poor functional results obtained with surgery. It is the proximity of the vagina to the female urethra and the rectum, particularly the nerve supply innervating the sphincters controlling the function of these organs, which makes any surgical procedure in the area very risky. A surgical procedure like an upper vaginectomy has been found to be effective for in situ and occult, superficially invasive carcinoma of the upper third of the vagina.[16]

For each individual case, a judicious combination of different radiation delivery modalities is selected so that a total tumoricidal dose of 6500–8000 cGy can be delivered to the tumor volume while restricting the dose to surrounding normal tissue and vital organs, especially the perineum, bladder, and rectum, to within their respective tolerance doses. The lower vaginal mucosa can tolerate about 9800 cGy of irradiation from all modalities while the upper vagina can accept almost 14,000 cGy before complications are encountered.[17] The modalities generally used are external beam radiotherapy (EBRT), intracavitary brachytherapy, and interstitial brachytherapy. The appropriate combination of techniques enables us to contribute an increasing dose to varying extents of tumor volume (Table 1).

Table 1.
General Radiotherapy Guidelines

	External Beam Radiotherapy	Intracavitary Brachytherapy	Interstitial Brachytherapy
Stage I:			
WD(<5 mm)	NO	YES	NO
WD(>5 mm)	NO	NO	YES
PD (<5 mm)	YES	YES	NO
PD (>5 mm)	YES	NO	YES
Stage II	YES	NO	YES
Stage III	YES	NO	YES
Stage IV	YES	NO	YES

PD = poorly differentiated; WD = well differentiated.

This has been demonstrated to improve local tumor control.[18,19]

Modes of Radiotherapy Delivery

A commonly used sequence of treatment is EBRT, followed by a 1- to 2-week break for recovery, which proceeds the brachytherapy. If no EBRT is planned then brachytherapy is implemented immediately.

External Beam Radiotherapy

EBRT is the initial radiation delivery technique used where there is disease extension beyond the vaginal mucosa or there is a significant risk of lymph node involvement. This would be applicable to stage I poorly differentiated disease and to stages II, III, and IV disease. All clinically involved sites and areas of significant potential microscopic involvement by tumor should receive a dose of about 4500 cGy in 180–200 cGy fractions. Those areas of microscopic involvement that are not incorporated into the target volume of the subsequent brachytherapy techniques to be utilized, should receive the entire dose of 4500 cGy with EBRT.

Tumors involving the upper third of the vagina are treated with EBRT portals similar to those used for carcinoma of the cervix except that, in this case, the entire vagina up to the introitus is included. A 4-field technique consisting of anteroposterior-posteroanterior (AP-PA) and laterally opposed portals is used. The target volume should include the external iliac, internal iliac, and common iliac lymph node chains.

The course of EBRT utilized for tumors involving the middle and lower thirds of the vagina covers the same target volume as for tumors of the upper third of the vagina with the addition of the inguinal and adjacent femoral lymph nodes. The simplest and often the most suitable means of accomplishing this is through an AP-PA pair of portals only. These portals should be enlarged to cover the inguinal lymph node regions. Use of separate anterior electron fields directed over these areas is inadvisable as the depth of the femoral vessels can range from 2.0–18.5 cm with an average of 6.1 cm.[20] The deep groin nodes are located adjacent to these vessels.[21]

If there is concern that the total dose to the bladder or rectum will exceed their respective tolerance dose when the entire course of irradiation, both EBRT and brachytherapy, is delivered, then other measures may be introduced. These include the introduction of a midline rectangular block followed by additional external irradiation delivered to the parametrial tissue. In this fashion the bladder and rectum are shielded from further external irradiation. This would permit these organs to remain within their respective dose tolerance after receiving additional radiation from the brachytherapy modalities used to boost the vagina and the adjacent tumor volume.

For clinically involved areas that are to be treated with EBRT alone, the dose delivered should be about 6500 cGy. One example is clinically involved inguinal lymph nodes where a small anteroposterior field of Co-60 or 12–15 MeV electrons is used to boost the area. A dose of 1500–2000 cGy, calculated at CT scan determined femoral vessel depth,[20] is delivered in addition to the initial 4500 cGy.

Intracavitary Brachytherapy

This is the technique of choice for carcinoma in situ and stage I superficially invasive carcinoma. For in situ disease, 6000 cGy of low-dose-rate (LDR) brachytherapy alone, at a dose rate of 1000 cGy per day, is delivered to the surface of the entire vagina due to the multicentric nature of the disease, while an additional 1500 cGy is deposited on the surface of the disease site. For superficially invasive carcinoma, 6500–8000 cGy is delivered to the surface of the entire vagina. For stage I tumors that are more than superficially invasive, or <0.5-cm thick, intracavitary brachytherapy can be the sole treatment modality if a dose of 7000 cGy can be delivered to the deep margin of the tumor volume while maintaining the dose to the vaginal mucosa under 10,000 cGy. If this cannot be achieved with intracavitary alone, then an interstitial approach should be used. The dose should be limited to avoid vaginal mucosal injury and preserve sexual function.

If the stage I lesion is poorly differentiated and there is concern about microscopic lymph node involvement, then the appropriate EBRT is used initially and the brachytherapy dose is reduced so that there is no change in the total dose delivered to the site of original involvement.

If one is using EBRT and high-dose-rate (HDR) intracavitary brachytherapy to treat vaginal cancer, then the dose prescription for brachytherapy can be 2000 cGy in four fractions, at 5 mm from the surface, given on a weekly basis.[22]

Interstitial Brachytherapy

For stage I lesions >0.5-cm thick, an interstitial single plane implant may be combined with intracavitary radiation, or an interstitial implant alone can be delivered using a template. In the latter instance, a single circumferential plane of needles would be positioned to cover the entire vaginal surface while an extra plane would be added at the clinically involved site. Whichever sequence is utilized, the intention is to deliver 6000 cGy of LDR brachytherapy to the entire vaginal mucosa, 8000–10,000 cGy to the involved vaginal mucosa, and about 8000 cGy to the tumor volume.[18]

For poorly differentiated stage I and all patients with stage II, III, and IV disease, the interstitial implant is used to deliver the extra boost of radiation to the tumor volume detected at the time of the original examination under anesthesia. It is difficult to deliver an adequate dose distribution enveloping the target volume with intracavitary means while limiting the dose to the bladder and rectum. The needles are positioned so as to cover the tumor volume plus a 0.5-cm margin. The dose delivered is dependent on the EBRT dose received by the tumor volume. The intent is to deliver a tumoricidal dose in total. For example, if 4500 cGy of EBRT is given, then the brachytherapy dose should be about 2500–3000 cGy at an isodose line that covers the gross tumor, delivered at 1000 cGy a day using the LDR approach. If HDR brachytherapy is to be used, 300 cGy is delivered twice daily for 4 consecutive days.[23]

Brachytherapy Technique

Intracavitary Brachytherapy

The fundamental reason for using intracavitary brachytherapy instead of interstitial is the ease of insertion of the applicator. As long as the target volume is covered, while keeping in mind the rapid fall-off in dose, intracavitary brachytherapy is the preferred technique. The dose fall-off can be diminished by increasing the active length of the linear source and increasing the distance between the sources and the irradiated vaginal mucosal surface. The latter is accomplished by fitting a vaginal cylinder with the largest diameter that the vagina can accommodate. This is done to improve the ratio of tumor-to-mucosal dose based on the inverse square law.

The patient is treated in a lithotomy position to facilitate the placement of the vaginal applicator. If a remote afterloading HDR technique is used, no sedation is required at any time. All applications are done on an out-patient basis. However, if the patient has an upper third vaginal lesion with an intact uterus, then the intracavitary application technique is similar to that used for cervical carcinoma. Localization radiographs are taken. Planning involves putting together a configuration of source strengths, at available source locations, that will deliver the target dose to points of interest chosen in and around the target as displayed in Figure 2. If there is only superficial, nonpalpable disease, the treatment dose is prescribed at points of interest along the vaginal surface, which corresponds to the applicator surface, or at a depth of 5 mm. Otherwise, the treatment is prescribed at points of interest along the maximum tumor depth. The principal radioactive isotope used for LDR applications is cesium-137, while for HDR remote afterloading, iridium-192 is generally used.

For the LDR approach, conventional vaginal cylinders do not provide a uniform dose rate to the vaginal surface, especially over the entire dome surface. To overcome this, one center uses a cylinder into which one can place specialized inserts with preselected cesium-137 sources, as shown in Figure 3.[24] Others use a contoured acrylic cylinder whose contours follow the isodose lines[25] while another center has developed a new ellipsoidal design for the dome component of the currently marketed Delclos uterine-vaginal afterloading dome (hemispherical) cylinder.[26]

None of the above modifications is neces-

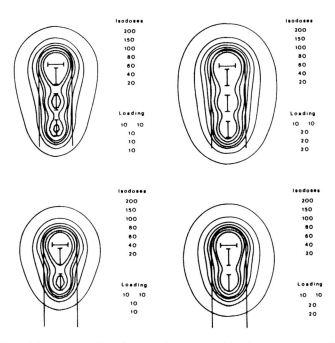

Figure 2. Examples of the variety of loadings and associated isodose curves available in the predefined library of 30 such loadings. Though the dose rates and vaginal dose gradient can be changed, the dose rates across the tip are reasonably uniform regardless of source loading. (From: Beach JL, Mendiondo OA, Martin JL. A rapid afterloading vaginal cylinder for ^{137}Cs brachytherapy. Int J Radiat Oncol Biol Phys 1991;21:1054.)

sary, however, with the advent of the single stepping source remote afterloader used for the HDR approach. Candidate source locations are distributed uniformly, at a specified increment, along a straight line.[27] By varying the dwell time of the source at each of the source locations, one is in effect adjusting the source strength. Having a cache of discrete radioactive sources of varying source strength is no longer required. Figure 4 illustrates how dwell time manipulation can lead to the delivery of the same dose at selected points of interest equidistant from the catheter. One must bear in mind though that there are limitations to this. The treatment distance selected cannot be too large.

If a shield is inserted into a vaginal cylinder, one must exercise caution in the dose prescription. The dose on the unshielded side can be significantly reduced with increasing distance from the source due to loss of scatter, while the dose on the shielded side is not totally eliminated due to scatter from the unshielded tissue.[28] To achieve almost unidirec-

tional irradiation, one may consider replacing the cesium-137 sources with americium-241.[29] The latter emits 60 keV photons rather than the 662 keV photons associated with cesium-137. The lower energy photons can be more effectively shielded by high atomic number materials.

Interstitial Brachytherapy

Interstitial brachytherapy is an invasive procedure and requires careful perioperative care to minimize morbidity and mortality rates.

Template Insertion

The night before the implant the patient is started on constipating medication and a fleet enema is given to clear the rectum of stool. Perioperative prophylactic antibiotics are administered. Since the patient is immobilized after the insertion of the needles, subcutaneous heparin is routinely given for the duration of the brachytherapy to diminish the risk of

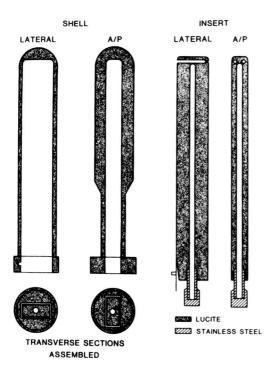

SHELL — INSERT
LATERAL A/P LATERAL A/P

LUCITE
STAINLESS STEEL

TRANSVERSE SECTIONS
ASSEMBLED

Figure 3. AP/PA, lateral, and transverse sections of the afterloading vaginal applicator. The cylindrical shell is shown on the left, tapered in the AP view to allow comfortable closure of the labia. The rectangular slot in the cylinder accepts the source-carrying insert, shown on the right, in a single motion insertion. Short cross-labeled Cs-137 sources fit snugly into the holes in the top and the capped shaft accepts small diameter Cs-137 sources in afterloading catheter, or standard diameter sources without the catheter. (From: Beach JL, Mendiondo OA, Martin JL. A rapid afterloading vaginal cylinder for ^{137}Cs brachytherapy. Int J Radiat Oncol Biol Phys 1991;21:1054.)

thromboembolic events. The implant procedure is performed in the operating room under spinal or general anesthetic. The patient is placed in a lithotomy position. A Foley catheter is inserted into the bladder and left in place for the duration of the interstitial treatment. The Foley baloon is filled with 1:10 diluted Hypaque dye for radiographic localization.

The implant needles can be inserted via a freehand technique and held in place by sutures or they can be inserted with the help of a template, as demonstrated in Figure 5.

However a template is preferred because this allows equal spacing of needles as well as accurate placement of needle tips using the obturator as a guide. The obturator is inserted into the vagina so that it is snug. The obturator has grooves along its surface to allow for needles to be placed along them. The template is then placed over the obturator and secured to it. The hollow needles are placed through the template into the cervix and parametria via the perineum. The needles are usually 17-gauge stainless steel. The template holes selected for needle insertion are based on the bimanual and rectovaginal examination prior to the initiation of EBRT. This enables one to tailor the implant to the patient's disease extent. Marking the tumor with an India ink "tattoo" at the initial presentation, followed by the placement of a purse-string suture and titanium hemoclips at the time of the implant may aid in tumor localization on implant localization films.[30]

If the superior margin of the target volume lies inferior to the apex of the vagina then the needles are inserted so that the tips lie at the level of the vaginal apex. The obturator position is used as a guide. If the target volume extends to the apex of the vagina, the implant needles must be inserted 1–2 cm beyond this. A laparotomy is used to assist in the needle positioning. The laparotomy also allows small bowel to be displaced superiorly away from the high dose area. The needle tips should not be inserted beyond the peritoneal floor.

A cover plate drilled in an identical pattern to the template, is superimposed onto the template and these plates are held together by tightening Allen head machine screws. This process locks the needles into position. The details of the technique vary with each applicator. The assembly is then sutured to the skin of the perineum. Finally, a rectal examinaton is performed to ensure that the needles have not penetrated the rectal mucosa. If they have, the needles are removed and repositioned. The patient is maintained on constipating medication, subcutaneous anticoagulation, antibiotic, and patient-controlled anesthesia for pain control throughout brachytherapy.

After the insertion of the needles in the operating room, the patient is transferred to the recovery room for routine postoperative care. After clearance by the anesthesiologist, the patient is taken to the radiation oncology de-

```
GAMMA MED II DWELL TIMES FOR CYLINDRICAL DOSE CONTOURS
        (by direct solution of linear equations)
```

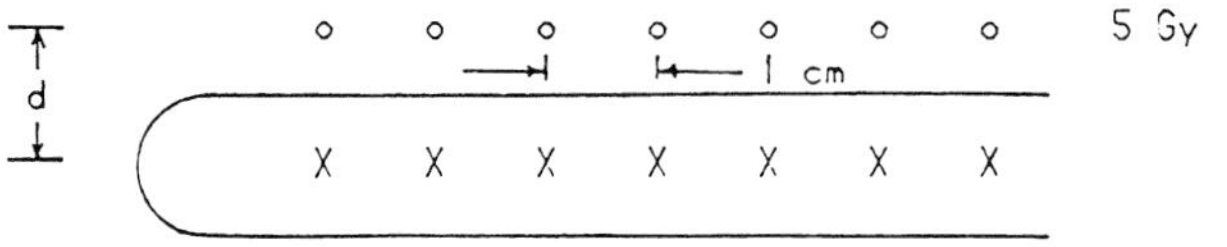

Treatment Distance d (cm)	Dwell Time (seconds)						
1.0	27	13	15	14	15	13	27
1.2	39	13	20	17	20	13	39
1.4	54	10	26	19	26	10	54
1.6	73	4	34	18	34	4	73
1.8	89	0	42	18	42	0	89
2.0	104	0	48	20	48	0	104

Figure 4. (From: Intracavitary brachytherapy planning and evaluation. In: Hilaris BS, Nori D, Anderson LL (eds). Atlas of Brachytherapy. Macmillan Publishing Company, New York, 1988, pp. 109.)

partment for planning. Localizing orthogonal radiographs are taken after inactive sources have been placed into the needles and a catheter containing inactive radiopaque sources is inserted into the rectum for localizing rectal points of interest.

The implant may be removed at the patient's bedside with only premedication given half an hour before removing the needles. The patient should then be examined for bleeding and lacerations from the removal process.

There are several advantages in using interstitial brachytherapy over the intracavitary technique. There is a better dose distribution and one can tailor the implant to the stage and tumor volume for each patient. One is able to increase the dose to the parametria, point A, by 33%, and to the pelvic side wall, point B, by 333% without having to increase the dose to the rectum and bladder.[31]

Low-Dose-Rate Manually Afterloaded Brachytherapy

Isodose distributions are calculated depending on the source activity. By varying the seed activity and active length of each Ir-192 ribbon, one can further conform the isodose distribution to the disease extent. Lower activity sources can be placed centrally to mini-

mize potential "hot spots" and the risk of complications. Alternatively, the Ir-192 ribbons can be unloaded at varying times. However, this would increase the radiation exposure to the medical personnel. The prescribed isodose line is often matched to the highest isodose line that encircles all the needles. The brachytherapy dose was already mentioned in the previous section. After the patient is returned to her room, the radioactive sources are afterloaded manually and subsequently removed at the appropriate time to achieve the prescribed dose.

High-Dose-Rate Brachytherapy

At McGill University, an HDR remote afterloading approach has been adopted for interstitial brachytherapy of the vagina.[32] The implant is performed in the operating room on a Monday morning. The localizing radiographs are done Monday afternoon. Computerized dosimetry is then used to determine the appropriate dwell times to enable the 300 cGy isodose curve to envelope the needles with a 5-mm margin and circumvent the rectum highlighted by the rectal catheter. This is illustrated in Figures 6 and 7, where it is noted that the rectum is included in the treatment volume when equal dwell times are prescribed. When the dwell times are manipu-

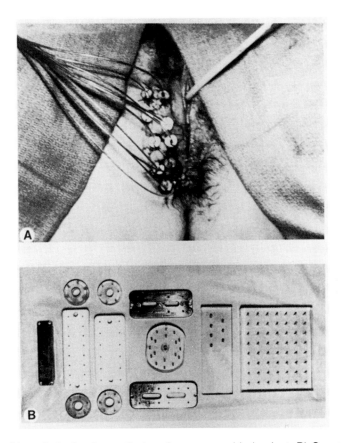

Figure 5. A) Position of afterloading catheters for a removable implant. B) Some of the templates used for removable implants in pelvic cancers. (From: Syed AMN, Puthawala A. Interstitial-intracavitary "Syed-Neblett" applicator in the treatment of carcinoma of the cervix. In: Hilaris BS, Nori D (eds). Radiation Therapy of Gynecological Cancer. Alan R. Liss, Inc, New York, 1987, p. 289.)

lated, the rectum can be excluded from the treatment volume. During the dosimetry process, the dose to the rectal catheter points are monitored and are kept under 200 cGy. If any portion of a needle lies adjacent to the rectum, the dwell time of the source position in that portion can be reduced to 0 seconds.

The treatment starts Tuesday morning and the patient receives two to three fractions a day spaced at least 5–6 hours apart. The recommended dose has been discussed in the previous section. The implant apparatus is then removed Friday afternoon after the final fraction.

Equipment

Some of the devices commonly used for interstitial volume implants of the vagina in-

clude the Syed-Neblett template[31] and the Martinez Universal Perineal Template (MUPIT).[33] Since the development of these devices there have been modifications to them to diverge the needles into the pelvic tissues as shown in Figure 8, and to customize the templates by computer.[34–36] One example is a modified Syed-Neblett type perineal template for HDR brachytherapy. Here, the template can be disassembled after needle insertion to allow cystoscopic and rectoscopic verification that there are no needles penetrating the bladder and rectum.[37]

Results of Therapy

Prophylactic Inguinal Node Irradiation

The lymphatic drainage of the vulva is similar to that of the lower third of the vagina.

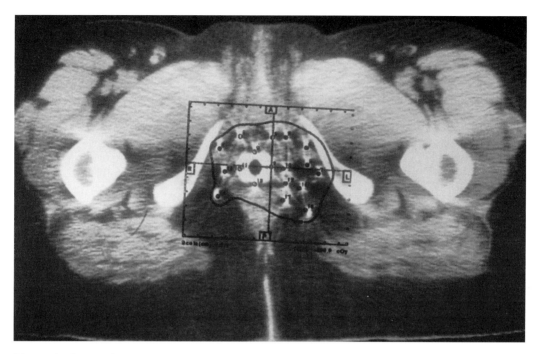

Figure 6. A 300 cGy isodose curve superimposed on a CT cut near the center of the implant: equal dwell times throughout. Note the inclusion of part of the rectum within the isodose curve. (From: Donath D, Clark B, Evans MDC. High dose rate interstitial brachytherapy of lower gynecological tract cancer. Proceedings of the Seventh International Brachytherapy Working Conference, 1992, p. 224.)

There is a great deal in the literature on the efficacy of prophylactic inguinal node irradiation in the treatment of vulvar cancer. Therefore data on prophylactic inguinal node irradiation for carcinoma of the lower third of the vagina is extrapolated, with caution, from data on vulvar cancer.

One of the most quoted series of results in this area stems from the Gynecologic Oncology Group (GOG) where patients with non-suspicious N0,N1 vulvar cancer were randomized between groin dissection and groin irradiation.[38] Radiation therapy consisted of 5000 cGy delivered in daily 200 cGy fractions to a depth of 3 cm below the anterior skin surface. The study closed prematurely due to an unusually high number of relapses among those receiving groin radiation. When the doses provided for five patients who failed prophylactic groin irradiation in the GOG study were recalculated based on new estimated deep femoral node depths, it was noted that they were underdosed.[20] This large

variation of inguinal lymph node depth in women was recently confirmed by a large study of 100 women whose lymph node depth ranged from 1.2–9.0 cm.[39] On the other hand, prophylactic inguinal node irradiation with parallel opposed photon portals to 5000 cGy results in a 91% actuarial control for vulvar cancer treated at the University of Wisconsin.[40] This is comparable to lymphadenectomy in this series although this is based on retrospective data.

Low-Dose-Rate Brachytherapy With or Without External Beam Radiotherapy

The survival rates of patients with carcinoma of the vagina range from 30%–90% according to the data from the Mallinckrodt Institute of Radiology (Figure 1).[8] Tumor control and survival rates exceed 90% for carcinoma in situ and stage I disease.[8,41] With increasing stage, the pelvic control rate decreased significantly.[8,42] The addition of EBRT

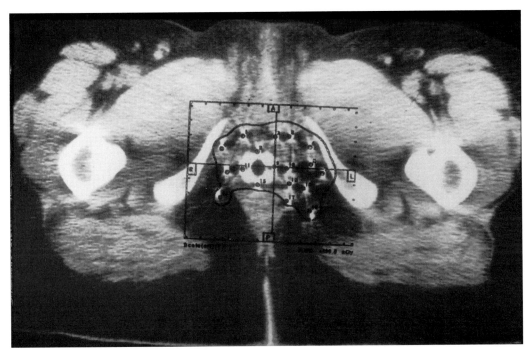

Figure 7. A 300 cGy isodose curve superimposed on a CT cut near the center of the implant: optimized dwell times. Note the exclusion of the rectum from the isodose curve. (From: Donath D, Clark B, Evans MDC. High dose rate interstitial brachytherapy of lower gynecological tract cancer. Proceedings of the Seventh International Brachytherapy Working Conference, 1992, p. 224.)

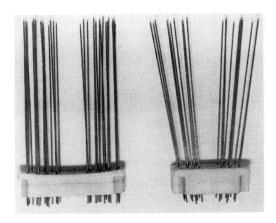

Figure 8. Anterior photograph of Syed-Neblett and diverging gynecological templates with needles in place. The diverging gynecological template is on the right. (From: John B, Scarbrough EC, Nguyen PD, et al. A diverging gynecological template for radioactive interstitial/intracavitary implants of the cervix. Int J Radiat Oncol Biol Phys 1988;15:463.)

to brachytherapy had no bearing on pelvic tumor control rates for stage I disease, while the combination of EBRT and brachytherapy achieved a better tumor control rate for stage II and III disease than brachytherapy alone (65% vs 40%).[43] This has been supported by other studies.[14,15] In one study,[15] the 2-year local control was 74% for combined EBRT and brachytherapy, 50% for brachytherapy alone, and 40% for EBRT alone. It was felt that a dose of 7500 cGy was required for tumor control. Other studies support the use of combination treatment over EBRT alone.[44,45] The analysis from Memorial Sloan-Kettering Cancer Center showed a significant increase in the 5-year actuarial survival for those patients who had brachytherapy as part of their treatment compared to those treated with EBRT alone (50% vs 9%) (P<0.001). In this series, the use of a temporary Ir-192 interstitial implant as part of the treatment for stage II and III disease demonstrated improved actuarial disease-free survival (80% vs 45%) (P=0.25) when compared to the use of intracavitary brachytherapy alone.

M.D. Anderson Cancer Center reported on their review of 167 patients with primary squamous cell carcinoma of the vagina treated with irradiation alone.[46] The local failure rate was 18% in stage I, 14% in stage II, 24% in stage III, and 30% in stage IVA. The individual selection of radiation therapy modalities had no bearing on outcome but the dose delivered with EBRT alone was 6000–7000 cGy.

Other studies observed improved control rates in stage III disease with interstitial brachytherapy at the expense of an increased complication rate.[15,47] Puthawala et al.[47] delivered a total tumor dose of 8000 cGy for stages I and II and 10,000 cGy for stages III and IV. At a median follow-up of 50 months, there was a local control rate of 80% and a 56% disease-free survival rate. The major drawback was a 15% severe complication rate. A series from the University of Florida noted a 91% local control rate when a dose of more than 8000 cGy was delivered with a combination of external radiotherapy and brachytherapy.[48] A multivariate analysis of their more recent data noted that the single most important predictor of pelvic control was overall treatment time.[49] If the entire course of radiotherapy (external beam and implant) was completed within 9 weeks, the pelvic control rate was 97%, otherwise it was 54% for treatment duration beyond 9 weeks.

In one series from India where only EBRT and intracavitary brachytherapy were used, the 2-year disease-free survival was 70% for stage II and 20% for stage III.[6] Whereas 30% of stage II failures had locally persistent or recurrent disease, 80% of stage III failures failed locally with either persistent or recurrent disease. Most recurrences occurred within 18 months. Less than 10% developed distant metastases or inguinal lymphadenopathy. For those who received EBRT alone, none of the patients with stage III or IV disease achieved a locoregional remission with a dose under 5000 cGy, while three of eight had local control with a dose of 5000–6000 cGy.

High-Dose-Rate Brachytherapy With or Without External Beam Radiotherapy

Information in this area is still sparse with short follow-up. Initial studies show encouraging results. One center used EBRT and intracavitary HDR brachytherapy for stage I and II vaginal cancer achieving a 100% complete response rate with 92% local control at a median follow-up of 2.6 years.[22] There was no grade 3 or 4 toxicity in the bladder and rectum while there was a 46% rate of moderate to severe vaginal stenosis. The latter occurred in those who were not sexually active.

The initial experience of using EBRT and HDR interstitial brachytherapy in one center to treat six patients with primary vaginal cancer revealed 50% control rate with three patients free of disease at 11, 15, and 30 months. The other three failed locally within 3 months of treatment.[23]

Sequelae of Therapy

Gynecological brachytherapy done under general or spinal anesthesia is associated with appreciable morbidity especially in patients with a history of cardiac disease and increased age.[50] Careful patient selection and vigilant perioperative care of the high risk patient should not be forsaken.

Perez et al.[8] reported grade 2–3 complications in 5% of stage I and 15% of stage II lesions. The major complications included fistula formation between the vagina and adjacent structures and proctitis. These events occurred mainly with the combination of EBRT and brachytherapy.

Radionecrosis of the vulva and distal vagina is difficult to manage. If hyperbaric oxygen is available, this should be implemented. In one center, 14 patients with radiation necrosis of the vagina alone, or in association with rectovaginal fistula, whose wounds failed to heal after 3 months of conservative therapy, had complete resolution of necrosis with hyperbaric oxygen.[51] Surgery with a myocutaneous flap is often required. Recurrent cancer must be ruled out; in one series, one third of patients undergoing excision of the radionecrotic site were found to have recurrent cancer.[52] For those with vaginal stenosis, delayed vaginal reconstruction, even years after initial therapy, can provide successful vaginal restoration with good function.[53]

When comparing complication figures among centers, one must bear in mind how the brachytherapy dose was prescribed, the dose rate of delivery, as well as the EBRT doses.

Follow-Up and Salvage

Most patients who recur do so within 16 months.[54] The pelvis is the first site of recurrence in 86% of all patients who recur.[54] The overall accuracy of MRI for recurrent vaginal cancer is 82%.[10] The ultimate goal is to differentiate between tumor and fibrotic tissue in patients suspected of having recurrent vaginal carcinoma. The key finding is the different signal intensity characteristics on T2-weighted images.[55] Recurrent vaginal tumors are relatively high in signal intensity and obliterate the low signal intensity vaginal muscularis. Salvage for local failure is poor, whether by surgery[15] or by chemotherapy.[12,13]

Conclusion

Many years ago primary carcinoma of the vagina was considered almost universally fatal.[56] Since then, the overall survival rates have risen from 28% in 1968[57] to 45% in 1977[58] to over 50% today.[45] Individualization of radiotherapy techniques and judicious use of intracavitary or interstitial brachytherapy have contributed to an enhanced survival rate and the preservation of reasonable functional integrity of the vagina.[27]

References

1. Daw E. Primary carcinoma of the vagina. J Obstet Gynecol Br Common 1971;78:853.
2. Gallup DG, Talledo OE, Shah KJ, et al. Invasive squamous cell carcinoma of the vagina: A 14-year study. Obstet Gynecol 1987;69:782–785.
3. Platz CE, Benda JA. Female genital tract cancer. Cancer 1995;75:270–294.
4. Perez CA, Arneson AN, Dehner LP, et al. Radiation therapy in carcinoma of the vagina. Obstet Gynecol 1974;44:862–872.
5. Plentl AA, Friedman EA. Lymphatic system of the female genitalia. In: The Morphologic Basis of Oncologic Diagnosis and Therapy. WB Saunders, Philadelphia, 1971, pp. 51–74.
6. Dixit S, Singal S, Baboo HA. Squamous cell carcinoma of the vagina: A review of 70 cases. Gynecol Oncol 1993;48:80–87.
7. Nori D. Principles of radiation therapy in the treatment of vaginal tumors. In: Hilaris BS, Nori D (eds). Radiation Therapy of Gynecological Cancer. Alan R. Liss, Inc, New York, 1987, pp. 173–190.
8. Perez CA, Camel HM, Galakatos AE, et al. Definitive irradiation in carcinoma of the vagina: Long-term evaluation of results. Int J Radiat Oncol Biol Phys 1988;15:1283–1290.
9. Benson RC. Cancer of the female genital tract. Cancer 1968;18:2–13.
10. Chang YC, Hricak H, Thurnher S, et al. Vagina: evaluation with MR imaging. Part II. Neoplasms. Radiology 1988;169:175–179.
11. Perez CA, Bedwinek JM, Breaux SR. Patterns of failure after treatment of gynecologic tumors. Cancer Treat Symp 1983;2:217.
12. Thigpen JT, Blessing JA, Homesley HD, et al. Phase II trial of cisplatin in advanced or recurrent cancer of the vagina: A Gynecologic Oncology Group study. Gynecol Oncol 1986;23:101–104.
13. Chu AM, Beechinor R. Survival and recurrence pattern in radiation treatment of carcinoma of the vagina. Gynecol Obstet 1984;19:298–307.
14. Kucera H, Vavra N. Radiation management of primary carcinoma of the vagina: Clinical and histopathological variables associated with survival. Gynecol Oncol 1991;40:12–16.
15. Peters WA, Kumar NB, Morley GW. Carcinoma of the vagina: Factors influencing treatment outcome. Cancer 1985;55:892–897.
16. Hoffman MS, DeCesare SL, Roberts WS, et al. Upper vaginectomy for in situ and occult, superficially invasive carcinoma of the vagina. Am J Obstet Gynecol 1992;166:30–33.
17. Hintz GL, Kagan AR, Chan P, et al. Radiation tolerance of the vaginal mucosa. Int J Radiat Oncol Biol Phys 1980;6:711–716.
18. Perez CA, Korba A, Sharma S. Dosimetric considerations in irradiation of carcinoma of the vagina. Int J Radiat Oncol Biol Phys 1977;2:639–649.
19. Spirtos NM, Doshi BP, Kapp DS, et al. Radiation therapy for primary squamous cell carcinoma of the vagina: Stanford University experience. Gynecol Oncol 1989;35:20–26.
20. Koh WJ, Chiu M, Stelzer KJ, et al. Femoral vessel depth and the implications for groin node radiation. Int J Radiat Oncol Biol Phys 1993;27:969–974.
21. Hacker NF, Eifel P, McGuire W, et al. Vulva. In: Hoskins WJ, Perez CA, Young RC (eds). Principles and Practice of Gynecologic Oncology. J.P. Lippincott Co., Philadelphia, 1992, pp. 537–566.
22. Nanavati PJ, Fanning J, Hilgers RD, et al. High-dose-rate brachytherapy in primary stage I and II vaginal cancer. Gynecol Oncol 1993;51:67–71.

23. Donath D, Roman TN, Clark B, et al. High dose rate interstitial brachytherapy of lower gynecological tract cancer. Eur J Cancer 1993;29A(6): 129.

24. Beach JL, Mendiondo OA, Martin JL. A rapid afterloading vaginal cylinder for Cs-137 brachytherapy. Int J Radiat Oncol Biol Phys 1991;21:1053–1055.

25. Johnson JM, Potish RA. The provision of a uniform vaginal surface dose rate by a novel afterloading cylinder. Med Dosim 1991;16: 193–198.

26. Sharma SC, Bhandare N. A new design of Delclos dome cylinders using standard Cs-137 sources. Int J Radiat Oncol Biol Phys 1991;21: 511–514.

27. Intracavitary brachytherapy planning and evaluation. In: Hilaris BS, Nori D, Anderson LL (eds). Atlas of Brachytherapy. Macmillan Publishing Company, New York, 1988, pp. 96–110.

28. Waterman FM, Holcomb DE. Dose distributions produced by a shielded vaginal cylinder using a high activity iridium source. Med Phys 1994;21:101–106.

29. Muench PJ, Nath R. Dose distributions produced by shielded applicatiors using AM-241 for intracavitary irradiation of tumors in the vagina. Med Phys 1992;19:1299–1306.

30. Finan MA, Hoffman MS, Greenberg H, et al. Interstitial radiotherapy for early stage vaginal cancer. A new method of tumor localization. J Reprod Med 1993;38:179–182.

31. Syed AMN, Puthawala A. Interstitial-intracavitary "Syed-Neblett" applicator in the treatment of carcinoma of the cervix. In: Hilaris BS, Nori D (eds). Radiation Therapy of Gynecologic Cancer. Alan R. Liss, Inc, New York, 1987, pp. 297–307.

32. Donath D, Clark B, Evans MDC. High dose rate interstitial brachytherapy of lower gynecological tract cancer. Proceedings of the Seventh International Brachytherapy Working Conference, 1992, pp. 219–225.

33. Martinez A, Edmundson GK, Cox RS, et al. Combination of external beam irradiation and multiple site perineal applicator (MUPIT) for treatment of locally advanced or recurrent prostatic, anorectal, and gynecologic malignancies. Int J Radiat Oncol Biol Phys 1984;11: 391–398.

34. John B, Scarbrough EC, Nguyen PD, et al. A diverging gynecological template for radioactive interstitial/intracavitary implants of the cervix. Int J Radiat Oncol Biol Phys 1988;15: 461–465.

35. Bentel GC, Oleson JR, Clarke-Pearson D, et al. Transperineal templates for brachytherapy

treatment of pelvic malignancies: A comparison of standard and customized templates. Int J Radiat Oncol Biol Phys 1990;19:751–758.

36. LaVigne ML, Schoeppel SL, McShan DL. The use of CT-based 3-D anatomical modeling in the design of customized perineal templates for intersitial gynecologic implants. Int J Radiat Oncol Biol Phys 1991;16:187–192.

37. Hockel M, Muller T. A new perineal template assembly for high-dose-rate interstitial brachytherapy of gynecologic malignancies. Radiat Oncol 1994;31:262–264.

38. Stehman FB, Bundy BN, Thomas G, et al. Groin dissection versus groin radiation in carcinoma of the vulva: A Gynecologic Oncology Group study. Int J Radiat Oncol Biol Phys 1992;24: 389–396.

39. McCall AR, Olson MC, Potkul RK. The variation of inguinal lymph node depth in adult women and its importance in planning elective irradiation for vulvar cancer. Cancer 1995;75: 2286–2288.

40. Petereit DG, Mehta MP, Buchler DA, et al. Inguinofemoral radiation of N0,N1 vulvar cancer may be equivalent to lymphadenectomy if proper radiation technique is used. Int J Radiat Oncol Biol Phys 1993;27:963–967.

41. Brown GR, Fletcher GH, Rutledge FN. Irradiation of in situ and invasive squamous cell carcinomas of the vagina. Cancer 1971;28: 1278–1283.

42. Prempree T, Amornmarn R. Radiation treatment of primary carcinoma of the vagina: Patterns of failure after definitive therapy. Acta Radiol Oncol 1985;24:51–56.

43. Perez CA, Camel HM. Long-term follow-up in radiation therapy of carcinoma of the vagina. Cancer 1982;49:1308–1315.

44. Leung S, Sexton M. Radical radiation therapy for carcinoma of the vagina-impact of treatment modalities on outcome: Peter MacCallum Cancer Institute experience 1970–1990. Int J Radiat Oncol Biol Phys 1993;25:413–418.

45. Stock RG, Mychalczak B, Armstrong JG, et al. The importance of brachytherapy technique in the management of primary carcinoma of the vagina. Int J Radiat Oncol Biol Phys 1992;24: 747–753.

46. Dancuart F, Delclos L, Wharton JT, et al. Primary squamous cell carcinoma of the vagina treated by radiotherapy: A failures analysis—the M.D. Anderson Hospital experience 1955–1982. Int J Radiat Oncol Biol Phys 1988; 14:745–749.

47. Puthawala A, Syed N, Nalick R, et al. Integrated external and interstitial radiation therapy for primary carcinoma of the vagina. Obstet Gynecol 1983;62:367–372.

48. Marcus RB, Million RR, Daly JW. Carcinoma of the vagina. Cancer 1978;42:2507–2512.

49. Lee WR, Marcus RB, Sombeck MD, et al. Radiotherapy alone for carcinoma of the vagina: The importance of overall treatment time. Int J Radiat Oncol Biol Phys 1994;29:983–988.

50. Dusenbery KE, Carson LF, Potish RA. Perioperative morbidity and mortality of gynecological brachytherapy. Cancer 1991;67:2786–2790.

51. Williams JA, Clarke D, Dennis WA, et al. The treatment of pelvic soft tissue radiation necrosis with hyperbaric oxygen. Am J Obstet Gynecol 1992;167:412–415.

52. Roberts WS, LaPolla JP, Greenberg H, et al. Management of radionecrosis of the vulva and distal vagina (meeting abstract). Proceedings of the Seventy-Second Annual American Radium Society Meeting, 1990, p. 11.

53. Berek JS, Hacker NF, Lagasse LD, et al. Delayed vaginal reconstruction in the fibrotic pelvis following radiation or previous reconstruction. Obstet Gynecol 1983;61:743–748.

54. Reddy S, Saxena VS, Lee MS, et al. Results of radiotherapeutic management of primary carcinoma of the vagina. Int J Radiat Oncol Biol Phys 1991;21:1041–1044.

55. Brown JJ, Gutierrez ED, Lee JK, et al. MR appearance of the normal and abnormal vagina after hysterectomy. Am J Roentgenol 1992;158: 95–99.

56. Taussig FJ. Early cancer of the vulva, vagina and female urethra: Five year results. Surg Gynecol Obstet 1935;60:477.

57. Frick HC, Jacox HW, Taylor HC. Primary carcinoma of the vagina. Am J Obstet Gynecol 1968; 101:695.

58. Prempree T, Viravathana T, Slawson RG, et al. Radiation management of primary carcinoma of the vagina. Cancer 1977;40:109–118.

Soft Tissue Sarcomas

David Donath, M.D., FRCP(C), Nora Janjan, M.D.,
Louis B. Harrison, M.D.

Introduction

Soft tissue sarcoma is a rare disease of unknown cause. Its incidence is approximately two out of 100,000. There is equal distribution between sexes and across age groups. Soft tissue sarcomas comprise a large number of different pathological diagnoses based on the cell of origin. Since they generally behave similarly with respect to clinical presentation and natural history, they are grouped together when their treatments are analyzed.

Soft tissue sarcomas are malignant tumors that originate from extraskeletal connective tissue. As a result, they often develop in the extremities. They have a tendency to extensively invade surrounding soft tissue and metastasize to the lungs. The soft tissue invasion is characterized by subclinical extension along lines of least tissue resistance, for example, parallel to fascial layers, along blood vessels and nerve sheaths, or between muscle fibers of adjacent grossly normal tissue. This has resulted in local recurrence rates of 60% when only a conservative resection, or local surgical excision of the gross tumor, was performed as the sole treatment.[1,2] It became obvious that an insufficient volume of tissue in the vicinity of the primary tumor was being treated. This led to the implementation of a radical compartmental excision or amputation in the treatment of this disease, with a subsequent reduction in the local recurrence rate to <30%.[1,2]

In selected cases, a conservative resection alone has proven to be sufficient in controlling loco-regional disease. A review at Memorial Sloan Kettering Cancer Center (MSKCC) revealed that at a median follow-up of 4 years, low grade, <5 cm in diameter, soft tissue sarcomas of the extremities had a local recurrence rate <10% following a conservative resection alone.[3] A review from Roswell Park Memorial Institute found the 5-year local recurrence rate in extremity sarcomas of varying size to be 6% for patients with minimal surgical margins 2 cm or greater.[4]

General Management

Postoperative External Radiotherapy

Over the past two decades, the treatment of several types of cancer has evolved to strategies that maximize functional and cosmetic outcome while achieving local control. To avoid the adverse impact that radical surgery may have on functional and cosmetic outcome, operations limited to the removal of the clinically or radiographically detectable mass are being implemented. They are then integrated with other therapeutic modalities designed to destroy subclinical extensions of sarcoma into the adjacent grossly normal tis-

From Nag S (ed): *Principles and Practice of Brachytherapy.* © Futura Publishing Co., Inc., Armonk, NY, 1997.

sue. This has resulted in local control and survival rates comparable to that achieved with radical surgery.

In keeping with this, limb sparing surgery and radiation therapy have supplanted amputation as the standard treatment for soft tissue sarcomas. One of the first studies to confirm this transition was a randomized prospective trial from the National Cancer Institute concerning the management of high grade extremity sarcomas. Radiation therapy was delivered in the form of postoperative external beam irradiation, with 5000 cGy directed towards all areas at risk for local tumor spread and 6000–7000 cGy delivered to the tumor bed. Daily treatments were given at 180–200 cGy per treatment resulting in a treatment period of about 7 weeks. This treatment regime followed a conservative surgical approach and was compared to amputation. Four of 27 in the limb-sparing approach recurred locally; whereas, none of the amputated patients did. However, there was no difference in actuarial disease-free survival rates (71% and 78% at 5 years; P = 0.75) or overall survival rates (83% and 88% at 5 years; P = 0.99) between the limb-sparing group and the amputation group.[5] The obvious additional benefit was the ability to preserve the limb.[6]

An additional finding of this study was that patients with positive resection margins had a higher likelihood of local recurrence compared with those with negative margins (P<0.0001). This difficulty in obtaining local control, after limb-sparing surgery and postoperative external beam irradiation for positive margins, has been experienced in other major centers as well. In a series from the Princess Margaret Hospital in Toronto, the local failure rate was 50% if any of the following criteria used to define histologic evidence of disease at the resection margin were met: 1) visualization of tumor tissue during the surgical procedure; 2) shelling out of tumor; or 3) a description by the pathologist of microscopic foci of tumor extending to the resection margin.[7] One of the first two criteria was always met when there was involvement of neurovascular structures, and the intent was to preserve these. Other studies have also confirmed the negative impact of positive resection margins on local control,[8–11] although one has found this feature to apply to only grossly positive margins, not microscopic.[11]

Preoperative External Radiotherapy

External beam radiation therapy given prior to a conservative surgical resection has also been shown to be effective in producing local control in over 80% of patients. The theoretical advantages of preoperative radiation therapy over postoperative external beam irradiation include decreased risk of tumor implantation in the surgical wound and tumor regression prior to surgery facilitating a surgical resection. As well, with postoperative external radiation, the entire operative bed, the surgical drain site, and a 5-cm margin must be included in the treatment volume. With preoperative radiation, only the gross tumor plus a 5-cm margin must be in the treatment volume.

In the most recent update of results from the Massachusetts General Hospital on preoperative radiation therapy, surgical margins of resection were also shown to be an area of concern. The 5-year actuarial local control rate was 97% for 104 tumors with negative margins and 82% for 28 tumors with positive margins.[12] A multivariate analysis of a series from the M.D. Anderson Cancer Center also showed diminished local control with microscopically positive margins or intraoperative tumor violation in patients with intermediate and high grade extremity sarcomas who received preoperative radiotherapy followed by surgery.[13]

Brachytherapy

Initial Results

At MSKCC in New York, brachytherapy has been studied as the adjuvant form of radiation therapy. Instead of using wide field external beam treatment, a more limited volume was treated with an interstitial implant placed at the time of surgery. The surgical procedure itself remained the same. The interstitial radiation was delivered via low-dose-rate manually afterloaded brachytherapy. Their pilot study involved 33 cases. The resection margin was positive in 30 and there was involvement of bone or neuro-vascular structures in 20. A median radiation dose of 4000 cGy was delivered over 4–5 days. With a median follow-up of 3 years, the local control rates were 100% for 17 patients with previously untreated tumors and 75% for 16 patients with recurrent tumors.[14] These results were impressive when compared to the results obtained with external beam irradiation for positive resection margins.

Rationale

There are several technical and radiobiological reasons cited for the early successes of this technique. When external beam irradiation is utilized, the radiation oncologist can only rely on preoperative CT/MRI images to plan the external beam portals. In comparison, the intraoperative placement of brachytherapy catheters over the tumor bed under direct visualization after the tumor has been removed results in a more accurate demarcation of the tumor site. This allows for increased precision in treating the target area with brachytherapy and sparing surrounding normal tissue. As the highest dose of radiation can now be more accurately localized to the region at greatest risk for microscopic disease, less of a margin is required. The brachytherapy target volume requires only a 1.5- to 2-cm margin beyond the intraoperative definition of the tumor bed while a 5-cm margin is required beyond radiologically defined tumor limits with external beam irradiation. Given the smaller treatment volume encountered with brachytherapy, one could expect a decrease in late tissue morbidity with a resulting improvement in functional outcome.

Second, the inverse square law effect ensures that doses higher than the prescription dose are delivered to the target volume, enabling better local control of positive microscopic resection margins often encountered around neuro-vascular bundles. Even with these higher doses, neurological function is rarely affected; and, when it is, the effect is transient following the application of aggressive physical therapy.[15] However, the main benefit of the inverse square law effect is that a diminished dose is delivered to normal tissue surrounding the target volume, further decreasing late tissue morbidity. This allows for the brachytherapy dose to be delivered in

4–5 days, unlike the 6–7 weeks required for external beam therapy, a distinct radiobiological advantage with respect to tumor control. In addition, the brachytherapy treatment begins within 5–7 days of surgery, anticipating a minimal tumor burden, as compared to 4–6 weeks later for external beam irradiation. Postoperative external radiation can be delayed even further if the wound heals slowly, potentially allowing the tumor cells to proliferate to a burden that could not be handled by the standard dose of postoperative radiation.

Finally, as the brachytherapy treatments are completed within 10 days following the operation, rather than the 10–12 weeks required for the completion of external beam irradiation, there is also the theoretical radiobiological advantage of treating the tumor cells prior to their entrapment in healed scar tissue that is hypoxic. In addition, adjuvant chemotherapy, if required, can be started much sooner after the surgery. As a result of all this and in keeping with clinical data, there is no need to treat the surgical wound, drain site, or tissue compartment, as is necessary with external beam therapy.[16]

These features make brachytherapy a more suitable adjuvant option in certain scenarios. One is the treatment of pediatric sarcomas.[17–19] Localization of the radiation dose is particularly important in children to reduce potential late radiation effects on cosmesis and growth and to prevent development of secondary tumors.

External Radiotherapy with Brachytherapy

Brachytherapy can be used to supplement the dose administered by external beam radiation in selected clinical presentations where higher doses are required for local control. It is often impossible to dissect locally advanced soft tissue sarcomas from neuro-vascular structures and bone, let alone achieve the desired 2-cm margin. Poor local control rates are obtained with limited surgery and external radiation in these situations. Brachytherapy would allow the administration of additional radiation to the site of residual tumor while sparing adjacent normal tissue.

Brachytherapy can also be used in situations where only a limited dose of external beam radiation can be given to the tumor bed. An example is tumors located in the paraspinous region where it is difficult to administer more than 50 Gy of external radiation to the tumor bed without exceeding the radiation tolerance of the adjacent spinal cord.[20] Brachytherapy (15–25 Gy) can be delivered to the tumor bed without exceeding the tolerance of the surrounding radiosensitive tissues.

Brachytherapy Technique

Initial Surgery

The ideal wide local excision should include the entire tumor specimen en block with a margin of normal tissue. The incision should be parallel to the long axis of the underlying principal muscle. There should be no disruption of this margin or of the pseudocapsule that lies just deep to the margin. All previous incisions and the access used for the biopsy should be excised along with an ellipse of surrounding normal skin. Excellent hemostasis should be obtained as a hematoma can spread tumor along its path. When there is involvement by tumor of functionally important structures such as neuro-vascular structures or bone, the emphasis should be placed on preserving normal limb function. The tumor should be dissected off these structures as well as is possible without interfering with the integrity of the structure.

Target Volume

The overlying and underlying surface surrounding the defect left following the excision of the specimen becomes the target area, the area where tumor cells are most likely to reside. Tissue lying within a depth of 0.5 cm beyond the target area is now considered the target volume, the volume to be incorporated in the prescription dose (Figure 1).[21] A single plane implant is sufficient to cover this volume. The dimensions of the target area includes those of the tumor specimen plus a 1.5- to 2.0-cm margin. Depending on the extent of the resection achieved around neuro-vascular structures, one may want to increase the margin along these structures.

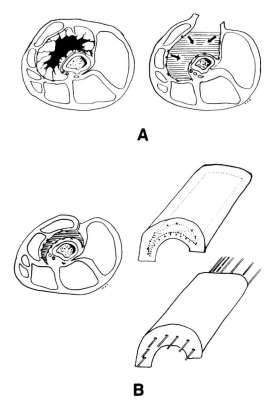

Figure 1. Brachytherapy of tumor bed. A) The tumor bed consists of the tissues around the tumor, bearing its microscopic ramifications. B) After excision of the tumor, the overlying skin and soft tissues including the repaired incision collapse into the underlying structures. This composite slab of tissues constitutes the tumor bed target for radiotherapy. (Reprinted with permission from Shiu MH, Brennan MF (eds). Surgical Management of Soft Tissue Sarcoma. Lea & Febiger, Philadelphia, PA, 1989.)

Low-Dose-Rate Manual Afterloaded Brachytherapy[22,23]

The dimensions of the target area are recorded. The limits of the target area are denoted by large metallic surgical clips. Using the New York-Memorial system of dosimetry, one determines the number of afterloading catheters that need to be implanted to deliver 1000 cGy per day to the target area. The catheters are placed parallel to the long axis of the extremity. Sealed-end catheters are usually used to avoid access between the catheter lumen and adjacent tissue.

The catheter insertion sites 1 cm apart are marked along a straight line using a sterile marker and ruler. This line is marked on the skin several centimeters away from the operative bed and perpendicular to the projected path of the catheter. A scalpel is used to pierce the skin at each site prior to inserting a trochar through the skin puncture and embedding the trochar in the operative bed. The catheter is threaded through the trochar until it emerges from the opposite end. While the catheter is held in place, the trochar is withdrawn until the catheter is in the proper position. If the catheter diameter is larger than the internal diameter of the trochar lumen, the thin leader attached to the catheter is threaded through the trochar. In this setting, the external diameter of the trochar is matched to the external diameter of the catheter. Therefore, when the trochar is withdrawn, no trauma is precipitated by the trailing catheter.

The tubes are then sutured in place to the operative bed using #2 or #3 absorbable suture material. A stainless steel button and a plastic hemispherical bead are then threaded over the exposed tail of the catheter. The stainless steel button is then fixed to the catheter by crimping the tubular segment of the button with a hemostat. The crimping is intended to hold the catheter firmly without permanently deforming the catheter lumen. To prevent the catheter from slipping out, a silk suture is inserted through each button hole and sutured to the skin.

Several days later when the patient is stable, localization radiographs are taken of the implant site with inactive radiopaque sources placed within the lumen of the catheters. The orientation of the radiographs will depend on the capabilities of the computerized planning system and image quality. Depending on the available Ir-192 source strength, the dose-rate distribution in several planes perpendicular to the axis of the catheters is then determined. The highest dose rate with a continuous isodose curve is then selected. Given a prescribed dose of 4500 cGy, the treatment time is then calculated. Tiny lead markers can be placed on the skin during the planning radiographs and then digitized on the planning system to determine the dose the skin receives. Ideally, 25 sq cm of skin should receive <4000 cGy and 100 sq cm, <2500 cGy. Iodine-125 radioactive sources, of an activity equivalent to the Ir-192 sources commonly used, are inserted if the setting dictates the least possible dose to adjacent structures. This would include the gonads in a child or a patient in the reproductive age group.

The brachytherapy dose is restricted to 15–25 Gy if external beam irradiation of 45–50 Gy is to be added.[24–27] The ideal time to load the catheters with radioactive Ir-192 sources is 5–7 days following the surgery. The stainless steel button is uncrimped. The ribbon containing radioactive sources is then inserted into the catheter. The ribbon is then secured in position by recrimping the tubular portion of the button. After the prescribed dose has been delivered, the Ir-192 sources and the catheters are removed at the bedside under sterile conditions. The catheter insertion sites are covered with antibiotic impregnated gauze, and the patient can be discharged the same day.

High-Dose-Rate Remote Afterloaded Brachytherapy

The basic procedure used to implant a patient for high-dose-rate brachytherapy is similar and only the differences will be discussed.

The number of catheters to be used is determined not by a dosimetry system but by the number that can be accommodated when placed at 1-cm intervals across the target width. Also, these catheters must have larger lumens to accommodate the high-dose-rate Ir-192 source of the remote afterloader. Once the catheters have been secured in the operative bed, a plastic hemispherical bead and a teflon button are threaded over the exposed portion of the catheter. The bead is similar to the one used for low-dose-rate and it easily slides over the catheter. The button is different. Its internal lumen is designed to hold the catheter firmly but it can be slid over the catheter when significant pressure is applied. The hemisphere and button are then sutured to the skin with a silk suture.

After the localizing radiographs have been digitized on the planning computer, dwell time optimization and manipulation are executed so that the prescription isodose curve covers the catheters in a continuous fashion with a 5- to 8-mm margin. This is determined on planes perpendicular to the long axis of the catheters.

Brachytherapy doses of 2–5 Gy per fraction are generally delivered on a BID basis starting 5–7 days after the operation. Total dose generally ranges from 35–50 Gy in 8–15 fractions if brachytherapy is given alone and 15–25 Gy if given as a boost to external beam, depending on the dose per fraction, external beam dose, and volume of residual tumor.[28,29] For each treatment, the catheters are connected to the accessory tubes of the remote afterloader. They are disconnected following the treatment. After the final treatment, the catheters are removed at the patient's bedside in a similar fashion to manually afterloaded techniques.

Results

Low-Dose-Rate Brachytherapy

Prospective Trial

In 1982, MSKCC embarked on a randomized prospective trial of limb-sparing surgery alone versus limb-sparing surgery and postoperative adjuvant low-dose-rate brachytherapy using Ir-192 to deliver 4200–4500 cGy over 4–6 days. Only those patients in whom limb-sparing surgery was viable with no more than microscopically positive margins were selected. One hundred and twenty-six patients were randomized between July 1982 and July 1987. Patients in each group were well matched with respect to age, sex, site, tumor size, depth, histologic type, and grade. At 5 years, the local control rate was 82% in the brachytherapy group and 67% in the group not receiving brachytherapy (P = 0.049). This decrease in the local recurrence rate was only observed in the high grade sarcomas, with a local control of 90% of those receiving brachytherapy versus 65% of those not receiving it (P = 0.013). However, this was not accompanied by any improvement in the disease specific survival or freedom from distant metastasis at 5 years.[30,31] The benefit of adjuvant brachytherapy was not demonstrated for low grade lesions.[32] Also, the status of the resection margin did not have any bearing on local control.[31] This is the only prospective randomized trial that questions the value of adjuvant radiation therapy after conservative resection. It clearly demonstrates that the addition of adjuvant radiation has led to an improvement in the local control of soft tissue sarcoma.

Functional Outcome

Further analysis of this randomized trial data-base also showed that there was no significant difference in the functional parameters of isometric muscle torque, gait velocity, cadence, stride length, and single limb stance time symmetry in the brachytherapy versus nonbrachytherapy groups.[33] This is in contrast to the external beam data. A similarly detailed review of the functional outcome with postoperative external beam radiation therapy showed decreasing function and strength with increasing tissue volume treated to at least 55 Gy.[34] In another study, external radiation doses in excess of 60 Gy resulted in increased fibrosis and a diminished functional outcome.[35]

Low Grade Tumors

A separate review from MSKCC concentrated on desmoid tumors or low grade fibrosarcoma. Most patients had very poor prognostic factors, including 75% with recurrent disease and 16% with gross residual disease. The local control rate was 66%, with one third of local failures occurring at the periphery of the implanted volume.[36]

Tumor Location

The MSKCC prospective trial data was obtained from patients with soft tissue sarcoma of the extremity and superficial trunk. A multivariate analysis of patients with soft tissue sarcoma treated with wide excision and interstitial brachytherapy at the Institut Gustave Roussy demonstrated that only tumor location was predictive of local failure (P<0.01), which in turn correlated with metastatic outcome (P<0.01). Sarcomas located in the extremity and head and neck fared better than those on the trunk.[37]

Locally Recurrent Tumors

A wide local excision and postoperative brachytherapy were also utilized for recurrent extremity sarcomas following conservative surgery and external beam irradiation.[38] With a median follow-up of 3 years, all patients with less than three prior recurrences achieved local control. In addition, all recurrent low grade tumors were controlled. Only 5 of 40 patients occurred complications requiring surgery, and this was usually limited to skin repair, with no impact on limb function. In comparison, the results of wide local excision and external radiotherapy for soft tissue sarcomas recurring following conservative surgery alone[10,39] or following conservative surgery and external radiotherapy[40] were much less favorable.

External Beam Radiotherapy and Brachytherapy

With postoperative external beam radiation therapy, as the tissue volume treated to at least 55 Gy increases, the functional outcome starts to deteriorate.[34] As a means of circumventing this limitation, some centers are decreasing the dose delivered with external irradiation and supplementing the difference with brachytherapy as it is more restrictive in the volume it treats to a significant dose. The overall intent is to deliver a high dose of localized radiation to the tumor bed and a relatively homogeneous dose to the larger anatomical area at risk. There has been concern expressed about giving brachytherapy alone due to the propensity of sarcomas to infiltrate surrounding tissue and cause marginal recurrences because of the rapid decrease in dose towards marginal sites. One study on the use of interstitial brachytherapy alone in 50 cases of soft tissue sarcoma over 20 years showed only 4% failed in the irradiated volume while 26% failed in marginal and local-regional sites.[41] Another concern about the use of brachytherapy alone is the potential for wound healing problems.

Local control rates exceed 80% when brachytherapy is used in combination with external beam irradiation.[24–27] Generally, the dose delivered with external beam was 30–50 Gy at 2 Gy per day while 15–25 Gy was given with a low-dose-rate implant at 10 Gy per day. One study determined that there was a significant increase in the local failure rate if the volume of tissue that received 65 Gy was less than the tumor volume.[25] This was irrelevant when the histologic margins were positive, as most of these cases failed locally regardless of the volume of tissue receiving 65 Gy. Another report was in agreement with this, as they showed a trend toward improvement in local control if the margin was negative versus microscopically versus grossly positive (92.3%, 76.9%, and 33%, respectively; P = 0.07).[24]

No difference in local control has been reported between preoperative and postoperative external beam therapy in combination with brachytherapy; however, 87% of the group undergoing preoperative external beam therapy compared to only 42% of postoperative group had tumors >5 cm in size in this report.[26] Wound complication rates for patients receiving preoperative irradiation and interstitial brachytherapy as a boost were quite significant ranging from 25%–40%, 15% of them severe.[9] In these series, the implants were loaded 3–4 days after the operation.

For patients with positive resection margins, the recent policy at MSKCC has been to use brachytherapy as a boost to a dose of 15–20 Gy, and then add 45–50 Gy of supplemental external beam radiation to cover a wider volume of tissue. When this combination is compared to brachytherapy alone for high grade tumors with positive margins, there would appear to be better local control (90% vs 59%).[42]

Complications

Although initial local control results with brachytherapy at MSKCC were encouraging, the complications that occurred, particularly to the wound and skin, were discouraging. Nine of 33 patients in the pilot study had serious wound complications, occasionally severe enough to require amputations.[14] This prompted further analysis of the randomized brachytherapy trial. It was discovered that the addition of brachytherapy was accompanied by a significant increase in the major and moderate wound complication rate, 48% versus 14% (P = 0.0006), and a significant increase in the median duration to complete resolution of these complications.[43]

One factor identified as a potential cause of this high complication rate was the early application of the radioactive implants. This was based on the consideration that previous animal experiments suggested delaying the application of radiation to 1 week after creating a wound, yielding a wound-breaking strength comparable to unirradiated controls. Most of these patients in the MSKCC series were loaded with the radioactive sources <5 days after surgery. A multivariate analysis of a series from the Massachusetts General revealed that the delivery of brachytherapy as a postoperative boost following preoperative external beam irradiation and surgery was a significant prognostic factor in determining wound morbidity.[44] Coincidentally, these patients were loaded with radioactive sources 3–5 days after the operation.

The MSKCC study was modified in 1985 to determine if wound-healing problems could be decreased if the radioactive sources were loaded 5–7 days after the operation. Reviewing the wound complications of these patients noted no difference in the complication rate between those who had surgery and brachytherapy and those patients who received surgery alone.[45] In contrast, a multivariate analysis at the Princess Margaret Hospital disclosed that the addition of preoperative "external beam" radiation to limb sparing surgery for soft tissue sarcomas was a significant risk factor (P = 0.04) leading up to major wound healing complications.[46]

Experience also exists regarding the risk for normal tissue complications between preoperative and postoperative external beam irradiation combined with supplemental brachytherapy. Higher rates of delayed wound healing have been reported with preoperative external beam therapy when combined with brachytherapy.[27,47] In keeping with basic principles, the volume of tissue irradiated is one of the critical factors related to normal tissue tolerance.[26,47] Eighty-six percent of major and moderate complications with brachytherapy, either alone or in combination with preoperative external beam irradiation, have been observed to occur when the irradiated area exceeded 100 sq cm[47]; major and moderate complications have been defined to include infection, persistent seroma/hematoma, and wound dehiscence treated conservatively or requiring operative revision.[43] On multivariate analysis, tumors located in the lower extremity, increasing age of the patient, and brachytherapy boost have been associated with major and moderate wound complications.[44] Myocutaneous flaps, placed at the time of tumor resection, have reduced the rate of wound complications by introducing unirradiated tissue in the surgical bed and decreasing the strain on the primary incision.[48]

Cost Comparison

Cost benefit analyses are progressively becoming very prominent features in the recommendation of the most appropriate therapy in cancer treatment. A study from M.D. Anderson compared treatment charges related to adjuvant irradiation for soft tissue sarcoma.[49] The charge assessment was restricted to the administration of radiotherapy and excluded costs due to unrelated intercurrent medical problems. The average cost incurred in delivering preoperative external beam irradiation, 50 Gy in 25 fractions with 6 MV photons, to 12 patients was compared to the cost of providing interstitial implantation to 23 patients. Hospital-based charges and professional fees were included. The total charge for external irradiation was $10,905; while, for brachytherapy, the charge was $9,345 for upper extremity lesions and $10,335 for lower extremity lesions. The cost of providing additional operating room time and hospital days for brachytherapy was included.

High-Dose-Rate Brachytherapy

The current standard treatment for soft tissue sarcoma is a wide local excision together with radiotherapy, given either preoperatively or postoperatively. In the postoperative setting, both external beam therapy alone and low-dose-rate manual afterloaded brachytherapy alone have proven to be successful; but each has serious limitations, particularly the latter.

For each individual case, the low-dose-rate radioactive sources must be procured and calibrated. The most important handicap, though, is radiation exposure of medical and nursing personnel. Daily visits by the assigned staff must be brief and held at a distance from the patient. As a result, an effective educational program must be organized for the staff to ensure that appropriate care of the implanted patient is sustained, that safe visitation procedures are in place, and that unusual situations (e.g., management of an unresponsive patient while catheters are loaded with radioactive sources) are properly planned for. Finally, personnel trained in the acquisition, handling, and calibration of the radioactive sources for each implant must be available. Understandably, the technical and financial resources necessary to provide this level of care are usually found only at major institutions and, therefore, limit the availability of this therapeutic option.

In addition, the MSKCC prospective trial on the use of low-dose-rate brachytherapy in the treatment of soft tissue sarcoma showed a significantly higher level of anxiety, depression, and appreciation of illness in the brachytherapy group.[33] It is believed that this was brought about by the required isolation policy endured during the brachytherapy treatment.

Several of these limitations have been overcome with the advent of the high-dose-rate, single stepping source, remote afterloading brachytherapy units. The brief exposure interval associated with each treatment has led to uncompromised nursing care and the elimination of visitor restrictions. This has turned out to be an important feature as it has enabled us to treat patients incapacitated from their surgery and requiring extensive postoperative nursing care. Another advantage of high-dose-rate brachytherapy is that only a single source is used and that source needs replacing only once every 3 months. Hence, source acquisition, handling, calibration, and storage are minimized. In addition, patients can be implanted with afterloading catheters at a hospital other than the center with the remote afterloading unit. They are then transported daily for their treatments without being admitted to that center. An additional advantage is that, in selected cases, treatment can be given on an out-patient basis, improving patient tolerance of the procedure and eliminating some of the costs of hospitalization.

The main area of apprehension is the possible morbidity associated with the delivery of large fractions of radiation. Initial results from two centers do not appear to justify this reservation about high-dose-rate brachytherapy.

Of 13 patients treated with conservative surgery, high-dose-rate brachytherapy with or without external beam radiotherapy, Wayne State University reported wound complications in only one patient. It consisted of hematoma and a healing delay that subsequently led to premature removal of the implant and skin debridement. Two patients who had skin graft prior to radiotherapy tolerated high-dose-rate brachytherapy well. Eight patients had high-dose-rate brachytherapy alone with a dose range of 3984 cGy/12 fractions to 4746 cGy/14 fractions. Five patients had 3000–5040 cGy of external beam radiation combined with a high-dose-rate brachytherapy dose of 2065–2394 cGy/7 fractions. With a median follow-up of 16 months, there were three local failures, and one patient died of disease.[50]

At McGill University and its affiliated hospitals, there is at least 1 year follow-up on 19 patients who underwent conservative surgery and high-dose-rate brachytherapy for soft tissue sarcoma. There were eight extremity lesions, four chest wall, four retroperitoneum, two head and neck, and one pelvis. Postoperative external radiation was not an option in 12 patients for various reasons including recurrent disease after conservative surgery and radiation, prior radiation for a different malignancy, and proximity to radiosensitive structures such as small bowel and spinal cord. Six to seven treatments of 500 cGy each were delivered on a BID basis over 4 days with a minimum of 5 hours between treatments. All patients started treatment 5 or more days following surgery. With a median follow-up of 2 years, ten are disease free. Six patients failed locally, particularly those who presented with what was considered to be a radiation-induced sarcoma. Three patients developed wound complications, two of which were due to external compression of the wound (for instance, patient lying on the pelvic wound after surgery.) Two of these resolved with nonsurgical measures.

Conclusions

A wide local excision and postoperative low-dose-rate brachytherapy have proven to be beneficial in the treatment of soft tissue sarcoma. Adjuvant treatment with brachytherapy improves local control in high grade tumors larger than 5 cm in diameter, but has no effect on low grade lesions, lesions under 5 cm, or on distant metastases. It has proven to be especially valuable in the management of soft tissue sarcoma where there has been intraoperative violation of the tumor or microscopic disease left behind. The combined treatment has also proven to be effective in the treatment of soft tissue sarcoma that has recurred after a prior course of surgery and radiation. Preliminary results with the use of high-dose-rate brachytherapy as an adjuvant treatment following a wide local excision have proven to be very encouraging.

Unlike that seen in preoperative external radiation, there has been no increase in the wound complication rate with the judicious use of brachytherapy, and extremity function, particularly neurological function, has not been compromised. Wide local excision and brachytherapy have proven to be convenient for patients in that all treatment is completed 10–14 days following surgery, and the patient is discharged from hospital.

Although brachytherapy as an adjuvant therapy to treat soft tissue sarcoma has been proven successful in terms of clinical outcome, functional outcome, and patient convenience, some difficulties related to its delivery have limited its application in North America. First, there are not many radiation oncologists trained in interstitial brachytherapy. Second, the problem of radiation exposure to medical staff and nursing personnel and the technical requirements and expense of dealing with radioactive source acquisition, handling, and safety are significant. As a result, many hospitals and radiation oncology departments have been reluctant to become involved with low-dose-rate, manually afterloaded brachytherapy.

The introduction of remote afterloading has eliminated the radiation exposure hazard and has made brachytherapy more accessible to even the outlying medical centers. Today, a patient at a peripheral hospital can undergo a brachytherapy implant at that hospital and then travel to the tertiary center for the appropriate brachytherapy treatment. Whether high-dose-rate remote afterloaded brachytherapy can provide similar excellent results as low-dose-rate brachytherapy in the adjuvant treatment of soft tissue sarcoma, however, remains to be seen.

References

1. Cantin J, McNeer GP, Chu FC, et al. The problem of local recurrence after treatment of soft tissue sarcoma. Ann Surg 1968;168:47–53.
2. Shiu MH, Castro EB, Hajdu SI, et al. Surgical treatment of 297 soft tissue sarcomas of the lower extremity. Ann Surg 1975;182:597.
3. Geer RJ, Woodruff J, Casper ES, et al. Management of small soft tissue sarcoma of the extremity in adults. Arch Surg 1992;127(11): 1285–1289.
4. Karakousis CP, Emrich LJ, Rao U, et al. Limb salvage in soft tissue sarcomas with selective combination of modalities. Eur J Surg Oncol 1991;17(1):71–80.
5. Rosenberg S, Tepper J, Glatstein E, et al. The treatment of soft tissue sarcomas of the extremities: Prospective randomized evaluations of (1) limb-sparing surgery plus radiation therapy compared with amputation and (2) the role of adjuvant chemotherapy. Ann Surg 1982; 196(3):305–315.
6. Rosenberg S, Glatstein E. Perspectives on the role of surgery and radiation therapy in the treatment of soft tissue sarcomas of the extremities. Semin Oncol 1981;8:190–200.
7. Bell RS, O'Sullivan B, Liu FF, et al. The surgical margin in soft tissue sarcoma. J Bone Joint Surg (Am) 1989;71(3):370–375.
8. Herbert SH, Corn BW, Solin LJ, et al. Impact of surgical margins on outcome after limb-preserving treatment for soft tissue sarcomas of the extremities. Abstract. Proc Am Radium Soc 75th Annual Meeting, 1993, p. 34.
9. Suit HD, Mankin HJ, Wood WC, et al. Preoperative, intraoperative, and postoperative radiation in the treatment of primary soft tissue sarcoma. Cancer 1985;55:2659–2667.
10. Avizonis VM, Sause WT, Menlove RL. Utility of surgical margins in the radiotherapeutic management of soft tissue sarcomas. J Surg Oncol 1990;45(2):85–90.
11. Pao WJ, Pilepich MV. Postoperative radiotherapy in the treatment of extremity soft tissue sarcomas. Int J Radiat Oncol Biol Phys 1990; 19(4):907–911.
12. Sadoski C, Suit HD, Rosenberg A, et al. Preoperative radiation, surgical margins, and local control of extremity sarcomas of soft tissues. J Surg Oncol 1993;52(4):223–230.
13. Tanabe KK, Pollock RE, Ellis LM, et al. Influence of surgical margins on outcome in patients with preoperatively irradiated extremity soft tissue sarcomas. Cancer 1994;73(6): 1652–1659.
14. Shiu M, Turnbull A, Nori D, et al. Control of locally advanced extremity soft tissue sar-

comas by function saving resection and brachytherapy. Cancer 1984;53:1385–1392.

15. Zelefsky MJ, Nori D, Shiu MH, et al. Limb salvage in soft tissue sarcomas involving neurovascular structures using combined surgical resection and brachytherapy. Int J Radiat Oncol Biol Phys 1990;19:913–918.

16. Harrison LB, Zelefsky MJ, Armstrong JG, et al. Brachytherapy and function preservation in the localized management of soft tissue sarcomas of the extremity. Semin Radiat Oncol 1993;3(1):260–269.

17. Curran WJ, Littman P, Raney RB. Interstitial radiation therapy in the treatment of childhood soft-tissue sarcomas. Int J Radiat Oncol Biol Phys 1988;14:169–174.

18. Fontanesi J, Kun L, Pao W, et al. Brachytherapy as primary or 'boost' irradiation in 18 children with solid tumors. Endocurie/Hypertherm Oncol 1991;7:195–200.

19. Gerbaulet A, Panis X, Flamant F, et al. Iridium afterloading curietherapy in the treatment of pediatric malignancies. Cancer 1985;56:1274–1279.

20. Armstrong JG, Fass DE, Bains M, et al. Paraspinal tumors: Techniques and results of brachytherapy. Int J Radiat Oncol Biol Phys 1991;20:787–790.

21. Shiu MH, Hilaris BS, Harrison LB, et al. Brachytherapy and function-saving resection of soft tissue sarcoma arising in the limb. Int J Radiat Oncol Biol Phys 1991;21:1485–1492.

22. Brachytherapy for soft tissue sarcomas. In: Hilaris BS, Nori D, Anderson LL (eds). Atlas of Brachytherapy. Macmillan Publishing Company, New York, 1988, pp. 170–182.

23. Hilaris BS, Shiu M, Nori D, et al. Limb sparing therapy for locally advanced soft tissue sarcomas. Endocurie/Hypertherm Oncol 1985;1:17–24.

24. Alekhteyar KM, Herskovic AM, Orton CG, et al. Combined brachytherapy and external beam radiotherapy in soft-tissue tumors. Endocurie/Hypertherm Oncol 1992;8:53–59.

25. Gemer LS, Trowbridge DR, Neff J, et al. Local recurrence of soft tissue sarcoma following brachytherapy. Int J Radiat Oncol Biol Phys 1991;20:587–592.

26. Schray MF, Gunderson LL, Sim FH, et al. Soft tissue sarcoma-integration of brachytherapy, resection and external irradiation. Cancer 1990;66:451–456.

27. O'Connor MI, Pritchard DJ, Gunderson LL. Integration of limb-sparing surgery, brachytherapy, and external beam irradiation in the treatment of soft tissue sarcoma. Clin Orthop 1993;289:73–80.

28. Donath D, Clark B, Pla C, et al. Post-operative adjuvant HDR brachytherapy in the treatment of poor prognosis soft tissue sarcoma. Abstract. Proc 16th Annual Mid-Winter Meeting of the American Endocuriether Soc, 1993, p. 28.

29. Alekhteyar KM, Porter AT, Ryan C, et al. Preliminary results of hyperfractionated high dose rate brachytherapy in soft tissue sarcoma. Abstract. Endocurie Hypertherm Oncol 1993;9:56.

30. Brennan MF, Casper ES, Harrison LB, et al. The role of multimodality therapy in soft-tissue sarcoma. Ann Surg 1991;214(3):328–336.

31. Harrison LB, Franzese F, Gaynor JJ, et al. Long-term results of a prospective randomized trial of adjuvant brachytherapy in the management of completely resected soft tissue sarcomas of the extremity and superficial trunk. Int J Radiat Oncol Biol Phys 1993;27(2):259–265.

32. Pisters PW, Harrison LB, Woodruff JM, et al. A prospective randomized trial of adjuvant brachytherapy in the management of low-grade soft tissue sarcomas of the extremity and superficial trunk. J Clin Oncol 1994;12(6):1150–1155.

33. Schupak KD, Lane JM, Weilepp AE, et al. The psychofunctional handicap associated with the use of brachytherapy in the treatment of lower extremity high grade soft tissue sarcomas. Abstract. Int J Radiat Oncol Biol Phys 1993;27(Suppl 1):293.

34. Karasek K, Constine LS, Rosier R. Sarcoma therapy: Functional outcome and relationship to treatment parameters. Int J Radiat Oncol Biol Phys 1992;24(4):651–656.

35. Robinson MH, Spuce L, Eeles R, et al. Limb function following conservative treatment of adult soft tissue sarcoma. Eur J Cancer 1991;27(12):1567–1574.

36. Zelefsky M, Harrison LB, Shiu M, et al. Combined surgical resection and iridium-192 implantation for locally advanced and recurrent desmoid tumors. Cancer 1991;67:380–384.

37. Habrand JL, Gerbaulet A, Pejovic MH, et al. Twenty years experience of interstitial brachytherapy in the management of soft tissue sarcomas. Int J Radiat Oncol Biol Phys 1991;20(3):405–411.

38. Nori D, Shupak K, Shiu MH, et al. Role of brachytherapy in recurrent extremity sarcoma in patients treated with prior surgery and irradiation. Int J Radiat Oncol Biol Phys 1991;20:1229–1233.

39. Robinson M, Barr L, Fisher C, et al. Treatment of extremity soft tissue sarcomas with surgery and radiotherapy. Radio Oncol 1990;18(3):221–233.

40. Essner R, Selch M, Eilber FR. Reirradiation for extremity soft tissue sarcomas: Local control

and complications. Proc Seventy-Second Ann Am Radium Soc Meeting. April 21–25, 1990, p. 21.

41. Habrand JL, Gerbaulet A, Durand S, et al. Twenty years experience of interstitial Iridium brachytherapy (IIB) in the management of soft tissue sarcomas (STS). Abstract. 17th International Congress of Radiology, Radiotherapy-Radiation Oncology Abstracts Book. Paris, France, July 1–8, 1989, p. 97.

42. Alekhteyar K, Leung DH, Brennan MF, et al. Is brachytherapy plus external beam radiotherapy better than brachytherapy alone in completely resected soft tissue sarcoma of the extremity with positive margins? Abstract. Int J Radiat Oncol Biol Phys 1994;30(Suppl 1):221.

43. Arbeit JM, Hilaris BS, Brennan MF. Wound complications in the multimodality treatment of extremity and superficial truncal sarcomas. J Clin Oncol 1987;5(3):480–488.

44. Bujko K, Suit HD, Springfield DS, et al. Wound healing after preoperative radiation for sarcoma of soft tissues. Surg Gyn Obst 1993; 176(2):124–134.

45. Ormsby MV, Hilaris BS, Nori D, et al. Wound complications of adjuvant radiation therapy in patients with soft tissue sarcomas. Ann Surg 1989;210(1):93–99.

46. Peat BG, Bell RS, Davis A, et al. Wound-healing complications after soft-tissue sarcoma surgery. Plas Recons Surg 1994;93(5):980–987.

47. Berkenstock K, Janjan NA, Hackbarth D, et al. Perioperative wound complications following brachytherapy alone or in combination with external beam irradiation in advanced soft-tissue sarcoma of the extremity. Endocurie/Hypertherm Oncol 1992;8:187–194.

48. Reece GP, Schusterman MA, Pollock RE, et al. Immediate versus delayed free-tissue transfer salvage of the lower extremity in soft-tissue sarcoma patients. Ann Surg Oncol 1993;1: 11–17.

49. Janjan NA, Yasko AW, Reece GP, et al. Comparison of charges related to radiotherapy for soft tissue sarcomas treated by preoperative external beam irradiation versus interstitial implantation. Ann Surg Oncol 1994;1(5): 415–422.

50. Alekhteyar KM, Porter AT, Ryan C, et al. Preliminary results of hyperfractionated high dose rate brachytherapy in soft tissue sarcoma. Abstract. Endocurie Hypertherm Oncol 1993;9: 56.

Brachytherapy for Pediatric Tumors

Subir Nag, M.D., Alain Gerbaulet, M.D.,
Eric Lartigau, M.D., Ph.D., James Fontanesi, M.D.

Introduction

External beam radiation therapy (EBRT) to the tumor, with generous margins and over a period of 5–6 weeks, is used to treat most pediatric tumors. This results in cosmetic deformity, altered dentition, altered organ function, and bone growth retardation,[1-3] especially in younger children. Multi-modality therapy including surgery, EBRT, and chemotherapy has improved survival in patients treated on the Intergroup Rhabdomyosarcoma Study.[4-6] However, decreased survival has been reported in infants with rhabadomyosarcoma (RMS). With increased survival achievable in the older children with multimodal therapy, it would be advisable to explore ways to reduce the dose to normal tissues and thereby preserve function (bone growth, sexual life, fertility, endocrine function) especially in younger children.

With brachytherapy, it is possible to deliver a high irradiation dose to a well defined tumor volume with a low dose to the normal surrounding tissues and thus to obtain a high tumor control with acceptable morbidity. These advantages of brachytherapy in comparison with EBRT are well known. Brachytherapy is routinely used in adults, but is less commonly used in children.[7-39] Typically, manually afterloaded low-dose-rate (LDR) brachytherapy has been used to obtain a high tumor control with an acceptable rate of complications.[7-27] However, the necessary close and frequent monitoring of these children provides a radiation exposure hazard to nursing staff and parents. This radiation hazard can be eliminated by the use of high-dose-rate (HDR) brachytherapy.[28-30] Doing this provides the additional advantages of eliminating the need for prolonged sedation or immobilizaton and allowing out-patient treatment.

Methods

It must be stressed that children are not small adults. Pediatric tumors are generally very sensitive to chemotherapy and radiotherapy and long-term toxicities (e.g., growth retardation) are of paramount importance. Hence, both the dose and the volume irradiated must be reduced so that growth function and organ preservation are maintained while obtaining a cure. Chemotherapy and organ preserving surgery are integral components of the treatment program. The patients are often initially treated with induction chemotherapy on an established protocol. Local control measures (surgery, brachytherapy)

From Nag S (ed): *Principles and Practice of Brachytherapy.* © Futura Publishing Co., Inc., Armonk, NY, 1997.

are then instituted, followed by maintenance chemotherapy. Mild chemotherapy (e.g., Vincristine) can be given during brachytherapy, while avoiding radiosensitizing chemotherapy such as Actinomycin-D and Adriamycin.

Surgery

Since organ preservation is a prime concern, enbloc resection of tumor (with a 2-cm margin of normal tissue wherever possible) or a debulking procedure is performed only if it can be done without causing significant cosmetic or functional deformity. Limited chest wall or rib resectons can be done; however, amputations and exenterations are avoided. A team approach is important; for a successful outcome, the extent of the surgery must be discussed by the surgeon, radiation oncologist, and the pediatric oncologist.

Brachytherapy Catheter Insertion

The brachytherapy techniques are modified from those used in adults. Preferably, the radiation oncologist should be present in the operating room at the time of tumor resection to observe the relationship of the tumor to the surrounding organs and to interact with the surgeon. Brachytherapy of the tumor (for grossly unresectable tumors) or tumor bed (for resected tumors with microscopic residual or questionable margins) can be performed at the time of original or second look surgery. If extensive surgical excision is performed, a delay of 3–7 days is often necessary for wound healing before start of brachytherapy.

Catheter Implant Techniques

A single plane implant is generallly used for resected tumor beds. A template, mesh, or applicator can be used to keep the catheters parallel. The peripheral (lateral) catheters should be placed just outside the target volume (area). The open ends should project 1–2 cm beyond the target volume to prevent dipping in of the isodose to ensure sufficient coverage. In our experience, most patients have been treated by a single plane implant to the tumor bed after gross resection. A double plane implant is performed for unresectable

tumors <2 cm thick. Larger tumors may require a volume (multiplane) implant. Catheters are usually implanted 1 cm apart throughout the tumor volume for these cases. For vaginal lesions with microscopic residual disease, a custom-made intracavitary vaginal cylinder or prosthesis with a central line source may be used. For gross residual disease in the vagina, an interstitial implant is preferable.

Mild sedation, arm or body immobilization restraints, papoose board, plaster cast, and the like may be used if the child cannot cooperate. However, general anesthesia can be avoided during the treatment time because slight movement of the patient is allowable. Gonadal shielding for boys is required whenever necessary and feasible.

Brachytherapy Volume

The late sequelae of brachytherapy depend not only on the dose given to the target volume, but more importantly on the volume irradiated (both within and outside of the target). Hence, the volumes implanted are generally smaller than those in adults. For example, in adult soft tissue sarcomas, the entire muscle compartment is implanted (from the origin to the insertion of the muscle group); however, in children, only the area at high risk for recurrence (usually the postchemotherapy residual volume with a variable margin) is implanted. The volume to be implanted is controversial and varies among institutions. The margin can be generous if there are no radiosensitive surrounding normal tissues, but the margins must be smaller if adjacent to critical normal tissues (e.g., bone growth plates).

Brachytherapy Dose and Dose Rates

The type of brachytherapy used depends on the patient's age, institutional preference, expertise, and availability of equipment. The doses used differ depending on the type of brachytherapy, the amount of residual tumor volume, the intended use of the brachytherapy—whether it is to be the sole treatment or a boost to EBRT. Manually afterloaded LDR doses of 45–50 Gy are commonly used as exclusive treatment; 15–25 Gy doses are used as boost doses. Dose rates of 0.4–0.6 Gy/hr (over 4–6 days) are preferable. However, higher dose rates (up to 1 Gy/hr) have been used to reduce the duration of radiation precaution that must be observed in these children who often require close attention. Iridium-192 is used for interstitial techniques, and cesium-137 for intracavitary techniques. Iodine-125 has been used to reduce the radiation exposure; LDR, HDR, or pulse-dose-rate (PDR) can eliminate these radiation hazards.

For HDR brachytherapy, it is very important that the dose be well fractionated to reduce late sequelae. The most common experience has been with 36 Gy total dose given in 12 fractions (3 Gy per fraction BID) over 6–8 days. The addition of HDR allows the use of optimized treatment plan, if required.

The dose is generally prescribed at 0.5-cm depth for resected tumor beds and at the periphery of the target volume for gross tumor. For intracavitary cylinders, the dose can be specified at various depths (2–5 mm, depending on the child's age and the diameter of the cylinder) to limit the vaginal surface dose to acceptable levels.

EBRT is generallly avoided if growth is a paramount consideration. EBRT (~40–50 Gy) can be added to treat extensive disease in older children. In these cases, brachytherapy can be used in limited doses as a boost (e.g., 15–25 Gy by LDR or 10–15 Gy by intropera-tive HDR techniques).

The details of brachytherapy doses used at various institutions are discussed in the specific sections on those institutions.

Institut Gustave-Roussy Experience

Patients

From 1972–1990, interstitial and intracavitary LDR brachytherapy have been carried out at the Institut Gustave-Roussy (IGR) in 127 young patients (excluding retinoblastomas). The tumor sites are shown in Table 1, and the pathological distribution in Table 2. The vast majority of the tumors treated were localized and not metastatic. In the head and neck area, regional clinical pathological nodes were diagnosed at the time of primary treatment in 21% of cases.

Table 1.
Tumor Sites

Pelvis:		57%
Cervix-vagina-vulva	76%	
Bladder-prostate	20%	
Anus-rectum	4%	
Head & neck		33%
Soft tissues		10%

Treatment Modalities

The primary aim was to achieve a cure with conservative treatment. For pelvic cancers, radical surgery like prostatectomy, cystectomy, hysterectomy, or pelvic exenteration was sometimes performed as a first line treatment; however, the challenge was to find a way of preserving function (sexual, hormonal, fertility) of the cured child.[9,10,13–16] For all histologic types except clear cell adenocarcinoma (CCA), the treatment was a combination of chemotherapy, surgery, brachytherapy, and in some cases, EBRT. For CCA, the treatment combined conservative surgery and brachytherapy with EBRT in some cases.

For all tumors, the type of surgery varied depending on the tumor location. This included tumor resection, lymphadenectomy, ovarian transposition, or additional intraoperative brachytherapy. Surgery also played a major role in the treatment of local failures.

Chemotherapy was used to reduce tumor volume in localized cases to facilitate surgery and/or brachytherapy and to prevent distant metastases. An average of six courses of chemotherapy (except in cases of the nonchemosensitive CCA) was generally used before surgery or radiation. Prior to 1984, VAC (Vincristine, Actinomycin D, and Cyclophosphamide) and VAD (Vincristine and Adriamycin) protocols were used to treat mesenchymal tumors. Then Ifosfamide was used in the place

Table 2.
Pathological Distribution

Rhabdosarcoma	53%
Clear cell adenocarcinoma	27%
Undifferentiated sarcoma	6%
Yolk sac tumor	6%
Others	14%

of Cyclophosphamide (IVA protocol).[9,10,14] In germ cell tumors (including Yolk sac), the MAC regimen (Methotrexate, Actinomycin D, Cyclophosphamide) was replaced at the same period by new active combinations with Cisplatinum, Vinblastine, and Bleomycin. For patients with a high metastatic risk, this chemotherapy was continued after the brachytherapy for a mean time of 1 year.

EBRT was not routinely prescribed in this combined treatment for childhood malignancies, as the irradiation of choice was represented by brachytherapy. In this series, brachytherapy alone was used in 90% of the cases, and combined brachytherapy-EBRT in 10% of the cases. The indications for adding EBRT were essentially bulky and extensive disease (for CCA) and/or nodal involvement.

LDR brachytherapy was more commonly used as the first line treatment (74%), rather than for recurrence as a salvage treatment (26%). The brachytherapy techniques used included plastic tubes, guide gutters, silk wires, hypodermic needles, and customized intracavitary mold applicators that were adapted from the corresponding techniques used in adults. Iridium-192 was used in the vast majority of the cases. Cesium-137 was reserved for some gynecological applications. The brachytherapy dose was between 45–65 Gy if given by brachytherapy only and 15–25 Gy if used as a boost to EBRT. Brachytherapy was performed using LDR (0.4–0.6 Gy/hr), and the total dose was delivered in one to three courses for gynecological tumors, and in one course for the other tumor sites. The computerized dosimetry was calculated according to the Paris system for interstitial brachytherapy and according to the International Commision of Radiological Units and Measurements (ICRU) recommendations for intracavitary brachytherapy.

Soft Tissue Sarcomas: Trunk and Limbs

Brachytherapy was mainly used as a salvage treatment in 10 of 13 patients with a sarcoma of the trunk or extremities. The disease-free survival (DFS) was 46% with a 61% local control rate and a 23% complication rate. An example of a plastic tube implant is shown in Figure 1.

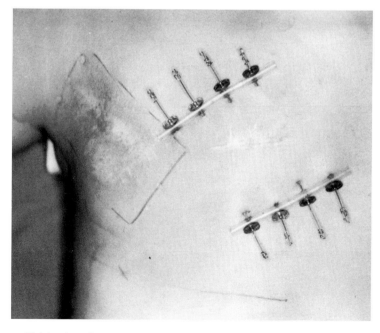

Figure 1. Interstitial implant for a recurrence of a rhabdomyosarcomas of the trunk. Plastic tube technique.

Table 3.
Results of Brachytherapy in Head and Neck Sarcomas

	Primary	Salvage
Number of patients	25	14
Mean dose (Gy)	69 Gy	57 Gy
Disease-free survival	76%	50%
5-year local control	84%	64%

Head and Neck Sarcomas

Thirty-nine patients (20 girls and 19 boys) were treated (Table 3). The mean age was 5.1 years. Tumor sites included the nasolabial sulcus (12) cases, the oral cavity (8), the neck (8), ear (4), lip (3), eye (2), and nasopharynx (2). The most common histology was rhabdomyosarcoma (27 cases). The results of treatment are summarized in Table 3. The complication rate was 23%; of these, 21% were considered moderate, 61% mild, and 18% severe.

Pelvic Tumors

These tumors were divided into gynecological tumors (76%), and bladder and prostate tumors (20%). Thirty cases of lower gynecological tract tumors (excluding CCA) were treated with brachytherapy, including:

1. Rhabdomyosarcoma of the vagina (17 patients): the site of origin was the vagina with spreading to the vulva in two cases, and to the cervix in one case. The FIGO stages were stage I in two cases, stage II in four, stage III in five, stage IV in one, and finally, five patients were treated for tumor recurrences (Table 4). The mean age was 24 months (8–43 months).

Table 4.
Gynecological Tumors: FIGO Staging

	I	II	III	IV	R
Rhabdomyosarcoma	2	4	5	1	5
Yolk sac tumors	2	1	3	1/M	1/M
Vulva	1	2	2	1	1
Clear cell adenocarcinoma	5	12	5	5	1/M

R = recurrences.

2. Endodermal sinus tumor of the vagina (6 patients): the site of origin was always the vagina with an extension to uterine cervix in two cases. The FIGO classification showed two tumors stage I, one tumor stage II, and three tumors stage III (Table 4). The mean age was 12 months (5–20 months).
3. Sarcoma of the vulva: seven tumors with one tumor stage I, two tumors stage II, two tumors stage III, one tumor stage IV, and one recurrence. The mean age was 7 years (8–13 years).

Twenty-seven patients with vaginal CCA were treated at IGR (Table 5). Diethylstilbestrol (DES) exposure during pregnancy was firmly documented in 16 cases (59%). The tumor was associated with local vaginal malformations in >40% of the cases. The first line surgery was an explorative laparotomy with pelvic lymphadenopathy and ovarian transposition. Ten of 17 having surgery before brachytherapy showed a nodal involvement at the time of lymphadenectomy (1 N+/8 tumors stage I or II proximal; 4 N+/14 tumors stage II distal or III, and 5 stage IVB). All patients had postsurgical intracavitary brachytherapy (Figures 2 and 3). Brachytherapy was delivered in one session in nine cases, two sessions in 14 cases, and three sessions in four cases. The intracavitary application covered the vagina only in three cases and the vagina plus the cervix in 24 cases. EBRT was used to treat bulky tumors, nodal involvement, or stage III and IV tumors. In this group, the survival varied greatly with T and N stage: survival at 5 years was 95% for N-tumors and 40% for N+ tumors. Twenty-two patients were alive, with 22 vaginal preservations, 20 uterine preservations, and 19 ovarian preservations: a 68% rate of complete conservation organ function. One of the treated women was able to conceive and gave birth to a child 6 years after her brachytherapy treatment.

Results of treatment of bladder and prostate tumors are summarized in Table 5.

Overall Results

The overall DFS for the whole population was 75% at 5 years (Table 6). The local control at 5 years was dependent on the type of

Table 5.
Results of Brachytherapy of Pelvic Tumors

	Bladder & Prostate Tumors	Vaginal Clear Cell Adenocarcinoma	
Number of patients	15	27	
FIGO stage	NS	IB	5
		II	12
		III	5
		IVB	5
Tumor site:	—		
Vagina alone		25%	
Cervix alone		21%	
Vagina + cervix		54%	
Disease-free survival	75%	78%	
5-year local control	60%	88%	
Complication rate	20%	Early	Late
Grade 1		37%	28%
Grade 2 or 3		11%	35%

brachytherapy with 81% for primary treatment versus 57% for salvage treatment. Two factors were associated with a higher local failure rate: brachytherapy used as a salvage procedure (43% vs 13%), and the site of the treated disease (limb and trunk 69%, ENT 26%, pelvis 12%). However, it must be said that the distribution of the treatment methods was not the same in all the tumor locations: brachytherapy was used as a salvage treatment in 10 of 13 extremity and truncal soft tissue sarcomas, but was used as a first

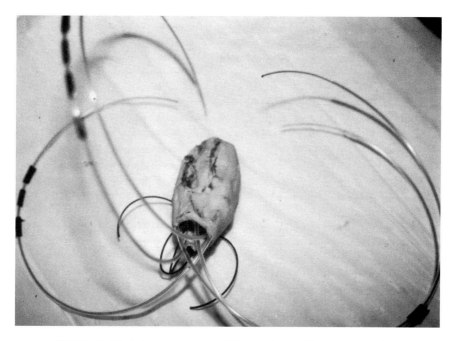

Figure 2. Rhabdomyosarcoma of the vagina: alginate impression.

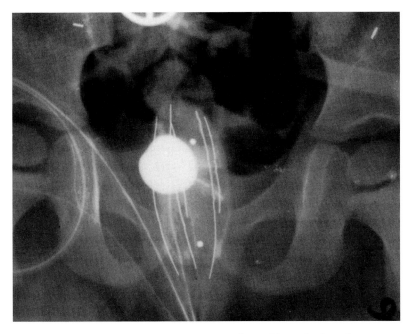

Figure 3. Control film for the same patient with vaginal applicator.

line treatment in 12 of 15 bladder-prostate tumors.

The overall complication rate was 22%. The rate of complication was higher in the early cases treated with a combination of surgery-chemotherapy and brachytherapy. This was mainly due to the large volume treated by the implant at a high dose (>70 Gy) after extensive surgery and local partial response obtained with first generation chemotherapy.[9] These late complications are now partially avoided with modern brachytherapy techniques (plastic tubes, iridium-192, computerized dosimetry, tumor imaging), and of course, with the increase in local tumor response achieved by modern chemotherapy.

In the IGR experience, brachytherapy, if feasible, is the modality of choice when radiotherapy is needed for the local control of pediatric malignancies. When used as a first line treatment, it increases local control, compared to that seen with EBRT, and decreases the probability of late complications.

St. Jude Experience

In the St. Jude Hospital experience using LDR either as a boost to external beam or as

Table 6.
Treatment Results

	Disease-Free Survival	Local Control
Soft tissue sarcomas	46%	61%
Gynecological tumors	83%	90%
Clear cell adenocarcinoma	78%	88%
Bladder-prostate sarcomas	73%	60%
Head & neck sarcomas	76% (first line)	84%
	50% (salvage)	64%

the sole radiotherapy modality in 18 pediatric patients, at a median follow-up of 44 weeks (range 6–432 weeks), local control in the implanted volume was maintained in 14 of the 18 patients.[11] Two of nine patients (in which brachytherapy was utilized as the sole radiation modality) required surgical treatment of soft tissue necrosis. Both of these patients were treated with Cs-137 vaginal molds, and the doses delivered were 47 Gy and 50 Gy, respectively. They remained with no evidence of disease (NED) at 42 and 45 months with only minimal residual complications.

In a recent update of the St. Jude experience, the results of local control, complications, and survival were presented on 46 children who received 50 brachytherapy applications in non-central nervous system sites.[12] Eleven sites received the entirety of their irradiation with brachytherapy, 16 sites received EBRT that was supplemented by a brachytherapy boost. The remaining 23 sites received treatment for recurrent disease or second malignant tumor that presented in previously irradiated sites or for metastatic disease. Local control was maintained in the implanted volume in 43 of 50 sites during follow-up ranging from 2–115 months (median = 41 months). The local failures all occurred by 20-months postimplant. Two patients were salvaged with surgical intervention. Complications were noted in 12 patients of which two were life-threatening.

Other Low-Dose-Rate Experiences

Curran et al.[8] reported that seven of eight children who received interstitial radiation during initial therapy for soft-tissue sarcomas at the University of Pennsylvania/Fox Chase Cancer Center demonstrated local control. Six of these children remained NED at a median follow-up of 5.8 years, but only one of the four patients treated for recurrent disease was alive. All of the patients developed self-limiting acute reactions, usually mucositis, but none required greater than a 2-week delay in the chemotherapy schedule. Functional and cosmetic effects from interstitial radiation were minimal at a median follow-up period of 6.5 years (range 2–16 years). Cherlow et al.[7] treated 11 pediatric patients with 40 Gy

iridium-192 brachytherapy. Eight patients have no evidence of disease at 11–62 months (median 38 months).

In an effort to reduce radiation exposure to the medical staff and parents, iodine-125, a low energy radionuclide, has been used.[20,27,36] Nechuskin et al.[23] have used LDR remote afterloading techniques of 30–35 Gy at 0.6–1.3 Gy/hr over 20–25 hours in four children to eliminate radiation exposure to the parents. However, it still required sedation or prolonged immobilization of small children.

There are several reports that detail the use of interstitial irradiation for the treatment of both primary and recurrent central nervous system (CNS) tumors.[31–36] The St. Jude Hospital experience was with 60 Gy brachytherapy in 6 days followed by 60–70 Gy EBRT (in selected cases, chemotherapy was also used). Nine of eleven newly diagnosed tumors demonstrate local control in follow-up of 15–48 months (median = 27 months).[31] However, radiation necrosis was noted in seven patients 1–17 months (median = 10 months) posttherapy. Gutin et al.[32] reported similar results in nine children (six primary, and three recurrent cases).[32] These series predominently used removable implantation for high grade lesions. There is little experience in the United States on the use of permanent brachytherapy. Experience with permanent brachytherapy from Europe documents 5-year local control rates similar to that reported for EBRT.[33–35] It still remains to be determined if the use of brachytherapy in the treatment of CNS tumors will increase local control and survival, although initial reports are promising.

The Ohio State University High-Dose-Rate Brachytherapy Experience

Thirteen young children with diverse sarcomas were treated with HDR brachytherapy between January 1990 and August 1993. The children ranged in age from 1–112 months (median = 19 months). Seven patients had rhabdomyosarcoma, and six had other histologies. Chemotherapy according to the Intergroup Rhabdomyosarcoma Study was used, except in the case of a Ewing's sarcoma of bone. In new cases, after initial cytoreduction with multiagent chemotherapy and function preserving surgery, HDR brachytherapy was given at a median of 3.5 months after diagnosis. The sites treated included the head and neck (3), pelvis (6), trunk (3), and extremity (1).

Fractionated High-Dose-Rate Brachytherapy Technique

Eleven patients were treated with brachytherapy alone. EBRT was avoided in these patients since a prime objective was preservation of organ and bone growth. The brachytherapy techniques used were similar to those used in adults. The plastic catheter loop techniques could not be used since the HDR source cannot negotiate sharp curves. Five patients had interstitial implantation of catheters in the operating room at the time of surgery. These catheters were left in the patient until the treatments were completed. The

other two patients were treated by a custom made intravaginal cylinder that was inserted into the vagina for each treatment. The post-chemotherapy residual tumor volume was implanted rather than the original tumor volume. The minimum peripheral dose was 36 Gy in 12 treatments (3 Gy each treatment given twice a day, 6 hours apart) over 8 elapsed days. Using the linear-quadratic (L-Q) model, the extrapolated response dose (ERD) was calculated to be equivalent to 50 Gy of continuous LDR given over 5 days. Each treatment lasted 2–5 minutes and was given on an out-patient basis. Since slight movement of the patient during treatment was allowable, the brachytherapy was given using either mild sedation or temporary body restraint (e.g., papoose board, arm splint) (Figure 4).

Intraoperative High-Dose-Rate Brachytherapy

Two patients (who were older) were treated with intraoperative HDR (IOHDR)

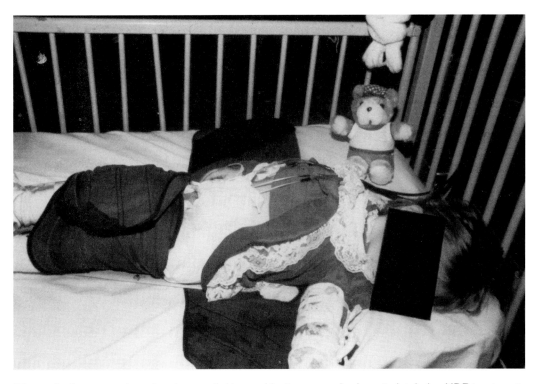

Figure 4. A papoose board and arm splint is used for temporary body restraint during HDR treatment.

brachytherapy. These patients had surgery in a shielded operating room, allowing delivery of HDR brachytherapy during the surgical procedure.[40] After resection, normal tissues were mobilized and retracted or shielded with lead to reduce radiation dose to radiosensitive tissues. HDR catheters placed within special intraoperative applicators were inserted on the tumor bed (Figure 5). The patients received 10–12.5 Gy intraoperatively in about 15 minutes. The catheters and applicators were then removed. Since the IOHDR was given as a single fraction, EBRT of 27 Gy was added about 4 weeks later.

Results

Grade 1 morbidity relating to HDR brachytherapy occurred in 46%, grade 2 in 15%, and grade 3 in 8% of the children. Of the 11 pa-

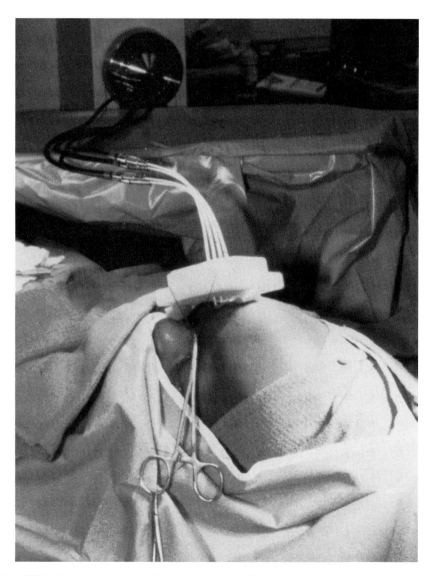

Figure 5. HDR catheters are placed in a template applicator and inserted on the tumor bed after resection of tumor to deliver HDR brachytherapy intraoperatively to superior orbit.

tients treated in first remission, there have been no recurrences. Nine patients have completed therapy. Disease-free follow-up ranges from 4–38 months (median = 32 months). Two patients with recurrent sarcoma were also treated. The patient with a recurrent rhabdomyosarcoma of the vagina had recurrence outside the HDR brachytherapy field. One patient treated for a local soft-tissue recurrence of Ewing's sarcoma of bone relapsed with pulmonary metastases and a local bone recurrence adjacent to the previously treated soft-tissue recurrence. The combination of conservative surgery, chemotherapy, and HDR brachytherapy offered the potential for good control of gross and microscopic residual disease in young children while preserving bone growth and organ function with acceptable morbidity. Further follow-up will be required to evaluate the long-term effect of this local control strategy.

Other High-Dose-Rate and Pulsed-Dose-Rate Brachytherapy Experience

Two other groups have reported their experience with HDR brachytherapy. Potter et al.[37] reported the combined experience of centers in Munster, Kiel, and Vienna with HDR and pulsed-dose-rate (PDR) brachytherapy in 18 children with soft tissue sarcoma (n = 12) and Ewing's sarcoma (n = 6). Of the 12 children with soft tissue sarcoma, seven received fractionated HDR brachytherapy of 15–43 Gy in 3–14 fractions; the other five were treated with PDR dose of 13–36 Gy in 12–45 fractions over 4–6 days. EBRT of 18–50 Gy in 9–25 fractions was used to supplement the brachytherapy dose in seven patients. In the six patients with Ewing's sarcoma, 10–12 Gy of IOHDR brachytherapy was used to boost 50–55 Gy of preoperative EBRT. The results were well tolerated except for transient acute morbidity in three patients.

The group at Memorial Sloan Kettering Cancer Center in New York have reported on IOHDR brachytherapy in eight patients with various pediatric tumors at various sites.[38] After gross resection, 12 Gy at 0.5–1.0 cm was delivered to the tumor bed. Supplemental EBRT was used in three patients. With this small number of patients, different diagnoses, inconsistent application of supplemental EBRT, and short follow-up, it is not possible to reach any conclusions about the efficacy of this approach.

Discussion

The standard treatment after surgery and chemotherapy in pediatric RMS is EBRT to the tumor with a generous (5 cm) margin for local control. This requires treatment over a 5- to 6-week period, the use of repeated deep sedation, and leads to unacceptable morbidity (especially organ and bone-growth retardation) in infants and younger children.[1-3]

Limited volume irradiation over a short duration (a few days) by brachytherapy may be sufficient therapy for children treated with aggressive chemotherapy, as shown by the use of LDR.[7-27] This allows high doses of radiation to be limited accurately to the tumor bed only while sparing the surrounding normal tissues, thus minimizing the late sequelae. Manually afterloaded removable iridium-192 has been the most commonly applied isotope, but iodine-125, gold-198, cesium-137, and californium-252 have also been used with good results.[7-27]

The major disadvantages of the LDR technique are that younger children must be sedated and immobilized during the entire period to prevent accidental removal of the implants. Radiation exposure to the medical personnel and the parents is another concern, although exposure can be reduced by placing a mobile lead shield at the bedside. The psychological effect of separating parents from their child can be significant and must be considered. The use of a low energy radionuclide like iodine-125, LDR remote brachytherapy, or PDR may reduce hazards of radiation exposure, but prolonged sedation and immobilization are still required.[20,23,27]

The use of HDR eliminates radiation exposure to the medical staff and the patients' families, and allows constant nursing care and interaction between the parents, nursing personnel, and the children. Each treatment takes only a few minutes and the treatment course can be completed in 1 week without requiring prolonged sedation or immobilization. The disadvantage is that the patient must be treated twice a day for 12 treatments versus a single treatment over 4–8 days for LDR brachytherapy. The patients treated with IOHDR brachytherapy have the advantage of a single treatment delivered over a few minutes, but usually they require additional EBRT.

The use of HDR can solve a logistic problem that may be present at some institutions. Cancer hospitals have brachytherapy facilities, but some are not equipped for prolonged pediatric care. Hence, LDR brachytherapy cannot be performed in young children at these cancer hospitals. Children's hospitals (which can be located several miles away) have surgical and in-patient facilities for young children, but may not have radioactive licensing or brachytherapy facilities. Hence, surgical catheter insertion and in-patient care (if required) are performed at the children's hospital, and the HDR treatments are performed on an out-patient basis at the cancer hospital.

The use of EBRT in large volume fields can be myelosuppressive and thus limit subsequent administration of systemic multiagent chemotherapy. Brachytherapy does not impede the later use of maintenance chemotherapy using alkylating agents. However, anthracycline-containing chemotherapy can cause an increase in the radiation reaction in some children treated by brachytherapy.[29,30,36] Therefore, it is recommended that anthracycline-containing chemotherapy be eliminated from the immediate postbrachytherapy maintenance chemotherapy regimen of these patients. A similar recommendation might be applicable to other radiosensitizing agents like Actinomycin D.

The selection of a patient for brachytherapy requires evaluation by a multidisciplinary team consisting of a pediatric surgeon, pediatric oncologist, and brachytherapist. The brachytherapist should preferably be present at the initial resective surgery for optimal placement of the brachytherapy catheters into the tumor bed. This could be done at a subsequent surgery, but the result might be suboptimal. The initial strategy for tumors that are unresectable by virtue of site or size is to achieve cyto-reduction with active multiagent chemotherapy. The second phase of this standard approach is to utilize an effective local control strategy, such as surgery and/or radiotherapy, when the tumor has the least number of viable cells. Patients with extensive residual tumor are not suitable candidates since marginal recurrence may result if small volumes are implanted or treatment-related sequelae may result if large volumes are implanted. An ideal candidate for brachytherapy would be a child with a soft tissue sarcoma in whom organ preservation and function is a priority and in whom the tumor can be reduced by a surgical procedure to microscopic residual. The experiences presented here demonstrate that organ-preserving surgery at selected sites in combination with brachytherapy can be accomplished without fear of jeopardizing local control. In this regard, brachytherapy has been used as an extension of the surgeon's scalpel without removing critical tissues.

Conclusions

The use of brachytherapy, if feasible, is the modality of choice when radiotherapy is needed for the local control of pediatric malignancies. When used as a first line treatment, it increases local control with a decrease in the probability of late complications (especially bone and organ growth) in comparison with EBRT. LDR with removable iridium-192 brachytherapy is more commonly used. Low energy radionuclides and remote afterloading technology has been used to reduce the radiation exposure hazards. The use of HDR, IOHDR, and PDR has extended treatment to infants and younger children, but their long-term effects need to be studied.

References

1. Fromm M, Littman P, Raney RB, et al. Late effects after treatment of twenty children with soft-tissue sarcomas of the head and neck. Cancer 1986;57:2070–2076.
2. Jaffe N, Toth BB, Hoan RE, et al. Dental and maxillofacial abnormalities in long-term survivors of childhood cancer: Effects of treatment with chemotherapy and radiation to the head and neck. Pediatrics 1984;73:816–823.
3. Pais RC, Ragab AH. Rhabdomyosarcomas in infancy. In: Maurer HM, Ruymann FB, Pochedly C (eds). Rhabdomyosarcoma and Related

Tumors in Children and Adolescents. CRC Press, Boca Raton, 1991, pp. 373–384.

4. Maurer HM, Beltangady M, Gehan EA, et al. Intergroup Rhabdomyosarcoma Study-I: A Final Report. Cancer 1988;61:209–220.

5. Maurer HM, Gehan E, Beltangady M, et al. The Intergroup Rhabdomyosarcoma Study-II. Cancer 1993;71:1904–1992.

6. Ragab A, Gehan E, Maurer H, et al. For the IRS Committee of CCSG, POG, & UKCCSG: Intergroup Rhabdomyosarcoma Study (IRS) III: Preliminary Report of the Major Results. Proc Am Soc Clin Oncol, San Diego, California, 1992, Volume 11, p. 1251.

7. Cherlow JM, Nisar Syed AM, Puthawala A, et al. Endocurietherapy in pediatric oncology. Am J Pediatr Hematol Oncol 1990;2:155–159.

8. Curran WJ, Littman P, Raney RB. Interstitial radiation therapy in the treatment of childhood soft-tissue sarcomas. Int J Radiat Oncol Biol Phys 1988;14:169–174.

9. Flamant F, Gerbaulet A, Nihoul-Fekete C, et al. Long-term sequelae of conservative treatment by surgery brachytherapy and chemotherapy for vulval and vaginal rhabdomyosarcoma in children. J Clin Oncol 1990;8:1847–1853.

10. Flamant F, Chassagne D, Cosset JM, et al. Embryonal rhabdomyosarcoma of the vagina in the children. Eur J Cancer 1979;15:527–532.

11. Fontanesi J, Kun L, Pao W, et al. Brachytherapy as primary or 'boost' irradiation in 18 children with solid tumors. Endocurie/Hypertherm Oncol 1991;7:195–200.

12. Fontanesi J, Rao BN, Fleming ID, et al. Pediatric brachytherapy. Cancer 1994;74:733–739.

13. Gerbaulet A. Pediatric neoplasms. In: Pierquin B, Wilson JF, Chassagne D (eds). Modern Brachytherapy. Masson Publishing USA, Inc, New York, 1987, pp. 315–316.

14. Gerbaulet AP, Esche BA, Haie CM, et al. Conservative treatment for lower gynecological tract malignancies in children and adolescents: The Institut Gustave-Roussy Experience. Int J Radiat Oncol Biol Phys 1989;16:655–658.

15. Gerbaulet A, Panis X, Flamant F, et al. Iridium afterloading curietherapy in the treatment of pediatric malignancies. Cancer 1985;56:1274–1279.

16. Gerbaulet A, Habrand JL, Haie C, et al. The role of brachytherapy in the conservative treatment of pediatric malignancies: Experience of the Institut Gustave-Roussy. Activity, Selec Brachyther J 1991;5:85–90.

17. Goffinet DR, Martinez A, Pooles D, et al. Pediatric brachytherapy. In: George FW III (ed). Modern Interstitial and Intracavitary Radiation Cancer Management. Masson Publishing USA, Inc, New York, 1981, pp. 57–70.

18. Hilaris BS, Nori D, Anderson LL. Brachytherapy in pediatric oncology. In: An Atlas of Brachytherapy. MacMillan Publishing Co, New York, 1988, pp. 294–302.

19. Knight PH, Doornbos JF, Rosen D, et al. The use of interstitial radiation therapy in the treatment of persistent, localized, and unresectable cancer in children. Cancer 1986;57:951–954.

20. Marquez CM, Larson DA, Roberts LW, et al. Iodine-125 implant of a rhabdomyosarcoma of the prostate in a 20-month-old boy. Endocurie/Hypertherm Oncol 1992;8:49–52.

21. Martinez A, Goffinet DR, Donaldson SS, et al. The use of interstitial therapy in pediatric malignancies. Front Radiat Ther Onc 1978;12:91–100.

22. Nag S, Rao B. Interstitial radiation implantation of pediatric solid tumors: Preliminary results. Abstract. Endocurie/Hypertherm Oncol 1985;1:138.

23. Nechuskin M, Androsov N, Durnov L, et al. Initial experience in the USSR in the treatment of paediatric cancers using the microSelectron-LDR. Selec Brachyther J 1990;4:78–79.

24. Novaes PE. Interstitial therapy in the management of soft tissue sarcomas in childhood. Med Ped Oncol 1985;13:221–224.

25. Pierquin B, Chassagne DJ, Chahbazian CM, et al. Embryonal sarcomas in children. In: Brachytherapy. Warren Green, St. Louis, 1978, pp. 207–208.

26. Plowman PN, Doughty D, Harnett AN. The role of brachytherapy in the multidisciplinary therapy of localized cancers. Br J Radiol 1989;62:218–222.

27. Zelefsky MJ, LaQuaglia MP, Harrison LB. Combination surgery and brachytherapy for pediatric soft tissue sarcomas. Endocurie Hypertherm Oncol 1993;9(1):50.

28. Nag S, Ruymann F, Su CM, et al. The use of high dose rate remote brachytherapy in paediatric tumors. Activity Selec Brachyther J 1990;4:22–23.

29. Nag S, Grecula JC, Ruymann F. Aggressive chemotherapy, organ-preserving surgery and high dose rate remote brachytherapy for the treatment of rhabdomyosarcoma in infants and young children. Cancer 1993;72:2769–2776.

30. Nag S, Olson T, Ruymann F, et al. High-dose rate (HDR) brachytherapy in childhood sarcomas: A local control strategy preserving bone growth and organ function. Med Pediat Oncol 1995;25:463–469.

31. Fontanesi J. Pediatric brachytherapy. Presented at the 16th Meeting of the American Endocurietherapy Society, Scottsdale, AZ, December 8–11, 1993.

32. Gutin PH, Edwards MSB, Wara WM, et al. Inter-

stitial brachytherapy for newly diagnosed patients with malignant gliomas: The UCSF experience. Int J Radiat Oncol Biol Phys 1992;24:593–597.

33. Etou A, Mundinger F, Mohadjer M, et al. Stereotactic interstitial irradiation of diencephalic tumors with iridium 192 and iodine 125: 10 years follow-up and comparison with other treatments. Childs Nerv Syst 1989;5:140–143.

34. Voges J, Sturm V, Berthold F, et al. Interstitial irradiation of cerebral gliomas in childhood by permanently implanted 125-iodine—preliminary results. Klin Padiatr 1990;202:270–274.

35. Thomson ES, Afshar F, Plowman PN. Paediatric brachytherapy. II. Brain implantation. Br J Radiol 1989;62:223–229.

36. Healey EA, Shamberger RC, Grier HE, et al. A 10-year experience of pediatric brachytherapy. Int J Radiat Oncol Biol Phys 1995;32:451–455.

37. Pötter R, Knocke TH, Kovacs G, et al. Brachytherapy in the combined modality treatment of pediatric malignancies. Principles and prelimi-

nary experience with treatment of soft tissue sarcoma (recurrence) and Ewing's sarcoma. Klin Pädiatr 1995;207:164–173.

38. Zelefsky MJ, LaQuaglia MP, Harrison LB. High dose rate intraoperative bachytherapy for pediatric tumors: Preliminary results of a prospective phase I/II study. Abstract. Proc 17th Am Brachyther Soc Meeting, Ft. Myers, FL, December 7–10, 1994, p. 22.

39. Rübe C, Hillmann A, Schmilowski GM, et al. Combination of preoperative external beam radiochemotherapy & intraoperative brachytherapy for children with Ewing's sarcoma. In: Bruggmoser G, Mould RF (eds). Brachytherapy Review: Proceedings of the German Brachytherapy Conference, Freiburg, November 1994. Albert-Ludwigs-University, Freiburg, FRG, Chapter 39.

40. Nag S, Orton C. Development of intraoperative high dose rate brachytherapy for treatment of resected tumor beds in anesthetized patients. Endocurie/Hypertherm Oncol 1993;9:187–193.

PART III

Special Topics

Chapter 32

Nursing Management of the Brachytherapy Patient

Debra Brown, R.N., B.S.N., O.C.N.,
Subir Nag, M.D., Lynda Petty, R.N.

Introduction

Brachytherapy refers to the treatment of tumors with radioactive sources (radionuclides) placed inside or close to tumors allowing the delivery of a large radiation dose to the tumor while sparing the surrounding normal tissues from the harmful effects of a high radiation dose. Unlike teletherapy where irradiation is delivered to the tumor from a distance outside the body, brachytherapy usually requires a surgical procedure for the insertion of the radionuclides. Hence, brachytherapy is very labor intensive and procedure oriented requiring specialized personnel and training for the needed intensive nursing care. Unfortunately, little information on the role of nursing in the brachytherapy patient has been published. This chapter will discuss the role of nurses in brachytherapy and the care of the brachytherapy patients.

Brachytherapy Treatment Modalities

Brachytherapy can be delivered using a variety of techniques with permanent or removable radioactive sources and inserting these sources either manually or by remote control. These procedures fall into three general cate-gories classified according to the process of placing the radioactive source: interstitial, intracavitary, and intraoperative. The choice of treatment method depends on the individual tumor type, stage of the disease, and location of the tumor.

Permanent Interstitial Brachytherapy

In permanent interstitial brachytherapy, encapsulated radioactive seeds are placed directly into the tumor and left there permanently; ultimately, the radioactivity decays completely (usually over a few weeks to months). Permanent interstitial brachytherapy may be performed after resection of as much tumor as can possibly and safely be removed (debulking), or when resection of the tumor is not the best option for the patient. Low energy radionuclides such as iodine-125 and palladium-103 are commonly used in permanent brachytherapy. The seeds are placed by the radiation oncologist using a mechanical needle applicator (e.g., Mick Applicator, Mick Radio-Nuclear Instruments, Inc., Bronx, NY, USA). The radiation oncologist consults with the surgeon in the operating room, assesses the tumor mass, and then determines the best treatment modality. The radiation oncology team (comprised of the brachythera-

From Nag S (ed): *Principles and Practice of Brachytherapy.* © Futura Publishing Co., Inc., Armonk, NY, 1997.

pist, physicist, and radiation technologist) then calculates the amount of radionuclide required and prepares for the intervention. Instrumentation and radioactive seeds are steam sterilized while the radiation oncologist performs a surgical hand scrub and is gowned and gloved in order to join the surgical team.

Removable Interstitial Brachytherapy

In removable interstitial brachytherapy, radionuclides are placed into catheters or applicators that have been inserted into the tumor. These procedures are generally performed in the operating room under general or spinal anesthesia. The brachytherapist is called to the operating room before tumor removal to visually ascertain the relationship of the tumor to the surrounding tissues and plan for placement of the implant. First, hollow needles or afterloading catheters are inserted into the tumor or tumor bed; the ends of these catheters extend outside the body cavity. The radioactive material (usually iridium-192 or cesium-137) is later inserted into the catheters or needles and left in place for the length of time necessary to deliver the radiation dose (typically a few days). The radioactive material and catheters are removed once the desired radiation dose has been delivered.

Remote Controlled High-Dose-Rate Brachytherapy

A major concern with most brachytherapy procedures has been the radiation exposure hazard to the medical caregivers. Remote controlled brachytherapy was introduced to eliminate radiation hazards. First, hollow afterloading applicators (or needles or catheters) are implanted into the tumor or tumor bed. Then the patient is placed in a shielded room and the applicators are connected to an afterloading machine by using transfer cables. The afterloading machine has a very high intensity iridium-192 source (of a nominal activity of 10 Ci) at the end of a steel cable. The operator then leaves the treatment room and, from the remote afterloading machine, controls the travel of the radioactive source through the transfer cables and applicator to the tumor site. Since the radioactive source has high intensity, the treatments can be performed in minutes. Once the source retracts, and the applicator removed, the patient is no longer radioactive. Usually these treatments can be performed on an out-patient basis with the need for minimal sedation, if any.

Intraoperative High-Dose-Rate Brachytherapy

Intraoperative high-dose-rate (HDR) brachytherapy involves the placement of brachytherapy catheters into a tumor mass or bed during the surgical procedure and after resection of as much tumor mass as is safe and possible for the patient. Normal tissues are then shielded or retracted from the area to be irradiated. A high dose of radiation is then delivered using the remote-controlled afterloading equipment to load the catheters with high energy radionuclides (iridium-192) while the patient is still under anesthesia. After the catheters are placed, all personnel vacate the operating room suite for remote-controlled loading of the radionuclide into the catheters. The patient is monitored by cameras and remote physiomonitoring equipment during the dosing period, which may vary from 5–20 minutes depending on the dosage calculations. Upon completion of the therapy and when radiation exposure is no longer a hazard (i.e., the radioactive source has been withdrawn into the remote afterloading machine), the surgical, anesthesia, and brachytherapy teams reenter the operating room. The surgical team and brachytherapist are regowned and gloved to comply with aseptic principles before moving to the sterile field. The catheters and templates are removed from the surgical field by the brachytherapist, and the patient's surgery is then continued.

Because of the complexity of the procedures involved and the physical facilities necessary, intraoperative brachytherapy is not a commonly available therapy alternative. Procedures for considerable planning and collaboration must be in place before a successful comprehensive intraoperative radiation oncology program can be successfully orchestrated. Intraoperative high-dose-rate (IOHDR) brachytherapy requires coordination of the efforts of the anesthesia, surgical, and brachytherapy teams. Operating room personnel require education and training as to the safety and use of radionuclides for the treatment of tumors. Policies and procedures must clearly delineate the patient safety issues as well as the issues related to the operating room environment.

Intracavitary Brachytherapy

Intracavitary implants are temporary implants that are done by placing an applicator into a body cavity (e.g., vagina or bronchus) adjacent to the tumor. The applicator is then loaded with the radionuclide either manually or by remote control. Placement of the applicator may be performed in the operating room. Newer techniques using HDR remote afterloading allow for placement of applicators without anesthesia.

Nursing Management of Brachytherapy Patients in Radiation Oncology

Patient and Family Education

Patient and family education is essential for any implant procedure to be successful and can require a great deal of time. Because brachytherapy procedures are unfamiliar to most patients, detailed teaching is needed to alleviate the fears and concerns of the unknown. The nurse is involved with the education process from the time the patient is consulted for treatment until treatment is completed and often into the follow-up phase. The nursing role in providing this education is outlined in Table 1.

Preimplant preparation of the patient involves doing an assessment of the patient/family needs so that the nurse knows what their needs are and how to address them. Teaching aids such as site specific booklets, self-care pamphlets, implant equipment or applicators, articles, and videotapes have been developed to assist the nurse in educating the patient. Whether the patient is receiving out-patient or in-patient brachytherapy treatment, he or she should be assessed before treatment for any questions, concerns, or side effects from the treatment. Being available to assist the in-patient staff nurses allows for better and consistent care for the patient.

Postprocedure teaching is also essential for the patient and family. Although the treatment may be completed, this can be a very emotional time for the patient. The patient or family may have many questions: Is the cancer gone? Will it come back again? Who's going to take care of me now? What radiation safety precautions may be necessary? Written discharge instructions and/or treatment completion instructions are helpful for the patient. They need to know what to do, what to expect, and how this all is going to affect them in the future. Therefore, the nurse needs to follow up with the patient after treatment, by telephone or follow-up visit, to assess the patient's status and reassure them about the normal expected healing process. It is also important to stress the need for follow-up with their oncologist on a routine basis.

Patient Care

Patient care is site specific and depends on the type of applicator used and the specific procedure done. The emotional care of the patient may not be as specific, but it should be addressed by the nurse whenever necessary. Nursing care may differ slightly depending on the type of the radioactive isotope used; whether the implant is temporary, permanent, interstitial, intracavitary, or remote or manually loaded; or whether the treatment is performed on an in-patient or out-patient basis.

Nursing Intervention for Brachytherapy Procedures (see Table 2)

The reader should refer to the individual chapters for detailed description of the brachytherapy techniques used.

Breast Implants

Breast implants can be done as boost therapy, after standard external beam radiation therapy (EBRT), or as primary therapy for certain types of breast cancer. The implant procedure is performed in the operating room under general or local anesthesia. A plastic template may be used to help the radiation oncologist guide the needles through the breast tissue. Plastic afterloading catheters are

Table 1.
Nursing Care Plan: Care of the Brachytherapy Patient

Nursing Diagnosis	Expected Outcome	Nursing Interventions
Knowledge deficit related to brachytherapy/internal radiation.	Patient will demonstrate a basic understanding of brachytherapy and how the treatment works.	Assess patient knowledge level and readiness to learn. Discuss basis principles of radiation therapy. Explain specific procedure that is to be done. Discuss potential side effects of implant treatment. Explain the course of the implant procedure, i.e. advance testing appointment, bowel prep, dietary restrictions, etc.
Anxiety/fear related to radiation therapy and the implant procedure.	Patient will verbalize fears and concerns regarding the brachytherapy procedure and will resolve any misconceptions regarding radiation therapy.	Assess patient/family's level of anxiety, knowledge and beliefs regarding radiation therapy and brachytherapy. Encourage patient to verbalize feelings, fears, and concerns. Explain treatment thoroughly: length of treatment, potential side effects; show patient equipment and treatment machine. Encourage patients to call and talk with family and friends when able. Encourage visitors as instructed for limited time. Make rounds on the inpatients daily. Consult support staff i.e., social work, pastoral care. Provide written educational materials if available. Re-evaluate learning and re-enforce teaching as indicated. Allow adequate time for discussion and questions. Discuss basic principles of radiation safety. Identify and support effective coping mechanisms.
Potential for complications/side effects related to specific brachytherapy procedure (site specific).	Patient will demonstrate understanding and learning of self-care measures for site specific and general side effects of brachytherapy treatment.	Explain that side effects of brachytherapy procedures are site specific; radiation treatments affect the only area treated.

Table 2.
Side Effects

General Side Effects: Altered skin integrity; Fatigue	
Assess skin integrity routinely to treated area. Assess level of fatigue and affect on activities of daily living. Instruct patient that it is normal for the side effects of treatment to continue for several weeks after treatment is completed.	Give written instructions to help re-enforce teaching. Reassure patient that side effects are temporary and usually resolve without medical intervention. Report any persistent problems to your physician.

Site Specific Side Effects	
Breast	Assess and teach patient signs and symptoms of infection. Instruct patient to support breast after implant. May need to pad bra for comfort. Patient may also feel shock like sensations in the treated breast tissues; reassure patient that this is normal.
Gynecological	Instruct patient regarding expected side effects: yellowish/white vaginal discharge, itching, changes in bowel or bladder habits. Instruct patient on vaginal douching. Instruct patient to use a vaginal dilator as indicated. Assess bowel and bladder functions. Monitor pain level and analgesics prescribed. Encourage routine follow up appointments for pelvic examinations and pap smears. Discuss return to normal sexual activities.
Endobronchial	Assess respiratory status—pulse rate, respiratory rate, any difficulty in breathing, shortness of breath, need for oxygen therapy, persistent cough, or hemoptysis. Assess for signs/symptoms of esophagitis—difficulty eating or swallowing.
Head and Neck	Instruct patient on expected side effects related to implant—taste alterations, mucositis, xerostomia, edema (swelling), sore throat. Assess and teach paitent signs/symptoms of infection. Inspect oral pharyngeal cavity routinely. Assess nutritional status and make dietary referral as needed—tube feedings, intravenous nutritional support. Monitor lab values. Discuss and provide pain management—oral analgesics, liquid solutions/gargles, topical applications. Identify any alterations in verbal communications. Provide alternative ways to communicate—paper and pencil, "magic" slates, chalk board, bell. Instruct patient on good oral hygiene—baking soda gargle, swish and swallow medications, mouth rinses. Provide artificial saliva products/solutions as indicated. Encourage routine follow-up with dentist.
Prostate	Instruct patient on expected side effects of implant: perineal soreness, bruising and/or swelling, hip or back soreness due to positioning during implant. Discuss any changes in bowel habits—diarrhea, constipation. Discuss any changes in urinary system—frequency, urgency, nocturia, dysuria, burning with urination. Encourage gradual increase in level of activity. Assess and teach patient signs/symptoms of infection. Instruct patient and family/signficant other on radiation safety measures with permanent implants; strain urine for specified duration; patient is minimally radioactive; visitors are allowed.
Esophagus	Instruct patient on the expected side effects of implant: sore throat, heartburn, nausea, esophagitis. Assess nutritional status—need for tube feedings temporarily, etc. Make dietary consult as needed. Provide medications as needed to control nausea and/or vomiting.

guided through the hollow needles and the needles are removed, leaving only the plastic catheters in place. The plastic catheters are secured at both ends with radio-opaque buttons. Stainless steel buttons are then crimped on one end of the catheters after the radioactive sources are placed. The patient may be taken to the simulation room for further treatment planning films. The radiation sources are placed into the plastic catheters once the patient is in a private hospital room. This technique, referred to as "afterloading," reduces the radiation exposure of health care providers. With this type of low-dose-rate (LDR) implant, the patient is hospitalized for 24–48 hours for boost therapy and for 72–96 hours for primary therapy. However, with the latest HDR remote afterloading techniques now available, breast implants can be performed on an out-patient basis with the treatment dose being delivered twice a day (BID) over 4–5 days.

Good skin care (cleansing with antibiotic ointment) is needed at the catheter insertion sites at least twice daily. Patients may also experience some slight pain or discomfort in the implanted breast, but generally the implants are well tolerated. The patients are allowed to be up and around but may not shower until the implant has been removed. In-patients are restricted to their private room until the radioactive sources are removed, and the time allotted for each visitor is limited.

Once the total radiation dose is completed and the radioactive source(s) secured, the afterloading catheters are removed in the patient's room or in the out-patient clinic exam room. Postprocedure care is site specific and should include information on skin care, support of the implanted breast tissue, and fatigue. The patient needs to be encouraged to follow up with their radiation oncologist on a regular basis. Table 3 lists the postimplant instructions for breast cancer patients.

Gynecological Implants

Gynecological (GYN) implants include implants of vaginal, cervix, and endometrial cancers. Although these implants are generally combined with EBRT, they may be used alone postoperatively as a prophylactic treatment or for local control of bulky or recurrent disease.

Table 3.
Post Implant Instructions for Breast Cancer Patients

We would like to explain some ways that you can assist in your recovery after your implant has been removed.

After the implant has been removed, you are no longer radioactive. The effects of the radiation may continue for a few weeks.

You may remove the dressing the day after you're discharged and may shower. Try to keep the area dry and expose it to the air when at all possible.

You may experience some uncomfortable feelings, perhaps sensations that feel like electric shocks, from time to time. Try not to let them frighten you. Your breast tissue is going through a healing process and these sensations are normal.

It is important too that the breast be supported but sometimes a bra can cause unnecessary friction. Padding the bra may help you feel more comfortable.

It is also important to watch for any signs of infection. If you notice any drainage from the implant area or if the skin becomes red and warm to touch, please notify us as soon as possible.

Please feel free to contact us if you have any further questions or concerns.

Adapted and edited with permission from William Beaumont Hospital, Department of Radiation Oncology-Nursing.

For LDR intracavitary treatments, the applicators are inserted under general or spinal anesthesia. The radiation oncologist secures the applicator in the vagina with gauze packing. Simulation films are taken to verify applicator placement. A dummy source is inserted into the tandem of the applicator for treatment planning for the bladder and rectal doses. Once the treatment planning is complete, the patient is returned to her room where the radioactive sources are loaded into the hollow applicator either manually or using remote afterloading techniques. The patient remains in the hospital on bed rest until the treatment is complete and the applicator can be removed. An indwelling catheter is placed in the bladder to maintain urine flow. A low residue diet and antidiarrheal medication are given to prevent the bowels from moving while the implant is in place. Although some discomfort is to be expected, severe, extreme pain is un-common. Mild analgesics will help to control the discomfort. Visitors are encouraged even though visitation time is limited.

Intracavitary GYN implants can also be done on an out-patient basis using HDR tech-niques, usually not requiring anesthesia. In some cases however, the initial application is performed under spinal anesthesia in the operating room. Usually subsequent applica-tions are performed without anesthesia, al-though mild sedation may be required before each treatment. The patient's vital signs are monitored, and placement of the applicator is verified fluoroscopically. Although these patients require several insertions, the proce-dures are generally tolerated very well.

Interstitial GYN implants, which can be manually or remotely afterloaded, are also done in much the same manner for some GYN tumors (usually for recurrent and/or bulky disease). Spinal or general anesthesia is used, and hollow needles are placed through the perineum and into the tumor area using a template as a guide. The patient is hospitalized for the duration of the implant and remains on complete bed rest.

Discharge or follow-up instructions should include discussion of the normal or expected side effects of the treatment. Changes in bowel habits, vaginal discharge, fatigue, uri-nary frequency, or urgency are all normal ex-pected side effects of GYN brachytherapy. Pa-tients are encouraged to increase their activity level gradually and may resume sexual activ-ity when they feel comfortable with it. Instruc-tions on the use of a vaginal dilator are given, if necessary. The patient is instructed on keeping the perineum clean and on vaginal douche. Regular follow-up with the physician is encouraged.

Endobronchial Implants

Intracavitary endobronchial implants are done for cancers of the lung and can be com-bined with EBRT for maximum local tumor control. Treatment catheters are placed using a bronchoscope. The patient is given sedation (e.g., valium or versed) intravenously and a local/topical anesthetic to numb the throat and nasal passages. The pulmonologist per-forms the bronchoscopy and the radiation on-cologist inserts the treatment catheter through the inner lumen of the bronchoscope. Cathe-ter placement is verified under fluoroscopy, and localization radiographs are taken for treatment planning. The patient is either sent to a private hospital room for LDR treatment or taken to a treatment room for out-patient HDR therapy. When the planning is com-pleted, the patient receiving LDR therapy undergoes loading of the radioactive sources and remains an in-patient until the therapy is completed. The patient receiving HDR ther-apy will be treated using the HDR remote af-terloader and sent home. Subsequent HDR treatments will be scheduled until the total dose prescribed is received.

The discharge instructions should include information about the normal expected side effects of this therapy, some of which include fatigue, sore throat, loss of appetite, and skin irritation. Patients should be reminded that these side effects are manageable and that their nurse and/or physician should be in-formed of them. Patients are encouraged to follow up routinely with their radiation oncol-ogist.

Head and Neck Implants

Cancers of the head and neck can include lesions at the base of the tongue, floor of the mouth, tonsil, and nasopharynx. Brachyther-apy for head and neck tumors is usually com-bined with EBRT as a boost therapy for better local control of the tumor. Permanent im-plants have been used for some deep-seated tumors, but more often interstitial or intracavi-tary removable implants are done.

The interstitial implant is performed in the operating room with the patient under gen-eral anesthesia. In some cases, the location of the tumor and subsequent edema of the tis-sues will necessitate that a tracheostomy be performed to provide an adequate airway. Hollow needles are carefully placed into the tumor area, avoiding vital structures such as the carotid vessels, mandible, and the gums. Plastic afterloading catheters are threaded through the hollow needles, and the needles are removed, leaving only the plastic cathe-ters in place. These are secured with radio-opaque and stainless steel buttons. Radio-graphs taken in the simulator room for treatment planning verify the placement of the catheters. The sources are loaded in the patient's hospital room. Alternatively, brachytherapy head and neck implants using preloaded or "hot" cesium implants may be performed in the radiation oncology unit with the patient under local anesthesia.

Interstitial head and neck implants tend to be very uncomfortable for the patients. Pain medication needs to be offered frequently to the patient. To decrease the swelling that is usually present, the patients are put on low doses of steroids. These patients require frequent (every 2–4 hours) oral irrigation with salt and soda or diluted hydrogen peroxide solution. The head of the patient's bed should be elevated to help with the swelling and secretions that may accumulate in the oral cavity. Tonsil suctioning equipment should be readily available at the bedside. The patients may be up out of bed in their room but are confined to their room while the sources are in place. Depending on the location of the implant, verbal communication may be a problem. The nurse should provide the patient with writing materials (paper and pen, chalk board, etc.) that the patient can use to communicate.

Depending on its location, the implant may be removed in the patient's room, in the radiation oncology department, or under general anesthesia in the operating room. The side effects that need to be addressed include: fatigue, localized pain, difficulty swallowing, loss of sense of taste, and decrease or loss of saliva. A referral to the dietitian may be needed to assist the patient with alternatives for good nutrition. The patient is often placed on high protein liquid or soft diet; a nasogastric tube insertion may be required. Frequent follow-up with their physicians is necessary and should be emphasized by the nurse.

Intracavitary implants are generally used for tumors of the nasal passages and nasopharyngeal region. Applicators are generally placed with minimal or no sedation. LDR or HDR techniques can be used. HDR treatments are generally fractionated over 2–3 weeks. Since the treatment time is short for the HDR patient, verbal communication is generally not a concern. The patient is watched closely and instructed to use hand gestures or a bell that is provided. Pain and swelling are mini-

mal and usually do not require medical intervention.

Prostate Implants

Temporary interstitial implants of the prostate gland have been done for a number of years, usually in conjunction with EBRT. These have also been used as sole therapy in the treatment of locally recurrent prostate disease. The temporary prostate implants are performed under general or spinal anesthesia using LDR and HDR techniques with manual or remote afterloading and may or may not require hospitalization.

HDR patients receive their treatment and are generally discharged the same day if there are no complications. LDR patients require a 3- to 5-day hospital stay. A template is used as a guide to place the hollow needles into the prostate. Transrectal ultrasound is used to visualize the needles as they are being placed. Once the needles are in place, x-ray films or a CT scan is done to verify placement and to assist with treatment planning. Radioactive seeds are placed into the needles either manually or using a remote afterloading machine. Once the prescribed dose is delivered, the implant is removed in the treatment room or in the patient's hospital room. The patient is either premedicated or still under spinal anesthesia, as in the HDR cases.

Permanent prostate implants using iodine-125 or palladium-103 are used as primary therapy and as supplemental boosts in some cases. The implant procedure is done with the patient under general or spinal anesthesia. With the patient in the lithotomy position, an ultrasound probe is introduced into the rectum, and the prostate gland is visualized. A plastic template is used to guide the needle placement. The needles are placed in the gland according to a preimplant plan using an applicator that pushes the seeds into the prostate tissue; the radioactive seeds are left in the prostate gland, and the needles are removed. Verification films and CT scans are taken to account for all the seeds placed and to accurately calculate the dose being delivered. Further verification films or a CT scan is obtained 2–4 weeks later to determine if any seeds have migrated. Because of this possibility, the patients are asked to strain their urine to retrieve any seeds that may have migrated out of the prostate gland.

In general, the patients may have some discomfort from the implant and may require mild narcotic analgesics. Patients may experience difficulty in urination, urinary frequency, and slight hematuria. These side effects generally resolve within a few days to weeks without medical intervention. Some patients may also experience changes in their bowel habits. These are usually related to the EBRT the patient may be receiving. Because the patient is discharged with the implant in place, the patient and family need to be reassured that only minimal radiation precautions are required. They need to understand that radioactive seeds decay over a period of time and that the type of isotope used will determine how long the patient will need to strain their urine and how long children and pregnant women should maintain a safe distance from the patient. Sexual activity may be resumed when the patient feels comfortable with it, but, during the first few weeks postimplant, a condom should be used. A medical alert bracelet is generally given to the patient to be worn during the period of radiation precaution. A written summary of the precautions and instructions are given to the patients. Routine follow-up with the radiation oncologist and urologist is recommended.

Esophageal Implants

Intracavitary implants of the esophagus are generally done as a boost therapy in combination with EBRT. They are usually performed using local anesthesia (xylocaine spray or jelly). The applicator or naso-gastric tube is placed with the patient in a sitting position. A mouth piece may be used to help guide and stabilize the applicator. When a naso-gastric tube is used, a 5Fr or 6Fr treatment catheter needs to be placed down the tube. If a problem occurs in passing the tube, it may be necessary to have the endoscopy department assist with placing the applicator or tube.

When the applicator/tube is in place, the placement is verified under fluoroscopy. The patient may be asked to swallow a contrast solution (e.g., barium) to better localize the esophageal obstruction. Once the position is verified, the patient is admitted to a private room and loaded with a radioactive source for LDR therapy or is treated with HDR therapy in the radiation oncology department. After the treatment, the tube is removed, and the patient may go home. Subsequent HDR treatments are scheduled on an out-patient basis until the total prescribed dose is delivered.

Discharge instruction should include information regarding the expected side effects of the treatment. They may include sore throat, decreased appetite, and nausea. Patients should notify their nurse or doctor about the side effects they are experiencing so that appropriate intervention can be taken. Routine follow-up with their physician is encouraged.

Nursing Considerations in the Operating Room

Care of the brachytherapy patient having intraoperative procedures adds additional considerations for the nursing staff in the operating room. The patient may have local, regional, or general anesthesia. The patient's position depends on the site and intended surgical approach. The patient may undergo tumor resection before the brachytherapy treatment or may have only the brachytherapy treatment performed under anesthesia. In all cases, both the attending surgeon and the radiation oncologist are present in the operating room to collaborate and support the plan of therapy.

The nursing staff in the operating room collaborate with the surgeon and brachytherapist to determine the patient care needs, instrumentation, and supplies necessary to perform the procedure. The nursing staff provide an aseptic field of instruments and supplies for the procedure and see that the mechanical applicators and radionuclide seeds are sterilized. In the case of tumor resection, the operating room nurse communicates the progress of the procedure to the radiation oncologist so that there is no delay in delivering the brachytherapy treatment while the patient is under general anesthesia.

Intraoperative Brachytherapy Plan of Care

The patient undergoing a scheduled intraoperative brachytherapy procedure is assessed by the operating room nurse in the preoperative holding area. A preoperative assessment includes:

1. accurate identification of the patient;
2. assessment of the patient's medical and surgical history;
3. assessment of the proposed surgical site with documentation of any findings for postoperative comparison;
4. assessment of the patient's understanding of the surgical procedure and postoperative events;
5. assessment of level of anxiety;
6. assessment of physical limitations;
7. assessment of past radiation therapy and chemotherapy regimens;
8. documentation of medications routinely taken at home and their purpose;
9. patient allergies to medications and other chemical substances such as latex or iodine.

The patient's chart is reviewed for the appropriate documents and diagnostic findings. Doctor's orders are reviewed for preoperative medications and application of antiemboli stockings or synchronous compression leggings. The events of the surgical experience are explained to the patient and emotional support is offered by means of establishing a professional, trusting relationship. Reassurance is given that the nurse will be with the patient throughout the surgery and that the patient's family will be kept informed of the progress. The operating room nurse confers with the anesthesia personnel as to the plan of care. The operating room is then prepared and arranged to receive the patient. Patient outcomes are formulated to guide the patient care interventions (see Table 4).

The patient enters the operating room via a transport cart and is assisted to the operating room table. The patient is positioned after anesthesia induction. Positioning aids and equipment are utilized in such a manner that fluoroscopic visualization or radiation dosimetry are not obstructed.

Site-Specific Needs

The site of brachytherapy treatment determines the supplies, instruments, and equip-

Table 4.
Sample Intraoperative Plan of Care for a Patient Having Surgical Brachytherapy

Nursing Diagnosis	Outcome Statement
Anxiety related to the patient's diagnosis of cancer and the lack of understanding of the treatment plan.	The patient will verbalize understanding of the surgical events and postoperative plan of care.
High risk for injury related to the surgical position.	The patient is free of injury related to surgical position as evidenced by the absence of neuromuscular impairment and tissue necrosis.
High risk for injury related to thermal hazards.	The patient is free of injury related to thermal hazards as evidenced by the absence of tissue damage secondary to hypothermia or hyperthermia.
High risk for impaired skin integrity.	The patient's skin integrity is maintained as evidenced by the absence of bruises, skin breakdown, discoloration, open skin lesions, or excoriation during the perioperative period (Rothrock, 1990).
High risk for infection related to surgical incision, catheter placement, and intravascular lines.	The patient is free from infection related to breaks in aseptic technique during surgery as evidenced by the absence of redness, edema, purulent incisional drainage, or postoperative temperature elevations above 100°F.

ment necessary for performing the procedure, as well as the patient's position and anesthesia alternatives. Brachytherapy delivered to the prostate, uterus, vagina, rectum, or perineum is usually performed with the patient in lithotomy position. The supine position is commonly used for tumor sites of the head, neck, breast, gastrointestinal, and pelvic areas. The patient may be positioned laterally for tumor sites in the thorax and kidney and in the prone position for anorectal tumors.

The size of the tumor determines the number of catheters or number of radionuclide seeds to be used. Templates are often used to guide the delivery of the brachytherapy catheters into the tumor and to stabilize the catheters during remote-controlled loading. Templates that are custom designed to the patient's tumor site are sterilized before the scheduled procedure.

The patient having brachytherapy of the prostate, vagina, rectum, or perineum may have the option of regional anesthesia achieved by spinal or epidural block. The patient remains awake with some intravenous sedation, if indicated. Placement of interstitial catheters may be performed under fluoroscopy to verify position. Plain radiographs are commonly taken to visualize the brachytherapy seed or catheter position before the patient's procedure is concluded.

The operating room nurse assesses the patient's understanding of the scheduled procedure before surgery and explains the procedure. It is very important that the patient understands that they may have tubes or catheters coming from the planned site after the procedure. Emotional support and reassurance are offered. If the patient undergoes the procedure under local or regional anesthesia, the nurse may frequently explain the progress of the procedure.

After surgery, the patient may be discharged from the operating room to the post-anesthesia care unit, surgical intensive care unit, or nursing unit. The operating room nurse accompanies the patient and reports the interventions to the nurse accepting the admission of the patient. The operating room nurse should identify all tubes and catheters that were placed during the procedure and document the location and description on the operating room record. If interstitial radionuclide seeds were placed, the site and approximate number are documented on the operating room record. This information and any radiation safety instructions are also communicated verbally to the nurse receiving the patient. (See Table 5 for summary of safety instructions).

Procedural Interventions

The operating room nurse, who knows the policies and procedures of intraoperative brachytherapy interventions, assesses the patient by conducting a preoperative interview to obtain the information necessary to plan for the individualized intraoperative care and positioning of the patient. The patient's age, anxiety level, nutritional status, size, medical history, surgical history, radiation therapy history, and chemotherapy history are reviewed, and a physical examination of the intended surgical site is performed. The patient's chart is reviewed for additional information. The patient should understand the intended procedure to the degree required for informed surgical consent. Laboratory results such as the patient's hemoglobin, hematocrit, white count, platelets, CEA, CA-125 or PSA, and electrolytes are reviewed. The nurse determines if blood products have been ordered and then confirms availability of the requested units. The nurse then contacts the patient's family to inform them that the patient will be going into the operating room.

The operating room nurse communicates pertinent patient care needs and develops a plan of care. Positioning aids and padding are prepared as necessary. The operating room is prepared by arranging and establishing a sterile field of instruments, supplies, and equipment. The patient enters the operating room, is transferred to the operating room table, and is given anesthesia. The patient is positioned for optimal access to the tumor site, and bony prominences and pressure areas are padded and limbs are restrained for safety. The principles of anatomical alignment are maintained so as to prevent neurovascular compromise.

The surgical site is prepped with antiseptic solutions, draped with sterile drapes to ensure isolation of the site and to prevent cross-contamination from other areas of the patient's body, and the sterile field is brought near to the patient. The procedure is initiated as planned.

Table 5.
Summary of Guidelines for Care of Radioactive Patients

Type of Implant	Radiation Exposure Level	Housing	Radiation Precautions
Removable Cesium-137 Removable Iridium-192 Permanent Gold-198	High	1	4–9, 12–14
Removable Iodine-125	Low	2	4, 11, 12, 14
Permanent Iodine-125 Permanent Palladium-103	Negligible	3	10, 17, 18, 19
Remote controlled high-dose-rate brachytherapy	None	3	10, 15
Iodine-131 solution administration	High	1	4–9, 13, 14, 16

1. Private corner room with private bath, preferably a shielded private room. Portable lead shield at bedside. Patient may not leave the room.
2. Any private room in hospital.
3. No restrictions. May be discharged home.
4. "Caution - Radiation Area" sign on door.
5. Nurses should wear film dosimeter badge while caring for the patient.
6. Nurses should not spend more than ½ hour daily within 3 feet of the patient.
7. Laundry should be placed in linen bag and saved. All items (e.g., dressings, linens) must remain in the room until approved by the Radiation Safety officer (or his designee) for disposal. (The radioactive source is sealed, unlike radiopharmaceutical therapy that involves sources that my be excreted in urine, feces, or body fluids.)
8. Housekeeping may not enter the room.
9. Each visit is limited to ½ hour per day. Visitors must remain at least 6 feet from the source, preferably behind the portable lead shield.
10. No visiting time restrictions.
11. No visiting time restrictions if lead patch is over the implanted area.
12. Do not touch the radioactive source with bare hands. If the source has been dislodged, retrieve it using long-handled forceps and deposit it in the lead container that is kept in the patient's room.
13. The paient may not have pregnant visitors or visitors under 18 years of age.
14. A dismissal survey must be performed before the patient is discharged. When the patient is discharged, the Radiation Safety officer should survey the room before its assignment to another patient.
15. No precaution after patient leaves the brachytherapy suite.
16. Excreted in urine, stool, saliva, and sweat. Toilet, sink, floor, etc. should be covered with disposable plastic or paper. Bedding, linens, trash, etc. are contaminated and should be disposed of according to radiation safety.
17. Strain urine (if implant is in prostate.)
18. After discharge, patient should wear medical alert bracelet for duration of radioactivity.
19. Children under 18 and pregnant women should not spend greater than 1 hour per day within 3 feet of patient for duration of radioactivity.

Upon completion of the brachytherapy procedure, the operating room is scanned with a hand-held gamma detection device to determine that no radioactive materials are left in the room. This inspection includes the instruments, drapes, operating room floors suction tubing, and canisters. All operating room personnel wear radiation detection badges for radiation exposure monitoring.

Permanent Interstitial Brachytherapy

The patient having intraoperative permanent interstitial brachytherapy is positioned and prepared for surgical intervention after anesthesia. If tumor is to be resected, the surgical team exposes the tumor site, and then the brachytherapist is called to visualize the tumor site before removal of the tumor. A plan of therapy is then established. Necessary implant devices, such as the Mick applicator and radionuclide seeds, are sterilized. The seeds are steam sterilized in shielded containers for 3 minutes at 30–32 psi pressure and at a minimum temperature of 270°F ($\approx$133°C). Sterilization for longer periods or at higher pressures may damage the seeds. The high dose of gamma radiation emitted at the surface of the seed results in virtual sterility of the surface. Autoclaving for 3 minutes ensures the sterility of the shielded containers.

The site is isolated by the surgical team and the brachytherapist places the needles into the tumor mass or bed of resection. The seeds are then transferred into the tumor mass with the Mick Applicator; the number and depth of seeds implanted are recorded by the brachytherapy team. After the application of seeds, the surgical wound is examined for any free seeds. The brachytherapist remains at the surgical field until hemostasis or other necessary intervention at the brachytherapy site has concluded. The room, drapes, instruments, sterile tables, garbage, linen, suction tubing, and suction containers are scanned with a hand-held radiation detecting device. Any tissue specimen removed from the brachytherapy site thereafter is scanned for radiation. A seed may be included in the fluid or tissue of the specimen and must be identified and removed before the specimen leaves the operating room. If a patient with permanently implanted seeds returns to surgery within the period of radioactivity (6 months for iodine-125 and 2 months for palladium-103), the operating room and tissue specimens must be monitored for any displaced radioactive seeds. If a drain is placed in the cavity of the brachytherapy site, the drain and reservoir must be monitored for free seeds. Although the low-dose radiation is attenuated by distance and tissue density, it is important to notify all health care personnel of the presence of permanent brachytherapy interstitial seeds.

Patients having permanent interstitial brachytherapy seeds do not require special radiation precautions and can be discharged to go home after surgical recovery. They are instructed, however, to minimize direct contact with children and pregnant women to <1 hour per day for 6 months if iodine-125 was used or for 2 months if palladium-103 was used. Pregnant nurses are not assigned to these procedures. Patients receive an information sheet that notes the date, isotope, and amount of radiation implanted and are required to wear a medical alert bracelet during the 2- or 6-month period stating radiation precautions.

Placement of Brachytherapy Catheters for Removable Brachytherapy

Brachytherapy catheters are surgically placed into a tumor or tumor bed of resection while the patient is anesthetized. The procedure may be performed under local, regional, or general anesthesia with the patient's position dependent on the site of the tumor. Placement of the catheters may be performed percutaneously under fluoroscopy or ultrasound guidance or under direct visualization during surgical exposure of the tumor site. The catheters protrude from the body cavity and are secured. Since the catheters are not radioactive, no specific radiation precautions are necessary until they are loaded with radioactive material. The catheters are placed so that safe and easy removal is possible after the therapy.

The patient will be admitted to a shielded room on the nursing unit for the treatment period. Once the radioactive material is loaded into the catheters, radiation precautions are enforced. The patient's room, bedding, garbage, linen, and other room contents are monitored with the hand-held survey meter to confirm that no radioactive materials have become dislodged. Isolation and visiting restrictions are calculated according to each patient's radioactivity measurement. The treatment may last for a few days, during which exposure of health caregivers, family, and friends is restricted from 30 minutes to a few hours per day. Portable lead shields are placed in the patient's room for visitors and caregivers to stand behind. After removal of the radioactive materials and catheters, the patient does not have residual radiation and can be transferred out of the shielded room or be discharged home.

Intraoperative High-Dose-Rate Remote Brachytherapy

When the brachytherapy team decides to use IOHDR brachytherapy to treat a site a plan of action is instituted. The circulating nurse confers with the brachytherapist as to the supplies and equipment (a variety of presterilized applicators are available) that will be required for the individual patient. The brachytherapist will select the applicator and number and type of catheters that will be placed at the tumor site. Transfer cables, "dummy" wires, check source, a sterile platform, and surgical clips are assembled for the radiation oncologist. Packing or suture is used to secure the catheters to the patient's body. If the radiation site is in an unusual location, the radiation oncologist may cut and sculpt sterile foam to provide a stabilizing structure for the placement of catheters. Once the catheters are placed and stabilized, localization radiographs are obtained with nonradioactive "dummy" wires to verify position of the applicators in the tumor bed.

All personnel leave the operating room and the patient is then monitored by camera and remote hemodynamic and cardiac monitors. The anesthesiologist, the surgeon, the scrub nurse, and the brachytherapy team remain in the adjacent monitoring room during the patient's treatment. The patient receives a pre-calculated radiation dose that may range in time/exposure from 5–20 minutes. The circulating nurse and all other operating room personnel stand by the door to prevent entry into the operating room during the radiation treatment. The operating room doors are lead-lined for radiation safety. When the door is opened, the radiation therapy is automatically discontinued due to a door interlock mechanism.

Upon completion of the brachytherapy, all members of the surgical scrub team reenter the operating room and are regowned and gloved by the scrub nurse. The radiation oncologist confirms the position of the catheters, then removes the catheters and templates and examines the site. The patient's surgery is then continued, or if all interventions have been achieved, the wound is closed.

Radiation Safety in Care of Brachytherapy Patients

In the past, radioactive implantation was performed with "hot" radium sources, which resulted in high radiation exposure. We now have modified techniques and new radioisotopes that have significantly lowered radiation exposure. However, the fear of radiation exposure continues. Although specific nursing care differs according to the implant site, nursing concerns regarding safety and protection are the same for all implants. The princi-

pal factors involved in minimizing radiation exposure are distance, shielding, and time.

Distance

Because radiation exposure is inversely proportional to the square of the distance from the source (e.g., one would receive 100 times less radiation at ten times the distance from the source), it is important to stay as far as possible from the radiation source. One should stand at either the head or foot of the bed of patients with intracavitary implants or at the side of the bed farthest from the implant for patients with head and neck implants. If not providing direct care, one should stop at the doorway when visiting or providing patient education.

Shielding

For brachytherapy patients with high energy removable implants, lead aprons provide little protection since they only minimally absorb high energy radiation (lead aprons do help in absorbing low energy x-rays such as those used for fluoroscopy). For these patients, a bedside lead shield can be used to reduce radiation exposure. When properly used, this shielding can provide additional protection from radiation exposure. However, shielding equipment is cumbersome, and its use may result in the nursing staff spending additional time in the patients' rooms maneuvering the shields. If nurses follow the guidelines for limiting time spent in patients' rooms maintaining maximum possible distance from the radioactive source, they can minimize their exposure regardless of the presence or absence of shielding.

Time

The length of time spent with the patient determines exposure. Guidelines posted on the chart and on the patient's door can indicate the length of time that nurses and visitors can safely spend with the patient. For nursing personnel, these guidelines can be exceeded if extra medical care is needed; however, radiation exposure should always be minimized by using time efficiently. After the patient returns to the room, the maximum amount of direct nursing care should be provided *before* the radioactive source is loaded. Vital signs and applicator site should be checked, comfort measures should be provided, and call button and personal objects should be placed within the patient's reach. The patient should be encouraged to care for himself/herself, and the nursing staff should be rotated. An explanation of the need to limit staff exposure should be explained to the patient. The patients should be reassured that adequate nursing care will be maintained.

In the following section, several categories of radiation sources and the precautions to be observed with each are listed. The typical radiation guidelines used at Ohio State University are summarized in Table 5.

Permanent Low Energy Implants

These are usually iodine-125 or palladium-103 implants. Palladium-103 is similar to iodine-125 except that it has a shorter half-life, making the period of radiation shorter. These implants require minimal precautions. Private room isolation, film badges, lead shields, and time restrictions are not needed. These patients may go home with their families, who are given an instruction sheet. To minimize risks to fetuses, pregnant nurses should not be assigned to these patients; however, there is no danger if a pregnant nurse accidentally enters the room for a short time.

Removable Iodine-125 Implants

These implants are most commonly used for eye plaques on patients with choroidal melanoma or in some breast implants. Private rooms are needed for these patients and time restrictions with these patients should be indicated on the patient's chart and door. If a lead patch is placed over the implanted area, then only minimal radiation precautions are necessary.

Removable High Energy Implants

Cesium-137 or iridium-192 is usually used for interstitial and intracavitary removable gynecological implants. These patients require private rooms. Since these sources are sealed, the risk of contamination is minimal.

A possible risk arises if the sources are damaged or lost. Since they cannot be excreted, no special precautions are needed for the excreta; however, the bedding should be surveyed to confirm that no radiation sources have been lost before it is removed from the room.

The dressings over the implanted area should be changed only by radiation oncology staff. If sources are dislodged or displaced, they should be picked up using long-handled forceps and placed in a shielded container in the room, and Radiation Oncology should be informed immediately. Before the patient's discharge, the room should be surveyed by Radiation Safety to confirm that there is no residual radioactivity.

High-Dose-Rate Remote Brachytherapy

These patients are not radioactive after they leave the procedure room and hence, require no radiation precautions.

Iodine-131 Solution Administration

These solutions are used for thyroid diseases and are usually administered by Nuclear Medicine personnel. Iodine-131 solution is not classified as a sealed source brachytherapy procedure. Because the radioactive material is in a solution, it is absorbed by the body and excreted in the urine, stool, sweat, and saliva. The toilet, sink, etc., should be covered with disposable plastic or paper. The bedding, linens, trash, and the like are contaminated and must be disposed of following radiation precautions.

Nursing Research

Cancer nursing research dates back to 1948 when the first published nursing research reported the number of cancer patients cared for by public health nurses. Historically, nursing involvement in research projects and protocols has been limited to providing nursing care to patients participating in clinical trials. The role of the nurse in research, since the early 1970s, has expanded. A number of research groups and institutions have developed their own protocols and guidelines for brachytherapy. Oncology nurses need to actively participate in these protocols focusing on patient care, monitoring toxicities and side effects, and providing documentation.

Nurses have become more visible in clinical nursing research over the past decade. Protocols have been developed by nurses and research is being conducted by nurses. Being involved in research helps to assist nurses and other health care providers to provide better care for cancer patients. All aspects of care should be explored, including home care, economics of cancer care, quality of life issues, detection and prevention, and symptom management. Nurses dramatically affect the quality of patient care delivered and patient's the overall well being and quality of life. Brachytherapy is one of the many areas for nursing researchers to explore. By doing so, we can provide better and safer care to the patients.

Conclusions

There are numerous brachytherapy procedures and techniques being used today that require highly skilled nursing intervention. The nursing care of brachytherapy patients encompasses many activities, including direct patient care, patient and family education, symptom management, and follow-up. Providing high quality nursing care for these patients presents a challenge to all nurses who choose to work in the specialty of oncology.

Acknowledgments: The authors thank Gail Havener, R.N., of the Nursing Staff Development Office and Robert Cannon, R.N., of the Division of Radiation Oncology at the Arthur G. James Cancer Hospital and Research Institute, Columbus, Ohio, for their valuable comments.

Useful Resources for Information on Brachytherapy Nursing

1. Dow K. Principles of brachytherapy. In: Dow K, Hilderley L (eds). Nursing Care in Radiation Oncology. W.B. Saunders Co., Philadelphia, PA, 1992.
2. Hubbard SM. Principles of clinical research. In: Johnson BL, Gross J (eds). Handbook of Oncology Nursing. John Wiley & Sons, New York, NY, 1985.
3. Brown D. The role of the nurse in brachytherapy. Act Selec Brachy J 1990;4(3):53–55.
4. Bucholtz JD. Radiation therapy. In: Johnson BL, Gross J (eds). Handbook of Oncology Nursing. Jones and Bartlett, Boston, MA, 1994.
5. Groenwald SL, Frogge MH, Goodman M, et al. Cancer Nursing Principles and Practice. Jones and Bartlett, Boston, MA, 1993, pp. 241–242, 264–267, 899, 1137.
6. Clarke DH, Martinez AA. Overview of brachytherapy in cancer management. Oncology 1990;4(9):39–46.
7. Baird SD, et al. (eds). A Cancer Resource Book for Nurses. American Cancer Society, Atlanta, GA, 1991, pp. 63–72.
8. Bucholtz JD. Implications of radiation therapy for nursing. In: Clark JC, McGee RF (eds). Core Curriculum for Oncology Nursing. W.B. Saunders, Philadelphia, PA, 1992, pp. 319–328.
9. Bucholtz JD. Radiation therapy. In: Ziegfield CR (ed). Core Curriculum for Oncology Nursing. W.B. Saunders, Philadelphia, PA, 1987, pp. 217–218.
10. Nag S, Petty L, Parrott S. Comprehensive surgical radiation oncology. AORN J 1994;60(1): 27–37.
11. Rothrock JC, Sculthorpe RH. Anesthesia and patient positioning. In: The RN First Assistant. Second Edition. JB Lippincott Co, Philadelphia, PA, 1993, pp. 116–142.
12. Meeker MH, Rothrock JC (eds). Alexander's Care of the Patient in Surgery. Tenth Edition. Mosby-Year Book, Inc, St. Louis, MO, 1995, pp. 96–111.
13. Hassey K. Care of patients with radioactive implants. Am J Nurs 1985;85:788–792.

Chapter 33

Pulsed Low-Dose-Rate Brachytherapy

Patrick S. Swift, M.D.

Introduction to Pulsed Brachytherapy

The routine use of interstitial brachytherapy by radiation oncologists for accessible malignancies has been restricted by an often low therapeutic ratio, the need for manual afterloading with its exposure risks to personnel, and the aggressive invasiveness of the procedures, especially in patients with gynecological or retroperitoneal malignancies. Two separate technological advancements have significantly altered these conditions over the past decade. The first is magnetic resonance imaging, with its superior ability to delineate tumor tissue form normal tissue in the extremities, pelvis, retroperitoneum, and brain. The second is the remote afterloading units developed for brachytherapy, specifically the pulsed low-dose-rate (PDR) Selectron unit (Nucletron Corporation, Columbia, MD, USA) with its isodose optimization capability. As in the case of external beam radiotherapy, where three-dimensional conformal therapy is being investigated in an attempt to deliver higher doses of radiation to abnormal tissues with a concomitant reduction of dose to surrounding normal tissues via multifield multiplanar techniques, interstitial pulsed brachytherapy is attempting to conform the desired isodose distributions more closely to the region of interest as seen on imaging studies.

The PDR Selectron (Figure 1) uses a single iridium-192 source of 1.1-mm diameter and 2.6-mm length (Figure 2), activity generally between 0.5–1.0 Ci, secured at the end of a cable-driven wire. This single source is programmed to move through a series of positions within catheters or needles placed previously in the tumor bed, stopping for variable lengths of time varying from 0–999.9 seconds per position per pulse ("dwell times") throughout the array. The position and dwell times are selected to deliver an average isodose distribution per pulse that most closely conform to the geometry of the region to be treated. One complete movement of the source through the entire array constitutes a single pulse. The total duration of the pulse, the dose delivered per pulse, and the interval between pulses all may be manipulated.

Advantages of Pulsed Brachytherapy

Pulsed brachytherapy has a number of advantages over manual afterloading techniques for interstitial treatment. First, only a single source of Ir is necessary, reducing the need for an extensive, expensive inventory of sources for use in various situations. With the intermediate half-life of Ir (74 days), the source may be kept for up to 3 months before

From Nag S (ed): *Principles and Practice of Brachytherapy.* © Futura Publishing Co., Inc., Armonk, NY, 1997.

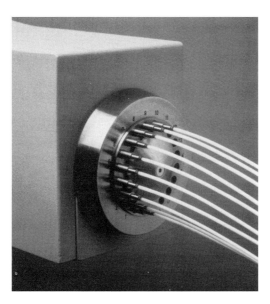

Figure 1. Photograph of remote afterloading PDR Selectron (from Nucletron Corporation, Columbia, MD, USA).

replacement is necessary, with storage of this source simplified by its location within the shielded unit. Since the maximum activity of the source is 1.0 Ci, additional shielding may be required to meet governmental standards in some rooms, but the source is only one tenth of that used in the high-dose-rate (HDR) units.

Second, as with any remote afterloading unit, the risk of exposure to radiation oncology personnel, nursing staff, physicians from other disciplines, or visiting family members is eliminated. Since the unit was designed to allow treatment for a fraction of each hour, the source would be safely isolated for the remainder of each hour, allowing the nursing staff to work more extensively with the patient. This becomes particularly important in the patient with extensive medical problems. The pulse is generally timed to end precisely at the hour to reduce confusion as to when the nursing staff may enter the room.

From a therapeutic standpoint, the main advantage of pulsed brachytherapy lies in the process of isodose optimization, the identical procedure that occurs in the use of the HDR remote afterloading unit. By carefully selecting the positions at which the source stops and dwell time of the source at each position, the average isodose distributions can be manipulated to reduce volumes that might be excessively irradiated in static implant arrays ("hot spots" secondary to decreased distances between needles or catheters in an implant) or to increase doses that might otherwise be

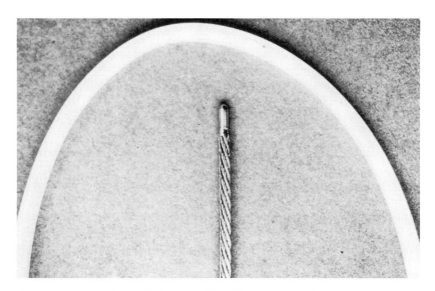

Figure 2. Ir-192 source on the end of steel cable with a plastic catheter above demonstrating the curvature of radius attainable by the cable.

inadequately dosed ("cold spots"). Within certain limits, dose homogeneity throughout an implant volume can be "optimized" in pulsed brachytherapy in a fashion not possible with static afterloading using ribbons with fixed sources. It must be pointed out, however, that even dose optimization cannot make a poorly implanted array good. There is no substitution for careful attention to uniform implantation of a volume with evenly spaced needles. The second benefit of optimization is that isodoses may be shaped to conform more closely to existing tumor geometry.

Pulsed brachytherapy has an additional advantage over standard continuous brachytherapy with other remote afterloading units in intraluminal or intracavitary insertions, (e.g., tandem and ovoid placements for cervix cancer, intraluminal catheters for esophageal and nasopharyngeal applications). In the continuous low-dose-rate (LDR) setting, any entry into the patient's room, for doctors visits or nursing attention, necessitates a break in the treatment as the source is removed automatically. The overall duration of the treatment is lengthened to account for these interruptions. In the pulsed setting, such visits ideally are timed to coincide with the breaks in treatment between pulses, keeping the overall duration of the implant constant. Through manipulation of dwell times, there is also an increased degree of flexibility found in determining the average dose per pulse (average dose per hour) compared to that possible with remote afterloaded fixed position sources. This last point will be discussed later in the chapter and must be approached cautiously.

Disadvantages of Pulsed-Dose-Rate Compared to High-Dose-Rate and Continuous Low-Dose-Rate

As with conventional continuous LDR brachytherapy, PDR treatments require several days to deliver the desired dose, thereby exposing the patient to spinal or general anesthetics and requiring prolonged hospital stays, compared to the out-patient nature of most HDR treatments. Risks of prolonged bedrest (e.g., deep venous thromboses, pulmonary emboli, stasis ulcers, etc.) exist with PDR. During the hospital stays, there is the potential for movement of the instrumentation out of the initial desired position (with tandem and ovoids for instance). Significant movement of the patient in the bed may result in disruption of the unimpeded transit of the cable-driven source with resultant treatment interruptions, requiring intervention to untwist the cables and catheters. Such events may occur after standard working hours, and, although not a danger to the patient, may lead to prolongation of the overall treatment time.

Compared to continuous LDR treatments, the main disadvantages are limited to the development of technical difficulties that are not seen with manual afterloading, and are far outweighed by the potential benefits.

Radiobiological Rationale

Several critical questions must be addressed before one can assume that PDR brachytherapy is equal to continuous LDR brachytherapy. Is a dose delivered to a volume as a brief pulse of a single stepping source at very high instantaneous dose rates biologically equivalent to the same average dose delivered constantly by a series of sources at a much lower instantaneous dose rate? Is the dose equivalent both in terms of its effect on early reacting tissues (including tumor) and late-reacting tissues? Is it equivalent over the range of half-times of tissue repair that are clinically relevant in the surrounding normal tissues?

Brenner and Hall[1] approached these questions by utilizing the linear-quadratic formalism of Lea and Catcheside[2] in the analysis of in vitro dose response data available for cell lines of human origin. Survival (S) at a dose D is a given by the following equation:

$$S(D) = \exp(-\alpha D - G\beta D^2)$$

where α is the portion of cell killing due to a single hit (the linear component), and β is that portion due to multiple hits (the exponential component). G is a function of the repair that occurs between successive hits of radiation and is dependent on the total time of irradiation, the spatial distribution of the radiation-induced events, and the repair capabilities of the particular cell line. Using 36 human cell lines, with their observed values for α, β, and t_o (characteristic repair time of the tissue), Brenner and Hall[1] set out to establish the condition under which pulsed therapy would be equivalent to continuous LDR therapy. The standard chosen for all comparisons was a total dose of 30 Gy delivered over 60 hours, representative of a typical continuous LDR implant. Various combinations of pulse widths and interval duration between pulses were examined to identify conditions under which the cell survival of early reacting tissues would be comparable to that seen with a continuous regimen. In further analysis, using the limited data available for late effects in humans, as well as animal data on late effects (mouse lung, rat spinal cord), the authors predicted the impact of a variety of pulsed regimens on late effects. Their conclusion was that 10-minute pulses, separated by 1-hour intervals, with the overall implant duration kept constant at 60 hours, would result in a similar cell survival for early reacting tissues and only a 2% increase in late effects when compared to the continuous regimen.

Increasing dose rates result in increasing biological effectiveness, but also inevitably lead to some decline in the therapeutic ratio according to Fowler and Hall et al.[3–6] If larger doses per pulse with increased intervals between pulses are used, the expected loss of therapeutic ratio would increase. Keeping the total duration of an implant static but increasing the interval between pulses, thereby increasing the dose per pulse, also increases the biological effectiveness of a dose. This increase in biological effectiveness is seen to be most significant in cell lines with a shorter half-time of repair ($t_{1/2}$). The amount of repair capacity is believed to be greater in late-reacting normal tissues than in early-reacting tissues (including most tumors). Therefore, at any level assumed for the half-time of repair, an increase in relative effectiveness would be expected to be more significant for late-reacting tissues than for early-reacting tissues, with a resultant decrease in the therapeutic ratio. If the $t_{1/2}$ for late-reacting tissues was known to be significantly longer than that of tumor tissues, the effect of pulsed therapy on the therapeutic ratio would be minimized. This, however, cannot be presumed to be uniformly the case.

Fowler and Mount[7] calculated the expected effect of various pulsed regimens (with dose rates in the pulse varying from 0.5–120 Gy/hr, pulses delivered every 1–4 hours) on early and late responding tissues, using a wide range of possible half-times of repair from 0.1–3 hours. The overall duration and total dose of the theoretic implant were kept constant at 70 Gy over 140 hours, and all effects were considered relative to a continuous regimen at 0.5 Gy/hr.

For early-reacting (tumor) tissues, biological effectiveness would not be expected to increase by >3% as long as dose rates remained in the 0.5–3 Gy/hr range and pulses were given hourly regardless of the assumed $t_{1/2}$. As the dose per pulse and interval duration increase, the biological effectiveness also increases for all $t_{1/2}$. This is true also for late-reacting tissues. As the pulse intervals increase to one pulse every 4 hours, the increase in biological effect in late tissue may rise as high as 15% (Figure 3). This becomes most pronounced in tissues with the shortest $t_{1/2}$ of repair and necessitates a decrease in the overall dose to sustain levels of late effects similar to that seen with continuous LDR regimens, a decrease which would result in a less-than-desired effectiveness for tumor control. Fowler and Mount,[7] therefore, arrived at a conclusion similar to that of Hall and Brenner[1]—keeping the repetition frequency at one pulse every 1 or 2 hours would be comparable to a continuous regimen with a negligible increase in late effects.

In Vitro Data

Armour et al.[8] compared continuous LDR irradiation (0.5 Gy/hr) to PDR (0.5 Gy/hr averages using 0.25 Gy/0.5 hour intervals, 1 Gy/2 hour intervals, 3 Gy/5 hour intervals) as treatment for rat 9L/SF gliosarcoma cells. Under separate tests at 37°C and 41°C, no appreciable differences were discernible between the pulsed and continuous regimens in the cell survival curves. However, when cells were treated with pulses of 6 Gy every 12 hours, an increase in cell killing (a relative decrease in D_o) was noted. Their conclusion was that cell killing is equivalent between pulsed and continuous techniques as long as the overall dose rate remains constant and the

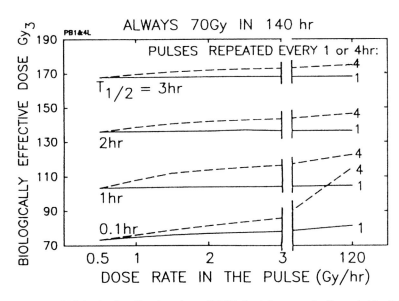

Figure 3. Increase of biologically effective dose (BED) for late complications ($a/\beta = 3$ Gy) with increasing dose rate in the pulses. Each pair of curves is for a different assumed $T_{1/2}$ of repair of sublethal damage. Full curves are for pulses of 0.5 Gy/hr. Dashed curves are for pulses of 2 Gy every 4 hours. To the left of the graph break is illustrated the pulsed brachytherapy region; to the right is illustrated the HDR or external beam dose rates up to 2 Gy/min. The common point for each pair of curves is for the continuous LDR of 0.5 Gy/hr given for 140 hours. This is the datum level for each value of assumed $T_{1/2}$.

dose per fraction is less than the width of the shoulder of the dose response curve.

In Vivo Data

Mason et al.[9] administered total body irradiation to mice using two continuous and two pulsed regimens to deliver a variety of doses over a range of 19–40 Gy. Mice were then sacrificed and the surviving cells per circumference of jejunum counted and plotted against the total dose for each regimen. In the continuous radiation schemas, average dose rates of 4.2 Gy/hr and 0.7 Gy/hr were used. For both of the pulsed schedules, average dose rates of 0.7 Gy/hr were used, with one pulse delivered in 10 minutes, one in 1 minute. The cell survival curves were identical for the continuous 0.7 Gy/hr and the 10-minute pulse of 0.7 Gy/hr. The shorter pulse duration of 1 minute (a 10-fold increase in dose rate), resulted in only a 3%– 4% shift in the cell survival curve to the left of the curve for the 10-minute pulse.

Martinez et al.[10] have carried out trials using Wistar rats subjected to pulsed and continuous brachytherapy schedules via transrectal applicators for comparisons of the early and late effects on normal rectal tissue. Total doses, duration of intraluminal applications, and average dose rates per hour were kept identical between the two treatment groups. Additional groups of animals were treated with a combination of external beam and brachytherapy to more closely recreate the clinical situation. The results of these initial studies are not yet published.

Clinical Results

The PDR remote afterloading units became available on the market in 1991 so that there is little clinical data to date. Between February 16, 1992 and April 22, 1994, 63 brachytherapy procedures were carried out in 56 patients using the Pulsed Low-Dose-Rate Selectron at the University of California at San Francisco. Any patient who was considered appropriate for standard afterloading brachytherapy procedures utilizing cesium-137 or iridium-192 in a continuous LDR fashion regardless of site, histology, or prior radiation was eligible for this study. For interstitial implants, MR scanning was routinely utilized in the preplanning stage to determine the number of needles or catheters necessary to uniformly cover the treatment volume with spacing of 1.0–1.2 cm between needles (Figures 4–6). The depth and lateral extent of coverage needed was also determined from the MR images. Standard stereo-shift images were obtained with the needles/catheters in place for dosimetric planning. Optimization was then carried out to conform the isodose lines to the geometry of the tumor. Based on the suggestions of Brenner, Hall, Fowler, and Mount, a single

pulse was administered every hour in a 24-hour period until the prescribed dose was delivered. When possible, treatment volume dose rates of between 40–80 cGy/hr were selected to approximate rates standardly used in continuous LDR procedures.

Twenty-six intracavitary procedures were performed as well as 28 perineal interstitial templates, eight interstitial catheters in other sites, and four intraluminal placements for esophageal and nasopharyngeal malignancies. Fifty patients had brachytherapy as a portion of their treatment for primary disease, and nine for recurrent disease (Table 1). Seven of the 59 patients had received prior radiation to the implanted area. Nine patients received concomitant chemotherapy, five concurrent hyperthermia, and eight pro-

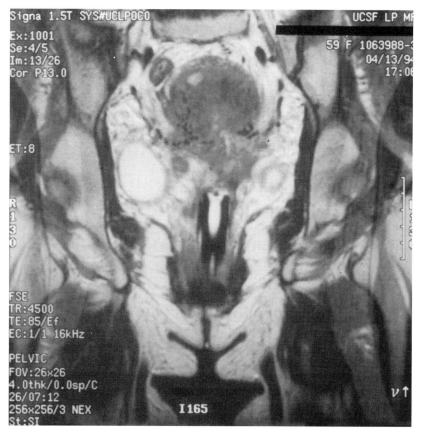

Figure 4. Coronal MR scan of stage IIIB cervix tumor, s/p 4000 cGy external beam therapy plus concomitant 5FU/platinum, with template and obturator in place for preplanning of perineal interstitial template placement.

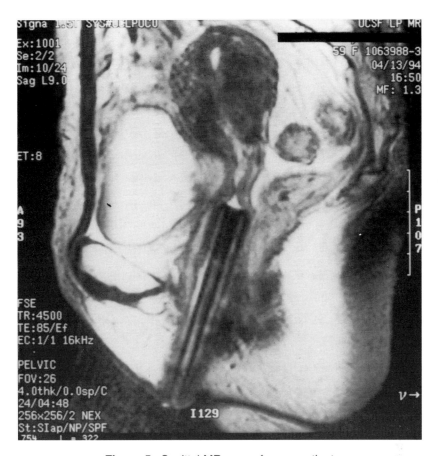

Figure 5. Sagittal MR scan of same patient.

ceeded to postradiation surgery as part of their planned course of treatment.

Total radiation doses ranged from 4000–10,000 cGy, with the brachytherapy doses to the prescribed region ranging from 500–6000 cGy. Mean follow-up was short at 7.4 months, and the initial report deals mainly with the incidence of acute toxicity, although some information is available on the late toxicity. Four acute or subacute complications requiring therapeutic intervention occurred for an incidence of 4/59 or 7%, an incidence similar to that seen with standard continuous LDR procedures. Two of these cases were patients with recurrent disease, who had received prior courses of radiation.

Six cases of delayed complications have been recorded: one esophageal stricture in a patient found later to have recurrent disease; two cases of soft tissue radionecrosis (primary oral tongue, recurrent neck node); a perineal pain syndrome requiring prolonged narcotics after perineal template; chronic cystitis with hematuria in the setting of HIV disease; a delayed wound infection requiring oral antibiotics and aggressive skin care after a cumulative dose of 10,000 cGy for recurrent sarcoma of the deltoid (4000 from the current implant, 6000 cGy external beam delivered 3 years prior); and a small fracture in the humerus at 6-months posttreatment in this same patient.

There does not appear to be any significant increase in acute toxicity associated with the pulsed approach when compared with the standard continuous LDR approach in the early results of this clinical study. It is essential to point out, however, that this is true under the conditions outlined, namely, hourly pulses of 40–80 cGy. Extrapolation of these conclusions to higher dose rates or longer in-

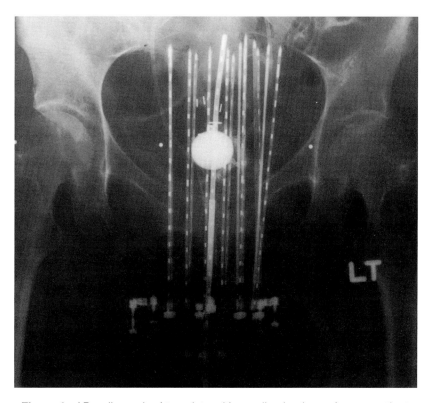

Figure 6. AP radiograph of template with needles in place of same patient.

Table 1.
Brachytherapy Procedures Performed at
UCSF Using the Pulsed Low-Dose-Rate
System, 1992-1994

Sites	Number
Cervix	37
Uterus	7
Tongue	4
Vagina	4
Esophagus	1
Rectum	2
Sarcoma	1
Breast	1
Neck node	1
Nasopharynx	1
Procedures	
Intracavitary	29
Templates	27
Catheters	7
Primary	47
Recurrent	12

UCSF = University of California at San Francisco.

tervals with increased doses per pulse cannot safely be made as indicated by radiobiological data.

Additional early information is available from centers in Toronto, Canada,[11] Sydney, Australia,[12] Kiel, Germany,[13] and Ghent, Belgium,[14] suggesting that the early complication rate with PDR is similar to that seen with conventional LDR therapy.

Future Directions

Further information must be accrued to show that the late toxicity of this treatment approach is similar to that seen with the continuous LDR regimens. An absence of appreciable increase in acute toxicity cannot be construed as proof that long-term toxicity will be acceptable. Further clinical studies must be carried out. An alternate approach is being investigated by Levendag (P. Levendag, personal communication) at the den Hoed Cancer Center in Rotterdam, using larger pulse sizes separated by 3-hour intervals, with 4–8 fractions per day. Such a schedule allows the physician to treat several patients concurrently with a single machine, disconnecting each individual patient between pulses. Results of this approach are not yet available. Great caution must be exercised in utilizing this approach due to the predicted loss in therapeutic ratio with increasing pulse intervals. Other investigational directions include increasing the dose per pulse while maintaining the same pulse interval, thereby shortening the overall duration of the implant.

References

1. Brenner DJ, Hall EJ. Conditions for the equivalence of continuous to pulsed low dose rate brachytherapy. Int J Radiat Oncol Biol Phys 1991;20(1):181–190.
2. Lea DE, Catcheside DG. The mechanisms of the induction by radiation of chromosome aberrations in tradescantia. J Genetics 1942;44:216–245.
3. Fowler JF. Why shorter half-times of repair lead to greater damage in pulsed brachytherapy. Int J Radiat Oncol Biol Phys 1993;26(2):353–356.
4. Hall EJ. Weiss lecture. The dose-rate factor in radiation biology. Int J Radiat Biol 1991;59(3):595–610.
5. Hall EJ, Brenner DJ. The dose-rate effect revisited: Radiobiological considerations of importance in radiotherapy. Int J Radiat Oncol Biol Phys 1991;21(6):1403–1414.
6. Hall EJ, Brenner DJ. The dose-rate effect in interstitial brachytherapy: A controversy resolved. Br J Radiol 1992;65:242–247.
7. Fowler J, Mount M. Pulsed brachytherapy: The conditions for no significant loss of therapeutic ratio compared with traditional low dose rate brachytherapy. Int J Radiat Oncol Biol Phys 1992;23(3):661–669.
8. Armour E, Wang ZH, Corry P, et al. Equivalence of continuous and pulse simulated low dose rate irradiation in 9L gliosarcoma cells at 37 degrees and 41 degrees C. Int J Radiat Oncol Biol Phys 1992;22(1):109–114.
9. Mason KA, Thames HD, Ochran TG, et al. Comparison of continuous and pulsed low dose rate brachytherapy: Biological equivalence in vivo. Int J Radiat Oncol Biol Phys 1994;28(3):667–671.
10. Martinez AA, White J, Armour E, et al. Continuous versus pulsed LDR: Preliminary analysis of rat rectal toxicity. In: Mould RF (ed). Brachytherapy from Radium to Optimization. Nucletron International B.V., Netherlands, 1994, pp. 260–269.
11. McLean M. Initial PDR brachytherapy experience at Toronto, Canada. Act Int Nucl Radiother J 1994;6–10.
12. Adler GF, Karolis C, Kramer W, et al. Initial PDR experience at Sydney, Australia. Act Int Nucl Radiother J 1994;11–14.
13. Kovacs G, Kohr P, Zimmermann J, et al. Initial PDR experience at Kiel, Germany. Act Int Nucl Radiother J 1994;15–21.
14. van Eijkeren M. Initial PDR experience at Ghent, Belgium. Act Int Nucl Radioth J 1994;22–23.

—— Chapter 34 ——————————————

Interstitial Thermo-Brachytherapy

Christopher T. Coughlin, M.D., FACP, FACR

Introduction

Interstitial implant techniques are a mainstay of treatment options within the field of radiation oncology. The implantation techniques involve the uniform spacing and placement of a variety of radioactive materials directly within a tumor mass. Virtually any primary site within the body can be implanted with proper surgical assistance and careful placement of silastic catheters throughout a tumor volume. The energy of the isotope utilized for the implant governs both the distance between catheters and the number of catheters used for provision of a uniform isodose distribution. Iridium-192 has become a popular isotope for implantation techniques. Iridium's 340-keV gamma ray emission dictates that a uniform dose distribution can be obtained by separating catheters by 0.5–1.0 cm. This coupled with a 74.5-day half-life enables the implant to be left in place for several days without significant decay of activity. Other isotopes have been used clinically but few have the advantages and simplicity of iridium-192.

Hyperthermia is a modality that utilizes heat to obtain selective tumor cell kill. A relative therapeutic window of between 42.5°C and 45°C has tantalized clinicians for years. If heat can be delivered closely in time with radiation, the hyperthermia has been noted to be synergistic with the irradiation cell killing effect. The difficulty has been development of delivery systems with adequate control to adequately heat a tumor volume uniformly for a requisite period of time.

Methods

Three major types of interstitial hyperthermia systems have been developed for clinical use. These include interstitial microwave hyperthermia, interstitial radiofrequency hyperthermia, and interstitial ferromagnetic seeds.

Microwave Hyperthermia

Interstitial microwave antennas as a means of providing localized hyperthermia arose in the late 1970s and early 1980s. Microwave power source can operate at frequencies between 433 and 2450 MHz. From the power source there is a power divider and a set of power controllers that deliver microwave energy to each of a variety of antennas that can be implanted with standard brachytherapy technique (Figure 1). Clinically, these antennas are normally inserted into catheters that have been implanted in a tumor (Figure 2). In practice these catheters are the same ones used in brachytherapy, making the hyperther-

From Nag S (ed): *Principles and Practice of Brachytherapy.* © Futura Publishing Co., Inc., Armonk, NY, 1997.

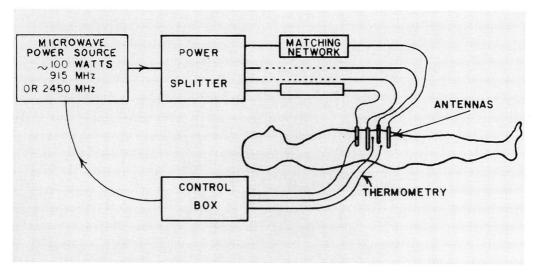

Figure 1. Schematic diagram of an Interstitial Microwave Antenna Array Hyperthermia (IMAAH) system with thermometry and feedback control to the power source.

mia compatible with the brachytherapy treatment. The temperature in the tumor volume is measured by a set of censors that feed the temperature information into a thermometry system. The temperature information is used to set the power levels going to each antenna automatically. The most common clinically useful frequency is 915 MHz. The radiation pattern along the longitudinal direction of an antenna is on the order of one-half wavelength in tissue. Therefore, different frequencies give longer or shorter heating patterns depending upon the power source used. Typical half wavelengths are 2.5 cm at 2450 MHz, 7 cm at 915 MHz, and 12 cm at 433 MHz. The majority of tumors that are implanted in clinical practice are in the 4- to 8-cm range, making the 915 MHz the most widely used.

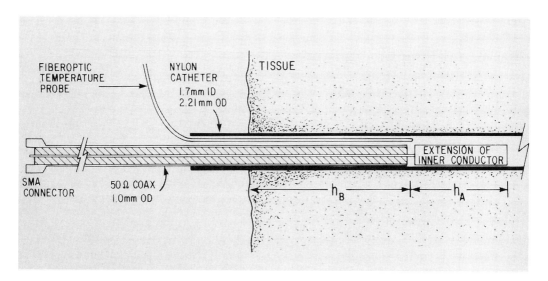

Figure 2. Schematic diagram of an antenna and its insertion into tissue with thermometry.

The power from the microwave generator goes through a power divider that splits the power to each antenna. The number of antennas that can be independently controlled range from 1–24. With the 915-MHz configuration the power from the divider then passes to the power controller, which sets the power to each antenna independently. The feedback thermometry power loop for this system allows automatic regulation of the power to each antenna on a second-by-second basis. This allows careful thermal configuration throughout a tumor volume that has heterogeneous blood flow. Since blood flow acts as a heat sink, poorly vascularized areas of a tumor heat with greater ease than well vascularized areas. The ability to have real time feedback to the power source is a major advantage for thermal configuration.

An alternative is to use a number of independent microwave power sources. If the number of antennas is equal to or less than the number of power sources, each antenna can be driven independently. If the number of antennas is greater than the number of power sources, each source can drive two or more antennas with groups of antennas under independent control. In the majority of systems the independent power sources are driven from a single oscillator, maintaining the "coherence" of the system.

Key to this type of system is the type of antenna utilized. Considerable effort has been expended in antenna design to allow shaping power deposition within tissue. The majority of antennas developed have been coaxial cables with an extension of the inner conductor on one end (Figure 3). The use of an electrically insulating catheter is essential to control power deposition. The length of the extension of the inner conductor (h_a) and the distance from the junction of the inner and outer conductor to the insertion point is h_b. The overall insertion depth of the antenna is $h_a + h_b$. The power deposition characteristics of each antenna are very sensitive to changes in these lengths. For example, the wall thickness of the catheter in which the antennas are implanted or the insertion depth alters the power distribution pattern in tissue. This is important as power deposition and temperature patterns produced may be considerably

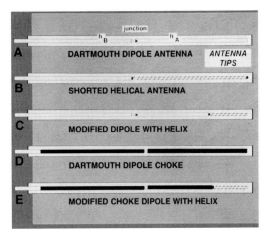

Figure 3. Schematic diagram of several antenna designs to preferentially manipulate power deposition.

different than one would expect. This would result in a poor heat treatment.

The theoretical and experimental power deposition patterns for both single antennas and various arrays have been well documented.[37] The specific absorption rate or power deposited per unit mass of tissue is called the SAR. The theoretical and experimental power deposition must be understood before implementation in the clinic. With a simple four element, 2x2 cm square array of 915-MHz antennas, the SAR pattern in the transverse plane perpendicular to the junction of each antenna reveals the coherent addition of the longitudinal component of the electric fields. This maximum SAR value is in the center of the array. The 50% contour is well inside this 2x2 cm square array. This distribution is particularly useful when combining hyperthermia delivery with iridium-192 irradiation. This longitudinal SAR pattern is very sensitive to the insertion depth for each antenna. Freely translated this means that for deep implants, there may be significant heating of the antenna backwards towards the insertion point. This can be adequately corrected with the appropriate preplanning so that the heat delivery can be optimally configured. An entire array of antennas have been designed to improve power deposition both near the tip of each antenna and along the length of each antenna.

Microwave hyperthermia techniques have been used in the clinical setting since the early 1980s. The majority of series that have been reported have used microwave antennas with a 915-MHz power source. The active length of heating is on the order of 5–7 cm in tissue. Typical implants would involve between 1–20 interstitial antennas and compatible thermometry devices. The ability to heat smaller tumors can be accomplished with a 2450-MHz power supply. This is particularly useful in brain implants. Masses with a cross-sectional diameter of approximately 5 cm can be adequately heated with five antennas, one in each corner of a box array with a central antenna. The corners of the array can be placed 0.5–1 cm within the margin of a tumor volume. This arrangement allows at most a 2-cm separation between antennas. Thermometry that can then be recorded at a variety of points within each catheter and at many points along a central catheter. A perpendicular catheter can be placed to allow further three-dimensional thermal mapping. This allows extensive thermal profiles to better describe heat distribution within the target volume. Single point thermometry is to be discouraged as virtually useless to describe the adequacy of a thermal treatment.

Most programs have utilized a target dose of 42°–43°C for 60 minutes. It is important to describe this target temperature through as many points in the tumor volume as is feasible. Proper thermal mapping will allow more adequate evaluation of the efficacy of a given treatment. This can be quantitated through a hyperthermia equipment performance rating (HEP). This defines the percentage of the tumor volume in which some specific thermal end-point was achieved. Unless this is done it is impossible to adequately correlate response rate with thermal delivery patterns.

There are several advantages to an implantable microwave system. It is compatible with the plastic catheters and brachytherapy techniques that are standard within the field of radiation oncology. Power can be deposited in tissue at some distance from the antennas and it has relatively few sources that need to be inserted to heat a region adequately. The actual dosimetry is governed by the separation of the catheters necessary to deliver a uniform iridium dose. A feedback control system provides better thermal distribution and power deposition than with other techniques. This feedback control to the power supply can be varied at each antenna dynamically during a treatment. Clinically there are relatively few disadvantages to this type of system. One potential disadvantage is in the use of deep-seated implants. There may be heating in fixed points along the shaft of the microwave antennas. This can be determined by measuring thermal dose at several points outside the tumor volume along the axis of the antenna. Particular care must be addressed to overheating an area where the antenna exits from the skin.

Most implants are left in place from 4–7 days in order to deliver the prescribed radiation dose. This allows sufficient time to elapse so that thermal tolerance is not a significant issue in this setting. Interstitial techniques allow relatively uniform heating within the implant volume, multipoint thermometry to define thermal mapping more accurately, and sparing of normal tissue, because the area implanted is the same as that to which the hyperthermia is delivered. Microwave antennas are compatible with standard brachytherapy techniques and can be used to deal with a wide variety of clinical circumstances. In development of antennas with insertion depth—independent heating has helped considerably in the clinic. A "family of antennas" can be obtained commercially such that with adequate preplanning, a useful therapeutic hyperthermia session can be administered for the majority of clinical situations that arise. Adequate three-dimensional heating and irradiation patterns can be accomplished.

Radiofrequency

Another type of interstitial heating involves the use of radiofrequency voltage between pairs of needle electrodes. This technique was described in the mid-1970s and in its simplest form involves two parallel planes of electrodes implanted on opposite sides of a tumor. Radiofrequency voltage is then applied between the two planes. Frequencies typically between 500 kHz and 13 MHz have been used. While the frequency is not very critical it does need to be high enough to avoid other biological effects in addition to heating, for example, depolarization of muscle or nerve fibers.

From a conceptual standpoint this system is similar to placing two capacitive electrode plates on opposite sides of a tumor mass and applying an hour of voltage between the two plates. The RF voltage across the resistive tumor creates an RF current in the tumor volume. This RF current causes joule heating and, hence, a rise in temperature. The interstitial needle system is similar except that the plates are replaced by planes of needles implanted on each side of the tumor volume. While the primary current path is between the two planes of needles, there are some important differences. Because these needles typically have a small diameter (approximately 1 mm), the currents must diverge from these small sources. Therefore, the current density in the neighborhood of the electrodes is very high. This high current density produces very high absorbed power density or SAR near the electrodes. As a result, thermal conduction is necessary for a smooth temperature distribution. In regions of very high blood flow there will tend to be large temperature gradients near the needles. To overcome this effect, implanting the electrodes at no more than 1 cm apart is practiced in the clinic.

To ensure a uniform temperature distribution it is important to keep the needles absolutely parallel to one another. If the needles either diverge or converge the current density will be much higher where the needles are close together resulting in overheating that area. Conversely they will be underheating in areas where the needles diverge.

Systems designed for clinical use are considerably more complicated than for microwave use. First, thermometry associated with this system requires extra needles to be inserted close to the electrodes for adequate thermal monitoring. Second, the needles are rigid and cannot be used to configure complex geometry adequately. Third, a simple two plane implant is rarely optimal for most clinical settings. One way to overcome the large temperature gradients has been to design a control system that controls power deposition at several points along each electrode. A "time-multiplex" system controls the voltage across pairs of electrodes. With this system the amount of time across any pair is con-

trolled with the object of maintaining the same temperature in the neighborhood of any pair of electrodes. A switching system that can connect across any two of the implanted electrode pairs has been developed through the use of complex computer algorithms.

The first electrodes developed were stainless steel needles that deposited power all along the length of the needle. This system was inadequate to implant tumors several centimeters below the skin. This problem was resolved by insulating the needle to the requisite depth. The insulation can be removed in the area of the tumor. Another problem with stainless steel needles is that they are rigid and can be very painful in the nonsedated patient. More flexible electrodes have been developed for use in the clinic. Electrodes have been developed that allow the use of radioactive seeds to be integrated into their use. Most of the clinically available resistive diathermy systems utilize radiofrequency currents in the range of 0.5–1 MHz. These electric currents are driven between pairs or arrays of implanted metallic needles. Virtually all reported implanted sites have been superficial with a typical distribution of 10–12 needles in at least two planes. Adequate hyperthermia treatments can be delivered and adequate multipoint thermal mapping has replaced single point temperature distribution. It is more difficult to obtain multiple point thermal mapping with the metallic needle system as many additional catheters need to be placed within a tumor volume.

Patient tolerance can be difficult with rigid steel needles although more flexible second generation applicators have been developed. The geometry of a tumor volume may pose some difficulty with RF heating as it does require the electrodes to be in parallel for adequate, uniform heating. While this system is easier to engineer than a microwave system, it has limited flexibility for clinical use. The substantial increase in the number of wires and thermometry probes may make a treatment session somewhat awkward for adequate hyperthermia control.

Ferromagnetic

A third alternative for interstitial hyperthermia has been the use of implantable ferromagnetic seeds. A patient can be placed in a large magnetic coil. This will create eddy currents that can be induced in the seeds that will produce a rise in temperature. Heat will then flow into the surrounding tissue due to thermal conduction. An advantage to this technique is that once the seeds are implanted, they can be heated noninvasively and at multiple times. The temperature rise in the seeds is proportional to a number of factors that include the strength of the magnetic field, the ferromagnetic material used, and separation of the seeds within the implant volume. Seeds have been developed whose Curie point is near the therapeutic temperature range. This material is alloyed with radioactive material and is compatible with dosimetry utilized with iodine-125. Curie point heating could self-adjust the heat deposition at all depths. A uniform seed distribution should be able to deliver uniform heating regardless of variable cooling provided that the seed distribution is of sufficient density within the tumor mass. Separation of the seeds by more than a few millimeters in each direction would result in cold spots within the tumor volume. As the tumor shrinks, this volume would be brought closer together and increase the efficiency and subsequent efficacy of a heat treatment. No external heat source connections are necessary. The seeds are permanent surgical implants and require only one manipulation with no other invasive procedures. Many heatings can be delivered over a long period of time. There is no restriction as to the actual number of heat sessions so that patient tolerance can be maximized. The dose along the seed implant would be uniform regardless of depth. Heat delivery is cylindrical as well as axially symmetrical and is independent of local tissue electrical properties. Trials with these techniques have been reported with very encouraging results.

This technique does have some disadvantages. First, there is no power deposited between the seeds. In order to change power deposition the spacing between the seeds would have to be manipulated. In general this would require spacing of <1 cm between seeds in each direction. Pretreatment planning is critical in this situation to optimize the number of sources and the potential temperature distributions. These cannot be adjusted once the seeds are in place. If thermal distributions were inadequate it would be impossible to redistribute the seeds. There is no real-time power control of individual seeds except through the Curie point regulation. If the heat treatment causes considerable pain, there would be no way to manipulate this during a treatment session. Electromagnetic shielding in a room is required due to the strong magnetic fields necessary to reach therapeutic temperature. This type of equipment is not portable and requires a higher initial investment. A high number of seeds would be required to cover a given tumor volume. For example, a 5x5x5 cm mass may require as many as 150 seeds with uniform spacing for adequate coverage. There is no way to correct for seed migration after completion of the implant. As a tumor mass shrinks, the system would become more efficient by bringing the seeds closer together.

Planning systems have been developed to optimize the use of multiple temperature ferromagnetic seeds within an array. However, the treatment plan would remain static over time and it would be impossible to correct for changes in blood flow. It is possible to place these seeds within catheters or strings that can be removed once a treatment is complete. This allows some degree of manipulation of thermal distribution over time.

Results

The ability to control various implantable tumors are listed below. Only complete responses are indicated. Partial responses are meaningless. Certain locations do not permit classic evaluation of complete versus partial response, i.e., brain or biliary. Responses are usually determined 3 months postimplant.

Table 1 indicates the extensive experience with microwave technology.[1–22] Most response rates are between 50%–90%. The results of radiofrequency heating (Table 2) are comparable and any decrement in tumor control may reflect difficulty in keeping the sources parallel.[23–33] Ferromagnetic technology has evolved recently (Table 3).[34–36]

Discussion

Each of the techniques described above has widespread applicability, but each is labor in-

Table 1.
Clinical Experience with Interstitial Microwave Hyperthermia

Authors & Year of Study	No. of Patients	Power (MHz)	Tumors Responses Complete %	Target Dose °C/min	No. of Sessions
Coughlin,[1] 1983	7	915	—	42°C/60 min	2
Salcman,[2] 1983	6	2450	—	—	1–2
Strohbehn,[3] 1984	6	915	(3) 50	42.5°C/60 min	2
Coughlin,[4] 1985	6	915	—	43°C/60 min	2
Emami,[5] 1985	24	915	(17) 71	42.5°C/60 min	1–2
Puthawala,[6] 1985	43	915	(32) 74	41–43°C/60 min	1–2
Roberts,[7] 1986	6	915	—	42.5°C/60 min	2
Roberts,[8] 1987	14	915	—	42.5°C/60 min	2
Emami,[9] 1987	46	915	(26) 57	42°C/60 min	1–2
Coughlin,[10] 1988	58	915	—	43°C/60 min	2
Lam,[11] 1988	27	915/630	(19) 70	42.5°C/45-60 min	1–2
Seegenschmiedt,[12] 1990	215	915	60	42.5°C/60 min	2
Sneed,[13] 1991	28	915/2450	—	42.5°C/30 min	2
Strohmaier,[14] 1991	20	915	—	42°C/60 min	4
Coughlin,[15] 1992	10	915	—	42.5°C/60 min	2
Sneed,[16] 1992	48	915	—	42.5°C/30 min	2
Kaplan,[17] 1992	15	—	—	<45°C/60 min	1
Seegenschmiedt,[18] 1993	26	915	76	41–44°C/60 min	2
Prevost,[19] 1993	24	915	84	—	1–2
Nakajima,[20] 1993	23	915	—	42°C/60 min	2
Seegenschmiedt,[21] 1994	90	915	66	41°C/60 min	2
Schreiber,[22] 1995	36	915	(93) 86	42°C/45 min	2

Table 2.
Clinical Experience with Industrial Radiofrequency Hyperthermia

Authors & Year of Study	No. of Patients	Power (MHz)	Tumor Responses Complete %	Temperature (°C/min)	No. of Sessions
Joseph,[23] 1981	7	0.5	(1) 14	41–43°C/30 min	1–2
Manning,[24] 1981	17	0.5–3	(12) 71	42.5–43°C/30 min	1–2
Oleson,[25] 1982–84	52	0.5	(20) 38	42°C/30 min	1–2
Vora,[26] 1982	16	0.5	(11) 69	41–45°C/30–40 min	1–2
Cosset,[27] 1984	11/14	0.5	(10) 91	44°C/45 min	1–2
Yabumoto,[28] 1984	7	0.5	(1) 14	—	1–2
Cosset,[29] 1985	29	0.5	(19) 66	44°C/45 min	1–2
Emami,[5] 1985	6	0.5	(5) 83	—	1–2
Vora,[30] 1988	19	0.5	(10) 53	42–43°C/30 min	1–2
Seegenschmiedt,[12] 1990	299	0.5	57	42.5°C/60 min	2
Shimm,[31] 1990	72	0.5	36	42°C/30 min	1–2
Koga,[32] 1993	6	8	—	—	
Prionas,[33] 1994	36	0.5	—	43°C/45 min	2

Table 3.
Clinical Experience with Interstitial Ferromagnetic Seeds

Authors & Year of Study	No. Patients	Tumor Responses Complete %	Target Dose °C/min	No. Sessions
Kobayashi,[34] 1991	25	—	—	many
Mack,[35] 1994	44	61	42°C/60 min	2
Stea,[36] 1994	25	—	42°C/60 min	2

tensive and requires considerable support for proper use. In experienced hands, interstitial hyperthermia offers adjunctive and often synergistic treatment to a wide variety of cancers. Do the benefits outweigh the cost? This question will only be answered as properly constructed multi-institutional clinical trials continue to mature.

Conclusion

Interstitial techniques for the delivery of hyperthermia have become very sophisticated in spite of the adverse clinical outcomes as reported by the RTOG. The European and Asian experience has been considerably more optimistic and this may relate to more compulsive control of hyperthermia equipment performance.

Extensive quality control and equipment performance characteristics have been developed in this country.[38] This has allowed the field to continue to develop though at a slower rate than in the early 1980s. As European data matures, enthusiasm for interstitial hyperthermia in this country may once again improve. Compatibility with standard brachytherapy techniques makes this an attractive supplement to currently utilized interstitial techniques.

References

1. Coughlin CT, Douple EB, Strohbehn JW, et al. Interstitial microwave-induced hyperthermia in combination with brachytherapy. Radiology 1983;148:285–288.
2. Salcman M, Samaras GM. Interstitial microwave hyperthermia for brain tumors. J Neuro-Oncol 1983;1:225–236.
3. Strohbehn JW, Douple EB. Hyperthermia and cancer therapy: A review of biomedical engineering contributions and challenges. IEEE Trans Biomed Eng BME 1984;31:779–787.
4. Coughlin CT, Wong TZ, Strohbehn JW, et al. Intraoperative interstitial microwave-induced hyperthermia and brachytherapy. Int J Radiat Oncol Biol Phys 1985;11:1673–1678.
5. Emami B, Perez A. Interstitial thermoradiotherapy: An overview. Hyperthermia Oncol 1985;1:35–40.
6. Puthawala AA, Nisar Syed AM, Sheikh KMA, et al. Interstitial hyperthermia for recurrent malignancies. Endocurie/Hypertherm Oncol 1985;1:125–131.
7. Roberts DW, Coughlin CT, Wong TZ, et al. Interstitial hyperthermia and iridium brachytherapy in treatment of malignant glioma. A phase I clinical trial. J Neurosurg 1986;64:581–587.
8. Roberts DW, Strohbehn JW, Coughlin CT, et al. Iridium-192 brachytherapy in combination with interstitial microwave-induced hyperthermia for malignant glioma. Appl Neurophysiol 1987;50:287–291.
9. Emami B, Perez C, Leybovich L, et al. Interstitial thermoradiotherapy in treatment of malignant tumours. Int J Hypertherm 1987;3(2):107–118.
10. Coughlin CT, Strohbehn JW, Ryan TP, et al. Interstitial hyperthermia for deep-seated malignancies. Presented at the Fifth International Hyperthermia Meeting, Kyoto, August, 1988.
11. Lam K, Astrahan M, Langholz B. Interstitial thermoradiotherapy for recurrent or persistent tumours. Int J Hypertherm 1988;4:259–266.
12. Seegenschmiedt MH, Brady LW, Sauer R. Interstitial thermoradiotherapy: Review on technical and clinical aspects. Am J Clin Oncol 1990;13(4):352–363.
13. Sneed PK, Stauffer PR, Gutin PH, et al. Interstitial irradiation and hyperthermia for the treatment of recurrent malignant brain tumors. Neurosurgery 1991;28(2):206–215.
14. Strohmaier WL, Bichler KH, Bocking A, et al. Histological effects of local microwave hyperthermia in prostatic cancer. Int J Hypertherm 1991;7(1):27–33.
15. Coughlin CT, Wong TZ, Ryan TP, et al. Intersti-

tial microwave-induced hyperthermia and iridium brachytherapy for the treatment of obstructing biliary carcinomas. Int J Hypertherm 1992;8(2):157–171.

16. Sneed PK, Gutin PH, Stauffer PR, et al. Thermoradiotherapy of recurrent malignant brain tumors. Int J Radiat Oncol Biol Phys 1992;23(4): 853–861.

17. Kaplan SA, Shabsigh R, Soldo KA, et al. Prostatic and periprostatic interstitial temperature measurements in patients treated with transrectal thermal therapy (local intracavitary microwave hyperthermia). J Urol 1992;147(6): 1562–1565.

18. Seegenschmiedt MH, Sauer R, Miyamoto C, et al. Clinical experience with interstitial thermoradiotherapy for localized implantable pelvic tumors. Am J Clin Oncol 1993;16(3):210–222.

19. Prevost B, De Cordoue-Rohart S, Mirabel X, et al. 915 MHz microwave interstitial hyperthermia. Part III: Phase II clinical results [published erratum appears in Int J Hypertherm 9(4):625, 1993]. Int J Hyperthermia 1993;9(3):455–462.

20. Nakajima T, Roberts DW, Ryan TP, et al. Pattern of response to interstitial hyperthermia and brachytherapy for malignant intracranial tumour: A CT analysis. Int J Hypertherm 1993; 9(4):491–502.

21. Seegenschmiedt MH, Martus P, Fletkau R, et al. Multivariate analysis of prognostic parameters using interstitial thermoradiotherapy (IHT-IRT): Tumor and treatment variables predict outcome. Int J Radiat Oncol Biol Phys 1994; 29(5):1049–1063.

22. Schreiber DP, Overett TK. Interstitial hyperthermia and iridium-192 treatment alone vs. interstitial iridium-192 treatment/hyperthermia and low dose cisplatinum infusion in the treatment of locally advanced head and neck malignancies. Int J Radiat Oncol Biol Phys 1995; 33(2):429–436.

23. Joseph C, Astrahan M, Lipsett J, et al. Interstitial hyperthermia and interstitial iridium-192 implantation: A technique and preliminary results. Int J Radiat Oncol Biol Phys 1981;7: 827–833.

24. Manning MR, Cetas TC, Miller RC. Clinical hyperthermia: Results of a phase I trial employing hyperthermia alone or in combination with external beam or interstitial radiotherapy. Cancer 1982;49:205–216.

25. Oleson JR, Sim DA, Manning MR. Analysis of prognostic variables in hyperthermia treatment of 161 patients. Int J Radiat Oncol Biol Phys 1984;10:2231–2239.

26. Vora N, Forell B, Joseph C, et al. Interstitial

implant with interstitial hyperthermia. Cancer 1982;50:2518–2523.

27. Cosset JM, Dutreix J, Dufour J, et al. Combined interstitial hyperthermia and brachytherapy: Institut Gustave Roussy technique and preliminary results. Int J Radiat Oncol Biol Phys 1984; 10:307–312.

28. Yabumoto E, Suyama S. In: Overgaard J (ed). Hyperthermic Oncology. Summary Papers, Vol 1. Taylor & Francis, London, 1984, p. 579.

29. Cosset JM, Dutreix Haie C, et al. Interstitial thermoradiotherapy: A technical and clinical study of 29 implantations performed at the Institut Gustave-Roussy. Int J Hypertherm 1985; 1:3–13.

30. Vora N, Luk K, Forell B, et al. Interstitial local current field hyperthermia for advanced cancers of the cervix. Endocurie/Hypertherm Oncol 1988;4:97–106.

31. Shimm DS, Kittelson JM, Oleson JR, et al. Interstitial thermoradiotherapy: Thermal dosimetry and clinical results. Int J Radiat Oncol Biol Phys 1990;18(2):383–387.

32. Koga H, Mori K, Tokunaga Y. Interstitial radiofrequency hyperthermia for brain tumors—Preliminary laboratory studies and clinical application. Neurol Med Chir (Tokyo) 1993;33(5):290–294.

33. Prionas SD, Kapp DS, Goffinet DR, et al. Thermometry of interstitial hyperthermia given as an adjuvant to brachytherapy for the treatment of carcinoma of the prostate. Int J Radiat Oncol Biol Phys 1994;28(1):151–162.

34. Kobayashi T, Kida Y. Interstitial hyperthermia of malignant brain tumors by an implant heating system using stereotactic techniques. Stereotactic Functional Neurosurg 1992;59: 123–127.

35. Mack CF, Stea B, Kittelson JM, et al. Interstitial thermoradiotherapy with ferromagnetic implants for locally advanced and recurrent neoplasms [published errata appear in Int J Radiat Oncol Biol Phys 28(3):793, 1994 and 29(5): 1209, 1994]. Int J Radiat Oncol Biol Phys 1993; 27(1):109–115.

36. Stea B, Rossman K, Kittelson J, et al. Interstitial irradiation versus interstitial thermoradiotherapy for supratentorial malignant gliomas: A comparative survival analysis. Int J Radiat Oncol Biol Phys 1994;30(3):591–600.

37. Ryan TP. Comparison of six microwave antennas for hyperthermia treatment of cancer: SAR results for single antennas and arrays. Int J Radiat Oncol Biol Phys 1991;21:403–413.

38. Emami B, Stauffer P, Dewhirst MW, et al. RTOG quality assurance guidelines for interstitial hyperthermia. Int J Radiat Oncol Biol Phys 1991;20:1117–1124.

Californium-252 Neutron Brachytherapy

Yosh Maruyama, M.D., FACR,[†]
Jacek G. Wierzbicki, Ph.D., Boris M. Vtyurin, M.D., Ph.D.,
Koichi Kaneta, M.D.

History

Californium-252 (Cf) is a radioactive transplutonium isotope that spontaneously emits neutrons. This led to the clinical trials that have evaluated its use for human cancer therapy. Cf was first prepared at the University of California at Berkeley using the cyclotron to bombard curium targets with helium ions.[1] The isotope Cf-252 was first found in the debris of a thermonuclear explosion[2] and later artificially produced in nuclear reactors capable of delivering high fluxes of neutrons.[3] Shlea and Stoddard[4] in 1965 first proposed that Cf could be used for neutron therapy as an alternative source for interstitial or intracavitary brachytherapy. Its neutron emissions were reported in an Atomic Energy Commission Report (DP-986) entitled "Radiation Properties of Californium-252," which compiled the properties of the reactor produced Cf.[5,6] Boulogne and Evans[7] made the first Cf needle for medical usage with the source designed after a radium needle. Wright, Boulogne, Reinig, and Evans[8] carried out the first dosimetry studies published in 1967.

Study of Cf has been the result of interest in more effective methods for treating advanced, bulky, or radioresistant neoplasms. The studies have been pursued mainly in the United States, Japan, and Russia where the largest clinical experiences have been carried out.[9] The studies to date have uniformly shown high efficacy in controlling tumors and overcoming radioresistance. Unlike neutron beam therapy, there have not been problems with normal tissue tolerance and local tumor control has been much better than photon radiation as would be expected based on the radiobiology of neutrons.[10,11] However, the outcome of therapy of advanced neoplasms is dependent on effective adjuvant therapy for distant minimal or micrometastatic disease. Those studies are just beginning.

Cf therapy possesses the biological properties of fast neutrons but delivers a much more localized dose that is very effective because the sources are positioned in the tumor and not in normal tissue. Clinical trials have shown that Cf is very effective for tumor control and is especially effective against localized advanced neoplasms and produces high rates of 5-year survivals without significant problems with late complications or induced secondary malignant neoplasms.[12]

[†] deceased; see "In Memoriam," pp. 719–720.

From Nag S (ed): *Principles and Practice of Brachytherapy.* © Futura Publishing Co., Inc., Armonk, NY, 1997.

The initial clinical trials treated only a few patients with tumors, usually of advanced stage, recurrent or metastatic.[13] Nearly all the patients failed soon after treatment. The treatment they used was designed to match the schedules, dose rates, time durations as Ra-226 and dose equivalents (i.e., relevant biological effectiveness [RBE] adjusted to the same total dose).[14] Those methods used low-dose-rate, long hospitalizations, and exposed the hospital environment and personnel to the hazards of Cf exposure.[13] Cf-252 was soon abandoned as an isotope for human cancer therapy with broad conclusions drawn without benefit of phase 1, 2, or 3 trials or sufficient experience to draw any reasonable conclusions. The major finding of this period was that RBE was very high, about 6–7.5. All the initial investigators had given up their efforts after a few patients were treated by the early 1970s after beginning their studies in the late 1960s. The early termination of studies and the conclusions drawn were premature.

This initial era yielded important data on Cf neutron dosimetry and the research by Krishnaswamy,[15] Colvett et al.,[16] and the review by Anderson[17] were most important. A large number of radiobiological studies were also carried out to assess RBE, the oxygen enhancement ratio (OER), and numerous radiobiological studies of mammalian cells to Cf irradiation. The radiobiology has been reviewed by Kal et al.[18–20] and Feola and Maruyama,[21] but high RBEs and low OERs were generally reported.

Several groups in three countries (United States of America, Japan, and Russia) began studies and clinical trials in the early 1970s and carried out their research with virtually no interaction or communication as the studies were carried out in widely separated sites in the world with major language, political, and related difficulties.[22] The studies were conducted in Lexington KY, USA, Tokyo, Japan, and in the Former Soviet Union. These groups met in Lexington KY, USA in 1985 for the first time and exchanged their separate technological developments and clinical experiences with Cf brachytherapy.[9] Great efficacy had been found for cervix cancers of all stages but most notable for the advanced stage III[23] and bulky IB cancers.[24] Endometrial adenocarcinomas[25] and vaginal cancers[26] were also very

sensitive and curable with Cf. Oral cavity,[27,28] cancers of the tongue,[27–29] floor of mouth,[27,30] tonsil,[31] buccal mucosa,[30] lip,[32] and recurrent tumors[33] were effectively treated. Radioresistant tumors such as melanoma, sarcoma, and glioblastoma were eradicated by Cf neutron brachytherapy.[9] The rationale, methodology, clinical experiences, treatment planning, radiobiology, physics, and dosimetry will be reviewed in this chapter. To date there have been about 3000 patients treated with Cf brachytherapy around the world. This chapter summarizes the findings of the American, Japanese, and Russian workers. A second International Workshop held in Lexington KY in 1990[34] confirmed the efficacy, high cure rates, and low rate of problems with tissue tolerance or late secondary malignant neoplasms. However, there have been political and economic problems in Cf production and only a very limited supply of Cf available, hence there is slow progress in marketing and clinical trials.

Rationale for Neutron Brachytherapy

The reason interest in Cf started and has continued is because Cf represents a compact, intense source of neutrons that can be fabricated into tiny, highly radioactive sources suitable for medical therapy. Among the advantages that have fostered the interest are its radiobiological properties such as:

1. High RBE advantage of neutrons.[18,21]
2. Low OER.[18,20]
3. Little cell-cycle age-dependent changes in sensitivity.[35]
4. Little or no repair of sublethal or potentially lethal damage (SLD or PLD).[36]

In addition, further advantages have become evident with clinical evaluation. These include:

1. Rapid regression and shrinkage of bulky tumor masses.[37]
2. Small volume dose possible with brachytherapy.[11]
3. Conformal therapy inherent in brachytherapy.[38]
4. Effectiveness of added photon ther-

apy for local and regional tumor control.[11,12]

5. Tumor/normal tissue advantage of neutron brachytherapy (tumors are hypoxic and normal tissues are oxygenated; RBE of hypoxic cells is larger for tumor than for oxic cells).[39]

These advantages, which have become evident, could not have been discovered without conducting the long-term clinical trials. Still, further advantages became evident that were unexpected. These include:

1. Schedule-dependence in use of neutrons.[40,41] Clinical studies of Cf brachytherapy discovered that the use of high linear energy transfer (LET) therapy was effective versus radioresistance and directly attacked hypoxic/radioresistant cells.

2. The up-front use of neutrons[41] increased the radiosensitivity of the remaining tumor to photons suggesting reduced residual radioresistance and emergence of resistant clones.[42] Advanced cervix tumors were cured better by the up-front schedule.[43]

3. Low rates of normal tissue complications.[43]

4. Low or nondetectable rates of second malignant neoplasms (SMN) in long-term cured patients (about 20-year follow-up of treated patients).[43]

5. Potential use of thermal neutron capture for adjuvant therapy and dose-enhancement (boron has been used for boron-neutron capture enhancement [BNCE]).[44]

Early Californium-252 Clinical Trials

Several groups undertook the early clinical trials using Cf: The M.D. Anderson Hospital in Houston, Texas,[45] the Oxford Hospital in Oxford, England,[46] the Memorial Sloan Kettering Cancer Center in New York,[47] the Villejuif Cancer Center in Paris, France, and the Radiation Therapy Oncology Group (RTOG) in the United States. Although the number of institutions was large, very few patients were actually treated and only about 52 patients were reported.[13] Most patients treated had metastatic, persistent, or recurrent tumors that had had prior radiotherapy in many cases.[13] No single anatomical site received adequate study to draw any conclusions. Still, the initial clinical trials upon later review revealed that 39% of the primary tumors (not recurrent, persistent, or metastatic) had 5-year cures including advanced vaginal and cervix cancers and a liposarcoma that was unresectable (cured over 10 years).[13]

In the USA the MDAH group treated 22 patients as reported by Castro et al.[45] The RBE was initially felt to be 7.5, but later concluded to be about 6.5 based on tissue and tumor reactions. The Memorial Sloan Kettering treated ten tumors in nine patients. Vallejo et al.[47] reported that tumors regressed more rapidly than after Ir-192 interstitial therapy in lymph node metastases in their patients. They concluded that RBE was 6.4 relative to Ir-192.

In the United Kingdom, Oxford Hospital treated 21 patients using interstitial or plaque techniques. Paine et al.[46] noted that breast cancers were sensitive to Cf and that the response pattern was similar to Ir-192. They concluded that RBE was about 7.0. In Villejuif, Paris, France, dosimetry and physics studies were carried out.[48]

As noted above, conclusions were made based on skimpy data and were premature. At the present time, we appreciate that the successful trials had addressed radiation safety as one of their principal concerns and hence were able to treat a large number of patients adequately.[49] Retrospectively and with the emergence of high-dose-rate (HDR) brachytherapy, the problems of controlling the environment, personnel exposure, and the need for dedicated facilities has become evident but were dealt with by Cf workers to deliver Cf therapy in Lexington, Japan, and Russia.[9]

In Japan, two groups began studies: 1) at the Japan Cancer Institute Hospital (JCIH), Tokyo, Japan under the direction of Drs. Tsuya and Kaneta,[50] and 2) at the Keio Cancer Center,[51] Tokyo, under the direction of H. Yamashita. JCIH carried out extensive studies on facility, remote afterloading, safety, storage and treatment room design using low-dose-rate (LDR) methods.[52] Yamashita et al. carried out the first studies of HDR Cf therapy[51,53] and developed a room, a remote afterloading machine, and techniques for the clinical use of large sources of Cf (500–900 μg). While the sources available to Yamashita were too large in size for clinical usage (they were nuclear reactor starter sources) they did demonstrate that RBE was less at HDR and that long-term cures were feasible without unusual late effects. These studies showed that total control of exposure was achievable and in fact was mandated by their authorities as after the atomic bombings of Hiroshima and Nagasaki, there was great public fear of exposure to any radiation. It was, therefore, not possible to perform brachytherapy procedures without remote afterloading.

In the Former Soviet Union, the evaluation of neutron effects in humans was supported by the "All Union Scientific Program on Californium-252," which conducted a broad scientific program aimed to evaluate neutron effects at Moscow Oncological Research Center, the Institute of Medical Radiology in Obninsk,[27] and several other sites. The Obninsk Center designed facilities (an entire hospital wing) and conducted extensive studies of LDR interstitial and plaque therapy especially of head and neck cancers.[27] Extensive facility, and equipment and physics studies were carried out.[54,55] Moscow carried out studies on the development of a remote afterloader machine and its use in gynecological patients. Elisyutin and his colleagues[56] were especially instrumental in the design and development of a remote afterloader and study of dosimetry for HDR Cf therapy. In Dimitrovgrad, Karelin et al. collaborated closely with Vtyurin in the design and manufacture of sources appropriate for medical therapy.[57] The programs in Russia led to additional programs in Lithuania,[58] Czechoslovakia,[59] and Eastern Europe.

In Lexington KY, a very active program was developed and has carried out the largest single institutional clinical experience. Lexington conducted the most focused research into the therapy of GYN, and especially bulky or advanced stage cervix cancers, malignant gliomas, as well as, carried out radiobiological research into cell, acute, and late effects tissue radiobiology and human cancer radiobiology.[21] Their study of medium-dose-rate (MDR) Cf therapy,[49] facility and equipment design,[49] and feasibility and clinical studies have enhanced understanding of neutron therapy in general. Their successful efforts to bring the international workers together for workshops[9,34] broke the isolation that language, distance, economics, politics, and the cold war had imposed on Cf research to that time. The present review will focus primarily on the studies at the Keio, JCIH, Obninsk, Moscow, and Lexington, their experiences, and the methods developed for clinical usage.

Properties and Production

Production of Cf-252 requires very special nuclear reactors that are capable of producing high fluxes of neutrons.[3,60,61] In the USA, the High Flux Isotope Reactor (HFIR) at the Oak Ridge National Laboratory produces Cf-252 and is the only facility in the Western world. In Russia, the only site is the SM-3 (formerly SM-2) reactor in Dimitrovgrad.[57] The chemical separation and purification requires a Transuranium Processing Plant (TRU) in Oak Ridge, which carries out the procedures necessary to obtain pure Cf-252 that is then fabricated into sources for further usage. The high flux of neutrons allows the production of transplutonium elements through a chain of neutron absorptions and beta decay. Cf-252 is produced by the irradiation of plutonium-242 for 12–15 months followed by processing of the targets and recovery of the transplutonium isotopes. To prepare pure Cf-252 requires separation from Cm by ion exchange. For fabrication of medical sources, the Cf is deposited uniformly on a thin wire that can be cropped into segments for each medical source and the sources doubly encapsulated and sealed in medical applicator tubes (AT), afterloading cell (ALC), or short afterloading cell (SALC). In Dimitrovgrad, a large[62] variety of medical sources has been manufactured from small seeds to multiseed ribbons (flexible) and applicator tubes that contain milligram amounts of Cf.[57] The Oak Ridge sources are capable of containing up to 33, 20, 5, and 2.5 micrograms.

Californium-252 Physics and Dosimetry

The radiation emitted from Cf-252 contain both gamma rays and fast neutrons, i.e., they

Table 1.
^{252}CF Properties

Half-life	2.65 years
Neutron emission	2.31 × 10^{12} n/s/g
Specific activity	536.3 C/g
SF branching fraction	3.092%
Neutron emission rate	3.77 n/s/fission
Mean fission neutron spectrum	2.14 MeV
Prompt γ-ray multiplicity (mean)	~10/fission
Average prompt γ-ray energy	0.8 MeV
Total prompt γ-ray energy	6.7–9.0 MeV
Decay mode	α

SF = spontaneous fission.

are mixed (Table 1). Dosimetry measurements of the mixed neutron/gamma ray fields have been done by Krishnaswamy,[15] Colvett et al.,[16] and others[17] by both direct measurement and by Monte Carlo simulation and analysis (Table 2). The most recent study was done by Yanch, et al.[63] using the Monte Carlo Neutron Program (MCNP) (Table 3), and for boron capture enhancement (BNCE).[64] Wierzbicki et al. carried out direct measurements using gold foils.[63,71,87] Cf-252 decays with a half-life of 2.65 years and emits neutrons at a rate of 2.31x10^{12} Bq g-1 and gamma rays (Table 1). The average neutron energy is 2.35 MeV. Cf-252 is a unique isotope that decays mostly by alpha-emission and the decay process produces neutrons with a fission spectrum and the gamma rays have energies between 0.5 and 1 MeV (Table 1). Very near the sources the ratio of dose from neutrons to gamma rays, i.e., the n/gamma ratio is 2. However in tissue at 5–10 cm from the source the ratio decreases and becomes about half. Cf source activity is expressed by the microgram content (or for HDR, as milligram content), which is 2.31x10^6 neutrons per second. The measurement of neutron dose by Colvett et al.[16] is regarded as the most accurate. They performed their measurements in large phantoms containing tissue equivalent fluid using small ion chambers with gas multiplication to enhance sensitivity. Total dose was measured using chambers with tissue equivalent walls filled with gas that was also tissue equivalent. Gamma ray dose was measured using chambers with aluminum walls filled with a mixture of 90% argon and 10% methane. Monte Carlo methods using computer were applied by Krishnaswamy[15] originally and more recently by Yanch et al.[63] (Table 3) using the MCNP code. Anderson[17,65] has reviewed the data of all the workers including Jones and Auxier, Stoddard, Windham, Anderson, Mahmoudi[48] (France), Kraitor et al.[66] (Russia) and Irifune et al.[67] (Japan). Yamashita et al.[68] have also carried out direct

Table 2.
Cf-252 Transverse Axis Specific Dose Rate Factor (cGy cm^2 μgh)$^{-1}$

Author: Method: Distance (cm)	Colvett et al. Ion Chamber Measurement		Krishnaswamy Monte Carlo Calculation	
	Neutrons	Gamma Rays	Neutrons	Gamma Rays
0.5	2.48	1.00	2.23	1.07
1.0	2.39	0.98	2.20	1.08
1.5	2.30	0.99	2.13	1.08
2.0	2.20	1.01	2.10	1.10
2.5	2.10	1.04	2.07	1.10
3.0	2.01	1.08	1.94	1.10
3.5	1.92	1.12	1.82	1.14
4.0	1.84	1.17	1.73	1.17
4.5	1.76	1.23	1.70	1.21
5.0	1.71	1.26	1.59	1.23

Modified from Anderson (65).

Measurements and calculations for an applicator tube source having an active length of 1.5 cm and an encapsulation of 0.7 mm P-Ir.

Table 3.

Along and Away Table: Neutron Dose Rate Distribution in cGy/h for a 1 μg Source ^{252}Cf

Distance Away	Distance Along										
	0.0 cm	0.5 cm	1.0 cm	1.5 cm	2.0 cm	2.5 cm	3.0 cm	3.5 cm	4.0 cm	4.5 cm	5.0 cm
0.500	5.8000	4.8000	2.5000	1.0000	0.5500	0.3400	0.2200	0.1600	0.1100	0.0830	0.0660
1.000	1.9000	1.7000	1.1000	0.7000	0.4500	0.2900	0.2000	0.1400	0.1000	0.0800	0.0630
1.500	0.9000	0.8000	0.6800	0.4800	0.3400	0.2400	0.1800	0.1300	0.1000	0.0780	0.0590
2.000	0.5000	0.4800	0.4100	0.3200	0.2600	0.2000	0.1500	0.1200	0.0900	0.0720	0.0570
2.500	0.3100	0.2700	0.2800	0.2300	0.2000	0.1500	0.1200	0.1000	0.0800	0.0640	0.0520
3.000	0.2100	0.2100	0.2000	0.1700	0.1500	0.1200	0.0970	0.0770	0.0650	0.0550	0.0450
3.500	0.1500	0.1500	0.1400	0.1300	0.1100	0.0950	0.8200	0.0660	0.0550	0.0470	0.0400
4.000	0.1100	0.1100	0.1000	0.0980	0.0860	0.0750	0.0670	0.0580	0.0480	0.0410	0.0350
4.500	0.0850	0.0820	0.0820	0.0730	0.0680	0.0600	0.0550	0.0500	0.0430	0.0350	0.0300
5.000	0.0660	0.0600	0.6200	0.0590	0.0560	0.0480	0.0430	0.0400	0.0370	0.0300	0.0250

Monte Carlo calculation: modified from Yanch, et al (64).

measurement studies and all the studies are in agreement with variation of only 3% with appropriate kerma adjustments.

The microdosimetry was studied by Beach and Harris,[69] who measured event size distributions in air and in infinite tissue equivalent phantoms. They used their microdosimetry data using small tissue equivalent proportional counters to predict the high LET event probabilities as a function of dose for Cf. They noted that the probability of clonogenic cells near the edge of the implant >1 cm from the nearest source containing no high LET events was large. They postulated that the scheduling of the delivery of the high LET components of the treatment as well as the dose per session and the addition of the external beam low LET dose would be important factors in the outcomes of Cf neutron brachytherapy. In addition, they found that the total number of high LET events is greater per cGy for Cf than for higher energy neutron beams (Figure 1). Microdosimetic spectra of energy deposition determined in tissue equivalent phantoms may be an important method to correlate with biological effects.

Fast neutrons are absorbed in tissue by interaction with nuclei by one or more of several primary mechanisms, i.e., elastic scattering, inelastic scattering, or neutron capture as neutrons are slowed to the thermal range. In elastic scattering, the neutron loses considerable energy by colliding with target nuclei, principally hydrogen, to produce recoil protons. These protons are responsible for the high LET effects. The fast neutron interactions

with hydrogen atoms account for >85% of the absorbed dose. The LET of the recoil protons from the fast neutrons is much higher than x- or gamma rays, hence the most important radiations of Cf are the low energy fast neutrons, which are responsible for the unique effectiveness of Cf against hypoxia or radioresistance. Low LET gamma rays are produced at LDR and are biologically much less potent. In inelastic scattering, fast neutrons interact with heavier atoms in tissue and after the collisions are scattered and lose energy but leave the nucleus in an excited state that is restored to a stable state by emitting ionizing radiation. Because of the loss of energy with interaction with hydrogen, the energy absorption from fast neutrons in different tissues depends on their hydrogen content. It is high with brain and breast and fat in subcutaneous tissues. The relative energy absorbed per gram is greatest in fatty tissue, which has the highest hydrogen content; it is least in bone, which has a low hydrogen content. The opposite is true for x- or gamma rays. Because of high fat content, late tissue reactions are frequent in brain and breast after neutron therapy.

In neutron capture, thermal neutrons are captured by atoms with high capture cross-section. The fast neutrons from Cf become thermalized with interactions with tissue nuclei and enhancement by neutron capture is possible. The target nucleus can fission with emission of an alpha particle and lithium nucleus if boron is the target atom.[70] Yanch et al.[63,64] have calculated the BNCE possible with Cf. Direct measurements have been

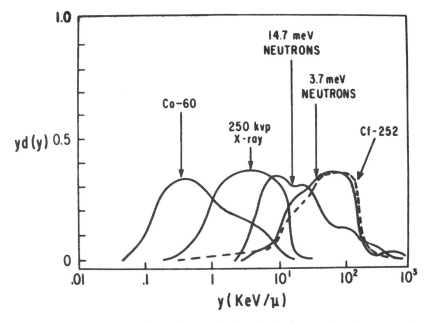

Figure 1. Lineal energy spectrum for various radiations including neutron beams and Cf-252. Cf has the highest LET spectrum. (Reproduced with permission from Nucl Sci Appl[49]).

made by Wierzbicki et al.[71] in tissue and in air with gold foils using clinical as well as milligram Cf sources. The degree of dose enhancement possible is increased as a function of the amount of boron present, the thermal neutron flux, and the target atom used (e.g., for gadolinium the secondary emissions are mainly electrons). BNCE is a unique advantage of Cf for the treatment of radiation resistant cancers because it allows boron neutron capture therapy in a hospital setting rather than at nuclear reactors, which are usually located far from urban (or medical) facilities.

Radiobiology

Neutron Lesions

Lethal lesions produced by neutrons in cells depend mainly on knock-on protons and are high LET events.[81] Contrasted to photon lesions, neutron lesions are less frequent but much more lethal for a given dose. Neutron biological effects such as RBE and OER differ greatly from photon or low LET effects and are much less sensitive to the absence of oxygen, dose rate, fractionation, time, or position

in the cell cycle.[35] Mainly sublethal, potentially lethal, nonlethal, and repairable lesions are produced by photons, but neutrons produce 1-hit cell killing. Cf has an RBE for cell killing of about 4–8, which varies with cell, tissue, and end-point, as well as a low OER of about 1.4.[11,49] The hypoxic RBE is much larger for neutrons.[39]

Cellular Effects

Cf survival curves for single mammalian cells are exponential[11,18,19,36,72] in contrast to photons (Figure 2). There is no dose rate or fractionation effect.[36] Cf radiobiology has been studied extensively[18–21,73,82] and is well understood.

Relative Biological Effectiveness

Cf survival curves are much steeper and have smaller shoulders than photon survival curves.[18,19] The RBE advantage varies with dose rate and is less at high-dose-rate (RBE ~3.0) than at low- or medium-dose-rate (RBE ~6.0).[18,21]

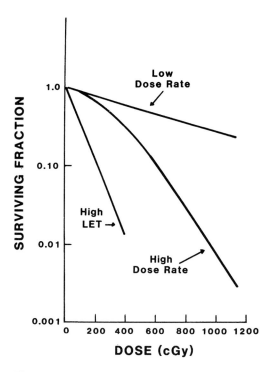

Figure 2. Survival curves for brachytherapy. Middle shouldered curve is for high-dose-rate photons (or for acute photon) irradiation; low-dose-rate curve (right) is for typical LDR; Cf neutrons curve is exponential left. (Reproduced with permission from Maruyama,[12] Adv Radiat Biol).

Concepts in the Use of Californium-252

1. *Dose Rate.* There is no dose-rate effect with neutrons.[36] For Cf the RBE is large because there is always a dose-rate effect for photons but neutron effects are the same regardless of dose rate. At very high-dose-rate, Cf neutron efforts become more like neutron beams.[68]

2. *OER.* Cf effects are much less sensitive to the presence of or absence of oxygen and is about 1.4[18,20] in contrast to photons where the OER is 2.5–3.5.

3. *Hypoxic Advantage Factor.* Hypoxic cells have a higher RBE than oxic cells.[39] This is an advantage for tumor control as Cf sources are placed directly in tumor using brachytherapy procedures and leads to a tumor/normal tissue advantage favoring tumor control and tissue tolerance. (Normal tissues are oxygenated).[39]

4. *SLD/PLD Repair.* There is little or no repair of SLD[36] or PLD damage[72,74] and both fractionation and low-dose-rate have little significant effect on Cf biological effects. A PLD neutron lesion can persist for many hours.[75] Total dose and acute tolerance, not fractionation, determine biological effect.[36]

5. *Cell Cycle.* The changes in sensitivity of cells with position in the cell cycle is large with photons but is minimal and insignificant with high LET.[35]

6. *Reoxygenation.* The reoxygenation of tumors appears to occur rapidly after neutrons and is facilitated by the rapid regression of bulky tumors.[37]

7. *Tumor Regression.* Neutrons early in the treatment course produce rapid regression of bulky tumor (Figure 3).[27,37,41,59] The quick shrinkage of tumors appears to improve its sensitivity to subsequent photon irradiation. A high RBE for tumor regression has been determined in experimental animal studies.[21,76,77]

8. *Inherent Cell Radiosensitivity.* Wide variations in inherent cellular sensitivity[78] is reduced for neutrons but still needs detailed study.

9. *Oxygen Gain Factor.* There is an oxygen gain factor for Cf[18–21] since OER is 1.4 compared to the OER for LDR photons of about 2.2.[12] An oxygen gain factor of 1.56 is obtained by the use of Cf versus LDR photon therapy.

10. *Schedule-Dependent Gain Factor.* Still poorly understood but recognized from the clinical studies is the fact that the early use of neutrons greatly enhances sensitivity to photons and rapidity of tumor regression.[11,23,37,41] Used in a delayed

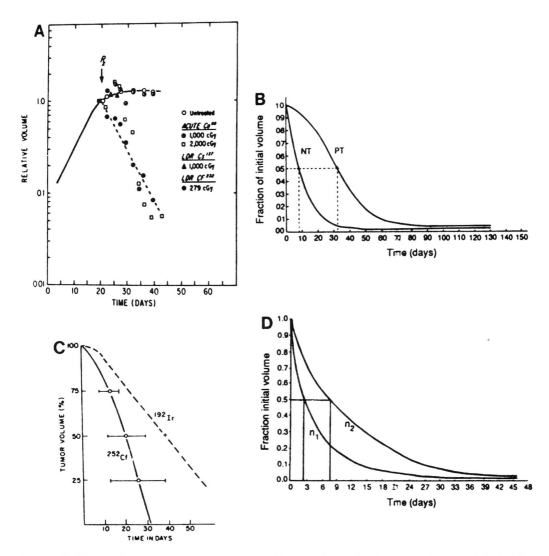

Figure 3. Regression curves for tumors observed in experimental animals or in human clinical trials. A) Nude mice bearing Hela cell (cervix) cancer tumor comparing acute Co-60, 20 Gy, LDR Cs-137 and Cf-252, 2.79 Gy; B) Human bulky/barrel carcinoma of cervix to Cf versus Cs-137 and radiation therapy (P<10[6]). (Reproduced with permission from Maruyama and Muir, Am J Clin Oncol [CCT][37]; C) Regression of lymph node metastasis after Cf or Ir-192 brachytherapy at Memorial Sloan Kettering Cancer Center, Vallejo, (reproduced with permission of Nucl Sci Appl[13]); and D) Regression of exophytic portions of tongue cancers after Cf versus Co-60 implant therapy, from Vtyurin and Tsyb.[27] (Reproduced with permission from Nucl Sci Appl.)

schedule, neutrons were less effective than when used early.[23] It was postulated that there was a microdosimetric basis for the observation based on the number and distribution of lethal cell lesions by Cf.[79]

Tacev et al.[59] have recently shown that human cervix tumor regression is significantly more rapid after an early or up-front Cf insertion than after delayed Ra-226 (conventional) treatment. Yaes et al.[80] have postulated that the use of the early schedule reduces the like-

Table 4.
Reasons for Brachytherapy Sequence in Radiation Therapy

Delayed (Conventional)	Early
1. Reduce tumor bulk to minimal and resistant core	1. Attack hypoxic tumor
2. Minimize regional tumor burden	2. Produce rapid reduction of tumor bulk
3. Attack residual tumor core	3. Allow tumor reoxygenation
4. Treat residual tumor core with high dose	4. Increase efficacy of low LET radiation
	5. Increase likelihood of residual tumor clearance by low LET

LET = linear energy transfer.

lihood for selection of mutant resistant clonogens (Table 4).

Facilities

The Cf workers who successfully conducted clinical trials recognized that facilities were important and designed and developed facilities where Cf treatments could be given. We describe in this section the type of treatments given and the type of facility developed to implement the therapy given.

Dose Rate for Californium-252 Brachytherapy

Low-Dose-Rate (Table 5)

LDR used needle, seed, pin, or flexible sources of low activity containing microgram amounts of Cf.[27,50] Various lengths between 2 and 5 cm and multiple sources were used in treatment sessions lasting from 48–120 hours. The dose rate is similar to Ra-226 therapy and the arrangement of sources is similar to those used for gamma ray emitting sources, i.e., fol-

lowing Manchester rules. LDR has been principally used for oral cavity, head and neck, and soft tissue using interstitial techniques. Dose rate is 5–10 cGy neutrons per hour and 10–100 micrograms are used per implant. RBE is 6.0. Tolerance and efficacy against tumor is good but this method has all the problems of LDR brachytherapy (time, environment, long hospitalization, personnel exposure, etc.). Therapeutic dose (neutrons only) is 8–10 Gy.

Medium-Dose-Rate

MDR utilizes multiple sealed sources containing 15–40 micrograms of Cf and the duration of the implant is hours i.e., ~4–10 hours in duration. The total amount of Cf used is 100–400 micrograms[12,49] per implant and the dose rate is 10–60 cGy/hr. MDR has been used mainly for GYN tumors but has also been successfully applied to brain, head and neck, and soft tissues. RBE is 6.0, and the treatment times and tolerance have been excellent with very good tumor control and low normal tissue complication rates. The procedures are performed on out-patients and are done in 1 working day (~8 hours). For GYN tumors, about 1/3 of the dose is neutrons and 2/3 is given later as photon beam therapy.

High-Dose-Rate

HDR Cf therapy requires special sources containing ~milligram quantities of Cf (500–2000 micrograms).[51,68,89] HDR requires remote afterloading machines and a totally controlled facility where the patient can be held for the time duration needed for treatment (minutes to hours). The dose rate is

Table 5.
Factors of Importance in Tumor Radiation Response to Low-Dose-Rate Neutrons

1. Tumor bulk and volume
2. Hypoxia and necrotic zones
3. Viable hypoxic tumor cells
4. Reoxygenation
5. Decreased tumor blood flow/increased with tumor shrinkage
6. Tumor microvascularity/revascularization
7. Kinetics of tumor cell killing and lysis

10–100 cGy/minute. The RBE decreases at these high-dose-rates and is about 2.5–4.[68,90] Further studies are needed to study the appropriate RBE factor more precisely. Safety and protection problems are of much greater concern and late effects and normal tissue complication rates still must be carefully documented. A single source is stepped through the treatment volume one centimeter at a time using a manual or remote afterloading machine (ANET-V or Toshiba).

There are several advantages in using HDR remote controlled afterloading methods:

1. Radiation exposure of medical and nursing personnel is eliminated.
2. Patient treatment and immobilization time is short with patient discomfort minimized and attendant medical problems reduced.
3. External fixation of applicator devices increases accuracy and reproducibility of applicator and source positioning.
4. Treatment dosimetry is more exact.
5. Out-patient treatments can be given, reducing costs.

Fractionation and control of dose in adjacent radiosensitive organs are important factors controlling the frequency of complications and outcome of therapy. At HDR the RBE of Cf neutrons goes from 6 to ~3 and, therefore, adjustments must be made in treatment prescription.[90] At least 2–4 insertions are probably optimal with a spacing of 1–2 weeks. With too long a time gap, rapid tumor shrinkage can bring adjacent organs closer to the sources thereby increasing their dose and the risk of late effects.[83] HDR Cf brachytherapy with remote afterloading will be increasingly used for the more advanced and bulky neoplasms of the GYN tract, e.g., of the cervix, uterus, and vagina. At the present time the level of understanding of optimal methods for usage of neutrons is still at an early stage.

General Design and Organization of Facilities (Table 6)

A shielded facility for storage and handling of sources as well as patient treatment allows

Table 6.
Special Personnel Requirements for Cf-252 Neutron Brachytherapy

1. Physician radiotherapist—requires special training and experience in neutron therapy.
2. Physicist—knowledge of neutron physics, measurements, and calibration.
3. Radiation safety officer—authority to control personnel exposure time.
4. Nurse(s)—implant suite experience. Patient care in neutron therapy holding suite.
5. Neutron curator—monitors sources, source selection, source strength in each application. Keeps records.
6. Radiotherapy technologist(s)—knowledge of special handling requirements of neutron emitting sources.
7. Radiobiologist—neutron and high LET, RBE, safety knowledge.
8. Engineer—building and maintenance of special equipment, devising and constructing special equipment requirements.
9. Other surgeons, gynecologists, and physicians—collaborators on joint study using protocols and orderly approaches to therapy.

LET = linear energy transfer; RBE = relative biological effectiveness.

use of Cf easily and safely and was a major aspect of all the successful long-term projects.[9,34,51,52,55,67,91] From the point of view of the potential user, the investment in developing a Cf facility offers considerable economic advantages over external beam neutron therapy. The neutron treatment involves the removal of sources from storage, delivery to the patient, insertion, retrieval, and return to storage. The use of afterloading was developed to reduce personnel exposure in the insertion and removal of sources. This can be done manually or using remotely controlled afterloading machines. To further reduce personnel exposure, bedside shields, instruments to allow increase in distance between sources and personnel, and thorough in-service instruction of personnel on appropriate operational procedures are essential so that time of exposures are minimal and completely controlled. Special neutron-sensitive personnel safety badges are needed to measure and keep records of exposure times of all personnel. A special team of well trained personnel is important to work together as a team to assure that the patient is well treated and no unusual deviations from the set procedures occur.[49]

The original neutron therapy room in most of the early facilities was an existing megavoltage therapy room. These are large rooms with heavily shielded walls and mazes designed for photon therapy. Provided with a bed and bedside shields and a Cf storage vault, one has the basic requirements for Cf neutron therapy. We added a TV camera, a monitor outside the room, a patient TV set, a voice communicator, a transport cart to transfer sources from the storage vault to the bedside, and a variety of handling tongs. Adjacent to the therapy room we added a minor surgery room with a radiographic machine so that the applicator position could be accurately simulated. An electronic link to the treatment planning computer allowed the planning of appropriate loadings to deliver individualized treatment to each patient. Sources were transported from the storage vault to the patients' bedside and loaded manually, or if a remote afterloader were available, using remote control, and then it was returned.

Low-Dose-Rate Facilities

Japan Cancer Institute Hospital, Tokyo, Japan[52,66] and the Institute of Medical Radiology in Obninsk, Russia developed LDR facilities[55] (Figure 4A). They developed facilities where sources of small size such as needles, seeds, pins, and flexible wire sources[62] or

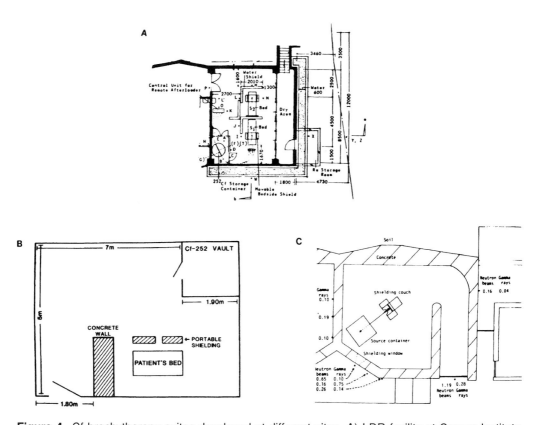

Figure 4. Cf brachytherapy suites developed at different sites. A) LDR facility at Cancer Institute Hospital, Tokyo Japan (after Irifune et al.[67]); B) MDR facility at Lexington, Kentucky (after Wierzbicki et al.[91]); and C) HDR facility at Keio Cancer Center, Tokyo, Japan.[51]

lightly loaded intracavitary tube sources could be used for implant periods of several days. The facility was a controlled room in a brachytherapy wing where both gamma and neutron brachytherapy were done. The patients remained in the controlled room during the entire procedure and sources were delivered to the bedside from the storage vault that could be in the room or in a separate room nearby. Sources could be inserted manually from behind a shielded barrier at the bedside (Figure 4A) or by remote controlled machine. Many of the cases treated were head and neck, either primary or recurrent cancers, and a wide variety of interstitial and intracavitary treatments were given using the LDR method. The long-term survival rates have been good and cure rates high in these feasibility trials in Russia,[89] at Keio,[92] and at JCIH.[50,93] Specially trained nurses and personnel monitored and cared for the patients during their hospitalization, which required several days. These persons worked from behind bedside shields that protected them during the loading and unloading or when they cared for the patient. Room time was controlled and limited.

High-Dose-Rate Facilities

Keio University Cancer Center, Tokyo, Japan[51] and the Moscow Oncological Research Center, Moscow, Russia developed HDR therapy methods. The initial trial and facility developed by Yamashita et al.[51] used sources of 500–900 micrograms that were moved through the treatment volume using a specially built remote afterloading machine. A specially shielded room was used as the treatment facility (Figure 4B). The machine, sources, and the remote afterloader were contained in the room and after applicator placement, only the patient was in the room under TV surveillance during treatment. Keio treated cervix[51] as well as head and neck and body surface cancers.[53] Yamashita et al. determined the RBE for HDR Cf therapy and found it was 2–3 for skin reaction in human and mouse skin and in sea urchin eggs by cleavage delay.[68] They used RBE values of 3–4 for clinical trials. This shows that at HDR the prescribed dose is not the same as for LDR or MDR where the RBE is 6. Ten-year survivors of therapy for Stage IIIB cervix cancers have been reported.[43,92]

Moscow Oncological Research Center developed the ANET afterloader[56] and have gradually upgraded the prototype from the earliest to the most advanced model. This machine in its most recent model contains a 2-mg source fabricated at Dimitrovgrad. The colpostats can be loaded using a 500-μg source; the uterine tandem is treated using the 2-mg (2000 μg) source that is stepped through the length of the tandem and treats an isodose surface selected for the tumor being treated. Treatment time is short (minutes to hours), is performed on out-patients, is computer-controlled, avoids personnel or hospital environment radiation safety problems, is well tolerated by patients, even medically ill, and is generally comparable to HDR photon GYN brachytherapy. RBE is ~3 and is less than for Cf using LDR.[68,90] The main tumors treated have been uterus, rectum, body surface, a few brain tumors, and other sites.[51,53,89,92] The ANET afterloader has been tested at other facilities including Obninsk[94] and Lithuania.[58] Rapid patient through-put is an advantage of HDR but requires more treatment sessions (4–5).

Medium-Dose-Rate Facilities[49]

Maruyama and the Lexington group developed MDR therapy for Cf treatments (Figure 4C) and have treated the largest number of patients (about 700) with outstanding results for long-term (to nearly 20 years) tumor control and cure with low (~5%) complication rates.[44] They applied these methods to treatment of cervix,[43] uterus,[25,95] vagina,[26,96] oral,[97] head and neck,[98,99] body surface,[97,99] and brain neoplasms.[100,107] Therapy is 4–10 hours long in most patients, who are treated with out-patient procedures. The patient enters the therapy facility at 7 AM and is discharged at around 5 PM. The brachytherapy center is a controlled and shielded facility with the following:

1. Cf storage vault.
2. Treatment bed (Figures 5A and B).
3. Bedside personnel shields (plastic).
4. Transport cart (plastic) (Figure 6).
5. Plastic eye goggles.
6. Remote afterloader-delivery machine.
7. TV, TV camera, voice communicator, radio, handling tongs, room neutron monitor, door interlock, etc.

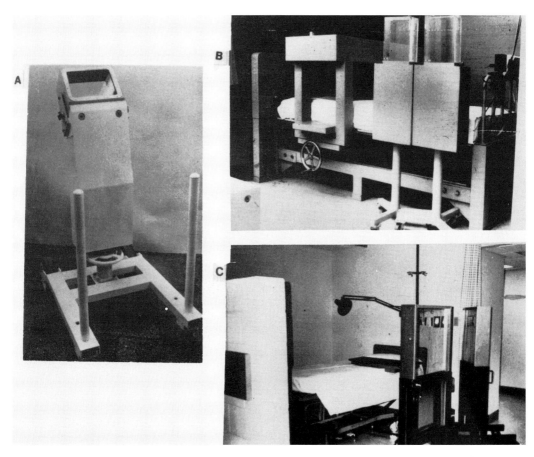

Figure 5. Bedside shields developed at different sites. A) Institute of Medical Radiol,[57] Obinsk, Russia; B) Cancer Institute Hospital, Tokyo, Japan; and C) Radiation Therapy Oncology Center, Lexington, Kentucky. All are movable to the bedside.

The brachytherapy center also has an operating suite with radiography, film developing and viewing facilities, a physics and radiobiology room, research irradiation facilities, offices for curator, physicist, and nearby, the radiation safety officer. A nursing station and treatment planning computer station, scrub room and supplies, film, record storage rooms, and clerical and waiting areas complete the Lexington facility.

The protocols followed in Lexington allowed the through-put of a large number of patients, rapidly and efficiently with excellent quality control. While the main procedures have focused on GYN, head and neck, and brain tumors, all types of procedures were performed, including intracavitary, interstitial, and plaque. The US DOE sources provided tubes, which were not appropriate for interstitial therapy (although they were tested using specially devised equipment). Nearly all the patients were treated using manual afterloading methods from behind shields, using rapid handling methods, very short times (minutes), distance, and trained teams of personnel. Since the prototype remote afterloader was not approved for patient therapy, it was tested as a bedside delivery system only. The RBE is ~6 for normal tissues and the antitumor RBE.

Floor Plan Design of Different Facilities

In Figure 4 we show representative floor plans and room designs for LDR, MDR, and

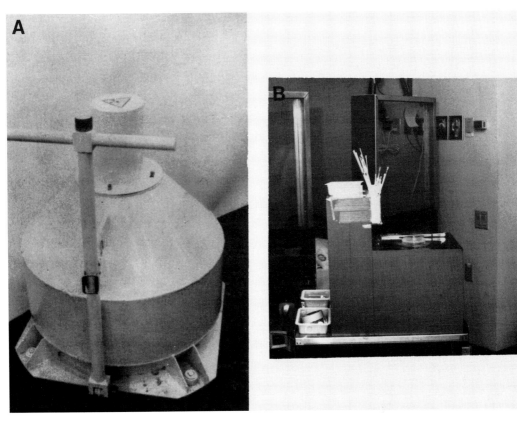

Figure 6. Transport carts developed at different sites. A) Institute of Medical Radiology, Obninsk, Russia; and B) Radiation Center, Lexington, Kentucky.

Radiation Safety and Late Effects

HDR facilities. A bedside shield is shown in Figure 5, and transport carts are shown in Figure 6.

Radiation safety has been a major concern of all the neutron brachytherapy programs.[49] All devised special facilities and protocols for handling the problems associated with use of Cf that have been effective within the constraints of the radiation safety regulations of the different countries. While traditional practices have used hospital operating rooms to insert the radioactive materials, held the patients in general hospital beds, and used general duty nurses to care for the radioactive patient, that has not been the practice of the active Cf programs.[9,34] Those neutron brachytherapy programs devised controlled access facilities and used specially trained staff to care for the patients in those facilities. The Cf was stored in the treatment room or in a nearby controlled room and the patients have remained in the treatment room during their treatment in the radiation oncology department. Sources were handled by trained personnel and generally curators kept records on source usage, removal from storage, and return. Transportation of sources was in shielded transportation carts, afterloading methods were used, and either remote controlled delivery-retrieval machines or very rapid handling systems from behind shields were used. Room monitors and neutron sensitive personnel badges were used to control exposure.

To summarize, the following characteristic considerations were used at all the Cf programs:

1. Strictly controlled treatment room (area).
2. Restricted personnel exposure times.
3. Distance.
4. Bedside shields made of plastic, water-extended plastic, plastic-water, some combined with lead.
5. Neutron dose monitors for area; personnel track-edge badges.
6. A trained and closely supervised staff.
7. Afterloading.

A responsible radiation safety officer is important to supervise and monitor the practices in the use of Cf.[49]

From the experience from the clinical use of Cf it is now possible to review the practices and hazards more objectively than was the case when more hysteria and less information[102] on neutron effects was prevalent. The Hiroshima-Nagasaki data on leukemogenic and carcinogenic risks of neutrons have been found to be in considerable error as well as the dose received by the exposed populations.[103] Those data had served as the basis of the early risk estimates. We also now have much more data on second tumors as well as complication rates in patients treated with Cf neutrons, cured of their tumors and followed for nearly 20 years.[43] Since no patient has developed leukemia, lymphoma, myeloma, or aplastic anemia it is not likely that RBE values of 10, 100, or 1000 (extrapolated from log-log dose-effect curves) apply to human risk estimates. In studies carried out in experimental C57BL mice exposed to Cf or Co-60 gamma rays, the RBE was found to lie between 1–2 for leukemogenesis.[104,105] In fact, the mixing of Cf neutrons with gamma rays shortened the latent period for induction and also the survival times of the mice.[105] This data is in agreement with the results of studies on leukemogenesis by other workers. Studies by Upton et al.,[106,107] and Ullrich et al.,[108,109] found low RBE values for leukemogenesis. More realistic and updated safety standards are needed based on better data for neutron safety.[110] Maisin et al.[111,112] have studied high energy d(50)-Be neutrons for late effects and reported RBE for life-shortening of 1–2 for single exposures and slightly higher values for fractionated neutrons. Results were not different for carcinomas, leukemias, or sarcomas. These studies did not support the very large values postulated earlier for neutrons. It may, therefore, be reasonable to use quality factors of about 10 for planning a program of radiation safety for Cf brachytherapy with the assurance that both personnel and patients will not have an unusual risk of hazards. Goud et al.[113,114] have carried out studies on sperm shape abnormalities and bone marrow micronuclei formation after Cf irradiation to assess risks for cell nuclear damage.

Clinical Observations of Effects

The initial anticipation was that Cf was just like Ra-226 in its properties and the protocols were set to exactly match the methods, equivalent doses, schedules, etc., of radium therapy. Only a few cases were treated in the early trials so that there was no opportunity to make many observations on Cf effects except for noting that acute tissue reactions were similar in intensity and duration to gamma therapy. Tumors regressed after treatment, but the generally held conclusion was that there were no advantages over gamma therapy. Much more accurate data has come from the later studies in Lexington, Tokyo, and Russia[9,34]; and more accurate data on clinical RBE has emerged, as well as better understanding of the high RBE compared to gamma emitter therapy, and the greater efficacy against bulky and radioresistant cancers. Some of the observations are detailed below.

1. Similar acute tissue effects as photon brachytherapy.[45–47] Skin, mucosa, and acutely reacting tissue responses all occur in the same time frame, severity, and time duration as photons. Similar late effects were also observed in the oral cavity.[115]
2. RBE. The RBE of normal tissue effects is larger than for photons[18,21,49] and the value is about 6 for equivalent tolerance dose. The exception is HDR where the RBE for tissue effects decreases to ~3.[68,90]
3. Therapeutic Dose. For Cf-only implant therapy, the neutron dose is 8–10 Gy.[27] For mixed Cf plus photon therapy, the dose should use an RBE

factor and also consider the other components of dose, i.e., the gamma rays.[49] Thus, therapeutic dose equivalent is $D = D_n \, RBE_n + D_{gamma}$. The RBE for gamma rays is 1.0. The total therapeutic dose should be 60–70 Gy-equivalents (Gy-eqs). The total therapeutic dose is the same regardless of the time period or the duration of the application.

4. Dose Rate Independence.[19,36] For Cf a variety of dose rates have been used and there is no adjustments necessary for total dose to correct for time. Implants have been done at LDR, MDR, and HDR. There was no difference whether a short (MDR—several hours) or a 1 week (LDR) implant was done as measured by efficacy or side effects. This has led to schedules favoring the shorter (MDR and HDR) schedules. Studies have shown that therapeutic efficacy is not dependent on duration of the application (20–96 hours) but depended instead on the total dose or fraction size.[84]

5. Rapid Tumor Regression. Tumor regression has been noted to be very rapid by Maruyama and Muir,[37] Vtyurin and Tsyb,[27] Tacev et al.,[84] and Vallejo et al.[47] Cervix, oral cavity tumors, and lymph node metastases all show quick regression (Figure 3).

6. Local Tumor Control. High efficacy for local control of tumor has been observed.[12,49] For oral, cervix, and uterus, local control of tumors has been very good. However, cure is determined by distant metastases and requires adjuvant therapy effective against minimal or microscopic remote disease.

7. Histologic Eradication of Tumor. In studies of cervix cancers it has been found that tumors are eradicated as a function of dose and schedule.[24,116,117] It has also been found that glioblastoma is eradicated from the brain using histologic study methods.[118] For cervix cancers, tumors are eradicated much more efficiently than photons and the RBE for destroying tumor is large.[119]

8. Tumor Cure. Patients have been cured for time period of up to 15–20 years using Cf brachytherapy.[9,23,34,43,92,93] The end-point of complete tumor regression (CR) has been found to reliably predict local tumor control; this, in turn, can lead to cure. However, since advanced tumors are being treated, ultimate outcome is dependent on the frequency of distant metastases and the efficacy of adjuvant therapy.

9. Schedule-Dependent Efficacy for Neutron Brachytherapy.[23,41] The use of the up-front or early implant schedule has been found to increase the efficacy of Cf therapy when used in combined neutron-photon therapy.[27,43] The increased efficacy is manifested by rapid tumor regression and the tumor regression is followed by high rates of CR response.

10. Tolerance Dose for Cf.[12] In phase I studies, it has been shown that brain tissue necrosis appears as critical doses are exceeded in brain implant therapy of malignant gliomas.[118] It has also been shown that tolerance can be exceeded when Cf is used in delayed schedules in treatment of cervix cancers.[83] When used in a delayed schedule, tumor shrinkage allows the adjacent sensitive organs to move closer to the radioactive sources and thus have greater risk of doses that can exceed normal tissue tolerance. Neutrons should not be used for the treatment of small, totally regressed tumors or for totally surgically resected tumors. Mixing Cf with photon beam therapy increases tissue tolerance.

11. Dose per Session. It has been found that dose per session is more effective when it is 10–20 Gy eqs per treatment rather than multiple sessions using small doses of 1.5 Gy eqs. Therapeutic RBE is high and tumor cell eradication more complete using larger doses, and it leads to quicker regression[37,77,117,119] and

reduces likelihood of tumor regeneration.[123]

12. Combined Chemo-Radiotherapy. A feasibility trial of chemo-neutron radiotherapy has been carried out using cisplatin + 5–Fluorouracil (5-FU) and hyperfractionated x-radiation therapy.[86] The combination was well tolerated for the treatment of advanced stage III-IV cervix cancers and it was found that the combined treatment produced good local tumor control as well as a 3-year survival of 90%. These results suggest that improved local control of localized advanced cancers can greatly increase the efficacy of systemic chemotherapy even when those agents have very limited antitumor efficacy.[122]

13. Low Rates of Normal Tissue Complications. There has been low complication frequencies observed after Cf therapy after the feasibility and phase I trials. Lexington reported a ~5% rate for patients treated with Cf for cervix cancers.[43] For oral cavity tumors more complications have been observed but this is due in part to the advanced tumors that frequently destroy large tissue volumes and invade bone and adjacent structures.[27,30,33,92,115]

14. Small Volume Dose. The low complication frequency is undoubtedly related to the small volume dose inherent in brachytherapy.[12]

15. Rapid Tumor Regeneration. For cervix cancer, there is rapid regeneration of tumor in ~9 days after Cf therapy.[123] This is evident by histologic study of hysterectomy specimens.

16. Low Rates of Second Malignant Neoplasms.[43] While SMNs have been observed, the tumors observed have been the same as those observed after photon brachytherapy. No hematological malignancies such as leukemia, lymphoma myeloma, or aplastic anemia have been reported to date, with follow-ups to 20 years.[43]

In general, the observations from all the investigators has been favorable with satisfactory responses of tumors of many different sites, stages, and histologic types.[9,34] Tumor regression has uniformly been noted to be quick as well as efficacious for hemostasis, reduction in pain, and patient toxicity. Local control has been excellent indicating that neutrons overcome factors that contribute to radioresistance. Regression of the exophytic portions of tumor is dramatic but has also been noted by serial volume measurement by clinical or CT observations. All histologic types of tumors respond including melanoma, glioblastoma, and sarcoma; the latter are generally regarded as radioresistant. It is notable that recurrent tumors also respond well after prior radiotherapy and surgery (objective responses in 93%).[33,89] This is notable as it is well known that these tumors are radioresistant. However, with prior heavy radiation and surgery, the complication rates can be high, which is the price for improved local control. The mechanism of rapid regression and improved control of the radioresistant histologies remains an important study for the future. Of special importance for future study is the biological basis of the effect of the early or up-front neutron schedule on the improved responses and local control of radioresistant tumors.

Clinical Experience with Different Tumors

Personnel for Californium Therapy

Table 6 summarizes the cadre of personnel needed for Cf therapy.[49] The physician must be a radiation oncologist with special training and interest in neutron therapy who can evaluate patients for the appropriateness of neutron therapy as well as deal with patient problems and their management. Patient selection is very important. Tumors must be selected so that they receive long-term benefit and optimal benefits from neutron therapy. The physicist must have a knowledge about neutron physics and properties and the measurement of neutrons. He/she must be able to calibrate sources. The radiation safety officer is important to monitor and control exposure of personnel and environment to neutrons and to implement a program of procedures for personnel working in the Cf program. The nurses need implant room training and experience to attend the patients, provide medication, carry out necessary procedures, and assist the radiation oncologists. The therapists must be able to load and unload patients and to work with afterloading equipment. The neutron curator must load and unload sources from storage, record usage, and return to storage, transport sources to usage sites, and keep files and film records of sources used in every implant. While others can serve as back-up, these personnel are absolutely essential to safe usage. A radiobiologist can help in research and the design of protocols and the safety practices and needs a knowledge of neutron radiobiology.

Sources

Only a limited number of source types and strengths have been available to date. The only producers are Oak Ridge, Tennessee in the USA,[60,61] and Dimitrovgrad in Russia.[57] Since the manufacture of Cf is a lengthy and complex process, and requires special sites and facilities, obtaining sources is still difficult. Dimitrovgrad produces the largest variety of sources and activities from seeds to needles to intracavitary sources to sources up to 2 milligrams[57] (Figure 7). They also produce the flexible wire source that allows interstitial therapy of any site. ORNL can produce only a limited variety of sources and have made lightly loaded seeds, needles, intracavitary sources, and the reactor starter sources. Lexington studied the use of the 33 μg intracavitary source for intracavitary as well as carried out assessment of usability of these sources for interstitial therapy (by necessity since proper sources were not available). While half-life of Cf is short and only 2.65 years, Lexington was able to double usable lifetime by developing double-loading methods for using the sources (e.g., instead of 3, using 6 sources) in a treatment session. This overcomes one of the problems of Cf usage.

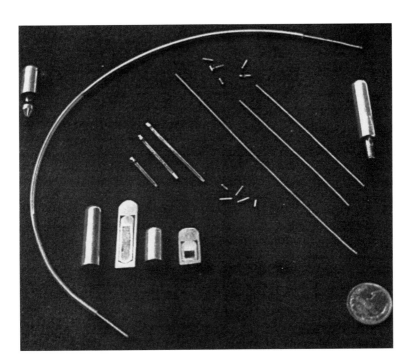

Figure 7. Cf sources designed and developed at Dimitrograd, Russia. Large sources are reactor starter sources. Cable has source of cylindrical type tube at end. Needles of different lengths, seeds, and intracavitary tube sources of different lengths shown next to seeds. Right lower reference is kopek coin (about the size of a penny).

Table 7.
Clearance of Tumors of Oral Cavity with Cf-252 and Co-60 Brachytherapy:
Early Results

Anatomic Site	Radionuclide	Stage	CR Response	%	Complication	%	2-Year Survival	%
Tongue	Cf-252	T_1	10/10	100	2	20	10	100
		T_2	11/12	96	4	31	10	83
Floor of mouth	Cf-252	T_1	10/10	100	4	40	5	50
		T_2	11/12	91	9	75	6	50
Oropharynx	Cf-252	T_2	4/5	80	1	20	2	40

CR = complete regression.
From Vtyurin (27).

As more users start programs and remote afterloading practices become routine, the problem of short supply and short half-life will be less because of the high efficiency of Cf and the need for only a few sessions and short treatment times. The high activity sources will have much longer usable half-lives (but will require longer and longer treatment times as the sources decay).

Head and Neck

Head and neck Cf brachytherapy studies were done principally at JCIH in Tokyo[50] and in Obninsk, Russia.[27,89,120] The largest series of patients with a wide variety of primary sites, stages, and either primary or recurrent status was done in Russia. The methods of treatment included Cf-only, Cf given in a delayed schedule after Co-60 beam therapy, and early Cf followed by Co-60 beam therapy. Standard interstitial techniques were used and generally LDR schedules were used. Lexington studied MDR methods[29,49,97] and had good results; Yamashita at Keio studied HDR methods[51] also with success but with technical difficulties because of the large source size. The latter two programs usually used surface plaque techniques because source size precluded most interstitial therapy. The sites treated have included tongue, floor of the mouth, lip, skin, oropharynx, buccal mucosa, tonsil, parotid gland, and lymph node metastases in the neck (Tables 7 and 8). For T1 and T2 tumors (classified by the UICC system), complete regression (CR), response, and local control was achieved in 80%–100%. Two- and 5-year survival rates were comparable to those achieved with conventional therapy.[27,89]

Table 8.
Clearance of Tumors in Various Sites with Cf-252 Brachytherapy: Early Results

Anatomic Site	Stage	CR Response	%	Complications	%	2-Year Survival	%
Lip	T_2	9/9	100	1	11	9	100
	T_3	3/3	100	—	—	3	100
Skin	T_2	4/4	100	—	—	4	100
	T_3	4/4	100	—	—	4	100
Melanoma	T_1	4/4	100	—	—	2	50
	T_2	3/3	100	—	—	2	66
Vulva	T_2	2/2	100	2	100	2	100
Penis	T_2	2/3	67	—	33	2	67
	T_3	4/5	80	1	20	3	60

CR = complete regression.
From Vtyurin (27).

Tongue

The tongue was treated with Cf-only using 8 Gy of LDR neutrons in Russia[27,124] (Table 7) using one- and two-plane or volume implants using needle, pin, or flexible sources. For T1 tumors, CR response was obtained in 92% and 3-year survival was 84% with 23% complications. For T2 tumors, there was 96% CR response, and 83% 2-year survivals. Complications occurred in 31%. Using early Cf followed by 40 Gy of Co-60 beam therapy, 58% CR response, and 50% 3-year survivals were observed with 8% complications in the treatment of T3 tumors.[27] Results were poorer when delayed Cf implants were done after 40 Gy of external Co-60 beam therapy. For T2 tumors, there were 72% CR responders and 55% 3-year survivals; for T3 there were 33% CR responders and 22% 3-year survivors. Russian experience supported the use of neutrons in the early schedule. Similar results were obtained in a much smaller series using MDR and larger sources in Lexington.[29] LDR to high dose was studied at JCIH in Japan.[50] Using data from the American, Russian, and Japanese trials, a dose-response curve was determined for Cf treatment of T2 tumors for mixed Cf plus photons or for pure Cf therapy that was sigmoid in shape.[29]

Floor of Mouth

Tumors of the floor of mouth were treated with Cf-only or using combined Co-60 and Cf (Table 7). Interstitial therapy used 8 Gy of LDR neutrons, which for T1 tumors led to 76% CR, 41% 3-year survival, and 29% complications.[27,89] When treated by the early implant schedule there was 100% CR response, 80% 3-year survivors with 20% complications. For T2 tumors, there was CR response in 67% and 83% survivors with 67% complications with the use of Cf-only. The patients treated with combined early Cf and Co-60, had 93% CR, 68% 3-year survivors, and 34% complications. For T3 and T4 tumors, there were 75% CR responses, 40% 3-year survivors, and 20% complications using combined early Cf plus Co-60. With delayed Cf, CR responses for the T3-T4 tumors were less and only 55%. This study indicates that tolerance and tumor control were improved by using combined Cf and Co-60 beam therapy.

Oropharynx

Tumors of the oropharynx have been treated with similar regimens in Russia[27,89] (Table 7). Cf-only implants led to 85% CR for T2 and 60% CR for T3 tumors. This produced 50% and 40% 5-year survivors with 17% complications.

Buccal Mucosa

Using Cf-only, Obinsk observed that the CR response rate was 89% with 55% 3-year survivors and no complications.[27,30,89] Lexington has also observed similar tumor control rates using MDR surface plaque therapy[97] with tumor control observed out to 10 years. Using similar combined modality methods of therapy, there were 100% local CR control, 57% 3-year survivors, and 0% complications.

Tonsil

Lexington first reported that T4 tonsillar tumors were readily controlled by Cf implant therapy in 1983 and the experience reviewed in 1991.[31] They treated large T3-T4 tumors with surface therapy using curved tubes sutured over the tonsillar-oropharyngeal region and followed this with 50–60 Gy of external beam Co-60 therapy. Patients that were of poor performance status and feeble or very elderly with large and bulky tumors, were noted to have CR tumor regression in 100% with 77% local control and 88% actuarial 2–year survivals. They reported that complete tumor responses were regularly observed and local control and survival rates were excellent. Further studies of combined Cf plus radiotherapy with adjuvant chemotherapy are indicated in the future.

Lip

Obninsk observed 100% CR responses of T1 and T2 lip tumors (Table 8) with 92% 3-year survivors with Cf brachytherapy only in 39 treated patients.[32] Even recurrent lip cancers responded well with 81% CR responses, 59% 3-year survivors, and 22% complications. For the primary tumors, there were only 10% complications. LDR brachytherapy was used in Russia.[83] Similar results were observed using MDR combined with photon therapy in Lexington.[97]

Nasopharynx

Tumors of the nasopharynx can sometimes be large tumors with base of skull invasion or be recurrent after prior radiotherapy. A small series of these tumors were treated in Lexington with favorable results observed. MDR was used with tubes inserted nasally into the nasopharynx and a brachytherapy treatment given before 50–60 Gy of external beam photon radiotherapy.[99] Treatment volume was selected to cover the walls of the nasopharynx to 15–20 Gy-eqs. Combination with cisplatin and 5-FU was well tolerated and effective.

Parotid

Parotid nonepithelial tumors are established to be sensitive to neutrons from observations around the world. Parotid tumors were treated with Cf neutrons in Lexington[97] and Obninsk[120] and it was found that these tumors are readily and effectively treated with Cf neutrons. There were 75% CR responses with recurrent tumors and 63% 2-year survivors. Generally, the Cf brachytherapist sees these patients only after multiple prior therapies including surgeries and radiation treatments. Since tumor size as well as treatment volume is usually small, therapy is effective with low complication rates. Both LDR therapy, LDR plus Co-60 beam therapy, and MDR plus photon therapy have been used successfully.

Skin (Including Melanomas) and Soft Tissues

One hundred percent of T2-T3 tumors involving the skin (Table 6) responded without complications with 100% 5-year survivors.[89] Ninety-three percent of 14 recurrent tumors responded completely with 16% complications and 71% 2-year survivors. Again tumors of the skin have usually had prior surgery and/or radiation before referral. Lexington reported complete response and cure of a massive tumor of the neck region using Cf (Figure

8) and radiation.[99] Interstitial, LDR, MDR, and HDR have been used with or without external beam photon or electron beam therapy.

Melanomas have been treated in Russia,[89] Japan,[53,121] and Lexington[125] with good local responses usually observed but with distant metastases and failures appearing all too frequently soon afterward. Obninsk noted 100% CR responses but only 57% 2-year survivals (Table 8). Raju et al.[125] reported 100% CR responses but only 20% 2-year survivals. Keio[53] and JCIH[121] have reported CR responses of acrallentiginous melanomas using Cf with long-term survivors but usually late distant metastases. LDR, MDR, plaque, interstitial, as well as HDR and combination with photon or electron therapy have been used.

Sarcomas

Sarcomas of soft tissues have been noted to be sensitive to Cf neutrons and effectively treated and locally controlled.[89,99] There were 75% CR responses with 62% 2-year survivals in Russia (Table 9) and dramatic regression responses have been reported from Lexington. However, these tumors can be of enormous size and few tumors have been treated owing to the limited availability of appropriate seed sources in suture, which could be used for unresectable tumors, e.g., of the retroperitoneum or other deep structures.

Recurrent Head and Neck Tumors

Recurrent tumors after prior surgery and radiation are common in the oral cavity. In 62% of tongue, 89% of floor of the mouth, 50% of oropharynx, 81% of lower lip, and 100% of skin and soft tissue tumors CR responses were obtained by Cf therapy[33] (Table 7). In about half, local control was obtained and long-term survivors up to 3, 5, or 10 years have been observed. For tongue, 3-year survival was 49%, floor of mouth 55%, oropharynx 50%, and lower lip 59%. For skin and soft tissue it was 86%. Cf treatment has been Cf-only used at LDR, MDR, HDR, and in combination with various doses of external beam radiation.[9,34] Vtyurin has written on the high efficacy of Cf for the treatment of the recurrent oral cavity/head and neck lesions (Table 9). While the treatment of recurrent tumors, particularly

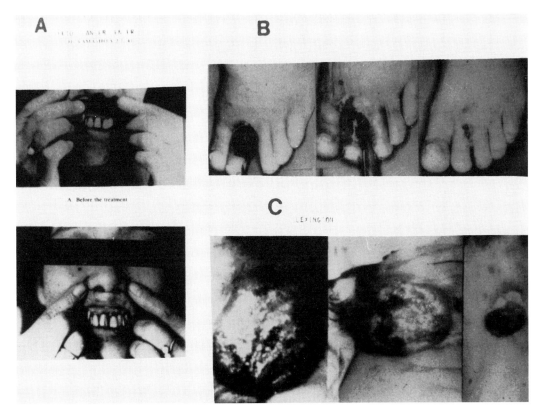

Figure 8. Response of melanoma at different centers. A) Before and after, response of melanoma of the upper lip from experience of H. Yamashita at Keio Cancer Center; B) Before and after, Cf treatment for toe melanoma at Cancer Institute Hospital from experience of Kaneta, et al., and C) Before and after Cf treatment for melanosarcoma of root of neck (15-cm tumor, from Maruyama, Radiation Center, Lexington). Regression led to ulceration for large tumors. This is a side effect and not a complication of therapy for bulky tumors.

Table 9.
Clearance of Recurrent Tumors with Cf-252 Brachytherapy

Anatomic Site	CR Response	%	Complications	%	2-Year Survival	%
Tongue	23/26	89	13	50	18	69
Floor of mouth	8/9	88	3	33	5	55
Lip	22/22	100	4	18	20	91
Skin	13/14	93	3	16	10	71
Soft tissue sarcomas	6/8	75	—	—	5	62
Parotid gland	4/6	66	—	—	3	50
Vulva	2/4	50	—	—	0	0
Metastases to lymph nodes of neck	3/4	75	—	—	2	50

CR = complete regression.
From Vtyurin (89).

those that have received prior courses of radical radiotherapy carries risks of side effects and normal tissue defects, these tumors left untreated will lead to similar problems with the added problem of local pain and uncontrolled progressive tumor. Surgery can be used to correct the tissue defects and once corrected, the long-term survivals and quality of life justify the Cf therapy.

The Russian researchers have been interested in and studied the immune status of patients with oral cavity tumors following neutron brachytherapy.[126]

Laryngeal Stomal Recurrence

Lexington has found that stomal recurrence of laryngeal cancers are very effectively treated with Cf using an intraluminal placement of Cf followed by external beam Co-60 therapy. There was 100% local CR response but the patients have high risk of failure from distant metastases.

Nasal Cavity and Antrum

Tumors of the maxillary antrum are resistant to external photon therapy and standard therapy is usually surgery followed by radiation. Neutron beam therapy has been found effective by Catterall and Bewley.[85,127] Lexington has reported implantation of Cf tubes in the antrum and delivering MDR Cf plus external photon therapy with CR response and long-term cure.[97] Similarly, results have been observed for nasal cavity tumors using similar methods.

Cervix and Female Genital Tract

Cervix cancers have been a model human tumor for brachytherapy.[128] Brachytherapy alone can be used for small tumors. As tumors get larger, they extend beyond the cervix into the parametrium and when very advanced, invade the bladder or rectum, or extend to the pelvic side wall. The natural history of the tumors is to stay localized for long periods of time before distant metastases occur.[128] A few patients were treated in the initial trials, but intensive study of the potential of Cf for treatment of cervix tumors did not begin until the studies carried out in Lexing-

ton.[23,24,37,41,43,83,86,116,119,123,128,132,135,136] The studies focused first on high stage cervix cancers but observation of very high efficacy very soon led to study of all stages (Table 10) and then to evaluation of Cf therapy for other GYN tumors of the uterus, vagina, vulva, and even of the urethra. This chapter will not attempt to review all the detailed studies on cervix cancers but will focus on important steps in the studies and outcomes (Table 11).

High Stage Cervix Cancers (Stage IIIB)

The initial studies of cervix cancers used conventional schedules and methods for intracavitary therapy. High-dose whole pelvis radiotherapy to 50–55 Gy was followed by a delayed brachytherapy implant and treated to point A as a reference point. It was found that efficacy was not very different from photon brachytherapy.[23] Maruyama et al.[131] postulated that the delayed schedule might be improved by the use of an up-front or "early" schedule for the use of the neutrons in order to attack the radioresistance in these advanced tumors immediately and combine the Cf with added large dose pelvic photon therapy. Complete tumor regression was observed in 90% of treated patients when the early schedule was used. The early schedule was significantly better than the delayed schedule or conventional Cs-137 photon brachytherapy (Figure 9) and produced quick regression of bulky tumors.[37,41] Its implications were not understood at once but by 1985, the meaning of the rapid regression was better understood. It was found that the use of the early implant schedule (and the quick CR response) led to much better 5-year survival and cure rates than the delayed schedule or the use of conventional photon therapy.[23,43,138] The quick regression of epithelial tumors by Cf was confirmed by Vtyurin[27] and Tacev et al.[84] Further study of bulky stage IB cervix cancers in Lexington and by Tacev et al.[84] has confirmed and further characterized tumor response using the half regression times of tumors.

For cervix tumors, the quick regression (Figure 3) has been further studied by the application of surgical[117] and histologic study methods to evaluate tumor responses.[24,116] This was done after a course of preoperative

Table 10.
Combination of External and Intracavitary Irradiation in Treatment of Carcinoma
of the Cervix Using Cf-252 Dose

Stage[a]	Tumor Size	Whole Pelvis* (cGy)	Intracavitary (cGy-eq)	Total Dose at Reference Point[b] Parametria‡ (cGy/cGy-eq)	Dose (Gy)	Comment
IB	any size	45	20–25 Cf (1×)	65–70 Gy at pt A[b]	50 Gy[b]	Cf is an alternate therapy for elderly or obese, medically poor risk patients.
IB Bulky or Barrel Shaped	>3 ≤ 6 with TAH-BSO	45	20 Cf (1×)	65–70 Gy-eq at pt A[b]	50[d]	Combined with extrafascial TAH-BSO.
	Without TAH-BSO	45	20–35 Cf (1×–2×)[c]	75–80 Gy-eq at pt A	50[d]	Larger dose for larger tumors. No extrafascial fascial TAH-BSO.
	>6 cm	45	20–35 Cf (1×–2×)[c]	75–80 Gy-eq at pt A	60[d]	With extrafascial TAH-BSO & abdominal staging.
IIAB	Generally, >4 cm	45‡	25-35 Cf (1×–2×)[c]	75–85 Gy-eq	60[d]	Usually radiation only. TAH-BSO for small tumors.
IIIAB	5–15 cm	55–60	25–35 Cf (1×–2×)[c]	80–85 Gy-eq	60[d]	No. of implants depends on tumor regression. Reduce pelvic field after 45 Gy.
IV	Any size	60	20–30 Cf-252 (1×)	75–85 Gy-eq	60[d]	For pelvic control.

* Standard fractionation.
† All Cf-252 done early before XRT; dose in Gy-eq (Cs-137, Ra-226, Ir-192 implants are done in delayed schedule).
‡ Overall field height reduced at 45 Gy and midline shaped block of entire central field.
[a] FIGO staging system.
[b] Treatment reference is point A or isodose curve.
[c] Second insertion in 2 weeks after early Cf intracavitary application.
[d] Sidewall boost with midline block.
TAH-BSO = total abdominal hysterectomy with bilateral salpingo-oophorectomy.

Table 11.
Worldwide Results of Californium-252 Brachytherapy For Cervix & Uterus Cancers

Site/Stage	Method	Results (5-Year Survival)	Center
Cervix			
Cervix IB	+ TAH-BSO	94%	Lexington
Cervix IB	Cf + RT only	91%	Lexington
Cervix II	Cf-NT + TAH-BSO	70%	Lexington
Cervix IIB	Cf-NT	80%	JCIH
Cervix IIIB	Early Cf-NT	54%	Lexington
Cervix IIIB	Cf-NT	44%	Keio
Cervix IIIB	Delayed Cf-NT	15%	Lexington
Cervix IVA	Cf-NT	18%	Lexington
Uterus			
Stage I–II	Cf-NT	75%	Soviet Union
Stage I	Cf-NT	83%	Lexington
Stage G1–2	Cf-NT	94%	Lexington
Stage II G–3	Cf-NT	21%	Lexington
Rectum			
Stage T2–3	Cf-NT ± Surgery	78%	Soviet Union

JCIH = Japan Cancer Institute Hospital.

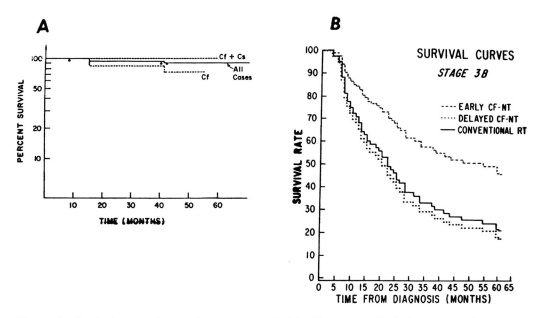

Figure 9. Survival curves for cervix cancer reported by Maruyama, Radiation Center, Lexington, KY, USA. A) Stage IB bulky tumors. Five-year survival was 91% with either Cf alone or mixed Cf plus Cs-137 implants; and B) Stage IIIB carcinoma of the cervix treated with early Cf implant (54% 5-year survivals), delayed Cf implant (20% 5-year survival), or delayed conventional Cs-137 implant (P<0.05). (Reproduced with permission from Cancer[133] and Int J Radiat Oncol Biol Phys[138].)

radiation using extrafascial hysterectomy 4–6 weeks later.[129] From these studies it was established that quick tumor shrinkage is the usual response of bulky tumors to neutrons.[27,37,41,84] The combined Cf and surgery was possible because the treatment volume exposed to high neutron dose is small, hence healing of tissues proceeds without problems. The tolerance by adjacent normal tissues has been excellent since those tissues never received high doses of neutrons (unlike neutron beam therapy). While different schedules and methods have been used in the different clinics, it is standard to combine external beam and brachytherapy for the treatment of advanced tumors. While different dose prescription methods can be used, the total biological dose using LDR or MDR should be 80–85 Gy-eqs at point A or the paracervical region.

Patient Evaluation Procedures

All patients are evaluated using standard history, general and pelvic examination, examination under anesthesia if necessary, bi-opsy, histologic study, blood tests for cell counts and chemistries, and radiological studies and the FIGO staging system.[130] We have used CT scanning to evaluate the abdomen and pelvis and urinary tract as well as chest x-rays. MRI has been used to evaluate the pelvis in more recent studies. Cystoscopy and proctoscopy has been used to evaluate the bladder and rectum if necessary. Stage is assigned using the FIGO system and is determined clinically. Laparoscopy has been used recently as well as fine needle aspiration studies of abnormal pelvic or abdominal densities detected by CT scanning.

Treatment Methods

All patients have received combined external beam and intracavitary therapy using Cf. Pure Cf implants plus external beam photon therapy is best for high stage or bulky disease. For low stage disease, mixed Cf plus Cs-137 or other photon-emitters can be used.[132] The external beam therapy has been whole pelvis therapy to doses of 45–60 Gy and we have generally not used central blocking. Cumulative doses of over 75 Gy-eqs to the anterior wall of the rectum or 80 Gy-eqs to the posterior wall of the trigone of the bladder are well tolerated. An RBE of 6 was used to calculate the dose equivalent to these normal tissues but, Cf implant therapy must be done early before the start of external radiation. Applicators are inserted into the uterus, cervix, and vagina and their position localized by orthogonal radiographs.[132] A single or double tandem is used with the double tandem used for large cavitary tumors of the cervix. Vaginal tubes rather than colpostats are used since it is better to place the sources closed to the tumor so neutron dose is high and not reduced by inverse square. Extra

vaginal tubes are used if there is excess distance between the tandem and the lateral vaginal tubes (Figure 10) or if tumor involves or extends down the vagina. Since tumors appropriate for Cf are usually bulky, more than one insertion is usually needed. The second should be performed about 2 weeks after the first since considerable tumor regression has occurred by that time and more remote tumor has shifted closer to the neutron sources. Waiting to the end of the external beam therapy course and delayed implant greatly increases the risks of complications since tumor shrinkage will be complete and sensitive organs now are much closer to the neutron sources and dose is high.[83]

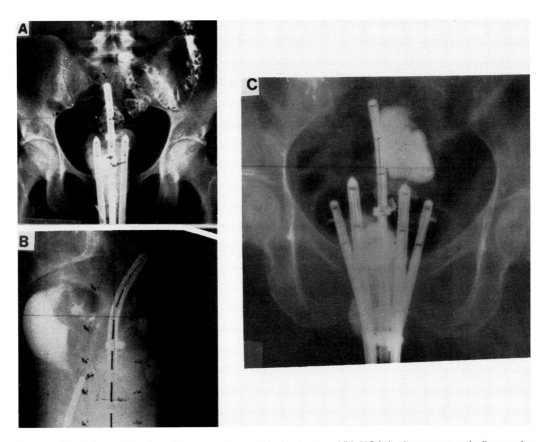

Figure 10. Intracavitary insertion as performed in Lexington, KY, USA for low stage or bulky cervix cancers. A) AP film for bulky IB cancer; B) Lateral implant simulation film for bulky IB cancer. All adjacent organs were localized to control dose at those organs; and C) AP film of bulky cervix cancer with large vaginal mass. Henschke applicators without are useful as there is no end effect for Cf sources. System surrounds the tumor mass without dosimetric "holes" in order to overcome limited range of Cf neutrons.

Table 10 shows our recommended treatment schedules and doses for Cf therapy of cervix cancers. We do not recommend Cf for small or minimal T1 tumors. These are easily treated with surgery or photons and there are no unusual risks or late hazards from such therapy. Cf can be an alternative therapy for elderly, obese, or medically poor risk patients or as tumors get larger and are 4–5 cm in diameter. For bulky IB or small IIB tumors, combined radiation and surgery or radiation therapy can be effective. For stages IIB-IV, Cf and radiation therapy is recommended. With the stage III and IV tumors, chemo-Cf-radiotherapy is recommended.[86,132] Cisplatin and 5-FU represent an effective regimen.[86]

Stage IB

For bulky stage I tumors we have treated patients using Cf alone or Cf[133] and radiation combined with extrafascial hysterectomy.[24,116,129] The 5-year cure rate has been 91% (Table 11) with 9% grade 2–3 complications treating a select group of poor-risk patients who were treated with Cf and radiation only[133] (Figure 11). For this group of patients,

mixed early Cf plus delayed Cs-137 is effective. Patients were treated with 40–45 Gy whole pelvis plus intracavitary insertion to a total point A dose of 30–35 cGy-eqs (70 Gy-eqs) and local control was 100%.

For the patients treated with Cf preoperatively,[24,116,129] the patients are treated with 45 Gy to the whole pelvis after an early Cf insertion that delivers 15–20 Gy-eqs to a total point A dose of 60–65 Gy-eqs. It was found that the presence of histologic tumor correlated with the dose given and tumor was eradicated as a function of dose given.[24] In some patients, two insertions were needed in order to deliver the appropriate dose. As the total dose was escalated, more specimens were cleared of tumor and at point A doses of 10–12 Gy-eqs about 25% of the specimens were positive but became <5% at doses of 18–20 Gy-eqs. The 5-year survival rate was 94% and complications minimal,[129] using the combined radiation-surgery procedure. It was found that survival and cure correlated with the histologic status of the specimen.[134] In patients where no tumor was found, survival was 95% and the survival curves were flat to over 10 years. If the specimen showed residual tumor, the

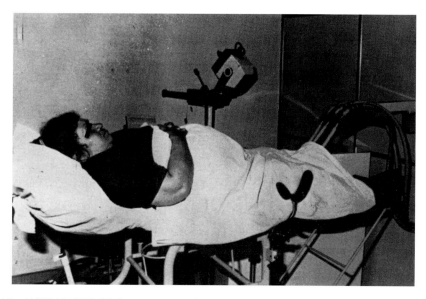

Figure 11. ANET-V HDR Cf therapy as performed in Moscow at oncologic center. Sources are stored behind barrier and are delivered with computer-controlled remote afterloading system to uterus, cervix, or vagina. Treatments require milligram activity Cf sources and is complete in minutes. (Courtesy of L. Marjina, Moscow Oncological Center, Russia.)

survival fell to 60% 5-year survival. This finding was the same for both Cf or Cs-137 brachytherapy.[116] Surgery was performed 4–6 weeks after completion of radiation and this time for sampling appeared to have prognostic significance.

Stage II Cervical Cancer

Similar methods were used to treat stage II tumors and were highly effective for local tumor control of >95% and the main problem was the later appearance of distant metastases.[135] For stage IIB tumors, the 5-year survival rate was 70% and failures were mainly distant in patients treated using an up-front Cf treatment protocol.[43] In a study group of stage II tumors treated with preoperative Cf therapy, the survival rate was 70% at 5-years.[135] It was found that 93% were cured if the surgical specimen was negative for tumor but fell to 46% if the specimen was positive. Local tumor was controlled more effectively by Cf than by Cs-137 by the use of an early or up-front schedule.[23,138] The efficacy of Cf for the therapy of advanced cervical cancers has been confirmed by JCIH[95] and Keio[94] in Japan, and in Russia, Czechoslovakia,[84] and Lithuania.[58] The initial trials showed that local control increased from 25%–30% with photons to 70%–80% using neutrons.[23,43]

Stage III and IV Cervical Cancer

Five-year survival for stage IIIB cancer was 54% using the early schedule, which was better than the delayed schedule or conventional Cs-137 photon. Lexington treated patients with stage IV tumors and reported a 5-year survival rate (Table 11) of ~20%.[136] These were patients who had received no other therapy and who had IVA disease with e.g., bladder invasion. Early Cf insertion was combined with 50–60 Gy of whole pelvis radiation. Stage IVB patients are patients who have distant metastases at diagnosis and long-term survivals would not be expected although there could be palliation of pelvic problems such as bleeding or pain.

Lexington has reported experiences and evaluation of parametrial interstitial implant methods for the treatment of stage IIIB and IVA tumors with favorable results and 5-year

cures.[137] Since the only sources available were of an intracavitary type, only a few cases were treated but the feasibility study results were favorable. To conduct a proper clinical trial, better sources (seeds) and remote afterloaders will be needed. Good results have been reported for stage III-IVA cancer.[138]

Bleeding and Hemorrhage from Advanced Pelvic Cancers[139]

Control of severe bleeding in advanced pelvic cancers of the GYN tract is a difficult problem. Deep pelvic infections can also be a difficult problem and associated with tubo-ovarian and deep pelvic abscess. Cf-252 has been found to be highly effective in controlling severe bleeding and facilitating drainage. The treatment is short and late radiation effects (external beam in large doses causes frequent severe delayed tissue effects). Lexington used short (hours) implants and readily controlled hemorrhage/infection problems associated with advanced bulky cancers.

For infections of the GYN tract, metronidazole was found to be a very potent antibiotic against anaerobic infections.[140] However, it was not effective as a radiation hypoxic sensitizer even with direct insertion of tablets into the tumor, combined with oral and intravenous drug administration.

Uterus

Both Lexington and the Russians have reported excellent results in the treatment of uterine cancers using Cf (Table 11). The first report came from Kentucky in 1980 and 1985[141] and was updated recently.[25] These were mainly patients who were obese, medically ill, and who had unfavorable presentations for surgery. They included many patients who had high grade, G3, and adenosquamous histology. Tumor was eradicated from the uterus in 36% of the specimens of surgically treated patients. Survival was 92% at 2 years and 83% at 5 years for stage I, 100% for G1, and 88% for G2. Russian experience has used the ANET HDR remote afterloading machine for the treatment of cancer of the uterine corpus.[142,143] Both Moscow and Obninsk report excellent results with 75% 5-year survivals after treatment of stage I and

II tumors using Cf.[89] These experiences indicate that uterine cancers are sensitive to neutrons and that Cf is an excellent treatment of choice for the patient with a medically inoperable corpus carcinoma.

Anal and Rectal Adenocarcinoma

Sixty-one patients with rectal malignant tumors were treated with HDR intracavitary Cf therapy in Russia using Cf[92] (Table 11). Combined Cf plus external radiation was followed by surgery in some of the cases. Forty patients were treated preoperatively and had T2-T3 tumors and the 5-year survival was 78% with 8% recurrences and 10% distant metastases. Lexington also reported a favorable experience using Cf on anal and low anal-rectal cancers.[144] There was 100% CR responses observed and 75% local control for anal region tumors. These experiences are encouraging and indicate that Cf therapy may be an alternative for adminoperineal resection (APR) and colostomy, which is the standard surgical therapy, for the patient who does not wish surgery. Adjuvant pelvic radiation to 45–55 Gy and as well as consolidative chemotherapy is indicated. HDR intracavitary experience has been reported from Russia.[145] Local tumor biopsy done 4–6 weeks after irradiation will establish whether a conservative or radical surgical procedure is indicated.

Lung and Bronchus

Kaneta and Tsuya at JCIH[121] reported that endobronchial Cf was effective for the treatment of central bronchial carcinoma obstructing the major bronchi or trachea. Sources were afterloaded into plastic catheters positioned under bronchoscopic control using local anesthesia. Treatment was effective for local control of tumors and failures were due to distant metastases. Further research will require seed sources, ribbons, and remote afterloaders capable of delivering MDR or HDR treatments. The treatment should reduce the number of treatment sessions now used and increase the efficacy of endobronchial therapy for palliation of recurrent cancers with obstructive pneumonitis, bleeding, atelectasis, or tumor stenosis.

Esophagus

Lexington, JCIH,[121] and Obninsk[146] have treated esophageal tumors using MDR or LDR methods and intracavitary methods. This has been combined with external beam photon therapy. Tumors treated have measured 1–14 cm in length and have usually been situated in the mid- or lower third. A plastic catheter has been inserted into the esophagus using topical anesthesia under fluoroscopic control, to the site of the tumor. Cf sources were then positioned at the tumor site. Anikin[146] reported the use of retrograde placement via a gastrostomy to position sources into the distal esophagus. Lexington researchers reported that tumor regression can be very rapid and there was risk of perforation since the esophagus is a very thin-walled organ. Further studies will require seed sources, remote afterloading, and use of MDR or HDR techniques. Local control is excellent but adjuvant chemotherapy and external radiation is necessary since mediastinal and mucosal spread and distant metastases are frequent. The addition of 50 Gy of x-radiation and cisplatin and 5-FU adjuvant therapy is indicated based on the favorable results reported recently.

Melanomas and Sarcomas

Cf has been found effective against tumors of different histologies. For melanomas, Lexington,[125] Keio,[53] JCIH,[121] and Russian[89] experiences have reported quick regression of these photon resistant tumors. Lexington, Keio, JCIH, and Obninsk have reported favorable responses in these tumors in the extremities, head and neck, i.e., acral-lentiginous tumors, as well as on other sites on the body surface.

Sarcomas of soft tissues respond well to Cf neutrons and CR responses have been noted to be rapid after treatment. However, the regression times were variable and this indicates the heterogeneity of these tumors.[89] Most of these tumors regress after 2–3 weeks and were complete in 82% of treated patients. A radiation-induced osteosarcoma[101] was noted to regress so rapidly after Cf neutron treatment in Lexington that it fell off leaving a large tissue defect that later needed surgical repair. Biopsies showed that the tumor had completely disappeared from the site of origin, and tissue grafts were needed to heal the effect.

Ocular Melanomas

Ocular melanomas have been proposed by Fontanesi (personal communication) as an appropriate tumor for Cf therapy since these tumors can be large and resistant to photon beam irradiation. The tumors respond favorably to brachytherapy. Proton and heavy ion beams have been used but lead to a 50% frequency of visual loss, hence brachytherapy methods can give superior quality of life outcomes.

Prostate

Lexington has reported favorable responses in the treatment of advanced and recurrent adenocarcinomas of the prostate gland or nonadenocarcinomas of the proximal male urethra region.[147] The treatment method utilized in the pilot study used an intraurethral catheter, much like the earliest method used for prostate cancer therapy in Europe, and seeds for proper therapy.

Female Urethra

The female urethra is an ideal site for intracavitary therapy using Cf. Lexington found that advanced tumors of this region were very effectively treated[99] using intraluminal placement of a catheter into which Cf could be afterloaded as well as interstitial sources. Cf therapy can be combined effectively with beam radiation as well as chemotherapy in this site.

Malignant Glioma, Glioblastoma Multiforme

The extremely poor prognosis of patients with malignant brain tumors is well documented.[148] There is a >50% mortality within 8.5 months and maximal radiation even with high doses, hyperaccelerated schedules, high-dose brachytherapy, and hyperthermia, and maximal chemotherapy in any combination or dosage has not significantly impacted on long-term survival or cure rates. The only

therapy that has been shown to consistently eradicate glioblastoma multiforme (GBM) is neutron therapy.[149,150] Those results led to the study of Cf neutrons for the treatment of GBM using interstitial techniques.[151]

Since 1980, feasibility followed by phase I clinical trials[118] have been conducted in Lexington for GBM.[152,153] Treatment focused on hemispheric tumors, histologically proven tumors, and interstitial therapy after debulking surgery. Initial study used a single applicator tube implant followed by 50–60 Gy of external beam radiation and used CT-guided tube placement.[152] The study advanced to use multiple tubes and then went on to the use of stereotactic implant methods, all combined with whole brain radiation therapy.[152] The initial studies showed that there was dramatic improvement in performance status and good tolerance of the implant and radiation procedures. Survival was improved by using multiple rather than a single tube.[152] Chin and Patchell reported on the patient survivals after Cf interstitial therapy[152,153] and it was noted that there were ~30% 2-year survivals. This led to the initiation of a phase 1 clinical trial to determine a dose of neutrons which eradicated tumor and produced no necrosis in normal brain using Cf interstitial therapy only. It has now been shown that 12 Gy of neutrons is the tolerance dose for Cf neutrons and at larger doses, brain necrosis begins to appear.[118,153,154] Despite the fact that this was a phase 1 study, long-term 4- to 5-year survivors have been observed already. Future trials await the production of appropriate seed sources to conduct the study using better conformal methods. BNCE can be used to enhance tumor dose[44] using neutron capture therapy.

The complications of the procedure have been remarkably few and intracranial hemorrhage has not occurred in any of the patients treated. We had no mortality attributable to brachytherapy. The major problems that occurred were cerebral edema (2%), infection (3%), and hemiplegia (1.5%), which occurred in a patient who was treated with a delayed implant after receiving external beam radiation to the skull. It was learned that high doses of neutrons should not be given to the scalp as it is a neutron-sensitive structure. Miller et al.[118] and Ciuba et al.[153] reported on the sensitivity of the scalp to neutrons as a side effect of Cf brachytherapy. Scalp necrosis was avoided if scalp neutron dose was kept below 10 Gy.[151] Hernandez et al.[155] have reported that Cf and accelerated hyperfractionated radiation[156] did not appear to increase efficacy of Cf brachytherapy.

Adjuvant Therapy for Californium-252 Neutron Therapy

Chemotherapy

The various ways in which radiation and chemotherapy can interact has been extensively studied and much has been written about the potential advantages and the promises of combining chemotherapy and radiation. In most sites the normal tissue side effects become much more severe and in conjunction with neutron beam therapy for lung cancer, there have been high rates of severe and fatal complications. However, the Lexington group reported that cisplatin plus 5-FU combined with high-dose hyperfractionated twice a day irradiation was well tolerated in the therapy of cervix cancers[86] (Table 2). Three cycles of chemotherapy, two during irradiation and one course 1 month later were given with the initial treatment with Cf done in week 0 to shrink the tumor. Cisplatin was given along with infusion of 5-FU for 4 consecutive days along with twice a day irradiation (weeks 1 and 4). The 90% 3-year survival rate supports further study and clinical evaluation of Cf chemoradiation for cervix cancers and perhaps for other cancers as well.

Boron Neutron Capture Enhancement Therapy[44]

In BNCE two agents are used: a thermal or epithermal beam of neutrons and a tumor-seeking boron containing compound that targets the tumor in high concentration and allows the high LET irradiation of target tumor cells.[63] The BNCE depends on the $B^{10}(n,\alpha)Li^7$ reaction. Beach et al.[44] postulated that Cf brachytherapy produced adequate thermal neutron flux in tissues to be able to treat tumors using BNCE. Wierzbicki et al.[71,87] have carried out detailed measurements of thermal neutrons produced in tissue-equivalent media and determined that enhancement would depend on distance from the sources. Schroy[74] studied Cf BNCE radiobiology. Yanch et al.[63] and Yanch and Zamenhof et al.[64] carried out Monte Carlo calculations of the radiations from Cf and produced along and away tables of the enhancement possible with different concentrations of B-10. From these studies it is clear that a potential exists for enhancement of Cf dose in tumor using B-10. While the enhancement is not large, and only about 10%–25%, it occurs mainly at the edges of the tumor (about 5–10 cm)[63,64] and it is postulated that malignant gliomas and advanced cervix cancers may be benefited by BNCE therapy. Matalka et al.[88] have carried out an experimental study in a nude rat brain tumor model using a human melanoma, MRA 27, implanted into the brain and irradiated with Cf plaque irradiation with or without prior B-10-boronophenylalanine administration. They reported that there was a doubling of the survival times of the BPA plus Cf treated rats compared to the those treated with Cf alone (Figure 12) showing that there was sufficient drug localization and thermal neutrons in the Cf irradiation to be detectable and to increase the therapeutic efficacy of Cf. Further experimental study is indicated in a variety of human tumor models using Cf as a source of thermal neutrons as well as uptake studies in human tumors where combined BNCE therapy may be applicable. Tumors that may be appropriate are melanoma, GBM, sarcomas, recurrent body surface breast and head and neck cancers, and advanced cervix and pelvic cancers such as rectal adenocarcinomas.[160]

Hyperthermia

Hyperthermia and Cf neutron therapy has been studied in the USA at Lexington[101] and in Obninsk. Hyperglycemia along with hyperthermia by glucose infusion has also been studied with Cf in Russia. Further research and phase II, III, and clinical trials will be needed to establish its role.

Summary and Conclusions

Cf therapy is readily usable by using a controlled facility in the Radiation Oncology de-

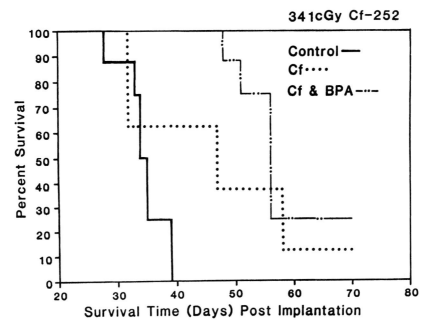

Figure 12. Boron Neutron Capture enhancement of Cf therapy as studied by Matalka et al.[88] using human MRA-27 tumor implanted intracerebrally in nude rats. Left solid curve is survival time of untreated control rats. Dotted central curve is survival of Cf treated rats. Right dot-dash curve is for B-10 boronphenylalanine plus Cf treated rats. Mean survival times were best for the BPA plus Cf treated animals (P<0.05).

partment. LDR, MDR, and HDR methods have been developed and tested by the different workers and found to be effective. Each method has advantages and disadvantages and the optimal method is one where antitumor RBE is large (i.e., about 6) and the treatment times short. The HDR methods are efficient but, may not be most effective since RBE is less and only about 3 for normal tissues. Because of this, adjacent normal tissue RBE may be higher (due to lower dose rate), and differential effect in tumor may be less. Time is not important in neutron therapy and hence short treatment times have been favored. MDR and HDR methods are best but the development of afterloading machines in the West has lagged behind Russia as well as the design of a variety of sources of different activities and sizes for medical usage. Multiple insertions are necessary and the initial investment costs are moderate.

The most important source size to develop for future brachytherapy is the high activity (3–10 μg) seed source. The seed source and afterloading machines would facilitate study of brain tumors, sarcomas, and a large variety of tumors. Based on the high antitumor efficacy of Cf against tumor, excellent normal tissue tolerance, high RBE, good patient acceptance and tolerance, a modified MDR may be the ideal system to use. With somewhat larger AT sources between 33–100 μg in size, treatment times could be shortened to a few hours (only slightly longer than HDR), but by using multiple sources, the number of insertions kept small (~2), RBE and efficacy high (RBE ~6), and overall treatment time short. Available remote afterloader equipment could be used for delivery or retrieval. Different remote afterloader machines and sources are needed for GYN or interstitial therapy using Cf. At the present time there is a need to carry out further radiobiological studies to evaluate the RBE and biological properties of Cf with different dose rates (between MDR and HDR) where the major biological changes take place and for combined modality and BNCE therapy. Further study of chemo-Cf-radiation

Table 12.
Methods of Increasing Efficacy of Radiotherapy

Technique	Method
Dose	Machines—megavoltage, Isocentric
	Conformal—3-D planning
	Particles
	Brachytherapy
Chemicals	Enhancers
	Radioprotectors
	Oxygen
	Oxygen-substitutes
Biology	Schedule
	Fractionation
	Dose rate
	Neutrons
Systemic	Hormones
	Cytotoxic
	Immunological
	Regulatory
Physical	Heat
	Dose Augmentation (BNCE)

therapy and BNCE are important and essential. Neutron brachytherapy represents the most promising avenue for radiation oncology to study in future trials for controlling locally advanced or radioresistant cancers. Table 12 presents methods that should be explored for use in future radiotherapy. Brachytherapy represents a powerful method to control dose delivery to tumor and neutrons and is a means of greatly increasing efficacy of therapy. Cf and neutron brachytherapy need further study and evaluation in the future of radiation medicine.

References

1. Thompson SG, Street K Jr, Ghiorso A, et al. The new element californium (atomic number 98). Phys Rev 1950;80:790–796.
2. Fields PR, et al. Transplutonium elements in thermonuclear debris. Phys Rev 1956;102:180–182.
3. Burch WD, Arnold ED, Chetham-Strode A. Production of the transplutonium elements. Nucl Sci Eng 1963;17:438–442.
4. Schlea CS, Stoddard DH. Californium isotopes proposed for interstitial and intracavitary radiation therapy with neutrons. Nature 1965;206:1058–1059.
5. Stoddard DH. Historical review of californium-252 discovery and development. Nucl Sci Appl 1986;2:189–199.
6. Stoddard DH. Radiation properties of californium-252. USAEC Rept. DP-986. EI DuPont de Nemours. Savanah River Lab. Aiken SC, 1965.
7. Boulogne AR, Evans AG. Californium-252 neutron sources for medical applications. Int J Appl Radiat Isotop 1969;20:453–461.
8. Wright CN, Boulogne AR, Reinig WC, et al. Implantable californium-252 neutron sources for radiotherapy. Radiol 1967;89:337–339.
9. Maruyama Y, Beach LJ, Feola JM. Californium-252 Brachytherapy and Fast Neutron Beam Therapy. Nucl Sci Appl 2. Chur. Harwood., 1986.
10. Fowler JF. Neutrons for radiotherapy of resistant tumors: Interaction with low LET. Nucl Sci Appl 1986;2:221–233.
11. Maruyama Y. Clinical radiobiology of Cf-252 for bulky tumor therapy. Nucl Sci Appl 1991;4:29–43.
12. Maruyama Y. Relative sensitivities of tumors to brachytherapy. Adv Radiat Biol 1992;15:71–152.
13. Maruyama Y, Peters L, Hilaris B, et al. Review of the early Cf-252 trials and the Lexington experience. Nucl Sci Appl 1986;2:201–217.
14. Hall EJ, Rossi H. The potential of californium-252 in radiotherapy. Preclinical measurements in physics and radiobiology. Br J Radiol 1975;48:777–790.
15. Krishnaswamy V. Calculation of the dose distribution about californium-252 needles in tissue. Radiology 1971;98:155–160.
16. Colvett RD, Rossi HH, Krishnaswamy V. Dose distributions around a californium-252 needle. Phys Med Biol 1972;17:356–364.
17. Anderson LL. Status of dosimetry for ^{252}Cf medical neutron sources. Phys Med Biol 1973;18:779–799.
18. Kal HB. Review of RBE and OER values for Cf-neutrons. Nucl Sci Appl 1986;2:303–316.
19. Fairchild RG, Atkins HL, Drew RM, et al. Biological effects of ^{252}Cf neutrons. Eur J Cancer 1974;10:305–308.
20. Kal HB, Barendsen GW. The OER at low dose-rates. Br J Radiol 1976;49:1049–1051.
21. Feola JM, Maruyama Y. Tumor and normal tissue effects and therapeutic gain for Cf-252. Nucl Sci Appl 1986;2:327–343.
22. Maruyama Y. Preface. In: Maruyama Y, Beach JL, Feola JM (eds). Californium-252 Brachytherapy and Fast Neutron Beam Therapy. Nucl Sci Appl 2. Chur. Harwood., 1986, pp. xiii-xviii.
23. Maruyama Y, Kryscio R, van Nagell JR, et al.

Neutron brachytherapy is better than conventional therapy in advanced cervical cancer. Lancet 1985;1:1120–1121.

24. Maruyama Y, van Nagell JR, Yoneda J, et al. Dose-response for californium-252 neutron brachytherapy by histological eradication of bulky stage IB cervical tumors. Endocurie Hypertherm Oncol 1989;5:111–120.

25. Maruyama Y, van Nagell JR, Yoneda J, et al. Clinical evaluation of ^{252}Cf neutron intracavitary therapy for primary endometrial adenocarcinoma. Cancer 1993;71:3920–3927.

26. Maruyama Y, Yoneda J, Krolikiewicz H, et al. Report of early responses in a clinical trial for advanced cervico-vaginal pelvic carcinoma using Cf-252 fast neutron therapy. Int J Radiat Oncol Biol Phys 1980;6:1629–1637.

27. Vtyurin BM, Tsyb AF. Brachytherapy with Cf-252 in USSR: Head and neck, GYN and other tumors. Nucl Sci Appl 1986;2:521–538.

28. Tsuya A, Kaneta K. Treatment of cancers of the tongue and oral cavity and lymph node metastases with Cf-252 at Cancer Institute Hospital, Tokyo, Japan. Nucl Sci Appl 1986; 2:539–553.

29. Maruyama Y, Patel P. Dose-effect for oral tongue cancer using Cf-252 neutron brachytherapy. Nucl Sci Appl 1991;4:251–258.

30. Medvedev VS, Vtyurin BM, Anikin VA, et al. Early and long term results of interstitial neutron Cf-252 brachytherapy of oral cavity mucosal cancers. Nucl Sci Appl 1991;4:235–238.

31. Stoll B, Maruyama Y, Patel P, et al. Cf-252 neutron brachytherapy for advanced tonsillar-oropharyngeal carcinoma. Nucl Sci Appl 1991;4:243–250.

32. Vtyurin BM, Medvedev V, Maksimov S, et al. Results of brachytherapy of lower lip cancer with Cf-252. Nucl Sci Appl 1991;4:231–234.

33. Vtyurin BM, Medvedev VS, Melin VS. Neutron brachytherapy of recurrent or persistent oral cavity tumors with Cf-252. Nucl Sci Appl 1991; 4:239–242.

34. Maruyama Y. International Neutron Therapy Workshop. Nucl Sci Appl v1–4. Chur. Harwood., 1991.

35. Gragg RL, Humphrey RM, Thames HD, et al. The response of Chinese hamster ovary cells to fast neutron radiotherapy beams. III. Variation in relative biological effectiveness with position in the cell cycle. Radiat Res 1978;76: 283–291.

36. Feola JM, Nava CA, Maruyama Y. Biological effects of Cf-252 neutrons at low dose rates. Int J Radiat Biol 1982;41:33–46.

37. Maruyama Y, Muir W. Human cervical cancer clearance after ^{252}Cf neutron brachytherapy vs. conventional photon brachytherapy. Am J Clin Oncol (CCT) 1984;7:347–352.

38. Wierzbicki JG, Maruyama Y. Treatment planning methods with Cf-252 at the University of Kentucky. Nucl Sci Appl 1991;4:19–27.

39. Maruyama Y, Feola JM, Beach JL. A tumor/normal tissue advantage for low dose rate neutron brachytherapy. Int J Radiat Oncol Biol Phys 1983;9:1715–1721.

40. Maruyama Y, Berner B, Feola J. Mixed sequence localized neutron brachytherapy plus photon radiation for tumor control in radiotherapy. Endocurie Hypertherm Oncol 1989; 5:39–48.

41. Maruyama Y. Rapid clearance of advanced pelvic carcinoma by low dose rate californium Cf-252 neutron therapy. Radiology 1979;133:473–475.

42. Yaes RJ, Berner B, Yoneda J, et al. Explanation for the efficacy of early vs. delayed californium brachytherapy for bulky cervix cancer. Nucl Sci Appl 1991;4:107–115.

43. Maruyama Y, van Nagell JR, Yoneda J, et al. A review of californium-252 neutron brachytherapy for cervical cancer. Cancer 1991;68: 1189–1197.

44. Beach JL, Schroy CB, Ashtari B, et al. Boron neutron capture enhancement of ^{252}Cf brachytherapy. Int J Radiat Oncol Biol Phys 1990;18:1421–1427.

45. Castro J, Oliver GD, Withers HR, et al. Experience with californium-252 in clinical radiotherapy. Am J Roentgenol 1973;117:182–194.

46. Paine CH, Berry RJ, Stedeford JB, et al. The use of californium-252 for brachytherapy of human tumours: A preliminary report. Eur J Cancer 1974;10:365–368.

47. Vallejo A, Hilaris BS, Anderson LL. ^{252}Cf for interstitial implantation: A clinical study at Memorial Hospital. Int J Radiat Oncol Biol Phys 1977;2:731–737.

48. Mahmoudi A. Contribution a la dosimetrie clinique des sources de californium-252 employees a l'Institut Gustave Roussy. Theses, Toulouse, 1977.

49. Maruyama Y. Cf-252 neutron brachytherapy: An advance for bulky localized cancer therapy. Nucl Sci Appl 1984;1:677–748.

50. Tsuya A, Kaneta K, Onai Y, et al. Clinical experience with californium-252 (first report). Nippon Acta Radiol 1977;37:238–247.

51. Yamashita H, Hashimoto S, Wada M, et al. Fast neutron therapy with high intensity Cf-252 sources by remotely controlled afterloading and clinical experiences in the treatment of gynecological cancers. Nucl Sci Appl 1986; 2:453–466.

52. Onai Y, Irifune T, Tomaru T, et al. Construction of storage, remote afterloader and treatment facility for californium-252 medical

sources and radiation protection survey. Nippon Acta Radiol 1978;38:643–653.

53. Yamashita H, Dokiya T, Hashimoto S. Experience at Keio University Hospial for Cf-252 radiation therapy of the head and neck and other sites. Nucl Sci Appl 1986;2:291–299.

54. Ivanov VN, Karelin EA, Elisyutin GP, et al. Dosimetry of Cf-252 radiation: Studies in the USSR. Nucl Sci Appl 1986;2:291–299.

55. Ivanov VN, Elisyutin GP, Komar V Ya, et al. Physical research into Cf-252 for brachytherapy in the USSR. Nucl Sci Appl 1991;4: 379–395.

56. Elisyutin GP, Komar V Ya. Dosimetry during contact therapy by ^{252}Cf isotope emission. Med Radiol 1977;10:54–59.

57. Karelin YE, Karasev VI, Berkutov VL. Californium sources of neutrons in medicine. Jaef Gkae Seminar on Radiation Utilization. Tokyo, Jpn, 30 Nov.-1 Dec., 1987, pp. 3–1 to 3–11.

58. Shpikalov VL, Atkochyus VB, Valuckas KK. The application of Cf-252 in contact neutron therapy of malignant tumors at the Scientific Research Institute of Oncology in Vilnius, Lithuania. Nucl Sci Appl 1991;4:419–424.

59. Tacev T, Strnad V, Vacek A, et al. Radiotherapy of cervix uteri carcinoma with Cf-252 implant and external hypoxyradiotherapy. Nucl Sci Appl 1991;4:201–212.

60. Keller OL. Californium-252: Properties and production. Nucl Sci Appl 1986;2:263–271.

61. Knauer JB, Alexander CW, Bigelow JE. Cf-252: Properties, production, source fabrication and procurement. Nucl Sci Appl 1991;4: 3–17.

62. Vtyurin BM, Medvedev VS, Ivanov VN, et al. Interstitial neutron therapy using flexible ^{252}Cf sources. Med Radiol 1984;6:7–16.

63. Yanch J, Zamenhof R, Wierzbicki J, et al. Comparison of dose distributions with ^{10}Boron augmented sources of ^{252}Cf obtained by Monte Carlo simulation and by experimental measurement. In: Allen BJ, Moore DE, Harrington BV (eds). Progress in Neutron Capture Therapy for Cancer. Plenum, New York, 1992, pp. 191–194.

64. Yanch J, Zamenhof R. Dosimetry of ^{252}Cf sources for neutron radiotherapy with and without augmentation by boron neutron capture therapy. Radiat Res 1992;131:249–256.

65. Anderson LL. Cf-252 physics and dosimetry. Nucl Sci Appl 1986;2:273–281.

66. Kraitor SN, Kuznetsova TV, Lumina NA, et al. Dosimetric characteristics of a neutron source. Med Radiol 1983;28:68–71.

67. Irifune T, Onai Y, Tomaru T, et al. Facility design, environmental protection and planning method for Cf-252 therapy at the Cancer Institute Hospital, Tokyo. Nucl Sci Appl 1986; 2:419–437.

68. Yamashita H, Wada T, Dokiya T, et al. Physical and biological dosimetries of Cf-252 radiation. Nucl Sci Appl 1986;2:345–367.

69. Beach JL, Harris MR. Microdosimetric studies of Cf-252. Nucl Sci Appl 1986;2:283–290.

70. Wierzbicki JG, Maruyama Y, Alexander CW. Cf-252 for teletherapy and thermalized Cf-252 neutrons for brachytherapy. Nucl Sci Appl 1991;4:361–366.

71. Wierzbicki JG, Alexander CW, Maruyama Y. Cf-252 neutron therapy and neutron capture therapy. In: Soloway AH, Barth RF, Carpenter DE (eds). Advances in Neutron Capture Therapy. Plenum, New York, 1991, pp. 139–141.

72. Todd P, Feola JM, Maruyama Y. Survival of cultured human cells exposed to californium-252 radiation at low dose rates. Am J Clin Oncol (CCT) 1984;7:495–498.

73. Vtyurin BM, Ivanov VN, Konoplyannikov AG, et al. Effects of ^{252}Cf source neutron and gamma-radiation. Moscow. Energoatomizdat, 1986, p. 128–179.

74. Schroy CB, Goud SN, Magura C, et al. Potentially lethal damage and radioprotection in human cells exposed to Cf-252. Nucl Sci Appl 1986;2:743–748.

75. Majima H, Ohara H, Urano M, et al. Repair of sublethal and potentially lethal damage in mouse squamous cell carcinoma cells following mixed neutron and x-ray irradiation: Relevance to early Cf-252 implant. Nucl Sci Appl 1991;4:47–56.

76. Maruyama Y, Feola J, Beach JL. Hela cell tumor response to Co-60, Cs-137, Cf-252 radiation and cis-platin chemotherapy in nude mice. Cancer 1984;54:247–252.

77. Parrish S, Feola JM, Maruyama Y. EMT6 tumor response to Co-60, Cs-137 and Cf-252 radiation in Balb/c mice. Endocurie Hypertherm Oncol 1987;3:3–9.

78. Malaise EP, Deschavanne PJ, Fertil B. Intrinsic radiosensitivity of human cells. Adv Radiat Biol 1992;15:37–70.

79. Beach JL, Milavickes LR, Maruyama Y. Microdosimetric considerations on the scheduling of combined neutron and photon radiation therapy. Proc. 7th ICRR. Broerse JJ, et al. (eds). Nijhoff, Amsterdam, 1983, p. D402.

80. Yaes RJ, Berner B, Yoneda J, et al. Explanation for the efficacy of early vs. delayed californium brachytherapy for bulky cervix cancer. Nucl Sci Appl 1991;4:107–115.

81. Maughan R. Fast neutron radiotherapy. Br J Radiol Suppl 1992;24:204–208.

82. Maruyama Y, Berner B, Feola JM. Mixed se-

quence localized neutron brachytherapy plus photon radiation for tumor control in radiotherapy. Endocurie Hypertherm Oncol 1989; 5:39–48.

83. Maruyama Y, van Nagell JR, Yoneda J, et al. Schedule in Cf-252 neutron brachytherapy: Complications after delayed implant therapy for cervical cancer in a phase II trial. Am J Clin Oncol (CCT) 1993;16:168–174.

84. Tacev T, Prokes B, Strnad V, et al. Effects of small doses of Cf-252 on the tumor regression in cervix uteri during combined radiotherapy. Strahlenther Onkol 1989;165:837–843.

85. Bessell E, Catterall M. The regression of tumors of the head and neck treated with neutrons. Int J Radiat Oncol Biol Phys 1983;9: 799–807.

86. Maruyama Y, Bowen MG, van Nagell JR, et al. A feasibility study of ^{252}Cf neutron brachytherapy, cis-platin + 5-FU chemoadjuvant and hyperaccelerated radiotherapy for advanced cervical cancer. Int J Radiat Oncol Biol Phys 1994, In Press.

87. Wierzbicki J, Maruyama Y, Porter AT. Measurements of augmentation of ^{252}Cf implants by ^{10}B and ^{157}Gd neutron capture. Med Phys 1994;21:787–790.

88. Matalka K, Barth RF, Bailey M, et al. Californium-252 brachytherapy of intracerebral melanoma with or without administration of boronophenylalanine utilizing a nude rat model. In: Soloway AH, Barth RF, et al. (eds). Advances in Neutron Capture Therapy. Plenum, NY, 1993, pp. 529–534.

89. Vtyurin BM, Tsyb AF, Mardynsky Yu S, et al. Tumor brachytherapy with Californium-252. Endocurie Hypertherm Oncol 1992;8:71–91.

90. Konoplyannikov AG, Vtyurin BM. Biological effects of Cf-252 gamma-neutron radiation: A summary of studies in the USSR. Nucl Sci Appl 1986;2:369–382.

91. Wierzbicki J, Maruyama Y, Mayfield M, et al. Facility and handling of californium-252 sources for brachytherapy. Endocurie Hypertherm Oncol 1992;8:131–136.

92. Yamashita H, Dokiya T, Yamashita S, et al. Comments on the results of remotely controlled high dose rate therapy of cancers of the uterine cervix using Cf-252. Nucl Sci Appl 1991;4:197–199.

93. Yamashita T, Kaneta K, Tsuya A, et al. Update on intracavitary radiotherapy with Cf-252 for uterine cervical carcinoma at Japan Cancer Institute Hospital. Nucl Sci Appl 1991;4: 193–196.

94. Vtyurin BM, Ivanov VN, Nikitenko VA, et al. Technique of contact neutron therapy with ^{252}Cf sources. Med Radiol 1981;5:7–13.

95. Maruyama Y, Kryscio RJ, Wood C, et al. Feasibility study: Results of treatment of primary and recurrent adenocarcinoma of the corpus uteri with Cf-252. Int J Radiat Oncol Biol Phys 1985;11:1199–1208.

96. Maruyama Y, Beach JL, van Nagell JR, et al. Californium-252: Isotope for modern radiotherapy of cervix, uterus and vaginal carcinomas. Strahlentherapie Onkol 1987;169: 373–381.

97. Maruyama Y. Experience with and potential of Cf-252 therapy for other tumors: Lexington clinical trials. Nucl Sci Appl 1986;2:601–614.

98. Maruyama Y, Beach L. Cf-252 neutron brachytherapy of short duration for bulky neck tumors. Int J Radiat Oncol Biol Phys 1986;12:761–770.

99. Maruyama Y, Wills C, Beach L, et al. Hyperthermia and Cf-252 neutron brachytherapy for bulky surface human neoplasms. Nucl Sci Appl 1986;2:713–718.

100. Chin HW, Maruyama Y, Young AB, et al. Cf-252 brain implantation for malignant glioma: Experience of the University of Kentucky, Lexington. Nucl Sci Appl 1986;2:585–600.

101. Patchell RA, Maruyama Y, Tibbs PA, et al. Neutron interstitial implant for malignant gliomas. J Neurosurg 1988;68:67–72.

102. Rossi H, Mays CW. Leukemia risk for neutrons. Health Phys 1978;34:352–360.

103. Loewe WW, Mendelsohn E. Revised dose estimates at Hiroshima and Nagasaki. Health Phys 1981;4:663–666.

104. Feola JM, Maruyama Y, Pattarasumunt A, et al. Cf-252 leukemogenesis in the C57BL mouse. Int J Radiat Oncol Biol Phys 1987;13: 69–74.

105. Maruyama Y, Feola JM, Wood C, et al. Californium-252 leukemogenesis in the C57BL mouse: Effect of mixed low dose rate ^{252}Cf and photon radiation schedule. Endocurie Hypertherm Oncol 1990;6:257–264.

106. Upton AC. Experimental radiation-induced leukemia. In: Duplan JF (ed). Radiation-Induced Leukemogenesis and Related Tumor Viruses. Inserm Symp. #4. North Holland, New York, 1977, pp. 37–50.

107. Upton AC, Randolph ML, Conklin CW. Late effects of fast neutrons and gamma rays in mice as influenced by the dose rate of irradiation-induction of neoplasia. Radiat Res 1970; 41:467–491.

108. Ullrich RL, Jernigan MC, Storer JB. Neutron carcinogenesis: Dose and dose-rate effects in Balb/c mice. Radiat Res 1977;72:487–498.

109. Ullrich RL, Jernigan MC, Cosgrove CE, et al. The influence of dose and dose-rate on the incidence of neoplastic disease in RFM mice

after neutron irradiation. Radiat Res 1976;68:
115–131.

110. Straume T. A radiobiological basis for setting
neutron radiation safety standards. Health
Phys 1985;49:883–896.

111. Maisin JR, Wambersie A, Gerber GB, et al.
Life-shortening and disease incidence in
C57BL mice after single and fractionated
gamma and high energy neutron exposure.
Radiat Res 1988;113:300–317.

112. Maisin JR, Wambersie A, Gerber GB, et al. Life
shortening and disease incidence in Balb/c
mice following a single d(50)-Be neutron of
gamma exposure. Radiat Res 1983;108:
374–389.

113. Goud SN, Feola JM, Maruyama Y. Sperm-
shape abnormalities in mice exposed to cali-
fornium-252 radiation. Int J Radiat Biol 1987;
52:755–760.

114. Goud SN, Feola JM, Maruyama Y. Micronuclei
in bone marrow cells of Balb/c mice after irradiation with Cf-252 or Co-60. Nucl Sci Appl
1986;2:781–786.

115. Severskaya LP, Nikitenko VA, Galantseva GV.
Changes in tooth-maxillary system during
treatment of mouth cavity tumors with ^{252}Cf
sources. In: Contact Radiation Therapy with
^{252}Cf Neutron Sources. Obninsk, 1982, pp.
103–106.

116. Maruyama Y, van Nagell JR, Yoneda J, et al.
Efficacy of brachytherapy with californium-
252 vs. cesium-137 photons for eradication of
bulky localized cervical cancer: Single institutional study. J Nat Cancer Instit 1988;80:
501–506.

117. Maruyama Y, Yoneda J, van Nagell JR, et al.
Tumor regression and histologic clearance
after neutron brachytherapy for bulky localized cervical carcinoma. Cancer 1982;50:
2802–2809.

118. Miller JP, Patchell R, Yaes R, et al. Preliminary
report on Cf-252 neutron interstitial implant
therapy for glioblastoma multiforme: A phase
I trial. Nucl Sci Appl 1991;4:281–289.

119. Maruyama Y, Feola JM, Wierzbicki J, et al.
Clinical study of relative biological effectiveness for cervical carcinoma treated by ^{252}Cf
and assessed by histological tumour eradication. Br J Radiol 1990;63:270–277.

120. Vtyurin BM, Medvedev VS, Ivanov VN, et al.
Perioperative neutron brachytherapy with
californium-252. Int J Radiat Oncol Biol Phys
1992;23:873–879.

121. Kaneta K, Tsuya A. Early experience with Cf-
252 brachytherapy for esophageal, bronchial,
skin cancers and malignant melanoma at the
Cancer Institute Hospital, Tokyo. Nucl Sci
Appl 1986;2:615–629.

122. Maruyama Y, Macdonald J, Patel P. Complete
response of metastatic squamous cell carcinoma after cisplatin chemotherapy without
sustained control following primary tumour
control by californium-252 brachytherapy. Br
J Radiol 1990;63:661–664.

123. Maruyama Y, Wierzbicki J, Feola J, et al. Regeneration in cervix cancer after ^{252}Cf neutron brachytherapy. Int J Radiat Oncol Biol
Phys 1990;19:61–67.

124. Vtyurin BM, Ivanov VK, Ivanov VN, et al.
Combined neutron and gamma therapy of
tongue cancer. Med Radiol 1986;9:14–19.

125. Raju P, Maruyama Y, Yoneda J. Experience
with treatment of melanoma using Cf-252
neutron therapy at the University of Kentucky. Nucl Sci Appl 1986;2:695–702.

126. Savina NP, Medvedev VS, Kuzina AA. Influence of contact neutron and gamma therapy
upon immunity of patients with mouth, mucous membrane tumors. Med Radiol 1986;11:
13–18.

127. Catterall M, Bewley D. Fast Neutrons in the
Treatment of Cancer. Academic, London,
1979.

128. Maruyama Y. Relative sensitivities of the female genital tract: Tumors of the cervix uteri.
Adv Radiat Biol 1990;14:23–110.

129. Van Nagell JR, Maruyama Y, Donaldson E,
et al. Phase II clinical trial using Cf-252 fast
neutron brachytherapy, external beam pelvic
radiation and extrafascial hysterectomy in the
treatment of bulky, barrel-shaped stage IB
cervical cancer. Cancer 1986;57:1918–1922.

130. International Federation of GYN and OB.
Classification and staging of malignant tumors in the female pelvis. Acta Obstet Gynecol Scand 1971;50:3–4.

131. Coffey CW, Yoneda J, Beach LJ, et al. Methods
for Cf-252 cervix cancer therapy and treatment for GYN malignancies in Lexington.
Nucl Sci Appl 1986;2:485–496.

132. Maruyama Y, Yoneda J, Wierzbicki J. Methods for treatment of cervix cancer using Cf-
252 neutron brachytherapy. Nucl Sci Appl
1991;4:213–227.

133. Maruyama Y, van Nagell JR, Yoneda J, et al.
Phase I-II clinical trial of californium-252:
Treatment of stage IB carcinoma of the cervix.
Cancer 1987;59:1500–1505.

134. Maruyama Y, van Nagell JR, Powell D, et al.
Predictive value of specimen histology after
preoperative radiotherapy in the treatment of
bulky barrel carcinoma of the cervix. Am J
Clin Oncol (CCT) 1992;15:150–156.

135. Maruyama Y, Donaldson E, van Nagell JR, et
al. Specimen findings and survival after preoperative ^{252}Cf neutron brachytherapy for

stage II cervical carcinoma. Gynecol Oncol 1991;43:252–259.

136. Maruyama Y, van Nagell JR, Donaldson E, et al. Feasibility study of californium-252 for the therapy of stage IV cervical cancer. Cancer 1988;61:2448–2452.

137. Boys J, Beach JL, Maruyama Y. Feasibility of parametrial interstitial implantation of advanced cervical cancer using californium-252. Endocurie Hypertherm Oncol 1986;2: 219–223.

138. Maruyama Y, Kryscio RJ, van Nagell JR, et al. Clinical trial of ^{252}Cf neutron brachytherapy vs. conventional radiotherapy for advanced cervical cancers. Int J Radiat Oncol Biol Phys 1985;11:1475–1482.

139. Maruyama Y, van Nagell JR, Yoneda J, et al. Efficacy of Cf-252 neutrons for control of hemorrhage/infection in advanced bulky gynecologic cancer. Nucl Sci Appl 1991;4: 429–434.

140. Maruyama Y, Martin A. Metronidazole in the treatment of cervical cancer using Cf-252 neutron brachytherapy. Nucl Sci Appl 1986;2: 719–726.

141. Maruyama Y, Kryscio R, Wood C, et al. Feasibility study: Results of treatment of primary and recurrent adenocarcinoma of the corpus uteri with californium-252. Int J Radiat Oncol Biol Phys 1985;11:1199–1208.

142. Kraus VS, Koryakina LP, Rykova VP, et al. Direct and short-term results of combined modality radiotherapy of uterine body cancer using neutron radiation of high energy ^{252}Cf sources. Med Radiol 1986;31:44–48.

143. Kiseleva VN, Savinova VF, Marina LA, et al. Treatment of endometrial carcinoma with neutrons from high energy ^{252}Cf sources. Voprosy Onkologiya (Voona) 1988;34: 1070–1074.

144. Cross B, Maruyama Y, Proudfoot W, et al. Brachytherapy for anal and ano-rectal carcinoma. Nucl Sci Appl 1986;2:703–706.

145. Berdov BA, Sidorchenkov VO, Yurchenko NI, et al. Combined preoperative radiation therapy using high activity ^{252}Cf neutron radiation for tumor therapy. In: Use of ^{252}Cf Radiation for Tumor Therapy. Obninsk, pp. 109–112.

146. Anikin VA. Neutron brachytherapy in the treatment of esophageal cancer. Nucl Sci Appl 1991;4:425–428.

147. Maruyama Y. Californium-252 neutron brachytherapy of prostatic cancer. In: Bruggmoser, Sommerkamp H, Mould RF (eds). Brachytherapy of Prostatic Cancer. Nucleotron, Veenendaal, Netherlands, 1991, pp. 153–167.

148. Chin HW, Young AB, Maruyama Y. Cf-252 neutron brachytherapy for malignant glioma: Retrospective and prospective views for future trials. Nucl Sci Appl 1991;4:261–272.

149. Parker RG, Berry HC, Gerdes A, et al. Fast neutron beam radiotherapy of glioblastoma multiforme. Am J Roentgenol 1976;127: 331–335.

150. Catterall M, Bloom HK, Ash DV, et al. Fast neutron compared with megavoltage x-rays in the treatment of patients with supratentorial glioblastoma: A controlled pilot study. Int J Radiat Oncol Biol Phys 1981;7:185–189.

151. Maruyama Y, Chin HW, Young AB. ^{252}Cf neutron brachytherapy for hemispheric malignant glioma. Radiology 1982;145:171–174.

152. Chin HW, Maruyama Y, Young AB, et al. Intracerebral neutron brachytherapy: The technique and application for malignant brain tumors. Endocurie Hypertherm Oncol 1985;1: 229–236.

153. Ciuba D, Yaes RA, Miller JP, et al. Preliminary report on californium-252 neutron brachytherapy for glioblastoma multiforme: A phase I trial. Endocurie Hypertherm Oncol 1991;7: 217–218.

154. Maruyama Y, Chin HW, Young AB, et al. Implantation of brain tumors with Cf-252: Use of CT and MRI to guide insertion and evaluate response. Radiology 1984;152:177–181.

155. Hernandez JC, Chin HW, Young AB, et al. Study of Cf-252 implant and accelerated hyperfractionated therapy for malignant glioma. Nucl Sci Appl 1991;4:291–295.

156. Maruyama Y. Californium-252 neutron brachytherapy: Accelerated high linear energy transfer radiotherapy for cancer. Endocurie Hypertherm Oncol 1991;7:161–169.

Chapter 36

Endovascular Brachytherapy

Ian Crocker, M.D., Ron Waksman, M.D.

Rationale

Angioplasty or balloon dilation of the coronary vessels was developed as a nonsurgical means of improving the vascular supply to the myocardium and as an alternative to coronary artery bypass grafting (CABG). There are approximately 450,000 coronary interventions (angioplasty, atherectomy, and intracoronary stent) carried out each year in the United States. Restenosis or renarrowing (Figure 1) after angioplasty of intracoronary vessels today remains the most common complication and limitation to the successful use of this clinical procedure.[1] A variety of pharmacological agents have been tested with little effect on the restenosis process.[2] Stenting of the intracoronary vessels was developed as a mechanical means of dealing with this problem.[3] In randomized comparisons of balloon angioplasty to directional atherectomy or intracoronary stents, angiographic restenosis occurs in about 42%–57% of cases following balloon angioplasty, 46%–50% following directional atherectomy, and 22%–32% of cases following stent placement.

Similar problems of restenosis following angioplasty or stent placement have been encountered within the peripheral vascular system. Information reported from several institutions report 5-year patency rates following femoro-popliteal balloon angioplasty of 50%–61%.[4,5] Recent studies of stents in femoral-popliteal vessels demonstrated rates of restenosis similar to those seen with balloon angioplasty.[6] This phenomenon seems less frequent in stented iliac and renal arteries. The incidence of restenosis in peripheral vessels seems highly dependent on the anatomical location of the original lesion, the morphology of the lesion, and the distal flow with lower restenosis rates occurring in larger vessels, and focal lesions with good distal flow.[7–10]

Restenosis is a complex process comprising immediate vascular recoil, neointimal hyperplasia, and late vascular remodeling.[11–16] The contribution of these elements to the restenotic process varies from case to case and among devices.

Immediate vascular recoil generally is thought of as the loss in luminal area that occurs immediately following angioplasty. It is measured from cineangiograms done immediately following balloon dilatation and those carried out at a point in time before the proliferative process would have had a chance to develop (30 minutes to 24 hours). In modern series, about 4% of angioplasty cases are immediate technical failures due to mechanistic vascular elastic recoil.

Neointimal hyperplasia has been thought to be the main culprit in the restenotic process. The pathogenesis of this process is incompletely understood. The lesion is composed largely of smooth muscle cells (SMCs) and develops within 3–6 months. Geometric remodeling resulting in a decrease of the

From Nag S (ed): *Principles and Practice of Brachytherapy.* © Futura Publishing Co., Inc., Armonk, NY, 1997.

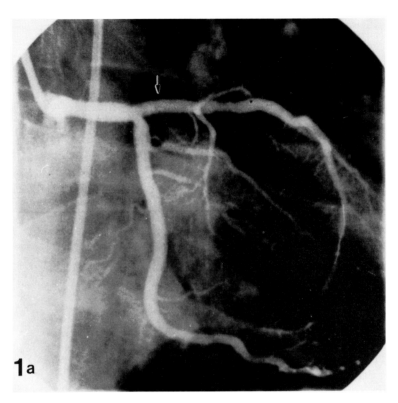

Figure 1a. Cineangiogram of dilated vessel. Arrow points to the dilated segment of coronary artery postballoon angioplasty.

overall cross-sectional arterial area has been seen mainly following atherectomy procedures and is significantly reduced by stenting. On serial studies of the vessel following angioplasty, Scott et al.[17] have described that adventitial myofibroblasts contribute to the process of neointima formation by proliferating and migrating into the neointima. These same cells that synthesize smooth muscle actin may also constrict the injured vessel and contribute to the process of arterial remodeling and late lumen loss.

Endovascular irradiation has been shown to have no effect on vascular reactivity.[18] Numerous authors have reported that it reduces neointimal hyperplasia. Its role on vascular remodeling is currently under investigation (Table 1). One desirable feature of radiation is that it interferes with the proliferative processes while the fixed postmitotic tissue is spared.

Preclinical Studies

The potential role of radiation in preventing restenosis following angioplasty or stent placement was first discussed by Dawson.[19] The first evaluation of radiation in the preclinical area was carried out by Schwartz et al.[20] in the porcine model of restenosis. In their study they administered radiation to the coronary vessels following stent placement with an orthovoltage x-ray unit. Despite the fact

Table 1.
Effect of Radiation on the Causes
of Restenosis

Mechanism	Effect of Radiation
Thrombosis	0
Vascular recoil	0
Neointimal hyperplasia	+ + +
Vascular remodeling	+

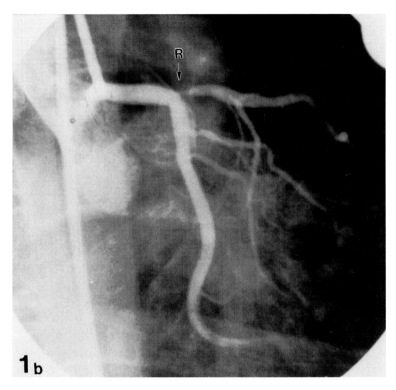

Figure 1b. Cineangiogram of restenotic vessel. Arrow points to restenosis at the angioplasty site at 3 months following the balloon dilatation.

that this study and a similar study from Yale using external orthovoltage x-rays revealed more neointimal hyperplasia in the irradiated group (Table 2) further evaluation of adjuvant irradiation with external techniques has revealed a benefit from treatment.[21–25]

More consistent evidence of benefit has come from groups using brachytherapy techniques. Groups led by Wiedermann et al.[26] from Columbia, Waksman et al.[27] from Emory, and Raizner et al.[28] from Baylor have evaluated the potential benefit of intraluminal

Table 2.
Preclinical Studies Performed Using Teletherapy

Author	Animal/Vessel	Radiation Source	Result
Abbas	Rabbit/iliac	Linac	6 Gy no benefit: 12 Gy benefit at 5 days post angioplasty
Schwartz	Pig/coronaries	Orthovoltage	Neointima significantly worse with radiation (4–8 Gy) post stent implantation
Gellman	Rabbit/iliacs	Orthovoltage	Increased neointima with 3 and 9 Gy post angioplasty
Hirai	Rabbit/femorals	Orthovoltage	2, 5 Gy no benefit; 10 and 20 Gy reduced neointimal post air drying
Shimatokahara	Rats/carotids	TeleCesium	Reduced neointima following balloon angioplasty

Table 3.
Studies with Catheter Based Therapy

Author	Animal/Vessel	Radiation Source	Result
Waksman	Pig/coronaries	Iridium-192	Decreased neointima with 3.5–14 Gy; sustained benefit at 6 months with 7/14 Gy
Wiederman	Pig/coronaries	Iridium-192	Decreased neointima with 15–20 Gy; worse with 10 Gy; benefit at 6 months with 20 Gy
Mazur	Pig/coronaries	Iridium-192 HDR	Decreased neointima with 10, 15, and 25 Gy following stent and angioplasty
Waksman	Pig/coronaries	Sr/Y-90	Benefit with 7 and 14 Gy post angioplasty similar results to Iridium-192
Verin	Rabbit/carotid + iliacs	Y-90	Decreased neointima with 18 Gy; no benefit with 6 and 12 Gy

iridium-192 (Ir-192) (Table 3). All three have shown the benefits of endovascular brachytherapy in the porcine model of restenosis. Some discrepancies exist among the groups regarding dose-response relationships, but all have shown that doses in the range of 14–25 Gy delivered following angioplasty or stent placement, significantly diminished the amount of neointimal hyperplasia in the short-term (2 weeks to 1 month). Waksman et al.[27] and Wiedermann et al.[29] have both shown that this effect appears to be durable with 6 months of follow-up.

Two groups (one from Emory and one from Geneva) have tested specially developed beta sources in the preclinical setting. Verin et al.[30] have shown the benefit of the use of endovascular Y-90 wire in the rabbit iliac model of restenosis. Waksman et al.[31,32] have shown that an Sr-90/Y-90 source train was as effective as Ir-192 in reducing neointimal hyperplasia following angioplasty and stent placement and was safer in terms of the exposures

to the patient and personnel. A thorough description of the Y-90 wire has been published by Popowski et al.[33]

Two additional groups have published on the use of radioactive stents in inhibiting restenosis (Table 4). Hehrlein et al.[34] were the first to demonstrate that a metallic stent (Palmaz-Schatz) made radioactive in a reactor could reduce restenosis when applied to rabbit iliac vessels. Laird et al.[35] subsequently showed that neointimal hyperplasia could be inhibited in the short-term by the application of a P-32 coated stent. These results have been seen with stents with total activities in the microcurie range as opposed to millicuries for the beta sources used with catheter-based therapy. The safety and durability of this therapy are currently being evaluated.

Technical Considerations in Endovascular Brachytherapy

Preclinical and clinical studies have utilized a variety of approaches in delivering dose to

Table 4.
Results of Radioactive Stents

Author	Animal/Vessel	Radiation Source	Result
Laird	Pig/iliac	P-32 coated stent	Decreased neointima at 6 weeks
Hehrlein	Rabbit/iliac	Radioactive steel stent (Palmaz-Schatz)	Decreased neointima at 12 weeks with 35μCi stent
Hehrlein	Rabbit/iliac	P-32 coated stent	Decreased neointima at 12 weeks with 13μCi stent

Table 5.
Delivery Techniques

Catheter Based Techniques	
Gamma Emitters	Beta Emitters
Iridium-192 MDR	Yttrium-90 wire
Iridium-192 HDR afterloader	Strontium-90/Yttrium-90 seeds
Radioactive Stents	
Mixed Gamma/Beta Emitters	
Radioactive Palmaz-Schatz stents	Beta Emitters
Radioactive Nitanol stents	P-32 coated stents

HDR = high-dose-rate; MDR = middle-dose-rate.

the vessel wall (Table 5). In addition to the above approaches, a number of different approaches have been the object of speculation. These include the use of liquid P-32 (a pure beta emitter) within an angioplasty balloon, or the use of low energy gamma emitters (iodine-125, palladium-103) as catheter-based radioisotopes. Balloon filled P-32 presents significant risks to the patient should the balloon burst, which makes this approach undesirable at the present time. Because of the low gamma factor with I-125 and Pd-103 there is a serious doubt as to whether sources of sufficient activity to deliver the treatment within a reasonable time frame (~5 minutes) could be developed. For these reasons these sources will not be discussed. Because of the inconsistent results with external techniques this discussion will be on the advantages and disadvantages of the different endovascular techniques and the radioactive sources that have been utilized in these approaches.

Catheter-Based Techniques

In evaluating the use of intracoronary irradiation using catheter-based techniques, the issues that must be addressed include:

1. treatment time
2. total body dose received by the patient
3. dose received by attending staff
4. the need for modification of current catheterization lab procedures.

Medium-Dose-Rate Iridium-192

Intracoronary irradiation using Ir-192 has been done within the research lab by two different groups (Waksman et al.,[27] Wiedermann et al.[29]) and in the clinical area by Tierstein et al.[36] This therapy can be safely carried out in the clinical catheterization lab according to early reports from Tierstein et al. but the treatment times are relatively long (20 minutes) during which time the source is continuously within the coronary artery. The total body dose absorbed by the patient is excessive when compared with that of beta emitters. In addition, the increased dose to the staff handling the sources compared to that seen with high-dose-rate afterloaders or beta sources, which are equally as effective and feasible is not compatible with ALARA principles. Medium-dose-rate Ir-192 has some advantage over Sr/Y-90 in that source centering is not as critical an issue.

High-Dose-Rate Iridium-192

The use of a conventional high-dose-rate afterloader would require either expensive modification of the cath lab for therapy to be undertaken there or transportation of the patient to Radiation Oncology for treatment (with a delivery catheter in the coronary artery). One alternative would be to provide shielding in close proximity to the patient. These issues are being examined by different groups. The prolonged time required by treatment planning with the current generation of high-dose-rate afterloaders may negate some of the advantages of high-dose-rate therapy compared to medium-dose-rate Ir-192. Additional problems to be solved include reducing the diameter of the source to allow delivery to normal size coronary arteries and navigating around the tight curves in these vessels. The advantage of the high-dose-rate afterloader is the precision with which dose can be delivered to the target volume, the extensive knowledge and experience with the dose distribution around these sources, and the flexibility in delivering the dose to lesions of different length.

Strontium-90/Yittrium-90

Beta emitting sources would seem to have an advantage over gamma emitters in terms of reduced dose delivered to normal tissues and radioprotection of the medical staff. Furthermore, because they are directly ionizing, it is possible to achieve very high-dose-rates with sources of modest activity. Strontium has a major advantage over Y-90 in terms of half-life (28.5 years vs 64 hours). Source handling is easily accomplished with both of these sources and they could easily be incorporated within the current cath lab environment. Both sources as currently described are of fixed length. To treat different length lesions would require a different wire or source train. The major disadvantage of these sources is the rapid fall-off in dose in radial distribution that would decrease the dose rate achievable in larger arteries. They would, however, seem to be sufficiently penetrating for irradiation of even the largest coronary arteries. Furthermore, if the clinical treatment volume is relatively thick, the dose received to the endothelial surface may be excessive. One additional concern is that the dosimetry around the sources is less well established than with Gamma sources.

High-Dose-Rate Phosphorus-32

A commercial company (Neocardia, Houston, TX, USA) has recently revealed plans to market a high-dose-rate afterloader with the source being encapsulated P-32. Although the half-life is somewhat shorter than other sources used in high-dose-rate afterloaders, the useful life of the source will be approximately 1 month according to the manufacturer. Whether the advantage of being able to customize the length of treatment warrants the use of a high-dose-rate afterloader remains to be determined.

Radioactive Stents

Radioactive stents have an advantage over catheter-based systems in that they are in direct contact with the tissues to which they deliver dose. There is, however, considerable heterogeneity of dose due to the irregular shape of the metallic portion of the stent that contains the radioisotope. Of these approaches, a stent containing a pure beta emitter would seem more desirable than a gamma emitting or mixed gamma/beta emitting stent, particularly if the gammas are penetrating or have a very long half-life. One major conceptual problem with stents is that the radiation dose should optimally be delivered over a relatively short period of time following placement of the stent, when proliferation of neointima is taking place. If one incorporates a short half-life radioisotope into the stent then the corresponding product has a short shelf-life. Additionally, not all stenotic patients can be stented nor does one necessarily want to insert a stent solely to deliver radiation. The length of the treatment volume with a stent-based approach is essentially confined to the length of the stent. If additional injury occurs beyond the stent in the longitudinal direction it may not be possible to deliver dose to this area. One additional concern is that unless the linear activity of the stent is increased at its ends, the dose rate and the resultant biological effect may be less at the proximal and distal margin.

Prescription of Dose

In prescribing endovascular radiation therapy for any of these purposes one needs to consider what the target tissue is and what dose will be delivered to it. Determining the target point for catheter-based therapy is problematic and a number of alternatives are possible (Figure 2). Issues that need to be addressed include whether to prescribe the dose to the luminal surface or the adventitia of the artery and whether the reference or treated vessel segment should be considered in prescribing treatment. Because different researchers have reported using different prescription points, the dose response relationships that are quoted often are not comparable from study to study. For example,

Prescription of Dose

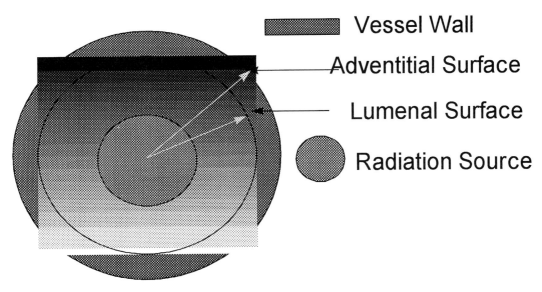

Figure 2. Diagram of an intraluminal radiation source illustrating the problems associated with the dose prescription point. Is the dose prescribed to the luminal surface or the adventitial surface or to an arbitrary point like 0.2 cm from the source?

in preclinical studies using Ir-192, Wiederman found benefit only with doses of 15 Gy and above whereas Waksman, using the same source, found benefit with doses of 3.5–14 Gy with both authors using Ir-192. In looking at the details of their dose prescription, the Emory group used the sources end-to-end without spacing and prescribed the dose at 2 mm (the adventitial surface of the artery), whereas Wiederman used a 1-mm spacing between sources and prescribed the dose at 1.5 mm. In fact, the 14 Gy prescribed by Waksman at 2 mm is the same as 20 Gy prescribed by Wiederman at 1.5 mm. Thus some, but not all, of the discrepancy between their results can be accounted for by examining the doses actually received by the target tissues. Most researchers feel that the target cell in the restenotic process migrates from the adventitia of the artery into the media. Delivering dose to this point would require the use of intravascular ultrasound, or IVUS, to establish the dis-

tance from the source to the prescription point. The American Association of Physicists in Medicine (AAPM) Task Group-60 (TG-60) is currently addressing issues regarding the prescription of dose in endovascular brachytherapy. The effect of curvatures, noncentering, and variability in the thickness of the clinical target volume are issues that have yet to be completely addressed (Figure 3).

Most stent therapy has been prescribed based on the activity of the radioactive stent with only rudimentary evaluation of the dose delivered to the target tissues. Because the dose delivered is variable depending on the degree of expansion and the geometric structure of the stent, it may be impossible to know in advance exactly what the absorbed dose will be in the target tissues.

Calibration of Sources

Calibration of iridium-192 or other gamma sources presents no new challenges to the ra-

Possible Dose Inhomogeneity Within CTV Despite Apposition to the Vessel Wall

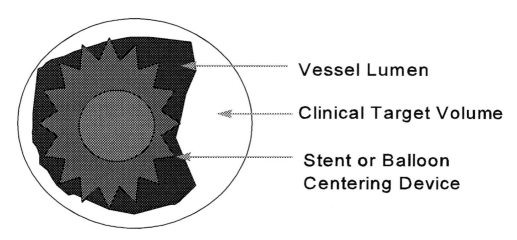

Vessel Lumen

Clinical Target Volume

Stent or Balloon Centering Device

Figure 3. Diagram illustrates the variability in the thickness of the clinical target volume.

diation physicist involved in a treatment program of this type. The measurement of the activity of pure beta emitters poses considerably greater difficulty. For both source types Monte-Carlo type calculations of the dose distribution surrounding these sources may be carried out. Physical measurement of the dose rate at distances <5 mm pose significantly greater problems and the guidance of TG-60 and the assistance of the National Institute of Standards (NIST) in establishing guidelines for use of these sources is currently under way.

Summary of Results in Peripheral Vessels

The first study done using radiation to prevent restenosis was carried out by Liermann et al.[37] in Frankfurt, Germany. In this study they selected patients for treatment who had a clinically relevant recurrent stenosis in the superficial femoral artery >4 cm in length that had occurred <6 months after the last percu-

taneous transluminal angioplasty (PTA). All the patients had undergone prior PTA or laser therapy and stent placement prior to or at the time of irradiation and all patients were 65 years or older. The patients received 12 Gy at the luminal surface with a high-dose-rate afterloader. With 25 patients treated as of their latest follow-up report and some patients with over 5 years of follow-up, they have not seen any evidence of restenosis in the treated segment. Not all of the patients have undergone systematic reevaluation with angiography so there is no information published or presented at this time as to any degree of luminal narrowing following treatment. One would have generally expected at least a 30% restenosis rate in these size vessels following primary angioplasty and this study provides strong evidence for the benefit of adjuvant irradiation. What is more important, however, is the fact that there was no late restenosis or other complications of the adjuvant irradiation. The authors point out that the source was not centered within the peripheral vessel and if the catheter had remained apposed to one of the coronary arteries for the duration of the treatment it is possible that the absorbed dose, based on minimum and maximum distances of the vessel wall, ranged from 8–28 Gy. This information gives us some indication that the dose range of effective treatment and safety could be quite broad.

The second clinical study of irradiation in peripheral vessels was carried out in Germany by Steidle[38] in Ravensburg. This was a randomized study of stent placement with and without adjuvant, fractionated external radiation treatment. The patients were treated with 12.5 Gy in 2.5 Gy fractions following stent placement in superficial femoral arteries. Of the 11 patients who received radiation treatment, there were only two episodes of occlusion with minimum 7-months follow-up. In the 13 control patients, there were five episodes of occlusion. Furthermore, there were no complications attributable to the radiation.

The only additional study carried out in peripheral arteries in humans is a preliminary report from our group at Emory involving adjuvant irradiation following angioplasty of stenosis within arteriovenous fistula grafts in dialysis patients. In most of these patients, angioplasty has proved to be very temporary palliation of the stenotic process. In the 12 patients treated at Emory with radiation following angioplasty, it has been our impression that the fistula have remained free from restenosis and the only threat to their long-term patency has been thrombosis.

Summary of Results in Coronary Vessels

The first study of intracoronary brachytherapy in humans was initiated in July 1994 by Condado and his colleagues[39] in Caracas, Venezuela. This study involved the administration of radiation by inserting a special small diameter Ir-192 wire into the vessel after angioplasty, rotoblator, or stent placement. In this study, 22 arteries in 21 patients were treated over a 5-month period of time. At the initiation of their study, the patients received 25 Gy at a standard depth of 1.5 mm from the source center. After the first ten arteries were treated, a further 12 arteries were treated with all but one of these patients receiving 20 Gy at

the luminal surface of the reference diameter. With a minimum of 6-months follow-up in the treatment groups, there have been four cases of restenosis. None of these have occurred in de novo lesions treated with 25 Gy. They observed no unexpected complications following treatment but did describe the occurrence of one pseudoaneurysm that they felt was secondary to a dissection with the initial angioplasty.

The second clinical trial is one by Tierstein et al.[36] at The Scripps Clinic in La Jolla, California, for which the preliminary results of a randomized trial of endovascular irradiation using a manually afterloaded Ir-192 source has been reported. In this trial, patients are randomized to receive or not receive endovascular irradiation following intracoronary stent placement. The prescribed dose is based on IVUS assessment of the maximum distance from the catheter to the coronary stent. Eight Gy is delivered to this point as long as the maximum dose to the intima does not exceed 30 Gy. As of November 1995, the authors had randomized 50 patients on this study and had reported only three cases of stenosis, all of these occurring in the nonirradiated group. The study is very preliminary and the significance of these findings remains to be determined. What is more important about this trial is that they have managed to use a manually afterloaded iridium source of up to ~140 mCi without any increased radiation exposure to the participating physicians. Furthermore, they have left the radiation source within the coronary artery for up to one-half hour without any increase in complications from this procedure. Two additional ongoing studies (one at Emory and a second in Geneva) using the specially developed beta sources described above have yet to report any data on their initial feasibility and safety studies.

Initiating a Clinical Program

The issues regarding the initiation of a clinical program in endovascular brachytherapy are complex involving both regulatory and clinical issues. At this point, studies of endovascular brachytherapy should be considered investigational and should be done under the auspices of a defined protocol approved by the responsible Human Investigation Committee (HIC). The FDA has made the determination that these procedures constitute "significant risk" to the patients and has mandated that all investigation in this area be carried out under an approved Investigational Device Exemption (IDE). As far as clinical issues are concerned, these studies are by their very nature multidisciplinary and involve coordinating activities between specialties without a long history of interaction or collaboration.

Radioactive stents are not commercially available, and therefore any new program at this time would involve catheter-based therapy.

Major differences exist between intracoronary brachytherapy (ICBT) and peripheral vessel brachytherapy (PVBT) in that:

1. ICBT needs to be undertaken in the cath lab immediately following placement of the delivery catheter in the coronary vessel. There is less urgency about initiating PVBT and these patients potentially could be transferred to the Radiation Oncology Department for treatment (as is done at Emory).
2. ICBT needs to be carried out quickly due to the potential adverse consequences of the treatment device within the coronary artery.
3. There is much greater variability in the length of the angioplastied lesion in peripheral arteries than in the coronary arteries where 90% of angioplasties are done with coronary balloons measuring 2 cm in length.

Intracoronary Brachytherapy

As beta systems are not commercially available and high-dose-rate devices are not well configured for this therapy, an ICBT program would most likely be based on the use of manually afterloaded Ir-192 ribbons of maximum commercially available activity (~145 mCi) in order to minimize treatment time. This treatment program will involve the close cooperation and involvement of the Radiation Oncologist, Radiation Physicist, Interventional Cardiologist, and Radiation Safety Officer. A clinical protocol governing the patient's treatment will need to be written and approved by the local HIC. Issues that will need to be discussed in advance by the team include:

1. Whether the team will deal only with scheduled patients or whether they will try to deal with patients undergoing catheterization who are found to have an appropriate lesion for treatment.
2. Who will get the patient's consent and when?
3. Indications for treatment, i.e., de novo ± recurrent lesions, native vessels ± vein grafts, angioplastied vessels ± stented vessels, maximum vessel diameter.
4. The prescription point for treatment and how it will be determined, i.e., by IVUS or QCA. How much margin will be given beyond the end of the angioplastied or stented lesion.
5. Maximum treatment time so that the radiation physicist can order new sources at appropriate intervals.
6. The choice of delivery catheter and whether the source and the individual handling the source needs to be sterile.

The radiation oncologist needs to come to the cath lab to gain familiarity with the procedure there. Knowledge about the procedure of cardiac catheterization and balloon angioplasty must be acquired, and an understanding of the terminology in use, including the vascular sheath, the guide wire, exchange wire, the guiding catheter, and the delivery catheter is necessary. But even more so the radiation oncologist will need to educate the cath lab staff about appropriate radiation safety procedures and often reassure them that radioisotopes can be used safely within this environment. A mock procedure with the radiation safety officer, radiation physicist, interventional cardiologist, radiation oncologist, and cath lab staff should be undertaken prior to the first patient treatment. It would be optimal if the team had the opportunity to perform an animal study first. Radiation oncologists by virtue of their training are familiar with developing procedures and solutions to specific problems. The process of collaboration with another department such as Cardiology is somewhat more complex as it involves disciplines not familiar with using sealed sources for treatment.

Peripheral Vessel Brachytherapy

This program will involve Interventional Radiology, Radiation Oncology, and Radiation Physics at a minimum. In some institutions the Interventional Cardiologist performs peripheral angioplasty and should be involved in the planning process as well. Many of these patients will be referred by Vascular Surgeons and their involvement may be critical. At Emory we have done endovascular irradiation following angioplasty of stenotic arteriovenous fistulae and it was crucial to involve the Renal Service early on to permit referral of these patients for treatment. High-dose-rate afterloaders, as currently configured, represent the optimal treatment device for peripheral vessels following angioplasty or stent placement as they allow one to treat variable vessel lengths. Furthermore, the delivery catheter can be inserted through the sheath across the patient's lesion and secured in position in the cath lab, allowing transportation of patients to the Radiation Oncology Department for treatment. Localization films can be taken either in the cath lab or on the simulator in the Radiation Oncology Department. Besides similar considerations as for ICBT, one issue for the Radiation Oncologist to decide will be the extent of treatment planning, i.e., whether to enter the actual radiographs, digitize the seed positions, and calculate optimized dwell times or whether to assume the catheter is straight and to use pre-planned dosimetry. A decision with the Interventional Radiologist about administration of anticoagulants prior to transfer to Radiation Oncology and details about removal of the sheath and compression of the wound will also need to be reviewed.

Conclusions

With any protocol therapy careful tabulation of the results and analysis of the outcomes are critical. This is an emerging field with an opportunity to provide clinically significant cost-effective treatment. It is incumbent on those involved with it to make sure studies are done carefully so that the marked benefits seen in preclinical studies are not lost. The expertise of an experienced brachytherapist is crucial to the initiation and continuation of a high quality program.

References

1. Holmes DR Jr, Vlietstra RE, Smith HC, et al. Restenosis after percutaneous transluminal coronary angioplasty (PTCA): A report from the PTCA registry of the National Heart, Lung and Blood Institute. Am J Cardiol 1984;53:77C-81C.
2. Popma JJ, Califf RM, Topol EJ. Clinical trials of restenosis after coronary angioplasty. Circulation 1991;84:1426–1436.
3. Mintz GS, Picharrd AD, Kent K, et al. Endovascular stents reduce restenosis by eliminating geometric arterial remodeling: A serial intravascular ultrasound study. J Am Coll Cardiol 1995;35A:701–705.
4. Zeiter E. Results of percutaneous transluminal angioplasty. Radiology 1983;146:57.
5. Waltman AC, Greenfield AJ, Noveline RA, et al. Transluminal angioplasty of the iliac and femoro-popliteal arteries: Current status. Arch Surg 1982;117:1218.
6. White GF, Liew SC, Waugh RC, et al. Early outcome of intermediate follow-up of vascular stents in the femoral and popliteal arteries without long term anticoagulation. J Vasc Surg 1995;21:279–280.
7. Schwarten DE, Cutcliff WB. Arterial occlusive disease below the knee: Treatment with percutaneous transluminal angioplasty performed with low profile catheters and steerable guide wires. Radiology 1988;169:71.
8. Hunink MFM, Magruder CD, Meyerovitz MF, et al. Risks and benefits of femoro-popliteal percutaneous balloon angioplasty. J Vasc Surg 1993;17:183–194.
9. Johnston KW. Femoral and popliteal arteries; Reanalysis of results of balloon angioplasty. Radiology 1992;183:767–771.
10. Murray RR Jr, Hewes RC, White RI Jr, et al. Long-segment femoro-popliteal stenoses: Is angioplasty a boon or bust? Radiology 1987; 162:473–476.
11. Austin GE, Ratliff MB, Hollman J. Intimal proliferation of smooth muscle cells as an explanation for recurrent coronary artery stenosis after percutaneous transluminal coronary angioplasty. J Am Coll Cardiol 1985;6:369–375.
12. Clowes AW, Reidy MA, Clowes MM. Mechanisms of stenosis after arterial injury. Lab Invest 1983;49:208–215.
13. Gravanis MB, Robinson KA, Santoian EC, et

al. The reparative phenomena at the site of balloon angioplasty in humans and experimental models. Cardiovasc Pathol 1993;2(4): 263–273.

14. Gravanis MB, Roubin GS. Histopathologic phenomena at the site of percutaneous transluminal coronary angioplasty: The problem of restenosis. Hum Pathol 1989;20:477–485.

15. Karas SP, Gravanis MB, Santoian EC, et al. Coronary intimal proliferation after balloon injury and stenting in swine: An animal model of restenosis. J Am Coll Cardiol 1992;20:467–474.

16. Liu MW, Roubin GS, King SB III. Restenosis after coronary angioplasty: Potential biologic determinants and role of intimal hyperplasia. Circulation 1989;79:1374–1387.

17. Scott NA, Cipolla GD, Ross CE, et al. Identification of a potential role for the adventitia in vascular lesion formation after balloon overstretch injury of porcine coronary arteries. Circulation 1996;93:2178–2187.

18. Wiedermann JG, Leavy JA, Amols H, et al. Effects of high-dose intracoronary irradiation on vasomotor function and smooth muscle histopathology. Am J Physiol 1994;(Heart Circ Physiol 35):H125-H132.

19. Dawson JT. Theoretical considerations regarding low-dose radiation therapy for prevention of restenosis after angioplasty. Texas Heart Inst J 1991;18:4–7.

20. Schwartz RS, Koval TM, Edwards WD, et al. Effect of external beam irradiation on neointimal hyperplasia after experimental coronary artery injury. J Am Coll Cardiol 1992;19: 1106–1113.

21. Gellman J, Healey G, Qingsheng, et al. The effect of very low dose irradiation on restenosis following balloon angioplasty. A study in the atherosclerotic rabbit. Circulation 1991; 118:331A-1319.

22. Shimatokahara S, Mayberg MR. Gamma irradiation inhibits neointimal hyperplasia in rats after arterial injury. Stroke 1994;25:424–428.

23. Hirai T, Korogi Y, Harada M, et al. Intimal hyperplasia in an atherosclerotic model: Prevention with radiation therapy. Radiology 1994; 872.

24. Abbas MA, Afshari NA, Stadius ML, et al. Effect of x-ray irradiation on neointimal proliferation following balloon angioplasty. Clin Res 1993; 41:79.

25. Shefer A, Eigler NIL, Whiting JS, et al. Suppression of intimal proliferation after balloon angioplasty with local beta irradiation in rabbits. J Am Coll Cardiol 1993;21:185.

26. Wiedermann JG, Marboe C, Schwartz A, et al. Intracoronary irradiation reduces restenosis after balloon angioplasty in a porcine model. J Am Coll Cardiol 1994;23:1491–1498.

27. Waksman R, Robinson KA, Crocker IR, et al. Endovascular low dose irradiation inhibits neointima formation after coronary artery balloon injury in swine: A possible role for radiation therapy in restenosis prevention. Circulation 1995;91:1553–1539.

28. Mazur W, Ali MN, Dabaghi SF, et al. High dose rate intracoronary radiation suppresses neointimal proliferation in the stented and ballooned model of porcine restenosis. Abstract. Circulation 1994;90:I-652.

29. Wiedermann JG, Marboe C, Amols H, et al. Intracoronary irradiation markedly reduces neointimal proliferation after balloon angioplasty in swine: Persistent benefit at 6-month follow-up. J Am Coll Cardiol 1995;25:1451–1456.

30. Verin V, Popowski Y, Urban P, et al. Intra-arterial beta irradiation prevents neointimal hyperplasia in a hypercholesterolemic rabbit restenosis model. Circulation 1995;92:2284–2290.

31. Waksman R, Robinson K, Crocker I, et al. Intracoronary radiation prior to stent implantation inhibits neointima formation in stented porcine coronary arteries. Circulation 1995;92: 1383–1386.

32. Waksman R, Robinson K, Crocker I, et al. Intracoronary low dose β-irradiation inhibits neointima formation after coronary artery balloon injury in the swine restenosis model. Circulation 1995;92:3025–3031.

33. Popowski Y, Verin V, Papirov I, et al. High dose rate brachytherapy for prevention of restenosis after percutaneous angioplasty: Preliminary dosimetric tests of a new source presentation. Int J Radiat Oncol Biol Phys 1995;33:211–215.

34. Hehrlein C, Gollan C, Donges K, et al. Low-dose radioactive endovascular stents prevent smooth muscle cell proliferation and neointimal hyperplasia in rabbits. Circulation 1995;92: 1570–1575.

35. Laird J, Carter A, Kufs W, et al. Inhibition of neointimal proliferation with a beta particle emitting stent. J Am Coll Cardiol.

36. Teirstein PS, Massullo V, Jani S, et al. Catheter-based radiation therapy to inhibit restenosis following coronary stenting. Circulation 1995;92: 543.

37. Bottcher HD, Schopohl B, Liermann D, et al. Endovascular irradiation—A new method to avoid recurrent stenosis after stent implantation in peripheral arteries: Technique and preliminary results. Int J Radiat Oncol Biol Phys 1994; 29:183–186.

38. Steidle B. Praventive perkutane Strahlentherapie zur Vermeidung von Intimahyperplasie nach Angioplastie mit Stentimplantation. Stra-

helntherapie und Onkologie 1994;170:151–154.

39. Condado JA, Gurdiel O, Espinoza R, et al. Percutaneous transluminal coronary angioplasty (PTCA) and intracoronary radiation therapy (ICRT): A possible new modality for the treatment of coronary restenosis: A preliminary report of the first 10 patients treated with intracoronary radiation therapy. J Am Coll Cardiol 1994;288A.

Additional Suggested Reading

1. Berner BM, Wright AE, Grant W, et al. Arterial brachytherapy. Medic Phys 1994;21:96.
2. Fischell TA, Kharma BK, Fuschell DR, et al. Low dose β-particle emission from stent wire results in complete, localized inhibition of smooth muscle cell proliferation. Circulation 1994;90:2956–2963.
3. Fischer-Dzoga K, Dimitrievich GS, Griem ML. Differential radiosensitivity of aortic cells in vitro. Radiat Res 1984;99:536–546.
4. Forrester JS, Fishbein M, Helfant R, et al. A paradigm for restenosis based on cell biology; clues for the development of new preventive therapies. J Am Coll Cardiol 1991;17:758–769.
5. Hehrlein C, Donges K, Gollan C, et al. Low-dose radioactive Palmaz-Schatz stents prevent smooth muscle cell proliferation and neointimal hyperplasia in rabbits. J Am Coll Cardiol 1995; 9ALy NC, Whiting JS, DeFrance A, et al. A novel brachytherapy source for treatment of coronary artery restenosis. Med Phys 1995;22:925.
6. Mintz GS, Popma JJ, Pichard AD, et al. Mechanisms of later arterial responses to transcatheter therapy: A serial quantitative angiographic and intravascular ultrasound study. Abstract. Circulation 1994;90:I24.
7. Prestwich WV, Kennett TJ, Kus FW. The dose distribution produced by a P32-coated stent. Med Phys 1995;22:313–320.
8. Rosen E, Goldberg K, Myrick K. Radiation survival properties of cultured vascular smooth muscle cells. Radiat Res 1984;100:182–191.
9. Verin V, Popowski Y, Urban P, et al. Intraarterial beta irradiation prevents neointimal hyperplasia in a hypercholesterolemic rabbit restenosis model. J Am Coll Cardiol 1995;2A:407–406.
10. Zeiter E. Results of percutaneous transluminal angioplasty. Radiology 1983;146:57.

Chapter 37

Brachytherapy in the New Millennium

Subir Nag, M.D., Arthur Porter, M.D., Dattatreyudu Nori, M.D.

Introduction

The current methodology used in brachytherapy has been expounded in this book. While we do not have a crystal ball to foresee the future, we feel comfortable in predicting that major developments in brachytherapy will be seen as a result of physical, radiobiological, clinical, and societal advances in the following areas:

1. Physical advances including: Low energy photons; Beta emitters; Optimization; Three-dimensional visualization; Dose-volume histograms; Newer delivery systems; Endovascular brachytherapy; Radiological imaging guidance; Endoscopic approaches; Radioimmunoguided brachytherapy; Radioimmunotherapy; Systemic radionuclides; Photon activation; Robot-controlled brachytherapy.
2. Radiobiological advances including: Remote-controlled brachytherapy; Radiosensitization and radioprotection.
3. Clinical advances including: Evolving concepts of resectability; Cytoreduction with chemotherapy/hormonal therapy; Brachytherapy in retreatment; Clinical trials.

4. Societal impact of brachytherapy including: Training and education; Official accreditation as a formal subspeciality; Standardization in brachytherapy; Socioeconomic benefits of brachytherapy; Radiation protection issues.

Low Energy Photons

Until recently, brachytherapy has generally been performed using high-energy emission radionuclides such as iridium-192 and cesium-137. A major disadvantage of this form of brachytherapy is the exposure of health care givers and the family of the patient to radiation and the fear this generates. Low energy radionuclides can reduce radiation exposure; I-125 has been used for this reason since 1965.[1] Although principally used as a permanent implant, I-125 can also be used for removable implants.[2–5] Exposure of personnel and the patient's family to radiation from removable I-125 implants can be almost entirely eliminated by covering the implanted area with lead foils. The most extensive experience in the use of I-125 for removable implants is in its use in eye plaques for treating choroidal melanomas.[4,5] The reader can refer

From Nag S (ed): *Principles and Practice of Brachytherapy.* © Futura Publishing Co., Inc., Armonk, NY, 1997.

to the chapter on eye tumors for further details.

The relatively long half-life of I-125 (60 days) results in an initial dose rate of 7 cGy/hr when I-125 is used as a permanent implant. Because of this low initial dose rate, I-125 may be less effective than shorter half-life radionuclides in treating rapidly-growing tumors. Recently, palladium-103, with a low energy like that of I-125 but a much shorter half-life (17 days), has been used for brachytherapy.[6–10] This shorter half-life allows treatment over a few weeks rather than months, and the higher initial dose rate it provides may make Pd-103 especially advantageous for poorly differentiated and presumably rapidly proliferating tumors. The short half-life of Pd-103 also results in a short shelf-life, requiring that Pd-103 be ordered on a case-by-case basis.

An ideal radioisotope for removable brachytherapy should have low energy emission that is generally attenuated by the surrounding tissues hence, reducing the radiation exposure to health care givers and patients' families; a thin lead foil can be used to further reduce the exposure if necessary. However, if the energy emitted by the radionuclide is too low and the seeds are spaced too far apart, there will be unacceptable dose heterogeneity ("cold spots") within the tumor volume. The half-life of the radionuclide source should be sufficiently long to eliminate the need for frequent calibration and to allow it to be reused many times. The source should have a high specific activity so that it can be contained within a very small volume, thus facilitating its insertion through narrow needles/tubes.

Although there is no radionuclide that meets all these criteria, a possible source is samarium-145.[10,11] It has a sufficiently long half-life of 340 days and a low energy of 38–45 keV. However, because samarium-145 is not readily available, is difficult to encapsulate, and does not have a high specific activity, it is not used clinically.

Another radionuclide for possible use as a removal implant is americium-241.[12] It has the advantage of a long half-life (432 years) and a reasonably low gamma emission (60 keV) to minimize radiation exposure hazards. However, it does not have a high specific activity; therefore, the source must be large. For this reason, americium-241 would be useful only for intracavitary radiation.

Ytterbium-169 (Yb-169) is a promising isotope because its intermediate half-life (32 days) and its photon energy (93 keV) make it suitable for dual application as a permanent or removable implant.[10,13] Its high specific activity will allow the manufacture of a small, narrow source. As a permanent implant, its half-life, which lies between that of I-125 and Pd-103, will produce an initial dose rate higher than that produced by I-125, and it will have a shelf-life longer than does Pd-103. Since its energy emission is higher than I-125 or Pd-103, its greater penetration may result in less dose inhomogeneity from slightly inhomogeneous seed distribution. However, the higher energy emission also means that radiation protection will be more problematic with Yb-169 when it is used for permanent implants. The use of Yb-169 in removable implants will involve fewer radiation exposure hazards than the use of Ir-192 or Cs-137; however, its shorter half-life will result in a short shelf-life.

Beta Emitters

Another alternative to the use of low energy photons to reduce radiation exposure is to use a β-emitter. Since electrons have limited penetration in tissue, there is minimal radiation exposure. However, their penetration may be so short as to limit their use to the treatment of very superficial tumors. Ruthenium-106 in eye plaques has been used to treat choroidal melanomas.[14] With the recent interest in intravascular irradiation, there is commercial interest in developing a narrow, sealed beta source for high-dose-rate (HDR) intravascular brachytherapy (personal communication, Nucletron Corp., Columbia, MD, USA; Neocardia, Houston, TX, USA). Possible radioisotopes include phosphorus-32 (P-32) and strontium-90 (Sr-90). These have high specific activity that allows HDR irradiation from a small source. Since the target tissue is the blood vessel wall, the limited penetration of beta sources seems to be ideal for this application.

Another novel method of using a beta source is to incorporate yttrium-90 (Y-90) into glass microspheres (TheraSphere, Theragenics, Atlanta, GA, USA). The Y-90 microspheres have been injected into the hepatic artery to treat hepatic metastases.[15,16]

Optimization

If the radiation sources are evenly distributed within the tumor volume, the highest dose is concentrated in the center, with the lowest dose in the periphery. Although this may be desirable in some tumors because the central core of the tumor can be hypoxic, it could also lead to increased complications if the high dose is close to critical radiosensitive structures (e.g., the urethra in prostate implants). Optimization can be used to provide more homogeneous dose distribution, which should produce a better therapeutic ratio. Optimization can be achieved by:

1. use of variable source strength so that higher intensity sources are used in the periphery and lower intensity sources are used in the center;
2. by variable source spacing with closer spacing of the sources in the periphery and more distant spacing of the sources toward the center;
3. by using a single high intensity stepping source of iridium-192 with variable dwell time as in HDR and pulsed-dose-rate (PDR) brachytherapy. The dose to a point is varied by varying the dwell times of the source in that position. Hence, it is possible to precisely shape the dose distribution within the target volume by changing the dwell times in each position. The source spends a greater time in the periphery and a shorter time in the center to achieve a more homogeneous dose distribution. In this way, "hot spots" within the tumor volume can be minimized while the dose to surrounding normal tissues is lowered. However, optimization must be used with caution and not be used as a substitute for improper anatomical positioning of the radionuclide within the tumor volume. It is said that "optimization can make a good implant better but optimization cannot be used to convert a bad implant into a good implant."

4. by using real-time optimization such as the ultrasound-based real-time optimization program developed at William Beaumont Hospital, Royal Oak, Michigan, for use in transperineal HDR prostate implantations.[17] A personal computer, used in the operating room, is connected to the treatment planning system. Each time a needle position is entered, the coordinates of the new dwell positions and an optimized isodose distribution are calculated and displayed in a few seconds. This is a significant improvement in that it allows the brachytherapist to visualize a three-dimensional isodose distribution within the tumor volume, and it allows the brachytherapist to perform optimum placement of radioactive sources.

Three-Dimensional Visualization

Conventional brachytherapy dose distribution is displayed in two dimensions. This does not adequately represent the complexities within an implanted volume. For a more accurate representation, one has to account for tissue inhomogeneity, the effects of neighboring radioactive sources, to compensate for the applicator/carrier material, and to display resultant dose distribution in three dimensions. Multiple CT scan images are obtained of the region of interest after the tumor has been implanted. These images are transferred to a three-dimensional reconstruction computer (using magnetic tapes or network or direct linkage). The computer then displays the isodose distribution three dimensionally in relation to the anatomical structures outlined. The use of three-dimensional dosimetry allows us to evaluate the isodose distribution produced by the radioactive sources in relation to the tumor and critical normal tissues. We are thus able to see if portions of the tumor are being underdosed or if critical tissues are being overdosed. This evaluation is critical, so that dose to the implant can be optimized to achieve a higher tumor control while morbidity is minimized. The isodoses can be rotated on any axis on the computer for further evaluation. This may additionally be combined with an optimization program for further benefit. The artifacts caused by the needles/sources can sometimes make it difficult to properly visualize the tumor boundaries on CT scans. These difficulties must be overcome before three-dimensional CT-based dosimetry is routinely implemented.[18]

Dose-Volume Histograms

The dose distribution from brachytherapy is inhomogeneous. Areas of high doses ("hot spots") within the treatment volume contribute to complications if they are close to critical normal tissues. Conversely, areas of low doses ("cold spots") reduce tumor control. Simply stating a single dose level (the reference dose) for an implant does not adequately describe the complex dose variation within the treatment volume. A dose-volume histogram more accurately describes this dose variation by specifying the volume irradiated at a certain dose level. Therefore, the first step to a better understanding of the effects of dose variation is for brachytherapists to systematically express the implant dosimetry using a dose-volume histogram. Dose-volume histograms have to be used to critically evaluate competing treatment plans and to optimize the therapeutic ratio of the treatment. The brachytherapist must then correlate their successes, failures, and complications with the dose-volume histograms. Meaningful indices (e.g., coverage index, dose inhomogeneity index, hyperdose sleeve, overdose volume index, etc.) must be developed and formally agreed upon to aid in this correlation.

Endovascular Brachytherapy

Balloon angioplasty and/or stent placement are alternatives to coronary artery bypass grafting for overcoming occluded coronary arteries. Restenosis after angioplasty or stent placement is the major limitation to the successful use of these procedures. In the coronary vessels it occurs in 30%–40% of unselected cases following angioplasty and in 20% of cases following stent placement. Restenosis is a complex process comprising immediate vascular recoil, neointimal hyperplasia, and vascular remodeling. At least neointimal hyperplasia, and possibly vascular remodel-

ing, are proliferative processes that may be potentially inhibited by irradiation, similar to the use of radiation to inhibit keloid formation.

A number of authors have shown in preclinical studies the potential role of endovascular irradiation of the arterial wall in preventing restenosis following coronary angioplasty or stent placement.[19–21] One clinical study in the peripheral arteries has shown long-term efficacy of endovascular HDR Ir-192 brachytherapy.[22] There are few ongoing clinical trials in the coronary vessels.[23,24] The advent of endovascular brachytherapy has created a number of special requirements for brachytherapy systems. These include:

1. High activity, narrow sources to allow delivery of the dose in a very short time within the narrow confines of the coronary artery.
2. Delivery systems that can ensure that the source can negotiate tortuous curves of the coronary vessels consistently.
3. Low energy photon or beta emitters to allow the use of a high activity radionuclide with minimal radiation exposure outside the confines of a shielded radiation therapy suite (e.g., in a cardiac catheterization lab or intraventional radiology suite).
4. New designs for incorporating a radioisotope within an intravascular stent.

Endovascular brachytherapy is set to explode onto the radiation oncology scene. An enormous potential exists for exploiting the benefits that radiation can offer in this setting. Although endovascular brachytherapy would be aimed at preventing restenosis in peripheral arteries, hemodialysis fistulae, renovascular hypertension, etc., the primary application of this modality is undoubtedly in the coronary arteries. With 450,000 angioplasties occurring each year in the United States, intravascular irradiation could represent the largest single application of brachytherapy, if these trials prove to be successful. However, care must be exercised in the design of controlled clinical trials to prove its efficacy since this is one of the few instances of the use of brachytherapy in nonmalignant diseases. The reader may refer to the chapter on intravascular brachytherapy for further details.

Radiological Imaging-Guided Implants

Traditionally, most implants have been performed under direct visualization. Thus tumors located in a deep organ, required surgical access. However, with the advancement in radiological techniques, implants can now be performed without surgical exposure even in deep organs. The most common example is the use of ultrasound for prostate implant. The prostate is scanned using transrectal ultrasound. Needles are then inserted into the prostate under ultrasound guidance, and iodine-125, palladium-103, or iridium-192 sources are implanted, or HDR brachytherapy is used.[6,25–28] Ultrasound guidance has also been used in pancreatic implants.[29]

Fluoroscopy is of great help and has been used usually in conjunction with transrectal ultrasound for implantation of the prostate.[30] It is of help in the use of transperineal parametrial implantation for gynecological malignancies. Fluoroscopy also aids in the localization of the intraluminal brachytherapy sources in implantation of esophagus and endobronchial tumors.

Another radiological modality with great potential is CT scan guidance, which can be used to insert needles for implantation of the prostate, lung, brain, and other organs.[31] The expertise of our interventional radiologist colleagues in CT-guided needle biopsy of various organs for diagnostic purposes can be very helpful in this regard.

Endoscopic Approaches

Another nonsurgical method of introducing radioisotopes into deep-seated tumors is to use an endoscopic access ("minimally invasive surgery"). This approach has commonly been used to treat endobronchial tumors via a bronchoscope, and the technique has been described in detail in the chapter on lung brachytherapy. This concept can be extended to the implantation of chest wall tumors through a thoracoscope or abdominal tumors via a laparoscope, thereby minimizing the morbidity and recovery time associated with major surgical procedures. However, the advantage of endoscopic access may be counterbalanced by the disadvantage of being unable to totally encompass the tumor volume when such a small opening is used. Development of special brachytherapy applicators may be necessary before this technique can be used on a routine basis.

Radioimmunoguided Brachytherapy

The effectiveness of brachytherapy depends upon adequately covering the tumor volume. The tumor volume to be implanted is traditionally demarcated by inspection/palpation or by using radiographic studies. However, if the tumor has been resected, demarcation of the area of residual microscopic disease by traditional techniques is difficult. The radioimmunoguided brachytherapy technique (RIGBY) was developed at The Ohio State University to allow precise demarcation of occult tumor or microscopic residual tumor for brachytherapy.[32,33]

In this technique, a monoclonal antibody (B72.3 or CC-49) radiolabeled with iodine-125 is injected into the patient systemically 2–3 weeks before surgery. The radiolabeled antibody circulates, binds to the tumor, thereby becoming a radioactive marker that can be detected intraoperatively with a hand-held gamma detection probe—the Neoprobe 1000 system. Maximal surgery is performed to remove all tumor possible. After all known disease has been resected, the probe is used to survey the tumor bed for residual radioactivity. Any areas of continued probe positivity presumably demarcate the margins of microscopic tumor. This is then the target volume for brachytherapy using either permanent iodine-125, removable low-dose-rate (LDR) iridium-192, or intraoperative HDR brachytherapy techniques. This is an exciting area currently undergoing evaluation at The Ohio State University. It is too early to say whether the more precise identification and demarcation of microscopic residual disease will ultimately lead to better tumor control and survival.[32,33]

Radioimmunotherapy

Conventional active immunotherapy introduces antigens to stimulate the individual immune system to produce antibodies. Antibodies (produced in animals) to tumor associated antigens may be labeled with radioisotopes (I-131, Y-90, etc.) to produce radiolabeled monoclonal antibodies (R-MAb) that may then be injected into patients. Tumor cells preferentially bind the R-MAb, since the malignant tumors have neovasculature with slower blood flow that allows a higher concentration of the antigen in or near tumor and thereby results in preferential binding. This process brings a high concentration of the radioisotope close to the tumor cells and allows destruction of the tumor cells while sparing normal tissue, which has a lower uptake of R-MAb.

A variety of antibodies have been radiolabeled with I-131 or Y-90 in clinical studies on non-Hodgkin's lymphoma patients as recently summarized by Knox.[34] I-131 also has a large gamma component (in addition to the therapeutic beta emission), which is advantageous since it allows easy imaging of its localization in the body. On the other hand, Y-90 is a pure β-emitter with a higher penetration than I-131 beta emissions and hence has a therapeutic advantage, but does not permit imaging. Radioimmunotherapy has great potential, and various methods of increasing its therapeutic results are being investigated.[35–37]

Systemic Radionuclides

Various bone seeking radionuclides given systemically have been used to palliate multiple areas of bony pain and to possibly increase survival. The bone seeking radioisotope is selectively taken up by the tumor in bone so that a highly localized dose of radiation can be delivered.

Initially, phosphorous-32 (P-32) was used. P-32 is a pure beta emitter with a maximum energy of 1.71 MeV, a mean energy of 0.7 MeV, and a half-life of 14.3 days. The average tissue penetration from P-32 beta particle is 2.5 mm, with a maximum range of 8 mm. Silberstein[38] recently reviewed 28 studies of P-32 used for relief of bony pain in cases of primary breast or prostate tumors. Eighty-four percent of the 342 patients with breast carcinoma and 77% of the 494 patients with prostate carcinoma responded to the P-32. A complete response to P-32 was noted in 20%–50% of the patients. There was no dose response relationship to the wide range of activity (4–24 mCi in single and divided doses) used. P-32 is not in common use primarily due its severe hematological toxicity.

Since P-32 produced significant bone marrow toxicity, Sr-89 has more recently been used for the systemic relief of bone pain.[39,40] Sr-89 is a pure beta emitter with a maximum beta energy of 1.4 MeV and half-life of 50.6 days. A calcium imitator, Sr-89 is not incorporated into the marrow and rapidly washes out of healthy bone, with a biological half-life of 14 days with retention of isotope at the site of metastasis.[39]

Porter et al.[40] reported on the randomized trans-Canada Sr-89 study. In eight Canadian cancer centers, 126 patients with endocrine refractory, metastatic prostate cancer were randomized to receive local field radiotherapy (30 Gy in ten fractions or 20 Gy in five fractions) and placebo versus local field radiotherapy with 10.8 mCi of Sr-89. Intake of analgesics was significantly reduced in patients treated with Sr-89. There was statistically significant reduction of new sites of pain or requirements for radiotherapy in patients treated with Sr-89. Quality of life was improved, and prostatic acid phosphatase, alkaline phosphatase, and PSA levels were reduced in the group receiving Sr-89. However, hematological toxicity (reduction in platelets and white cells) was significantly greater in the group receiving Sr-89 compared to the group receiving placebo. Clinical bleeding, pneumonia, and hemorrhage were more common in the Sr-89 treated group. There was no significant statistical improvement in survival benefit with the Sr-89 treatment.[40]

Nag[41] recently summarized the results of multiple clinical trials showing that intravenous administration of Sr-89 produces a response rate of 70%–80% of patients treated (especially breast and prostate primary), with 10%–25% of patients remaining pain free. The major toxicity (dose dependent) is hematological. Sr-89 has recently been approved for clinical use in the United States and is currently the radionuclide commonly used for treating symptomatic, widespread bone pain.

Samarium-153 (Sm-153), rhenium-186 (Re-186), and iodine-131 (I-131) are other radioisotopes used for systemic radiotherapy. These radioisotopes emit beta particles suitable for therapy and gamma rays suitable for diagnostic imaging that are used to verify localization in areas causing pain and to quantitate the radiation dose to be delivered to the tumor site. Sm-153 is a beta emitter with a maximum energy of 810 keV with an average penetration range of 0.8 mm. It also emits 103 keV of gamma photons and has a half-life of 46 hours. Re-186 has a beta energy of 1.07 MeV and a gamma energy of 138 keV. The half-life of Re-186 is 3.8 days, which allows for shipment, processing, and convenient disposal. I-131 is easily available; however, its lower beta energy has a shorter penetration. The use of I-131 is well established for treatment of thyroid carcinoma. Because radioactive iodine is concentrated by the follicular thyroid cells, I-131 has been used for palliation of painful bony metastases in patients with this disease.[42] Sm-153 and Re-186 are currently undergoing clinical trials in the systemic management of widespread bony metastasis and early results are encouraging.[43,44]

It may be possible to increase the response rate and duration of pain relief by increasing the dose of radionuclide administered while supporting bone marrow suppression by the administration of colony stimulating factors.[45] Biphosphonates may possibly increase radioisotope retention.[46] Low-dose infusion Cisplatinum has also been used to potentiate the action of Sr-89.[47] Another possibility is to combine hemibody irradiation with systemic radionuclide therapy[48] so that systemically administered radionuclide could give a greater radiation dose to areas of bony metastases while hemibody radiation could also treat areas of soft tissue metastases not treated by the administered radionuclide. Further investigations are needed in this field to firmly establish the role of brachytherapy for systemic treatment of disseminated malignancies.

Photon Activation

Photon activation therapy (PAT) is a binary system that combines two weak therapies to produce a highly tumoricidal treatment. Iododeoxyuridine (IUdR) is a weak radiosensitizer. When IUdR is injected into patients, it is preferentially incorporated into the DNA of tumor cells. When the tumor is implanted with a radionuclide with photon emission just above the K absorption spectrum of iodine (33 keV), Auger electrons are released. Auger electrons are high linear energy transfer (LET) radiation with a short ($\approx$8–14 μ or roughly the diameter of a cell) range. Thus, the highly lethal dose of cellularly localized radiation released by this process destroys the DNA of tumor cells while sparing nearby, slower growing normal tissues that have not incorporated the IUdR into their DNA. Radionuclides proposed for PAT include samarium-145 (38–45 keV) and americium-241 (60 keV).[11,49,50]

Robot-Controlled Brachytherapy

With advances in computerization and robotic engineering, we foresee brachytherapy being delivered by robotic control to allow access to clinical sites with a precision that is not possible by manual control. The patient is placed in a stereotactic head-holder, and a CT scan and/or MRI is performed. The coordinates of the tumor volume can be mapped relative to the stereotactic frame. An optimized treatment plan can be performed by digitizing the radioactive source positrons precisely at various points within the stereotactic coordinates. A robot can then be used to place the radioactive sources at the designated coordinates with a precision not currently possible. Although this technique has immediate application for brain tumors, with modifications, similar approaches may be used at other sites.

Remote-Controlled Brachytherapy

With the trend toward reducing radiation exposure by adhering to the ALARA principle, remote-controlled brachytherapy will be the area that will undergo maximum development in the coming decade. Although there will be advances in remote-controlled LDR and PDR brachytherapy, we feel the major area of interest will be HDR brachytherapy. This is because, in addition to the elimination of radiation exposure due to remote control, HDR has the advantage of short treatment times and administration as out-patient therapy, making the treatments more convenient and cost effective.

However, HDR therapy is not without its disadvantages. A practical disadvantage of current HDR using Ir-192 is the requirement of a shielded treatment room, which is expensive and not easily available. The use of beta emitters such as strontium-90 or phosphorus-32 or a low energy gamma emitter will solve this problem and allow HDR to be performed in a nonshielded room, making brachytherapy available in a conventional operating room or angiography suite for example. Narrower source size (achieved by using high specific activity radionuclides) will be required to permit entry into narrow lumens, for use in intravascular and percutaneous brachytherapy. The use of HDR has inherent radiobiological disadvantages since there is no repair of sublethal damage or reoxygenation during the short duration of treatment. To overcome these and reduce late morbidity effects, the treatments must be adequately fractionated. If multiple fractions are not an option, the dose to normal tissues must be reduced by tissue displacement or shielding, as in intraoperative HDR brachytherapy.[51] HDR afterloaders are expensive both in capital expenditure and manpower. Hence, individual institutions need a certain treatment load to justify the purchase of an HDR afterloader. However, a number of smaller treatment centers that do not individually have the work volume to justify the purchase of a dedicated HDR afterloader can share the use of a mobile HDR unit. Such units have only recently become available, and their use will extend the availability of HDR to smaller centers.

Currently, HDR is most commonly used in the endobronchial treatment of lung cancer; however, we believe that HDR brachytherapy will have wider applicability in the new millennium and will be used extensively in intracavitary, interstitial, and intraoperative implantations.

Radiosensitization and Radioprotection

Hypoxia is one of the causes of radioresistance and failure of clinical radiation therapy. A hypoxic sensitizer like IUdR has only limited cytotoxicity when used alone; however, when it is incorporated into the DNA and then irradiated, it is highly toxic. IUDR is incorporated almost exclusively into the DNA of proliferating cells. In the case of a rapidly growing tumor in the vicinity of nonproliferating normal tissues, the IUDR will be preferentially incorporated in the tumor DNA rather than that of the normal tissues, thus sensitizing the tumor to the effects of radiation from the brachytherapy sources while the normal tissues are spared. This radiosensitizing effect is even more useful to overcome the effect of hypoxia and radioresistance in the use of single fraction brachytherapy (e.g., intraoperative HDR brachytherapy).

Hyperthermia is another modality that can be used to sensitize tumor cells to the effects of brachytherapy. Although hyperthermia can be cytotoxic on its own, there is some synergism between hyperthermia and radiation therapy, probably because hypoxic and poorly nourished (and, therefore, more radioresistant) cells are more sensitive to hyperthermia. Cells in the radioresistant S phase of the mitotic cycle are also more sensitive to hyperthermia. The weakness of hyperthermia is that effective delivery of heat to deeper structures is difficult. To overcome this difficulty, catheters implanted for interstitial brachytherapy can be used to deliver interstitial hyperthermia, as has been detailed in the chapter by Dr. Coughlin in this book. This approach has much promise and deserves further investigation in controlled clinical trials.

An alternative strategy to increase the effectiveness of brachytherapy is to use radioprotectors that are taken up by normal cells. This will reduce the toxicity of brachytherapy in the normal tissues but will not reduce the response of the tumor cells to the effects of brachytherapy. Naturally occurring sulfhydryl compounds, such as glutathione (GSH), protect cells from radiation damage by acting as scavengers of hydroxyl radicals produced by radiation. An analogue of cysteamine, WR-

2721, has been used for selective radioprotection of normal tissues. Its use allows the delivery of a higher brachytherapy dose and thereby produces an increased tumor effect without increasing morbidity.

Evolving Concepts of Resectability

There has been a move toward organ conservation and function preservation leading to changing concepts in surgical resectability. A small tumor can be treated by brachytherapy alone or, if resectable, by a surgical excision alone. When large tumors are close to critical structures (nerves, blood vessels, etc.) and a function preserving surgical excision is done, microscopic disease is often left behind after the resection. These cases benefit by the use of a combined modality treatment in which the core of the tumor (which may be hypoxic and, therefore, radioresistant) is removed by surgery and brachytherapy is added to deliver a high dose of radiation to the tumor bed. In these circumstances, brachytherapy acts very much like an extension of the surgeon's scalpel. A common example of this combination is in the treatment of soft tissue sarcomas[52] and pediatric tumors.[53] Most commonly, catheters are inserted on the tumor bed at the time of surgery. These catheters are later loaded with radioactive material after waiting a few days for wound healing. A refinement of this technique is the use of intraoperative HDR brachytherapy, which has additional advantages including the ability to temporarily displace or shield radiosensitive tissues from the high-dose area of radiation, as well as elimination of delay between the surgery and delivery of the radiation. Also, the problems of catheter displacement or geographical miss are eliminated.[51]

Cytoreduction with Chemotherapy or Hormonal Therapy

Generally, large tumors are not suitable for brachytherapy. However, chemotherapy or hormonal therapy may be used to reduce the size of large tumors sufficiently to allow them to be implanted. In addition, chemotherapy may have either an additive or synergistic effect on the tumor and since it is a systemic agent, may prevent micrometastasis of tumor. Chemotherapy and brachytherapy have been used in combination to treat pediatric tumors while preserving normal functions.[53] Hormonal therapy may be used to reduce the size of borderline prostate tumors so that transperineal brachytherapy may be used.

Brachytherapy for Retreatment

Brachytherapy can be used as the sole modality or as a boost to external beam radiation therapy (EBRT) in the treatment of primary tumors. However, for tumors that recur after previous radiation therapy, EBRT is not an option because of the expected morbidity. Brachytherapy alone is an excellent alternative in the treatment of small, localized recurrent tumors, since high dose can be delivered to the tumor whereas a limited dose is delivered to the surrounding normal tissues. To limit the late normal tissue effects, LDR brachytherapy is the preferred modality in these cases. If HDR is used, the brachytherapy should be highly fractionated.

Clinical Trials in Brachytherapy

A major obstacle to the development of brachytherapy has been the lack of modern clinical trial data support. Most of the trials and published results in brachytherapy are phase I and II retrospective studies evaluating the technique; there are very few phase III trials. As a result, the lack of confirmation of clinically demonstrated efficacy by randomized studies has contributed to the undervaluing of brachytherapy at the same time that other oncological specialities have flourished. The Radiation Therapy Oncology Group (RTOG) currently has conducted only one brachytherapy trial, a feasibility trial of HDR and LDR brachytherapy in carcinoma of the esophagus. It is clear that properly designed brachytherapy trials are needed to consolidate the position of brachytherapy as a modality for treating cancer. Although useful data can be obtained from phase I and II studies, it is the randomized, phase III, national and international cooperative clinical trials that will identify the appropriate place for brachytherapy in the treatment of oncological diseases. In reality, while most current phase III trials evaluate survival, local control, and morbidity, in the modern era of managed health care, the cost effectiveness and quality of care will also have to be concurrently evaluated in the design of future trials.

Brachytherapy is often thought to be more of an art rather than a science, dependent on the skill of the brachytherapist. The American Brachytherapy Society (ABS) has established the Clinical Research Committee to promote clinical research and to establish guidelines in brachytherapy. This committee has surveyed the brachytherapy practice in the United States and has also reported on consensus guidelines in brachytherapy.[54,55] While this is an initial step in the right direction, much has yet to be done. Many obstacles must be overcome in conducting brachytherapy trials. There is a steep learning curve that must be overcome before embarking on a large scale trial. Quality assurance is difficult to control, especially because there is great variation in terminology, methodology, dose specification, dosimetry, and reporting methods; and there are few national or international standards. These difficulties must be surmounted and effective clinical trials instituted if credibility with the medical community is to be established.

Training and Education in Brachytherapy

Although most radiation oncologists have some knowledge of brachytherapy, in many centers, brachytherapy training is limited primarily to intracavitary brachytherapy for gynecological malignancies. The narrow scope of this training is one of the greatest obstacles in brachytherapy. Insufficient training leads to increased errors, poor outcomes, and a reluctance to perform brachytherapy procedures. To increase the knowledge of radiation oncologists regarding brachytherapy, we must require more brachytherapy training for residents in radiation oncology. Centers that have inadequate brachytherapy experience should provide additional brachytherapy training to their residents by mandatory rotation at centers with brachytherapy expertise. More brachytherapy fellowships should be created for graduating radiation oncology residents to provide in-depth training and research experience. These fellowships will also be appropriate for practicing radiation oncologists who wish to become more familiar and comfortable with brachytherapy.

The annual meetings of the ABS and the European Curietherapy Group (GEC) serve to disseminate recent advancements in brachytherapy to the radiation oncology community. This information is supplemented by workshops organized by GEC and the recently instituted "Brachytherapy Schools" of the ABS. The recent successful joint meeting of the GEC, ABS, and brachytherapists from Latin America (GLAC) held at Tours, France, is a welcome move to foster international education in brachytherapy. It may interest the readers that the final brush strokes to this chapter were laid during this first international joint meeting. These joint meetings are scheduled to be held every 4 years, with the next one planned be held in the United States in the year 2000. This promises to become a truly international event in preparation for "Brachytherapy in the New Millennium."

Official Accreditation as a Formal Subspecialty

Although it is true that with technological advances in the last decades, brachytherapy has become very sophisticated, the brachytherapy skills required for a general radiation oncology board certification are rather rudimentary. Currently, any radiation oncologist can attempt intricate brachytherapy procedures without being formally trained in these complex procedures. If brachytherapy is to be performed safely and with optimal results, the practitioners performing advanced brachytherapy procedures should be trained and certified to perform them. Therefore, the time has come for those currently involved in the practice of brachytherapy to move to recognize brachytherapy as a subspecialty with requirements for certification like those of other subspecialties. Only those who are fully trained in brachytherapy and officially recognized as such (for example, by completing a brachytherapy fellowship) should be permitted to perform advanced brachytherapy procedures.

Official accreditation is necessary to maintain a high quality of treatment. A first step would be for the ABS to issue a certificate of competency in brachytherapy. In time, this should lead to a subspecialty board certification in brachytherapy. Brachytherapy will flourish once it is formally recognized as a subspecialty. As a formal society, we must find our political voice and network with other national societies to get our message out to the general public and to the primary physicians so that the role that brachytherapy can play in the arsenal of an integrated cancer treatment program is evident to those who can benefit from its application.

Standardization in Brachytherapy

Brachytherapy is regarded by many as more of an art than a science. Because brachytherapy has evolved from several different schools, the treatment regimes, techniques, terminology, methodology, dose specification, and dosimetry used by different brachytherapists vary widely, and controversy exists regarding the radionuclide and techniques, as well as dosing, dose rate, and fractionation of brachytherapy to be used. The methodologies for dosimetry and prescription point also vary as well. This lack of standardization in the application of brachytherapy limits communication between investigators and hinders discussion of technique and results. The current paucity of national or international standards or consensus underscores the urgent need to develop a common language in the field of brachytherapy and to come to some preliminary consensus. Although initial steps have been taken by the International Commission on Radiation Units and Measurements (ICRU), the High Dose Rate Brachytherapy Working Group (HIBWOG), and the ABS[55–57] to develop some consensus in brachytherapy, there is an urgent need to establish uniform standards of dose prescription and dose reporting, including a requirement to clearly describe the dose variation within the relevant volume of tissue irradiated. It is highly recom-

mended that these uniform guidelines and standards be followed by radiation oncologists as they become available.

Socioeconomic Benefits of Brachytherapy

Brachytherapy is a highly effective local treatment modality. However, with contemporary changes in the health care delivery system and the advent of managed health care, we will be required to demonstrate and quantify the cost effectiveness of these brachytherapy procedures to justify their use. Although brachytherapy has always been associated with an attendant hospitalization cost, the advent of HDR brachytherapy has ushered in out-patient brachytherapy. This development provides a clear socioeconomic benefit since hospitalization is no longer required. Further, the therapy provides a better quality of life to the patient. To truly analyze the socioeconomic benefits of brachytherapy, we must compare the social costs and problems associated with uncontrolled, progressive, or recurrent tumor growth with the financial costs of an effective brachytherapy treatment. Obviously, this is difficult to do. We must also critically compare the costs of these brachytherapy procedures with those of surgery and a protracted course of EBRT, including the costs of hospitalization and recovery time from surgical procedures and the hidden cost of loss of productive work hours. Finally, we must be flexible and consider reengineering to try to "do the best with less."

Radiation Protection Issues

A basic concept in brachytherapy is the ALARA ("as low as reasonably achievable") principle to reduce radiation exposure to the medical staff and general public. The previous yearly limit for whole-body exposure of 0.5 REM has recently been decreased to 0.1 REM. We will, therefore, be continually challenged to reduce or eliminate radiation exposure from brachytherapy procedures during the coming decade. We will see manual brachytherapy techniques being replaced by remote-controlled brachytherapy techniques (especially HDR brachytherapy with its added advantage of out-patient therapy), and high energy gamma emitters will be replaced by safer, low energy radionuclides or beta emitting radionuclides. We believe the regulatory bodies will continue to issue stricter guidelines regarding radiation safety issues and that these guidelines will be enforced more stringently. Severe penalties will be imposed on those not following these guidelines. Radiation oncologists should therefore become familiar with techniques to ensure adherence to the ALARA principle so that they will be adequately prepared to meet these challenges in the new millennium.

Radiation protection issues will also require consideration outside the narrow confines of the radiation oncology department. With the increasing use of intraoperative brachytherapy and the emerging interest in endovascular brachytherapy, radioprotection considerations will become relevant in and critical to operating rooms, cardiac catheterization labs, and interventional radiology suites. These new personnel, who are not familiar with brachytherapy, require education about brachytherapy procedures and methods to reduce radiation exposure.

Conclusions

It is likely that substantial developments in the physical and radiobiological framework of brachytherapy and its clinical base will occur. In physics, the use of new isotopes, optimized treatment planning, and better imaging for visualization of tumors to be treated will enhance our ability to perform brachytherapy. The introduction of novel delivery systems such as RIGBY, systemic radionuclides, and yttrium microspheres increases the possibilities for using brachytherapy to treat a wide range of tumor conditions, including the disseminated metastatic patient. Delivery systems such as robotic brachytherapy may allow the access to clinical sites with precision that was impossible with manual systems.

The development of endoscopic access techniques, such as laparoscopy and ventriculoscopy, extends the limits of brachytherapy to virtually every clinical site within the body. The acceptance of the multidisciplinary, and therefore multi-modality, approach to oncology has led to the integration of surgical, hormonal, and chemotherapeutic debulking with EBRT and brachytherapy. These complementary oncological procedures may allow improved sterilization of tumors.

The integration of the concepts of surgery (to reduce the tumor burden), HDR brachytherapy (high radiation dose, reduced normal tissue dose, elimination of radiation hazard, short treatment times), and intraoperative radiation therapy (displacement of normal tissue, avoidance of geographical miss) leading to the birth of intraoperative HDR brachytherapy is a dramatic development that will surely come to play an important role in cancer treatment in the new millennium.

In terms of an understanding of tumor biology and interaction of agents, including radiation at different dose rates, hyperthermia, radiation protectors, and sensitizers, there will be an increasing ability to use these agents in ways that will best provide for a therapeutic gain to tumor versus normal tissue.

It is clear that brachytherapy remains the optimum way of delivering conformal radiotherapy tailored to the shape of the tumor while sparing normal tissues. Compared to any other curative cancer treatment modality, it has the least morbidity with maximal organ preservation potential. As the application of brachytherapy gains broader acceptance and the spectrum of major clinical sites in which its efficacy can be demonstrated increases, the field of brachytherapy will become an integral part in the management of cancer, either on its own or in combination with external beam brachytherapy, surgery, and/or chemotherapy. And with the increasing emphasis placed on cost effective patient care, the economies in time possible for practitioner, patient, and treatment center with the use of brachytherapy will contribute to the growing interest in this modality.

There is a need for rigorous and well conducted clinical trials to establish fully the place of brachytherapy within the armamentarium of competing therapies. Clearly, this is a challenge that is just beginning to be answered. As the role of brachytherapy in these studies is more clearly defined, the credibility of brachytherapy as a therapeutic modality will be enhanced within the medical community. Fully using the new developments that are on the horizon in brachytherapy will require that the discipline of radiation oncology broaden its training and strengthen its emphasis on educational experiences in brachytherapy in order to adequately train the physicians of the future.

It must still be remembered that brachytherapy in many ways bears considerable similarities to surgery, as the difference between a well conducted and successful implant and a poor outcome can often be reflected in the operator's skill. There is no substitute in brachytherapy for hands-on clinical operative experience. This textbook, therefore, can only serve as a guide to broaden the experience of those practitioners who choose to practice brachytherapy.

References

1. Hilaris BS, Henschke VK, Holt JG. Clinical experience with long half-life and low-energy encapsulated radioactive sources in cancer radiation therapy. Radiology 1968;91: 1163–1167.
2. Clarke DH, Edmundson CK, Martinez A, et al. The utilization of I-125 seeds as a substitute for Ir-192 seeds in temporary interstitial implants. An overview and a description of the William Beaumont Hospital technique. Int J Radiat Oncol Biol Phys 1988;15:1027–1033.
3. Vicini FA, White J, Gustafson G, et al. The use of iodine-125 seeds as a substitute for iridium-192 seeds in temporary interstitial breast implants. Int J Radiat Oncol Biol Phys 1993;27(3): 561–566.
4. Fontanesi J, Nag S. Brachytherapy for ocular disease. In: Nag S (ed). Principles and Practice of Brachytherapy. Futura Publishing Company, Inc, Armonk, NY, 1997, pp. 291–304.
5. Packer S, Rotman M, Salanitro P. Iodine-125 irradiation of choroidal melanoma. Clinical experience. Ophthalmology 1984;91:1700–1708.
6. Nag S, Scaperoth DD, Badalament R, et al. Transperineal palladium-103 prostate brachytherapy: Analysis of morbidity and seed migration. Urology 1995;45:87–92.
7. Nag S, Sweeney PJ, Wientjes MG. Dose response study of iodine-125 and palladium-103 brachytherapy in a rat prostate tumor (Nb A1–1). Endocurie/Hypertherm Oncol 1993;9: 97–104.
8. Porrazzo MS, Hilaris BS, Mourthy CR, et al. Permanent interstitial implantation using palladium-103: The New York Medical College preliminary experience. Int J Radiat Oncol Biol Phys 1992;23:1033–1036.
9. Finger P, Lu D, Buffa A, et al. Palladium-103 versus iodine-125 for ophthalmic plaque radiotherapy. Int J Radiat Oncol Biol Phys 1993;27: 849–854.
10. Nath R. New directions in radionuclide sources for brachytherapy. Semin Radiat Oncol 1993; 3:278–289.
11. Fairchild RG, Kalef-Ezra J, Packer S, et al. Samarium-145: A new brachytherapy source. Phys Med Biol 1987;32:847–858.
12. Nath R, Peschel RE, Park CH, et al. Development of an ^{241}Am applicator for intracavitary irradiation of gynecologic cancers. Int J Radiat Oncol Biol Phys 1988;14:969–978.
13. Mason DLD, Battista JJ, Barnett RB, et al. Ytterbium-169: Calculated physical properties of a new radiation source for brachytherapy. Med Phys 1992;19:695–703.
14. Lommatzsch PK. Results after B-Irradiation (^{106}Ru/^{106}Rh) of choroidal melanoma. Am J Clin Oncol 1987;10:146–151.
15. Shepherd FA, Rotstein LE, Yip TK, et al. A phase I dose escalation trial of Yttrium-90 microspheres in the treatment of primary hepatocellular carcinoma. Cancer 1992;70: 2250–2254.
16. Marn CS, Andrews JC, Francis IR, et al. Hepatic parenchymal changes after intraarterial Y-90 therapy: CT findings. Radiology 1993;187: 125–128.
17. Edmundson GK. Ultrasound in treatment planning: A prototype real-time planning system. In: International Brachytherapy. Programme & Abstracts, 7th International Brachytherapy Working Conference, Baltimore, MD, 6–8 September, 1992. Nucletron International B.V., Veenendaal, The Netherlands, 1992, pp. 119–121.
18. Hilaris BS, Tenner M, High M, et al. Three-dimensional brachytherapy treatment planning. In: International Brachytherapy. Programme & Abstracts, 7th International Brachytherapy Working Conference, Baltimore, MD, 6–8 September, 1992. Nucletron International B.V., Veenendaal, The Netherlands, 1992, pp. 117–118.
19. Hehrlein C, Gollan C, Donges K, et al. Low-dose radioactive endovascular stents prevent smooth muscle cell proliferation and neointimal hyperplasia in rabbits. Circulation 1995;92: 1570–1575.
20. Fischell TA, Kharma BK, Fischell DR, et al. Low-dose, beta-particle emission from 'stent' wire results in complete, localized inhibition of smooth muscle cell proliferation. Circulation 1994;90:2956–2963.
21. Wiedermann JG, Marboe C, Amols H, et al. Intracoronary irradiation markedly reduces

neointimal proliferation after balloon angioplasty in swine: Persistent benefit at 6-month follow-up. J Am Coll Cardiol 1995;25: 1451–1456.

22. Liermann DD, Boettcher HD, Kollatch J, et al. Prophylactic endovascular radiotherapy to prevent intimal hyperplasia after stent implantation in femoro-popliteal arteries. Cardiovasc Intervent Radiol 1994;17:12–16.

23. Condado JA, Gurdiel O, Espinoza R, et al. Percutaneous transluminal coronary angioplasty (PTCA) and intracoronary radiation therapy (ICRT): A possible new modality for the treatment of coronary restenosis: A preliminary report of the first 10 patients treated with intracoronary radiation therapy. J Am Coll Cardiol 1994;288A.

24. Teirstein PS, Massullo V, Jani S, et al. Catheter-based radiation therapy to inhibit restenosis following coronary stenting. Circulation 1995; 92:543.

25. Holm HH, Juul N, Pedersen JF, et al. Transperineal ^{125}iodine seed implantation in prostatic cancer guided by transrectal ultrasonography. J Urol 1983;130:283–286.

26. Blasko JC, Grimm PD, Radge H. Brachytherapy and organ preservation in the management of carcinoma of the prostate. Semin Radiat Oncol 1993;3:240–249.

27. Syed AMN, Puthawala A, Austin P, et al. Temporary iridium-192 implant in the management of carcinoma of the prostate. Cancer 1992;69: 2515–2524.

28. Mate TP, Kovács G, Martinez A. High dose rate brachytherapy of the prostate. In: Nag S (ed). High Dose Rate Brachytherapy. Futura Publishing Company, Inc, Armonk, NY, 1994, pp. 355–371.

29. Joyce F, Burcharth F, Holm HH, et al. Ultrasonically guided percutaneous implantation of iodine-125 seeds in pancreatic carcinoma. Int J Radiat Oncol Biol Phys 1990;19:1049–1052.

30. Nag S. Transperineal iodine-125 implantation of the prostate under transrectal ultrasound and fluoroscopic control. Endocurie/Hypertherm Oncol 1985;1:207–211.

31. Arterbery VA, Wallner K, Roy J, et al. Short-term morbidity form CT-planned transperineal I-125 prostate implants. Int J Radiat Oncol Biol Phys 1993;25:661–667.

32. Nag S, Hinkle G, Martin E, et al. Radioimmunoguided Brachytherapy (RIGBY)—A new technique for implantation of occult tumors. Antib Immunoconjug Radiopharm 1993;6(1):29–37.

33. Nag S, Ellis RJ, Martin EW, et al. Radioimmunoguided iodine-125 brachytherapy for metastatic colorectal cancer. Radiat Oncol Investig 1995;2:230–236.

34. Knox SJ. Radioimmunotherapy of the non-Hodgkin's lymphomas. Semin Radiat Oncol 1995;5:331–341.

35. Press OW, Eary JF, Appelbaum FR, et al. Radiolabeled antibody therapy of lymphomas. Biologic Therapy of Cancer Updates 1994;4:1–13.

36. Wahl RL. Experimental radioimmunotherapy. A brief overview. Cancer 1994;73:989–992.

37. Meredith RF, Khazaeli MB, Liu T, et al. Dose fractionation of radiolabeled antibodies in patients with metastatic colon cancer. J Nucl Med 1992;33:1648–1653.

38. Silberstein EB. The treatment of painful osseous metastases with phosphorus-32-labeled phosphates. Semin Oncol 1993;20:10–21.

39. Blake GM, Gray JM, Zivanovic MA, et al. Strontium-89 radionuclide therapy: A dosimetric study using impulse response function analysis. Br J Radiol 1987;60:685–692.

40. Porter AT, McEwan AJB, Powe JE, et al. Results of a randomized phase-III trial to evaluate the efficacy of strontium-89 adjuvant to local field external beam irradiation in the management of endocrine resistant metastatic prostate cancer. Int J Radiat Oncol Biol Phys 1993;25: 805–813.

41. Nag S. Radiotherapeutic techniques for cancer pain management. In: Parris W (ed). Cancer Pain Management. Butterworth-Heinemann, Newton, MA, 1997, pp. 413–427.

42. Eisenhut M, Berberich R, Kimming B, et al. I-131-labeled biphosphonates for palliative treatment of bone metastases: Preliminary clinical results with iodine-131 BDP3. J Nucl Med 1986;27:1255–1261.

43. Turner JH, Claringbold PG. A phase II study of treatment of painful multifocal skeletal metastases with single and repeated dose samarium-153 ethylenediamine-tetramethylene phosphonate. Eur J Cancer 1991;27:1084–1086.

44. Maxon HR, Thomas SR, Hertzberg VS, et al. Rhenium-186 hydroxyethylidene biphosphonate for the treatment of painful osseous metastases. Semin Nucl Med 1992;22:33–40.

45. Mertens WC. Radionuclide therapy of bone metastases: Prospects for enhancement of therapeutic efficacy. Semin Oncol 1993; 20(Suppl 2):49–55.

46. Fleisch H. Bisphosphonates: Pharmacology and use in the treatment of tumor-induced hypercalcemic and metastatic bone disease. Drugs 1991;42:919–944.

47. Mertens WC, Porter AT, Reid RH, et al. Strontium-89 and low-dose infusion cisplatin for patients with hormone refractory prostate carcinoma metastatic to the bone: A progress

report. Abstract. Nucl Med Commun 1992;13: 212.

48. McEwan AJB, Porter AT, Venner PM, et al. An evaluation of the safety and efficacy of treatment with strontium-89 in patients who have previously received wide field radiotherapy. Antibody Immunoconj Radiopharm 1990;3: 91–98.

49. Laster BH, Thomlinson WC, Fairchild RG. Photon activation of iododeoxyuridine: Biological efficacy of auger electrons. Radiat Res 1993; 133:219–224.

50. Nath R, Bongiorni P, Rockwell S. Iododeoxyuridine radiosensitization by low- and high-energy photons for brachytherapy dose rates. Radiat Res 1990;124:249–258.

51. Nag S, Lukas P, Thomas DS, et al. Intraoperative high dose rate remote brachytherapy. In: Nag S (ed). High Dose Rate Brachytherapy: A Textbook. Futura Publishing Company, Inc, Armonk, NY, 1994, pp. 427–445.

52. Nag S, Porter AT, Donath D. The role of high dose rate brachytherapy in the management of adult soft tissue sarcomas. In: Nag S (ed). High Dose Rate Brachytherapy: A Textbook. Futura Publishing Company, Inc, Armonk, NY, 1994, pp. 393–398.

53. Nag S, Ruymann FB, Fontanesi J. High dose rate remote brachytherapy in the treatment of pediatric tumors. In: Nag S (ed). High Dose Rate Brachytherapy: A Textbook. Futura Publishing Company, Inc, Armonk, NY, 1994, pp. 399–408.

54. Nag S, Owen JB, Farnan N, et al. Survey of brachytherapy practice in the United States: A report of the clinical research committee of The American Endocurietherapy Society. Int J Radiat Oncol Biol Phys 1995;31:103–107.

55. Nag S, Abitbol A, Anderson LL, et al. Consensus guidelines for high dose rate remote brachytherapy (HDR) in cervical, endometrial, and endobronchial tumors. Int J Radiat Oncol Biol Phys 1993;27:1241–1244.

56. Nag S, Abitbol A, Clark D, et al. High dose rate brachytherapy working group (HIBWOG) of North America. In: International Brachytherapy. Programme & Abstracts, 7th International Brachytherapy Working Conference, Baltimore, MD, 6–8 September, 1992. Nucletron International B.V., Veenendaal, The Netherlands, 1992, pp. 525–526.

57. El-Mahdi A. International high dose rate cooperative group. 7th International Brachytherapy Conference and GammaMed User Meeting, Luzern, Switzerland, 6–9 May 1992, Abstract No. 64.

In Memoriam

Chapter 35, "Californium-252 Neutron Brachytherapy," is dedicated to its author, Dr. Yosh Maruyama, who died before the chapters final publication.

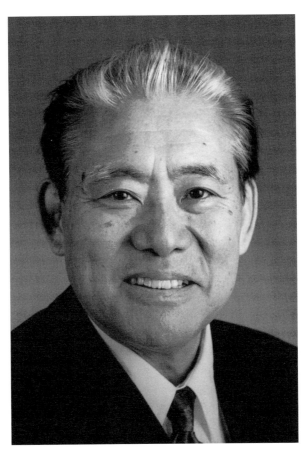

With deep regret we announce the death of Yosh Maruyama, M.D., FACP, Director of Neutron Therapy at the Gershenson Radiation Oncology Center at Harper Hospital, Detroit, Michigan, Professor of Radiation Oncology at Wayne State University School of Medicine, and a senior attending physician at the Detroit Medical Center. Dr. Maruyama died unexpectedly on January 10, 1995. He was one of the most respected radiation oncologists in the United States and was recognized both nationally and internationally as an authority on neutron brachytherapy.

Dr. Maruyama graduated in biochemistry from the University of California, San Francisco, and completed his residency in radiation oncology at Harvard University. After his training as a radiation oncologist, he completed fellowships at Oak Ridge Institute for Nuclear Sciences, Stanford University, the Karolinska Institute, and Hammersmith Hospital. In 1964, he accepted an appointment as assistant professor at the University of Minnesota and became director of the division of radiotherapy there in 1968, serving in that capacity until 1970 when he was appointed professor, chairman of Radiation Medicine, and Director of the Radiation Cancer Center at the University of Kentucky. He built that center into one of the premier radiation therapy centers in the southern United States. During his tenure at the University of Kentucky, he developed new techniques to treat malignant tumors, particularly gynecological tumors. He also advanced the use of new radiation isotopes for cancer treatment, including the neutron producing isotope, californium-252.

In 1993, Dr. Maruyama was appointed director of clinical neutron therapy at the Gershenson Radiation Oncology Center. During his short tenure there, he developed several key laboratory and clinical programs, and, under his leadership, Wayne State University was recently approved as a center for research in neutron brachytherapy as a treatment for radioresistant cancer.

In June of 1993, Dr. Maruyama visited the former Soviet Union as a member of a special scientific panel, appointed by the United States Department of Energy, to assess transuranium element research. The team visited previously secret nuclear reactor facilities where production of transplutonium isotopes had been carried out. Among those facilities was the V.I. Lenin Research Institute of Atomic Reactors (in Dimitrograd, Volga Region), one of the two most powerful reactors in the world and a producer of californium-252, the neutron emitting isotope that Dr. Maruyama had advocated for use in cancer therapy. As the biomedical expert on the panel, Dr. Maruyama also visited the Institute of Medical Radiology at the Academy of Medical Sciences in Oninsk and the Oncological Research Center at the Academy of Medical Sciences in Moscow: centers where neutron brachytherapy has been used and continues to be used as a treatment for cancer. Dr. Maruyama vigorously promoted communication between the United States and Soviet medical scientists regarding clinical trials of neutron brachytherapy.

Dr. Maruyama will be remembered as an enlightened scholar, a diligent teacher, and a dedicated clinician who contributed significantly to improving cancer therapy in the United States and internationally.

Subir Nag, M.D.
Jacek Wierzbicki, Ph.D.

Index

A Message from the Editor

Thank you for reading **Principles and Practice of Brachytherapy**. Any comments, suggestions, or criticisms you can contribute will be extremely helpful to us in preparing future editions. Please rate each category or chapter from unacceptable (1) to outstanding (5) or not applicable (NA). Your name is optional. Thank you.

Regarding the book overall:

1. Clinical relevance	1	2	3	4	5	NA
2. Quality of Printing	1	2	3	4	5	NA
3. Format (size)	1	2	3	4	5	NA
4. Organization	1	2	3	4	5	NA
5. Value for price	1	2	3	4	5	NA

Regarding individual chapters:

1. Principles of Brachytherapy	1	2	3	4	5	NA
2. History of Brachytherapy	1	2	3	4	5	NA
3. Radiobiology	1	2	3	4	5	NA
4. Basic Physics	1	2	3	4	5	NA
5. Instrumentation & Equipment	1	2	3	4	5	NA
6. Calibration	1	2	3	4	5	NA
7. Quality Assurance	1	2	3	4	5	NA
8. Treatment Planning	1	2	3	4	5	NA
9. Imaging Techniques	1	2	3	4	5	NA
10. Radiation Safety	1	2	3	4	5	NA
11. Skin	1	2	3	4	5	NA
12. Brain	1	2	3	4	5	NA
13. Head & Neck	1	2	3	4	5	NA
14. Eye	1	2	3	4	5	NA
15. Esophagus	1	2	3	4	5	NA
16. Lung	1	2	3	4	5	NA
17. Breast	1	2	3	4	5	NA
18. Bile Duct & Liver	1	2	3	4	5	NA
19. Pancreas	1	2	3	4	5	NA
20. Ano-colorectal	1	2	3	4	5	NA
21. Prostate	1	2	3	4	5	NA
22. Bladder	1	2	3	4	5	NA
23. Female Urethra	1	2	3	4	5	NA
24. Penis	1	2	3	4	5	NA
25. Cervix: LDR	1	2	3	4	5	NA
26. Cervix: HDR	1	2	3	4	5	NA
27. Cervix: Interstitial	1	2	3	4	5	NA
28. Endometrium	1	2	3	4	5	NA
29. Vagina & Vulva	1	2	3	4	5	NA
30. Soft-tissue Sarcomas	1	2	3	4	5	NA
31. Pediatric Tumors	1	2	3	4	5	NA
32. Brachytherapy Nursing	1	2	3	4	5	NA
33. Pulsed Dose Rate	1	2	3	4	5	NA

(continued)

34. Interstitial Thermo-brachytherapy	1	2	3	4	5	NA
35. Neutron Brachytherapy	1	2	3	4	5	NA
36. Intravascular Brachytherapy	1	2	3	4	5	NA
37. Future Directions	1	2	3	4	5	NA

Was the overall length of the book:

Short _____ Long _____ About Right _____

Best Feature:

Worst Feature:

Chapters to add:

Chapters to delete:

Additional comments (particularly on those items rated 1 or 2):

Are you a:

Resident, Radiation Oncologist, Physicist, Radiobiologist, Physician (non-radiation oncologist), Therapist, Other _____

Name (optional)

_____

Return to:
Subir Nag, M.D., Chief of Brachytherapy
Arthur G. James Cancer Hospital & Research Institute
The Ohio State University
300 W. Tenth Avenue
Columbus, Ohio 43210
Tel: 614-293-8415
Fax: 614-293-4044